Accessing the E-book edition

Using the VitalSource® ebook

Access to the VitalBook™ ebook accompanying this book is via VitalSource® Bookshelf – an ebook reader which allows you to make and share notes and highlights on your ebooks and search across all of the ebooks that you hold on your VitalSource Bookshelf. You can access the ebook online or offline on your smartphone, tablet or PC/Mac and your notes and highlights will automatically stay in sync no matter where you make them.

1. **Create a VitalSource Bookshelf account at** *https://online.vitalsource.com/user/new* or log into your existing account if you already have one.

2. **Redeem the code provided in the panel below to get online access to the ebook.**
   Log in to Bookshelf and select **Redeem** at the top right of the screen. Enter the redemption code shown on the scratch-off panel below in the **Redeem Code** pop-up and press **Redeem**. Once the code has been redeemed your ebook will download and appear in your library.

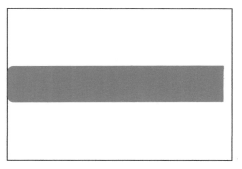

No returns if this code has been revealed.

DOWNLOAD AND READ OFFLINE

To use your ebook offline, download BookShelf to your PC, Mac, iOS device, Android device or Kindle Fire, and log in to your Bookshelf account to access your ebook:

On your PC/Mac

Go to *https://support.vitalsource.com/hc/en-us* and follow the instructions to download the free **VitalSource Bookshelf** app to your PC or Mac and log into your Bookshelf account.

On your iPhone/iPod Touch/iPad

Download the free **VitalSource Bookshelf** App available via the iTunes App Store and log into your Bookshelf account. You can find more information at *https://support. vitalsource.com/hc/en-us/categories/200134217-Bookshelf-for-iOS*

On your Android™ smartphone or tablet

Download the free **VitalSource Bookshelf** App available via Google Play and log into your Bookshelf account. You can find more information at *https://support.vitalsource.com/ hc/en-us/categories/200139976-Bookshelf-for-Android-and-Kindle-Fire*

On your Kindle Fire

Download the free **VitalSource Bookshelf** App available from Amazon and log into your Bookshelf account. You can find more information at *https://support.vitalsource.com/ hc/en-us/categories/200139976-Bookshelf-for-Android-and-Kindle-Fire*

N.B. The code in the scratch-off panel can only be used once. When you have created a Bookshelf account and redeemed the code you will be able to access the ebook online or offline on your smartphone, tablet or PC/Mac.

SUPPORT

If you have any questions about downloading Bookshelf, creating your account, or accessing and using your ebook edition, please visit *http://support.vitalsource.com/*

Maternal-Fetal Evidence Based Guidelines

SERIES IN MATERNAL-FETAL MEDICINE
Published in association with the
Journal of Maternal-Fetal & Neonatal Medicine

Edited by
Gian Carlo Di Renzo and Dev Maulik

Howard Carp, *Recurrent Pregnancy Loss*, ISBN 9780415421300

Vincenzo Berghella, *Obstetric Evidence Based Guidelines*,
ISBN 9780415701884

Vincenzo Berghella, *Maternal-Fetal Evidence Based Guidelines*,
ISBN 9780415432818

Moshe Hod, Lois Jovanovic, Gian Carlo Di Renzo, Alberto de Leiva,
Oded Langer, *Textbook of Diabetes and Pregnancy, Second Edition*,
ISBN 9780415426206

Simcha Yagel, Norman H. Silverman, Ulrich Gembruch,
Fetal Cardiology, Second Edition, ISBN 9780415432658

Fabio Facchinetti, Gustaaf A. Dekker, Dante Baronciani,
George Saade, Stillbirth: *Understanding and Management*,
ISBN 9780415473903

Vincenzo Berghella, *Maternal-Fetal Evidence Based Guidelines,
Second Edition*, ISBN 9781841848228

Vincenzo Berghella, *Obstetric Evidence Based Guidelines, Second Edition*,
ISBN 9781841848242

Howard Carp, *Recurrent Pregnancy Loss: Causes, Controversies, and
Treatment, Second Edition*, ISBN 9781482216141

Moshe Hod, Lois G. Jovanovic, Gian Carlo Di Renzo, Alberto De Leiva,
Oded Langer, *Textbook of Diabetes and Pregnancy, Third Edition*,
ISBN 9781482213607

Vincenzo Berghella, *Maternal-Fetal Evidence Based Guidelines,
Third Edition*, ISBN 9781841848228

Vincenzo Berghella, *Obstetric Evidence Based Guidelines, Third Edition*,
ISBN 9781841848242

MATERNAL-FETAL EVIDENCE BASED GUIDELINES

THIRD EDITION

EDITED BY

VINCENZO BERGHELLA, MD, FACOG

Director, Division of Maternal-Fetal Medicine
Professor, Department of Obstetrics and Gynecology
Sidney Kimmel Medical College of Thomas Jefferson University
Philadelphia, Pennsylvania, USA

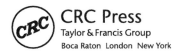

CRC Press
Taylor & Francis Group
Boca Raton London New York

CRC Press is an imprint of the
Taylor & Francis Group, an **informa** business

CRC Press
Taylor & Francis Group
6000 Broken Sound Parkway NW, Suite 300
Boca Raton, FL 33487-2742

© 2017 by Taylor & Francis Group, LLC
CRC Press is an imprint of Taylor & Francis Group, an Informa business

No claim to original U.S. Government works

Printed on acid-free paper
Version Date: 20161111

International Standard Book Number-13: 978-1-4987-4744-8 (Pack - Book and Ebook)

Visit the Taylor & Francis Web site at
http://www.taylorandfrancis.com

and the CRC Press Web site at
http://www.crcpress.com

To Paola, Andrea, Pietro, Mamma, and Papá,

*For giving me the serenity, love, and strength at home now, then,
and in the future to fulfill my dreams and spend my talents as best as possible.*

To all those who loved the first and second editions

*To my mentors and to my mentees who have been so passionate
and supportive about these books*

To the health of mothers and babies

And—as I often toast—to the next generation!

Contents

Introduction .... *x*
How to "Read" This Book .... *xiii*
List of Abbreviations .... *xiv*
Contributors .... *xx*

1. **Hypertensive disorders** 1
   Amanda Roman

2. **Cardiac disease** 24
   Meredith Birsner and Sharon Rubin

3. **Obesity** 32
   Kathryn Shaia and Maria Teresa Mella

4. **Pregestational diabetes** 50
   A. Dhanya Mackeen and Michael J. Paglia

5. **Gestational diabetes** 59
   A. Dhanya Mackeen and Melisa Lott

6. **Hypothyroidism** 73
   Sushma Jwala

7. **Hyperthyroidism** 80
   Sushma Jwala

8. **Prolactinoma** 86
   Katherine Husk

9. **Nausea/vomiting of pregnancy and hyperemesis gravidarum** 92
   Rupsa C. Boelig

10. **Intrahepatic cholestasis of pregnancy** 103
    Giuliana Simonazzi and Steven K. Herrine

11. **Inflammatory bowel disease** 110
    Priyadarshini Koduri

12. **Gallbladder disease** 119
    Priyadarshini Koduri

13. **Pregnancy after liver and other transplantation** 124
    Ignazio R. Marino, Lucio Mandalà, and Augusto Lauro

14. **Maternal anemia** 131
    Marcela C. Smid and Robert A. Strauss

15. **Sickle cell disease** 139
    Mariam Naqvi and Jeffrey Ecker

16. **von Willebrand disease** 145
    Dawnette Lewis and Srikanth Nagalla

17. **Renal disease** 150
    Rebekah McCurdy

18. **Headache** 162
    Stephen Silberstein and Shuhan Zhu

19. **Seizures** 167
    Sally Mathias and Meriem K. Bensalem-Owen

20. **Spinal cord injury** 173
    Megan Gooding and Leonardo Pereira

21. **Mood disorders** 177
    *Madeleine A. Becker, Tal E. Weinberger, Ann Chandy, Nazanin E. Silver,
    and Elisabeth J. S. Kunkel*

22. **Smoking** 196
    Jorge E. Tolosa and David M. Stamilio

23. **Drug abuse** 206
    Neil S. Seligman

24. **Respiratory diseases: asthma, pneumonia, influenza, and tuberculosis** 225
    Lauren A. Plante and Ryan K. Brannon

25. **Systemic lupus erythematosus** 246
    Maria A. Giraldo-Isaza

26. **Antiphospholipid syndrome** 254
    Tracy A. Manuck

27. **Inherited thrombophilia** 260
    Robert M. Silver and James A. Airoldi

28. **Venous thromboembolism and anticoagulation** 269
    Melissa Chu Lam and James A. Airoldi

29. **Hepatitis A** 283
    Neil Silverman and Steven K. Herrine

30. **Hepatitis B** 285
    Neil Silverman and Steven K. Herrine

31. **Hepatitis C** 291
    Neil Silverman, Raja Dhanekula, and Jonathan M. Fenkel

32. **HIV** 297
    William R. Short

33. **Gonorrhea** 305
    A. Marie O'Neill

34. **Chlamydia** 310
    Rebecca J. Mercier

35. **Syphilis** 315
    A. Marie O'Neill

36. **Trichomoniasis** 322
    Tino Tran

37. **Group B *Streptococcus*** 325
    Laura Carlson and M. Kathryn Menard

38. **Vaccination** 332
    Amber S. Maratas, Edward M. Buchanan, and Joshua H. Barash

39. **Trauma** 339
    Lauren A. Plante

40. **Critical care** 349
    Lauren A. Plante

41. **Amniotic fluid embolism** 365
    Antonio F. Saad and Luis D. Pacheco

42. Cancer 373
    Elyce Cardonick

43. Dermatoses of pregnancy 386
    Dana Correale, Joya Sahu, and Jason B. Lee

44. Multiple gestations 398
    Edward J. Hayes and Michelle R. Hayes

45. Fetal growth restriction 412
    Shane Reeves and Henry L. Galan

46. Fetal macrosomia 432
    Oscar A. Viteri and Suneet P. Chauhan

47. Cytomegalovirus 436
    Timothy J. Rafael

48. Toxoplasmosis 442
    Corina N. Schoen and Timothy J. Rafael

49. Parvovirus 447
    Timothy J. Rafael

50. Herpes 451
    Timothy J. Rafael

51. Varicella 456
    Timothy J. Rafael

52. Fetal and neonatal alloimmune thrombocytopenia 460
    Kelly M. Orzechowski

53. Hemolytic disease of the fetus/neonate 467
    Danielle L. Tate, Jacques E. Samson, and Giancarlo Mari

54. Nonimmune hydrops fetalis 477
    Katherine Connolly and Joanne Stone

55. Fetal death 488
    Nahida Chakhtoura and Uma M. Reddy

56. Antepartum testing 496
    Nora Graham and Christopher R. Harman

57. Sonographic assessment of amniotic fluid: oligohydramnios
              and polyhydramnios 513
    Ibrahim A. Hammad and Suneet P. Chauhan

58. Fetal maturity testing 521
    Paniz Heidari and Sarah Poggi

Index 526

Introduction

Welcome to the third edition of our evidence-based books on obstetrics and maternal-fetal medicine! I am indebted for your support! I can't believe how much praise we have gotten for these companion volumes. Your words of encouragement have kept me and all the collaborators, past and present, going now for well over a decade (we are indebted to contributors to previous editions of this text for their work). It has been extremely worthwhile and fulfilling. You are making me happy! In return, I hope we are helping you and your patients toward ever better evidence-based care of pregnant women and their babies and, therefore, better outcomes. Indeed, maternal and perinatal morbidities and mortalities throughout the world are improving.

To me, pregnancy has always been the most fascinating and exciting area of interest as care involves not one, but at least two persons—the mother and the fetus—and leads to the miracle of a new life. I was a third-year medical student when, during a lecture, a resident said, "I went into obstetrics because this is the easiest medical field. Pregnancy is a physiologic process, and there isn't much to know. It is simple." I knew from my "classical" background that "obstetrics" means to "stand by, stay near," and that indeed pregnancy used to receive no medical support at all.

After more than 25 years of practicing obstetrics, I now know that although physiologic and, at times, simple, obstetrics and maternal-fetal medicine can be the most complex of the medical fields: Pregnancy is based on a different physiology than for nonpregnant women, can include any medical disease, require surgery, etc. It is not so simple. In fact, ignorance can kill—in this case, with the health of the woman and her baby both at risk. Too often, I have gone to a lecture, journal club, rounds, or other didactic event to hear presented only one or a few articles regarding the subject without the presenter reviewing the pertinent best review of the total literature and data. It is increasingly difficult to read and acquire knowledge of all that is published, even just in obstetrics, with about 3000 scientific manuscripts published monthly on this subject. Some residents or even authorities would state at times that "there is no evidence" on a topic. We indeed used to be the field with the worst use of randomized trials [1]. As the best way to find something is to look for it, my coauthors and I searched for the best evidence. On careful investigation, indeed there are data on almost everything we do in obstetrics, especially on our interventions. Indeed, our field is now the pioneer for numbers of meta-analyses and extension of work for evidence-based reviews [2]. Obstetricians are now blessed with lots of data and should make the best use of it.

The aims of this book are to summarize the best evidence available in the obstetrics and maternal-fetal medicine literature and make the results of randomized controlled trials (RCTs) and meta-analyses of RCTs easily accessible to guide clinical care. The intent is to bridge the gap between knowledge (the evidence) and its easy application. To reach these goals, we reviewed all trials on effectiveness of interventions in obstetrics. Millions of pregnant women have participated in thousands of properly conducted RCTs. The efforts and sacrifice of mothers and their fetuses for science should be recognized at least by the physicians' awareness and understanding of these studies. Some of the trials have been summarized in more than 600 *Cochrane* reviews with hundreds of other meta-analyses also published on obstetrical topics (Table 1). All of the *Cochrane* reviews, as well as other meta-analyses and trials in obstetrics and maternal-fetal medicine, were reviewed and referenced. The material presented in single trials or meta-analyses is too detailed to be readily translated to advice for the busy clinician who needs to make dozens of clinical decisions a day. Even the Cochrane Library, the undisputed leader for evidence-based medicine efforts, has been criticized for its lack of flexibility and relevance in failing to be more easily understandable and clinically readily usable [3]. It is the gap between research and clinicians that needed to be filled, making sure that proven interventions are clearly highlighted and are included in today's care. Just as all pilots fly planes under similar rules to maximize safety, all obstetricians should manage all aspects of pregnancy with similar, evidenced-based rules. Indeed, only interventions that have been proven to provide benefit should be used routinely. On the other hand, *primum non nocere*: interventions that have clearly been shown to be not helpful or indeed harmful to mother and/or baby should be avoided.

Table 1   Obstetrical Evidence

More than 600 current *Cochrane* reviews
Hundreds of other current meta-analyses
More than 1000 RCTs
Millions of pregnant women randomized

Another aim of this book is to make sure the pregnant woman and her unborn child are not marginalized by the medical community. In most circumstances, medical disorders of pregnant women can be treated as in nonpregnant adults. Moreover, there are several effective interventions for preventing or treating specific pregnancy disorders.

Evidence-based medicine is the concept of treating patients according to the best available evidence. Although George Bernard Shaw said, "I have my own opinion, do not confuse me with the facts," this can be a deadly approach, especially in medicine, and compromise two or more lives at the same time in obstetrics and maternal-fetal medicine. What should be the basis for our interventions in medicine? Meta-analyses of RCTs provide a comprehensive summary of the best research data available. As such, they provide the best guidance for "effective" clinical care [4]. It is unscientific and unethical to practice medicine, teach, or conduct research without first knowing all that has already been proven [4]. In the absence of trials or meta-analyses, lower-level evidence is reviewed. This book aims at providing a current systematic review of all the best evidence so that current practice and education as well as future research can be based on the full story from the best-conducted research, not just the latest data or someone's opinion (Table 2).

These evidence-based guidelines cannot be used as a "cookbook" or a document dictating the best care. The knowledge from the best evidence presented in the guidelines needs to be integrated with other knowledge gained from clinical judgment, individual patient circumstances, and patient preferences to lead to best medical practice. These are guidelines, not rules. Even the best scientific studies are not always perfectly related to any given individual, and clinical judgment must still be applied to allow the best "particularization" of the best knowledge for the individual, unique patient. Evidence-based medicine informs clinical judgment but does not substitute it. It is important to understand, however, that greater clinical experience by the physician actually correlates with inferior quality of care if not integrated with knowledge of the best evidence [5]. The appropriate treatment is given in only 50% of visits to general physicians [5]. At times, limitations in resources may also limit the applicability of the guidelines but should not limit the physician's knowledge. Guidelines and clinical pathways based on evidence not only point to the right management, but also can decrease medicolegal risk [6]. We aimed for brevity and clarity. Suggested management of the healthy or sick mother and child is stated as straightforwardly as possible for everyone to easily understand and implement (Table 3). If you find the *Cochrane* reviews, scientific manuscripts, and other publications difficult to "translate" into care of your patients, this book is for you. We wanted to prevent information overload.

Table 2   Aims of This Book

Improve the health of women and their children
"Make it easy to do it right"
Implement the best clinical care based on science
   (evidence), not opinion
Education
Develop lectures
Decrease disease, use of detrimental
   interventions, and therefore costs
Reduce medicolegal risks

Table 3   This Book Is For

Obstetricians
Midwives
Family medicine and others (practicing obstetrics)
Residents
Nurses
Medical students
Maternal-fetal medicine attendings
Maternal-fetal medicine fellows
Other consultants on pregnancy
Lay persons who want to know "the evidence"
Politicians responsible for health care

On the other hand, "everything should be made as simple as possible, but not simpler" (A. Einstein). Key management points are highlighted at the beginning of each guideline and in bold in the text. The chapters are divided into two volumes, one on obstetrics and one on maternal-fetal medicine; cross-references to chapters in *Obstetric Evidence Based Guidelines* have been noted in the text where applicable. Please contact us (vincenzo.berghella @jefferson.edu) for any comments, criticisms, corrections, missing evidence, etc.

I have the most fun discovering the best ways to alleviate discomfort and disease. The search for the best evidence for these guidelines has been a wonderful, stimulating journey. Keeping up with evidence-based medicine is exciting. The most rewarding part, as a teacher, is the dissemination of knowledge. I hope, truly, that this effort will be helpful to you, too.

REFERENCES

1. Cochrane AL. 1931–1971: A critical review, with particular reference to the medical profession. In: Medicines for the Year 2000. London: Office of Health Economics, 1979: 1–11. [Review]
2. Dickersin K, Manheimer E. The Cochrane Collaboration: Evaluation of health care and services using systematic reviews of the results of randomized controlled trials. *Clinic Obstet Gynecol* 1998; 41: 315–31. [Review]
3. Summerskill W. Cochrane Collaboration and the evolution of evidence. *Lancet* 2005; 366: 1760. [Review]
4. Chalmers I. Academia's failure to support systematic reviews. *Lancet* 2005; 365: 469. [III]
5. Arky RA. The family business—To educate. *NEJM* 2006; 354: 1922–6. [Review]
6. Ransom SB, Studdert DM, Dombrowski MP et al. Reduced medico-legal risk by compliance with obstetric clinical pathways: A case-control study. *Obstet Gynecol* 2003; 101: 751–5. [II-2]

How to "Read" This Book

The knowledge from RCTs and meta-analyses of RCTs is summarized and easily available for clinical implementation. Relative risks and 95% confidence intervals from studies are quoted sparingly. Instead, the straight recommendation for care is made if one intervention is superior to the other with the percentage improvement often quoted to assess degree of benefit. If there is insufficient evidence to compare to interventions or managements, this is clearly stated.

References: Cochrane reviews with 0 RCT are not referenced, and instead of referencing a meta-analysis with only one RCT, the actual RCT is usually referenced. RCTs that are already included in meta-analyses are not referenced for brevity and because they can be easily accessed by reviewing the meta-analysis. If new RCTs are not included in meta-analysis, they are obviously referenced. Each reference was reviewed and evaluated for quality according to a modified method as outlined by the U.S. Preventive Services Task Force (http://www.ahrq.gov):

I	Evidence obtained from at least one properly designed randomized controlled trial.
II-1	Evidence obtained from well-designed controlled trials without randomization.
II-2	Evidence obtained from well-designed cohort or case-control analytic studies, preferably from more than one center or research group.
II-3	Evidence obtained from multiple time series with or without the intervention. Dramatic results in uncontrolled experiments could also be regarded as this type of evidence.
III (Review)	Opinions of respected authorities, based on clinical experience, descriptive studies, or reports of expert committees.

These levels are quoted after each reference. For RCTs and meta-analyses, the number of subjects studied is stated, and, sometimes, more details are provided to aid the reader to understand the study better.

List of Abbreviations

AA	artery-to-artery
AAN	American Academy of Neurology
AAP	American Academy of Pediatrics
AASLD	American Association for the Study of Liver Diseases
Ab	antibody
AC	abdominal circumference
ACA	anticardiolipin antibody
ACCM	American College of Critical Care Medicine
ACE	angiotensin-converting enzyme
ACOG	American College of Obstetricians and Gynecologists
ACR	acute cellular rejection
ACR	American College of Rheumatology
ACS	acute chest syndrome
ADHD	attention deficit hyperactivity disorder
ADP	atopic dermatitis of pregnancy
ADR	autonomic dysreflexia
AED	antiepileptic drug
AEDF	absent end-diastolic flow
AEP	atopic eruption of pregnancy
AF	amniotic fluid
AFE	amniotic fluid embolism
AFI	amniotic fluid index
AFP	alpha-fetoprotein
AFV	amniotic fluid volume
Ag	antigen
AGA	appropriate for gestational age
AHA	American Heart Association
aHR	adjusted hazard ratio
AIDS	acquired immune deficiency syndrome
AII	angiotensin type II
AIT	alloimmune thrombocytopenia
ALI	acute lung injury
ALT	alanine aminotransferase
ANA	antinuclear antibodies
APA	American Psychiatric Association
APS	antiphospholipid syndrome
aPT	activated prothrombin time
aPTT	activated partial thromboplastin time
ARDS	adult respiratory distress syndrome
AROM	artificial rupture of membranes

ARPV	airway pressure release ventilation
ART	antiretroviral therapy
ART	assisted reproductive technologies
ASA	aspirin
ASD	atrial septal defect
ASD	autism spectrum disorder
AST	aspartate aminotransferase
ATIII	antithrombin III
ATLS	Advanced Trauma Life Support
ATS	American Thoracic Society
AV	artery-to-vein
AVD	assisted vaginal delivery
AZT	zidovudine
BAD	bipolar disorder
BCG	bacille Calmette-Guerin
BHI	biphasic human insulin
BIAsp	biphasic insulin aspart
bid	"bis in die," i.e., twice per day
BMI	body mass index
BP	blood pressure
BPD	biparietal diameter
BPD	bronchopulmonary dysplasia
bpm	beats per minute
BPP	biophysical profile
BPS	biophysical profile score
BUN	blood urea nitrogen
CAP	community-acquired pneumonia
CBC	complete blood count
CCAM	congenital cystic adenomatoid malformation
CCTG	computerized cardiotocography
CD	cesarean delivery
CD	Crohn's disease
CDC	Centers for Disease Control
CDH	congenital diaphragmatic hernia
CF	cystic fibrosis
CFC	chlorofluorocarbon
CFU	colony-forming unit
cGH	comparative genomic hybridization
CGRP	calcitonin gene-related peptide
CHB	congenital heart block
CHD	congenital heart defect
CHF	congestive heart failure
CHIPS	Control of Hypertension in Pregnancy Study
CHTN	chronic hypertension
CL	cervical length

CLIA	Clinical Laboratory Improvement Amendments	ECT	electroconvulsive therapy
CMV	cytomegalovirus	ECV	external cephalic version
CNS	central nervous system	ED	emergency department
CPAM	congenital pulmonary airway malformation	EDC	estimated date of confinement
CPAP	continuous positive airway pressure	EDD	estimated date of delivery (synonym of EDC)
CPR	cardiopulmonary resuscitation	EDF	end-diastolic flow
CPR	cerebroplacental ratio	EFW	estimated fetal weight
CPS	capsular polysaccharide	EIA	enzyme immunoassay
CPS	complex partial seizure	EKG	electrocardiogram
CRF	chronic renal failure	ELISA	enzyme-linked immunosorbent assay
CRI	chronic renal insufficiency	EM	electron microscopy
CRL	crown-rump length	EM	expectant management
CS	corticosteroid	EN	enteral nutrition
CSD	cortical spreading depression	EPCOT	European Prospective Cohort on Thrombophilia
CSE	combined spinal epidural	EPDS	Edinburgh Postnatal Depression Scale
CSF	cerebrospinal fluid	EPS	extrapyramidal symptom
CSII	continuous subcutaneous insulin infusion	EPT	expedited partner therapy
CST	contraction stress test	ERCP	endoscopic retrograde cholangiopancreatography
CT	computerized tomography	ESLD	end-stage liver disease
CT	connective tissue	ESRD	end-stage renal disease
CTG	cardiotocography	FAST	focused abdominal sonogram for trauma
CTPA	computed tomography pulmonary angiography	FBS	fetal blood sampling
		FD	fetal distress
CTZ	chemo-receptor trigger zone	FDA	Food and Drug Administration
CVS	chorionic villus sampling	FDC	fixed-dose combination
CVS	congenital varicella syndrome	FEV1	forced expiratory volume in one second
D&E	dilation and evacuation	FFN	fetal fibronectin
DAA	direct-acting antiviral agent	FGR	fetal growth restriction
DBP	diastolic blood pressure	FHM	familial hemiplegic migraine
DC/DA	dichorionic/diamniotic	FHR	fetal heart rate
DES	diethylstilbestrol	FHT	fetal heart tracing
DHHS	Department of Health and Human Services	FISH	fluorescent in situ hybridization
DIC	disseminated intravascular coagulation	FKCG	fetal kinetocardiogram/ tissue Doppler echocardiography
DIF	direct immunofluorescence	FLM	fetal lung maturity
DM	diabetes mellitus	FMAIT	fetal maternal alloimmune thrombocytopenia
DMPA	depot medroxyprogesterone acetate	FNAIT	fetal and neonatal alloimmune thrombocytopenia
DNA	deoxyribonucleic acid	FOB	father of baby
DNS	dysplastic nevus syndrome	FPG	fasting plasma glucose
DPI	dry powder inhaler	FPR	false positive rate
DPL	diagnostic peritoneal lavage	FSBS	fetal scalp blood sampling
DRVVT	dilute Russell's viper venom time	FSE	fetal scalp electrode
		FSI	foam stability index
DV	ductus venosus	FTS	first-trimester screening
DVP	deepest vertical pocket	FVC	forced vital capacity
DVT	deep vein thrombosis	FVL	factor V Leiden
DZ	dizygotic	g	grams
EASL	European Association for the Study of the Liver	GA	gestational age
EBV	Epstein-Barr virus	GBS	group B streptococcus
ECDC	European Centre for Disease Prevention and Control	GBS	Guillain–Barré syndrome
		GDM	gestational diabetes
ECMO	extracorporeal membrane oxygenation	GERD	gastroesophageal reflux disease
EC-MPS	enteric-coated mycopheno-late sodium	GFR	glomerular filtration rate
		GHB	gamma-hydroxybutyrate

GHTN	gestational hypertension	IUGR	intrauterine growth restriction (synonym of FGR)
GI	gastrointestinal		
GISP	Gonococcal Isolate Surveillance Project	IUPC	intrauterine pressure catheter
GTC	generalized tonic clonic		
GTT	glucose tolerance test	IV	intravenous
GWG	gestational weight gain	IVC	inferior vena cava
HAART	highly active antiretroviral therapy	IVDU	intravenous drug use
		IVF	intravenous fluids
HAV	hepatitis A virus	IVH	intraventricular hemorrhage
HBsAg	hepatitis B surface antigen		
		L&D	labor and delivery
HBV	hepatitis B virus	L/S	lecithin/sphingomyelin
HC	head circumference	LA	lupus anticoagulant
HCG	human chorionic gonadotroponin	LABA	long-acting β-agonist
		LAGB	laparoscopic adjustable gastric baning
Hct	hematocrit		
HCV	hepatitis C virus	LB	lamellar body
HD	hemodialysis	LBW	low birth weight
HD	Hodgkin's disease	LBW	low birth weight (infants)
HDU	high-dependency unit	LCR	ligase chain reaction
HELLP	hemolysis, elevated liver enzymes, and low platelet count	LFT	liver function tests
		LGA	large for gestational age
		LGV	lymphogranuloma venereum
HES	hydroxyethyl starch		
HFA	hydrofluoroalkane	LMP	last menstrual period
HG	hyperemesis gravidarum	LMW	low molecular weight
Hgb	hemoglobin	LMWH	low-molecular-weight heparin
HIE	hypoxic-ischemic encephalopathy		
		LR	likelihood ratio
HIT	heparin-induced thrombocytopenia	LSD	lysergic acid diethylamide
		LSD	lysosomal storage disease
HIV	human immunodeficiency virus	LTRA	leukotriene receptor antagonist
HLA	human leukocyte antigen	MA/MC	monoamniotic
HPA	hypothalamic–pituitary–adrenal	MAC	mycobacterium avium complex
HPA	human platelet antigen	MAOI	monoamine oxidase inhibitor
HR	heart rate		
HSV	herpes simplex virus	MAS	meconium aspiration syndrome
HTN	hypertension		
IAAT	immunosorbent agglutination assay test	MC/DA	monochorionic diamniotic
		MCA	middle cerebral artery
IALE	International League Against Epilepsy	MCV	mean corpuscular volume
		MD	mean difference
IBD	inflammatory bowel disease	MDD	major depressive disorder
		MDI	metered-dose inhaler
IBW	ideal body weight	MDI	multiple-dose insulin
ICH	intracranial hemorrhage	MDQ	Mood Disorders Questionnaire
ICP	intrahepatic cholestasis of pregnancy		
		MDR	multidrug-resistant
ICS	immunochromatographic strip	MFM	maternal–fetal medicine
		MHC	major histocompatibility complex
ICS	Intensive Care Society		
ICU	intensive care unit	MI	myocardial infarction
IDSA	Infectious Diseases Society of America	MM	malignant melanoma
		MMF	myco-phenolate mofetil
IGRA	interferon gamma-release assay	MMR	measles–mumps–rubella
		MOM	multiple of the median
IH	impetigo herpetiformis	MPA	mycophenolic acid products
IM	intramuscular	MRCP	magnetic resonance cholangiopancreatography
INR	international normalized ratio		
		MRI	magnetic resonance imaging
IOL	induction of labor		
IPAA	ileal pouch–anal anastomosis	MRU	magnetic resonance urography
IPV	inactivated polio vaccine	MSAFP	maternal serum alpha-fetoprotein
ISS	injury severity score		
IUD	intrauterine device	MSH	melanocyte-stimulating hormone
IUFD	intrauterine fetal demise		

MTHFR	methylenetetrahydrofolate reductase	NVP	nausea and vomiting of pregnancy
MTX	methotrexate	OB	obstetrician
MVI	prenatal multivitamin	OCT	oxytocin challenge test
MVP	maximum vertical pocket	OCT	oxytocin contraction test
MZ	monozygotic	OGTT	oral glucose tolerance test
n/v	nausea and/or vomiting	OPV	oral live polio vaccine
NA	not available	OR	odds ratio
NA-ACCORD	North American AIDS Cohort Collaboration on Research and Design	OR	operating room
		OSA	obstructive sleep apnea
		OTC	over the counter
NAAED	North American Antiepileptic Drug	PAPP-A	pregnancy-associated plasma protein-A
NAAT	nucleic acid amplification test	PC	platelet count
		PC	protein C
NAEPP	National Asthma Education and Prevention Program	PCA	patient-controlled analgesia
		PCI	percutaneous coronary intervention
NAIT	neonatal alloimmune thrombocytopenia	PCP	phencyclidine
NAS	neonatal abstinence syndrome	PCP	Pneumocystis carinii pneumonia
NBPP	neonatal brachial plexus palsy	PCR	polymerase chain reaction
		PCWP	pulmonary capillary wedge pressure
NCHS	National Center for Health Statistics	PD	peritoneal dialysis
NEC	necrotizing enterocolitis	PDA	patent ductus arteriosus
NG	nasogastric	PE	pulmonary embolus
NHL	Non–Hodgkin's lymphoma	PEA	pulseless electrical activity
NICU	neonatal intensive care unit	PEFR	peak expiratory flow rate
		PEP	polymorphic eruption of pregnancy
NIH	National Institutes of Health	PER	prophylaxis effective rate
NIH	nonimmune hydrops	PET	positron emission tomography
NIS	National Inpatient Sample		
NNRTI	non-nucleoside reverse transcriptase inhibitor	PFP	pruritic folliculitis of pregnancy
NODM	new-onset diabetes mellitus	PFT	pulmonary function tests
		PG	pemphigoid gestationis
NOTES	natural orifice translumenal endoscopic surgery	PG	phosphatidylglycerol
		PG	plasma glucose
		PGL	persistent generalized lymphadenopathy
NPH	neutral protamine Hagedorn	PGM	prothrombin gene mutation
NRFHR	nonreassuring fetal heart rate	PI	protease inhibitor
		PI	pulsatility index
NRFHT	nonreassuring fetal heart testing	PICC	peripherally inserted central catheter
NRFS	nonreassuring fetal status	PID	pelvic inflammatory disease
NRI	norepinephrine reuptake inhibitor	PK	pharmacokinetic
		PL	pregnancy loss
NRT	nicotine replacement therapy	PlGF	placental growth factor
NRTI	nucleoside reverse transcriptase inhibitor	PMCD	perimortem cesarean delivery
NS	nephrotic syndrome	PN	parenteral nutrition
NS	normal saline	PNC	prenatal care
NSAIDS	nonsteroidal anti-inflammatory drugs	PNM	perinatal mortality
NSCIA	National Spinal Cord Injury Association	po	"per os," i.e., by mouth
		PP	prurigo of pregnancy
NST	nonstress test	PP-13	placental protein-13
NSVD	normal spontaneous vaginal delivery	PPD	purified protein derivative
		PPH	postpartum hemorrhage
NT	nuchal translucency	PPHN	persistent pulmonary hypertension of the newborn
NTD	neural tube defect		
NTDB	National Trauma Data Banks	PPI	proton-pump inhibitor
NTPR	National Transplantation Pregnancy Registry	PPROM	preterm premature rupture of membranes

PR	per rectum	SLE	systemic lupus erythematosus
pRBC	packed red blood cells		
PRCD	planned repeat cesarean delivery	SLICC	Systemic Lupus International Collaborating Clinics
PROM	preterm rupture of membranes	SNRI	serotonin-norepinephrine reuptake inhibitor
PS	protein S		
PS	pulmonic stenosis	SPTB	spontaneous preterm birth
PSI	Pneumonia Severity Index	SQ	subcutaneous
PSV	peak systolic velocity	SSC	Surviving Sepsis Campaign
PT	prothrombin time		
PTB	preterm birth	SSKI	saturated solution of potassium iodide
PTL	preterm labor		
PTT	partial thromboplastin time	SSRI	selective serotonin reuptake inhibitor
PTU	propylthiouracil	STD	sexually transmitted diseases (synonym of STI)
PUBS	percutaneous umbilical blood sampling	STI	sexually transmitted infections
PUPPP	pruritic urticarial papules and plaques of pregnancy	STS	second-trimester screening
PUQE	pregnancy-unique quantification of emesis/nausea	SUDEP	sudden unexpected death in epilepsy
PVR	pulmonary vascular resistance	SVC	superior vena cava
		SVR	systemic vascular resistance
PW	pulsed wave	SVR	sustained virologic response
qd	once a day		
qhs	before bedtime	TB	tuberculosis
qid	four times per day	TBG	thyroid-binding globulin
QS	quadruple screen	TBII	thyroid-stimulating hormone-binding inhibitory immunoglobulin
RBC	red blood cell		
RCT	randomized controlled study		
		TCA	tricyclic antidepressant
RCVS	reversible cerebral vasoconstriction syndrome	TDD	total daily dose
		TG	*Toxoplasma gondii*
RDS	respiratory distress syndrome	TH	therapeutic hypothermia
		THC	tetrahydrocannabinol
RDW	red blood cell distribution width	tid	three times per day
REDF	reverse end-diastolic flow	TIV	trivalent inactivated vaccine
RI	resistive index		
RNA	ribonucleic acid	TMA	transcription-mediated amplification
ROM	rupture of membranes		
ROSC	return of spontaneous circulation	TNF	tumor necrosis factor
		TOL	trial of labor
RPR	rapid plasma reagin	TOLAC	trial of labor after cesarean
RR	relative risk	TPO	thyroid peroxidase
RR	respiratory rate	TRAb	TSH receptor antibody
RR	risk ratio	TRALI	transfusion-related acute lung injury
Rx	treatment		
S/D	systolic/diastolic	TRAP	twin reversal arterial perfusion
SAB	spontaneous abortion		
SABA	short-acting β-agonist	TSH	thyroid-stimulating hormone
SBP	systolic blood pressure		
SC	subcutaneous	TSI	thyroid-stimulating immune globulins
SCI	spinal cord injury		
SCRN	Stillbirth Collaborative Research Network	TST	tuberculin skin testing
		TTTS	twin–twin transfusion syndrome
SD	striae distensae		
SDA	strand-displacement amplification	TVU	transvaginal ultrasound
		U/S (or u/s)	ultrasound
SDP	single deepest pocket	UA	umbilical artery
SEE	Syphilis Elimination Effort	UC	ulcerative colitis
SFDT	Sabin–Feldman dye test	UDCA	ursodeoxycholic acid
SG	striae gravidarum	UFH	unfractionated heparin
SGA	small for gestational age	UPC	urinary protein creatinine
SIDS	sudden infant death syndrome	USPSTF	U.S. Preventative Services Task Force
SJS	Stevens–Johnson syndrome	UTI	urinary tract infection
		V/Q	ventilation/perfusion

VAS	vibroacoustic stimulation	**VTE**	venous thromboembolism
VBAC	vaginal birth after cesarean	**VV**	vein-to-vein
		vWD	von Willebrand disease
VC	vital capacity	**vWF**	von Willebrand factor
VDRL	venereal disease research laboratory	**VZIG**	varicella zoster immune globulin
VEGF	vascular endothelial growth factor	**VZV**	varicella zoster virus
		WBC	white blood cell
VIG	vaccinia immune globulin	**WHO**	World Health Organization
VKA	vitamin K antagonist		
VL	viral load	**WIHS**	Women's Interagency HIV Study
VPA	valproic acid		
VSD	ventricular septal defect	**XDR**	extensively drug-resistant

Contributors

James A. Airoldi Department of Obstetrics and Gynecology, Division of Maternal-Fetal Medicine, St Luke's University Health Network, Bethlehem, Pennsylvania

Joshua H. Barash Department of Family and Community Medicine, Thomas Jefferson University Hospital, Philadelphia, Pennsylvania

Madeleine A. Becker Department of Psychiatry and Human Behavior, Division of Consultation-Liaison Psychiatry, Psychosomatic Medicine Fellowship, Thomas Jefferson University Hospital, Philadelphia, Pennsylvania

Meriem K. Bensalem-Owen University of Kentucky, Lexington, Kentucky

Vincenzo Berghella Department of Obstetrics and Gynecology, Division of Maternal-Fetal Medicine, Sidney Kimmel Medical College of Thomas Jefferson University, Philadelphia, Pennsylvania

Meredith Birsner Department of Obstetrics and Gynecology, Division of Maternal-Fetal Medicine, Sidney Kimmel Medical College of Thomas Jefferson University, Philadelphia, Pennsylvania

Rupsa C. Boelig Department of Obstetrics and Gynecology, Division of Maternal-Fetal Medicine, Sidney Kimmel Medical College of Thomas Jefferson University, Philadelphia, Pennsylvania

Ryan K. Brannon Drexel University College of Medicine, Philadelphia, Pennsylvania

Edward M. Buchanan Department of Family and Community Medicine, Thomas Jefferson University Hospital, Philadelphia, Pennsylvania

Elyce Cardonick Division of Maternal-Fetal Medicine, Robert Wood Johnson Medical School New Brunswick, New Jersey

Laura Carlson Department of Obstetrics and Gynecology, Division of Maternal-Fetal Medicine, University of North Carolina School of Medicine, Chapel Hill, North Carolina

Nahida Chakhtoura Eunice Kennedy Shriver National Institute of Child Health and Human Development, Bethesda, Maryland

Ann Chandy Department of Psychiatry and Human Behavior, Thomas Jefferson University Hospital, Philadelphia, Pennsylvania

Suneet P. Chauhan Eunice Kennedy Shriver NICHD Maternal-Fetal Medicine Units Network, Bethesda, Maryland and McGovern Medical School, University of Texas Health Science Center, Houston, Texas

Melissa Chu Lam Department of Obstetrics and Gynecology, St. Luke's University Health Network, Bethlehem, Pennsylvania

Katherine Connolly Department of Obstetrics, Gynecology and Reproductive Sciences, Division of Maternal Fetal Medicine, Icahn School of Medicine at Mount Sinai, New York, New York

Dana Correale Private Practice, Cheshire Dermatology, Cheshire, Connecticut

Raja Dhanekula Department of Medicine, Division of Gastroenterology, Sidney Kimmel Medical College, Thomas Jefferson University, Philadelphia, Pennsylvania

Jeffrey Ecker Department of Obstetrics and Gynecology, Division of Maternal Fetal Medicine, Massachusetts General Hospital, Boston, Massachusetts

Jonathan M. Fenkel Department of Medicine, Division of Gastroenterology, Sidney Kimmel Medical College, Thomas Jefferson University, Philadelphia, Pennsylvania

Henry L. Galan Department of Obstetrics and Gynecology, Division of Maternal-Fetal Medicine, Colorado Institute for Maternal and Fetal Health, University of Colorado Hospital, Aurora, Colorado

Maria A. Giraldo-Isaza Florida Perinatal Associates, Obstetrix Medical Group, Inc, Tampa, Florida

Megan Gooding College of Health and Human Services, George Mason University, Fairfax, Virginia

Nora Graham Department of Obstetrics and Gynecology, Thomas Jefferson University Hospital, Philadelphia, Pennsylvania

Ibrahim A. Hammad Department of Obstetrics and Gynecology, Division of Maternal Fetal Medicine, University of Utah Health Sciences Center, Salt Lake City, Utah

Christopher R. Harman Department of Obstetrics, Gynecology and Reproductive Sciences, University of Maryland Medical Center, Baltimore, Maryland

Edward J. Hayes Department of Obstetrics and Gynecology, Division of Maternal-Fetal Medicine, Aurora Baycare Medical Center, Greenbay, Wisconsin

Michelle R. Hayes Department of Obstetrics and Gynecology, Division of Maternal-Fetal Medicine, Aurora Baycare Medical Center, Greenbay, Wisconsin

Paniz Heidari Department of Obstetrics and Gynecology, Sidney Kimmel Medical College of Thomas Jefferson University, Philadelphia, Pennsylvania

Steven K. Herrine Division of Gastroenterology and Hepatology, Thomas Jefferson University, Philadelphia, Pennsylvania

Katherine Husk Department of Urogynecology and Reconstructive Pelvic Surgery, University of North Carolina, Chapel Hill, North Carolina

Sushma Jwala Department of Obstetrics and Gynecology, Division of Maternal-Fetal Medicine, Obstetrix Medical Group of Washington, Seattle, Washington

Priyadarshini Koduri Division of Maternal-Fetal Medicine, Antenatal Resource Center, Advocate Illinois Masonic Medical Center, Chicago, Illinois

Elisabeth J. S. Kunkel Division Consultation-Liaison Psychiatry, Department of Psychiatry and Human Behavior, Thomas Jefferson University, Philadelphia, Pennsylvania

Augusto Lauro Liver and Multiorgan Transplant Unit, St. Orsola University Hospital, Bologna, Italy

Jason B. Lee Department of Dermatology and Cutaneous Biology, Sidney Kimmel Medical College, Thomas Jefferson University, Philadelphia, Pennsylvania

Dawnette Lewis Division of Maternal-Fetal Medicine, Department of Obstetrics and Gynecology, Mount Sinai St. Luke's Hospital, New York

Melisa Lott Division of Maternal-Fetal Medicine, Women's and Children's Institute, Geisinger Health System, Danville, Pennsylvania

A. Dhanya Mackeen Division of Maternal-Fetal Medicine, Women's and Children's Institute, Geisinger Health System, Danville, Pennsylvania

Lucio Mandalà HPB Unit, La Maddalena Cancer Center, Palermo, Italy

Tracy A. Manuck Department of Obstetrics and Gynecology, Division of Maternal-Fetal Medicine, University of North Carolina, Chapel Hill, North Carolina

Amber S. Maratas Department of Family and Community Medicine, Thomas Jefferson University Hospital, Philadelphia, Pennsylvania

Giancarlo Mari Department of Obstetrics and Gynecology, University of Tennessee Health Science Center, Memphis, Tennessee

Ignazio R. Marino Department of Surgery, Sidney Kimmel Medical College, Thomas Jefferson University, Philadelphia, Pennsylvania

Sally Mathias Department of Neurology, University of Kentucky, Lexington, Kentucky

Rebekah McCurdy Department of Obstetrics and Gynecology, Division of Maternal-Fetal Medicine, Sidney Kimmel Medical College, Thomas Jefferson University, Philadelphia, Pennsylvania

Maria Teresa Mella Department of Obstetrics, Gynecology and Reproductive Sciences, Division of Maternal Fetal Medicine, Icahn School of Medicine at Mount Sinai, New York

M. Kathryn Menard Department of Obstetrics and Gynecology, Division of Maternal-Fetal Medicine, University of North Carolina School of Medicine, Chapel Hill, North Carolina

Rebecca J. Mercier Department of Obstetrics and Gynecology, Division of General Obstetrics and Gynecology, Sidney Kimmel Medical College Thomas Jefferson University, Philadelphia, Pennsylvania

Srikanth Nagalla Department of Medicine, Division of Hematology/Oncology, UT Southwestern Medical Center, Dallas, Texas

Mariam Naqvi Department of Obstetrics and Gynecology, Division of Maternal Fetal Medicine, Massachusetts General Hospital, Boston, Massachusetts

A. Marie O'Neill Rowan University School of Osteopathic Medicine, Stratford, New Jersey

Kelly M. Orzechowski Department of Obstetrics and Gynecology, Division of Maternal Fetal Medicine, Virginia Hospital Center, Arlington, Virginia

Luis D. Pacheco Department of Obstetrics/Gynecology, Division of Maternal Fetal Medicine and Department of Anesthesiology, Division of Surgical Critical Care, The University of Texas Medical Branch, Galveston, Texas

Michael J. Paglia Division of Maternal-Fetal Medicine, Women's and Children's Institute, Geisinger Health System, Danville, Pennsylvania

Leonardo Pereira Department of Obstetrics and Gynecology, Division of Maternal-Fetal Medicine, Oregon Health and Science University, Portland, Oregon

Lauren A. Plante Department of Obstetrics and Gynecology, Division of Maternal-Fetal Medicine and Department of Anesthesiology, Drexel University College of Medicine, Philadelphia, Pennsylvania

Sarah Poggi The Brock Perinatal Diagnostic Center Alexandria, Virginia

Timothy J. Rafael Division of Maternal-Fetal Medicine, Department of Obstetrics and Gynecology, Mount Sinai Beth Israel Hospital, New York

Uma M. Reddy Eunice Kennedy Shriver National Institute of Child Health and Human Development, Bethesda, Maryland

Shane Reeves Division of Maternal-Fetal Medicine, Colorado Institute for Maternal and Fetal Health, University of Colorado, Aurora, Colorado

Amanda Roman Department of Obstetrics and Gynecology, Division of Maternal-Fetal Medicine, Sidney Kimmel Medical College, Thomas Jefferson University, Philadelphia, Pennsylvania

Sharon Rubin Department of Internal Medicine, Division of Cardiology, Pennsylvania Hospital, University of Pennsylvania, Philadelphia, Pennsylvania

Antonio F. Saad Department of Obstetrics/Gynecology, Division of Maternal Fetal Medicine, The University of Texas Medical Branch, Galveston, Texas

Joya Sahu Department of Dermatology and Cutaneous Biology, Sidney Kimmel Medical College, Thomas Jefferson University, Philadelphia, Pennsylvania

Jacques E. Samson Department of Obstetrics and Gynecology, University of Tennessee Health Science Center, Memphis, Tennessee

Corina N. Schoen Department of Obstetrics and Gynecology, Division of Maternal Fetal Medicine, Baystate Medical Center, Springfield, Massachusetts

Neil S. Seligman Division of Maternal Fetal Medicine, Strong Memorial Hospital, University of Rochester, Rochester, New York

Kathryn Shaia Department of Obstetrics, Gynecology and Reproductive Sciences, Icahn School of Medicine at Mount Sinai, New York

William R. Short Division of Infectious Diseases, Perelman School of Medicine, University of Pennsylvania, Philadelphia, Pennsylvania

Stephen Silberstein Jefferson Headache Center, Thomas Jefferson University, Philadelphia, Pennsylvania

Nazanin E. Silver Department of Psychiatry and Human Behavior, Thomas Jefferson University Hospital, Philadelphia, Pennsylvania

Robert M. Silver Department of Obstetrics and Gynecology, University of Utah, Salt Lake City, Utah

Neil Silverman Department of Obstetrics and Gynecology, Division of Maternal-Fetal Medicine, David Geffen School of Medicine at UCLA, Los Angeles, California

Giuliana Simonazzi Department of Medical and Surgical Sciences, Division of Obstetrics and Prenatal Medicine, St. Orsola Malpighi Hospital, University of Bologna, Bologna, Italy

Marcela C. Smid Department of Obstetrics and Gynecology, Division of Maternal-Fetal Medicine, University of North Carolina, Chapel Hill, North Carolina

David M. Stamilio Department of Obstetrics and Gynecology, Division of Maternal Fetal Medicine, University of North Carolina, Chapel Hill, North Carolina

Joanne Stone Department of Obstetrics, Gynecology and Reproductive Sciences, Division of Maternal Fetal Medicine, Icahn School of Medicine at Mount Sinai, New York, New York

Robert A. Strauss Department of Obstetrics and Gynecology, Division of Maternal-Fetal Medicine, University of North Carolina, Chapel Hill, North Carolina

Danielle L. Tate Department of Obstetrics and Gynecology, University of Tennessee Health Science Center, Memphis, Tennessee

Jorge E. Tolosa Department of Obstetrics and Gynecology, Division of Maternal-Fetal Medicine, Oregon Health and Science University, Portland, Oregon and Departamento de Obstetricia y Ginecologia, Centro Nacer, Salud Sexual y Reproductiva, Facultad de Medicina, Universidad de Antioquia, Medellín, Colombia

Tino Tran Department of Obstetrics and Gynecology, Crozer-Keystone Medical Center, Chester, Pennsylvania

Oscar A. Viteri Department of Obstetrics, Gynecology and Reproductive Sciences, Division of Maternal-Fetal Medicine, McGovern Medical School, University of Texas Health Science Center, Houston, Texas

Tal E. Weinberger Thomas Jefferson University Hospital, Philadelphia, Pennsylvania

Shuhan Zhu Department of Neurology, Boston University School of Medicine, Boston, Massachusetts

Hypertensive disorders*

Amanda Roman

CHRONIC HYPERTENSION
Key Points
- Chronic hypertension (CHTN) is defined as either a history of hypertension preceding the pregnancy or a blood pressure (BP) ≥140/90 prior to 20 weeks gestation.
- Severe CHTN has been defined as systolic blood pressure (SBP) ≥160 mmHg or diastolic blood pressure (DBP) ≥110 mmHg.
- High-risk CHTN has been defined in pregnancy as that associated with secondary hypertension, target organ damage (left ventricular dysfunction, retinopathy, dyslipidemia, microvascular disease, prior stroke), maternal age >40, previous pregnancy loss, SBP ≥180, or DBP ≥110 mmHg.
- Maternal complications of CHTN include worsening HTN, superimposed preeclampsia, severe preeclampsia, eclampsia, HELLP (Hemolysis, Elevated Liver enzymes, and Low Platelet count) syndrome, cesarean delivery, and (uncommonly) pulmonary edema, hypertensive encephalopathy, retinopathy, cerebral hemorrhage, and acute renal failure.
- Fetal complications of CHTN: fetal growth restriction (FGR), oligohydramnios, placental abruption, preterm birth (PTB), and perinatal death.
- Prevention (mostly preconception) consists of exercise, weight reduction, proper diet, and restriction of sodium intake.
- In addition to history and physical examination, initial evaluation may include liver function tests (LFTs), platelet count, creatinine, urine analysis, and 24-hour urine for total protein (and creatinine clearance). Women with high-risk, severe, or long-standing HTN may need an electrocardiogram (EKG) and echocardiogram as well. If hypertension is newly diagnosed and has not been evaluated previously, a medical consult may be indicated to assess for possible etiologic factors (renal artery stenosis, pheochromocytoma, hyperaldosteronism, etc.).
- There is insufficient evidence to assess bed rest for managing CHTN in pregnancy.
- Blood pressure decreases physiologically in the first and second trimester in pregnancy, especially in women with CHTN. As blood pressure is usually <140/90 mmHg at the first visit for hypertensive women, often antihypertensive drugs do not need to be increased. BP will usually increase again in the third trimester, leading to a workup for preeclampsia and, if absent, restarting of antihypertensive drugs.

- Antihypertensive medications in pregnancy are recommended in cases with severe HTN: SBP ≥160 or DBP ≥100 on two occasions. The goal is usually to maintain a BP of around 140–150/90–100 mmHg. With end-organ damage, such as renal disease, diabetes with vascular disease, or left ventricular dysfunction, these thresholds should probably be lowered to <140/90.
- On the basis of limited trial data, labetalol and nifedipine are the current antihypertensive drugs most used by experts. Labetalol dosing can start at 100 mg twice a day with a maximum dose of 2400 mg a day. Nifedipine is started at 10 mg twice a day or 30 mg XL once a day with a maximum dose of 120 mg/day. Angiotensin-converting enzyme (ACE) inhibitors are contraindicated in pregnancy.

Diagnosis/Definition (Table 1.1)
Chronic hypertension in pregnancy (CHTN) is defined as either a history of hypertension preceding the pregnancy or a blood pressure ≥140/90 prior to 20 weeks gestation. Though controversial, the 5th Korotkoff sound is used for the diastolic reading. Blood pressure measurements can be obtained using a manual or an automated cuff with the patient in the sitting position. Severe CHTN is defined as SBP ≥160 mmHg or DBP ≥110 mmHg. In non-pregnant adults, BP <120/80 mmHg is normal, BP 120–139/80–89 mmHg is prehypertension, BP 140–159/90–99 is stage 1 hypertension, and BP ≥160/100 mmHg is stage 2 hypertension.

Epidemiology/Incidence
CHTN occurs in about 1% to 5% of pregnant women. CHTN in pregnancy is the second leading cause of maternal mortality in the United States, accounting for about 15% of such deaths. Hypertensive disorders, such as CHTN, gestational hypertension, preeclampsia with or without severe features, or HELLP syndrome, occur in 12% to 22% of pregnancies.

Etiology/Basic Pathophysiology
CHTN mostly develops as a complex quantitative trait affected by both genetic and environmental factors. Most women have essential or primary hypertension, and around 10% may have underlying renal or endocrine disease.

Classification
Severe CHTN has been defined as SBP ≥160 mmHg or DBP ≥110 mmHg [1]. High-risk CHTN has been defined in pregnancy as that associated with secondary hypertension, target organ damage (left ventricular dysfunction, retinopathy, dyslipidemia, maternal age >40 years, microvascular

---

* Hypertensive disorders of pregnancy include chronic hypertension, gestational hypertension, preeclampsia, HELLP syndrome, and eclampsia.

Table 1.1   Definitions and Diagnostic Criteria for Hypertensive Disorders of Pregnancy

Chronic hypertension in pregnancy
Either a history of hypertension (HTN) preceding the pregnancy with or without antihypertensive medication or a blood pressure ≥140/90 prior to 20 weeks gestation.

Gestational Hypertension
Sustained (on at least two occasions, six hours apart) BP ≥140/90 after 20 weeks without proteinuria, other signs or symptoms of preeclampsia, or a prior history of HTN.

Preeclampsia without severe features ("mild preeclampsia")
Sustained (at least twice, six hours but not >7 days apart) BP ≥140/90 mmHg and proteinuria (≥300 mg in 24 hours in a woman without prior proteinuria) after 20 weeks of gestation in a woman with previously normal blood pressure.

Superimposed preeclampsia
One or more of the following criteria:
- New onset of proteinuria (**≥300 mg in 24 hours without prior proteinuria**) after 20 weeks in a woman with chronic HTN or sudden increase in proteinuria in a woman with known proteinuria before or early in pregnancy
- A sudden increase in hypertension previously well controlled or escalation of antihypertensive medication to control BP

Superimposed preeclampsia with severe features
Superimposed preeclampsia and one or more of the following criteria:
- Severe range of BP (≥160/110 mmHg) despite escalation of antihypertensive medication
- Platelet count <100,000/mm³
- Increased hepatic transaminases (AST and/or ALT) two times the upper limit of normal concentration at a particular laboratory
- New onset or worsening renal insufficiency (creatinine ≥1.1 mg/dL or a doubling of the serum creatinine)
- Pulmonary edema
- Persistent neurological symptoms (e.g., headache, visual changes)

Preeclampsia with severe features ("severe preeclampsia")
Preeclampsia with any one of the following criteria:
- BP ≥160/110 mmHg (two occasions, >4 hours apart)
- Thrombocytopenia (platelets <100,000/mm³) and/or evidence of microangiopathic hemolytic anemia
- Increased hepatic transaminases (AST and/or ALT) two times of the upper limit of normal concentration for the particular laboratory
- Progressive renal insufficiency (creatinine ≥1.1 mg/dL or a doubling of the serum creatinine or oliguria (<500 mL urine in 24 hours)) in absence of other renal disease
- Persistent headache or other cerebral or visual disturbances (including grand mal seizures)
- Persistent epigastric (or right upper quadrant) pain
- Pulmonary edema or cyanosis

HELLP syndrome
Tennessee Classification (most commonly used)
- **Hemolysis** as evidenced by an abnormal peripheral smear in addition to either serum LDH >600 IU/L or total bilirubin ≥1.2 mg/dL (≥20.52 μmol/L)
- **Elevated liver enzymes** as evidenced by an AST or ALT two times the upper limit of normal concentration at a particular laboratory
- **Platelets <100,000 cells/mm³.**
If all the criteria are met, the syndrome is defined "complete"; if only one or two criteria are present, the term "partial HELLP" is preferred.

Subclassification: Mississippi HELLP Classification System
- Class 1: HELLP syndrome (severe thrombocytopenia): platelet count ≤50,000 cells/mm³ + LDH >600 IU/L and AST or ALT ≥70 IU/L
- Class 2: HELLP syndrome (moderate thrombocytopenia): platelet count >50,000 but ≤100,000 cells/mm³ + LDH >600 IU/L and AST or ALT ≥70 IU/L
- Class 3: HELLP syndrome (mild thrombocytopenia): platelet count >100,000 but ≤150,000 cells/mm³ + LDH >600 IU/L and AST or ALT ≥40 IU/L

Eclampsia
- Seizures (grand mal) in the presence of preeclampsia and/or HELLP syndrome.

Abbreviations: ALT, alanine aminotransferase; AST, aspartate aminotransferase; BP, blood pressure; HELLP, hemolysis, elevated liver enzymes, low platelets; LDH, lactase dehydrogenase.

disease, prior stroke), previous loss, SBP ≥180 mmHg or DBP ≥110 mmHg or other maternal diseases, such as obesity [2] and/or diabetes mellitus. For gestational HTN, see below.

Risk Factors/Associations

Renal disease (the most common cause of secondary CHTN); collagen vascular disease; antiphospholipid syndrome; diabetes; and other disorders such as thyrotoxicosis, Cushing's disease, hyperaldosteronism, pheochromocytoma, or coarctation of the aorta.

Complications

Maternal
Worsening CHTN, superimposed preeclampsia (20%) with or without severe features, eclampsia, HELLP syndrome, and cesarean delivery. Pulmonary edema, hypertensive encephalopathy, retinopathy, cerebral hemorrhage, and acute renal failure are uncommon but are more common with severe CHTN [3].

Fetal
Growth restriction (8%–15%); oligohydramnios, placental abruption (0.7%–1.5%, about a twofold increase), **PTB**

(12%–34%), and **perinatal death** (two- to fourfold increase). All of these complications have higher incidences with severe or high-risk CHTN.

Management
Principles
Pregnancy is characterized by increased blood volume, decreased colloid oncotic pressure (see also Chapter 3 in *Obstetric Evidence Based Guidelines*). Physiologic BP decreasing in the first and second trimester may mask CHTN.

Initial Evaluation/Workup
History. Antihypertensive drugs, prior workup, end-organ damage, prior obstetrical history, family history of renal or cardiac disease.

Physical examination. Blood pressure, cardiac murmurs, edema.

Laboratory tests. Baseline values may be useful to be able to compare in cases of possible later preeclampsia, liver function test (**LFT), platelets, creatinine, urine analysis, 24-hour urine for total protein (and creatinine clearance)** (see also Chapter 23). An early glucose challenge test may be indicated. Coagulation studies (especially fibrinogen) are usually not indicated except in specific severe cases. Creatinine clearance (mL/min) is calculated as follows:

$$\frac{\text{Urine creatinine}(mg/dL) \times \text{Total urine volume}(mL)}{\text{Serum}(mg/dL) \times 1440\,\text{minutes}}$$

Other tests. Maternal **EKG, echocardiogram, and ophthalmological examination** are suggested, especially in women with long-standing, high-risk, or severe hypertension. Renal ultrasound to rule out polycystic kidney disease or obstructive disease causing renal failure may be considered in cases of suspected obstructive uropathy or strong family history of kidney disease.

Workup
It is important to identify cardiovascular risk factors or any reversible cause of hypertension and assess for target organ damage or cardiovascular disease. Reversible causes include chronic kidney disease, coarctation of the aorta, Cushing's syndrome, drug-induced/related causes, pheochromocytoma, hyperaldosteronism, renovascular hypertension (renal artery stenosis), thyroid/parathyroid disease, and sleep apnea. If hypertension is newly diagnosed and has not been evaluated previously, a medical consult may be indicated to assess for any of these factors. Secondary hypertension, target organ damage (left ventricular dysfunction, retinopathy, dyslipidemia, renal disease, microvascular disease, prior stroke), maternal age >40 years, previous loss, SBP ≥180 or DBP ≥110 mmHg are associated with higher risks in pregnancy.

Prevention
A baby aspirin is recommended starting at 12 week or at least before 24 week to decrease the incidence of preeclampsia.In women with mild hypertension, gestational hypertensive disorders, or a family history of hypertensive disorders, 30 minutes of **exercise** three times a week may decrease DBP, as per a very small trial [4]. **Maintaining ideal body weight and preconception weight reduction** is recommended for overweight or obese women. A **proper diet** should be rich in fruits, vegetables, and low-fat dairy foods with reduced saturated and total fats. **Restriction of sodium intake** to <2.4 g sodium daily intake, recommended for essential hypertension, is beneficial in nonpregnant adults. Use of alcohol and tobacco is strongly discouraged.

Screening/Diagnosis
Initial BP evaluation may help to identify women with chronic hypertension, and third-trimester blood pressure readings aid in preeclampsia screening. **A BP of ≥120/80 mmHg in the first or second trimester is not normal** and associated with later risks of preeclampsia. **Blood pressure should be taken properly**. Appropriate measurement of BP includes using Korotkoff phase V, appropriate cuff size (length 1.5 × upper-arm circumference, or a cuff with a bladder that encircles ≥80% of the arm), and position so that the woman's arm is at the level of the heart (sitting up) at rest.

Preconception Counseling
There are significant risks associated with hypertension and preeclampsia in pregnancy. All women should be counseled appropriately regarding the possible complications and preventive and management strategies for hypertensive disorders in pregnancy. ACE inhibitors and angiotensin type II (AII) receptor antagonists should be discontinued. A complete evaluation and workup, as described above, should be done, especially if she has a several-year history of hypertension and/or hypertension never fully evaluated. Baseline tests can also be obtained for later comparison. Abnormalities should be addressed and managed appropriately (see specific chapters). If, for example, serum creatinine (Cr) is >1.4 mg/dL, the woman should be aware of increased risks in pregnancy (pregnancy/fetal loss, reduced birth weight, preterm delivery, and accelerated deterioration of maternal renal disease). Even mild renal disease (Cr = 1.1–1.4 mg/dL) with uncontrolled HTN is associated with 10 times higher risk of fetal loss (see Chapter 17).

Prenatal Care
Often BP monitoring at home is suggested in pregnancies with CHTN. At present, the possible advantages and risks of ambulatory blood pressure monitoring during pregnancy, in particular in hypertensive pregnant women, cannot be defined because there is no randomized controlled trial (RCT) evidence to support the use of ambulatory BP monitoring during pregnancy [5].

Therapy
Lifestyle changes and bed rest. There are no trials to assess lifestyle changes other than bed rest in pregnancy. Weight reduction is not recommended. The diet should be rich in fruits, vegetables, and low-fat dairy foods with reduced saturated and total fats and with sodium intake restricted to <2.4 g sodium daily.

There is **insufficient evidence** to demonstrate any differences between bed rest (in or out of the hospital) for reported outcomes overall. Compared with routine activity at home, some bed rest in the hospital for **nonproteinuric hypertension** is associated with a 42% reduced risk of severe hypertension and a borderline 47% reduction in risk of PTB in one trial [6]. The trial did not address possible adverse effects of bed rest. Three times more women in the bed rest group opted **not** to have the same management in future pregnancies, if the choice is given. There are no significant differences for any other outcomes [6].

Antihypertensive drugs
Common types

- *Labetalol (alpha- and beta-blocker)*: On the basis of limited trial data (see below), labetalol is the **current drug of choice** of many experts [1,7]. It has a rapid onset of action (within two hours). Dosing can start at 100 mg twice a day with maximum dose of 2400 mg a day. As with other drugs, generally a different agent should not be added until maximum doses of the first drug are achieved. Labetalol has been associated with elevated liver enzymes in rare cases (which may be confused with HELLP syndrome) as well as lethargy, fatigue, sleep disorders, and bronchoconstriction. Labetalol should be avoided in women with asthma, heart disease, or congestive heart failure.
- *Calcium channel blockers*: Calcium channel blockers are frequently used as **first or second option** for CHTN in pregnancy. There is no known association with birth defects with reassuring long-term follow-up of babies up to 1.5 years. Nifedipine is not associated with adverse perinatal outcome [8]. Nifedipine can be started at 10 mg twice a day with a maximum dose of 120 mg/day. Long-acting nifedipine XL can be started at 30 mg with 120 mg as a maximum dose. Very rare cases of neuromuscular blockade have been reported when nifedipine is used simultaneously with magnesium sulfate. This blockade is reversible with 10% solution of calcium gluconate. Although amlodipine is widely used in nonpregnant individuals with hypertension, there are sparse data of its use in pregnancy [9]. Other calcium antagonists, such as verapamil and diltiazem, have been used.
- *Beta-blockers*: The safety of beta-adrenergic blockers is somewhat controversial due to reports of premature labor, FGR, neonatal apnea, bradycardia, and hypoglycemia in pregnancy compared to placebo and with higher mortality in nonpregnant adults compared to other agents and **should probably be avoided**. There is insufficient evidence to assess if other drugs in this class (or even other classes) are associated with the same effect (see below).
- *Diuretics*: Women who use diuretics from early in pregnancy do not have the physiologic increase in plasma volume, which poses a theoretical concern because preeclampsia is associated with reduced plasma volume. Nonetheless, the reduction in plasma volume associated with diuretics has not been associated with adverse effects on outcomes. Diuretics are not contraindicated in pregnancy except in settings in which uteroplacental perfusion is already reduced (i.e., preeclampsia and FGR). This is usually the drug of first choice for some nonpregnant adults and should be considered as a secondary option in pregnant women. The initial dose of hydrochlorothiazide is usually 12.5 mg twice a day with a maximum dose of 50 mg/day. Dose should be adjusted to prevent hypokalemia.
- *ACE inhibitor (or AII receptor antagonists)*: These drugs are **contraindicated** in the first trimester because they might be associated with a twofold increase in malformations and are contraindicated also later in pregnancy because they are associated with FGR, oligohydramnios, neonatal renal failure, and neonatal death. Postpartum complications include oliguria and anuria.
- *Methyldopa (Aldomet)*: This drug was the preferred first-line agent historically because it is associated with stable

uteroplacental blood flow and fetal hemodynamics, and no long-term adverse effects are seen in exposed children (up to 7.5 years; best documentation of fetal safety of any antihypertensive drug). It is a mild antihypertensive agent and has a slow onset of action (three to six hours). Liver disease is a contraindication. Initial dose is usually 250 mg two to three times a day with the highest dose 500 mg four times a day (2 g/day). Side effects include dry mouth and drowsiness/somnolence.

Effectiveness
Mild-to-moderate HTN. Mild-to-moderate HTN is usually defined in trials as a SBP of 140 to 159 mmHg or a DBP of 90 to 109 mmHg. A Cochrane review published in 2014 included 49 trials (4723 women) to evaluate the management in pregnant women with **mild-to-moderate hypertension** (all diagnoses included). Antihypertensive drugs vs. placebo were associated with a **50% reduction in the risk of developing severe hypertension but no differences in the risk of developing preeclampsia, PTB, small for gestational age (SGA), perinatal death, or any other outcomes [10]**. Of the included studies, only six had dedicated inclusion of women with CHTN: Similar to the overall findings, in this subgroup of women, there was a 43% reduction in the risk of developing severe hypertension but no changes in other maternal or perinatal outcome. Beta-blockers and calcium channel blockers used together instead of methyldopa have a 46% reduction in the risk of severe hypertension and a 27% overall risk of developing proteinuria/preeclampsia. **However, there is insufficient evidence to conclude that one antihypertensive is better than another** [10]. Other meta-analyses have suggested that women receiving **beta-blockers** had a significant 38% increase risk in SGA and a threefold **increase in birth weight <5th percentile** [11–13] A recent multicenter international RCT compared "less tight control" to "tight control" of BP for pregnant women with mild-to-moderate hypertension [14]. The study reported outcomes for 987 women who were enrolled at 14–33 weeks of gestation; participants had either chronic (75%) or gestational (25%) nonproteinuric hypertension. Women were randomized to either less tight control (target DBP 100 mmHg) or tight control (target DBP 85 mmHg) during pregnancy. The primary outcome of pregnancy loss or need for high-level neonatal care for ≥48 hours did not differ between groups (31.4% vs. 30.7%). The frequency of severe hypertension was higher with less-tight control but was not associated with any adverse pregnancy outcome, such as preeclampsia, abruption, or composite of "serious maternal complications." The overall risk of SGA (<10th percentile) was not different between groups, aOR:0.78; (0.56–1.08). In the subgroup with chronic hypertension, the risk of SGA was 34% lower with less-tight control (13.9% vs. 19.7%; aOR:0.66; 95% CI 0.44–1.00) although this study was underpowered to examine subgroup differences [14]. In the absence of strong evidence of benefits and risks of pharmacologic treatment and SGA, management of pregnant women with mild-to-moderate chronic hypertension remains uncertain [1,7].

The task force of hypertension in pregnancy recommends that women with mild to moderate hypertension (SBP ≥140 mmHg but <160 mmHg or DBP ≥90 mmHg but <110 mmHg) without end-organ damage should not be treated with pharmacologic agents [1].

In women with known CHTN well controlled on antihypertensive medications, discontinuation of the medication during the first trimester is a reasonable alternative **as blood** pressure is usually <140/90 at the first visit. Often BP will increase again in the third trimester, leading to a workup for preeclampsia, and if preeclampsia is absent, antihypertensive drugs can be restarted.

For women with CHTN and end-organ damage (renal disease, diabetes with vascular disease, or left ventricular dysfunction), these thresholds should probably be lowered to <140/90 mmHg to avoid progression of the disease during pregnancy and associated complications.

Severe HTN. Severe HTN is defined as **SBP ≥160 mmHg or DBP ≥110 mmHg [1]**. There is insufficient evidence to assess the benefits and risks of different antihypertensive drugs for severe CHTN as most studies that address this question have not been limited to women with CHTN and also have included gestational HTN and preeclampsia. A Cochrane systematic review of 35 trials, 3573 women, evaluated the drug treatment for severe HTN during pregnancy [15]. Drug therapy was initiated for DBP ≥100–110 mmHg mostly during the third trimester. They included a few women with CHTN, but subgroup analysis was not performed. The task force on hypertension in pregnancy recommends **starting antihypertensive therapy at SBP >160 mmHg or DBP >105 mmHg on at least two occasions with a goal of SBP between 120 and 160 mmHg and DBP between 80 and 105 mmHg**, avoiding overly aggressive BP lowering due to concerns of decreased uteroplacental blood flow [1]. This is to decrease the risk of cerebrovascular accidents and cardiovascular (e.g., congestive heart failure) and renal complications. **The goal is to maintain BP around 140–150/90–100 mmHg.**

There are two indications of antihypertensive medications for women with CHTN: 1) acute lowering of severe HTN in the hospital (Table 1.3), or 2) chronic treatment in an outpatient setting (Table 1.4). Based on findings of the Cochrane systematic review [15], there is **no clear evidence that one antihypertensive is preferable to the others for improving outcomes for women with very high blood pressure during pregnancy**. Therefore, **the choice of antihypertensive should depend on the experience and familiarity of an individual clinician with a particular drug and on what is known about adverse maternal and fetal side effects.** Three drugs—**high-dose diazoxide [16], ketanserin, and nimodipine—have serious disadvantages and so should probably be avoided** for women with very high blood pressure during pregnancy.

Antepartum Testing

Increased perinatal morbidity and mortality is mainly attributed to severe CHTN and high-risk CHTN with end-organ damage or secondary HTN. The risk of FGR with uncomplicated CHTN is 8% to 15%, and with severe and high-risk CHTN, the risk increases up to 40%. Early detection of FGR can decrease the risk of stillbirth by 20% [17], and the addition of umbilical artery Doppler on those with suspected FGR decreases perinatal mortality by 29% [18]. Initial **dating ultrasound**, preferably in the first trimester (FTS at 11–14 weeks), **anatomy ultrasound** at around 18 to 20 weeks, and **ultrasound for growth** at 28 to 32 weeks are suggested for women with uncomplicated CHTN and every month after anatomy ultrasound on those with severe and high-risk CHTN (see also Chapter 4 in *Obstetric Evidence Based Guidelines*).

Antenatal testing (usually with weekly nonstress tests) is suggested starting around 32 weeks, especially if poorly controlled, severe HTN, high-risk CHTN, FGR, or

superimposed preeclampsia is indicated. Umbilical artery Doppler is recommended in cases of FGR (see Chapter 44). For uterine artery Doppler, see the section titled "Preeclampsia."

Delivery

Often PTB (either spontaneous or iatrogenic) occurs because of complications. In the uncomplicated pregnancy with CHTN, the pregnancy should probably be delivered by the estimated date of confinement (EDC). Unfortunately, there are no RCTs evaluating timing of delivery for women with chronic HTN. In a large population-based cohort study, among women with otherwise uncomplicated chronic hypertension, **delivery at 38 or 39 weeks** appears to provide the optimal trade-off between the risk of adverse fetal and adverse neonatal outcomes. The risk of stillbirth is significantly higher at 41 weeks [19].

Anesthesia

See the section titled "Preeclampsia" and also Chapter 11 in *Obstetric Evidence Based Guidelines*.

Postpartum/Breast-Feeding

Methyldopa, labetalol, beta-blockers, calcium channel blockers, and most other agents are safe with breast-feeding, with the possible exception of ACE inhibitors, because even low concentrations in breast milk could affect neonatal renal function.

GESTATIONAL HYPERTENSION
Definition (Table 1.1)

Gestational hypertension (GHTN), formerly known as pregnancy-induced hypertension, is defined as sustained (on at least two occasions, 6 hours apart) BP ≥140/90 after 20 weeks, without proteinuria, other signs or symptoms of preeclampsia, or a prior history of HTN. Severe GHTN is defined similarly except that the cutoffs are ≥160/110 mmHg.

Incidence

About 6% to 17% healthy nulliparous women.

Risk Factors

Most risk factors are similar to preeclampsia (Table 1.2).

Complications

Progression to preeclampsia usually is seen in 1–3 weeks. Severe GHTN is associated with higher morbidities than mild preeclampsia with incidences of abruption, PTB, and SGA, similar to severe preeclampsia. If GHTN develops before 30 weeks or is severe, there is a high (50%) rate of progression to preeclampsia.

Antenatal Management

GHTN is usually associated with good outcomes, similar to low-risk pregnant women [20], so that **close surveillance for development of preeclampsia** but no other intervention is usually needed. **Before 37 weeks**, in **the absence of severe GHTN, preeclampsia with severe features** or preterm labor and in the presence of reassuring fetal testing, **expectant management** is suggested. Outpatient management with close surveillance of maternal symptoms, BP (suggest daily as outpatient with personal BP cuff), proteinuria, and laboratory

Table 1.2 Selected Clinical Risk Factors for Preeclampsia

Primiparity
Primipaternity
Previous preeclamptic pregnancy
Chronic hypertension
Chronic renal disease
History of thrombophilia
In vitro fertilization
Family history of preeclampsia
Pregestational diabetes mellitus
Obesity
Systemic lupus erythematosus
Advanced maternal age (>40 years)

tests is suggested. Antihypertensive medications for BP <160/110 mmHg or bed rest are not recommended. Antepartum surveillance also should include daily fetal kick counts, ultrasonographic fetal growth assessment every 3–4 weeks, BPP or modified BPP every week starting at the onset of diagnosis.

Severe GHTN usually requires admission to the hospital at diagnosis to increase maternal fetal surveillance. Antihypertensive medications are recommended in women with SBPs ≥160 mmHg or DBPs ≥110 mmHg to avoid maternal complications (stroke, cardiac failure, pulmonary edema, renal impairment, and death). Drugs of choice for both oral or intravenous administration, and doses, are described in Table 1.3 and Table 1.4 (same recommendations as above in CHTN section).

Delivery

For women at or beyond 37 weeks with GHTN, delivery is recommended rather than continued observation. Compared to expectant management, induction of labor in women with mostly (about 66%) gestational hypertension (or preeclampsia without severe features) at 36 to 41 weeks gestation is associated with a trend for lower incidence of maternal

Table 1.3 Antihypertensive Medications for Urgent Blood Pressure Control in the Hospital

Drug	Dose	Comments
Labetalol	10–20 mg IV, then 20–80 mg every 20–30 minutes to a maximum dose of 300 mg or constant infusion 1–2 mg/min IV	Considered first-line agent Tachycardia is less common and fewer adverse effects Contraindicated in patients with asthma, heart disease, or congestive heart failure
Hydralazine	5 mg IV or IM, then 5–10 mg IV every 20–40 minutes to maximum dose of 30 mg or constant infusion 0.5–10 mg/h	Higher or frequent dosage associated with maternal hypotension, headaches, and fetal distress—maybe more common than other agents
Nifedipine	10–20 mg orally, repeat in 30 minutes if needed; then 10–20 mg every 2–6 hours	May observe tachycardia and headaches

Source: American College of Obstetricians and Gynecologists, Task Force on Hypertension in Pregnancy. *Obstet Gynecol*, 122, 5, 1122–31, 2013.
Abbreviations: IM: intramuscular; IV, intravenous.

Table 1.4 Oral Antihypertensive Medications in Pregnant Patients (Outpatient)

Drug	Dosage	Comments
Labetalol	200–2400 mg/d orally in two or three divided doses	Well tolerated Partial broncho-constrictive effects Avoid in patients with asthma and congestive heart failure
Nifedipine	30–120 mg/day orally of a slow release preparation	Do not use sublingual form
Methyldopa	0.5–3 g/day orally in two to three divided doses	Childhood safety data up to 7 years of age May not be as effective in control of severe hypertension
Thiazide diuretics	Depends on the agent	Not first line agent Risk of hypokalemia
Angiotensin-converting enzyme inhibitors/ angiotensin receptor blockers		Associated with fetal anomalies Contraindicated in pregnancy and preconception period Postpartum oliguria and anuria

Source: American College of Obstetricians and Gynecologists, Task Force on Hypertension in Pregnancy. *Obstet Gynecol*, 122, 5, 1122–31, 2013.

complications (e.g., HELLP, severe HTN, and pulmonary edema) (RR 0.81, 95% CI 0.63–1.03), and lower incidence of neonatal pH <7.05 with induction of labor ≥37 weeks [21]. Trends were seen for benefit of induction associated with less cesarean delivery and maternal ICU admission. Magnesium sulfate for seizure prophylaxis is not indicated in GHTN. **There is no strict recommendation of when to deliver women with severe GHTN in absence of severe features.** If any of the criteria for severe features of preeclampsia are present, delivery is indicated at 34 weeks or after (see below).

Postpartum management of women with GHTN requires continued observation of BPs for 72 hours postpartum and outpatient follow up in 7–10 days as there is an increased risk of postpartum preeclampsia/eclampsia and CHTN in these women [1].

PREECLAMPSIA
Key Points

- **Preeclampsia** is defined as sustained (at least twice, 6 hours but not >7 days apart) new onset of **SBP ≥140 mmHg or DBP ≥90 mmHg and new onset of proteinuria (≥300 mg in 24 hours or protein creatinine ratio ≥0.3 or dipstick reading of more than 1+ only if other methods are not available), after 20 weeks of gestation in a woman with previously normal blood pressure.**
- **Preeclampsia** can be diagnosed as well **if there is** new onset of **SBP ≥140 mmHg or DBP ≥90 mmHg in absence**

of proteinuria but with new onset of any of the following: platelets <100,000/mm³, serum creatinine level ≥1.1 mg/dL or doubling of the previous creatinine level in absence of other renal disease, elevated aspartate aminotransferase (AST) and/or alanine aminotransferase (ALT) twice the reference level, pulmonary edema or persistent headache or other cerebral or visual disturbances.

- **Superimposed preeclampsia (in a woman with known well-controlled CHTN)** is defined as the new onset of proteinuria **(≥300 mg in 24 hours or protein/creatinine ratio ≥0.3)** after 20 weeks or significant increase in pre-existing proteinuria or sudden exacerbation of BPs or worsening HTN requiring increased dose of antihypertensive medications on more than two occasions.

- **Preeclampsia with severe features** ("severe preeclampsia") is defined as preeclampsia with any of the following: SBP ≥160 mmHg or DBP ≥110 mmHg or higher in two occasions at least 4 hours apart while on bed rest, platelets <100,000/mm³, progressive renal disease as diagnosed by elevated serum creatinine level ≥1.1 mg/dL or doubling of the previous creatinine level in absence of other renal disease, impaired liver function as indicated by elevated AST and/or ALT twice the reference level, severe right upper quadrant or epigastric pain not accounted for by other etiologies, pulmonary edema or new onset of persistent headache, or other cerebral or visual disturbances.

- **HELLP syndrome** is defined as **hemolysis,** elevated liver enzymes **(AST or ALT)** twice the reference level, and **platelets** <100,000/mm³.

- **Eclampsia** is defined as new onset of grand mal seizures in the presence of preeclampsia and/or HELLP syndrome. Eclampsia can occur before, during, and after labor.

- **Maternal complications** of preeclampsia include (maternal) **HELLP syndrome,** disseminated intravascular coagulation **(DIC), pulmonary edema, abruptio placentae, renal failure, cardiac failure, seizures** (eclampsia), **cerebral hemorrhage, liver hemorrhage,** and **maternal death.**

- **Fetal complications** of preeclampsia include FGR, PTB, perinatal death, hypoxemia, or neurologic injury.

- **Low-dose aspirin (75–150 mg/day)** given to women with **risk factors for preeclampsia** is associated with a **17% reduction** in the risk of **preeclampsia,** a small **(8%) reduction** in the risk of **PTB <37 weeks,** a **10% reduction** in **SGA** babies, and a **14% reduction in perinatal deaths.**

- If low-dose aspirin is given anyway because of a history of preeclampsia, then uterine artery Doppler screening may not be necessary or beneficial. It is recommended to start **low-dose aspirin early (≤16 weeks)** in women with high risk for preeclampsia as it is associated with a **90% reduction in severe preeclampsia, a 69% reduction in gestational hypertension, and a 49% reduction in intrauterine growth restriction (IUGR).**

- **Calcium supplementation** is associated with a 35% **reduction in the incidence of high blood pressure** and a 55% **reduction in the risk of preeclampsia.** This effect is greatest in women with low baseline calcium intake or high risk of preeclampsia, in which calcium supplementation (1.5–2 g/day) may be indicated.

- **Antioxidant therapy with vitamin C** 1000 mg/day and **vitamin E** 400 IU/day starting in the early second trimester is not associated with a **reduction** in the risk of preeclampsia. Antioxidant therapy is **not recommended for prevention of preeclampsia.**

- Diuretics or dietary salt restriction during pregnancy are not associated with reduction in the incidence of preeclampsia.

- Bed rest or the restriction of other physical activity should not be used for the primary prevention of preeclampsia and its complications.

- In women with risk factors for preeclampsia, the **baseline values** should be obtained **at first prenatal visit:** complete history and physical examination (BP), **AST** and **ALT, platelets,** creatinine, **24-hour urine for total protein** (and creatinine clearance), and/or protein/creatinine ratio.

- **Indications for delivery:** Preeclampsia without severe features at ≥37 weeks. Preeclampsia with severe features (severe preeclampsia) at ≥34 weeks warrants expeditious delivery after maternal stabilization. Before 34 weeks, delivery within 48 hours after completion of corticosteroid administration is suggested for uncontrollable BP in spite of continuing increase in antihypertensive drugs, **persistent headache and/or visual/ CNS symptoms, epigastric pain, vaginal bleeding, persistent oliguria, preterm labor, premature preterm rupture of membranes (PPROM), platelets <100,000/ mm³ or elevated liver enzymes (partial or complete HELLP syndrome), nonreassuring fetal heart rate, or reversed umbilical artery end-diastolic flow ≥32 weeks. Immediate delivery** even before completion of steroids is recommended in case of **eclampsia, pulmonary edema, acute renal failure, DIC, suspected abruptio placentae, or nonreassuring fetal status.**

- **Magnesium is the drug of choice for prevention of eclampsia,** as it is superior to phenytoin and diazepam. Magnesium is associated with a 59% **reduction in** the risk of **eclampsia,** a 36% reduction in **abruption,** and a nonstatistically significant but clinically important 46% reduction in **maternal death. The reduction is similar regardless of severity of preeclampsia** with about 400 women who need to be treated to prevent eclampsia for mild preeclampsia, 71 for severe preeclampsia, and 36 for preeclampsia with central nervous system (CNS) symptoms.

- Magnesium is recommended in women with preeclampsia with severe features. The **intravenous** route is recommended, initiating with a loading dose of 4–6 g followed by maintenance dose of **1–2 g/hr, usually given at least in active labor and 24 hours postpartum** without mandatory serum monitoring. When cesarean delivery is indicated, it is recommended to continue magnesium during the procedure as discontinuing magnesium may increase the risk of postpartum eclampsia.

- **Antihypertensive drugs** for the treatment of preeclampsia with **severe HTN (SBP ≥160 and/or DBP ≥110)** are usually **labetalol, nifedipine, or hydralazine.**

- Antihypertensive therapy may decrease progression to severe hypertension by 50%, but there is no effect on the risk of developing severe preeclampsia and it may also be associated with impairment of fetal growth.

- There is **insufficient evidence to recommend the use of dexamethasone or other steroids for therapy specific for HELLP syndrome.**

- In **about 15% of cases, hypertension or proteinuria** may be **absent before eclampsia. A high index of suspicion for eclampsia** should be maintained in **all cases of hypertensive disorders in pregnancy,** in particular those with **CNS symptoms** (e.g., headache and visual disturbances).

- In **eclampsia** (see below), the first priorities are **airway, breathing, and circulation.**
- Women with **prior preeclampsia or its complications are** not only at **increased risk of recurrence,** but also at **increased risk of cardiovascular disease in the future.**

Diagnoses/Definitions (Table 1.1)

Preeclampsia
Sustained (at least twice, 6 hours but not >7 days apart) **BP ≥140 or ≥90 mmHg** and **new onset of proteinuria (≥300 mg in 24 hours or urinary protein creatinine ratio [UPC] ≥0.3) after 20 weeks of gestation** in a woman with previously normal blood pressure and normal protein in the urine [1,22,23]. BP should be measured with adequate cuff size, position of the heart at arm level, and with calibrated equipment. The accuracy of dipstick urinalysis with a 1+ (0.1 g/L) threshold in the prediction of significant proteinuria by 24-hour urine is poor [24]. Preeclampsia without severe features ("mild preeclampsia") is usually defined as preeclampsia not meeting severe criteria (see below). "Toxemia" is a lay term. The "30–15 rule" and edema have been eliminated as criteria to diagnose preeclampsia [23].

Superimposed Preeclampsia
One or more of the following criteria:

- New onset of proteinuria **(≥300 mg in 24 hours without prior proteinuria)** after 20 weeks in a woman with chronic HTN or sudden increase in proteinuria in a woman with known proteinuria before or early in pregnancy.
- A sudden increase in hypertension previously well controlled or escalation of antihypertensive medication to control BP.

Superimposed preeclampsia with severe features
One or more of the following are present

- Severe range of BP (≥160/110 mmHg) despite escalation of antihypertensive medication
- Platelet count <100,000/mm³
- Increased hepatic transaminases (AST and/or ALT) two times of the upper limit of normal concentration at a particular laboratory
- New onset or worsening renal insufficiency (creatinine ≥1.1 mg/dL or a doubling of the serum creatinine)
- Pulmonary edema
- Persistent neurological symptoms (e.g., headache, visual changes)

Severe preeclampsia or preeclampsia with severe features
Any of the following criteria:

- BP ≥160/110 mmHg (two occasions, ≥4 hours apart)
- Thrombocytopenia, Platelets <100,000/mm³ (and/or evidence of microangiopathic hemolytic anemia)
- Increased hepatic transaminases (AST and/or ALT) two times of the upper limit of normal concentration at a particular laboratory
- Progressive renal insufficiency (creatinine ≥ 1.1 mg/dL or a doubling of the serum creatinine or oliguria (<500 mL urine in 24 hours) in absence of other renal disease
- Persistent headache or other cerebral or visual disturbances (including grand mal seizures)

- Persistent epigastric (or right upper quadrant) pain
- Pulmonary edema or cyanosis

Proteinuria ≥5 g/24 hours was removed as criteria of severe preeclampsia as expectant management was not associated with worsening maternal or neonatal outcome, and resolution of renal dysfunction occurred in all women after delivery [25,26].

HELLP Syndrome
HELLP syndrome can have an antepartum or postpartum onset, and it is associated with increased maternal morbidity and mortality. For HELLP syndrome to be diagnosed, there must be micro-angiopathic hemolysis, thrombocytopenia, and abnormalities of liver function. There is no consensus, however, on the classification criteria and the specific thresholds of hematologic and biochemical values to use in establishing the diagnosis of HELLP syndrome. The following criteria are most commonly used (*Tennessee Classification*): **hemolysis** as evidenced by an abnormal peripheral smear in addition to either serum lactate dehydrogenase (LDH) >600 IU/L or total bilirubin ≥1.2 mg/dL (≥20.52 μmol/L); **elevated liver enzymes,** (AST and/or ALT) two times of the upper limit of normal concentration at a particular laboratory, and **platelets <100,000 cells/mm³** [27]. If all the criteria are met, the syndrome can be also called "complete"; if only one or two criteria are present, the term "partial HELLP" is preferred.

Eclampsia
New onset of grand mal seizures in the presence of preeclampsia and/or HELLP syndrome.

Symptoms
Persistent headache or other cerebral or visual disturbances, altered mental status (including grand mal seizures), persistent epigastric (or right upper quadrant) pain, severe range of BPs. Massive proteinuria and/or edema may be present.

Epidemiology/Incidence
In healthy nulliparous women, about 7% (most occur at term and are mild).

Etiology/Basic Pathophysiology
Preeclampsia is a **systemic** disease of unknown etiology. It is associated with **endothelial disease** with **vasospasm** and **sympathetic overactivity. Trophoblastic invasion** by the placenta into the spiral arteries of the uterus is **incomplete,** resulting in **reduced perfusion.** Hypoxia, free radicals, oxidative stress, and activation of endothelium are characteristic. Thromboxane (which is associated with vasoconstriction, platelet aggregation, and decreased uteroplacental blood flow) is increased, and prostacyclin (which has opposite effects) is decreased. FGR is also theorized to develop as a result of defective placentation and the imbalance between prostacyclin and thromboxane.

Alterations of the immune response.

- *Vascular*: vasospasm and subsequent hemoconcentration are associated with contraction of intravascular space; capillary leak and decreased colloid oncotic pressure may predispose to pulmonary edema.
- *Cardiac*: usually reduced cardiac output, decreased plasma volume, increased systemic vascular resistance.

- *Hematological*: thrombocytopenia and hemolysis with HELLP syndrome (also elevated LDH), disseminated intravascular coagulation (DIC).
- *Hepatic*: elevated AST, ALT; subcapsular hematoma and liver rupture.
- *CNS*: eclampsia, intracranial hemorrhage, headache, blurred vision, scotomata, hyperreflexia, temporary blindness.
- *Renal*: vasospasm, hemoconcentration, and decreased renal blood flow resulting in oliguria (rarely leading to acute tubular necrosis, possibly leading to acute renal failure), proteinuria, and hematuria.
- *Fetal*: impaired uteroplacental blood flow (FGR, oligohydramnios, abruption, and nonreassuring fetal heart rate testing [NRFHT]).

Classification
See without severe features ("mild") versus with severe features ("severe"), discussed above.

Risk Factors/Associations
Nulliparity, limited sperm exposure, primipaternity, "dangerous father" (for preeclampsia), donor eggs and/or sperm, multifetal gestation, prior preeclampsia, chronic HTN, diabetes, vascular and connective tissue disease, nephropathy, antiphospholipid syndrome (APS), obesity, insulin resistance, young maternal age or advanced maternal age, African-American race, family history of preeclampsia, maternal low birth weight, low socioeconomic status, increased soluble fms-like tyrosine kinase 1 (sFlt-1), reduced placental growth factor, and higher fetal cells in maternal circulation (Table 1.2). A change in partner is usually associated with a protective effect if prior pregnancy had preeclampsia. Previous pregnancy with the same partner seems to be protective, albeit for a short (one to three years) time. Smoking is associated with decreased incidence of preeclampsia. The presence of inherited thrombophilias, such as factor V Leiden, prothrombin 20210, and Methylene tetrahydrofolate reductase (MTHFR), has not been associated with preeclampsia when the best studies (prospective, large, etc.) are evaluated (see Chapter 27 and Table 27.3). Although antiphospholipid antibodies, in particular ACA, are associated with an increased risk of preeclampsia, screening is not suggested as no therapy has been evaluated in these cases (see Chapter 26).

Prediction
Despite the variety of methods studied, there are still **no sensitive prediction tests for preeclampsia** shown to alter outcome. No single test or combination of tests reliably predicts preeclampsia, early onset of preeclampsia, or progression of GHTN or mild preeclampsia into severe preeclampsia.

Uterine artery Doppler velocimetry has been studied, especially in pregnant women who are at high risk for preeclampsia [28]. Abnormal **uterine artery Doppler** findings in the second trimester have a sensitivity of 20% to 60% and a positive predictive value of 6% to 40%, depending on prevalence of preeclampsia. According to recent meta-analyses, an increased pulsatility index alone or combined with notching is the best predictor of preeclampsia in women with risk factors (positive likelihood ratios = 21.0 in high-risk women), but it is not so predictive in low-risk populations (positive likelihood ratio = 7.5) [29]. Uterine artery Doppler evaluation alone has a low predictive value for the development of early onset of preeclampsia. Furthermore, the studies included in the meta-analysis are heterogeneous in severity of disease and outcomes, timing of uterine artery Doppler assessment, and inclusion of other screening tests.

A variety of blood tests to predict the risk of preeclampsia have been studied. Some of the metabolites that have been proposed as early biochemical markers of preeclampsia are beta-human chorionic gonadotropin (β-hCG), α-fetoprotein; first-trimester serum levels of the biomarkers placental protein-13 (PP-13), pregnancy-associated plasma protein-A (PAPP-A), soluble Flt-1 (soluble vascular endothelial growth factor receptor-1), placental growth factor (PlGF), vascular endothelial growth factor (VEGF), and soluble endoglin. Some of these markers are altered 4–5 weeks prior to the onset of preeclampsia and cannot be detected earlier in pregnancy. An algorithm developed by logistic regression that combined the logs of **uterine artery pulsatility index, mean arterial pressure, PAPP-A, serum-free PlGF, body mass index, and presence of nulliparity or previous preeclampsia** revealed that at a 5% false positive rate, the detection rate for early preeclampsia was 93.1%; more impressively, the positive LR was 16.5, and the negative LR was 0.06 [30]. However, **none of these studies have demonstrated improvement in maternal or fetal outcome** or both in women who had undergone uterine artery Doppler assessment or biomarker testing or both. Some of these biomarkers are not approved in the United States by the Food and Drugs Administration (FDA), and they are not endorsed by ACOG [31].

Currently, there is no reliable predictive test for preeclampsia. Further research is needed to identify the ideal timing of uterine artery Doppler and the possible combination with other predictors of preeclampsia, such as measurement of maternal serum biomarkers, to improve perinatal outcomes. **A complete medical history and physical exam to evaluate for risk factors and strict surveillance and education are currently the only strategies for clinical prediction.**

Complications
Complications depend on gestational age at time of diagnosis, severity of disease, presence of other medical conditions, and, of course, management. Most cases of mild preeclampsia, at term, do not convey significant risks. Rates of complications **for severe preeclampsia** are given in the following subsections in the parentheses [32].

Maternal
HELLP syndrome (20%), **DIC** (10%), **pulmonary edema** (2%–5%), **abruptio placentae** (1%–4%), **renal failure** (1%–2%), **seizures** (eclampsia, <1%), **cerebral hemorrhage** (<1%), **liver hemorrhage** (<1%), death (rare).

Fetal/Neonatal
PTB (15%–60%), **FGR** (10%–25%), **perinatal death** (1%–2%), **hypoxemia-neurologic injury** (<1%), long-term cardiovascular morbidity (rate unknown—fetal origin of adult disease).

Management
(Figures 1.1 and 1.2) [32–35]

Principles
Preeclampsia is one of the most common and perhaps most typical obstetric complications. The only interventions associated with significant prevention of preeclampsia are

antiplatelet agents, primarily low-dose aspirin, and calcium supplementation. It is important to understand that pre-eclampsia's **only cure is delivery.** As such, preeclampsia is a temporary disease, which resolves usually 24 to 48 hours after delivery. Remember that there are two patients: delivery is always good for the mother but not always for the baby, especially if very premature. In general, most patients with preeclampsia are otherwise healthy.

Prevention

Aspirin. Aspirin acts to inhibit thromboxane synthesis while maintaining vascular wall prostacyclin synthesis, which could theoretically improve uteroplacental blood flow and fetal growth.

Compared to placebo or no treatment, antiplatelet agents, such as **low-dose aspirin (75–150 mg/day),** given to women **with risk factors for preeclampsia** (especially early onset or severe preeclampsia in previous pregnancies) are associated with a **17% reduction** in the risk of **preeclampsia** [36]. Low-dose aspirin is also associated with a small **(8%) reduction** in the risk of **PTB <37 weeks,** a **10% reduction** in **SGA** babies, and a **14% reduction** in **perinatal deaths** [36].

Compared with trials using 75 mg or less of aspirin, there is a significant reduction in the risk of preeclampsia in trials using **higher doses** (e.g., 150 mg). Although there is evidence that higher doses of aspirin may be more effective, this requires careful evaluation as risks may also be increased [36]. Low-dose aspirin use has been shown to be safe for the fetus even in the first trimester [37].

There is some evidence that **the earlier low-dose aspirin is started in pregnancy, the greater the benefits are,** as shown in a meta-analysis of 34 RCTs [38]. Low-dose aspirin initiated **before 16 weeks** is associated with a significant decrease in the incidence of gestational hypertension (69%), preeclampsia (53%), severe preeclampsia (90%), IUGR (54%), and PTB (78%) in women identified to be at risk for preeclampsia; therefore, **it is recommended to start prior to 16 weeks** of gestation. However, other two meta-analyses (Cochrane [36] and USPSTF [39]) found no difference in outcome when the gestational age at the initiation of ASA was evaluated. There is still benefit when ASA is started later in pregnancy. According to ACOG and the United States Preventive service task Force (USPSTF), **indications for low-dose aspirin** include women with a **history of preeclampsia, multifetal gestation, CHTN, Type I or II diabetes mellitus, renal disease, and autoimmune disease** (antiphospholipid syndrome, systemic lupus erythematosus). The American Heart Association and American Stroke Association for women recommend low-dose aspirin >12th week of gestation until delivery to women with CHTN or history of preeclampsia [40].

Low-dose aspirin appears to be of little or no benefit in women who already have developed preeclampsia [41–43]. Aspirin does not prevent progression to severe features and may increase the risk of bleeding in patients with HELLP syndrome.

Aspirin prophylaxis should be discontinued before delivery by 37 to 38 weeks.

Prevention with abnormal uterine Doppler ultrasound. Impedance to flow in the uterine arteries normally decreases as pregnancy progresses. Increased impedance for gestational age reflects high downstream resistance due to defective differentiation of trophoblast, leading to preeclampsia and placental insufficiency. Abnormal uterine artery Doppler in the second trimester has been associated with an increased

risk of preeclampsia. The only intervention studied if this screening test is abnormal is low-dose aspirin. **If low-dose aspirin is given anyway because of a history of preeclampsia or other indications (see above), then uterine artery Doppler screening may not be necessary or beneficial.**

A meta-analysis of nine RCTs (n = 1317) comparing **low-dose** (50–150 mg/day) **aspirin** to placebo or no treatment in women **with abnormal uterine Doppler ultrasound at 14 to 24 weeks** reveals that **preeclampsia is decreased by 52% when aspirin treatment starts before 16 weeks** with no significant reduction when started later in pregnancy. Early start of the treatment in women with abnormal uterine Doppler also significantly **reduces the incidence of severe preeclampsia by 90%, gestational hypertension by 69%, and IUGR by 49%** [44]. There are **insufficient data to assess other important outcomes**, such as abruption and perinatal death.

The combination of abnormal uterine artery Doppler at 22 and 24 weeks of gestation and low dose aspirin in nulliparous women without risk factors for preeclampsia versus no Doppler and placebo was evaluated in a large French trial [45] trying to assess this intervention with a different study design from the others; this trial is not included in the meta-analysis. Women in this trial were randomized to having the uterine Doppler examination between 22 and 24 week of gestation and always getting aspirin if abnormal or not receiving the Doppler screening. This trial confirmed the predictive value of uterine artery Doppler for preeclampsia but failed to demonstrate the value of routine screening followed by low-dose aspirin therapy for a positive test compared to routine prenatal care [45]. The late initiation of treatment reported in this trial may explain the negative results obtained, confirming that aspirin treatment may not be effective in preventing preeclampsia if started late in pregnancy. A meta-analysis including only women with abnormal uterine artery Doppler at first trimester who were randomized to low-dose aspirin vs. placebo at or before 16 weeks of gestation (three trials, 346 women) showed that aspirin reduced the risk of preeclampsia by 40% and severe preeclampsia by 70% [46]. These data require further investigation as the sample sizes were small, and they included some women with increased risk for preeclampsia as CHTN, pregestational diabetes, etc.

Heparin. A meta-analysis including eight studies comparing heparin (alone or in combination with dipyridamole or low-dose aspirin) versus no treatment showed no significant differences in the risk of developing preeclampsia in women at risk of placental dysfunction. The use of heparin was associated with 60% reduction in risk of perinatal mortality; 54% and 28% reduction in preterm birth before 34 and 37 weeks gestation, respectively; and 50% reduction in SGA. However, there is no information regarding serious adverse events in infants and long-term childhood outcomes [47]. Further trials are needed to evaluate the potential benefits of heparin in preventing preeclampsia. Therefore, LMWH is not recommended at this time as a prophylaxis for recurrence for women with a history of preeclampsia [48,49].

Calcium. Compared with placebo or no treatment, calcium supplementation is associated with a 35% **reduction in the incidence of high blood pressure and a 55% reduction in the risk of preeclampsia** as shown in a meta-analysis of 13 studies, 15,730 women [50]. The reduction is greater among women at high risk of developing hypertension (78%) and in those with low baseline calcium intake (64%). Although the risk of preeclampsia is reduced, this is not clearly reflected in any reduction in severe preeclampsia, eclampsia, or admission to intensive care. One of the largest trials reported no reduction in the rate or severity of preeclampsia and no delay in its onset [51]. Optimum dosage and the effect on some substantive outcomes require further investigation.

Calcium supplementation is also associated with a 24% reduction in the risk of PTB overall and by 55% in women at high risk of preeclampsia. There is no evidence of any effect on admission to NICU, fetal death, or death before discharge from the hospital. The risk ratio of the composite outcome "maternal death or severe morbidity" is reduced by 20% for women receiving calcium supplementation. Maternal death alone was not significantly different. In one study, childhood systolic blood pressure >95th percentile is reduced by 41%.

Overall, these results **support the use of calcium supplementation during pregnancy, especially for women at high risk of developing preeclampsia and for those with low dietary intake** [50]. For most studies, the intervention was **1.5 to 2 g/day of calcium**. Nonetheless, some experts still doubt calcium benefit in these settings as the data and the selection factors are not homogeneous (e.g., several different risk factors for preeclampsia included), and final results are mostly due to the influence of smaller and lower quality studies [52].

Antioxidant therapy. Preeclampsia has been associated in some studies (but not in others) with oxidative stress. Antioxidative therapy (in particular vitamins C and E) has been tested as a preventative intervention. Evidence from a meta-analysis of 10 trials does not support routine antioxidant supplementation during pregnancy to reduce the risk of preeclampsia and its complications [53]. Comparing antioxidant use with placebo or no treatment, **there is no significant difference in the risk of preeclampsia**, PTB, SGA infants, or fetal or neonatal death. Two more recent meta-analyses confirmed previous results [54–56], which do not show any maternal or fetal benefit, including no reduction in preeclampsia, eclampsia, or gestational hypertension among high- and low-risk women receiving daily supplementation with 1000 mg of vitamin C and 400 IU of vitamin E, starting in the early second trimester. In one of the trials [56], the intervention is associated with an increased risk of fetal loss or perinatal death, PROM, and PPROM (an increased risk of PPROM is observed in another previous trial) [57]. Given these results, antioxidant therapy should **not be recommended for prevention of preeclampsia. In two studies in which women already had preeclampsia [58,59], antioxidants were not associated with any clinical benefit.**

Magnesium. There is insufficient evidence to assess magnesium as a preventive intervention for preeclampsia.

Diuretics. There is insufficient evidence to support the use of diuretics on prevention of preeclampsia and its complications. Diuretics for preventing preeclampsia are not associated with benefits but have adverse effects, and so their use for this purpose cannot be recommended [60].

Salt intake. Compared to advice to continue a normal diet, advice to reduce dietary salt intake is associated with similar outcomes, including incidence of preeclampsia [61]. In the absence of evidence that advice to alter salt intake during pregnancy has any beneficial effect for prevention of preeclampsia or any other outcome, either reliance on the nonpregnancy data on a beneficial salt-restricted diet or personal preference can guide salt intake.

Fish oil. The use of omega-3 fatty acids contained in fish oil is not associated with significant prevention of preeclampsia in a meta-analysis of four studies [62].

Garlic. There is not enough evidence to recommend increased garlic intake for preventing preeclampsia and its complications [63].

Rest/exercise. There is insufficient evidence to support recommending rest or reduced activity to women for preventing preeclampsia and its complications [64]. It has been suggested that exercise may help prevent preeclampsia in women at moderate-to-high risk, but current evidence is insufficient to draw reliable conclusions about this effect [65].

Progesterone. There is insufficient evidence for reliable conclusions about the effects of progesterone for preventing preeclampsia and its complications. Therefore, progesterone should not be used for this purpose in clinical practice at present [66].

Nitric oxide. There is insufficient evidence to draw reliable conclusions about whether nitric oxide donors and precursors prevent preeclampsia or its complications [67].

Preconception Counseling
Preventive measures are as per chronic hypertension, identification of secondary CHTN, decrease weight as described above, plus avoidance of risk factors if feasible.

Diagnosis
Diagnosis is described above (see Table 1.1).

History
Headache, blurry vision, "spots in front of eyes," abdominal pain.

Physical Examination
Vital signs (BP, HR, RR, O_2 saturation, urinary output), auscultate lungs: look for pulmonary edema, RUQ tenderness, edema (especially in hands, face, lower abdomen; excessive quick weight gain), increased reflexes. Period when hypertension is first documented (before or after 20 weeks) is important.

Workup
Laboratory tests: **CBC** (hemoconcentration/hemolysis, **platelet count**), **AST** and **ALT**, creatinine, **24-hour urine for total protein** (and creatinine clearance). It is **important to know the baseline values** of these tests in the woman when either not pregnant or at least in the beginning of the pregnancy to be able to compare in women being evaluated for preeclampsia or its complications. Therefore, these tests should be obtained **at first prenatal visit** in women with significant risk factors (e.g., chronic hypertension, diabetes, renal disease, collagen disorders, APS, prior preeclampsia, and HELLP). Coagulation studies (especially fibrinogen) can be obtained only in severe cases. Uric acid is neither sensitive nor specific and has not been shown to be helpful in management. **Repeat** laboratory tests can be performed at least once a week or as clinically indicated. Fetal assessment: dating ultrasound, biometry (to rule out IUGR); if IUGR is diagnosed, include umbilical artery Doppler, amniotic fluid, nonstress test, biophysical profile as needed.

Evaluate for symptoms and laboratory tests to distinguish preeclampsia from superimposed preeclampsia in patients with chronic HTN and to assess disease progression and severity.

Counseling
Delivery (the only definite treatment) is always appropriate for the mother but may not be so for the fetus. The woman

should be instructed on the signs and symptoms of pre-eclampsia and severe preeclampsia. The management plan should always consider gestational age, maternal and fetal status, and presence of labor or PPROM. Expectant management aims to palliate the maternal condition to allow fetal maturation and cervical ripening. Consider **corticosteroid administration** to accelerate fetal lung maturity between 24 and 33 6/7 weeks. BP (several times a day), urine for protein, fluid input and output, weight, laboratory tests (as above), and fetal status should be closely monitored.

Admission
Management of gestational hypertension or preeclampsia without severe features (proteinuric and nonproteinuric hypertension) in **day care units** has **similar clinical outcomes** and costs but **greater maternal satisfaction** compared to hospital admission [68–70]. Admission for 24 hours observation is acceptable to establish diagnosis and rule out severe features. Hospitalization may be indicated in cases in which the woman is unreliable. Admission is indicated in cases of preeclampsia with severe features (Figure 1.2).

Magnesium Prophylaxis
Magnesium is the drug of choice for prevention of eclampsia; it is superior to phenytoin and diazepam. Compared with placebo or no anticonvulsant, magnesium sulfate is associated with a **59% reduction in** the risk of **eclampsia** (number needed to treat for an additional beneficial outcome: 100), a 36% reduction in **abruption,** and a nonstatistically significant but clinically important 46% reduction in **maternal death** [71].

The **reduction of the risk of eclampsia** is consistent across the subgroups. In particular, **the reduction is similar regardless of severity of preeclampsia.** As eclampsia is more common among women with severe preeclampsia than among those with mild preeclampsia, **the number of women who would need to be treated to prevent one case of eclampsia** is greater for (mild) preeclampsia without severe features (i.e., **400 for mild preeclampsia, 71 for severe preeclampsia, and 36 in those with CNS symptoms**) [72]. In women with **mild preeclampsia**, the incidence of eclampsia may be only <1/200, and magnesium has not been shown to affect perinatal outcome, possibly because too few (n = 357) women with mild preeclampsia have been enrolled in the two specific trials [72]. In women with **severe preeclampsia,** the incidence of eclampsia decreases 61%, **from 2% in the placebo group to 0.6% in the magnesium group** (four trials) [71,72].

Magnesium is also associated with a trend for a 33% decrease in abruption in women with severe preeclampsia. Women allocated to magnesium sulfate have a **small increase (5%) in the risk of cesarean section.** There is no overall difference in the risk of fetal or neonatal death.

Side effects, in particular flushing, occur in 24% of women on magnesium, compared to 5% of controls. Almost all the data on side effects and safety come from studies that used either the intramuscular (IM) regimen for maintenance therapy or the **intravenous** (IV) route with **1 g/hr** and for around 24 hours. One trial compared a low-dose regimen with a standard-dose regimen over 24 hours. This study was too small for any reliable conclusions about the comparative effects [73]. Other toxicities and their associated magnesium serum levels are shown in Table 1.5.

Intravenous administration is preferable, where there are appropriate resources, as side effects and injection site problems are lower. Magnesium is recommended in women

Table 1.5 Maternal Serum Magnesium Concentrations Associated with Toxicity

	mmol/L	mEq/L	mg/dL
Loss of patellar reflexes	3.5–5	7–10	8.5–12
Respiratory depression	5–6.5	10–13	12–16
Altered cardiac conduction	>7.5	>15	>18
Cardiac arrest	>12.5	>25	>30

with preeclampsia with severe features and **usually given at least in active labor,** initiating with a loading dose of 4–6 g followed by a maintenance dose of **1–2 g/hr and for 12 to 24 hours postpartum but can be given for a shorter or longer period depending on the severity of preeclampsia** (maintenance dose depends on renal function and maternal urine output). Three trials compared short maintenance regimens postpartum (e.g., 12 hours), continuing for 24 hours after the birth, but even taken together, these trials were too small for any reliable conclusions [73]. Most trials managed magnesium **without serum monitoring** but with clinical monitoring of respiration, tendon reflexes, and urine output. If serum levels are used, Table 1.5 shows the correlations with side effects. Monitoring of patellar reflexes can be used to avoid toxicity. The use of higher doses and longer duration cannot be supported by trial data. Magnesium sulfate for preeclampsia prophylaxis does not significantly affect labor but is associated with higher use of oxytocin [74].

Compared to **phenytoin,** magnesium sulfate is associated with a **92% better reduction in the risk of eclampsia** with a 21% increased risk of cesarean section [71]. Compared to **nimodipine,** magnesium sulfate is associated with a **67% better reduction in the risk of eclampsia.** There is insufficient evidence on other agents, such as diazepam or methyldopa [71].

Magnesium sulfate does not appear to affect blood loss intrapartum and postpartum in women with preeclampsia. A recent meta-analysis including five trials showed that the incidence of postpartum hemorrhage was similar between the two groups (magnesium sulfate: 17% vs. no magnesium sulfate: 18%, RR 0.97, 95% CI 0.88–1.06). There was no statistical difference between any of the other blood loss outcomes reported in the included studies. The rate of eclampsia with magnesium sulfate was decreased by 60% when compared to placebo. Magnesium sulfate, therefore, should be continued during CD, given the benefit of seizure prophylaxis without any increased risk of hemorrhage [75].

Plasma Volume Expansion
Blood plasma volume increases gradually in women during pregnancy. The increase is usually greater for women with multiple pregnancies and less for those with small babies. Plasma volume is reduced in women with preeclampsia. There is insufficient data to assess any effect of plasma volume expansion on outcomes in women with preeclampsia. Three small trials compared a colloid solution with no plasma volume expansion. For every outcome reported, the confidence intervals are very wide and cross the no-effect line [76].

Antihypertensive Therapy
Patients with SBP consistently ≥160 mmHg and/or DBP ≥110 (severe HTN) should be placed on antihypertensive medication; this includes those women with preeclampsia or its complications (HELLP, etc.). As stated above, it is appropriate

to initiate therapy at lower blood pressures in patients with evidence of end-organ damage (renal, cardiovascular, etc.) and diabetes. Target BP should be 140–150 mmHg systolic and about 90 mmHg diastolic. ACE inhibitors are contraindicated in pregnancy. Any patient requiring antihypertensive agents may be placed on home BP monitoring if managed as an outpatient. There are no trials on this intervention in preeclampsia.

Most antihypertensive drugs are effective at reducing blood pressure with little evidence that one is any better or worse than another [15,77]. Types of medications for acute management of hypertension include the following: (Table 1.3)

- *Labetalol*: 20-mg IV bolus, then 40, 80, 80 mg as needed, every 10 minutes (maximum 220 mg total dose).
- *Hydralazine*: 5 to 10 mg IV (or IM) every 20 minutes. Change to another drug if no success by 30 mg (maximum dose). Hydralazine may be associated with more maternal side effects and NRFHT than IV labetalol or oral nifedipine [78].
- *Nifedipine*: 10 to 20 mg orally, may repeat in 30 minutes. This drug is associated with diuresis when used postpartum. Nifedipine and magnesium sulfate can probably be used simultaneously.
- *Sodium nitroprusside* (rarely needed): start at 0.25 μ/kg/min to a maximum of 5 μ/kg/min.

Antiplatelet Agents

Five trials compared antiplatelet agents with placebo or no antiplatelet agent for the **treatment** of preeclampsia. There are insufficient data for any firm conclusions about the possible effects of these agents when used for treatment of preeclampsia [79] (meta-analysis, now withdrawn).

Antepartum Testing

Antenatal testing (usually with nonstress tests) is done at diagnosis and repeated once or twice weekly; twice weekly for FGR or oligohydramnios. Umbilical artery Doppler ultrasound is recommended at least weekly if FGR is present. Ultrasound for fetal growth and amniotic fluid assessment should be performed at diagnosis and every three weeks if still pregnant.

Anesthesia

(See also Chapter 11 of *Obstetric Evidence Based Guidelines*.) Regional anesthesia is preferred but contraindicated with coagulopathy or platelets <75,000/mm³. Patients with hypertension may benefit from epidural analgesia as it may improve uterine perfusion through several pathways (localized neuraxial vasodilatory effect, reduced catecholamine release). **Epidural analgesia is the analgesia of choice in hypertensive pregnant women**. Patients with hypertension, preeclampsia, and eclampsia are at increased risk for hemodynamic instability during both labor and surgical anesthesia. Some, but not all studies, have found a higher incidence of hypotension in parturients receiving a spinal versus epidural anesthesia. Methods to prevent hypotension should be employed. The prevention, rather than treatment, of hypotension has been associated with better outcomes for the fetus. In women with severe preeclampsia, a careful approach is necessary for either regional or general anesthesia. Provided this is followed, they are associated with similar good outcomes

in a small trial [80]. Women with severe preeclampsia who must undergo **general anesthesia** are **at risk for an extremely exaggerated hypertensive response to intubation** and often benefit from pretreatment with an antihypertensive, such as labetalol, immediately prior to induction. Prophylaxis with magnesium sulfate for preeclampsia/eclampsia can potentiate neuromuscular blockade in patients receiving general anesthesia, so care must be taken in using intermediate- to long-acting nondepolarizing muscle relaxants.

Delivery (Figures 1.1 and 1.2)

Timing

Before 37 weeks, in **the absence of severe criteria** or preterm labor and in the presence of reassuring fetal testing, expectant management is suggested with delivery for development of any severe criteria (see below).

Compared to expectant management, induction of labor in women with gestational hypertension or mild preeclampsia at 36 to 41 weeks gestation is associated with a 29% reduction in composite maternal outcome (e.g., HELLP, severe HTN, severe preeclampsia, eclampsia, abruptio placentae, and pulmonary edema) and lower incidence of neonatal pH <7.05 with induction of labor ≥37 weeks but no differences in rates of neonatal complications or cesarean delivery [21].

Therefore, even **with gestational hypertension and "mild" preeclampsia, delivery (usually by induction) at ≥37 weeks is recommended**.

Mode

Vaginal delivery is preferred with induction of labor if necessary [81]. Women with GHTN or preeclampsia without severe features benefit most from induction if the cervix is unfavorable [82]. With severe preeclampsia, the chances of a successful induction vary from 34% to more than 90% in different studies [83–89]. Table 1.6 shows the rate of cesarean delivery in induced labors at different gestational ages and should be helpful with counseling and management. If the woman is stable and accepts a low incidence of success, induction may be reasonable, especially in a woman desiring a large family.

Hemodynamic Monitoring

Invasive hemodynamic monitoring in preeclamptic women, even with severe cardiac disease, renal disease, refractory HTN, pulmonary edema, or unexplained oliguria, is usually unnecessary, especially because Swan–Ganz catheters have been associated with complications and no improvements in outcomes in nonpregnant critically ill adults (see Chapter 40). There are no trials on this intervention in pregnancy.

Table 1.6 Rate of Cesarean Delivery in Induced Labors in Women with Severe Preeclampsia at 24 to 34 Weeks Gestation

Author	24–28 Weeks % (*n*)	28–32 Weeks % (*n*)	32–34 Weeks % (*n*)
Nassar [64]	68 (13/19)	55 (47/86)	38 (15/40)
Blackwell [61]	96 (26/27)	65 (33/51)	31 (23/73)
Alanis [58]	93 (14/15)	53 (84/158)	31 (34/109)
Mashiloane [63]		35 (14/40)	
Overall	**87** (53/61)	**53** (178/335)	**32** (72/222)

PREECLAMPSIA COMPLICATIONS
Superimposed Preeclampsia

Prognosis may be much worse for mother and fetus than with either diagnosis (chronic hypertension or preeclampsia) alone. Complications are similar to preeclampsia but more common and severe (e.g., PTB 50%–60%, FGR 15%, abruption 2%–5%, perinatal death 5%). There are no specific trials to guide management; therefore, management should follow as per preeclampsia (Figures 1.1 and 1.2) with even more caution given the higher morbidity and mortality [90,91].

Management [1]
CHTN with superimposed preeclampsia without severe features

- Antihypertensive medications for SBP >160 mmHg or >105 mmHg
- Maintain BPs between >120/80 mmHg and <160/105 mmHg
- Consider outpatient management in selected populations with easy access to the health system [90]

- Home BP measurement
- Close follow-up in clinic every week with NST
- Fetal growth evaluation every 3 weeks
- Delivery no less than 37 weeks
- Close postpartum BP surveillance for first 72 hours
- Close follow-up 7–10 days after delivery

CHTN with superimposed preeclampsia with severe features

- Admission to the hospital for evaluation
- Antihypertensive medications for SBP >160 mmHg or >105 mmHg
- Magnesium sulfate for maternal seizure prevention
- Expectant management until no more than 34 weeks
- Delivery by 34 weeks
- Close postpartum BP surveillance for first 72 hours
- Close follow-up 7–10 days after delivery

Preeclampsia with Severe Features
See also the section titled "Preeclampsia."

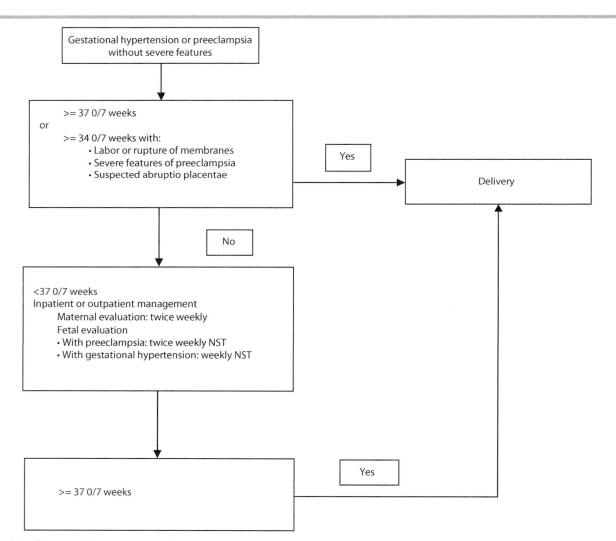

Figure 1.1 Suggested management of gestational hypertension and preeclampsia without severe features. *Developing any of the severe features. (Adapted from American College of Obstetricians and Gynecologists, Task Force on Hypertension in Pregnancy. *Obstet Gynecol*, 122, 5, 1122–31, 2013.)

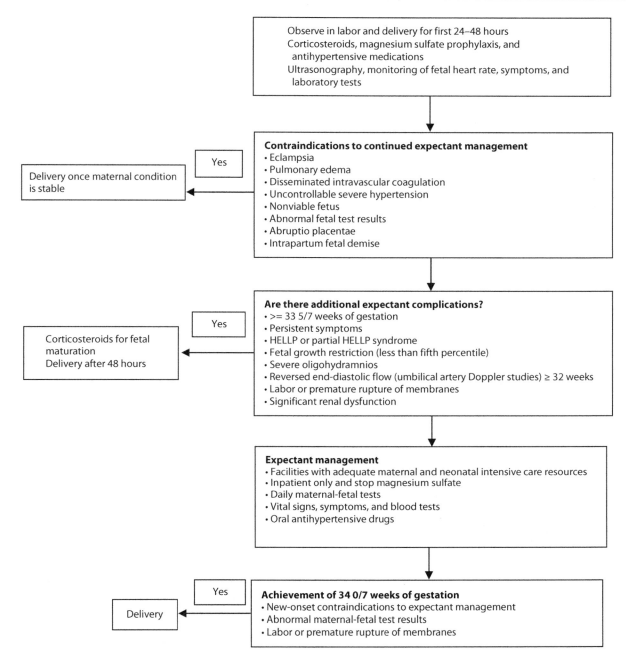

Figure 1.2 Suggested management of severe preeclampsia <34 weeks. (Adapted from American College of Obstetricians and Gynecologists, Task Force on Hypertension in Pregnancy. *Obstet Gynecol*, 122, 5, 1122–31, 2013.)

Diagnostic Criteria (Table 1.1)

If one or more of the following are present: (1) BP ≥160/110 mm on two occasions at least four hours apart while the patient is on bed rest (unless antihypertensive therapy is initiated before this time); (2) thrombocytopenia <100,000 platelets/mL; (3) impaired liver function AST or ALT twice normal concentration, severe persistent right upper quadrant or epigastric pain unresponsive to medication and not accounted for by alternative diagnoses or both; (4) progressive renal insufficiency (serum creatinine concentration >1.1 mg/dL or a doubling of the serum creatinine concentration in the absence of other renal disease); (5) pulmonary edema; and (6) cerebral or visual disturbances.

Severe proteinuria (>5 g) has been eliminated from the consideration of preeclampsia as severe feature as several studies indicated that expectant management was not associated with worse maternal or fetal outcome [92–94]. As fetal growth restriction is managed similarly in pregnant women with and without preeclampsia, it has been removed as well as criteria of severe features of preeclampsia.

Management (Figure 1.2)

Magnesium sulfate. See section titled "Preeclampsia."

Plasma volume expansion. The addition of **plasma volume expansion** as a temporizing treatment does not improve maternal or fetal outcome in women with early preterm severe preeclampsia [95].

Timing of delivery (Figure 1.2). In the presence of preeclampsia with severe features at ≥34 weeks, **expeditious delivery** is recommended given the high maternal incidence of complications with expectant management. Timing the delivery of a very premature infant <34 weeks in the presence of severe preeclampsia is a difficult clinical decision. When the mother's life is in danger, there is no doubt that delivery is the only correct course of action. This situation is rare. More usually, the risks of maternal morbidity if the pregnancy is continued have to be constantly balanced against the hazards of prematurity to the fetus if it is delivered too early. The **options are expeditious delivery, delivery after completion of corticosteroids, or expectant management** to improve perinatal outcome, but there are only three trials comparing these approaches at 28 to 32–34 weeks [96–98]. In general, an interventionist approach with **immediate delivery before 48 hours and before completion of corticosteroid administration ("aggressive management")** is suggested **with eclampsia, pulmonary edema, DIC, abruptio placentae, abnormal fetal testing, uncontrollable BP** in spite of continuing increase in antihypertensive drugs, fetal demise, or nonviable fetus. Delivery after 48 hours **after completion of corticosteroids** is suggested in women **with persistent headache and/or visual/CNS symptoms, epigastric pain, renal dysfunction (Cr >1.1, double creatinine value or persistent oliguria), preterm labor, PROM, AST/ALT more than twofold normal value, platelets <100,000/mm³ (partial or complete HELLP syndrome), severe oligohydramnios, or reversed umbilical artery end-diastolic flow ≥32 weeks** [33,99].

There are insufficient data for reliable conclusions comparing these policies for outcome for the mother. For the baby, there is insufficient evidence for reliable conclusions about the effects on fetal or neonatal death. Babies whose mothers are allocated to **an interventionist** group have 2.3-fold **more hyaline membrane disease** and 5.5-fold **more necrotizing enterocolitis** and are 32% **more likely to need admission to neonatal intensive care** unit (NICU) than those allocated to an expectant policy [99]. Nevertheless, babies allocated to the interventionist policy are 64% less likely to be SGA. There are no statistically significant differences between the two strategies for any other outcomes.

In observational studies, expectant care of severe preeclampsia <34 weeks is associated with pregnancy prolongation of 7 to 14 days and few serious maternal complications (<5%), similar to interventionist care [100].

Expectant management. **Expectant management (prolonging pregnancy beyond 48 hours)** is possible only if none of the conditions described above is present. At any time during expectant management, the development of any sign described above necessitates delivery (Figure 1.2) [33]. Expectant management is not recommended beyond 34 weeks because maternal risks outweigh perinatal benefits.

Expectant management of severe preeclampsia remote from term warrants hospitalization at a tertiary facility [101], daily antenatal testing, and laboratory studies at frequent intervals with the decision to prolong pregnancy determined day to day. Expectant management was associated with increased risk of abruptio and SGA in an RCT from Latin America [98].

In cases of severe HTN, such as those with severe preeclampsia, in which expectant management is appropriate, we suggest adding labetalol 200 to 800 mg orally every eight hours to the antihypertensive therapy described above. An alternative is nifedipine 10 to 20 mg orally every four to six hours (Table 1.4).

Women with renal disease, systemic lupus erythematosus, insulin-dependent diabetes, or multiple gestations require very careful management if expectantly managed. Massive proteinuria, even >10 g in 24 hours, is not associated per se with worse maternal or neonatal outcomes compared with proteinuria of <10 or even <5 g and so should probably not be a criterion for delivery by itself. The presence of FGR requires even closer monitoring and is associated with worse outcomes but is usually not in itself a criterion for delivery [102,103].

HELLP Syndrome

Epidemiology
HELLP syndrome is a severe manifestation of preeclampsia and complicates approximately 0.5% to 0.9% of all pregnancies and 10% to 20% of cases with severe preeclampsia [104]. Approximately 72% of cases are diagnosed antepartum and 28% postpartum (of which 80% <48 hours and 20% ≥48 hours postpartum). Of the antepartum cases, about 70% occur at 28 to 36 weeks, 20% >37 weeks, and about 10% <28 weeks. HELLP syndrome detected before fetal viability may identify a pregnancy complicated by partial mole/triploidy, trisomy 13, antiphospholipid syndrome, autoantibodies to angiotensin AT(1)-receptor or severe preterm preeclampsia with "mirror" syndrome [27].

Diagnosis
See above and Table 1.1. Patients presumptively diagnosed with HELLP syndrome can have other disorders concurrent with HELLP syndrome or other disorders altogether. The diseases that may imitate HELLP syndrome and that have to be considered in the differential diagnosis are shown in Table 1.7 [27].

Signs and Symptoms
The presenting symptoms are usually right upper abdominal quadrant or epigastric pain, nausea, and vomiting. Headache and visual symptoms can occur. Malaise or viral syndrome-like symptoms may be present with advanced HELLP syndrome. It is important to note that 15% have no hypertension and 13% no proteinuria (Table 1.8) [105].

Complications
Complications (Table 1.9) of HELLP syndrome are somewhat similar in incidence and severity to those of severe preeclampsia once gestational age is controlled [105]. If profound hypovolemic shock occurs, suspect liver hematoma. If confirmed, liver hematoma is best managed conservatively. Contributing factors to deaths of women with HELLP syndrome are, in order of decreasing frequency, stroke, cardiac arrest, DIC, adult respiratory distress syndrome, renal failure, sepsis, hepatic rupture, hypoxic encephalopathy [27].

Management
See Figure 1.3 for management [106].

Workup. Laboratory tests as per severe preeclampsia, plus peripheral smear evaluation.

Corticosteroids. Eleven trials (550 women) have assessed corticosteroids versus placebo/no treatment for HELLP syndrome and are summarized in a meta-analysis [107]. The dose of dexamethasone was usually 10 mg IV every six to 12 hours for two to three doses, followed by 5 to 6 mg IV six to 12 hours later for two to three more doses. There is **no**

Table 1.7 Differential Diagnosis of HELLP Syndrome

Acute fatty liver of pregnancy (AFLP)
Lupus flare: Exacerbation of systemic lupus erythematosus
Thrombotic thrombocytopenic purpura (TTP)
Hemolytic uremic syndrome (HUS)
Immune thrombocytopenic purpura (ITP)
Thrombophilias (e.g., antiphospholipid syndrome)
Severe folate deficiency
Cholangitis/cholecystitis/pancreatitis/ruptured bile duct
Gastric ulcer
Cardiomyopathy
Dissecting aortic aneurysm
Systemic viral sepsis (herpes, cytomegalovirus)
SIRS/sepsis
Hemorrhagic or hypotensive shock
Stroke in pregnancy or puerperium
Paroxysmal nocturnal hemoglobinuria
Pheochromocytoma
Advanced embryonal cell carcinoma of the liver
Acute cocaine intoxication
Myasthenia gravis
Pseudocholinesterase deficiency

Source: Martin JN Jr., Rose CH, Briery CM. *Am J Obstet Gynecol*, 195, 4, 914–34, 2006.

Table 1.8 Signs and Symptoms of HELLP Syndrome

Condition	Frequency (%)
Hypertension	85
Proteinuria	87
Right upper quadrant or epigastric pain	40–90
Nausea or vomiting	30–85
Headaches	35–60
Visual changes	10–20
Mucosal bleeding	10
Jaundice	5

Source: Sibai BM. *OBG Management*, 4, 52–69, 2005.
Abbreviation: HELLP, hemolysis, elevated liver enzymes and a low platelet count.

difference in the risk of maternal death, maternal death or severe maternal morbidity, or perinatal/infant death. The only significant effect of treatment on individual outcomes is improved platelet count: This effect is strongest if the treatment is started antenatally.

In two trials comparing dexamethasone with betamethasone, there is no clear evidence of a difference between groups in respect to perinatal morbidity or mortality. Maternal death and severe maternal morbidity is not reported. Regarding platelet count, dexamethasone is superior to betamethasone when treatment is commenced both antenatally and postnatally [108,109].

The two largest and only placebo-controlled trials [110,111] failed to show any significant difference between dexamethasone and placebo with respect to duration of hospitalization, recovery time for laboratory or clinical parameters, complications, or need for blood transfusion. These results remained unchanged, even following analysis stratified according to whether the patients were still pregnant or postpartum. A subgroup analysis according to the severity of disease shows a shorter platelet recovery and duration

Table 1.9 Complications of HELLP Syndrome

Complication	Frequency (%)
Maternal death	1
Adult respiratory distress syndrome (ARDS)	1
Laryngeal edema	1–2
Liver failure or hemorrhage	1–2
Acute renal failure	3
Pulmonary edema	6–8
Pleural effusions	10–15
Abruptio placentae	10–15
Disseminated intravascular coagulopathy	10–15
Marked ascites	10–15
Perinatal death	7–20
PTB	70

Source: Sibai BM. *OBG Management*, 4, 52–69, 2005.
Abbreviations: HELLP, hemolysis, elevated liver enzymes and low platelets; PTB, preterm birth.

of hospitalization in the subgroup with class 1 HELLP who received dexamethasone [72].

There is only one randomized placebo-controlled trial evaluating the effect of prolonged administration of high-dose prednisolone in 31 pregnant women with early-onset (<30 weeks) HELLP syndrome during expectant management (mean prolongation of about seven days) [112]. The results show a reduced risk of recurrent HELLP syndrome exacerbations (presence of at least two of the following three criteria: right upper abdominal or epigastrical pain, a platelet count decrease below 100,000/mm³, and an increase of AST/ALT more than twofold normal value) in the prednisolone group as compared to the placebo group (hazard ratio 0.3, 95% CI 0.3–0.9). Nevertheless, expectant management for >48 hours in women with HELLP syndrome, even with early onset, is not recommended.

Given no significant improvements in important maternal and fetal outcomes, there is still **insufficient evidence to recommend the routine use of steroids for therapy specific for HELLP syndrome**, and this approach should be considered experimental. The use of corticosteroids may be justified in clinical situations in which increased rate of recovery in platelet count is considered clinically worthwhile.

Anesthesia
Regional anesthesia is usually allowed by anesthesiologists in cases with platelet counts ≥75,000/mm³. General anesthesia may be safer in cases with lower platelet counts.

Delivery
Timing (Figure 1.3). Prompt delivery is indicated if HELLP is diagnosed at ≥34 weeks or even earlier if multiorgan dysfunction, DIC, liver failure or hemorrhage, renal failure, possible abruption, or NRFHT are present. Delivery can only be delayed for a maximum of 48 hours between 24 and 33 6/7 weeks to give steroids for fetal maturity, but even this management is not tested in trials. Although some women may have improvement in laboratory values in these 48 hours, delivery is still indicated in most cases.

Mode. Mode of delivery should generally follow obstetrical indications with HELLP syndrome not being an indication for cesarean per se. No randomized trial compared maternal and neonatal outcome after vaginal delivery or cesarean section in women with HELLP syndrome.

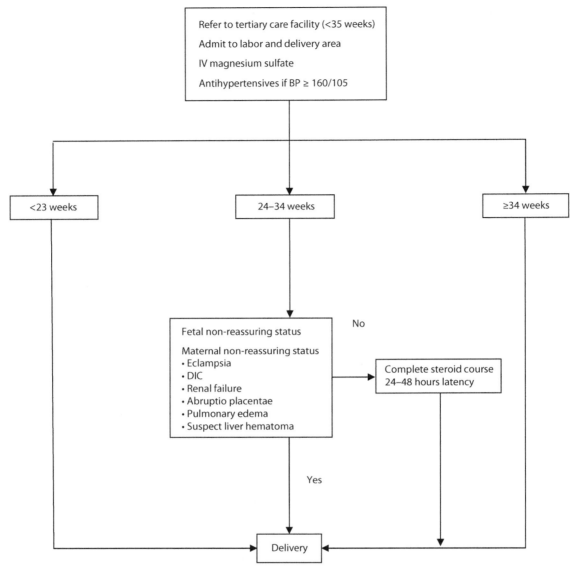

Figure 1.3   Suggested management of HELLP syndrome. (Adapted from Sibai BM. *Obstet Gynecol*, 103, 5 Pt. 1, 981–91, 2004.)

Counseling and management should include the information that the incidence of cesarean delivery in the trial of labor with HELLP at <30 weeks is high.

With platelet count <100,000/mm³, a drain may be indicated under and/or over the fascia in cases of cesarean delivery.

Eclampsia

Incidence

The incidence is about two to three cases per 10,000 births in Europe and other developed countries and 16 to 69 cases per 10,000 births in developing countries [113]. The onset can be antepartum (40%–50%), intrapartum (20%–35%), or postpartum (10%–40%). Late postpartum eclampsia (>48 hours but <4 weeks after delivery) is rare but can occur.

Definition

Eclampsia is the occurrence of new onset of ≥1 grand mal seizure(s) in association with preeclampsia.

Complications

The risk of **maternal death** is around **1% to 2%** in the developed world and up to **10%** in developing countries. An estimated 50,000 women die each year worldwide having had an eclamptic convulsion. **Perinatal mortality** is 6% to 12% in the developed world and up to 25% in developing countries. Other complications are similar and possibly more severe than severe preeclampsia cases (maternal abruption 7%–10%, DIC 7%–11%, HELLP 10%–15%, pulmonary edema 3%–5%, renal failure 5%–9%, aspiration pneumonia 2%–3%, cardiopulmonary arrest 2%–5%; perinatal PTB 50%) [72].

Management

Principles. **In about 15% of cases, hypertension or proteinuria may be absent before eclampsia. A high index of suspicion for eclampsia should be maintained in all cases of hypertensive disorders in pregnancy, in particular those with CNS symptoms (headache, visual disturbances).** Up to 50% or more of cases of eclampsia, occurring in women with no diagnosis of preeclampsia or only mild disease preterm or before hospitalization, may not be preventable.

The first priorities are **airway, breathing, and circulation**. Multidisciplinary care is essential as several people are needed for immediate stabilization. Interventions include airway assessment and placing the patient in the lateral decubitus position (to avoid aspiration). Maintain oxygenation with supplemental oxygen via 8 to 10 L/min mask. Obtain vital signs and assess pulse oximetry. Supportive care includes inserting a tongue blade between the teeth (avoiding inducing a gag reflex) and preventing maternal injury.

Workup. Cerebral imaging is usually not necessary for the diagnosis and management of most women with eclampsia. It might be helpful in cases complicated by neurologic deficits, coma, refractory to magnesium, or seizures >48 hours after delivery.

Therapy. **Magnesium sulfate is the drug of choice to treat eclampsia and prevent recurrent convulsions** as it is associated with maternal and fetal/neonatal benefits compared to all interventions against which it has been tested. The standard intravenous regimen widely used in many countries consists of a loading dose of 4 g, followed by an infusion of 1 g/hr [73]. Increasing the loading dose to 6 g and the infusion rate to 2 g/hr has also been suggested [72].

Trials comparing alternative treatment regimens (loading dose alone vs. loading dose plus maintenance therapy for 24 hours or low-dose regimen vs. a standard-dose regimen over 24 hours) are too small for reliable conclusions [73].

Serum monitoring of magnesium levels is not absolutely necessary. The effectiveness and safety of magnesium sulfate has been demonstrated with clinical monitoring alone [73].

Trials comparing magnesium sulfate with other anticonvulsants for treating eclampsia demonstrate that it is more effective than diazepam, phenytoin, or lytic cocktail [114–116].

Magnesium vs. diazepam. Compared with diazepam, magnesium sulfate is associated with **reductions** in **maternal death** by 41%, in **further convulsions** from eclampsia by 57%, in **Apgar scores <7 at five minutes** by 30%, in the need of intubation at the place of birth by 33%, and in **length of stay in special care baby unit >7 days** by 34% [114]. There was no clear difference in perinatal deaths.

Magnesium vs. phenytoin. Compared with phenytoin, magnesium sulfate is associated with **reduction** in maternal complications, such as the **recurrence of convulsions** by 66%, **maternal death** by 50% (nonsignificant because of small numbers: RR 0.50, 95% CI 0.24 to 1.05), **pneumonia** by 56%, ventilation by 32%, and **admission to the intensive care unit** by 33%. For the baby, magnesium sulfate is associated with 27% **fewer admissions to a special care baby unit** and 23% **fewer babies who died or were in special baby care unit for >7 days** [115].

Magnesium vs. lytic cocktail. Lytic cocktail is usually a mixture of Thorazine (chlorpromazine), Phenergan (promethazine), and Demerol (meperidine). Compared to a lytic cocktail, magnesium sulfate is associated with an **86% reduction in maternal death** and a **94% reduction in subsequent convulsions**. Magnesium sulfate is also associated with **88% less maternal respiratory depression and 94% less coma without any clear difference in the risk of neonatal death** [116].

Other issues About 10% of women will have a **second seizure** even after receiving magnesium sulfate. In that case, another bolus of 2 g of magnesium sulfate can be then

given intravenously over three to five minutes, and, rarely, if another convulsion occurs, sodium amobarbital 250 mg IV over three to five minutes is necessary [72].

Blood pressure should be maintained at about 140–159/90–109 by antihypertensive agents as described for preeclampsia.

Antepartum Testing
NRFHT occurs in many cases of eclampsia, but it usually resolves spontaneously in three to 10 minutes by **fetal in utero resuscitation** with maternal support. Therefore, **NRFHT is not an indication for immediate cesarean delivery in case of eclampsia** unless it continues >10 to 15 minutes despite normal maternal oxygenation.

Delivery
Delivery should occur expeditiously, but only **when the mother is stable.** This requires a **multidisciplinary, efficient, and timely** effort.

Postpartum Management
Eclampsia prophylaxis. **Magnesium** should be continued for at least 12 hours and often for about 24 hours or at least improvement in maternal urinary output (e.g., >100 mL/hr). In some cases of severe preeclampsia, eclampsia, HELLP or continuing oliguria, or other complications, magnesium may need to be continued for >24 hours. Preeclampsia can worsen postpartum. Edema always worsens, and the woman should be aware of this. Eclampsia can still occur, especially in the first 48 hours post-delivery and even up to ≥14 days postpartum.

Management of hypertension. There are no reliable data to guide management of women who are hypertensive postpartum or at increased risk of becoming so. Women should be informed that they will require long-term surveillance (and possible therapy) for hypertension at their postpartum visit.

For prevention in women who had antenatal preeclampsia, there is **insufficient data** to assess outcomes comparing furosemide or nifedipine with placebo/no therapy [117]. Compared to no therapy, postpartum **furosemide** 20 mg orally for five days does not affect any outcomes in women with mild or superimposed preeclampsia [118]. In women with severe preeclampsia, this intervention normalizes blood pressure more rapidly and reduces the need for antihypertensive therapy but does not affect the incidence of delayed complications or the length of hospitalization [118]. L-**Arginine** therapy does hasten recovery in postpartum preeclampsia [119]. Therefore, **for women with antenatal hypertension, even that of preeclampsia, it is unclear whether or not they should routinely receive postpartum antihypertensive therapy.** Although blood pressure peaks on days 3 to 6 postpartum, whether or not routine postpartum treatment can prevent transient severe maternal hypertension and/or prolongation of the maternal hospital stay has not been established [117].

For treatment, there is insufficient data to assess the antihypertensives studied: these are oral timolol or hydralazine compared with oral methyldopa for treatment of mild-to-moderate postpartum hypertension, and oral hydralazine plus sublingual nifedipine compared with sublingual nifedipine [117]. Oral **nifedipine** (10 mg every eight hours short-acting or 30 mg daily long-acting; maximum dose 120 mg/day) is a reasonable choice, with **ACE inhibitors for women with diabetes or nephropathy. If a clinician feels that**

hypertension is severe enough to treat, the agent used should be based on his or her familiarity with the drug.

Long-Term Counseling

Because a history of early-onset hypertensive disorders of pregnancy increases the risk of recurrence in subsequent pregnancies, long-term counseling should involve review of recurrence and preventive measures (see above). The risk of complications in the subsequent pregnancy depends on how early in gestation and how severe the complications were, other underlying medical conditions, age of the woman at future pregnancy, same versus different partner, and many other variables (see section titled "Risk Factors" above). Several studies tried to identify prediction tests for recurrent hypertensive disease in pregnancy, but there is insufficient evidence to assess the clinical usefulness of these tests [120].

In a large cohort study, the **recurrence risk** of preeclampsia is around **15%** in the second pregnancy for women who had preeclampsia in their first pregnancy and 30% for women who had preeclampsia in the previous two pregnancies [121,122]. In a systematic review of seven studies, the pooled risk of recurrence of hypertension, preeclampsia, or HELLP syndrome resulting in a delivery before 34 weeks is 7.8% [123]. In two recent large cohort studies, the recurrence rate of preeclampsia associated with delivery before 34 weeks' gestation is 6.8% and 17%, respectively [122,124].

Women with a history of the HELLP syndrome have an increased risk of at least 20% (range 5%–52%) that some form of hypertension will recur in a subsequent gestation [104], about 5% for recurrence of HELLP, 30% to 40% of PTB, 25% of SGA, and up to 5% to 10% of perinatal death [125].

Moreover, **women with prior preeclampsia and related hypertensive disorders are at increased risk of cardiovascular disease in the future**, even premenopause if the preeclampsia occurred early in pregnancy, is recurrent, associated with IUGR, as a multipara, or in menopause if it happened at term in a primipara. These cardiovascular risks equal the risk associated with obesity or smoking. In 2011, the American Heart Association added preeclampsia to risk factors to cardiovascular disease. For prevention of this cardiovascular disease and its complications, early intervention is suggested [126].

REFERENCES

1. American College of Obstetricians and Gynecologists, Task Force on Hypertension in Pregnancy. Report of the American College of Obstetricians and Gynecologists' Task Force on Hypertension in Pregnancy. *Obstet Gynecol* 2013; 122(5): 1122–31. [Guideline]
2. Willett WC, Dietz WH, Colditz GA. Guidelines for healthy weight. *N Engl J Med* 1999; 341: 427. [Guideline]
3. American College of Obstetricians and Gynecologists. ACOG Practice Bulletin No. 125: Chronic hypertension in pregnancy. *Obstet Gynecol.* 2012 Feb; 119(2 Pt. 1): 396–407. PubMed PMID: 22270315. [Guideline]
4. Yeo S, Steele NM, Chang MC. Effect of exercise on blood pressure in pregnant women with a high risk of gestational hypertensive disorders. *J Reprod Med* 2000; 45(4): 293–8. [RCT, *n* = 16; I]
5. Bergel E, Carroli G, Althabe F. Ambulatory versus conventional methods for monitoring blood pressure during pregnancy. *Cochrane Database Syst Rev* 2002; (2): CD001231. [Review; III]
6. Meher S, Abalos E, Carroli G. Bed rest with or without hospitalisation for hypertension during pregnancy. *Cochrane Database Syst Rev* 2005; (4): CD003514. [Meta-analysis; 4 RCTs, *n* = 449; I]
7. Committee SP. SMFM Statement: Benefit of antihypertensive therapy for mild-to-moderate chronic hypertension during pregnancy remains uncertain. *Am J Obstet Gynecol* 2015; 213(1): 3–4. [Guideline]
8. Nifedipine versus expectant management in mild to moderate hypertension in pregnancy. Gruppo di Studio Ipertensione in Gravidanza. *British Journal of Obstetrics and Gynaecology* 1998; 105(7): 718–22. [II-1]
9. Ahn HK, Nava-Ocampo AA, Han JY et al. Exposure to amlodipine in the first trimester of pregnancy and during breastfeeding. *Hypertension in Pregnancy* 2007; 26(2): 179–87. [II-2]
10. Abalos E, Duley L, Steyn DW. Antihypertensive drug therapy for mild to moderate hypertension during pregnancy. *Cochrane Database Syst Rev* 2014; 2: CD002252. [Meta-analysis; 46 RCTs, *n* = 4282; 28 of which compared an antihypertensive drug with placebo/no antihypertensive drug (*n* = 3200); I]
11. Magee LA, Duley L. Oral beta-blockers for mild to moderate hypertension during pregnancy. *Cochrane Database Syst Rev* 2003; (3): CD002863. [Meta-analysis; 29 RCTs, *n* = 2500; I]
12. von Dadelszen P, Ornstein MP, Bull SB, Logan AG, Koren G, Magee LA. Fall in mean arterial pressure and fetal growth restriction in pregnancy hypertension: A meta-analysis. *Lancet* 2000; 355(9198): 87–92. [Meta-analysis; 15 RCTs; *n* = 1,782; I]
13. Nakhai-Pour HR, Rey E, Berard A. Antihypertensive medication use during pregnancy and the risk of major congenital malformations or small-for-gestational-age newborns. *Birth Defects Research Part B, Developmental and Reproductive Toxicology* 2010; 89(2): 147–54. [II-2]
14. Magee LA, von Dadelszen P, Rey E et al. Less-tight versus tight control of hypertension in pregnancy. *N Engl J Med* 2015; 372(5): 407–17. [I]
15. Duley L, Meher S, Jones L. Drugs for treatment of very high blood pressure during pregnancy. *Cochrane Database Syst Rev* 2013; 7: CD001449. [Meta-analysis; 24 RCTs, *n* = 2949]
16. Hennessy A, Thornton CE, Makris A. A randomised comparison of hydralazine and mini-bolus diazoxide for hypertensive emergencies in pregnancy: The PIVOT trial. *Aust N Z J Obstet Gynaecol* 2007; 47(4): 279–85. [RCT, *n* = 124, hydralazine vs. mini-bolus diazoxide; not included in *Cochrane* by Duley; I]
17. Imdad A, Yakoob MY, Siddiqui S, Bhutta ZA. Screening and triage of intrauterine growth restriction (IUGR) in general population and high risk pregnancies: A systematic review with a focus on reduction of IUGR related stillbirths. *BMC Public Health* 2011; 11 Suppl 3: S1. [Review]
18. Alfirevic Z, Stampalija T, Gyte GM. Fetal and umbilical Doppler ultrasound in normal pregnancy. *Cochrane Database Syst Rev* 2010; (8): CD001450. [Meta-analysis]
19. Hutcheon JA, Lisonkova S, Magee LA. Optimal timing of delivery in pregnancies with pre-existing hypertension. *BJOG* 2011; 118 (1): 49–54. [Population-based cohort study, *n* = 171,669; II-2]
20. Sibai BM. Diagnosis and management of gestational hypertension and preeclampsia. *Obstet Gynecol* 2003; 102(1): 181–92. [Review; III]
21. Koopmans CM, Bijlenga D, Groen H. Induction of labour versus expectant monitoring for gestational hypertension or mild preeclampsia after 36 weeks' gestation (HYPITAT): A multicentre, open-label randomised controlled trial. *Lancet* 2009; 374 (9694): 979–88. [RCT, *n* = 756; I]
22. ACOG practice bulletin. Diagnosis and management of preeclampsia and eclampsia. Number 33, January 2002. *Obstet Gynecol* 2002; 99(1): 159–67. [Review III]
23. Report of the National High Blood Pressure Education Program Working Group on High Blood Pressure in Pregnancy. *Am J Obstet Gynecol* 2000; 183(1): S1–22. [Guideline]
24. Waugh JJ, Clark TJ, Divakaran TG. Accuracy of urinalysis dipstick techniques in predicting significant proteinuria in pregnancy. *Obstet Gynecol* 2004; 103(4): 769–77. [Review; III]
25. Schiff E, Friedman SA, Kao L, Sibai BM. The importance of urinary protein excretion during conservative management of severe preeclampsia. *Am J Obstet Gynecol* 1996; 175: 1313–6. [II-2]

26. Newman MG, Robichaux AG, Stedman CM, Jaekle RK, Fontenot MT, Dotson T et al. Perinatal outcomes in preeclampsia that is complicated by massive proteinuria. *Am J Obstet Gynecol* 2003; 188: 264–8. [II-2]

27. Martin JN Jr., Rose CH, Briery CM. Understanding and managing HELLP syndrome: The integral role of aggressive glucocorticoids for mother and child. *Am J Obstet Gynecol* 2006; 195(4): 914–34. [Review; III]

28. Rath W, Fischer T. The diagnosis and treatment of hypertensive disorders of pregnancy: New findings for antenatal and inpatient care. *Dtsch Arztebl Int* 2009; 106(45): 733–8. [Review; III]

29. Cnossen JS, Morris RK, ter Riet G. Use of uterine artery Doppler ultrasonography to predict pre-eclampsia and intrauterine growth restriction: A systematic review and bivariable meta-analysis. *CMAJ* 2008; 178(6): 701–11. [Meta-analysis, 74 studies, n = 79,547; I]

30. Poon LC, Kametas NA, Maiz N, Akolekar R, Nicolaides KH. First-trimester prediction of hypertensive disorders in pregnancy. *Hypertension* 2009; 53: 812–8. [II-2]

31. First-trimester risk assessment for early-onset preeclampsia. Committee Opinion No. 638. American College of Obstetricians and Gynecologists. *Obstet Gynecol* 15; 126: e25–7. [Guideline]

32. Sibai B, Dekker G, Kupferminc M. Pre-eclampsia. *Lancet* 2005; 365(9461): 785–99. [Review; III]

33. Haddad B, Sibai BM. Expectant management in pregnancies with severe pre-eclampsia. *Semin Perinatol* 2009; 33(3): 143–51. [Review; III]

34. Sibai BM. Expectant management of preeclampsia. *OBG Management* 2005; 3: 18–36. [Review; III]

35. Sibai BM, Barton JR. Expectant management of severe preeclampsia remote from term: Patient selection, treatment, and delivery indications. *Am J Obstet Gynecol* 2007; 196(6): 514–9. [Review; III]

36. Duley L, Henderson-Smart DJ, Meher S. Antiplatelet agents for preventing pre-eclampsia and its complications. *Cochrane Database Syst Rev* 2007; (2): CD004659. [Meta-analysis; 59 RCTs, n = 37,560; I]

37. Kozer E, Nikfar S, Costei A. Aspirin consumption during the first trimester of pregnancy and congenital anomalies: A meta-analysis. *Am J Obstet Gynecol* 2002; 187(6): 1623–30. [Meta-analysis; 22 RCTs; I]

38. Bujold E, Roberge S, Lacasse Y. Prevention of preeclampsia and intrauterine growth restriction with aspirin started in early pregnancy: A meta-analysis. *Obstet Gynecol* 2010; 116(2 Pt. 1): 402–14. [Meta-analysis; 34 RCTs, n = 11,348; I]

39. Henderson JT, Whitlock EP, O'Conner E, Senger CA, Thompson JH, Rowland MG. Low-dose aspirin for the prevention of morbidity and mortality from preeclampsia: A systematic evidence review for the U.S. Preventive Services Task Force [Internet]. Rockville (MD): Agency for Healthcare Research and Quality (US); 2014 Apr. Available from http://www.ncbi.nlm.nih.gov/books/NBK196392/PubMed PMID: 24783270. [Review]

40. Bushnell C, McCullough LD, Awad IA et al. American Heart Association Stroke Council, Council on Cardiovascular and Stroke Nursing, Council on Clinical Cardiology, Council on Epidemiology and Prevention, Council for High Blood Pressure Research. Guidelines for the prevention of stroke in women: A statement for healthcare professionals from the American Heart Association/American Stroke Association. *Stroke* 2014; 45(5): 1545. [Guideline]

41. Dekker GA, Sibai BM. Low-dose aspirin in the prevention of preeclampsia and fetal growth retardation: Rationale, mechanisms, and clinical trials. *Am J Obstet Gynecol* 1993; 168(1 Pt. 1): 214. PMID 8420330. [Review]

42. CLASP (Collaborative Low-dose Aspirin Study in Pregnancy) Collaborative Group. CLASP: A randomised trial of low-dose aspirin for the prevention and treatment of pre-eclampsia among 9364 pregnant women. *Lancet* 1994; 343(8898): 619. PMID 7906809. [RCT]

43. Schiff E, Barkai G, Ben-Baruch G, Mashiach S. Low-dose aspirin does not influence the clinical course of women with mild pregnancy-induced hypertension. *Obstet Gynecol* 1990; 76 (5 Pt. 1): 742. PMID 2216216. [I]

44. Bujold E, Morency AM, Roberge S. Acetylsalicylic acid for the prevention of preeclampsia and intra-uterine growth restriction in women with abnormal uterine artery Doppler: A systematic review and meta-analysis. *J Obstet Gynaecol Can* 2009; 31(9): 818–26. [Meta-analysis; 9 RCTs, n = 1317; I]

45. Subtil D, Goeusse P, Houfflin-Debarge V. Randomised comparison of uterine artery Doppler and aspirin (100 mg) with placebo in nulliparous women: The Essai Regional Aspirine Mere-Enfant study (Part 2). *BJOG* 2003; 110(5): 485–91. [RCT, n = 1253; I]

46. Villa PM, Kajantie E, Räikkönen K, Pesonen AK, Hämäläinen E, Vainio M, Taipale P, Laivuori H, PREDO Study group. Aspirin in the prevention of pre-eclampsia in high-risk women: A randomised placebo-controlled PREDO Trial and a meta-analysis of randomised trials. *BJOG* 2013; 120(1): 64. [RCT, and meta-analysis]

47. Dodd JM, McLeod A, Windrim RC, Kingdom J. Antithrombotic therapy for improving maternal or infant health outcomes in women considered at risk of placental dysfunction. *Cochrane Database Syst Rev* July 24, 2013; 7: CD006780. doi: 10.1002/14651858 .CD006780.pub3 [Meta-analysis, 10 RCTs, n = 1139; I]

48. Rey E, Garneau P, David M. Dalteparin for the prevention of recurrence of placental-mediated complications of pregnancy in women without thrombophilia: A pilot randomized controlled trial. *J Thromb Haemost* 2009; 7(1): 58–64. [RCT, n = 116; I]

49. Bates SM, Greer IA, Pabinger I. Venous thromboembolism, thrombophilia, antithrombotic therapy, and pregnancy: American College of Chest Physicians Evidence-Based Clinical Practice Guidelines (8th Edition). *Chest* 2008; 133(6 Suppl.): 844S–86S. [Guidelines]

50. Hofmeyr GJ, Lawrie TA, Atallah AN, Duley L, Torloni MR. Calcium supplementation during pregnancy for preventing hypertensive disorders and related problems. *Cochrane Database Syst Rev* 2014; 6: CD001059. [Meta-analysis, 13 RCTs, n = 15,730; I]

51. Levine RJ, Hauth JC, Curet LB. Trial of calcium to prevent preeclampsia. *N Engl J Med* 1997; 337(2): 69–76. [RCT]

52. Sibai BM. Calcium supplementation during pregnancy reduces risk of high blood pressure, pre-eclampsia and premature birth compared with placebo? *Evid Based Med* 2011; 16(2): 40–1. [Review; III]

53. Rumbold A, Duley L, Crowther CA. Antioxidants for preventing pre-eclampsia. *Cochrane Database Syst Rev* 2008; (1): CD004227. [Meta-analysis; 10 RCTs, n = 6533; I]

54. Basaran A, Basaran M, Topatan BSO. Combined vitamin C and E supplementation for the prevention of preeclampsia: A systematic review and meta-analysis. *Obstet Gynecol Surv* 2010; 65(10): 653. [9 studies]

55. Conde-Agudelo A, Romero R, Kusanovic JP, Hassan SS. Supplementation with vitamins C and E during pregnancy for the prevention of preeclampsia and other adverse maternal and perinatal outcomes: A systematic review and metaanalysis. *Am J Obstet Gynecol* 2011; 204(6): 503.e1. [Nine trials involving a total of 19,810 women]

56. Xu H, Perez-Cuevas R, Xiong X. An international trial of antioxidants in the prevention of preeclampsia (INTAPP). *Am J Obstet Gynecol* 2010; 202(3): 239. [RCT, n = 2363; I]

57. Spinnato JA, Freire S, Pinto e Silva JL. Antioxidant supplementation and premature rupture of the membranes: A planned secondary analysis. *Am J Obstet Gynecol* 2008; 199(4): 433–8. [RCT, n = 697; I]

58. Stratta P, Canavese C, Porcu M et al. Vitamin E supplementation in preeclampsia. *Gynecol Obstet Invest* 1994; 37(4): 246. [I]

59. Gülmezoğlu AM, Hofmeyr GJ, Oosthuisen MM. Antioxidants in the treatment of severe pre-eclampsia: An explanatory randomised controlled trial. *Br J Obstet Gynaecol* 1997; 104(6): 689. [RCT]

60. Churchill D, Beevers GD, Meher S. Diuretics for preventing preeclampsia. *Cochrane Database Syst Rev* 2007; (1): CD004451. [Meta-analysis; 5 RCTs, n = 1836; I]

61. Duley L, Henderson-Smart D, Meher S. Altered dietary salt for preventing pre-eclampsia, and its complications. *Cochrane Database Syst Rev* 2005; (4): CD005548. [Meta-analysis; 2 RCTs, *n* = 603; I]

62. Makrides M, Duley L, Olsen SF. Marine oil, and other prostaglandin precursor, supplementation for pregnancy uncomplicated by pre-eclampsia or intrauterine growth restriction. *Cochrane Database Syst Rev* 2006; 3: CD003402. [Meta-analysis; 6 RCTs, *n* = 2783; I]

63. Meher S, Duley L. Garlic for preventing pre-eclampsia and its complications. *Cochrane Database Syst Rev* 2006; 3: CD006065. [Meta-analysis; 1 RCT, *n* = 100; I]

64. Meher S, Duley L. Rest during pregnancy for preventing pre-eclampsia and its complications in women with normal blood pressure. *Cochrane Database Syst Rev* 2006; (2): CD005939. [Meta-analysis; 2 RCT, *n* = 106; I]

65. Meher S, Duley L. Exercise or other physical activity for preventing pre-eclampsia and its complications. *Cochrane Database Syst Rev* 2006; (2): CD005942. [Meta-analysis; 2 RCTs, *n* = 45]

66. Meher S, Duley L. Progesterone for preventing pre-eclampsia and its complications. *Cochrane Database Syst Rev* 2006; (4): CD006175. [Meta-analysis; 2 RCTs, *n* = 296; I]

67. Meher S, Duley L. Nitric oxide for preventing pre-eclampsia and its complications. *Cochrane Database Syst Rev* 2007; (2): CD006490. [Meta-analysis, 6 RCTs, *n* = 310]

68. Kroner C, Turnbull D, Wilkinson C. Antenatal day care units versus hospital admission for women with complicated pregnancy. *Cochrane Database Syst Rev* 2001; (4): CD001803. [Meta-analysis; 1 RCT, *n* = 54]

69. Tuffnell DJ, Lilford RJ, Buchan PC. Randomised controlled trial of day care for hypertension in pregnancy. *Lancet* 1992; 339(8787): 224–7. [RCT, *n* = 54; included in Cochrane by Kroner; I]

70. Turnbull DA, Wilkinson C, Gerard K. Clinical, psychosocial, and economic effects of antenatal day care for three medical complications of pregnancy: A randomised controlled trial of 395 women. *Lancet* 2004; 363(9415): 1104–9. [RCT, *n* = 395; not included in *Cochrane* by Kroner; I]

71. Duley L, Gulmezoglu AM, Henderson-Smart DJ. Magnesium sulphate and other anticonvulsants for women with preeclampsia. *Cochrane Database Syst Rev* 2010; 11: CD000025. [Meta-analysis; 15 RCTs, *n* = 11,444; I]

72. Sibai BM. Diagnosis, prevention, and management of eclampsia. *Obstet Gynecol* 2005; 105(2): 402–10. [Review; III]

73. Duley L, Matar HE, Almerie MQ. Alternative magnesium sulphate regimens for women with pre-eclampsia and eclampsia. *Cochrane Database Syst Rev* 2010; (8): CD007388. [Meta-analysis; 6 RCTs, *n* = 866; of which 2 compared regimens for women with eclampsia and 4 for women with pre-eclampsia; I]

74. Witlin AG, Friedman SA, Sibai BM. The effect of magnesium sulfate therapy on the duration of labor in women with mild preeclampsia at term: A randomized, double-blind, placebo-controlled trial. *Am J Obstet Gynecol* 1997; 176(3): 623–7. [RCT, *n* = 135; I]

75. Graham NM, Gimovsky AC, Roman A et al. Blood loss at cesarean delivery in women on magnesium sulfate for preeclampsia. *Matern Fetal Neonatal Med* 2015 Sep 2: 1–5. [Epub ahead of print] [II-1]

76. Duley L, Williams J, Henderson-Smart DJ. Plasma volume expansion for treatment of women with pre-eclampsia. *Cochrane Database Syst Rev* 2000; (2): CD001805. [Meta-analysis; 3 RCTs, *n* = 61; I]

77. ACOG Committee Opinion No. 623. Emergent therapy for acute-onset, severe hypertension during pregnancy and the postpartum period. *Obstet Gynecol* 2015; 125: 521–5 [Guideline]

78. Magee LA, Cham C, Waterman EJ. Hydralazine for treatment of severe hypertension in pregnancy: Meta-analysis. *BMJ* 2003; 327 (7421): 955–60. [Meta-analysis; 1 RCTs, *n* = 893, of which eight compared hydralazine with nifedipine and five with labetalol; I]

79. Knight M, Duley L, Henderson-Smart DJ. Withdrawn: Antiplatelet agents for preventing and treating pre-eclampsia.

Cochrane Database Syst Rev 2007; (2): CD000492. [Meta-analysis; 42 RCTs, *n* = 32,000; I]

80. Wallace DH, Leveno KJ, Cunningham FG. Randomized comparison of general and regional anesthesia for cesarean delivery in pregnancies complicated by severe preeclampsia. *Obstet Gynecol* 1995; 86(2): 193–9. [RCT, *n* = 80; I]

81. Tajik P, van der Tuuk K, Koopman CM et al. Should cervical favorability play a role in the decision for labour induction in gestational hypertension or mild preeclampsia at term? An exploratory analysis from the HYPITAT trial. *BJOG* 2012; 119: 1123–30. [Secondary analysis of RCT, *n* = 756; I]

82. Tajik P, van der Tuuk K, Koopman CM et al. Should cervical favorability play a role in the decision for labour induction in gestational hypertension or mild preeclampsia at term? An exploratory analysis from the HYPITAT trial. *BJOG* 2012; 119: 1123–30. [Secondary analysis of RCT, *n* = 756; I]

83. Alanis MC, Robinson CJ, Hulsey TC. Early-onset severe preeclampsia: Induction of labor vs. elective cesarean delivery and neonatal outcomes. *Am J Obstet Gynecol* 2008; 199(3): 262–6. [Level II-3]

84. Alexander JM, Bloom SL, McIntire DD. Severe preeclampsia and the very low birth weight infant: Is induction of labor harmful? *Obstet Gynecol* 1999; 93(4): 485–8. [Level III]

85. Berkley E, Meng C, Rayburn WF. Success rates with low dose misoprostol before induction of labor for nulliparas with severe preeclampsia at various gestational ages. *J Matern Fetal Neonatal Med* 2007; 20(11): 825–31. [Level III]

86. Blackwell SC, Redman ME, Tomlinson M. Labor induction for the preterm severe pre-eclamptic patient: Is it worth the effort? *J Matern Fetal Med* 2001; 10(5): 305–11. [Level III]

87. Hall DR, Odendaal HJ, Steyn DW. Delivery of patients with early onset, severe pre-eclampsia. *Int J Gynaecol Obstet* 2001; 74(2): 143–50. [Level III]

88. Mashiloane CD, Moodley J. Induction or caesarean section for preterm pre-eclampsia? *J Obstet Gynaecol* 2002; 22(4): 353–6. [Level III]

89. Nassar AH, Adra AM, Chakhtoura N. Severe preeclampsia remote from term: Labor induction or elective cesarean delivery? *Am J Obstet Gynecol* 1998; 179(5): 1210–3. [Level III]

90. Schoen CN et al. Is outpatient management safe for women with superimposed preeclampsia without severe features? *American Journal of Obstetrics & Gynecology* 2016; 214(1): S411. [II-1]

91. Schoen et al. Predictors of progression of preterm preeclampsia without severe features to severe disease. 2016 *ACOG* abstract (full reference pending). [II-2]

92. Schiff E, Friedman SA, Kao L, Sibai BM. The importance of urinary protein excretion during conservative management of severe preeclampsia. *Am J Obstet Gynecol* 1996; 175(5): 1313. [II-2; 66 cases]

93. Hall DR, Odendaal HJ, Steyn DW, Grové D. Urinary protein excretion and expectant management of early onset, severe pre-eclampsia. *Int J Gynaecol Obstet* 2002; 77(1): 1. [74 cases]

94. von Dadelszen P, Payne B, Li J et al. Prediction of adverse maternal outcomes in pre-eclampsia: Development and validation of the full PIERS model. PIERS Study Group. *Lancet* 2011; 377(9761): 219. [Prospective, *n* = 2023; I] [II-3]

95. Ganzevoort W, Rep A, Bonsel GJ. A randomised controlled trial comparing two temporising management strategies, one with and one without plasma volume expansion, for severe and early onset pre-eclampsia. *BJOG* 2005; 112(10): 1358–68. [Meta-analysis; 2 RCTs, *n* = 216; I]

96. Odendaal HJ, Pattinson RC, Bam R. Aggressive or expectant management for patients with severe preeclampsia between 28 to 32 weeks' gestation: A randomized controlled trial. *Obstet Gynecol* 1990; 76(6): 1070–5. [RCT, *n* = 28; included in *Cochrane* by Churchill, 2002; I]

97. Sibai BM, Mercer BM, Schiff E. Aggressive versus expectant management of severe preeclampsia at 28 to 32 weeks' gestation: A randomized controlled trial. *Am J Obstet Gynecol* 1994; 171(3): 818–22. [RCT, *n* = 95; included in *Cochrane* by Churchill, 2002; I]

98. Vigil-De Gracia, P., Reyes-Tejada, O., Calle Miñaca, A et al. Expectant management of severe preeclampsia remote from term: The MEXPRE Latin Study, a randomized, multicenter clinical trial. *American Journal of Obstetrics & Gynecology*, 2013; 209(5): 425.e1–8. [RCT, *n* = 267]

99. Churchill D, Duley L. Interventionist versus expectant care for severe pre-eclampsia before term. *Cochrane Database Syst Rev* 2002; (3): CD003106. [Meta-analysis; 2 RCTs, *n* = 133; I]

100. Magee LA, Yong PJ, Espinosa V. Expectant management of severe preeclampsia remote from term: A structured systematic review. *Hypertens Pregnancy* 2009; 28(3): 312–47. [Review; 72 studies; III]

101. American College of Obstetricians and Gynecologists and Society for Maternal–Fetal Medicine, Menard MK, Kilpatrick S, Saade G, Hollier LM, Joseph GF Jr, Barfield W, Callaghan W, Jennings J, Conry J. Levels of maternal care. *Am J Obstet Gynecol* 2015 Mar; 212(3): 259–71. doi: 10.1016/j.ajog.2014.12.030. Epub Jan 22, 2015. PubMed PMID: 25620372. [Guideline]

102. Publications Committee, Society for Maternal-Fetal Medicine, Sibai BM. Evaluation and management of severe preeclampsia before 34 weeks' gestation. *Am J Obstet Gynecol* 2011 Sept; 205(3): 191–8. doi: 10.1016/j.ajog.2011.07.017. Epub Jul 20, 2011. Review. PubMed PMID: 22071049. [Guideline]

103. Society for Maternal-Fetal Medicine Publications Committee, Berkley E, Chauhan SP, Abuhamad A. Doppler assessment of the fetus with intrauterine growth restriction. *Am J Obstet Gynecol* 2012 Apr; 206(4): 300–8. doi:10.1016/j.ajog.2012.01.022. Erratum in: *Am J Obstet Gynecol* 2015 Feb; 212(2): 246. *Am J Obstet Gynecol* 2012 Jun; 206(6): 508. PubMed PMID: 22464066. [Guideline]

104. Haram K, Svendsen E, Abildgaard U. The HELLP syndrome: Clinical issues and management. A review. *BMC Pregnancy Childbirth* 2009; 9: 8. [Review; III]

105. Sibai BM. A practical plan to detect and manage HELLP syndrome. *OBG Management* 2005; 4: 52–69. [Review; III]

106. Sibai BM. Diagnosis, controversies, and management of the syndrome of hemolysis, elevated liver enzymes, and low platelet count. *Obstet Gynecol* 2004; 103(5 Pt. 1): 981–91. [Review; III]

107. Woudstra DM, Chandra S, Hofmeyr GJ. Corticosteroids for HELLP (hemolysis, elevated liver enzymes, low platelets) syndrome in pregnancy. *Cochrane Database Syst Rev* 2010; (9): CD008148. [Meta-analysis; 11 RCTs, *n* = 550; I]

108. Isler CM, Barrilleaux PS, Magann EF. A prospective, randomized trial comparing the efficacy of dexamethasone and betamethasone for the treatment of antepartum HELLP (hemolysis, elevated liver enzymes, and low platelet count) syndrome. *Am J Obstet Gynecol* 2001; 184(7): 1332–7. [RCT, *n* = 40. Dexamethasone versus betamethasone; I]

109. Isler CM, Magann EF, Rinehart BK. Dexamethasone compared with betamethasone for glucocorticoid treatment of postpartum HELLP syndrome. *Int J Gynaecol Obstet* 2003; 80(3): 291–7. [RCT, *n* = 36; Dexamethasone versus betamethasone I]

110. Fonseca JE, Mendez F, Catano C. Dexamethasone treatment does not improve the outcome of women with HELLP syndrome: A double-blind, placebo-controlled, randomized clinical trial. *Am J Obstet Gynecol* 2005; 193(5): 1591–8. [RCT, *n* = 132; I]

111. Katz L, de Amorim MM, Figueiroa JN. Postpartum dexamethasone for women with hemolysis, elevated liver enzymes, and low platelets (HELLP) syndrome: A double-blind, placebo-controlled, randomized clinical trial. *Am J Obstet Gynecol* 2008; 198(3): 283–8. [RCT, *n* = 105; I]

112. van Runnard Heimel PJ, Huisjes AJ, Franx A. A randomised placebo-controlled trial of prolonged prednisolone administration to patients with HELLP syndrome remote from term. *Eur J Obstet Gynecol Reprod Biol* 2006; 128(1–2): 187–93. [RCT, *n* = 31; I]

113. Duley L. The global impact of pre-eclampsia and eclampsia. *Semin Perinatol* 2009; 33(3): 130–7. [Review; III]

114. Duley L, Henderson-Smart DJ, Walker GJ. Magnesium sulphate versus diazepam for eclampsia. *Cochrane Database Syst Rev* 2010; 12: CD000127. [Meta-analysis; 7 RCTs, *n* = 1396; I]

115. Duley L, Henderson-Smart DJ, Chou D. Magnesium sulphate versus phenytoin for eclampsia. *Cochrane Database Syst Rev* 2010; (10): CD000128. [Meta-analysis; 7 RCTs, *n* = 972; I]

116. Duley L, Gulmezoglu AM, Chou D. Magnesium sulphate versus lytic cocktail for eclampsia. *Cochrane Database Syst Rev* 2010; (9): CD002960. [Meta-analysis]

117. Magee L, Sadeghi S. Prevention and treatment of postpartum hypertension. *Cochrane Database Syst Rev* 2005; (1): CD004351. [Meta-analysis; 6 RCTs: 3 RCTs on prevention, *n* = 315; 3 RCTs on treatment, *n* = 144; I]

118. Ascarelli MH, Johnson V, McCreary H. Postpartum preeclampsia management with furosemide: A randomized clinical trial. *Obstet Gynecol* 2005; 105(1): 29–33. [RCT, *n* = 264; I]

119. Hladunewich MA, Derby GC, Lafayette RA. Effect of L-arginine therapy on the glomerular injury of preeclampsia: A randomized controlled trial. *Obstet Gynecol* 2006; 107(4): 886–95. [RCT, *n* = 45; I]

120. Sep S, Smits L, Prins M. Prediction tests for recurrent hypertensive disease in pregnancy, a systematic review. *Hypertens Pregnancy* 2010; 29(2): 206–30. [Review, 33 studies; III]

121. Van Oostwaard MF, Langenveld J, Schiut E et al. Recurrence of hypertensive disorders of pregnancy: An individual patient data metaanalysis. *AJOG* 2015; 212: 624.e1-17. [II-1]

122. Hernandez-Diaz S, Toh S, Cnattingius S. Risk of pre-eclampsia in first and subsequent pregnancies: Prospective cohort study. *BMJ* 2009; 338: b2255. [Cohort analytic study, *n* = 763,795; II-2]

123. Langenveld J, Jansen S, van der Post J. Recurrence risk of a delivery before 34 weeks of pregnancy due to an early onset hypertensive disorder: A systematic review. *Am J Perinatol* 2010; 27(7): 565–71. [Meta-analysis; 7 RCTs, *n* = 2188; I]

124. Langenveld J, Buttinger A, van der Post J. Recurrence risk and prediction of a delivery under 34 weeks of gestation after a history of a severe hypertensive disorder. *BJOG* 2011; 118(5): 589–95. [Cohort analytic study, *n* = 211; II-2]

125. Chames MC, Haddad B, Barton JR. Subsequent pregnancy outcome in women with a history of HELLP syndrome at < or = 28 weeks of gestation. *Am J Obstet Gynecol* 2003; 188(6): 1504–7. [II-2]

126. Magnussen EB, Vatten LJ, Smith GD. Hypertensive disorders in pregnancy and subsequently measured cardiovascular risk factors. *Obstet Gynecol* 2009; 114(5): 961–70. [Observational study, *n* = 15,065; II-3]

2

Cardiac disease

Meredith Birsner and Sharon Rubin

KEY POINTS

- Normal pregnancy physiology—particularly increased intravascular volume, hypercoagulability, and decreased systemic vascular resistance—can severely exacerbate cardiac disease during pregnancy.
- **For many cardiac conditions**, especially pulmonary hypertension and aortic stenosis, **relative hypervolemia**, rather than fluid restriction, and **avoidance of hypotension** are the **key intrapartum management principles**. Mitral stenosis and some cases of cardiomyopathy are the main exceptions to this principle.
- Women with congenital heart disease should have a **fetal echocardiogram** at around 22 weeks.
- **Most cardiac diseases in pregnancy do** *not* **benefit from cesarean delivery**, and this can be reserved for usual obstetrical indications.
- **Pulmonary hypertension, Marfan syndrome with aortic root >4 cm, and severe cardiomyopathy** are associated with **high maternal mortality**, and should be counseled prepregnancy of this risk and provided alternatives to their own pregnancy.

BACKGROUND

For "cardiac disease in pregnancy," this guideline reviews *maternal* cardiac disease. These women are at higher risk for cardiovascular complications, neonatal complications, and even maternal death [1,2]. Concern for cardiac decompensation occurs when the heart, either from acquired or congenital physiologic or structural defects, is unable to accommodate pregnancy physiology or dynamics of parturition. **There are no trials of intervention specific for cardiac disease in pregnancy.**

SYMPTOMS/SIGNS

Symptoms can include fatigue, limitation of physical activity, palpitations, tachycardia, shortness of breath, chest pain, dyspnea on exertion, and cyanosis. These symptoms and signs of cardiac disease can often be confused with common pregnancy complaints.

EPIDEMIOLOGY/INCIDENCE

Cardiac disease complicates 1% to 4% of pregnancies, but accounts for 10% to 25% of maternal mortality [3–5]. Cardiac disease is a leading cause of ICU admission in the obstetric population [6]. In the United States, congenital heart defect (CHD) is more common than rheumatic heart disease as a result of medical care and surgical advances. Despite significant medical and surgical advances over the past two decades, cardiac disease remains a significant cause of maternal mortality.

GENETICS

When the mother has a congenital heart defect, the fetus is at increased risk for a congenital heart defect (generally 3%–5%, but ranges from 1% to 15%). Therefore, fetal-echocardiography (best if done at around 22 weeks) is recommended. DiGeorge syndrome (chromosomal deletion in 22q11), Marfan syndrome, and hypertrophic obstructive cardiomyopathy are all autosomal dominant.

ETIOLOGY/BASIC PATHOPHYSIOLOGY/PREGNANCY CONSIDERATIONS

The main function of the heart is to provide oxygen (and other nutrients) and remove carbon dioxide (and other wastes) to and from all end organs of the body, which include the uterus and fetus during pregnancy. The chief determinants of oxygen delivery include the amount carried by the blood (determined by the amount of hemoglobin and degree of saturation) and the delivery of that blood: primarily cardiac output (determined by preload, afterload, cardiac contractility, and heart rate). Any disease process or pregnancy physiology that interferes with this main function of the heart can result in maternal and fetal morbidity and mortality.

Five principal physiologic changes of pregnancy can complicate cardiac disease during pregnancy. See also Chapter 3 of *Obstetric Evidence Based Guidelines* [7]:

1. *Decreased systemic vascular resistance (SVR).* For example, ventricular septal defects (VSDs) result in the shunting of blood from the left ventricle to the right ventricle because the systemic blood pressure is greater than the pulmonary blood pressure. Over time, this will result in pulmonary hypertension that can approach systemic blood pressures. Pregnancy, with its associated 20% decrease in SVR, can allow pulmonary pressures to equal or exceed systemic pressures resulting in a reversal or right to left shunting of blood. This would result in deoxygenated right ventricular blood entering the left ventricle, resulting in decreased oxygen delivery to the body and even cyanosis and death [8].
2. *Increase in intravascular volume.* This occurs throughout pregnancy (50% increase), and is maximal by 32 weeks gestation. Women with severe myocardial dysfunction, such as cardiomyopathy, may not be able to accommodate this physiologic demand and may experience congestive heart failure and pulmonary edema.
3. *Postpartum increase in intravascular volume from "autotransfusion" of blood from the contracted uterus and mobilization of third spaced fluid.* Women with mitral stenosis have restricted left ventricular filling. This postpartum vascular load could result in pulmonary edema [9].
4. *Hypercoagulability.* This well-characterized pregnancy adaptation can dramatically heighten the risk for thromboembolism in at-risk patients. Pregnant women with

artificial mechanical heart valves, for example, can develop fatal thromboses despite adequate anticoagulation as a result of this physiology [10,11].

5. *Marked increase in cardiac output during parturition* [12]. This increase occurs during pregnancy and is both necessary for and partly "worsened" by labor and delivery and the postpartum volume shift described above. In women whose cardiac output is fixed and very dependent on preload, such as aortic stenosis, these volume shifts are poorly tolerated. A negative volume shift from postpartum hemorrhage can result in a precipitous drop in cardiac output and lead to inadequate coronary and cerebral perfusion [13].

Understanding these pathophysiologic interactions forms the basis for understanding, anticipating, and managing patients with cardiac disease during pregnancy.

CLASSIFICATION

Patients with heart disease are symptomatically classified by their clinical functional class (New York Heart Association [NYHA] system). **Women who have prepregnant NYHA III or IV functional capacity tend to tolerate pregnancy poorly**, but even less symptomatic women are at risk during pregnancy because up to 40% of those who develop congestive heart failure during gestation begin their pregnancy without symptoms (class I) [14] (Table 2.1), and 15% to 55% of pregnant women with heart disease show deterioration by this system.

RISK FACTORS

Predictors of maternal complications include prior cardiac events, NYHA class III or IV (Table 2.1), left heart obstruction (mitral stenosis, aortic stenosis), mechanical heart valve, Marfan syndrome, aortic root dilatation, and significant left ventricular systolic dysfunction [15–17]. The modified WHO classification (Table 2.2) [18] is the best available assessment model for estimating cardiovascular risk in pregnant women with congenital heart disease; this model integrates all knowledge about maternal risk, including known contraindications for pregnancy that are not addressed in other risk scores as well as known predictors found in other studies, underlying heart disease, and other morphological and clinical variables [19].

Table 2.1   New York Heart Association Classification

Class I
No symptoms or limitations.
Ordinary physical activity does not cause undue fatigue, dyspnea, or palpitations.
Class II
Slight limitation of physical activity.
Comfortable at rest.
Ordinary physical activity (e.g., carrying heavy packages) may result in fatigue, palpitations, or dyspnea.
Class III
Marked limitation of physical activity.
Comfortable at rest.
Less than ordinary physical activity (e.g., getting dressed) leads to symptoms.
Class IV
Severe limitation of physical activity.
Symptoms of heart failure or angina are present *at rest* and worsen with any activity.

Expert knowledge is sometimes required for use of this model, especially when choosing between WHO class II and III.

COMPLICATIONS

Today, with proper management, maternal mortality is predominantly restricted to patients with **severe pulmonary hypertension, coronary artery disease (CAD), cardiomyopathy, endocarditis, and sudden arrhythmia** [4,20]. These groups can be used to determine general treatment principles. Neonatal complications mostly derive from preterm birth, miscarriage, and growth restriction.

MANAGEMENT
Preconception Counseling

Women with **cardiac diseases that can be ameliorated** (invasively or noninvasively) **should be advised to do so before pregnancy** to decrease their pregnancy-related morbidity and mortality. These include severe mitral, aortic, or pulmonic stenosis; uncorrected tetralogy of Fallot; CAD; coarctation of the aorta; large intracardiac shunt from atrial septal defect (ASD); or VSD with mild or moderate pulmonary hypertension [21]. Coexisting disorders, such as anemia, thyroid disease, or hypertension, should be treated and controlled before pregnancy.

On the other hand, certain women should be advised to complete their childbearing before their cardiac condition requires repair, which could further complicate pregnancy management. For example, a woman with moderately severe valvular disease may ultimately require a prosthetic valve in the future. During pregnancy, some of these valves carry very high thromboembolic and anticoagulant risk [10,11].

Counseling should include diet and activity modifications, infection prevention and control, and review of prognosis, possible complications, and management in a future pregnancy.

Patients with group III lesions or significant dilated cardiomyopathy (including peripartum cardiomyopathy with residual left ventricular dysfunction) should be advised not to conceive because they have an increased risk of mortality. Contraception and sterilization counseling should be offered. If such patients present postconception, pregnancy termination should be offered [21].

Prenatal Care/Antepartum Testing

The patient should be questioned and examined during frequent prenatal visits for cardiac failure. **Maternal echocardiogram** allows assessment of heart function. Pulmonary hypertension is often unreliable when estimated noninvasively by echocardiogram and may need to be confirmed by cardiac catheterization. EKG shows physiologic changes such as QRS axis shift to left (because of elevated diaphragm), and minor ST and T-wave changes in lead III. Fetal growth ultrasounds should be performed every four to six weeks when there is concern for developing intrauterine growth restriction. This can be coupled with serial antenatal testing at 34 weeks [22]. Finally, future contraceptive plans, including sterilization, should be reviewed [23,24].

General Management

Certain general principles apply to most women with cardiac disease:

1. *Antepartum activity restriction.* This can be used to minimize maternal exertion and oxygen demand in the

Table 2.2 Maternal Risk Associated with Pregnancy: Modified WHO Classification (see further ref. [18])

	WHO I	WHO II	WHO II–III	WHO III	WHO IV
Caveat		If otherwise well and uncomplicated	Depending on individual		
Definition	No detectable increased risk of maternal mortality and no/mild increase in morbidity.	Small increased risk of maternal mortality or moderate increase in morbidity.		Significantly increased risk of maternal mortality or severe morbidity; expert counseling required. If pregnancy is decided upon, intensive specialist cardiac and obstetric monitoring needed throughout pregnancy, childbirth, and the puerperium.	Extremely high risk of maternal mortality or severe morbidity; pregnancy is contraindicated. If pregnancy occurs, termination should be discussed. If pregnancy continues, care as for class III.
Conditions	Uncomplicated, small or mild: Pulmonary stenosis Patent ductus arteriosus Mitral valve prolapse Successfully repaired simple lesions (atrial or ventricular septal defect, patent ductus arteriosus, anomalous pulmonary venous drainage) Atrial or ventricular ectopic beats, isolated	Unoperated atrial or ventricular septal defect Repaired tetralogy of Fallot Most arrhythmias	Mild left ventricular impairment Hypertrophic cardiomyopathy Native or tissue valvular heart disease not considered WHO I or IV Marfan syndrome without aortic dilatation Aorta <45 mm in aortic disease associated with bicuspid aortic valve Repaired coarctation	Mechanical valve Sytemic right ventricle Fontan circulation Cyanotic heart disease (unrepaired) Other complex congenital heart disease Aortic dilatation 40–45 mm in Marfan syndrome Aortic dilatation 45–50 mm in aortic disease associated with bicuspid aortic valve	Pulmonary arterial hypertension of any cause Severe systemic ventricular dysfunction (LVEF <30%, NYHA III–IV) Previous peripartum cardiomyopathy with any residual impairment of left ventricular function Severe mitral stenosis, severe symptomatic aortic stenosis Marfan syndrome with aorta dilated >45 mm Aortic dilatation >50 mm in aortic disease associated with bicuspid aortic valve Native severe coarctation

pregnant patient with limited cardiac output or cyanotic heart disease [24]. Strict bed rest should be avoided to prevent thromboembolism.

2. *Treat coexisting medical conditions.* The morbidity of cardiac disease can be compounded by medical conditions such as anemia, hypertension, or thyroid disease. Therefore, these conditions should be optimized to minimize their comorbidity [21].

3. *Collaborative care by multiple specialists.* Pregnant patients with cardiac disease are very complex, and should be **managed by a multidisciplinary team of specialists from a variety of areas**, including obstetrics, maternal-fetal medicine, cardiology, and anesthesiology [25].

4. *Labor in the lateral decubitus position.* This maximizes blood return to the heart by decreasing vena caval compression by the gravid uterus and, therefore, maximizes cardiac output [26,27]. This preload preservation can be critical to women with cardiac compromise [23,24].

5. *Epidural anesthesia.* This minimizes pain, sympathetic stress, oxygen utilization, and fluctuations in cardiac output. Sometimes "just" a narcotic epidural should be used, avoiding the sympathetic blockade (and consequent hypotension) of local anesthetics. Spinal anesthesia should be avoided, and epidural should be dosed slowly with adequate prehydration (intravenous fluids) to minimize risk of hypotension and its consequent drop in preload leading to decreased cardiac output [24,28–30].

6. *Oxygen, particularly during labor and delivery, as necessary.* Keeping maternal PaO_2 ≥70 mmHg allows for adequate maternal and fetal hemoglobin oxygen saturation [23,30].

7. *Bacterial endocarditis prophylaxis.* **Antibiotics are recommended only for** *those patients deemed to be at highest* risk for infective endocarditis: **prosthetic heart valve, prior infective endocarditis, unrepaired CHD, repaired CHD with prosthetic material during the first six months after the procedure (during endothelialization), and repaired CHD with residual defect(s)** (Table 2.3) [31]. Some experts have even suggested that no prophylaxis is needed at all [32]. The usual recommended antibiotic regimen for cardiac prophylaxis is a single dose of

Table 2.3 Cardiac Conditions for Which Antibiotic Prophylaxis for Bacterial Endocarditis is Reasonable (see further ref. [31])

Prosthetic cardiac valve or prosthetic material used for cardiac valve repair
Previous infective endocarditis
Congenital heart defect (CHD):
   Unrepaired cyanotic CHD, including palliative shunts and conduits
   Completely repaired CHD with prosthetic material or conduits (where placed by surgery or catheter intervention within six months of procedure)
   Incompletely repaired CHD with residual defects at or near the site of prosthetic patch or device

ampicillin 2.0 g IV preprocedure. Cefazolin, ceftriaxone, or clindamycin can be substituted in the penicillin-allergic patient [33].

8. *Cesarean delivery is usually reserved for obstetrical indications.* Operative delivery is associated with greater blood loss, increased pain, thromboembolism, and prolonged bed rest compared to vaginal delivery and therefore can complicate the gravida with heart disease. Although labor induction and/or assisted second stage may be necessary for certain maternal or fetal indications, **cesarean delivery should be used for usual obstetrical reasons** [22,23,29]. Contraindications to trial of labor to be considered are Marfan syndrome with root >4 cm, aortopathy, and maternal therapeutic anticoagulation with warfarin that cannot be interrupted.

9. *Invasive hemodynamic monitoring with a pulmonary artery catheter.* Although the safety and utility of pulmonary artery catheters in critically ill nonpregnant patients have been questioned [34–36], they may be helpful in managing certain high-risk conditions that are preload dependent, such as critical aortic stenosis or pulmonary hypertension [23,24].

10. *Most patients benefit from avoiding hypotension during labor and delivery.* Although not true for all patients, most with group II and III cardiac lesions will benefit from avoiding hypotension or hypovolemia. **To avoid hypotension, keep the woman on the "wetter" side, avoid hemorrhage, replenish blood loss adequately, avoid spinal anesthesia, hydrate at least 1 L of intravenous fluids before "slow" epidural, and avoid supine hypotension.**

11. *Postpartum contraceptive management is imperative.* Many women with cardiac disease use inadequate or inappropriate contraception [37]. The widely available Medical Eligibility Criteria for Contraceptive Use document from the World Health Organization can assist in reproductive planning [38].

Pregnancy Management of Specific Diseases

Palpitations

Workup should be similar to the nonpregnant patient and include thyroid function and ruling out drugs, alcohol, caffeine, or smoking as well as an EKG and echocardiogram. The woman can be counseled that premature atrial and ventricular contractions are increased in pregnancy and usually benign.

VSD

Pregnancy outcome is usually good. Rule out pulmonary hypertension, especially in large, long-standing cases. In the absence of pulmonary hypertension, mortality is unlikely [39]. Intrapartum, avoid fluid overload [24].

Pulmonary Hypertension

It is important to avoid false positive diagnosis of pulmonary hypertension by echocardiogram as up to 30% of women with this diagnosis (pulmonary artery systolic pressure >30–40 mmHg) by echocardiography have normal pulmonary pressures by pulmonary artery catheterization.

Over time, in women with unrepaired VSD, ASD, or patent ductus arteriosus (PDA), the congenital left to right shunt leads to pulmonary hypertension, **right to left shunt**, and consequently decreased pulmonary perfusion and hypoxemia. Although recent data suggests improved outcomes [40], even with modern management, a high risk of maternal death remains [41]. Some of this mortality is secondary to thromboembolic events [42]. Delayed postpartum death can be seen four to six weeks after delivery, possibly secondary to loss of pregnancy-associated hormones and increased pulmonary vascular resistance (PVR) [24,42].

The main physiologic difficulty in pulmonary hypertension is maintenance of adequate pulmonary blood flow. Any situation that decreases venous return to the heart decreases right ventricular preload and consequently pulmonary blood flow. Therefore, as hypovolemia and **hypotension** can fatally precipitate decreased pulmonary perfusion and oxygenation (and reverse the left to right cardiac shunt in cases of Eisenmenger's syndrome; see section titled "Etiology/Basic Pathophysiology/Pregnancy Considerations"), leading to sudden death, it **must be avoided**. Such situations are common intrapartum (vasodilation from regional anesthesia or pooling of blood in the lower extremities from vena caval compression) and sometimes unanticipated (hemorrhage). As such, patients are better managed on the "wet" side even at the expense of mild pulmonary edema. This allows a margin of safety against unexpected hemorrhage or drug-induced hypotension [42]. Pulmonary artery catheterization may be useful in this regard [24]. Avoid increase in PVR and myocardial depressants. Anticoagulant prophylaxis may be useful in preventing thromboembolic risk, and intravenous prostacyclin (or its analogues) or inhaled nitric oxide may be helpful in reducing PVR while sparing the SVR [43,44].

Route of delivery for women with severe pulmonary hypertension remains controversial. Although vaginal delivery is associated with less risk of hemorrhage, infection, and venous thromboembolism, emergency cesarean without proper cardiac anesthesia personnel or maternal hemodynamic monitoring is associated with an increased risk of complications; scheduled cesarean can allow optimization of delivery conditions with multidisciplinary team involvement and resources [45].

Coarctation of the Aorta

If surgically corrected, maternal outcome is good. Women with smaller aortic dimensions are more likely to experience hypertensive complications related to pregnancy, and conversely, those with larger aortic dimensions have a lower risk of adverse cardiovascular, obstetric, and fetal/neonatal events; cardiovascular magnetic resonance imaging can aid in risk stratification [46]. There is increased risk for maternal mortality when associated with aneurysmal dilation or associated cardiac lesions (VSD, PDA) [47]. **Avoid hypotension, myocardial depression, and bradycardia** [48].

Tetralogy of Fallot

It consists of VSD, pulmonary stenosis, hypertrophy of right ventricle, and overriding aorta. Corrected lesions do well, but uncorrected ones are still associated with high maternal mortality [49]. Because of the VSD-associated shunting in uncorrected cases, **hypotension**, myocardial depressants, and bradycardia **should be avoided** [24].

Mitral Stenosis

Women with >1.5 cm² mitral valve area usually have good outcomes. When **significant (valve area <1.5 cm²) mitral stenosis** is present, left ventricular filling is limited, which leads to fixed cardiac output. If the pregnant patient is unable to accommodate the volume shifts that occur during gestation and puerperium, pulmonary edema can result (see pathophysiology above). Antenatally, this risk is greatest at 30 to 32 weeks when maternal blood volume peaks. In that scenario, percutaneous balloon valvuloplasty may be relatively safely performed in certain patients [50]. Although it appears safer for the fetus than open mitral commissurotomy, it should be reserved for women who are unresponsive to aggressive medical therapy [51,52]. As cardiac output is dependent on adequate diastolic filling time, **tachycardia** can result in hemodynamic decompensation (hypotension and fall in cardiac output) and should be **avoided**. Intrapartum, therefore, short-acting beta-blockers should be considered when pulse exceeds 90 to 100 bpm [24,53]. Although inadequate preload will decrease cardiac output, too much will result in pulmonary edema, particularly postpartum when pulmonary capillary wedge pressure (PCWP) can rise up to 16 mmHg [9]. Invasive hemodynamic monitoring via pulmonary artery catheterization with cautious, individualized intrapartum diuresis to a predelivery target of 14 mmHg (although normal is 6 to 9 mmHg, mitral stenosis patients often need elevated wedge pressures to maintain left ventricular filling) may be desirable in some patients [24]. Patients with moderate stenosis with only mild fluid overload can often be managed with just fluid restriction to complement their insensible loss during labor [24]. Avoid decrease in SVR and increase in PVR.

Aortic Stenosis

The major issue is fixed and limited cardiac output through a restricted valve area. Mortality is related to degree of stenosis with **>100 mmHg of mean shunt gradient associated with 15% to 20% mortality**. Congestive heart failure (CHF), syncope, and previous cardiac arrest are other contraindications to pregnancy. Hypotension and decreased preload can lead to a precipitous drop in cardiac output. Consequently, **hypotension should be avoided** [54]. Intrapartum, invasive hemodynamic monitoring may be helpful to increase the PCWP to the range of 15 to 17 mmHg to maintain a margin of safety against unexpected blood loss or hypotension (although the data is insufficient for an evidence-based recommendation) [23,24]. This range of PCWP minimizes risk of frank pulmonary edema even with normal postpartum fluid shifts, and furthermore, hypovolemia is potentially more dangerous in these patients than pulmonary edema. Avoid decrease in venous return and tachycardia.

Pulmonic Stenosis

Congenital pulmonic stenosis (PS) is a lesion for which survival to adulthood is high. It is generally well tolerated during pregnancy. **Balloon valvuloplasty should be considered prior to conception in patients with asymptomatic severe PS (peak gradient >60 mmHg) or symptomatic patients with peak gradient >50 mmHg** (in association with less than moderate pulmonic regurgitation) [55]. In patients with functional capacity NYHA class I–II, pulmonic stenosis does not appear to adversely affect maternal outcomes [56]. **Adequate preload** is needed to maintain right ventricular cardiac output. Very severe PS (>80 mmHg) may be associated with maternal and fetal complications, including hypertension-related disorders, preterm delivery, and offspring mortality [57]. Percutaneous pulmonary valvuloplasty has been successfully performed in cases of severe symptomatic obstruction during pregnancy.

Mitral and Aortic Insufficiency

These lesions are usually well tolerated in pregnancy unless associated with NYHA III or IV symptoms at baseline. Avoid arrhythmia, bradycardia, increase in SVR, and myocardial depressants.

Mechanical Heart Valves

Women with mechanical heart valves are at increased risk of adverse outcomes in pregnancy, including valve thrombosis (4.7%), hemorrhage (23.1%), and death (1.4%), making prepregnancy counseling and centralization of care imperative [58]. Those women who anticipate ultimately needing valve replacement surgery should be encouraged to complete childbearing before valve replacement. For women with mechanical heart valves, optimal anticoagulation during pregnancy is controversial. The highest risk is with first-generation mechanical valves (Starr–Edwards, Bjork–Shiley) in the mitral position, followed by second-generation valves (St. Jude) in the aortic position. These women need to be **therapeutically anticoagulated throughout pregnancy and postpartum with blood levels frequently (usually weekly) checked to ensure therapeutic levels of anticoagulation.** The 2012 CHEST Guidelines [59] indicate, "For pregnant women with mechanical heart valves, the decision regarding the choice of anticoagulant regimen is so value- and preference-dependent (risk of thrombosis vs. risk of fetal abnormalities) that we consider the decision to be completely individualized." Women of childbearing age and pregnant women with mechanical valves should be counseled about potential maternal and fetal risks associated with various anticoagulant regimens. The Guidelines specify one of the following regimens over no anticoagulation for pregnant women with mechanical valves:

1. Adjusted-dose bid low-molecular weight heparin (LMWH) throughout pregnancy with dose adjusted to achieve peak anti-Xa four hours postinjection.
2. Adjusted-dose unfractionated heparin (UFH) throughout pregnancy administered subcutaneously every 12 hours in doses adjusted to keep the mid-interval aPTT at least twice control or attain an anti-XA heparin level of 0.35–0.70 units/mL.
3. UFH or LMWH (as above) until the 13th week with substitution by vitamin K antagonists until close to delivery when UFH or LMWH is resumed.

In women judged to be at very high risk of thromboembolism in whom concerns exist about the efficacy and safety of UFH or LMWH as dosed above (e.g., older generation prosthesis in the mitral position or history of thromboembolism), the Guidelines suggest vitamin K antagonists throughout pregnancy with replacement by UFH or LMWH (as above) close to delivery rather than one of the regimens above; women who place a higher value on avoiding fetal risk than on avoiding maternal complications (e.g., catastrophic valve thrombosis) are likely to choose LMWH or UFH over vitamin K antagonists. Warfarin throughout pregnancy and postpartum may be the regimen associated with the least maternal risks of thromboembolism, but in the first trimester, warfarin is associated with a 10% to 15% teratogenic risk (nasal hypoplasia, optic atrophy, digital anomalies, mental impairment). On the other hand, UFH throughout can be ineffective [10,11]. Regarding delivery, therapeutic anticoagulation should be stopped during active labor and for delivery, with therapeutic heparin restarted about 6 to 12 hours after delivery when adequate hemostasis is assured, and warfarin restarted in an overlapping fashion (to avoid paradoxical thrombosis) 24 to 36 hours after delivery. Last, for pregnant women with prosthetic valves at high risk of thromboembolism, the addition of low-dose aspirin, 75 to 100 mg/day, is suggested.

Marfan Syndrome

Marfan syndrome is an autosomal-dominant generalized connective tissue disorder with 80% of affected women having a family history of this condition. Its main risk in pregnancy is aortic aneurysm, leading to rupture and dissection. Women with personal or family history of Marfan syndrome should have an **echocardiogram**, possibly a slit lamp examination to look for ectopia lentis, and **genetic counseling**. Prognosis is reasonable when there is no aortic root involvement (<5% mortality) although mortality can still occur. There is a risk of aortic rupture, dissection, and mortality (up to 50%) in pregnancy when the **aortic root is dilated beyond 4 cm**, such that pregnancy is contraindicated in these women before repair. This may result from the "shearing force" of normal pregnancy because of increase in blood volume and cardiac output [60–62]. Prenatally, serial maternal echocardiograms to follow the cardiac root should be performed [61]. **Hypertension should be avoided**, and **beta-blockade therapy** should be considered. Although pregnancy data are limited for this last recommendation, long-term use in nonpregnant patients has been shown to slow the progression of aortic root dilation [63]. Avoid positive inotropic drugs, and plan epidural (watch for dural ectasia, present in about 90% of patients with Marfan syndrome) to reduce cardiovascular stress. If cesarean delivery is required, retention sutures should be considered because of generalized connective tissue weakness [24].

Hypertrophic Cardiomyopathy

(Previously called idiopathic hypertrophic subaortic stenosis.) It can be inherited as autosomal dominant with variable penetrance. It can result in left ventricular hypertrophy, leading to obstruction of the left ventricular outflow. The decrease in SVR of pregnancy can worsen outflow obstruction. Also, tachycardia decreases diastolic filling time, compromising cardiac output. Peripartum management focuses on avoiding tachycardia (treatment with beta-blockade), hypovolemia, and hypotension [64,65].

Dilated Cardiomyopathy

Patients with preexisting dilated cardiomyopathy with symptomatic, moderate to severe left ventricular dysfunction (ejection fraction <45%) have an increased risk of cardiovascular events during pregnancy and postpartum. Therefore prepregnancy counseling is imperative. Additionally, pregnancy may negatively impact ventricular function possible due to the hemodynamic burden of pregnancy or discontinuation of medical therapy during pregnancy [66].

Peripartum Cardiomyopathy

This is defined as cardiomyopathy (with **EF <45%**) occurring **during last four weeks of pregnancy or within five months postpartum** (peaks at 2 months postpartum) without other cause. The incidence is 1/3000 to 4000 live births. Risk factors are older maternal age, multiparity, African-American race, multiple gestations, and hypertensive disorders of pregnancy. Serial echocardiography, medical management (**digoxin, diuretics**, afterload reduction—**hydralazine** and/ or **beta-blockers** in pregnancy, ACE inhibitors postpartum), anticoagulation if EF is <35%, and possible intrapartum PAC in severely decompensated patients may be needed for management [24,67–70]. The addition of bromocriptine to standard heart failure therapy appears to improve left ventricular EF and a composite clinical outcome in women with acute severe peripartum cardiomyopathy, but the number of patients studied was too small to make any recommendation [71].

The majority of patients with peripartum cardiomyopathy have favorable outcomes. Severity of left ventricular dysfunction and the degree of left ventricular enlargement at presentation are associated with less likelihood of recovery of ventricular function [72].

Regarding future pregnancies after a diagnosis of peripartum cardiomyopathy, **persistent dilated cardiomyopathy with abnormal EF predicts a high risk (19%) of mortality and symptoms of cardiac failure (44%) with subsequent gestation** and should be discouraged. Of women with EF <25%, 57% require a cardiac transplant or are on a transplant list because of progressive symptoms of heart failure at a mean of 3.4 years of follow-up postpartum [73]. Even **women with "normal" echocardiograms (EF ≥45%–50%) after recovering from peripartum cardiomyopathy can have persistent "subclinical" low contractile reserve [68]** with up to 21% risk of developing **symptoms of CHF but no mortality** reported in one study [70].

Coronary Artery Disease

Underlying risks factors, such as diabetes, obesity, hypercholesterolemia, smoking, hypertension, and stress, should be individually addressed and treated, ideally before conception. Women with pre-established coronary artery disease or an acute coronary syndrome/myocardial infarction prior to pregnancy are at risk for serious adverse maternal cardiac events (10%) during pregnancy; the highest rates of nonfatal ischemic cardiac complications during pregnancy occur in women with atherosclerotic coronary disease [74]. Stable angina can be treated with nitrates, calcium channel blockers, and/or beta-blockers in pregnancy. With unstable angina, the woman should be counseled regarding severe risks and offered termination if early enough in pregnancy. Myocardial infarction (MI) is rare in reproductive-age women with a 1/10,000 incidence in pregnancy. When it occurs in the third trimester or within two weeks of labor, there is a high (20%) maternal mortality risk [75]. Women with prior MI with recovered heart function and optimally controlled coronary artery disease can anticipate a successful pregnancy [76]. Management of MI during pregnancy is similar to management principles in nonpregnant patients, including percutaneous coronary intervention (PCI) with placement of coronary stents or coronary angioplasty; thrombolytic therapy is a relative contraindication [23,75,77] but may be used in hospitals with no PCI capability [78]. Heparin and beta-blockers are recommended. If labor occurs within four days of an MI, cesarean delivery is often advocated [79]. Women with a prior MI should wait at least one year and ensure normal cardiac function before pregnancy. In such circumstances, a future pregnancy is associated with low risk of maternal or fetal morbidity or mortality.

CONCLUSION

With medical and surgical advances and advancing maternal age, heart disease complicating pregnancy is increasingly common. Understanding the physiologic changes of pregnancy and their effect on specific cardiac conditions forms the basis for management during pregnancy. Prepregnant cardiavascular assessment and counseling should be a primary goal. Heightened awareness to optimize cardiac status, close perinatal surveillance, and a coordinated management team are critical to improve maternal and fetal outcome.

REFERENCES

1. Siu S, Colman J, Sorenson S. Adverse neonatal and cardiac outcomes are more common in pregnant women with cardiac disease. *Circulation* 2002; 105: 2179. [II-3]
2. Berg C, Callaghan W, Syverson C et al. Pregnancy-related mortality in the United States, 1998 to 2005. *Obstet Gynecol* 2010; 116: 1302–9. [II-3]
3. Koonin LM, Atrash HK, Lawson HW et al. Maternal mortality surveillance, United States 1979–1986. *MMWR CDC Surveill Summ* 1991; 40: 1–13. [II-3]
4. DeSweit M. Maternal mortality from heart disease in pregnancy. *Br Heart J* 1993; 69: 524. [II-3]
5. Berg CJ, Atrash HK, Koonin LM et al. Pregnancy-related mortality in the United States, 1987–1990. *Obstet Gynecol* 1996; 88: 161–7. [II-3]
6. Small MJ, James AH, Kershaw T et al. Near-miss maternal mortality: Cardiac dysfunction as the principal cause of obstetric intensive care unit admissions. *Obstet Gynecol* 2012 Feb; 119(2 Pt. 1): 250–5. [II-3]
7. American College of Obstetricians and Gynecologists. Cardiac Disease in Pregnancy. ACOG Technical Bulletin No. 168—June 1992. *Int J Gynaecol Obstet* 1993; 41(3): 298–306. [III]
8. Sinnenberg RJ. Pulmonary hypertension in pregnancy. *South Med J* 1980; 73: 1529–31. [III]
9. Clark SL, Phelan JP, Greenspoon J et al. Labor and delivery in the presence of mitral stenosis: Central hemodynamic observations. *Am J Obstet Gynecol* 1985; 152: 984–8. [II-3]
10. Oakley CM, Doherty P. Pregnancy in patients after heart valve replacement. *Br Heart J* 1976; 38: 1140–8. [II-3]
11. Golby AJ, Bush EC, DeRook FA et al. Failure of high-dose heparin to prevent recurrent cardioembolic strokes in a pregnancy patient with a mechanical heart valve. *Neurology* 1992; 42: 2204–6. [III]
12. van Oppen ACC, Stigter RH, Bruinse HW. Cardiac output in normal pregnancy: A critical review. *Obstet Gynecol* 1996; 87: 310–8. [III]
13. Arias F, Pineda J. Aortic stenosis and pregnancy. *J Reprod Med* 1978; 20: 229–32. [II-3]
14. Sciscione AC, Callen NA. Pregnancy and contraception: Congenital heart disease in adolescents and adults. *Cardiol Clin* 1993; 11: 701–9. [III]
15. Siu S, Sermer M, Colman J et al. Prospective multicenter study of pregnancy outcomes in women with heart disease. *Circulation* 2001; 104(5): 515–21. [II-2]
16. Bonow R, Carabello B, Chatterjee K et al. 2008 Focused update incorporated into the ACC/AHA 2006 guidelines for the management of patients with valvular heart disease: A report of the American College of Cardiology/American Heart Association Task Force on Practice Guidelines (Writing Committee to Revise the 1998 Guidelines for the Management of Patients With Valvular Heart Disease): Endorsed by the Society of

17. Vahanian A, Baumgartner H, Bax J et al. Guidelines on the management of valvular heart disease: The Task Force on the Management of Valvular Heart Disease of the European Society of Cardiology. *Eur Heart J* 2007; 28: 230. [III]
18. European Society of Gynecology (ESG); Association for European Paediatric Cardiology (AEPC); German Society for Gender Medicine (DGesGM), Regitz-Zagrosek V, Blomstrom Lundqvist C et al., ESC Committee for Practice Guidelines. ESC Guidelines on the management of cardiovascular diseases during pregnancy: The Task Force on the Management of Cardiovascular Diseases during Pregnancy of the European Society of Cardiology (ESC). *Eur Heart J* 2011 Dec; 32(24): 3147–97. [III]
19. Balci A, Sollie-Szarynska KM, van der Bijl AG, Ruys TP, Mulder BJ, Roos-Hesselink JW et al., ZAHARA-II investigators. Prospective validation and assessment of cardiovascular and offspring risk models for pregnant women with congenital heart disease. *Heart* 2014 Sep; 100(17): 1373–81. [II-2]
20. Jacob S, Bloebaum L, Shah G et al. Maternal mortality in Utah. *Obstet Gynecol* 1998; 91: 187–91. [II-3]
21. Blanchard DG, Shabetai R. Cardiac diseases. In: Creasy RK, Resnik R, Iams JD, eds. *Maternal Fetal Medicine Principles and Practice.* 5th ed. Philadelphia, PA: Saunders, 2004; 815–44. [III]
22. McFaul PB, Dornan JC, Lamki H et al. Pregnancy complicated by maternal heart disease: A review of 519 women. *BJOG* 1988; 95: 861–7. [III]
23. Tomlinson MW. Cardiac disease. In: James DK, Steer PJ, Weiner CP et al. eds. *High Risk Pregnancy Management Options.* 3rd ed. Philadelphia, PA: Saunders, 2006. [III]
24. Foley MR. Cardiac disease. In: Dildy GA, Belfort MA, Saade GR et al. eds. *Critical Care Obstetrics.* 4th ed. Molden, MA: Blackwell Publishing Company, 2004; 252–74. [II-3]
25. Surgue D, Blake S, MacDonald D. Pregnancy complicated by maternal heart disease at the National Maternity Hospital, Dublin, Ireland, 1969–1978. *Am J Obstet Gynecol* 1981; 139: 1–6. [III]
26. Ueland K, Novy MJ, Peterson EN et al. Maternal cardiovascular dynamics IV. The influence of gestational age on maternal cardiovascular response to posture and exercise. *Am J Obstet Gynecol* 1969; 104: 856. [II-3]
27. Clark SL, Cotton DB, Pivarnik JM et al. Position change and hemodynamic profiling during normal third-trimester pregnancy and postpartum. *Am J Obstet Gynecol* 1991; 164: 883. [II-3]
28. Vadhera RB. Anesthesia for the critically ill parturient with cardiac disease and pregnancy induced hypertension. In: Dildy GA, Belfort MA, Saade GR et al. eds. *Critical Care Obstetrics.* 4th ed. Malden, MA: Blackwell Publishing, 2004. [III]
29. Siu S, Sermer M, Colman J et al. Prospective multicenter study of pregnancy outcome in women with heart disease. *Circulation* 2001; 104: 515–21. [II-3]
30. Sobrevilla LA, Cassinella MT, Carcelen A et al. Human fetal and maternal oxygen tension and acid–base status during delivery at high altitude. *Am J Obstet Gynecol* 1971; 111: 1111–8. [III]
31. Antibiotic prophylaxis for infective endocarditis. ACOG Committee Opinion No. 421. American College of Obstetricians and Gynecologists. *Obstet Gynecol* 2008; 112: 1193–4. [Review]
32. Tower C, Nallapena S, Vause S. Prophylaxis against endocarditis in obstetrics: New NICE guideline: a commentary. *BJOG* 2008; 115: 1601–4. [III]
33. Wilson W, Taubert K, Gewitz M et al. Prevention of infective endocarditis: Guidelines from the AHA. *Circulation* 2007; 116:1736–54. [III]
34. Bernard G, Sopko G, Cerra F et al. Pulmonary artery catheterization and clinical outcomes: National Heart, Lung, and Blood Institute and Food and Drug Administration Workshop Report. *JAMA* 2000; 283: 2568–72. [III]
35. Sandham JD, Hull RD, Brant RF et al. A randomized, controlled trial of the use of pulmonary-artery catheters in high-risk surgical patients. *N Engl J Med* 2003; 348: 5–14. [I]

36. Parson PE. Progress in research on pulmonary-artery catheters. *N Engl J Med* 2003; 348: 66–8. [III]

37. Vigl M, Kaemmerer M, Seifert-Klauss V, Niggemeyer E, Nagdyman N, Trigas V et al. Contraception in women with congenital heart disease. *Am J Cardiol* 2010 Nov 1; 106(9): 1317–21. [III]

38. *Medical Eligibility Criteria for Contraceptive Use.* 5th edition. Geneva: World Health Organization; 2015. [III]

39. Schaefer G, Arditi LI, Solomon HA et al. Congenital heart disease and pregnancy. *Clin Obstet Gynecol* 1968; 11: 1048–63. [III]

40. Jaïs X, Olsson KM, Barbera JA, Blanco I, Torbicki A, Peacock A et al. Pregnancy outcomes in pulmonary arterial hypertension in the modern management era. *Eur Respir J* 2012 Oct; 40(4): 881–5. [II-3]

41. Avila WS, Grinberg M, Snitcowsky R et al. Maternal and fetal outcome in pregnant women with Eisenmenger's syndrome. *Eur Heart J* 1995; 16: 460–4. [III]

42. Weiss BM, Zemp L, Seifert B et al. Outcome of pulmonary vascular disease in pregnancy: A systematic overview from 1978–1996. *J Am Coll Cardiol* 1998; 31: 1650–7. [III]

43. Stewart R, Tuazon D, Olson G et al. Pregnancy and primary pulmonary hypertension. *Chest* 2001; 119: 973–5. [III]

44. Lam JK, Stafford RE, Thorp J et al. Inhaled nitric oxide for primary pulmonary hypertension in pregnancy. *Obstet Gynecol* 2001; 98: 895–8. [II-3]

45. Curry RA, Fletcher C, Gelson E, Gatzoulis MA, Woolnough M, Richards N, Swan L, Steer PJ, Johnson MR. Pulmonary hypertension and pregnancy—A review of 12 pregnancies in nine women. *BJOG* 2012 May; 119(6): 752–61. [II-3]

46. Jimenez-Juan L, Krieger EV, Valente AM et al. Cardiovascular magnetic resonance imaging predictors of pregnancy outcomes in women with coarctation of the aorta. *Eur Heart J Cardiovasc Imaging* 2014 Mar; 15(3): 299–306. [II-3]

47. Deal K, Wooley CF. Coarctation of the aorta and pregnancy. *Ann Intern Med* 1973; 78: 706–10. [III]

48. Koszalka, MF. Cardiac disease in pregnancy. In: Foley MR, Strong TH. *Obstetric Intensive Care: A Practical Manual.* Philadelphia, PA: Saunders, 1997. [III]

49. Shime J, Mocarski EJM, Hastings D et al. Congenital heart disease in pregnancy: Short and long term implications. *Am J Obstet Gynecol* 1987; 156: 313–22. [III]

50. Iung B, Cormier B, Elias J et al. Usefulness of percutaneous balloon commissurotomy for mitral stenosis during pregnancy. *Am J Cardiol* 1994; 73: 398–400. [III]

51. Elkayam U, Bitar F. Valvular heart disease in pregnancy. Part I: native valves. *J Am Coll Cardiol* 2005; 46: 223. [III]

52. de Souza J, Martinez E, Ambrose J et al. Percutaneous balloon mitral valvuloplasty in comparison with open mitral valve commissurotomy for mitral stenosis during pregnancy. *J Am Coll Cardiol* 2001; 37(3): 900–3. [II-3]

53. Al Kasab SM, Sabag T, Al Zailbag M et al. b-Adrenergic receptor blockade in the management of pregnant women with mitral stenosis. *Am J Obstet Gynecol* 1990; 163: 37–40. [III]

54. Lao TT, Stemmer M, Magee L et al. Congenital aortic stenosis and pregnancy: A reappraisal. *Am J Obstet Gynecol* 1993; 169: 540–5. [III]

55. *ACC/AHA 2008 Guidelines for the Management of Adults With Congenital Heart Disease/Executive Summary Circulation.* 2008; 118: 2395–451 [III]

56. Hameed AB, Goodwin T, Elkayam U. *American Heart Journal* 2007; 154: 852–4. [II-2]

57. Drenthen W, Pieper PG, Roos-Hesselink JW et al. Non-cardiac complications during pregnancy in women with isolated congenital pulmonary valvar stenosis. *Heart* 2006; 92(12): 1838–43. [III]

58. Van Hagen IM, Roos-Hesselink JW, Ruys TP et al. Pregnancy in women with a mechanical heart valve: Data of the European Society of Cardiology Registry of Pregnancy and Cardiac Disease (ROPAC). *Circulation* 2015: 132(2): 132–42. [II-2]

59. Bates SM, Greer IA, Middeldorp S, Veenstra DL, Prabulos AM, Vandvik PO, American College of Chest Physicians. VTE, thrombophilia, antithrombotic therapy, and pregnancy: Antithrombotic Therapy and Prevention of Thrombosis, 9th ed: American College of Chest Physicians Evidence-Based Clinical Practice Guidelines. *Chest* 2012 Feb; 141(2 Suppl.): e691S–736S. [I for subject of valves]

60. Pyeritz RE. Maternal and fetal complications of pregnancy in the Marfan syndrome. *Am J Med* 1981; 71: 784–90. [III]

61. Rossiter JP, Repke JT, Morales AJ et al. A prospective longitudinal evaluation of pregnancy in the Marfan syndrome. *Am J Obstet Gynecol* 1995; 173: 1599–606. [III]

62. Lipscomb KJ, Smith JC, Clarke B et al. Outcome of pregnancy in women with Marfan's syndrome. *BJOG* 1997; 104: 201–6.

63. Shores J, Berger KR, Murphy EA et al. Progression of aortic dilatation and the benefit of long term b-adrenergic blockade in Marfan's syndrome. *N Eng J Med* 1994; 330: 1335–41. [II-3]

64. Maron BJ. Hypertrophic cardiomyopathy: A systematic review. *JAMA* 2002; 287: 1308–20. [III]

65. Fairley CJ, Clarke JT. Use of esmolol in a parturient with hypertrophic obstructive cardiomyopathy. *Br J Anaesth* 1995; 74: 801–4. [III]

66. Grewal J, Siu SC, Ross HJ et al. Pregnancy outcomes in women with dilated cardiomyopathy. *J Am Coll Cardiol* 2009; 55: 45–52. [II-3]

67. Demakis JG, Rahimtoola SH, Sutton GC et al. Natural course of peripartum cardiomyopathy. *Circulation* 1971; 44: 1053–61. [III]

68. Lampert MB, Weinert L, Hibbard J et al. Contractile reserve in patients with peripartum cardiomyopathy and recovered left ventricular function. *Am J Obstet Gynecol* 1997; 176: 189–95. [II-3]

69. Witlin AG, Mabie WC, Sibai BM. Peripartum cardiomyopathy: an ominous diagnosis. *Am J Obstet Gynecol* 1997; 176: 182–8. [III]

70. Elkayam U, Tummala PP, Rao K et al. Maternal and fetal outcomes of subsequent pregnancies in women with peripartum cardiomyopathy. *N Eng J Med* 2001; 344: 1567–71. [II-3]

71. Sliwa K, Blauwet L, Tibazarwa K et al. Evaluation of bromocriptine in the treatment of acute severe peripartum cardiomyopathy: A proof-of-concept pilot study. *Circulation* 2010; 121(13): 1465–73. [RCT, n = 20]

72. McNamara DM, Elkayam, U, Alharethi R et al. Clinical outcomes for peripartum cardiomyopathy in North America. *J Am Coll Cardiol* 2015; 66: 905–14. [II-2]

73. Elkayam U. Risk of subsequent pregnancy in women with a history of peripartum cardiomyopathy. *J Am Coll Cardiol* 2014; 64(15): 1629–36 [III]

74. Burchill LJ, Lameijer H, Roos-Hesselink JW, Grewal J, Ruys TP, Kulikowski JD et al. Pregnancy risks in women with pre-existing coronary artery disease, or following acute coronary syndrome. *Heart* 2015 Apr; 101(7): 525–9. [II-2]

75. Roth A, Elkayam RA. Acute myocardial infarction associated with pregnancy. *Ann Intern Med* 1996; 125: 751–62. [III]

76. Vinatier D, Virelizier S, Depret-Mosser S et al. Pregnancy after myocardial infarction. *Eur J Obstet Gynecol Reprod Biol* 1994; 56: 89–93. [III]

77. Garry D, Leikin E, Fleisher AG et al. Acute myocardial infarction in pregnancy with subsequent medical and surgical management. *Obstet Gynecol* 1996; 87: 802–4. [III]

78. Pacheco LD, Saade GR, Hankins GD. Acute myocardial infarction during pregnancy. *Clin Obstet Gynecol* 2014 Dec; 57(4): 835–43. [review]

79. Mabie WC, Anderson GD, Addington MB et al. The benefit of cesarean section in acute myocardial infarction complicated by premature labor. *Obstet Gynecol* 1988; 71: 503–6. [III]

3

Obesity

Kathryn Shaia and Maria Teresa Mella

KEY POINTS

- The preconception visit may be the single most important health care visit when viewed in the context of its effect on pregnancy. Height in meters and weight in kilograms should be recorded for all women at each doctor visit to allow for calculation of BMI. The BMI category should be reviewed with the patient, making sure she understands that her category is not normal.
- Obesity is a risk factor for cardiovascular disease; diabetes; hypertension; stroke; osteoarthritis; gall stones; increased incidence of endometrial, breast, or colon cancer; cardiomyopathy; fatty liver; obstructive sleep apnea; urinary tract infections; other complications; and, most importantly, mortality. Prepregnancy obesity and excessive gestational weight gain are associated with increased risk of childhood obesity.
- **Preconception weight loss with diet, exercise, behavior change**, and, if necessary, pharmacotherapy is recommended. Weight loss of at least 5% to 10% will help reduce the incidence of obesity-related comorbidities.
- Preconception (and at first prenatal visit), check **BP with a large cuff, fasting lipid profile and blood sugar, thyroid function tests**, and **overnight polysomnogram**. In obese patients with chronic hypertension or type 2 diabetes, it is advisable to obtain an **EKG** and an **echocardiogram**.
- Women with BMI ≥40 kg/m² or ≥35 kg/m² with comorbidities are candidates for **bariatric surgery** in the preconception or interconception period. Incidences of gestational diabetes and hypertension are reduced after gastric bypass surgery, especially if BMI is back to less than obese levels. Pregnant patients with bariatric surgery can be started on **vitamin B12, folate, iron, and calcium if deficient**.
- Obesity is strongly correlated with impaired fertility, miscarriage, congenital malformations, gestational diabetes, hypertension, preeclampsia, stillbirth, cesarean birth, labor abnormalities, macrosomia, anesthesia complications, wound infection, and thromboembolism.
- **Discussion and education about obesity and its comorbidities and poor perinatal outcomes are recommended.**
- Optimal gestational weight gain in the obese remains unclear. Some data **suggest no weight gain or even some weight loss in obese (especially class III obesity) gravidas for optimal obstetric outcomes**.
- **Serial fetal growth ultrasounds should be performed starting at 28 to 32 weeks.**
- **Obese women with a BMI >35 kg/m² should undergo a screening fetal echo between 20 and 24 weeks.**
- **At cesarean, the subcutaneous layer should be closed with sutures if depth is >2 cm, and the subcuticular layer should be closed with suture in order to reduce wound infection and separation.**
- **Early mobilization** after delivery and **graduated compression stockings** during and after cesarean are recommended.
- Postpartum, women should be strongly encouraged and helped to **return to a normal BMI** through **counseling, diet, exercise, and breast-feeding**.

DEFINITION AND CLASSIFICATION

Obesity is defined as **BMI ≥30 kg/m²**, and extreme obesity is defined as BMI ≥40.0 kg/m² (Table 3.1) [1]. Super obesity is a term originally used by bariatric surgeons to describe patients with BMIs of ≥50 kg/m² or more than 225% above ideal body weight [2]. BMI is defined as weight in kilograms divided by height in meters squared. BMI correlates best with body fat mass. It is a simple clinical tool with online calculators available (http://www.nhlbisupport.com/bmi/). Increasing severity of class of obesity in pregnancy is associated with greater risks of adverse perinatal outcomes (Table 3.2) [3–67] and other health risks (Table 3.3) [4]. A waist circumference >88 cm or 35 inches measured at the level of the iliac crest in expiration is an indicator of central obesity that identifies obese women at higher risk for cardiovascular disease and metabolic disorders.

EPIDEMIOLOGY/INCIDENCE

WHO describes **obesity** as "one of the most blatantly visible, yet neglected, public-health problems that threatens to overwhelm both more and less developed countries." As of 2014, the WHO estimates that more than 1.9 billion adults are overweight, including 600 million who are obese [68]. By 2030, more than 2.16 billion people worldwide are projected to be overweight with an additional 1.12 billion people projected to be obese [69,70]. In 2008, obesity-related health care utilization cost an estimated $147 billion. Medical costs for obese patients were $1429 higher than those of normal weight [71]. At all ages and throughout the world, women are generally found to have higher mean BMI and higher rates of obesity than men [72]. These numbers are increasing as the obesity epidemic explodes on the public health stage.

The prevalence of overweight, obese, and extremely obese women aged 20–74 has continued to increase since 1960. As of 2012, the prevalence of obesity and extreme obesity in women was 36.6% and 8.6%, respectively, compared to 15.8% and 1.4% in 1960 [73]. Population data indicates that 50% of women are overweight or obese at the start of pregnancy [74]. The incidence of super obesity is estimated to be 1.8%–2.2% in the obstetric population [2,75,76].

There are racial differences with **non-Hispanic black women** having the highest prevalence of obesity (56.6%) when compared to Hispanic (44.4%), non-Hispanic white (32.8%), and non-Hispanic Asian (11.4%) women [73].

Table 3.1 The International Classification of Adult Underweight, Overweight, and Obesity According to BMI, WHO

Classification	BMI (kg/m²)
Underweight	<18.5
Normal range	18.5–24.9
Overweight	25.0–29.9
Obese	≥30.0
Obese class I	30.0–34.9
Obese class II	35.0–39.9
Obese class III	≥40.0

Source: World Health Organization. *Obesity: Preventing and managing the global epidemic*. Geneva, Switzerland: World Health Organization: 2000. WHO Technical Report Series 894: 1–253, 2000.

GENETICS

A heritability of about 50% to 90% has been shown in adoptive and biological relationships [77]. Role of chromosome 2 p 21 with serum leptin levels in human pregnancies has been identified in some ethnic groups [77]. The risk of childhood obesity is significantly increased if one parent is obese, but the risk is even higher if both parents are affected (adjusted odds ratio [aOR] 10.4, 95% confidence interval [CI] 5.1–21.3) [78]. Many other single mutations in different genes have been identified [79–81]. Maternal obesity results in in utero programming and childhood obesity due to the effects of a maternal high-fat diet leading to insulin resistance, hyperinsulinemia, and increased fat accumulation in the offspring. Additionally, environmental factors, such as diet, play a role in obesity [79].

ETIOLOGY/BASIC PATHOPHYSIOLOGY

White adipose tissue produces proteins with endocrine function called adipokines. A state of relative hypoxia occurs in the adipocytes in obesity, which sets a chronic inflammatory response, causing the release of adipokines. Leptin, adiponectin, resistin, and ghrelin are the most studied adipokines [82].

The name "leptin" is derived from the Greek, which means the "thinning factor." Leptin is a neuroendocrine hormone that acts as a satiety factor, inducing a reduction in food intake and an increase in energy utilization [83]. Leptin is produced by the adipocytes, placenta, and fetal adipose tissue. Endometrium and ovarian follicles also have leptin receptors. Adiponectin is an endogenous insulin sensitizer that is present in lower circulating concentrations in obesity [83].

Maternal leptin levels increase throughout pregnancy from six weeks onward and decrease rapidly after parturition. Conversely, adiponectin levels appear to decrease throughout pregnancy and are especially low in patients with prepregnancy obesity [83]. High levels of serum leptin in pregnancy are similar to that seen in obesity [84]. Leptin appears to be an independent regulator of fetal growth, and leptin levels are a marker for fetal fat mass. The majority of leptin (98%) produced by the placenta is released into maternal circulation. This increased level stimulates increased production of cytokines, such as interleukin-6, interleukin-1, and alpha tumor necrosis factor, that lead to a chronic inflammatory state, further resulting in structural and vascular damage [85,86]. Epigenetic modification in the preimplantation stage, alteration in very early metabolism of the embryo, and endometrial abnormalities seen on biopsy in obese patients could result in low implantation rates, birth defects, and fetal growth aberrations [87].

RISK FACTORS

Older, multiparous women from lower socioeconomic backgrounds, limited resource environments especially for good nutrition, unsafe neighborhoods for unrestricted physical activity, lack of access to medical care, minority status, and family history, all are risk factors for obesity in general and for its associated complications in pregnancy [86].

PREGNANCY COMPLICATIONS

Table 3.2 summarizes the long list of pregnancy complications associated with obesity in pregnancy. **The higher the patient's BMI, the greater the chance of complications.**

Obesity is associated with an **increased risk of congenital anomalies**. Maternal obesity is an independent risk factor for **congenital heart defects** (CHD) with an aOR of 1.16 (95% CI 1.05–1.29), 1.15 (95% CI 1.00–1.32), and 1.31 (95% CI 1.11–1.56) for overweight, obese, and morbidly obese (>35 kg/m²) patients, respectively [34,88]. Prepregnancy BMI >25 kg/m² and increasing levels of obesity are associated with several phenotypes of CHD, such as conotruncal defects, total anomalous pulmonary venous return, hypoplastic left heart syndrome, right ventricular outflow tract defects, and septal defects [34,35]. Maternal obesity (BMI >30 kg/m²) also increases the risk for other congenital anomalies including **neural tube defects** (NTD) (OR 4.08; 95% CI 1.87–7.75), hydrocephaly, orofacial clefts (OR 1.90; 95% CI 1.27–2.86), anal atresia, hypospadias, cystic kidney, talipes, omphalocele, and diaphragmatic hernia [37,89]. Neural tube defects may be due to folate deficiency or local endometrial and placental factors, leading to altered angiogenesis related to leptin or altered carbohydrate metabolism with undetected hyperglycemia. This higher rate of anomalies persists in obese women even after controlling for diabetes.

Excluding women with hypertension, the risk of **preeclampsia** is doubled with each 5 to 7 kg/m² increase in prepregnancy BMI [12]. When compared to a BMI of 21 kg/m², the risk is doubled with a BMI of 26 kg/m² and almost tripled when the BMI is >30 kg/m² [90,91]. Women with class III obesity had a higher incidence of preeclampsia, antepartum stillbirth, cesarean delivery, instrumental delivery, shoulder dystocia, meconium aspiration, fetal distress, early neonatal death, and large babies as compared to normal-weight women [13,90,91].

Increased BMI is a risk factor for **impairment of carbohydrate tolerance**. Fasting and postprandial plasma insulin concentrations are higher in obese pregnant women than in those who are not obese.

Each 1-unit increase in pregravid BMI (5 lb) increases the risk of **cesarean delivery** by about 7% [92]. Success rates of vaginal birth are low in the obese population and infectious morbidity, such as chorioamnionitis, is increased particularly after labor [29,30,93]. Antepartum complications of obesity largely account for this higher cesarean delivery rate as well as macrosomia-associated cephalopelvic disproportion, nonreassuring fetal testing, and failed induction.

Operative risks are also high in obese patients, including **increased total operative time, blood loss, endometritis, and wound disruptions and infections** [94]. **Fetal deaths** are mostly unexplained and are thought to be secondary to placental dysfunction and related comorbidities [40,41]. Suggested pathophysiological mechanisms include placental dysfunction, placental inflammation, impaired glucose tolerance and insulin resistance, and excessive hyperlipidemia.

Table 3.2 Complications of Obesity Related to Pregnancy (see also text) [4–67]

	Risk (%) or OR	Comments	Ref.
Infertility	OR 1.7–2	Smoking is a risk factor in the obese	4–6
Miscarriage rates	OR 1.31		4, 7, 8, 50
Recurrent miscarriage	OR 1.71		50
Prenatal/medical			
Chronic hypertension	OR 2–3		4, 9, 10
Gestational hypertension	OR 2.5–3.2		11, 51
Preeclampsia	OR 1.44–14.14	Risk increases with increasing class of obesity	8, 11–15, 51–54
Gestational diabetes	OR 1.4–20		4, 9, 16, 17, 51
Venous thromboembolism	OR 1.30–2.65		4, 55, 56
Obstructive sleep apnea	OR 1.12		18–21
Respiratory issues (e.g., asthma exacerbations)	OR 1.3		22
Depression	OR 1.12	OR 4.9 class III	23, 24
Urinary tract infections	OR 1.4		5
Obstetric			
Spontaneous pregnancy loss	OR 1.7		7, 16
Indicated preterm birth	OR 1.3	Includes overweight	25
Spontaneous preterm birth	OR 1.24		25
Lower accuracy of ultrasound	25%–48% detection Residual anomaly risk after ultrasound in obese 1%	Progressively worse with increasing BMI	26
Difficulty with fetal testing (e.g., FH monitoring)		No definite recommendation for invasive monitoring	27
Failure to progress	OR 2.6	Class II	28
Induction of labor	OR 2.2		9, 14
Fetal distress	OR 1.3	Class II (BMI >35)	28
Lower success of TOLAC	OR 0.53–2.0	Excessive weight gain lowers success—Class III	29, 30
Rupture/dehiscence after TOLAC	OR 5.6		30
Post-term birth (less likely to go into spontaneous labor)	OR 1.7		31
Lower rates of breast-feeding (Failure to start and sustain)	OR 2.6	Class III	5
Late prenatal care	OR 1.56		9
Fetus/neonate			
Congenital fetal defects			
NTD	OR 1.7–2.8	OR 3–4 class II–III	32, 33, 57
CHD	OR 1.3–1.5		33–37
Cleft lip/palate	OR 1.2–1.9		33, 37
Anorectal atresia	OR 1.5		33, 37
Hydrocephalus	OR 1.7		37
Limb reduction defects	OR 1.3		33
Down syndrome	1.12–1.56		58
IUGR	2.1		59
Gastroschisis	OR 0.17	Reduced risk in the obese	33
Macrosomia (>4000 g)	OR 1.7–2.36		5, 9, 10, 38, 39
Birth injury, shoulder dystocia	OR 1.51–3.1	Associated most with macrosomia	13, 39, 61
Low Apgar scores	OR 1.4–13.4		5, 52, 62
Fetal death	OR 2.0–3.6		13, 40, 41–43
Neonatal mortality	OR 1.15–1.3	OR 3.4 class III	13, 33, 63
Childhood obesity BMI >95th percentile and metabolic syndrome	OR 1.62–2.2	Increases with increasing levels of obesity and GWG	5, 64
NICU admission	OR 1.28–1.34		9, 10, 61
Intrapartum			
Earlier admission			
Longer labor	7 hours (obese) vs. 5.4 hours (normal)	Slow labor to 7 cm	44
Anesthesia complications	8.4% composite morbidity	6/8 maternal deaths were in obese gravida	45–47
Difficult regional anesthesia placement	OR 19.4		48
Difficult intubations (general anesthesia)	OR 2.1		48

(Continued)

Table 3.2 (Continued) Complications of Obesity Related to Pregnancy (see also text) [4–67]

	Risk (%) or OR	Comments	Ref.
Need for cesarean delivery	OR 1.46–3.0	47% in class II–III (especially failure to progress)	11, 51–53, 60, 61, 65
Increase operative time >60 minutes;	OR 9.3		13, 46, 48
Emergency cesarean	OR 4.7		48
Wound infections/disruptions	OR 2.24–3.4		9, 66
Hemorrhage	OR 5.2	Morbid obesity >300 lb	48
Postpartum hemorrhage	OR 1.4–2.11		9, 44, 67
Longer hospitalization	OR 1.48		9
ICU admissions	OR 3.8	BMI >50	15
Hormonal contraceptive failure	OR 1.91	BMI >25; limited studies, may still be the best if used properly	49

Abbreviations: BMI, body mass index; CHD, congenital heart disease; GWG, gestational weight gain; NTD, neural tube defect; OR, odds ratio; TOLAC, trial of labor after cesarean.

Table 3.3 Health Risks Associated with Obesity

• Premature death	• Cancer
• Type 2 diabetes	• High cholesterol
• Metabolic syndrome	• Hirsutism
• Heart disease	• Stress incontinence
• Stroke	• Surgical risk
• Hypertension	• Osteoarthritis
• Gallbladder disease	• Asthma
• Sleep apnea	• Social stigma
• Depression	

Source: U.S. Department of Health and Human Services. *The Surgeon General's Call to Action to Prevent and Decrease Overweight and Obesity.* Rockville, MD: U.S. Department of Health and Human Services, Public Health Service, Office of the Surgeon General, 2001.

Prepregnancy obesity and excessive gestational weight gain are associated with **indicated preterm birth**, and obesity seems to protect against spontaneous preterm birth [25,31,95–100]. Nulligravid obese women are likely at greater risk than the multiparous women.

Obstructive sleep apnea (OSA) has a higher incidence in obese women, especially with neck circumference >38 cm. OSA has been associated with preeclampsia, gestational diabetes, and pulmonary hypertension [101–103]. It is also associated with fetal heart rate decelerations during periods of maternal hypoxia. Lower Apgar scores, low birth weight, and increased admission to neonatal intensive care units are seen in infants of obese women with OSA [102,104]. OSA may complicate anesthesia and postoperative care [18–20]. Continuous positive airway pressure (CPAP) has been shown to improve blood pressure control in pregnant women with chronic hypertension [105].

Prepregnancy obesity is an independent risk factor for large for gestational age (LGA) fetuses and **macrosomia** and is correlated with increasing categories of obesity and gestational weight gain. Maternal excess weight with BMI >25 kg/m² before pregnancy has been shown to be a determinant of fetal macrosomia (OR 2.0; 95% CI 1.72, 2.32) [106]. Macrosomic fetuses are at high risk for childhood obesity and adult metabolic syndrome. Excessive weight gain during pregnancy can increase the risk of macrosomia by 30%. The incidence of shoulder dystocia remains undefined with some reporting a higher incidence and others no difference in the obese population versus the nonobese. Shoulder dystocia is associated with birth weight rather than increasing levels of obesity [38,39].

Obesity is associated with **greater health care usage** with more prenatal visits with physicians, fetal testing, obstetrical ultrasound, medications, telephone calls, longer length of stay, increased cesarean deliveries, and medical conditions associated with obesity [69]. It is estimated that 5.7% of the total U.S. health expenditure is from obesity-related illness [70].

Close to 300,000 deaths annually are attributed to a diagnosis of obesity [2]. About 24% deaths in adult women aged 25 to 64 years are due to obesity [71].

PRECONCEPTION CARE/PREVENTION
Preconception Evaluation

The preconception visit may be the single most important health care visit when viewed in the context of its effect on pregnancy (Chapter 1 of *Obstetric Evidence Based Guidelines*). Height in meters and weight in kilograms should be recorded for all women at each doctor visit to allow for calculation of BMI (http://www.nhlbisupport.com/bmi) (Figure 3.1). Identification and awareness by both patient and health care worker of obesity is the first step in prevention of complications and appropriate management. The BMI category should be reviewed with the patient, making sure she understands that her category is not normal (Table 3.1).

Once obesity is confirmed, a **waist circumference** can be measured at the end of expiration at the level of the iliac crest. This, as well as the exact BMI, should be documented. A risk assessment of cardiovascular disease by taking **BP with a large cuff**, dyslipidemia by obtaining a **fasting lipid profile** and diabetes evaluation with a **fasting blood sugar**, thyroid disease with **thyroid function tests**, and OSA requiring a standard **overnight polysomnogram** should be initiated. In obese patients with chronic hypertension or type 2 diabetes, it is advisable to obtain an **EKG** and an **echocardiogram** [107]. Obese women are more likely to experience congestive heart failure and cardiomyopathy. Family history should be elicited. History of weight cycling is important and indicates poor compliance and may be associated with an increased risk of comorbidities.

Discussion and education about obesity and its comorbidities and poor perinatal outcomes should be provided (e.g., give a copy of Tables 3.2 and 3.3). An assessment should be made to see if the patient is ready for intervention with diet and exercise. **Motivational interviewing** is defined as a "directive, client-centered counseling style for eliciting behavior change by helping clients explore and resolve ambivalence" (Table 3.4) [108,109].

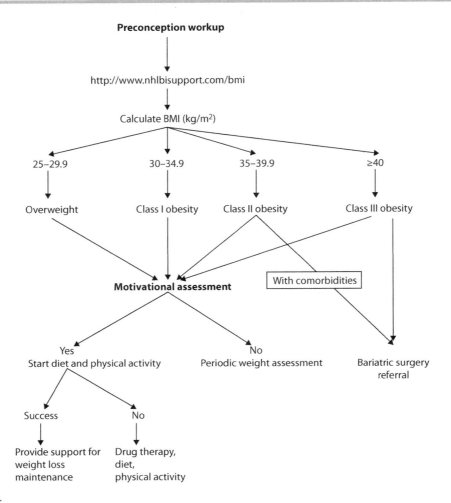

Figure 3.1   Algorithm.

Table 3.4   Stages of Change Model to Assess Readiness for Weight Loss

Stage	Characteristic	Appropriate Intervention	Sample Dialogue
Precontemplation	Unaware of problem, no interest in change	Provide information about health risks and benefit of weight loss	"Would you like to read some information about the health aspects of obesity?"
Contemplation	Aware of problem, beginning to think of changing	Help resolve ambivalence; discuss barriers	"Let's look at the benefits of weight loss as well as what you may need to change."
Preparation	Realizes benefits of making changes and thinking about how to change	Teach behavior modification; provide education	"Let's take a closer look at how you can reduce some of the calories you eat and how to increase your activity during the day."
Action	Actively taking steps toward change	Provide support and guidance with a focus on the long term	"It's terrific that you are working so hard. What problems have you had? How have you solved them?"
Maintenance	Initial treatment goals reached	Relapse control	"What situations continue to tempt you to overeat? What can be helpful for the next time you face the situation?"

Source: Modified from ACOG Committee Opinion No. 319 and from American Medical Association—Roadmaps for Clinical Practice series: Assessment and management of adult obesity. Available at http://www.ama-assn.org/ama/pub/category/10931.html.

Women with increased BMI are known to have a three-fold greater risk of infertility due to disturbances in the hypothalamic-pituitary axis, menstrual cycle alterations, and anovulation [110]. An abnormal BMI is associated with significantly reduced live-birth rate and increased miscarriage rate after IVF treatment [110]. Fertilization rates and clinical pregnancy rates are reported to be lower in obese women [111].

The most effective intervention in the adult obese population is diet, physical activity, and behavior modification (http://www.nhlbi.nih.gov/guidelines/obesity/ob_home .htm). **The most important interventions in the management of obesity in reproductive-age women are weight reduction prior to conception and prevention of excessive gestational weight gain** (Table 3.5) [38,112].

Table 3.5 Suggested Management of the Obese Gravida

Preconception
Calculate and record BMI and category
Review history and comorbidities
Counseling of pregnancy complications (show, review, and give a copy of Table 3.2)
Counseling of medical long-term complications (show, review, and give a copy of Table 3.3)
Glucose screen with 2-hour glucose tolerance test or hemoglobin A1c
Consider lipid screening
Counsel and plan regarding weight loss and exercise before considering pregnancy—behavior modification
Nutrition counseling
Exercise counseling
Document blood pressure
Baseline 24-hour urine for proteinuria; LFTs, platelets
Evaluation for possible long-term complications
(especially if BMI >35)
   Echocardiogram
   EKG
   Sleep apnea evaluation
Consider referral to bariatric surgery program

Pregnancy
First trimester
   All recommendations as **Preconception** except weight loss
   Confirm pregnancy with first-trimester ultrasound for dating
   Nuchal translucency and serum screening for chromosomal abnormalities
   Early 1-hour glucose screen
   Review weight gain goals (Table 3.7) and address throughout prenatal care
Second/third trimester
   Counsel regarding limitations of fetal ultrasound
   Fetal echocardiogram, if pregestational diabetes or BMI >35
   Consider fetal growth ultrasound in third trimester (e.g., 32 weeks)
   Repeat as needed if suspected macrosomia
   Repeat 1-hour glucose screen if negative in first trimester
   Begin antepartum testing ≥32 weeks
   Anesthesia consult in third trimester

Intrapartum
Secure early venous access
Ultrasound to confirm fetal presentation
Early placement of regional anesthesia with extra-long spinal/epidural needles and fiberoptic bronchoscope
Cross for appropriate blood products
Consider AROM and IUPC to assess contractions
Early application of FSE if unable to evaluate FHT externally
Large blood pressure cuff
Large speculums
OR tables that accommodate ≥160 kg (standard OR tables support 130–160 kg)
Lithotomy stirrups with capacity of 230 kg (i.e., Yellofins® Stirrups and Yellofins Elite®, respectively, Allen Medical Systems, Acton, MA, USA)
Long instrument tray
   Closure of subcutaneous fat ≥2 cm with sutures during cesarean
   Closure of subcuticular layer with stitches
   Appropriately sized graduated compression stockings
   Extra staffing to assist with patient transfer
   Labor beds and stretchers rated for morbidly obese patients
   Bariatric wheelchairs

Postpartum
Incentive spirometry
Graduated compression stockings and prophylactic heparin until ambulation
Early mobilization and hydration
Compression boots and/or prophylactic heparin during prolonged bed rest
75-mg, 2-hour glucose challenge test >6 weeks postpartum
Referral to nutritional and behavioral counselors for weight loss
Contraceptive counseling
Encourage breast-feeding
Establish a plan for postpartum weight loss

Source: Di Lillo M, Hendrix N, O'Neill M et al. *Cont Obstet Gynecol*, 11, 48–53, 2008.
Note: Routine screening offered to all pregnant women (e.g., sequential screening) not included.
Abbreviations: AROM, artificial rupture of membranes; BMI, body mass index; DM, diabetes mellitus; FHT, fetal heart tracing; FSE, fetal scalp electrode; IUPC, intrauterine pressure catheter; LFT, liver function test.

Prepregnancy Weight Reduction

Diet

Use of a low-calorie diet that creates a deficit of 500 to 1000 kcal/day will cause a weight loss of 1 to 2 lb/week and a 10% weight loss over six months [108]. There is good evidence that such a weight loss can be sustained over long periods of time, at least one year. This level of weight loss will improve the BP, lipid profile, and blood glucose levels. Patients can be referred to a nutritionist or can visit websites such as http://www.mypyramid.gov.

Physical Activity

Exercise contributes only modestly to weight loss, but it may decrease visceral fat; it increases cardiorespiratory fitness and helps with all weight loss maintenance programs. **Moderate exercise for 30 to 45 minutes for at least three to five days initially and followed by accumulation of at least 30 minutes daily on most days** should be an integral part of weight loss and weight maintenance [108].

Behavior Therapy

Specific strategies include self-monitoring of eating habits and physical activity, stress management, stimulus control, problem solving, contingency management, cognitive restructuring, and social support [108].

Pharmacotherapy

Weight loss drugs should only be used when concomitant lifestyle modifications have not obtained sufficient results. Orlistat (Xenical) and Chitosin are two drugs currently marketed for weight loss with questionable efficacy [113–115]. Indications for use are BMI >30 kg/m² or BMI >27 kg/m² with comorbidities despite maximal efforts at diet, exercise, and behavior therapy. Weight loss produced by antiobesity drugs has not been shown to be any better than weight loss through lifestyle modification in reducing related comorbidities. However, **weight loss pharmacotherapy is contraindicated in pregnancy.**

Bariatric Surgery

Women with BMI >40 kg/m² or BMI >35 kg/m² with comorbidities are candidates for bariatric surgery when diet, physical activity, and behavior modification (and possible drug therapy) have failed (Table 3.6). The weight loss following surgery is in the range of 10 to 105 kg and is sustained for as long as eight years. Approximately 80% of bariatric surgery recipients are of reproductive age [116].

Bariatric surgery procedures are generally categorized into **three groups: 1) restrictive procedures, 2) malabsorptive procedures, and 3) restrictive and malabsorptive procedures.** Restrictive procedures (e.g., laparoscopic adjustable gastric banging [LAGB], sleeve gastrectomy) reduce gastric capacity, which consequently restricts energy intake [117–119]. Malabsorptive procedures (e.g., biliopancreatic diversion, jejunoileal bypass) cause weight loss by restricting absorption of nutrients; however, these procedures are rarely performed as they have been associated with long-term complications such as hepatic failure [120,121]. Last, malabsorptive and restrictive procedures (e.g., Roux-en-Y gastric bypass) reduce stomach capacity causing malabsorption and a restriction of food intake. Intragastric balloon appears to have little benefit in weight loss therapy over diet, behavior modification, and

Table 3.6 Special Considerations for Preconception and Prenatal Care after Bariatric Surgery

Preconception
- Fertility often resumes after bariatric surgery
- Bariatric surgery should not be considered a treatment for infertility
- Oral contraception is often ineffective because of potential malabsorption; consider injectable forms of hormonal contraception as needed. Use reliable contraception until period of maximal weight loss (at least 12 months) is over
- Consider waiting 12 months or more after bariatric surgery before conception
- Evaluate and treat comorbidities

Prenatal
- Monitor for nutritional deficiencies (especially after Roux-en-Y) such as
  - Vitamin B12 (if needed, 500–1000 µg daily)
  - Folate (up to 5 mg daily)
  - Iron (check ferritin; if needed, ferrous fumarate)
  - Vitamin D (if needed, do not exceed pregnancy RDA of 400 IU maximum)
  - Calcium (if needed, 1200 mg calcium citrate)
- Be aware that nausea, vomiting, abdominal pain, etc., may be signs of bariatric surgery complications, such as intestinal obstruction, GI hemorrhage, anastomic leaks, hernias, band erosions and migrations, and even maternal death. Early consultation with bariatric surgeon is suggested.
- Avoid glucola screening given risk of dumping syndrome. Use fasting and 2-hour postprandial blood sugar monitoring as an alternative.
- If BMI is still 30 kg/m², risks remain as in Tables 3.2 and 3.3, and management in general as in Table 3.5.
- Bariatric surgery is not an indication for cesarean delivery.

motivation [122]. Adjustable gastric band management during pregnancy is not well defined, but almost 20% may need adjustment or removal of band for nausea and vomiting [123].

A weight maintenance program consisting of diet, physical activity, and behavior therapy should be a priority after the initial 6 to 12 months of weight loss therapy. Lifelong medical surveillance after surgical therapy is a necessity. Almost 20% of patients who undergo bariatric surgery experience some complication although they are usually minor, and the postoperative mortality is <1%. There is a 5% failure rate from use of OCP following bariatric surgery [124]. After the surgical procedure, there is typically a rapid weight loss in the first 6–18 months [125]. Thus, pregnancy during this period may be complicated by nutritional deficiencies that could be detrimental to the growing fetus [126–129]. Patients should be advised to **delay pregnancy for at least 12 months** [16,130]. There is little evidence to support the duration of delay for conception with regard to birth weight, cesarean delivery, or congenital malformation. Weight loss usually plateaus after 12 to 18 months.

Prognosis for a future pregnancy depends mostly on the BMI that has been attained. There is a **significant decrease in incidence of gestational diabetes** (OR 0.31; 95% CI 0.15–0.65), **hypertensive disorders** (OR 0.42; 95% CI 0.23–0.78), **and macrosomia** (OR 0.40; 95% CI 0.24–0.67) **following bariatric surgery,** especially for women capable of starting the pregnancy with a BMI <30 kg/m² compared to before bariatric surgery or to obese (often morbidly) women who have not had bariatric surgery [117,123,130–133]. Often the studies are not matched for BMI, a major shortcoming.

Nutritional supplementation should be recommended because there is good evidence of increased incidences of maternal and neonatal deficiencies of **vitamin B12, vitamin D, iron, and calcium** in women post bariatric surgery [134] (Table 3.6). Preconception issues mentioned above should be reviewed, including an increased likelihood of small-for-gestational age newborns among bariatric surgery recipients (OR 2.16; 95% CI 1.28–3.66) [117,131,132] as well as possible increased risk of stillbirth or neonatal death [131] (Table 3.6). Patients with bariatric surgery should be started on **vitamin B12, folate, iron, and calcium if deficient** [130]. **Vitamin D supplement 10 mg daily** during pregnancy and breast-feeding can be recommended as per the Royal College of Obstetricians and Gynaecologists (RCOG) guidelines [135]. A bariatric surgeon should be involved during prenatal care should the gastric band need some adjustments. Seemingly insignificant or normal prenatal complaints warrant attention as patients who have had bariatric surgery are at risk for postoperative complications. During pregnancy, patients who present with signs and symptoms of intestinal obstruction, perforation, or hemorrhage should have a CT scan done to establish diagnosis because this can be associated with 20% maternal mortality.

Folic Acid Supplementation and Other Necessary Vitamins

Proper general preconception care should be provided (Chapter 1 of *Obstetric Evidence Based Guidelines*). Because almost 50% of pregnancies are unplanned, all patients capable of childbearing should be placed on folic acid 0.4 to 0.8 mg (400–800 µg) supplementation at least one month before conception and continue daily supplements through the first two to three months of pregnancy [136]. Folate levels have been noted to be low in the obese population [137]. Although obesity is considered a risk factor for a NTD, the folic acid supplementation in the United States has remained the same [136]. However, both the RCOG [135] and the Society of Obstetricians and Gynaecologists of Canada (SOGC) [27] have **recommended a dose of 5 mg daily** for the obese population (**BMI >35 kg/m²**) starting from one to three months preconception through the first trimester. The use of periconception multivitamins has not been associated with reduction of the increased risk of CHD in the overweight and obese population [13]. Drug history should be reviewed to identify any potential teratogens.

PRENATAL CARE

Preconception management, except for large weight loss, should be followed (Table 3.5) [112,138].

Ideal Weight Gain

There is lots of evidence to make recommendations regarding weight changes in the obese gravida. One should remember that the total weight of an average fetus, placenta, and amniotic fluid at term is about 4 to 5 kg. In the last 20 years, both the Institute of Medicine (IOM) and American College of Obstetricians and Gynecologists (ACOG) have suggested 5 to 9 kg (11–20 lb) as total weight gain in pregnancy for obese women [139]. This suggestion does not account for differences in class of obesity. Significant weight loss during pregnancy is not recommended by ACOG and IOM.

More recent data suggest that lower weight gain in the obese gravida is associated with maternal and fetal benefits [38,140–144]. **For obese women, weight gain has no benefit. The lowest risks for mother and baby seem to occur with weight gain of 0 to 9 lb for class II obese women (or even some minimal weight loss), and weight loss of 0 to 9 lb for class III obese women** [14,28,140,142,145]. On the basis of these data, new guidelines should be considered for obese women (Table 3.7).

Nutritional consult may be sought to prevent excessive gestational weight gain. Charts to outline the patient's progress should be a permanent part of the prenatal record. Excessive weight retention self-perpetuates the obesity cycle for subsequent pregnancies [38]. Almost three fourths of all women will weigh more at a subsequent pregnancy [146]. Excessive gestational weight gain is associated with childhood obesity [147].

Diet

A balanced diet, rich in high fiber and complex carbohydrates with low glycemic intake, is suggested. **Up to 5 mg of folic acid** should be continued from the prepregnancy period until at least 10 weeks gestation [27,135]. Education about weight gain, healthy eating, and exercise decreases the percentage of women who exceed weight gain recommendations [148]. The evidence for antenatal dietary and lifestyle interventions in overweight and obese pregnant women to decrease complications is still insufficient to make recommendations [149].

Exercise

Physical activity during pregnancy is successful in restricting gestational weight gain [150]. Physical activity intervention assessed by pedometer is associated with lower gestational weight gain compared to controls [151]. Physical activity should be encouraged as per ACOG recommendations [152]. During pregnancy, women can be encouraged to maintain an active lifestyle as long as there are no risks to the pregnancy. Class III obesity is considered a relative contraindication to aerobic exercise during pregnancy [152].

Table 3.7 Weight Gain Suggestions for Overweight and Obese Women

Prepregnancy Weight Category	Our Suggested Total Weight Gain Range (Lb)	IOM Recommendations (lb)
Overweight (BMI 25–29.9 kg/m²)	6–20 (2.7–9.0 kg)	15–25 (6.8–11.4 kg)
Class I Obesity (BMI 30–34.9 kg/m²)	5–15 (2.3–6.8 kg)	11–20 (5–9.1 kg)
Class II Obesity (BMI 35–39.9 kg/m²)	−9 to 9 (−4.0 to 4.0 kg)	11–20 (5–9.1 kg)
Class III Obesity (BMI >40 kg/m²)	−15 to 0 (−6.8 to 0 kg)	11–20 (5–9.1 kg)

Sources: Bianco AT, Smilen SW, Davis Y et al. *Obstet Gynecol*, 91, 97–102, 1998; Siega-Riz AM, Viswanathan M, Moos MK et al. *Am J Obstet Gynecol*, 201, 4, 339.e1–14, 2009; Livingston EH. *Am J Surg*, 184, 2, 103–13, 2002; Fernandes MAP, Atallah AN, Soares BG et al. *Cochrane Database Syst Rev*, 1, CD004931, 2007; Maggard M, Li Z, Yermilov I et al. *Evid Rep Technol Assess (Full Rep)*, 169, 1–51, 2008; Robinson JA, Burke AE. *Women's Health (London, England)*, 9, 5, 453–66, 2013; Wax J, Cartin A, Wolff R et al. *Obes Surg*, 18, 12, 1517–21, 2008.

General Issues

Diabetic screening should be done at the first visit. If this is negative, it should be repeated at 24 to 28 weeks [153]. Baseline data to evaluate renal function and liver status, such as liver function tests **(LFTs), 24-hour urine for protein and creatinine clearance** can be obtained. Reassessment of risk and the need for **EKG and echocardiogram** can be made. Excess weight has an effect on biochemical serum aneuploidy screening, so adjustment has to be made according to maternal weight to achieve similar detection rates as in other women.

Equipment in the office or clinic to accommodate the needs of this population, such as wide chairs, sit-on weighing scales, tables, and large BP cuffs, should be available. The professional team should undertake a discussion of pregnancy and maternal and fetal outcomes. Educational materials should be provided. Pharmacotherapy for obesity is contraindicated in pregnancy. Although the RCOG recommends more frequent prenatal visits every 3 weeks from 24 to 32 weeks and then every 2 weeks until delivery, there is insufficient level I data to make this an evidence-based recommendation [154].

Fetal Ultrasound

Gestational age should be established with early (e.g., **first trimester** is optimal) **ultrasound** (Chapter 4 of *Obstetric Evidence Based Guidelines*).

Data from the FaSTER trial found that the ability to obtain a nuchal translucency (NT) is significantly decreased with increasing BMI. In women with Class II obesity, the failure rate for NT is 7.8% compared to 1.0% in normal weight gravida [155]. Multiple techniques can be used by the ultrasonographer to improve visualization, including changing ultrasound probes to improve resolution and penetration, adjusting the tissue harmonics index and frequency, increasing the gain, elevating the patient's pannus, placing the patient on their side, or scanning through the umbilicus [156].

A detailed fetal survey is recommended between 20 and 24 weeks to rule out any fetal anomalies. Ultrasound detection of fetal abnormalities is limited in obese women because of the increased depth of abdominal adipose tissue and increased angle of insonation [157–159]. This leads to **lower prenatal detection of fetal anomalies** via ultrasonography (aOR 0.77; 95% CI 0.60–0.99) [33,160]. For normal BMI; overweight; and class I, II, and III obesity, detection with standard ultrasonography was 66%, 49%, 48%, 42%, and 25%, respectively, and with targeted ultrasonography 97%, 91%, 75%, 88%, and 75%, respectively [26]. Obese gravida should also be counseled that the ultrasound duration will be longer with a high likelihood of having to return for repeat ultrasounds [155]. Women with a **BMI >35 kg/m² should undergo a screening fetal echo between 20 and 24 weeks**.

Because obese gravidas are at an increased risk for LGA infants, and fetal growth is difficult to assess clinically, **ultrasounds are recommended every 4 weeks from 28 to 36 weeks to assess fetal growth and amniotic fluid** [161].

Antepartum Fetal Testing

There is insufficient evidence that fetal heart rate testing would benefit the perinatal outcomes in the obese population; however, because the risk of fetal demise is high, antepartum testing may be considered. Fetal kick counts are also encouraged.

INTRAPARTUM CARE

A multidisciplinary approach to the intrapartum management of an obese gravida should be undertaken. The RCOG recommends that women with a prepregnancy BMI of ≥30 kg/m² have an informed and clearly documented **discussion about the possible complications** that can occur as a result of obesity [162]. The hospital facility should be notified so that appropriate equipment, pneumatic compression devices, beds, transfer equipment, hoists, wide corridors, and stretchers are available. Early venous access is suggested. The obese gravida is at an **increased risk for induction of labor** (26.2% in normal weight and 34.4% in obese women), **failed induction** (13% in normal weight vs. 29% in obese women), **prolonged first stage of labor** (up to 5 hour difference while second stage length is not dependent on BMI), **greater oxytocin requirements, operative vaginal deliveries, failed anesthesia, and postpartum hemorrhage** (two- to threefold increase) [67,163–171].

There may be **limitations to monitoring uterine contractions and fetal heart rate** in labor. Invasive tocomonitoring may become necessary if there are no other contraindications. Active management of the third stage would help reduce the incidence of postpartum hemorrhage.

For the neonate, there is an **increased risk of shoulder dystocia** (two- to threefold increase), **malpresentation, lower Apgar scores, and greater risk of NICU admission** [27,172].

Vaginal birth after cesarean (VBAC) section rates are also lower in obese women with a failure rate of 45% compared to 30% in nonobese gravida with a greater risk of uterine rupture [30,173].

A planned cesarean section in the morbidly obese does not decrease maternal or neonatal morbidity and is not recommended [174]. A **scheduled cesarean at 39 weeks**, however, **should be planned if the estimated fetal weight is >4500 g in a diabetic patient and >5000 g in a nondiabetic obese patient** [16].

ANESTHESIA

If an anesthesia consult was not obtained antepartum, then it should be obtained early in labor. Regional anesthesia is the anesthetic of choice. **A combined spinal epidural is preferred.** Distorted anatomic landmarks, difficult maternal positioning, and excessive layers of adipose tissue make regional anesthesia more challenging. Obesity is associated with increased regional anesthesia failure rates, higher incidences of dural puncture, and greater need for general anesthesia [175]. **More attempts at placement of epidural or spinal anesthesia** have to be made in the obese population as compared to the nonobese. The initial failure rate of epidural catheter placement can be as high as 42% in the morbidly obese. Obese women can be a challenge because of related OSA and asthma. Positioning and placement of the panniculus can impair respiratory function [45]. In a morbidly obese patient (BMI >40 kg/m²) undergoing a planned cesarean delivery, the overall conductive anesthesia complication rate is about 8%. General anesthesia in the obese pregnant woman also poses its own challenges including difficult endotracheal intubation due to excessive tissue and edema and intraoperative respiratory events from failed or difficult intubation [176]. **General anesthesia** is used more frequently in morbidly obese patients and intraoperative hypotension can be a problem [46]. Of about 1% maternal deaths that were anesthesia related, 75% were noted to be obese [47]. The incidence of partially obliterated oropharyngeal anatomy among obese parturients is double that among nonobese parturients. This leads to an increased risk of **difficult intubations, gastric aspiration, and difficulty in maintaining adequate mask ventilation** [45]. Mask ventilation tends to be difficult because of low chest wall compliance and increased intra-abdominal pressure. The anesthesiologist should have long epidural needles and equipment such as a laryngeal mask ventilation or ultrasound available for these challenging cases [16,177].

Cesarean Delivery

Obesity is a risk factor for complications from cesarean section. As BMI increases, the time from incision to delivery and total operative time (43 vs. 48 and 55 minutes in normal weight, obese, and morbidly obese, respectively, $p < 0.001$) also increases. **Increased operative time** leads to worse outcomes [66,178]. **Wound complications** (separation and infection) are as high as 30% in obese women compared to a 3%–17% overall population risk with the vast majority occurring 8–10 days post cesarean section [179]. Tissue oxygenation is poor in the obese population. Increased oxygen supplementation perioperatively may enhance wound healing, as per non-pregnancy data, but there is insufficient evidence to recommend it in the obese obstetric population [180–183]. (See also Chapter 13 in *Obstetric Evidence Based Guidelines*.)

Surgical techniques that have been proven to reduce wound infection and separation include **closure of the subcutaneous layer with suture if the depth is >2 cm and subcuticular closure with suture over staples** [184–186]. A more controversial recommendation includes placement of the skin incision either vertically or transverse although the literature states that a **transverse skin incision is likely preferred and associated with less morbidity** [179,187–190]. This decision should be individualized as this may differ depending on the category and type (e.g., central) of obesity. **Placing the incision above the panniculus, which at times means above the umbilicus, may be necessary in the woman with extreme obesity** [185].

Prophylactic antibiotics should be administered (e.g., with cefazolin 2 g IV) at least 30 minutes prior to the skin incision. Some studies suggest that 4 g of IV cefazolin leads to higher tissue concentrations than 2 g, which may result in decreased surgical site infections and endometritis [191–193]. A recently published double-blind RCT demonstrated that although 3 g of cefazolin administered preoperatively results in significantly higher adipose tissue concentrations at the time of hysterotomy and fascial closure and greater umbilical cord blood concentrations compared to 2 g, both doses achieved sufficient adipose tissue concentrations to provide prophylaxis against Gram-positive and Gram-negative bacteria [194]. Other recent studies have produced conflicting data in regards to reaching adequate adipose tissue concentrations with higher doses of prophylactic cefazolin (2 g vs. 3 g) in obese women [195,196]. **Further studies are needed to evaluate alterations in maternal dosing before changing the currently recommended dose of 2 g.**

POSTPARTUM
Venous Thromboembolism

Obese women have an up to fourfold increased risk of venous thromboembolism compared to normal-weight women [197].

Because of this increased risk, ACOG recommends early mobilization and placement of **pneumatic compression devices before surgery in all cases of anticipated prolonged labor and then continued until ambulation is established postpartum** [16,198,199]. More recently, non-RCT evidence supports the use of **pharmacologic thromboprophylaxis for seven days postpartum in obese women with additional risk factors for thromboembolism (age >35, weight >80 kg, ≥para 4, preeclampsia, immobility >4 days prior to surgery, major illness, emergency cesarean section, current infection, antiphospholipid syndrome, prior thromboembolic event, or family history of thromboembolism) or in all women who are morbidly obese (BMI >40 kg/m²)** [200–202]. One study suggests that weight-based dosing of low-dose heparin, e.g., enoxaparin (0.5 mg/kg SQ every 12 hours) to be better than traditional prophylactic dosing (40 mg SQ daily); however, this has not been sufficiently studied [203]. Women who meet criteria for pharmacologic prophylaxis should at the very least be started on enoxaparin (lovenox) 40 mg SQ daily for 1 week postpartum although weight-based dosing is also acceptable.

Other Complications

In the postpartum period, obese women are also at a greater risk of requiring longer hospital stays, resulting in increased medical costs, maternal ICU admissions (OR 3.50; 95% CI 2.72–4.51), wound infections (OR 3.4; 95% CI 1.4–1.8), postpartum endometritis, emergency department visits (aOR 2.2; 95% CI 1.03–4.9), and maternal death (OR 2.9; 95% CI 1.1–8.1) [15,66,166,177,204]. Specifically, one study found that for every 9091 obese pregnant patients, one patient will experience death at delivery hospitalization. About 24% of deaths in adult women aged 25 to 64 years are due to obesity [205]. Because of these increased postpartum risks, special care should be given to the postpartum obese patient by experienced physicians and nursing staff.

Psychological Implications: Compared to normal-weight women, obese gravida are at an increased risk of depression during pregnancy and postpartum (OR 1.43; 95% CI 1.27–1.61 and OR 1.30; 95% CI 1.20–1.42, respectively). They are also at an increased risk for anxiety (OR 1.68; 95% CI 1.34–2.12) [206]. Eating disorders and arthritic pain together with psychosocial factors (e.g., social stigmatization) could account for this increase [23]. The patient should be provided with resources for counseling and social work prior to discharge home with consideration to have them return sooner than the routine six-week postpartum visit.

Breast-Feeding

Women should be strongly encouraged and helped to **return to a normal BMI** through **counseling, diet, exercise, and breast-feeding**. Breast-feeding is encouraged because it benefits both the mother and infant. In particular, it helps accelerate the return to prepregnancy weight and decreases the risk of chronic diseases such as type 2 diabetes and breast and ovarian cancer. For the infant, breast-feeding reduces the risk of obesity [207,208].

Obese women are less likely to initiate breast-feeding or exclusively breast-feed compared to normal-weight women. In order to increase the rates of breast-feeding, obese women would benefit from consultation with a lactation specialist [209].

CONTRACEPTION

The contraceptive **intrauterine device (IUD), implant**, ring, depot medroxyprogesterone acetate injectable contraception, and the progestin-only contraceptive pill appear to be as effective in obese and nonobese women and should be encouraged for postpartum use. Some studies indicate that **oral hormonal contraception may not be as effective as in the nonobese** [49,210]. Oral contraceptives may also not be as effective in women who undergo bariatric surgery because of the malabsorptive effects. Pregnancy rates are high after weight loss surgery; therefore, effective contraception should be discussed prior to the procedure [211]. Additionally, **body weight >90 kg is a risk factor for failure of the contraceptive patch and should thus not be offered** [212].

LONG-TERM MATERNAL AND OFFSPRING RISKS

Obesity during pregnancy is an independent risk factor for long-term **cardiovascular morbidity** (aHR 2.6; 95% CI 2.0–3.4), specifically ischemic stroke (aHR 2.63; 95% CI 1.41–1.91) and myocardial infarction (aHR 1.89; 95% CI 1.25–2.84). So too, there is a greater risk of **all-cause mortality** in obese women (HR 1.35; 95% CI 1.02–1.77) compared to women of normal pregnancy BMI [213–216].

    Offspring of obese mothers are at increased risk for significant health conditions later in life as a result of in utero programming, which may work through environmental, genetic, and epigenetic mechanisms. The biggest risks include **obesity, lower childhood cognitive scores, autism** (OR 1.58; 95% CI 1.26–1.98), **type 2 diabetes mellitus, cancer, and cardiovascular disease** [217–221]. The key is to identify and intervene early and to potentially reverse the known future adverse consequences associated with maternal obesity.

FUTURE

Future research should assess the degree of intensiveness and contact with a health care provider during management with diet and exercise, drug therapy to target different biological pathways to obesity, the mechanisms of fetal macrosomia, fetal demise secondary to obesity, and childhood obesity, among many others. Controlling maternal prepregnancy obesity and excessive gestational weight retention will help control the obesity epidemic. Food industry companies, insurance companies, public education, school education, tax breaks, premium breaks, fitness programs, and many others should work together to end this vicious cycle, leading to now earlier mortality than previous generations because of obesity.

RESOURCES

ACOG Committee Opinion #319 [107]
ACOG Committee Opinion #315 [16]
ACOG Practice Bulletin #120 [191]
ACOG Practice Bulletin #123 [198]
American Medical Association. Roadmaps for Clinical Practice Series: Assessment and management of adult obesity: http://www.ama-assn.org/ama/pub/category/10931.html
American Society for Bariatric Surgery: http://www.asbs.org
ACOG Clinical Updates in Women's Health Care–Weight control: Assessment and management: http://www.clinicalupdates.org

National Heart, Lung, and Blood Institute–Clinical guidelines on the identification, evaluation, and treatment of overweight and obesity in adults: http://www.nhlbi.nih.gov/guidelines/obesity/ob_home.htm
The Surgeon General's call to action to prevent and decrease overweight and obesity: http://www.surgeongeneral.gov/topics/obesity
U.S. Preventive Services Task Force–Screening for obesity in adults: http://www.ahrq.gov/clinic/uspstf/uspobes.htm

Patient Resources

American Obesity Association: http://www.obesity.org
American Society of Bariatric Physicians: http://www.asbp.org
MedlinePlus: Weight loss and dieting: http://www.nlm.nih.gov/medlineplus/weightlossanddieting.html
National Heart, Lung, and Blood Institute. Obesity education initiative: http://www.nhlbi.nih.gov/about/oei/index.htm
Overeaters Anonymous: http://www.overeatersanonymous.org
TOPS: Take Off Pounds Sensibly: http://www.tops.org
Weight-control Information Network: http://www.win.niddk.nih.gov

REFERENCES

1. World Health Organization. *Obesity: Preventing and managing the global epidemic.* Geneva, Switzerland: World Health Organization: 2000. WHO Technical Report Series 894: 1–253. [III: Review]
2. Marshall N, Guild C, Cheng Y et al. Maternal superobesity and perinatal outcomes. *Am J Obstet Gynecol* 2012; 206: 417.e1–6. [II-2: retrospective cohort study, BMI >50 kg/m², n = 1185]
3. Yogev Y, Catalano P. Pregnancy and obesity. *Obstet Gynecol Clin North Am* 2009; 36: 285–300. [III: Review]
4. U.S. Department of Health and Human Services. *The Surgeon General's Call to Action to Prevent and Decrease Overweight and Obesity.* Rockville, MD: U.S. Department of Health and Human Services, Public Health Service, Office of the Surgeon General, 2001. [III: Review]
5. Nohr EA, Timpson NJ, Anderson CS et al. Severe obesity in young women and reproductive health: The Danish National Birth Cohort. *PloS One* 2009; 4(12): e8444. [II-2: Danish National Birth Cohort, prospective cohort, n = 4901, obese BMI >30 kg/m², n = 2451]
6. Bolumar F, Olsen J, Rebagliato M et al. Body mass index and delayed conception: A European Multicenter Study on Infertility and Subfecundity. *Am J Epidemiol* 2000; 151: 1072–9. [II-2: European multicenter prospective study, n = 4035]
7. Metwally M, Ong KJ, Ledger WL et al. Does high body mass index increase the risk of miscarriage after spontaneous and assisted conception? A meta-analysis of the evidence. *Fertil Steril* 2008; 90: 714–26. [II-2: 16 studies meta-analysis n = 5545, BMI >25 kg/m²]
8. Lashen H, Fear K, Sturdee DW. Obesity is associated with increased risk of first trimester and recurrent miscarriage: Matched case-control study. *Hum Reprod* 2004; 19:1644–6. [II-2: BMI >30 kg/m², n = 1644]
9. Sebire NJ, Jolly M, Harris JP et al. Maternal obesity and pregnancy outcome: A study of 287,213 pregnancies in London. *Int J Obes* 2001; 25: 1175–82. [II-3: UK observational study 1989–1997, n = 287,213; BMI >30 kg/m², n = 31,276]
10. Kumari A. Pregnancy outcome in women with morbid obesity. *Int J Gynaecol Obstet* 2001; 73: 101–7. [II-2: United Arab Emirates, retrospective case control study, n = 488, BMI >40 kg/m², n = 180]
11. Weiss JL, Malone FD, Emig D et al. Obesity, obstetric complications and cesarean delivery rate—A population-based screening study. FASTER Research Consortium. *Am J Obstet Gynecol* 2004; 190: 1091–7. [II-1: Prospective multicenter population-based screening study, n = 16,102; BMI 30–35 kg/m², n = 1473; BMI >35 kg/m², n = 877]

12. O'Brien TE, Ray JG, Chan W-S. Maternal body mass index and the risk of preeclampsia: A systematic overview. *Epidemiology* 2003; 14: 368–74. [II-2: 13 studies, 4 prospective cohort, 9 retrospective cohort, *n* = 1,390,226]

13. Cedergren MI. Maternal morbid obesity and the risk of adverse pregnancy outcome. *Obstet Gynecol* 2004; 103: 219–24. [II-2: Prospective population cohort study, *n* = 3480 with BMI >40 kg/m²]

14. Jensen DM, Damm P, Sørensen B et al. Pregnancy outcome and prepregnancy body mass index in 2459 glucose-tolerant Danish women. *Am J Obstet Gynecol* 2003; 189: 239–44. [II-2: Retrospective cohort study, *n* = 2459]

15. Knight M, Kurinczuk JJ, Spark P et al. on behalf of the UK Obstetric Surveillance System Extreme Obesity in Pregnancy in the United Kingdom. Extreme obesity in pregnancy in the United Kingdom. *Obstet Gynecol* 2010; 115: 989–97. [II-2: Population-based cohort study, BMI >50 kg/m², *n* = 665]

16. American College of Obstetricians and Gynecologists. Obesity in pregnancy. ACOG Committee Opinion No. 315, Sept. 2005. *Obstet Gynecol* 2005; 106: 671–5. [III: Review]

17. Baeten JM, Bukusi EA, Lambe M. Pregnancy complications and outcomes among overweight and obese nulliparous women. *Am J Public Health* 2001; 91: 436–40. [II-2: Population-based cohort study *n* = 96,801]

18. Sahin FK, Koken G, Cosar E et al. Obstructive sleep apnea in pregnancy and fetal outcome. *Int J Gynaecol Obstet* 2008; 100: 141–6. [II: Prospective observational study, *n* = 35]

19. Lefcourt LA, Rodis JF. Obstructive sleep apnea in pregnancy. *Obstet Gynecol Surv* 1996; 51: 503–6. [III: Review]

20. Louis JM, Auckley D, Sokol RJ et al. Maternal and neonatal morbidities associated with obstructive sleep apnea complicating pregnancy. *Am J Obstet Gynecol* 2010; 202(3): 261.e1–5. [II-3: Retrospective cohort, *n* = 114]

21. Olivarez SA, Maheshwari B, McCarthy M et al. Prospective trial on obstructive sleep apnea in pregnancy and fetal heart rate monitoring. *Am J Obstet Gynecol* 2010; 202(6): 552.e1–7. [II- 3, Prospective study, *n* = 100]

22. Hendler I, Schatz M, Momirova V et al., for the National Institute of Child Health and Human Development Maternal–Fetal Medicine Units Network. Association of obesity with pulmonary and nonpulmonary complications of pregnancy in asthmatic women. *Obstet Gynecol* 2006; 108: 77–82. [II-2, Secondary analysis of prospective cohort, *n* = 2566].

23. Atlantis E, Baker M. Obesity effects on depression: Systematic review of epidemiological studies. *Int J Obes (Lond)* 2008; 32: 881–91. [Systematic review, 4 prospective cohort studies, 20 cross-sectional, 10 from the United States]

24. Ma J, Xiao L. Obesity and depression in US women: Results from the 2005–2006 National Health and Nutritional Examination Survey. *Obesity (Silver Spring)* 2010; 18: 347–53. [II-2: Population-based study, *n* = 1875, average age 48 years].

25. McDonald SD, Han Z, Mulla S et al., on behalf of the Knowledge Synthesis Group. Overweight and obesity in mothers and risk of preterm birth and low birth weight infants: Systematic review and meta-analyses. *BMJ* 2010; 341: c3428. doi:10.1136/bmj.c3428. [Systematic review and meta-analysis, cohort studies, *n* = 64, case control studies, *n* = 20]

26. Dashe JS, McIntire DD, Twickler DM. Effect of maternal obesity on the ultrasound detection of anomalous fetuses. *Obstet Gynecol* 2009; 113: 1001–7. [II-2: Retrospective cohort study, *n* = 11,210]

27. Davies GAL, Maxwell C, McLeod L et al. Obesity in pregnancy. SOGC Clinical Practice Guidelines. *Int J Gynaecol Obstet* 2010; 110(2): 165–73. [III: Clinical guideline, 79 references]

28. Bianco AT, Smilen SW, Davis Y et al. Pregnancy outcome and weight gain recommendations for the morbidly obese woman. *Obstet Gynecol* 1998; 91: 97–102. [II-2, U.S. retrospective cohort study, *n* = 11,926]

29. Gabor J, Gyamfi C, Gyamfi P et al. Effect of body mass index and excessive weight gain on success of vaginal birth after cesarean delivery. *Obstet Gynecol* 2005; 106: 741–6. [II-2: Retrospective study, *n* = 1213]

30. Hibbard JU, Gilbert S, Landon MB et al., for the National Institute of Child Health and Human Development Maternal–Fetal Medicine Units Network. Trial of labor or repeat cesarean delivery in women with morbid obesity and previous cesarean delivery. *Obstet Gynecol* 2006; 108(1): 125–33. [II-2: Multicenter, prospective study, *n* = 28,442]

31. Stotland NE, Washington AE, Caughey AB. Prepregnancy body mass index and the length of gestation at term. *Am J Obstet Gynecol* 2007; 197(4): 378.e371–5. [II-2: Retrospective study, US, one center, *n* = 9336]

32. Rasmussen SA, Chu SY, Kim SY et al. Maternal obesity and risk of neural tube defects: A metaanalysis. *Am J Obstet Gynecol* 2008; 198: 611–9. [II-2: 4 cohort studies, 8 case control studies]

33. Stothard KJ, Tennant PWG, Bell R et al. Maternal overweight and obesity and risk of congenital anomalies: A systematic review and meta-analysis. *JAMA* 2009; 301: 636–50. [II-2: Systematic review 39 studies mostly from the United States, meta-analysis 18 studies]

34. Gilboa SM, Correa A, Botto LD et al., and the National Birth Defects Prevention Study. Association between prepregnancy body mass index and congenital heart defects. *Am J Obstet Gynecol* 2010; 202(1): 51.e1–10. [II-2: US population-based observational study, *n* = 11,113]

35. Waller DK, Shaw GM, Rasmussen SA et al. Prepregnancy obesity as a risk factor for structural birth defects. *Arch Pediatr Adolesc Med* 2007; 161: 745–50. [II-2: Case-control, National Birth Defects Prevention Study, *n* = 10,249]

36. Watkins ML, Botto LD. Maternal prepregnancy weight and congenital heart defects in the offspring. *Epidemiology* 2001; 11: 439–46. [II-2: Atlanta Birth Defects Case-Control Study, *n* = 1049]

37. Blomberg MI, Källén B. Maternal obesity and morbid obesity: The risk for birth defects in the offspring. *Birth Defects Res A Clin Mol Teratol* 2010; 88(1): 35–40. [II-2: Swedish Medical Health Registries, *n* = 1,049,582]

38. Siega-Riz AM, Viswanathan M, Moos MK et al. A systematic review of outcomes of maternal weight gain according to the Institute of Medicine recommendations: Birthweight, fetal growth, and postpartum weight retention. *Am J Obstet Gynecol* 2009; 201(4): 339.e1–14. [III: Systematic review of 35 studies from 1990 to 2007]

39. Robinson H, Tkatch S, Mayes DC et al. Is maternal obesity a predictor of shoulder dystocia? *Obstet Gynecol* 2003; 101(1): 24–7. [II-2: Canada, case control study, *n* = 45,877]

40. Nohr EA, Bech BH, Davies MJ et al. Prepregnancy obesity and fetal death: A study within the Danish National Birth Cohort. *Obstet Gynecol* 2005; 106(2): 250–9. [II-2: Retrospective, population-based cohort study, *n* = 54,505]

41. Chu SY, Kim SY, Lau J et al. Maternal obesity and risk of stillbirth: A meta-analysis. *Am J Obstet Gynecol* 2007; 197(3): 223–8. [II-3: Meta-analysis of 9 observational studies]

42. Salihu HM, Alio AP, Wilson RE et al. Obesity and extreme obesity: New insights into the black–white disparity in neonatal mortality. *Obstet Gynecol* 2008; 111: 1410–6. [II: Missouri state 1978–1997 population-based cohort study, *n* = 1,405,698]

43. Cnattingius S, Bergstrom R, Lipworth L et al. Pregnancy weight and the risk of adverse pregnancy outcome. *N Engl J Med* 1998; 338(3): 147–52. [II-2: Sweden 1992–1993, population-based cohort study, *n* = 167,750]

44. Vahratian A, Zhang J, Troendle JF et al. Maternal prepregnancy overweight and obesity and the pattern of labor progression in term nulliparous women. *Obstet Gynecol* 2004; 104(5 Pt. 1): 943–51. [II-2: US prospective cohort study, *n* = 612]

45. Saravanakumar K, Rao SG, Cooper GM. The challenges of obesity and obstetric anaesthesia. *Curr Opin Obstet Gynecol* 2006; 18: 631–5. [III: Review]

46. Vricella LK, Louis JM, Mercer BM et al. Anesthesia complications during scheduled cesarean delivery for morbidly obese women. *Am J Obstet Gynecol* 2010; 203(3): 276.e1–5. [II-2: Retrospective cohort study, *n* = 578]

47. Mhyre JM, Riesner MN, Polley LS et al. A series of anesthesia-related maternal deaths in Michigan, 1985–2003. *Anesthesiology* 2007; 106: 1096–104. [II-2: Michigan Maternal Mortality Surveillance 1985–2003, retrospective study, $n = 855$]

48. Perlow JH, Morgan MA. Massive maternal obesity and perioperative cesarean morbidity. *Am J Obstet Gynecol* 1994; 170: 560–5. [II-2: $n = 43$ patients >300 lb]

49. Lopez LM, Grimes DA, Chen-Mok M et al. Hormonal contraceptives for contraception in overweight or obese women. *Cochrane Database Syst Rev* 2010; 7: CD008452. [III: Reviews, 11 trials, $n = 39,531$]

50. Boots C, Stephenson M. Does obesity increase the risk of miscarriage in spontaneous conception: A systematic review. *Semin Reprod Med* 2011; 29(6): 507–13. [II-2: 6 retrospective studies meta-analysis, BMI >28 kg/m^2, $n = 3800$]

51. Athukorala C, Rumbold A, Wilson K et al. The risk of adverse pregnancy outcomes in women who are overweight or obese. *BMC Pregnancy and Childbirth* 2010; 10–56. [I: Australian Collaborative Trial of Supplements, secondary analysis $n = 1661$; BMI >25 kg/m^2, $n = 446$, BMI >30 kg/m^2, $n = 272$]

52. Ovesen P, Rasmussen S, Kesmodel U. Effect of prepregnancy maternal overweight and obesity on pregnancy outcome. *Obstet Gynecol* 2011; 118(2 Pt. 1): 305e12. [II-2: Danish Medical Birth Registry, prospective cohort 2004–2010, $n = 369,347$]

53. Hyperglycaemia and Adverse Pregnancy Outcome (HAPO) study: Associations with maternal body mass index. *BJOG* 2010; 117(5): 575e84 [II-2: Observational cohort study, 15 centers, 9 countries, $n = 23,316$]

54. Samuels-Kalow ME, Funai EF, Buhimschi C et al. Prepregnancy body mass index, hypertensive disorders of pregnancy, and long-term maternal mortality. *Am J Obstet Gynecol* 2007; 197(5): 490.e1e6. [II-2: Retrospective cohort study, $n = 13,722$]

55. Jensen TB, Gerds TA, Gron R et al. Risk factors for venous thromboembolism during pregnancy. *Pharmacoepidemiol Drug Saf* 2013; 22(12): 1283e91. [II-2: Retrospective cohort study, Denmark national registers, $n = 299,810$]

56. Knight M. Antenatal pulmonary embolism: Risk factors, management and outcomes. *BJOG* 2008; 115(4): 453e61. [II-2: Case-control study, UK Obstetric Surveillance System, $n = 143$ cases of pulmonary embolism matched with 259 controls, BMI >30 kg/m^2]

57. Ray JG, Wyatt PR, Vermeulen MJ et al. Greater maternal weight and the ongoing risk of neural tube defects after folic acid flour fortification. *Obstet Gynecol* 2005; 105(2): 261e5. [II-2: Retrospective population-based study, $n = 420,362$]

58. Hildebrand E, Kallen B, Josefsson A et al. Maternal obesity and risk of Down syndrome in the offspring. *Prenat Diagn* 2014; 34(4): 310e5. [II-2: Population-based cohort study, Study Group I, $n = 1,568,604$, Study Group II, $n = 10,224$]

59. Gupta M, Lauring J, Kunselman AR et al. Fetal growth restriction may be underestimated in obese patients. *Obstet Gynecol* 2014; 123(Suppl. 1): 98se9s. [II-2: Retrospective cohort study comparing $n = 150$ normal weight (BMI <25 kg/m^2) and $n = 150$ obese (BMI >30 kg/m^2)]

60. Catalano PM, McIntyre HD, Cruickshank JK et al. The hyperglycemia and adverse pregnancy outcome study: Associations of GDM and obesity with pregnancy outcomes. *Diabetes Care* 2012; 35(4): 780e6. [II-2: HAPO observational cohort study, 15 centers, 9 countries, $n = 28,562$]

61. Crane JM, Murphy P, Burrage L et al. Maternal and perinatal outcomes of extreme obesity in pregnancy. *J Obstet Gynaecol Can* 2013; 35(7): 606e11. [II-2: Population based cohort study, $n = 5,788$; BMI >50 kg/m^2 $n = 71$]

62. Sekhavat L, Fallah R. Could maternal pre-pregnancy body mass index affect Apgar score? *Arch Gynecol Obstet* 2013; 287(1): 15e8. [II-2: Retrospective cohort study, single-center, $n = 3120$]

63. Aune D, Saugstad OD, Henriksen T et al. Maternal body mass index and the risk of fetal death, stillbirth, and infant death: A systematic review and meta-analysis. *JAMA* 2014; 311(15): 1536e46. [II-3: Meta-analysis: 38 studies, $n = 10,147$ fetal deaths, $n = 16,274$ stillbirths, $n = 4311$ perinatal deaths, $n = 11,294$ neonatal deaths, and $n = 4983$ infant deaths were included]

64. Curhan GC, Chertow GM, Willett WC et al. Birth weight and adult hypertension and obesity in women. *Circulation* 1996; 94(6): 1310e5. [II-2: population-based cohort study, Nurses' Health Study Part I, $n = 71,100$ and Part II, $n = 92,940$]

65. Bautista-Castano I, Henriquez-Sanchez P, Aleman-Perez N et al. Maternal obesity in early pregnancy and risk of adverse outcomes. *PLoS One* 2013; 8(11): e80410. [II-2: Population-based cohort study, single-center study, $n = 6887$]

66. Stamilio DM, Scifres CM. Extreme obesity and postcesarean maternal complications. *Obstet Gynecol* 2014; 124(2 Pt. 1): 227e32. [II-2: Retrospective cohort analysis of a previous randomized control trial, $n = 585$]

67. Fyfe EM, Thompson JM, Anderson NH et al. Maternal obesity and postpartum haemorrhage after vaginal and caesarean delivery among nulliparous women at term: A retrospective cohort study. *BMC Pregnancy and Childbirth* 2012; 12: 112. [II-2: Retrospective cohort study, National Women's Health Clinical Database, $n = 11,363$]

68. World Health Organization. *Obesity and overweight.* Geneva, Switzerland: World Health Organization: 2015. WHO Fact Sheet. Updated 2015. [III: Review]

69. Kelly T, Yang W, Chen C et al. Global burden of obesity in 2005 and projections to 2030. *Int J Obesity* 2008; 32: 1431–7. [II-3: Pooling analysis of representative population samples from 106 countries]

70. Han J, Lawlor D, Kimm S. Childhood obesity. *Lancet* 2010; 375(9727): 1737–48. [III: Review].

71. Centers for Disease Control. *Adult Obesity Facts.* Division of Nutrition, Physical Activity, and Obesity. Updated September 21, 2015. Accessed October 2015.

72. James WPT, Jackson-Leach R, Ni Mhurchu C. Overweight and obesity (high body mass index). In: Ezzati TM, ed. *Comparative Quantification of Health Risks Global and Regional Burden of Disease Attributable to Selected Major Risk Factors.* Vol 1. Geneva: World Health Organization 2004: 497–596. [III: Review]

73. Fryar C, Carroll M, Ogden C. *Prevalence of overweight, obesity, and extreme obesity among adults: United States, 1960–1962 through 2011–2012.* Division of Health and Nutrition Examination Surveys. September 2012: 1–8. [III: Review]

74. Scheil W, Scott J, Catcheside B et al. *Pregnancy Outcome in South Australia 2012.* Adelaide: Pregnancy Outcome Unit, SA Health, Government of South Australia, 2014. [III: Review]

75. Swank ML, Marshall NE, Caughey AB et al. Pregnancy outcomes in the super obese, stratified by weight gain above and below Institute of Medicine Guidelines. *Obstetrics & Gynecology* 2014; 124(6): 1105–10. [II-2: Retrospective cohort study, $n = 1034$]

76. Alanis MC, Goodnight WH, Hill EG et al. Maternal super-obesity (body mass index > or = 50) and adverse pregnancy outcomes. *Acta Obstet Gynecol Scand* 2010; 89: 924–30. [II-2: Cross-sectional study, single-center study, $n = 19,700$]

77. Barsh GS, Farooqi IS, O'Rahilly S. Genetics of body-weight regulation. *Nature* 2000; 404: 644–51. [III: Review]

78. Reilly JJ, Armstrong J, Dorosty AR et al., for the Avon Longitudinal Study of Parents and Children Study Team. Early life risk factors for obesity in childhood: Cohort study. *BMJ* 2005; 330(7504): 1357. [II-2: Prospective cohort observational study, $n = 8234$]

79. Centers for Disease Control and Prevention. *Obesity and genomics.* Available at: http://www.cdc.gov/genomics/resources/diseases/obesity/obesedit.htm. Accessed 02/07/11.

80. Willer CJ, Speliotes EK, Loos RJ, for the Genetic Investigation of Anthropometric Traits Consortium et al. Six new loci associated with body mass index highlight a neuronal influence on body weight regulation. *Nat Genet* 2009; 41: 25–34. [II-3: Meta-analysis: 15 genome-wide association studies for BMI ($n > 32,000$) and followed up top signals in 14 additional cohorts ($n > 59,000$)]

81. Savona-Ventura, C. The inheritance of obesity. *Best Practice & Research Clinical Obstetrics & Gynaecology* 2015; 29(3): 300–8. [III: Review]

82. Metwally M, Ledger WL, Li TC. Reproductive endocrinology and clinical aspects of obesity. *Ann N Y Acad Sci* 2008; 1127: 140–6. [III: Review]

83. Luo, ZH. Maternal and fetal leptin, adiponectin levels and associations with fetal insulin sensitivity. *Obesity* 2013; 21: 210–6. [II-2: Prospective cohort study, n = 248]

84. Kratzsch J, Hockel M, Kiess W. Leptin and pregnancy outcome. *Curr Opin Obstet Gynecol* 2000; 12: 501–5. [III: Review]

85. Hauguel-de Mouzon S, Lepercq J, Catalano P. The known and unknown of leptin in pregnancy. *Am J Obstet Gynecol* 2006; 194(6): 1537–45. [III: Review]

86. American College of Obstetricians and Gynecologists. Challenges for overweight and obese urban women Challenges for overweight and Obese Women. ACOG Committee on Health Care for Underserved Women. *Obstet Gynecol* 2014; 123(3): 726–30. [III: Review]

87. Jungheim ES, Moley KH. Current knowledge of obesity's effects in the pre- and periconceptional periods and avenues for future research. *Am J Obstet Gynecol* 2010; 203(6): 525–30. [III: Review]

88. Brite J, Laughon SK, Troendle J, Mills J. Maternal overweight and obesity and risk of congenital heart defects in offspring. *Int J Obes* 2014; 38(6): 878–82. [II-2: Cohort study, the Consortium on Safe Labor, n = 121, 815 deliveries with 1388 infants with CHD]

89. Rankin J, Tennant PW, Stothard KJ, Bythell M, Summerbell CD, Bell R. Maternal body mass index and congenital anomaly risk: A cohort study. *Int J Obes* 2010; 34: 1371–80. [II-2: prospective cohort study, n = 682]

90. Schummers L, Hutcheon JA et al. Risk of adverse pregnancy outcome by prepregnancy body mass index. A population-based study to inform prepregnancy weight loss counseling. *Obstetrics & Gynecology* 2015; 125(1): 133–43. [II-2: Population-based cohort study, n = 226,958]

91. Swank M, Marshall N, Caughey A et al. Pregnancy outcomes in the super obese stratified by weight gain above and below Institute of Medicine guidelines. *Obstetrics & Gynecology* 2014; 124(6): 1105–10. [II-2: Retrospective cohort study, n = 1034]

92. Santangeli L, Sattar N, Huda S. Impact of maternal obesity on perinatal and childhood outcomes. *Best Practice & Research Clinical Obstetrics and Gynaecology* 2014; 29: 438–48. [III: Review]

93. Brost BC, Goldenberg RL, Mercer BM et al. The Preterm Prediction Study: Association of cesarean section with increases in maternal weight and body mass index. *Am J Obstet Gynecol* 1997; 177(2): 333–7. [II-2: Prospective study, n = 2809]

94. Chauhan SP, Magann EF, Carroll CS et al. Mode of delivery for the morbidly obese with prior cesarean delivery: Vaginal versus repeat cesarean section. *Am J Obstet Gynecol* 2001; 185: 349–54. [II-2: Prospective study, n = 69, maternal weight >300 lb]

95. Hendler I, Goldenberg RL, Mercer BM et al., for the National Institute of Child Health and Human Development, Maternal–Fetal Medicine Units Network, National Institutes of Health. The Preterm Prediction Study: Association between maternal body mass index and spontaneous and indicated preterm birth. *Am J Obstet Gynecol* 2005; 192(3): 882–6. [II-1: US 10 centers, prospective observational study, n = 2910, BMI >30 kg/m^2, n = 597]

96. Salihu HM, Lynch O, Alio AP et al. Obesity subtypes and risk of spontaneous versus medically indicated preterm births in singletons and twins. *Am J Epidemiol* 2008; 168(1): 13–20. [II-2: US population cohort study, n = 459,913]

97. Dietz PM, Callaghan WM, Cogswell ME et al. Combined effects of prepregnancy body mass index and weight gain during pregnancy on the risk of preterm delivery. *Epidemiology* 2006; 17: 170–7. [II: Prospective observational cohort (PRAMS) US study 21 states, n = 113,019]

98. Ehrenberg HM, Iams JD, Goldenberg RL et al., for the Eunice Kennedy Shriver National Institute of Child Health and Human Development (NICHD), Maternal–Fetal Medicine Units Network. Maternal obesity, uterine activity, and the risk of spontaneous preterm birth. *Obstet Gynecol* 2009; 113: 48–52. [II: US multicenter, case control, n = 253]

99. Zhong Y, Cahill A, Macones G. The association between pre-pregnancy maternal body mass index and preterm delivery. *Am J Perinatology* 2010; 27(4): 293–98. [II-2: Retrospective cohort study, n = 44,421]

100. Wang T, Zhang J, Lu X et al. Maternal early pregnancy body mass index and risk of preterm birth. *Arch Gynecol Obstet* 2011; 284: 813–9. [II-2: Population-based cohort study, China 1993–2005, n = 353,477]

101. Yinon D, Lowensteing L. Pre-eclampsia is associated with sleep-disordered breathing and endothelial dysfunction. *Eur Respir J* 2006; 27(20): 328–33. [II-2: Case-control study, single center, n = 17 women with preeclampsia]

102. Sahin FK. Obstructive sleep apnea in pregnancy and fetal outcome. *Int J Gynecol Obstet* 2008; 100: 141–6. [II-2: Prospective observational study, n = 35]

103. Boujeily G, Ankner G. Sleep-disordered breathing in pregnancy. *Clin Chest Med* 2011; 32: 175–89. [III: Review]

104. Chen YH, Kang JH, Lin CC, Wang IT, Keller, JJ, Lin HC. Obstructive sleep apnea and risk of adverse pregnancy outcomes. *Am J Obstet Gynecol* 2012; 206(20): 136, e131–5. [II-2: Cross-sectional study, n = 218,776 women, n = 791 had been diagnosed with OSA]

105. Poyares D, Guilleminault C. Pre-eclampsia and nasal CPAP: Part 2: Hypertension during pregnancy, chronic snoring, and early CPAP nasal intervention. *Sleep Medicine* 2007; 9: 15–21. [I: Randomized control trial, n = 16]

106. Gaudet L, Ferraro ZM, Wen SW, Walker M. Maternal obesity and occurrence of fetal macrosomia: A systematic review and meta-analysis. *BioMed Research International* [II-3: Meta-analysis: 30 studies, multicenter, multicountry review, n = 162,183 obese patients versus normal or underweight control group n = 1,072,397]

107. ACOG Committee on Gynecologic Practice. The role of the obstetrician–gynecologist in the assessment and management of obesity. ACOG Committee Opinion No. 319. *Obstet Gynecol* 2005; 106(4): 895–9. [III: Review]

108. National Institutes of Health. Clinical guidelines on the identification, evaluation, and treatment of overweight and obesity in adults—The Evidence Report 1998. *Obes Res* 1998: 6(Suppl. 2): 51S–209S. [III: Review]

109. American College of Obstetricians and Gynecologists. Motivational interviewing: A tool for behaviour change. ACOG Committee Opinion No. 423. *Obstet Gynecol* 2009; 113: 234–6. [III: Review]

110. Rittenburg V, Seshadri S, Sunkara, S et al. Effect of body mass index on IVF treatment outcome: An updated systematic review and meta-analysis. *Reproductive Biomedicine Online* 2011; 23: 421–39. [II-3: Meta-analysis: 33 studies analyzing 47,967 treatment cycles]

111. Vural F, Vural B, Çakıroğlu Y. The role of overweight and obesity in in vitro fertilization outcomes of poor ovarian responders. *BioMed Research International* 2015; 2015: 781543. doi:10.1155/2015/781543. [II-2: Retrospective cohort study: Single center design, normal weight (18.5–24.9 kg/m^2, n = 96); Group 2 was overweight (25.0–29.9 kg/m^2, n = 52); and Group 3 was obese (≥30.0 kg/m^2, n = 40)]

112. Di Lillo M, Hendrix N, O'Neill M et al. Pregnancy in obese women: What you need to know. *Cont Obstet Gynecol* 2008; 11: 48–53. [III: Review]

113. Bray GA, Tartaglia LA. Medicinal strategies in the treatment of obesity. *Nature* 2000; 404: 672–7. [III: Review]

114. Perrio MJ, Wilton LV, Shakir SAW. The safety profiles of orlistat and sibutramine: Results of prescription-event monitoring studies in England. *Obesity (Silver Spring)* 2007; 15(11): 2712–22. [II-2: Observational cohort study, n = 28,357]

115. Jull AB, Ni Mhurchu C, Bennett DA et al. Chitosan for overweight or obesity. *Cochrane Database Sys Rev* 2008, 3: CD003892. doi:10.1002/14651858. CD003892.pub3. [II-3: metaanalysis]

116. Ducarme G, Parisio L, Santulli P et al. Neonatal outcomes in pregnancies after bariatric surgery: A retrospective multi-centric cohort study in three French referral centers. *J Maternal-Fetal & Neonatal Medicine* 2013; 26(3): 275–8. [II-2: Retrospective cohort study, multicenter study, laparoscopic adjustable gastric banding (LAGB, n = 63) or Roux-en-Y gastric bypass (RYGB, n = 31), BMI class (n = 72 women with BMI ≥30 kg/m²)]

117. Yi X, Li Q, Zhang J et al. A meta-analysis of maternal and fetal outcomes of pregnancy after bariatric surgery. *Int J Gynaecol Obstet* 2015; 130(1): 3–9. [II-3: Meta-analysis, 21 cohort studies reviewed]

118. Guelinckx I, Devlieger R, Vansant G. Reproductive outcome after bariatric surgery: A critical review. *Hum Reprod Update* 2009; 15(2): 189–201. [III: Review]

119. Buchwald H, Oien D. Metabolic/bariatric surgery worldwide 2008. *Obes Surg* 2009; 19(12): 1605–11. [III: Review]

120. Scopinaro N, Gianetta E, Civalleri D, Bonalumi U, Bachi V. Bilio-pancreatic bypass for obesity: II. Initial experience in man. *Br J Surg* 1979; 66(9): 618–20. [II-2: Prospective cohort study in initial patients undergoing bilio-pancreatic bypass, n = 18]

121. Livingston EH. Obesity and its surgical management. *Am J Surg* 2002; 184(2): 103–13. [III: Review]

122. Fernandes MAP, Atallah AN, Soares BG et al. Intragastric balloon for obesity. *Cochrane Database Syst Rev* 2007; (1): CD004931. [II-3: Meta-analysis, 9 RCTs, n = 395, high level of bias, nonpregnant participants]

123. Maggard M, Li Z, Yermilov I et al. Bariatric surgery in women of reproductive age: Special concerns for pregnancy. *Evid Rep Technol Assess (Full Rep)* 2008; (169): 1–51. [III: Review 57 studies; 23 case reports, 21 case series, 12 cohort, 1 case control]

124. Robinson JA, Burke AE. Obesity and hormonal contraceptive efficacy. *Women's Health (London, England)* 2013; 9(5): 453–66. [III: Review]

125. Wax J, Cartin A, Wolff R et al. Pregnancy following gastric bypass for morbid obesity: Effect of surgery-to-conception interval on maternal and neonatal outcomes. *Obes Surg* 2008; 18(12): 1517–21. [II-2: Retrospective cohort study, n = 50]

126. Agnolo C, Cyr C, Montigny F et al. Pregnancy after bariatric surgery: Obstetric and perinatal outcomes and the growth and development of children. *Obes Surg* 2015; Published online April 20, 2015. [II-2: Retrospective cross-sectional study, n = 19]

127. Parikh R, Lavoie M, Wilson L, Maranda L, Leung K, Simas TM. Timing of pregnancy after bariatric surgery. *Obstet Gynecol* 2014; 123(Suppl. 1): 165S. [II-2: Retrospective cohort study, n = 52]

128. Martin LF, Finigan KM, Nolan TE. Pregnancy after adjustable gastric banding. *Obstet Gynecol* 2000; 95(6 Pt. 1): 927–30. [II-1: Clinical trial evaluating adjustable gastric banding, n = 359 obese women]

129. Wittgrove AC, Jester L, Wittgrove P, Clark GW. Pregnancy following gastric bypass for morbid obesity. *Obes Surg* 1998; 8(4): 461–4. [II-2: Retrospective cohort study, n = 41]

130. American College of Obstetricians and Gynecologists. Bariatric surgery and pregnancy. ACOG Practice Bulletin No. 105. *Obstet Gynecol* 2009; 113: 1405–13. [III: Review]

131. Johannson K, Cnattinius S, Naslund I et al. Outcomes of pregnancy after bariatric surgery. *N Engl J Med* 2015; 372: 814–24. [II-2: Retrospective cohort study using Swedish Medical Birth Register, n = 628,778, women who had undergone bariatric surgery n = 1755]

132. Adams T, Hammoud A, Davidson L et al. Maternal and neonatal outcomes for pregnancies before and after gastric bypass surgery. *Int J Obes (Lond)* 2015; 39(4): 686–94. [II-2: Retrospective matched-control cohort study, RYGB (group 1; n = 295 matches) and women with pregnancies after RYGB (group 2; n = 764 matches)]

133. Catalano PM. Management of obesity in pregnancy. *Obstet Gynecol* 2007; 109: 419–33. [III: Review]

134. Shekelle PG, Morton SC, Maglione MA et al. Pharmacological and surgical treatment of obesity. *Evid Rep Technol Assess (Summ)* 2004; (103): 1–6. [II-3: Meta-analysis: 28 trials of orlistat; 147 total studies for surgery, 89 for weight loss analysis, 134 for mortality analysis, 128 for complication analysis]

135. Centre for Maternal and Child Enquiries/Royal College of Obstetricians and Gynaecologists. Management of women with obesity in pregnancy. *RCOG Guidelines* 2010. [III: Clinical guideline, 77 references]

136. U.S. Preventive Services Task Force. Folic acid for the prevention of neural tube defects: U.S. Preventive Services Task Force recommendation statement. *Ann Intern Med* 2009; 150(9): 626–31. [III: 5 studies from 1995–2008; RCT = 1]

137. Mojtabai R. Body mass index and serum folate in childbearing women. *Eur J Epidemiol* 2004; 19: 1029–36. [II-1: US population based cohort study National Health and Nutrition Examination Survey (NHANES) from 1988 to 1994 and 1999 to 2000, n = 5018]

138. Ghaffari N, Srinivas SK, Durnwald CP. The multidisciplinary approach to the care of the obese parturient. *Am J Obstet Gynecol* 2015; 318–25. [III: Review]

139. Rasmussen KM, Yaktine AL, for Institute for Medicine and National Research Council (US) Committee to Reexamine IOM Pregnancy Weight Guidelines. *Weight gain during pregnancy: Reexamining the guidelines.* Washington, DC: National Academic Press 2009. [III: Consensus Report]

140. Oken E, Kleinman KP, Belfort MB et al. Association of gestational weight gain with short- and longer-term maternal and child health outcomes. *Am J Epidemiol* 2009; 170: 173–80. [II-2: Project Viva, Massachusetts 1999–2002 US observational study, n = 2012]

141. Cedergren MI. Optimal gestational weight gain for body mass index categories. *Obstet Gynecol* 2007; 110(4): 759–64. [II-2: Swedish Medical Birth Register, population-based cohort study, n = 298,648]

142. Kiel DW, Dodson EA, Artal R et al. Gestational weight gain and pregnancy outcomes in obese women. How much is enough? *Obstet Gynecol* 2007; 110: 752–8. [II-2: Population-based cohort, n = 120,251]

143. Nohr EA, Vaeth M, Baker JL et al. Pregnancy outcomes related to gestational weight gain in women defined by their body mass index, parity, height, and smoking status. *Am J Clin Nutr* 2009; 90: 1288–94. [II-2: Danish population based observational study, n = 59,147]

144. Dietz PM, Callaghan WM, Smith R et al. Low pregnancy weight gain and small for gestational age: A comparison of the association using 3 different measures of small for gestational age. *Am J Obstet Gynecol* 2009; 201: 53.e1–7. [II-2: Retrospective cohort study, Pregnancy Risk Assessment Monitoring System (PRAMS), n = 104,980]

145. Kominiarek MA, Seligman NS, Dolin C et al. Gestational weight gain and obesity: Is 20 pounds too much? *Obstet Gynecol* 2013; 209: e1–11. [II-1: Prospective cohort study, high weight gain was associated with increased large for gestational age infants (class I OR, 2.4; 95% CI, 1.9–2.9; class II OR, 1.7; 95% CI, 1.3–2.1; class III OR, 1.6; 95% CI, 1.3–2.1) n = 20,950]

146. Gore S, Brown DM, Smith-West D. The role of postpartum weight retention in obesity among women: A review of evidence. *Ann Behav Med* 2003; 26: 149–59. [III: Review]

147. Oken E, Taveras EM, Kleinman KP et al. Gestational weight gain and child adiposity at age 3 years. *Am J Obstet Gynecol* 2007; 196: 322. [II-2: Prospective cohort study, n = 1044]

148. Polley BA, Wing RR, Sims CJ. Randomized controlled trial to prevent excessive weight gain in pregnant women. *Int J Obesity Relat Metab Disord* 2002; 26: 1494–502. [I: RCT, n = 120]

149. Dodd JM, Grivell RM, Crowther CA et al. Antenatal interventions for overweight or obese pregnant women: A systematic review of randomized trials. *BJOG* 2010; 117: 1316–26. [II-3: Meta-analysis; 9 RCTs, n = 743]

150. Streuling I, Beyerlein A, Rosenfeld E et al. Physical activity and gestational weight gain: A meta-analysis of intervention trials. *BJOG* 2011; 118: 278–84. [II-3: Meta-analysis; 12 RCTs, *n* = 1073]

151. Renault KM, Norgaard K, Nilas L et al. The treatment of obese pregnant women (TOP) study: A randomized controlled trial of the effect of physical activity intervention assessed by pedometer with or without dietary intervention in obese pregnant women. *Am J Obstet Gynecol* 2014; 210: 134.e1–9. [I: RCT, *n* = 389]

152. American College of Obstetricians and Gynecologists. Exercise during pregnancy and the postpartum period. ACOG Committee Opinion No. 267. *Obstet Gynecol* 2002; 99: 171–3. [III: Review]

153. American Academy of Pediatrics and the American College of Obstetrics and Gynecologists. *Guidelines for Perinatal Care.* 6th ed. October 2007: 191–2. [III: Review]

154. Centre for Maternal and Child Enquiries/Royal College of Obstetricians and Gynaecologists. *Management of women with obesity in pregnancy.* RCOG Guidelines. 2010. [III: Clinical guideline, 77 references]

155. Aagaard-Tillery KM, Flint Porter T, Malone FD, Nyberg DA, Collins J. Influence of maternal BMI on genetic sonography in the FaSTER trial. *Prenat Diagn* 2010; 30: 14–22. [II-2: Prospective cohort, *n* = 8555]

156. Tsai PJS, Loichinger M, Zalud I. Obesity and the challenges of ultrasound fetal abnormality diagnosis. *Best Practice Res Clin Obstet Gynecol* 2015; 29: 320–7. [III: Review]

157. Tsai LJ, Ho M, Pressman EK et al. Ultrasound screening for fetal aneuploidy using soft markers in the overweight and obese gravida. *Prenat Diagn* 2010: 30: 821–6. [II-2: Retrospective review, *n* = 5690]

158. Maxwell C, Dunn E, Tomlinson G et al. How does maternal obesity affect the routine fetal anatomic ultrasound? *J Matern Fetal Neonatal Med* 2010; 23: 1187–92. [II-2: Retrospective review, *n* = 100]

159. Fuchs F, Houllier M, Voulgaropoulos A et al. Factors affecting feasibility and quality of second-trimester ultrasound scans in obese pregnant women. *Ultrasound Obstet Gynecol* 2013; 41: 40–6. [II-2: Prospective study, *n* = 283]

160. Best KE, Tennant PW, Bell R et al. Impact of maternal body mass index on the antenatal detection of congenital anomalies. *BJOG* 2012; 119(12): 1503–11. [II-2: Population-based register study, *n* = 3096]

161. Harper LM, Jauk VC, Owen J et al. The utility of ultrasound surveillance of fluid and growth in obese women. *Am J Obstet Gynecol* 2014; 211(5): 524:e1–8. [II-2: Retrospective cohort, *n* = 1164]

162. Royal College of Obstetricians and Gynecologists. CMAE/ RCOG Joint Guideline. *Management of women with obesity in pregnancy.* England and Wales: Centre for Maternal and Child Enquiries. Royal College of Obstetricians and Gynecologists; 2010. [III: Review]

163. Kbayashi N, Lim BH. Induction of labour and intrapartum care in obese women. *Best Practice Research Clin Obstet Gynecol* 2015; 29: 394–405. [III: Review]

164. Arrowsmith S, Wray S, Quenby S. Maternal obesity and labor complications following induction of labor in prolonged pregnancy. *BJOG* 2011; 118: 578–88. [II-2: Retrospective cohort, *n* = 29, 224]

165. Wolfe KB, Rossi RA, Warshak CR. The effect of maternal obesity on the rate of failed induction of labor. *Am J Obstet Gynecol* 2011; 205(125): 1–7. [II-2: Population based cohort study, Ohio Department of Health birth certificate data, *n* = 279,521]

166. Wolfe H, Timofeev J, Tefera E et al. Risk of caesarean in obese nulliparous women with unfavorable cervix: Elective induction vs. expectant management at term. *Am J Obstet Gynecol* 2014; 210: e1–5. [II-2: Retrospective cohort, *n* = 470]

167. Tonidandel A, Booth J, D'Angelo R, Harris L, Carlhall S, Kallen K, Blomberg M. Maternal body mass index and duration of labor. *Eur J Obstet Gynecol Repro Biol* 2013; 17: 49–53. [II-2: Historical prospective cohort study, *n* = 63,829]

168. Soni S, Chivan N, Cohen WR. Effect of maternal body mass index on oxytocin treatment for arrest of dilatation. *J Perinat Med* 2013; 41(5): 517–21. [II-2: Retrospective analysis, *n* = 118]

169. Vinayagam D, Chandraharan E. Clinical study: The adverse impact of maternal obesity on intrapartum and perinatal outcomes. International Scholarly Research Network. *Obstet Gynecol* 2012. Article ID 939762. [II-2: Retrospective case-control analysis, the study group (BMI >40 kg/m²) *n* = 100 women and a control group (BMI 20–25 kg/m²) *n* = 100]

170. Poobalan AS, Aucott LS, Gurun T, Smith WC et al. Obesity as an independent risk factor for elective and emergency cesarean delivery in nulliparous women-systematic review and meta-analysis of cohort studies. *Obes Rev* 2009; 10: 28–35. [II-3: Meta-analysis, *n* = 209,193]

171. Clark-Ganheart CA, Reddy UM, Kominiarek MA, Huang C-C et al. Pregnancy outcomes among obese women and their offspring by attempted mode of delivery. *Obstet Gynecol* 2015; 126(5): 985–93. [II-2: retrospective cohort study, *n* = 47,372]

172. Gunatilake RP, Perlow JH. Obesity and pregnancy: Clinical management of the obese gravida. *Am J Obstet Gynecol* 2011; 204(2): 106–19. [III: Review]

173. Belogolovkin V, Crisan L, Lynch O, Weldeselasse H et al. Neonatal outcomes of successful VBAC among obese and super obese mothers. *J Matern Fetal Neonatal Med* 2012; 25: 714–8. [II-2: Missouri maternally linked cohort data, *n* = 30,017]

174. Subramaniam A, Jauk VC, Goss AR, Alvarez MD et al. Mode of delivery in women with class II obesity: Planned cesarean compared with induction of labor. *Am J Obstet Gynecol* 2014; 211: 700.e1–9. [II-2: Retrospective cohort study, *n* = 661]

175. Tan T, Sia AT. Anesthetic considerations in the obese gravida. *Semin Perinatol* 2011; 35: 350–5. [III: Review]

176. Obestetric Anaesthetic Association and the Association of Anaesthetists of Great Britain and Ireland) (Royal College of Obstetricians and Gynecologists. CMAE/RCOG Joint Guideline. *Management of women with obesity in pregnancy.* England and Wales: Centre for Maternal and Child Enquiries. Royal College of Obstetricians and Gynecologists; 2010. [III: Review]

177. Tonidandel A, Booth J, D'Angelo R, Harris L, Tonidandel S. Anesthetic and obstetric outcomes in morbidly obese parturients: A 20 year follow-up retrospective cohort study. *Inl J Obstet Anesthesia* 2014; 23P357–364. [II-2: Retrospective cohort, *n* = 460]

178. Girsen AI, Osmundson SS, Naqvi M, Garabedian MJ et al. Body mass index and operative times at cesarean delivery. *Obstet Gynecol* 2014; 124(4): 684–9. [II-2: Cohort study, Maternal Fetal Medicine Units Network Cesarean Registry, *n* = 21,372]

179. Alanis MC, Villers MS, Law TL, Steadman EM et al. Complications of cesarean delivery in the massively obese parturient. *Am J Obstet Gynecol* 2010; 203: 271.e1–7. [II-2: Retrospective cohort, *n* = 194]

180. Kabon B, Nagele A, Reddy D et al. Obesity decreases perioperative tissue oxygenation. *Anesthesiology* 2004; 100: 274–80. [Clinical investigation, *n* = 46]

181. Scifres CM, Leighton BL, Fogertey PJ et al. Supplemental oxygen for the prevention of postcesarean infectious morbidity: A randomized controlled trial. *Am J Obstet Gynecol* 2011; 205: 267.e1–9. [I: RCT, *n* = 585]

182. Gardella C, Goltra LB, Laschansky E, Drolette L et al. High-concentration supplemental perioperative oxygen to reduce the incidence of postcesarean surgical site infection. *Obstet Gynecol* 2008; 112(3): 545–52. [I: double-blind RCT, *n* = 143]

183. Duggal N, Poddatoori V, Noroozkhani S, Siddik-Ahmad Ri et al. Perioperative oxygen supplementation and surgical site infection after cesarean delivery: A randomized trial. *Obstet Gynecol* 2013; 122(1): 79–84. [I: RCT, *n* = 831]

184. Hellums EK, Lin MH, Ramsey PS. Prophylactic subcutaneous drainage for prevention of wound complications after cesarean delivery- a metaanalysis. *Am J Obstet Gynecol* 2007; 197: 229–35. [II-3: Meta-analysis, 6 RCTs included]

185. Dahlke JD, Mendez-Figueroa H, Rouse DJ, Berghella V et al. Evidence-based surgery for cesarean delivery: An updated systematic review. *Am J Obstet Gynecol* 2013; 294–306. [III: Systematic Review, 73 RCTs, 10 metaanalyses and/or systematic reviews, and 12 *Cochrane* reviews]

186. Mackeen AD, Schuster M, Berghella V. Suture versus staples for skin closure after cesarean: A metaanalysis. *Am J Obstet Gynecol* 2015; 212(5): 621.e1010. [II-3: Meta-analysis, 12 RCTs, n = 3112]

187. Marrs CC, Moussa HN, Sibai BM, Blackwell SC. The relationship between primary cesarean delivery skin incision type and wound complications in women with morbid obesity. *Am J Obstet Gynecol* 2014; 210: 319.31-4. [II-2: Secondary analysis of a multicenter cesarean registry of the Eunice Kennedy Shriver National Institute of Child Health and Human Development Maternal-Fetal Medicine Units Network, n = 3200]

188. Thornburg LL, Linder MA, Durie DE, Walker B et al. Risk factors for wound complications in morbidly obese women undergoing primary cesarean delivery. *J Mat-Fet Neonatal Med* 2012; 25(9): 1544–8. [II-2: Retrospective cohort, n = 623]

189. McLean M, Hines R, Polinkovsky M, Stuebe A et al. Type of skin incision and wound complications in the obese parturient. *Am J Perinatol* 2012; 29: 301–6. [II-2: Secondary analysis of the Pregnancy, Infection and Nutrition study, which was a large observational cohort study, n = 238]

190. Conner SN, Verticchio JC, Tuuli MG, Odibo AO et al. Maternal obesity and risk of post cesarean wound complications. *Am J Perinatol* 2014; 31: 299–304. [II-2: Retrospective cohort, n = 2444]

191. Use of Prophylactic Antibiotics in Labor and Delivery. ACOG Practice Bulletin No. 120. American College of Obstetricians and Gynecologists. *Obstet Gynecol* 2011; 117: 1472–83. [III: Review]

192. Pevzner L, Swank M, Krepel C, Wing D et al. Effects of maternal obesity on tissue concentrations of prophylactic cefazolin during cesarean delivery. *Obstet Gynecol* 2011; 117(4): 877–82. [II: descriptive study with prospective collection, n = 29]

193. Stitely M, Sweet M, Slain D, Alons L et al. Plasma and tissue cefazolin concentrations in obese patients undergoing cesarean delivery and receiving differing pre-operative doses of drug. *Surgical Infections* 2013; 14(5): 455–9. [I: RCT, n = 23]

194. Young OM, Shaik IH, Twedt R et al. Pharmacokinetics of cefazolin prophylaxis in obese gravidae at time of cesarean delivery. *Am J Obstet Gynecol* 2015; 213: 541.e1–7. [I: Double-blind RCT, n = 26]

195. Swank ML, Wing DA, Nicolau DP, McNulty JA. Increase 3-gram cefazolin dosing for cesarean delivery prophylaxis in obese women. *Am J Obstet Gynecol* 2015; 213(3): 415.e1–8 [II-2: Prospective cohort, n = 28].

196. Maggio L, Nicolau DP, DaCosta M, Rouse DJ et al. Cefazolin prophylaxis in obese women undergoing cesarean delivery: A randomized controlled trial. *Obstet Gynecol* 2015; 125(5): 1205–10) [I: double-blind RCT, n = 57]

197. Robinson HE, O'Connell CM, Joseph KS, McLeod NL. Maternal outcomes in pregnancies complicated by obesity. *Obstet Gynecol* 2005; 106: 1357–64. [II-2: Population-based cohort study, Nova Scotia Atlee Perinatal Database, n = 142,404]

198. Thromboembolism in pregnancy. Practice Bulletin No. 123. American College of Obstetricians and Gynecologists. *Obstet Gynecol* 2011; 118: 718–29. [III:Review]

199. Tepper NK, Boulet SL, Whiteman MK, Monsour M et al. Postpartum venous thromboembolism: Incidence and risk factors. *Obstet Gynecol* 2014; 123(5): 987–96. [II-2: Truven Health MarketScan Commercial and Multi-State Medicaid databases, n = 2,456 venous thromboembolisms]

200. Cavazza S, Rainaldi MP, Adduci A, Palareti G. Thromboprophylaxis following cesarean delivery: One site prospective pilot study to evaluate the application of a risk score model. *Throm Res* 2012; 129: 28–31. [II-2: n = 501]

201. Royal College of Obstetricians and Gynaecologists. Reducing the risk of thrombosis and embolism during pregnancy and the puerperium. Green-top Guideline No. 37a. London: *RCOG* 2009. [III: Review]

202. Drife J. *Best practice and research clinical obstetrics and gynaecology* 2015: 29; 365–76. [III: Review]

203. Overcash RT, Somers AT, LaCoursiere Y. Enoxaparin dosing after cesarean delivery in morbidly obese women. *Obstet Gynecol* 2015; 125(6): 1371–6. [II-2: Prospective sequential cohort study, n = 42]

204. Campbell KH, Savitz D, Werner EF, Pettker CM et al. Maternal morbidity and risk of death at delivery hospitalization. *Obstet Gynecol* 2013; 122(3): 627–33. [II-2: Restrospective cohort, Birth certificate data and the Statewide Planning and Research Cooperative System database, n = 1,084,862 live singleton births and n = 132 maternal deaths]

205. Flegal KM, Williamson DF, Pamuk ER et al. Estimating deaths attributable to obesity in the United States. *Am J Public Health* 2004; 94: 1486–9. [III: Review]

206. Molyneaux E, Poston L, Ashurst-Williams S, Howard LM. Obesity and mental disorders during pregnancy and postpartum: A systematic review and meta-analysis. *Obstet Gynecol* 2014; 123(4): 857–67. [II-3: Meta-analysis, 62 studies, n = 540,373]

207. Verret-Chalifour J, Giguere Y, Forest JC, Croteau J et al. Breastfeeding initiation: Impact of obesity in a large Canadian perinatal cohort study. *PLoS ONE* 10(2): e0117512. doi:10.1371/journal.pone.0117512. [II-2: Retrospective cohort, n = 7866]

208. Rothberg BEG, Magriples U, Kershaw TS, Rising SS. Gestational weight gain and subsequent postpartum weight loss among young, low-income, ethnic minority women. *Am J Obstet Gynecol* 2011; 204: 1–11. [II-2: Retrospective cohort, n = 427]

209. Baker JL, Michaelson KF, Sorenson TIA, Rasmussen KM. High prepregnant body mass index is associated with early termination of full and any breastfeeding in Danish women. *Am J Clin Nutr* 2007; 86: 404. [II-2: Retrospective cohort, n = 37,459]

210. Merki-Feld GS, Skouby S, Serfaty D, Lech M et al. European Society of Contraception Statement on Contraception in Obese Women. *Eur J Contracep Reprod Health Care* 2015; 20(1): 19–28. [III: Review]

211. Merhi ZO. Revisiting optimal hormonal contraception following bariatric surgery. *Contraception* 2013; 87(2): 131–3. [III: Review]

212. Yamazaki M, Dwyer K, Sohban M, Davis D et al. Effect of obesity on the effectiveness of hormonal contraceptives: An individual participant data meta-analysis. *Contraception* 2015 (Article in Press) [II-3: Meta-analysis, 7 clinical trials (n = 14,024: 2707 obese and 11,317 nonobese]

213. Yaniv-Salem S, Shoham-Vardi I, Kessous R, Pariente G, Sergienko R, Sheiner E. Obesity in pregnancy: What's next? Long-term cardiovascular morbidity in a follow-up period of more than a decade. *J Matern Fetal Neonatal Med* 2015. doi:10.2109/14767058.2015.1013932. [II-2: Population based retrospective cohort, n = 46,688]

214. Schmiegelow MD, Anderson C, Kober L, Anderson SS et al. Prepregnancy obesity and associations with stroke and myocardial infarction in women in the years after childbirth: A nationwide cohort study. *Circulation* 2014; 113: 330–7. [II-2: Cohort, Danish Medical Birth Register, n = 273,101]

215. Mongraw-Chaffin ML, Anderson CA, Clark JM, Bennett WL. Prepregnancy body mass index and cardiovascular disease mortality: The Child Health and Development Studies. *Obesity* 2014; 22(4): 1149–56. [II-2: Retrospective cohort, California Vital Status Records, n = 1839]

216. Lee KK, Raja EA, Lee AJ, Bhattacharya S et al. Maternal obesity during pregnancy associated with premature mortality and major cardiovascular events in later life. *Hypertension* 2015; pii: HYPERTENSIONAHA.115.05920. [Epub ahead of print]. [II-2: Retrospective cohort, n = 18,873]

217. Krakowiak P, Walker CK, Bremer AA, Baker AS et al. Maternal metabolic conditions and risk for autism and other neurodevelopmental disorders. *Pediatrics* 2012; 129(5): e1121–8. [II-2: Population-based cohort study, *n* = 517 ASD, *n* = 172 DD, *n* = 315 controls]

218. Li YM, Ou JJ, Zhang D, Zhao JP et al. Association between maternal obesity and autism spectrum disorder in offspring: A meta-analysis. *J Autism Dev Disord* 2015; doi:10.1007/s10803-015 -2549-8. [II-3: Meta-analysis, 5 observational studies]

219. Reynolds RM, Allan KM, Raja EA, Bhattacharya S et al. Maternal obesity during pregnancy and premature mortality from cardiovascular event in adult offspring: Follow-up of 1,323,275 person years. *BMJ* 2013; 347: f453. [II-2: Record linkage cohort analysis, Aberdeen Maternity and Neonatal databank, *n* = 37,709]

220. Starling AP, Brinton JT, Glueck DH, Shapiro AL et al. Associations of maternal BMI and gestational weight gain with neonatal adiposity in the Health Start study. *Am J Clin Nutri* 2015; 101: 302–9. [II-2: Prospective cohort, *n* = 1132]

221. Eriksson JG, Sandboge S, Salonen MK, Kajantie E et al. Long-term consequences of maternal overweight in pregnancy on offspring later health: Findings from the Helsinki Birth Cohort Study. *Ann Med* 2014; 46: 434–8. [II-2: Cohort study, Helsinki Birth Cohort Study, *n* = 13,345]

4

Pregestational diabetes

A. Dhanya Mackeen and Michael J. Paglia

KEY POINTS

- **Poorly controlled** diabetes in pregnancy is associated with **increased risks** of first-trimester miscarriage, congenital malformations (especially cardiac defects and CNS anomalies), fetal death, preterm birth, preeclampsia, ketoacidosis, polyhydramnios, macrosomia, operative (both vaginal and cesarean) delivery, birth injury (including brachial plexus), delayed lung maturity, respiratory distress syndrome, jaundice, hypoglycemia, hypocalcemia, and perinatal mortality as well as long-term consequences for the children, such as obesity, type II diabetes, and lower IQ.
- **Preconception counseling should include weight loss, exercise, appropriate diet, and optimization of blood sugar control.** Normalization of glucose levels (**hemoglobin A1c <6%**) prevents most, if not all, of the complications of diabetes in pregnancy.
- In pregestational diabetics, **fasting glucose ≤95 mg/dL and two-hour postprandial ≤120 mg/dL (or one-hour postprandial ≤140 mg/dL)** should be achieved and maintained at all times with diet, exercise, and insulin therapy as necessary.
- There is insufficient evidence to assess the efficacy of oral hypoglycemic agents in pregestational diabetes.
- **Diabetic ketoacidosis is treated with aggressive hydration and intravenous insulin.**
- In pregestational diabetics with good glycemic control, timing of delivery should occur between 39 0/7–39 6/7 weeks; cesarean delivery should be offered if estimated fetal weight is ≥4500 g.

Diagnosis/Definition

Diabetes mellitus (DM) is defined as a metabolic abnormality characterized by elevated circulating glucose. **The diagnoses of diabetes and impaired glucose tolerance outside of pregnancy are established on the basis of formal laboratory criteria** (Table 4.1) [1–4]. As different countries use either mmol/L or mg/dL for glucose values, a comparison is provided (Table 4.2).

Symptoms

Often asymptomatic, but classic symptoms of uncontrolled diabetes are polydipsia, polyuria, and polyphagia.

Epidemiology/Incidence

Though the prevalence of pregestational DM continues to increase in many high-income countries, specific incidence is difficult to calculate due to the inconsistent inclusion of gestational diabetes. Diabetes was noted to complicate 6% of all pregnancies in the United States in 2013 although the majority of these are likely gestational [5,6].

Basic Pathophysiology

The etiology of the disease varies and includes a primary insulin production defect, insulin receptor abnormalities, end-organ insulin resistance, and diabetes secondary to another disease process, such as cystic fibrosis [3]. *Type I* diabetics are insulin deficient secondary to the autoimmune destruction of the pancreatic islet beta cells [3]. These individuals develop disease early in life, require insulin replacement, and become acutely symptomatic with ketoacidosis if no therapy is initiated. In contrast *type II* diabetics continue to produce insulin, but do so at diminished levels. They are often hyperinsulinemic, at least in the early stages; relative hypo-insulinemia may (or may not) develop later [3]. Insulin resistance is the cardinal feature of type II diabetics and many exhibit insulin resistance at the level of the end-organ receptor. The onset of disease is usually later in life, the course is gradual but progressive, and the disease is linked to obesity [3]. The onset of disease is rapidly changing: type II diabetes is now being seen at earlier ages, including childhood and adolescence. Both groups can be further subclassified on the basis of the presence of vascular complications, such as hypertension, renal disease, and retinopathy. The same physiologic changes of pregnancy that cause gestational diabetes (see Chapter 5) also complicate the achievement of optimal glucose control in the pregestational diabetic. In a meta-analysis, women with type II diabetes had a 1.5 times increased risk of perinatal mortality, decreased risk of diabetic ketoacidosis, and decreased cesarean delivery rate as compared to those with type I diabetes; however, there were no significant differences between the two groups in the frequency of major congenital malformation, stillbirth, or neonatal mortality [7].

Classification

To facilitate the management of these patients, the classification of diabetes has undergone recent revisions to reflect the physiology and implications of the disease process. Classification as type I and type II diabetes (as defined above) is still commonly used, especially in nonpregnant patients. Presence of vascular disease, defined as chronic hypertension (HTN), renal insufficiency, retinopathy, coronary artery disease, or prior cerebrovascular accident, is a better predictor of adverse pregnancy outcome than is White's classification [8,9]. Therefore, the White's classification is no longer recommended for management.

Risk Factors/Associations

Obesity, hypertension, advanced maternal age, non-white race, family history (type II diabetes), metabolic syndrome, among others.

Table 4.1   Criteria for the Diagnosis of Diabetes Mellitus in the Nonpregnant State

Normal Values	Impaired Fasting Glucose or Impaired Glucose Tolerance	Diabetes Mellitus
FPG: <100 mg/dL 75 g, 2-hour OGTT: 2-hour PG <140 mg/dL	FPG: 100–125 mg/dL 75 g, 2-hour OGTT: 2-hour PG 140–199 mg/dL Hemoglobin A1c 5.7%–6.4%	FPG: ≥126 mg/dL (7.0 mmol/L)[a] 75 g, 2-hour OGTT: 2-hour PG ≥200 mg/dL (11.1 mmol/L)[a] Hemoglobin A1c ≥6.5%[a] Symptoms of hyperglycemia and PG (without regard to time since last meal) ≥200 mg/dL (11.1 mmol/L)

Source: American Diabetes Association. Diabetes Management guidelines 2015. 2015, http://www.ndei.org/ADA-diabetes -management-guidelines-diagnosis-A1C-testing.aspx.
Abbreviations: FPG, fasting plasma glucose; OGTT, oral glucose tolerance test; PG, plasma glucose.
[a]Unless unequivocal hyperglycemia is present, the diagnosis of diabetes mellitus should be confirmed on a separate day by any of these three tests.

Table 4.2   Glucose Equivalents

mmol/L	mg/dL
5.9	105
6.7	120
7.8	140
8.0	144
11.0	198

Table 4.3   Diabetes Workup in Pregnancy

Workup
- Careful history (review of glucose control and therapy; history of end-organ disease)
- Laboratory tests (preconception or first trimester if feasible):
  - Hemoglobin A1c
  - Metabolic profile (glucose, creatinine)
  - Urine culture: repeat each trimester
  - 24-hour urine collection for protein and creatinine clearance
  - TSH for type I diabetics
- Consider EKG, especially if concomitant hypertension
- Consider ophthalmologic consult to assess for any retinopathy, especially if long-standing or poorly controlled diabetes mellitus

Abbreviation: EKG, electrocardiogram.

Complications

Incidence of complications is **inversely proportional to glucose control** with minimal complications if glucose control is optimal [10]. Pedersen first proposed that the exaggerated fetal response to insulin is provoked by fetal hyperglycemia that results from maternal hyperglycemia [11]. Poorly controlled DM is associated with increased risks of the following: *first-trimester miscarriage; congenital malformations* [12] (most common malformations are cardiac defects and CNS anomalies, especially neural tube defects [13]; most pathognomonic are sacral agenesis/ caudal regression); *intrauterine fetal demise; preterm birth* (both iatrogenic and spontaneous); *preeclampsia; ketoacidosis; polyhydramnios; macrosomia* (increased fetal insulin acts as growth factor; the degree of macrosomia is correlated with fasting and postprandial blood glucose values outside of the suggested parameters); *operative delivery* (both vaginal and cesarean) and *birth injury* (including brachial plexus) (both related to macrosomia); *delayed lung maturity; respiratory distress syndrome; jaundice* (because of polycythemia), *hypoglycemia, hypocalcemia* and *polycythemia* in the neonate, all related to elevated glucose levels and consequent hyperinsulinemia antenatally; and *perinatal mortality* [14,15]. Long-term follow-up has shown higher rates of *obesity, type II DM,* and *lower IQ* in children of mothers with poorly controlled DM in pregnancy [14–18].

Pregnancy Considerations

It is always important to consider the effect of maternal disease on pregnancy and, conversely, the effect of pregnancy on maternal end organs (Table 4.3), especially because pregestational diabetes affects the micro- and macrovascular systems. Diabetic **retinopathy** is the leading cause of blindness in reproductive years. Background retinopathy is characterized by retinal microaneurysms and dot-blot hemorrhages and proliferative retinopathy by neovascularization. Proliferative diabetic retinopathy may progress as tightened glycemic control is achieved [19]. However, clinicians should not be deterred from achieving optimal glucose control as the risk of subsequent progression of retinopathy is overall decreased as compared to patients not managed with intensive therapy [19]. Diabetic **nephropathy** occurs in 5% to 10% of pregestational diabetics and can progress to end-stage renal disease, especially in women with creatinine of ≥1.4 mg/dL or 24-hour proteinuria of ≥3 g (see Chapter 17). Proteinuria increases in diabetic patients as they approach term, particularly in those who have baseline nephropathy. Women with baseline nephropathy are at increased risk of iatrogenic preterm birth and uteroplacental insufficiency. Progression of renal insufficiency is not clearly linked to the physiologically increased glomerular filtration rate of pregnancy although those with nephrotic range proteinuria and moderate-to-severe renal insufficiency may progress to end-stage renal disease [20,21]. Diabetic **neuropathy** is not worsened, per se, in pregnancy although decreased gastrointestinal motility related to progesterone and mechanical factors may exacerbate underlying gastroparesis [21]. The presence of **hypertension** (in 5%–10% of women with pregestational DM) further increases the risks of preeclampsia, fetal growth restriction, and fetal death [20]. Progression of **cardiovascular** disease in the diabetic pregnant patient has not been reported, but symptomatic coronary artery disease is a contraindication to pregnancy in these diabetic women [21].

Management (Table 4.4)

Principles
Strict glycemic control, aiming for HgbA1c of <7%.

Workup
See Table 4.3.

Table 4.4   Management of the Pregestational Diabetic

Preconception counseling
- Weight loss
- Exercise
- Glucose testing
- Treatment of hyperglycemia as appropriate
- Strict glucose control

Preconception evaluation (Table 4.5)
- Normalization of the hemoglobin A1c to within 1% of normal (<7%)
- Evaluate the presence of vascular disease
  - Ophthalmologic exam with retinal evaluation
  - 24-hour urine for protein and creatinine clearance
  - EKG
- Nutritional counseling (Table 4.7)
  - 30–35 kcal/kg/day if normal weight
- Institute glucose testing to include fasting and postprandial values (Table 4.8)
- Incorporate exercise regimen
- Start or refine insulin regimen (Figures 5.1 and 5.2)

Antepartum management
- Insulin therapy adjusted by weight and pregnancy trimester as guided by glucose monitoring (Tables 4.8 and 5.4; Figures 5.1 and 5.2)
- Viability/dating scan
- Fetal surveillance and antepartum testing (Table 4.11)
  - Alpha-fetoprotein screening at 16–20 weeks
  - Detailed anatomic survey at 18–20 weeks
  - Fetal echocardiogram (at 14–16 weeks especially if hemoglobin A1c >8%) and at 20–22 weeks
  - Serial ultrasounds for growth in the second and third trimester
  - Antenatal assessments with NST or BPP weekly or twice weekly from 32 to 35 6/7 weeks, then twice weekly until delivery
    - Start at 28 weeks if diabetes is poorly controlled

Intrapartum management (Figure 4.1)
- Trial of labor unless clinical or ultrasound estimated fetal weight greater than 4500 g
- Delivery at: 39 0/7–39 6/7 weeks if pregestational diabetes is well controlled; 37 0/7–39 6/7 weeks if pregestational diabetes is complicated by vascular disease; 34 0/7–39 6/7 weeks (individualized to situation) if diabetes is poorly controlled [22]
- IV insulin therapy to maintain blood sugar between 70 and 110 mg/dL
- IV dextrose solution if blood sugars fall <70 mg/dL or with development of ketonuria
- For scheduled cesarean section, administer the dose of long-acting insulin in p.m. and withhold the a.m. short-acting dose
- Monitor blood glucose hourly

Postpartum management
- Reduce the antepartum insulin dose by half and administer it with the resumption of oral intake
- Supplement breast-feeding mothers with extra 500 kcal compared to nonpregnant levels

Abbreviations: BPP, biophysical profile; EKG, electrocardiogram; IV, intravenous; NST, nonstress test.

Prevention
Weight loss, exercise, and optimization of blood sugar control can prevent most, if not all, of the complications of DM in pregnancy.

Preconception Counseling

The care of the pregestational diabetic is best instituted in the preconception period. The objectives of prepregnancy care are shown in Table 4.5. The frequency of maternal hospitalizations, length of NICU admission, congenital malformations, and perinatal mortality are reduced in women with DM who seek consultation in preparation for pregnancy; unfortunately, only about one third of these women receive such consultation [23].

The evaluation should emphasize the importance of tight glycemic control with **normalization of the hemoglobin A1c (aim for at least <7%)** (Tables 4.4, 4.5, and 4.6) [8,24,25]. Decreased spontaneous miscarriage, congenital anomalies, and other complications have been demonstrated in multiple studies, including RCTs, when optimal glucose control is attained via multiple daily insulin doses adjusted to glucose monitoring ≥4 times per day [26,27]. Optimal glucose control also prevents future obesity, DM, and its complications in the offspring. In addition to advocating the use of at least 400 micrograms of folic acid for at least one month prior to conception, this consultation affords the opportunity to screen for end-organ damage (Table 4.3). Ophthalmologic evaluation, EKG, and renal evaluation via a 24-hour urine collection for total protein and creatinine clearance will ascertain end-organ damage and determine ancillary pregnancy risks. As 40% of young women with type I diabetes have hypothyroidism, thyroid-stimulating hormone (TSH) should be checked. Proliferative retinopathy should be treated with laser before pregnancy. Women compliant with insulin pumps may continue this regimen. Sexually active diabetic adolescents benefit from preconception counseling [28,29].

Prenatal Care

Optimizing health outcomes can be achieved by a combination of diet, exercise, glucose monitoring, and insulin therapy. Women with type I DM and glucose levels of >200 mg/dL

Table 4.5   The Objectives of Diabetes Prepregnancy Care

- Patient education
- Assessment of patient's medical condition
- Optimize glycemic control (hemoglobin A1c <6% *prior to conception*)
- Folic acid supplementation (at least 400 µg) for at least one month *prior* to conception

Table 4.6   Risk of Congenital Malformations Based on Hemoglobin A1c

HbA1c (%)	Risk
<7	No increased risk
7–10	3%–7%
10–11	8%–10%
≥11	10%–20% or more

Source: Guerin A, Nisenbaum R, Ray JG. *Diabetes Care*, 30, 7, 1920–5, 2007.

should check their urine ketones and immediately alert their health care provider if positive [8]. A glass of milk is preferable to juice for hypoglycemia. Glucagon should be immediately available.

Diet

Nutritional requirements are adjusted on the basis of maternal body mass index (BMI); women with normal BMI require 30 to 35 kcal/kg/day (Table 4.7) [8]. Individuals <90% of their ideal body weight (IBW) may increase this by an additional 5 kcal/kg/day, and those >120% of their IBW should decrease this value to 24 kcal/kg/day [8]. The content should be distributed as 45% complex, high-fiber carbohydrates, 20% protein, and 35% primarily unsaturated fats (Table 4.7) [8,23]. The calories are distributed over three meals and three snacks with breakfast receiving the smallest allotment at 15%, and the other two meals receiving near equal distribution. Saccharin, aspartame, acesulfame-K, maltodextrin, and sucralose may be used safely in moderate amounts. Carbohydrate counting and the assistance of a registered dietitian may provide benefit, but these two interventions have been insufficiently studied in pregnancy [30].

Exercise

Moderate exercise decreases the need for insulin therapy in type II diabetics by increasing the glucose uptake in skeletal muscle and, therefore, should be strongly encouraged for diabetic patients although it is important to take into consideration any preexisting comorbidities, including class III obesity [31].

Glucose Monitoring

Frequent home glucose monitoring, both pre- and postprandially, has been associated with enhanced glucose control and shorter interval to achieve target blood sugars. Capillary blood glucose ("finger stick") measurements using a glucometer should be obtained at least four times a day—fasting and two hours (or one hour) postprandial [32,33]. There are no RCTs comparing one- versus two-hour postprandial glucose monitoring in pregnancy. Target levels are

Table 4.7 Diabetic Diet

30–35 kcal/kg/day (usually 2000–2400 kcal/day)	
3 meals, 3 snacks	
Composition	
Carbohydrate (complex)	45%
Protein	20%
Fat (<10% saturated)	35%

Source: ACOG practice bulletin. Pregestational diabetes mellitus. *Obstet Gynecol*, 105, 675–84, 2005.

Table 4.8 Target Venous Plasma Glucose Levels

Timing of Measurement	Ideal Glucose Range (mg/dL)
Fasting	60–90
Preprandial	60–100
One-hour postprandial	≤140
Two-hour postprandial	≤120
3 a.m.	60–90

Source: Landon MB, Catalano PM, Gabbe SG. Diabetes mellitus complicating pregnancy. In: Gabbe SG, Niebyl JR, Simpson JL, eds. *Obstetrics: Normal and problem pregnancies.* 5th ed. Elsevier, 976–1005, 2007.

in Table 4.8 [34]. Some women will require another assessment at 3 a.m. for prevention of hypoglycemic episodes.

Glycosylated hemoglobin A1c <6% is normal [35]. Hemoglobin A1c of 6% reflects a mean glucose level of 120 mg/dL; each 1% increment in hemoglobin A1c is equal to a change in mean glucose level of 30 mg/dL. There is evidence that blood sugars (and hemoglobin A1c measurements) should be maintained within normal limits throughout gestation and not just in a particular trimester to decrease the risk of poor pregnancy outcomes [36]. Although earlier studies [37,38] suggested some benefit to continuous glucose monitoring, more recent studies showed no improvement in glycemic control or in maternal/fetal outcomes in women using continuous (measurements every 10 seconds for up to 288 measurements daily) glucose monitoring intermittently (for six days at various time points in pregnancy) versus routine monitoring [39] or constant continuous monitoring [40].

Oral Hypoglycemic Agents

Although overall considered safe to use in pregnancy [41,42], **there is insufficient evidence to assess the effectiveness of oral hypoglycemic agents in women with pregestational diabetes**. Therefore, even in women on oral hypoglycemic control before pregnancy, insulin therapy is suggested for glucose control. Occasionally, a woman well controlled on either glyburide or metformin prepregnancy and with a normal hemoglobin A1c can be managed by continuing these medications as long as glycemic control remains optimal [27,41,43]; although newer evidence suggests that metformin is preferred over glyburide when oral hypoglycemic agents are employed (at least for GDM management) [44]. Improved maternal glycemic control and reduced neonatal hypoglycemia, respiratory distress syndrome, and NICU admission were noted when metformin was added to an insulin regimen in women with poor control despite daily insulin dose of ≥1.12 units/kg [45].

Insulin

Multiple-dose insulin (MDI) injection therapy is the mainstay in the management of pregestational diabetes. All subcutaneous insulin types have been approved during pregnancy.

A review of the types of insulin, their onset, and duration of action are listed in Table 4.9. Human insulin is preferred to animal insulin [46]. Women, particularly those new to insulin therapy, need to be counseled about the differences in the various insulins in order to use them to their greatest efficacy. Close monitoring with **at least weekly contact with a provider** is suggested to maximize insulin adjustment. The goals of therapy are shown in Table 4.8 [34]. Both fasting and postprandial blood sugars are correlated with fetal

Table 4.9 Types of Insulin and Their Pharmacokinetics [see further Ref. 47]

Type	Onset	Peak	Duration
Lispro/ aspart	15–30 minutes	0.5–3 hours	≤5 hours
Regular	30 minutes	2.5–5 hours	4–12 hours
NPH	1–2 hours	4–12 hours	14–24 hours
Detemir	3–4 hours	3–9 hours	6–23 hours (dose dependent)
Glargine	3–4 hours	none	24 hours

macrosomia, especially elevated postprandials (see Chapter 5) [48,49]. Hypoglycemia can cause significant maternal morbidities but has not been associated with embryopathy [50]. *Glucagon* should be available for home use in emergency situations.

Although satisfactory glucose control may be obtained solely with an intermediate-acting insulin rather than a short-acting insulin [51], we suggest optimizing metabolic control with one evening injection of **long-acting** insulin **(e.g., insulin glargine)** and meal-time (three daily) injections of **short-acting insulin (e.g., lispro or aspart)** (Figures 5.1 and 5.2). Glargine cannot be mixed in the same syringe with other insulins. Intermediate-acting insulin (e.g., neutral protamine Hagedorn [NPH]) twice daily can also be used instead of insulin glargine. Studies have shown that short-acting insulin is as effective as regular insulin and may result in improved postprandial glucose control and less preterm deliveries [52,53]. Insulin lispro should be given immediately before eating. As compared to two daily insulin injections, additional doses are associated with improved glycemic control [54]. A meta-analysis of cohort studies comparing insulin glargine to NPH did not reveal any significant differences in outcomes, including infant birth weight, congenital anomalies, and respiratory distress [55]. A large randomized trial, including 310 pregnancies compared insulin detemir with NPH and found no differences between maternal HgA1c, the frequency of major hypoglycemic episodes [56], early fetal loss, congenital anomalies or adverse events [57].

Subcutaneous insulin pump therapy (continuous subcutaneous insulin infusion therapy [CSII]) may be continued in women already compliant with this mode of therapy. In nonpregnant adults, women compliant with insulin pumps have increased satisfaction, decreased episodes of severe hypoglycemia, and better control of hyperglycemia [8]. Basal infusion rates tend to increase, and carbohydrate-to-insulin ratios decrease during the course of pregnancy [58]. There is currently insufficient evidence to recommend CSII versus MDI in pregnancy in women not already on pumps [59,60]. Inhaled insulin has been tested in nonpregnant adults, but there are yet insufficient data for pregnancy management [61].

Carbohydrate counting and the use of an insulin-to-carbohydrate ratio of 1 unit of insulin for every 15 g of carbohydrate in early gestation can allow for greater flexibility in eating but has not been studied in a trial. As pregnancy advances with its concomitant increased insulin resistance, an increased ratio is required with 1 unit covering a lower amount of carbohydrates, for example, 1 unit/3 g of carbohydrate [58].

Useful sample calculations for the total daily insulin requirement and insulin regimen are in Table 5.4 and Figures 5.1 and 5.2.

Very Tight vs. Tight Control

There are limited data to assess the effect of moderately tight versus very tight glycemic control in women with type I pregestational diabetes, but there is some evidence to suggest **very tight control** (either fasting and 2 hour pp <5.6 mmol/L or fasting <4.4 mmol/L and 1.5 hour pp <6.7 mmol/L) **improves neonatal metabolic outcomes including hypoglycemia** [62]. **Loose control (fasting blood glucose above 7.0 mmol/L) is associated with increased incidences of preeclampsia,**

cesarean deliveries, and infants that were large for gestational age [63]. There are no data to assess the clinical impact for prevention of significant long-term neonatal morbidity. Patients with type I diabetes may be at increased susceptibility to hypoglycemia during pregnancy than in the prepregnant state; early pregnancy hypoglycemia was not associated with an increased risk of early pregnancy loss or malformations, which is consistent with other studies [50].

Diabetic Ketoacidosis

Diabetic ketoacidosis occurs in 5% to 10% of pregnant women with pregestational type I diabetes. It is defined by elevated glucose (usually >250 mg/dL), positive serum ketones, and acidosis. Risk factors include type I diabetes, new onset diabetes, infections (e.g., urinary or respiratory tract infections), poor compliance, insulin pump failure, and treatment with beta-mimetics or steroids [8]. Symptoms include abdominal pain, nausea, vomiting, and altered sensorium. Laboratory tests should include an arterial blood gas (pH <7.3), electrolytes (serum bicarbonate <15 mEq/L and elevated anion gap), serum and urinary ketones (elevated). **Aggressive hydration, intravenous insulin, and correction of the underlying etiology are the most important interventions,** with close electrolyte (especially glucose and potassium) monitoring (Table 4.10) [8,64,65]. Fetal mortality may be up to 10%, even with aggressive management.

Table 4.10 Management of Diabetic Ketoacidosis in Pregnancy

IV hydration: Use isotonic saline (0.9% NS)
- First hour: Give 1 L NS
- Hours 2–4: 0.5–1 L NS/hour
- Thereafter (24 hours): Give 250 mL/hour 0.45% NS until 80% deficit corrected
- Body water deficit = {[0.6 body weight (kg)] + [1−(140/ serum sodium)]} ≈ 100 mL deficit/kg body weight

Insulin: Mix 50 units of regular insulin in 500 mL of NS and flush IV tubing prior to infusion
- Loading: 0.2–0.4 units/kg
- Maintenance: 2–10 units/hour
- Continue insulin therapy until bicarbonate and anion gap normalize

Potassium replacement: Maintain serum K^+ at 4–5 mEq/L
- If K^+ is initially normal or reduced, consider an infusion of up to 15–20 mEq/hour
- If K^+ is elevated, do not add supplemental potassium until levels are within normal range, then add 20–30 mEq/L

Phosphate: Consider replacement if serum phosphate <1.0 mg/ dL or if cardiac dysfunction present or patient obtunded

Bicarbonate: If pH is <7.1, add one ampule (44 mEq) of bicarbonate to 1 L of 0.45% NS

Laboratory tests: Check arterial blood gas on admission; check serum glucose, ketones, and electrolytes every one to two hours until normal
- Consider doubling insulin infusion rate if serum glucose does not decrease by 20% within the first two hours
- When blood glucose reaches 250 mg/dL, change IVF to D5NS
- Continue insulin drip until ketosis resolves and the first subcutaneous dose of insulin is administered

Sources: Carroll MA, Yeomans ER. *Crit Care Med*, 33, 10 Suppl., S347–53, 2005; ACOG practice bulletin. Pregestational diabetes mellitus. *Obstet Gynecol*, 105, 675–84, 2005.
Abbreviations: IVF, intravenous fluids; kg, kilograms; K^+, potassium; NS, normal saline.

Antepartum Testing

Fetal surveillance is required to determine whether congenital anomalies are present and to minimize perinatal mortality (Table 4.11). The nature of this surveillance is by convention and expert consensus rather than supported by well-performed trials. Because of the increased risk of birth defects, particularly cardiac and neural tube defects, patients should be offered alpha-fetoprotein screening at 16 to 18 weeks gestation, targeted ultrasonography at 18 to 20 weeks, and **fetal echocardiography at 20 to 22 weeks**. Some suggest an earlier first anatomic fetal sonographic survey at around 14 to 16 weeks as well as early fetal echocardiography at this time, especially in women with poor glycemic control in the first trimester (e.g., hemoglobin A1c >10 mg/dL). Serial ultrasounds in the third trimester to evaluate fetal growth and frequent prenatal visits to review glucose control are also advocated. The use of fetal surveillance with nonstress test (NST) and/or biophysical profile is recommended by expert opinion [23], but the frequency and nature of the testing cannot be determined, since there is no randomized trial to direct effective screening. For women with good glycemic control, antepartum testing can start at 32 weeks with once or twice weekly NSTs, increased to twice weekly at 36 weeks, and continued until delivery [8]. For women with poor glycemic control, antepartum testing may need to begin earlier [8].

Delivery

Timing
Timing of delivery in women with pregestational DM in good control is usually at about 39 0/7–39 6/7 weeks (unless maternal or fetal factors dictate earlier intervention) as perinatal mortality increases after 40 weeks. In general, indicated delivery before 39 weeks, if truly indicated, should not require assessment of fetal maturity. If assessment of fetal maturity is done, laboratory tests are interpreted as in nondiabetic patients, with phosphatidylglycerol ≥3% accepted by most authorities as the lab value indicating the least risk for fetal respiratory insufficiency in diabetic women; patients

Table 4.11 Antepartum Testing

A. Assessment of viability and exact GA: first-trimester ultrasound
B. Detection of congenital malformations
   1. If hemoglobin A1c is elevated, consider transvaginal ultrasound at about 14 weeks to rule out structural defects, including cardiac
   2. Maternal serum alpha-fetoprotein level at 16 weeks
   3. Level II ultrasound at 18–20 weeks
   4. Fetal echocardiogram at 20–22 weeks
C. Assessment of fetal growth
   1. Serial growth ultrasounds in third trimester every 3–4 weeks
D. Assessment of fetal well-being
   1. Maternal assessment of fetal activity ("fetal kick counts")
   2. Once or twice weekly NSTs/BPPs starting at 32 weeks until 36 weeks, then twice weekly until delivery. Begin at 32 weeks if maternal glycemic control is satisfactory, fetal growth is appropriate, and there are no coexisting maternal medical or obstetric complications. Begin earlier (~28 weeks) with increased frequency if the above conditions are not met

Abbreviations: BPP, biophysical profile; NST, nonstress tests.

should be cautioned that a positive test does not preclude infant morbidities (see Chapter 57). Compared to expectant management until 42 weeks, induction of labor at 38 completed weeks in women with insulin-dependent diabetes (of which >90% were gestational) is associated with reduced incidences of macrosomia [66,67]. However, the sample size was too small to evaluate the impact on perinatal mortality, which is a concern in women with diabetes who are delivered prior to 39 weeks [66].

Mode
Mode of delivery is generally vaginal. **Cesarean** is indicated if estimated **fetal weight is ≥4500 g** (see Chapter 45) [8]. The diagnosis of macrosomia is inexact by ultrasound and clinical estimation, confounding the ability to make a clear recommendation. Induction for macrosomia is not recommended due to lack of evidence for benefit [68,69].

Intrapartum Glucose Management
The usual subcutaneous long-acting (e.g., glargine) or intermediate-acting insulin (e.g., NPH) is given at bedtime the evening before delivery, and the usual subcutaneous morning insulin is withheld on the day of delivery. Intrapartum management (Figure 4.1) [34] is targeted to maintain maternal glucose levels between 70 and 110 mg/dL. Often the insulin requirement is decreased because of the energy requirements of labor. Intravenous insulin, dextrose solution, frequent (usually every one hour) glucose monitoring, and evaluation of urinary ketones are required to prevent a catabolic state and the development of ketoacidosis. Once active labor begins or glucose is <70 mg/dL, IV 5% dextrose at 125 cc/hour can be started. Once glucose level is ≥100 mg/dL, short-acting (e.g., lispro or regular) IV insulin should be started. IV 5% dextrose and insulin infusions should be separate and often should occur at the same time to prevent ketonuria. Adjustments to the basal infusion rates are based on hourly finger stick blood sugars while in labor. The use of the insulin pump, maintaining the basal rate, rather than using an IV insulin infusion, is an accepted alternative. A small, randomized controlled trial did not show any benefit to using real-time continuous glucose monitoring versus hourly monitoring during labor to reduce the likelihood of neonatal hypoglycemia [70].

With cesarean delivery, use of a single injection of long-acting insulin, an IV insulin infusion, or subcutaneous pump at a low basal rate are equal alternatives until oral intake is assured and more standard dosing can be reinstituted. Insulin requirements are diminished postpartum and are generally half of the antepartum requirement.

Anesthesia
No specific adjustments necessary.

Postpartum/Breast-Feeding
Usual diabetic diet should be restarted after delivery with one half of the predelivery dose or the full prepregnancy dose (if this achieved euglycemia) restarted [34]. If food intake cannot be restarted soon, then glucose levels of >140 mg/dL should be treated with proper coverage. Breast-feeding has increased maternal caloric demands and an additional 500 kcal/day needs to be added to the diet to avoid hypoglycemia. All

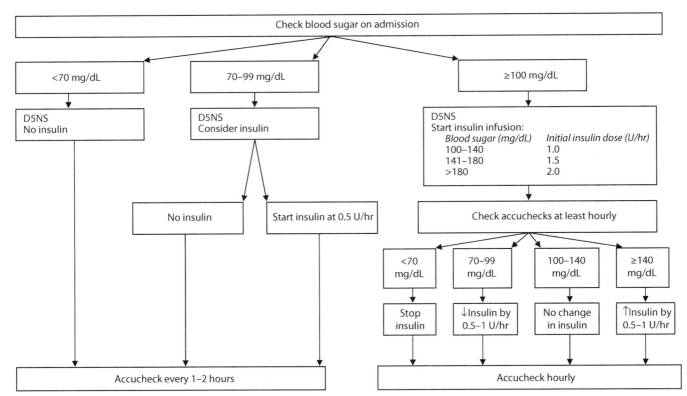

Please note:
• These are suggestions, and patients should be managed on a case-by-case basis.
• Insulin should be mixed as follows: Mix 10 units of short-acting insulin in 1000 mL of D5NS.
• Intravenous fluids should be infused at a rate of 100–150 cc/h (2.5 mg/kg/min).
• If patients persistently have blood sugars >180 mg/dL, consider normal saline (NS) instead of D5NS and evaluate for DKA.
• We suggest having two lines, one running NS and one running D5NS, so that rate of NS infusion can be changed as per L&D needs and D5NS can be consistently infused.

Figure 4.1   Intrapartum management of diabetes (GDMA2 and pregestational). *Abbreviations*: DKA, diabetic ketoacidosis; L&D, labor and delivery; NS, normal saline. (Adapted from ACOG practice bulletin. *Obstet Gynecol*, 105, 675–84, 2005; Landon MB, Catalano PM, Gabbe SG. Diabetes mellitus complicating pregnancy. In: Gabbe SG, Niebyl JR, Simpson JL, eds. *Obstetrics: Normal and problem pregnancies*. 5th ed. Elsevier, 976–1005, 2007.)

forms of contraception are available to diabetics, providing they have no contraindications, such as hypertension or vascular disease (see Chapter 27 of *Obstetrics Evidence Based Guidelines*).

Future

New therapeutic approaches include pancreatic islet cell transplant.

REFERENCES

1. Galernau F, Inzucchi SE. Diabetes mellitus in pregnancy. *Obstetrics and Gynecology Clinics of North America* 2004; 31: 907–33. [Review]
2. Expert Committee on the Diagnosis and Classification of Diabetes Mellitus. Report of the expert committee on the diagnosis and classification of diabetes mellitus. *Diabetes Care* 2003; 26(Suppl. 1): S5–20. [Review, Guideline]
3. American Diabetes Association. Diagnosis and classification of diabetes mellitus. *Diabetes Care* 2010; 33(Suppl. 1): S26–69. [Review, guideline]
4. American Diabetes Association. Diabetes Management guidelines 2015. 2015, http://www.ndei.org/ADA-diabetes-management-guidelines-diagnosis-A1C-testing.aspx. [Guideline]
5. Martin JA, Hamilton BE, Osterman MJ, Curtin SC, Matthews TJ. Births: Final data for 2013. *Natl Vital Stat Rep* 2015; 64(1): 1–68. http://www.cdc.gov/nchs/data/nvsr/nvsr64/nvsr64_01.pdf. [Data review]
6. American Diabetes Association. Management of diabetes in pregnancy. *Diabetes Care* 2015; 38: S77–9. [Review]
7. Balsells M, Garcia-Patterson A, Gich I, Corcoy R. Maternal and fetal outcome in women with type 2 versus type 1 diabetes mellitus: A systematic review and meta-analysis. *J Clin Endocrinol Metab* 2009; 94(11): 4284–91. [Meta-analysis, 33 RCTs, *n* ≥ 11,000]
8. ACOG practice bulletin. Pregestational diabetes mellitus. *Obstet Gynecol* 2005; 105: 675–84. [Review, guideline]
9. Cormier CM, Martinez CA, Refuerzo JS et al. White's classification of diabetes in pregnancy in the 21st century: Is it still valid? *Am J Perinatol* 2010; 27(5): 349–52. [II-2]
10. Jovanovic L, Druzin M, Peterson CM. Effect of euglycemia on the outcome of pregnancy in insulin-dependent diabetic women as compared with normal control subjects. *Am J Med* 1981; 71(6): 921–7. [Level II-2]
11. Pedersen J. Diabetes and pregnancy. Blood sugar of newborn infants during fasting and glucose administration. *Nordisk Medicin* 1952; 2: 1049. [Level III]
12. Correa A, Giloba SM, Besser LM, Botto LD, Moore CA, Hobbs CA, Cleves MA, Riehle-Colarusso TJ, Waller K, Reece A. Diabetes mellitus and birth defects. *Am J Obstet Gynecol* 2008; 199(3): 237.e1–9. [Review]

13. Yazdy MM, Liu S, Mitchell AA, Werler MM. Maternal dietary glycemic intake and the risk of neural tube defects. *Am J Epidemiol* 2010; 171(4): 407–14. [Case control, *n* = 1394]

14. Tyrala EE. The infant of the diabetic mother. *Obstet Gynecol Clin North Am* 1996; 23(1): 221–41. [Review]

15. Boulet SL, Alexander GR, Salihu HM, Pass M. Macrosomic births in the United States: Determinants, outcomes, and proposed grades of risk. *Am J Obstet Gynecol* 2003; 188(5): 1372–8. [Case control, *n* = 8.2 million]

16. Van Assche FA, Holemans K, Aerts L. Fetal growth and consequences for later life. *J Perinat Med* 1998; 26(5): 337–46. [Review]

17. Rizzo T, Metzger BE, Burns WJ, Burns K. Correlations between antepartum maternal metabolism and child intelligence. *N Engl J Med* 1991; 325(13): 911–6. [Observational, *n* = 223]

18. Dabelea D, Knowler WC, Pettitt DJ. Effect of diabetes in pregnancy on offspring: Follow-up research in the Pima Indians. *J Matern Fetal Med* 2000; 9(1): 83–8. [II-3]

19. The effect of intensive treatment of diabetes on the development and progression of long-term complications in insulin-dependent diabetes mellitus. The diabetes control and complications trial research group. *N Engl J Med* 1993; 329(14): 977–86. [RCT, *n* = 1441]

20. Simpson LL. Maternal medical disease: Risk of antepartum fetal death. *Semin Perinatol* 2002; 26(1): 42–50. [Data review]

21. Kitzmiller JL, Block JM, Brown FM et al. Managing preexisting diabetes for pregnancy: Summary of evidence and consensus recommendations for care. *Diabetes Care* 2008; 31(5): 1060–79. [Review]

22. Spong CY, Mercer BM, D'alton M, Kilpatrick S, Blackwell S, Saade G. Timing of indicated late-preterm and early-term birth. *Obstet Gynecol* 2011; 118(2 Pt. 1): 323–33. [Review, guideline]

23. Koerenbrot CC, Steinberg A, Bender C et al. Preconception care: A systematic review. *Maternal and Child Health Journal* 2002; (6): 75–88. [Review of seven studies addressing the value of preconceptional care in the diabetic patient]

24. Jensen DM, Korsholm L, Ovesen P et al. Peri-conceptional A1C and risk of serious adverse pregnancy outcome in 933 women with type 1 diabetes. *Diabetes Care* 2009; 32(6): 1046–8. [Prospective, *n* = 933]

25. Guerin A, Nisenbaum R, Ray JG. Use of maternal GHb concentration to estimate the risk of congenital anomalies in the offspring of women with prepregnancy diabetes. *Diabetes Care* 2007; 30(7): 1920–5. [II-2]

26. Pregnancy outcomes in the diabetes control and complications trial. *Am J Obstet Gynecol* 1996; 174(4): 1343–53. [RCT, *n* = 180]

27. Tieu J, Middleton P, Crowther CA. Preconception care for diabetic women for improving maternal and infant health. *Cochrane Database Syst Rev* 2010; 12: CD007776. [1 RCT, *n* = 53]

28. Fischl AF, Herman WH, Sereika SM et al. Impact of a preconception counseling program for teens with type 1 diabetes (READY-girls) on patient-provider interaction, resource utilization, and cost. *Diabetes Care* 2010; 33(4): 701–705. [RCT, *n* = 88]

29. Charron-Prochownik D, Ferons-Hannan M, Sereika S, Becker D. Randomized efficacy trial of early preconception counseling for diabetic teens (READY-girls). *Diabetes Care* 2008; 31(7): 1327–30. [RCT, *n* = 53]

30. McCance DR, Holmes VA, Maresh MJ et al. Vitamins C and E for prevention of pre-eclampsia in women with type 1 diabetes (DAPIT): a randomised placebo-controlled trial. *Lancet* 2010; 376(9737): 259–66. [RCT, *n* = 761]

31. Committee opinion no. 650: Physical activity and exercise during pregnancy and the postpartum period. *Obstet Gynecol* 2015; 126(6): e135–42. [Review, guideline]

32. de Veciana M, Major CA, Morgan MA et al. Postprandial versus preprandial blood glucose monitoring in women with gestational diabetes mellitus requiring insulin therapy. *N Engl J Med* 1995; 333(19): 1237–41. [RCT, *n* = 66]

33. Landon MB, Gabbe SG. Gestational diabetes mellitus. *Obstet Gynecol* 2011; 118(6): 1379–93. [Review]

34. Landon MB, Catalano PM, Gabbe SG. Diabetes mellitus complicating pregnancy. In: Gabbe SG, Niebyl JR, Simpson JL, eds. *Obstetrics: Normal and problem pregnancies.* 5th ed. Elsevier, 2007: 976–1005. [Review]

35. Gabbe SG, Graves CR. Management of diabetes mellitus complicating pregnancy. *Obstet Gynecol* 2003; 102(4): 857–68. [III]

36. Damm P, Mersebach H, Rastam J et al. Poor pregnancy outcome in women with type 1 diabetes is predicted by elevated HbA1c and spikes of high glucose values in the third trimester. *J Matern Fetal Neonatal Med* 2014; 27(2): 149–54. [RCT, *n* = 322]

37. Murphy HR, Rayman G, Lewis K et al. Effectiveness of continuous glucose monitoring in pregnant women with diabetes: Randomised clinical trial. *BMJ* 2008; 337: a1680. [RCT, *n* = 71]

38. McLachlan K, Jenkins A, O'Neal D. The role of continuous glucose monitoring in clinical decision-making in diabetes in pregnancy. *Aust N Z J Obstet Gynaecol* 2007; 47(3): 186–90. [Descriptive study, *n* = 68]

39. Secher AL, Ringholm L, Andersen HU, Damm P, Mathiesen ER. The effect of real-time continuous glucose monitoring in pregnant women with diabetes: A randomized controlled trial. *Diabetes Care* 2013; 36(7): 1877–83. [RCT, *n* = 149]

40. Petrovski G, Dimitrovski C, Bogoev M, Milenkovic T, Ahmeti I, Bitovska I. Is there a difference in pregnancy and glycemic outcome in patients with type 1 diabetes on insulin pump with constant or intermittent glucose monitoring? A pilot study. *Diabetes Technology & Therapeutics* 2011; 13(11): 1109–13. [Pilot RCT, *n* = 25]

41. Tieu J, Coat S, Hague W, Middleton P. Oral anti-diabetic agents for women with pre-existing diabetes mellitus/impaired glucose tolerance or previous gestational diabetes mellitus. *Cochrane Database Syst Rev* 2010; 10(10): CD007724. [Meta-analysis, RCTs = 0]

42. Feig DS, Briggs GG, Koren G. Oral antidiabetic agents in pregnancy and lactation: A paradigm shift? *Ann Pharmacother* 2007; 41(7): 1174–80. [Review]

43. Tieu J, Crowther CA, Middleton P. Dietary advice in pregnancy for preventing gestational diabetes mellitus. *Cochrane Database Syst Rev* 2008; 2(2): CD006674. [Meta-analysis, 2 RCTs, *n* = 82]

44. Balsells M, Garcia-Patterson A, Sola I, Roque M, Gich I, Corcoy R. Glibenclamide, metformin, and insulin for the treatment of gestational diabetes: A systematic review and meta-analysis. *BMJ* 2015; 350: h102. [Meta-analysis, 15 RCTs, *n* = 2509]

45. Ibrahim MI, Hamdy A, Shafik A, Taha S, Anwar M, Faris M. The role of adding metformin in insulin-resistant diabetic pregnant women: A randomized controlled trial. *Arch Gynecol Obstet* 2014; 289(5): 959–65. [RCT, *n* = 90]

46. Jovanovic-Peterson L, Kitzmiller JL, Peterson CM. Randomized trial of human versus animal species insulin in diabetic pregnant women: Improved glycemic control, not fewer antibodies to insulin, influences birth weight. *Am J Obstet Gynecol* 1992; 167(5): 1325–30. [RCT, *n* = 43]

47. Drug result page - MICROMEDEX®. http://www.micromedex solutions.com/micromedex2/librarian/ND_T/evidencexpert /ND_PR/evidencexpert/CS/3F59D1/ND_AppProduct/evi dencexpert/DUPLICATIONSHIELDSYNC/A04EE9/ND_PG /evidencexpert/ND_B/evidencexpert/ND_P/evidencexpert /PFActionId/evidencexpert.DoIntegratedSearch?SearchTerm =Insulin+Human+Regular&fromInterSaltBase=true&false=nul l&false=null&=null#. Accessed December 3, 2015.

48. Durnwald CP, Mele L, Spong CY et al. Glycemic characteristics and neonatal outcomes of women treated for mild gestational diabetes. *Obstet Gynecol* 2011; 117(4): 819–27. [Secondary analysis, RCT, *n* = 460]

49. Prutsky GJ, Domecq JP, Wang Z et al. Glucose targets in pregnant women with diabetes: A systematic review and meta-analysis. *J Clin Endocrinol Metab* 2013; 98(11): 4319–24. [Meta-analysis, 34 RCTs, *n* = 9433]

50. Rosenn BM, Miodovnik M, Holcberg G, Khoury JC, Siddiqi TA. Hypoglycemia: The price of intensive insulin therapy for pregnant women with insulin-dependent diabetes mellitus. *Obstet Gynecol* 1995; 85(3): 417–22. [Prospective, *n* = 84]

51. Nor Azlin MI, Nor NA, Sufian SS, Mustafa N, Jamil MA, Kamaruddin NA. Comparative study of two insulin regimens in pregnancy complicated by diabetes mellitus. *Acta Obstet Gynecol Scand* 2007; 86(4): 407–8. [RCT, *n* = 68]

52. Hod M, Damm P, Kaaja R et al. Fetal and perinatal outcomes in type 1 diabetes pregnancy: A randomized study comparing insulin aspart with human insulin in 322 subjects. *Am J Obstet Gynecol* 2008; 198(2): 186.e1–7. [RCT, *n* = 322]

53. Mathiesen ER, Kinsley B, Amiel SA et al. Maternal glycemic control and hypoglycemia in type 1 diabetic pregnancy: A randomized trial of insulin aspart versus human insulin in 322 pregnant women. *Diabetes Care* 2007; 30(4): 771–6. [RCT, *n* = 322]

54. Nachum Z, Ben-Shlomo I, Weiner E, Shalev E. Twice daily versus four times daily insulin dose regimens for diabetes in pregnancy: Randomised controlled trial. *BMJ* 1999; 319(7219): 1223–7. [RCT, *n* = 392]

55. Pollex E, Moretti ME, Koren G, Feig DS. Safety of insulin glargine use in pregnancy: A systematic review and meta-analysis. *Ann Pharmacother* 2011; 45(1): 9–16. [Meta-analysis, *n* = 702]

56. Mathiesen ER, Hod M, Ivanisevic M et al. Maternal efficacy and safety outcomes in a randomized, controlled trial comparing insulin detemir with NPH insulin in 310 pregnant women with type 1 diabetes. *Diabetes Care* 2012; 35(10): 2012–7. [RCT, *n* = 310]

57. Hod M, Mathiesen ER, Jovanovic L et al. A randomized trial comparing perinatal outcomes using insulin detemir or neutral protamine hagedorn in type 1 diabetes. *J Matern Fetal Neonatal Med* 2014; 27(1): 7–13. [RCT, *n* = 310]

58. Mathiesen JM, Secher AL, Ringholm L et al. Changes in basal rates and bolus calculator settings in insulin pumps during pregnancy in women with type 1 diabetes. *J Matern Fetal Neonatal Med* 2014; 27(7): 724–8. [Prospective, *n* = 27]

59. Farrar D, Tuffnell DJ, West J. Continuous subcutaneous insulin infusion versus multiple daily injections of insulin for pregnant women with diabetes. *Cochrane Database Syst Rev* 2007; 3(3): CD005542. [Meta-analysis, RCT 2, *n* = 60]

60. Mukhopadhyay A, Farrell T, Fraser RB, Ola B. Continuous subcutaneous insulin infusion vs. intensive conventional insulin therapy in pregnant diabetic women: A systematic review and meta-analysis of randomized, controlled trials. *Am J Obstet Gynecol* 2007; 197(5): 447–56. [Meta-analysis, 6 RCTs or quasi-RCTs, *n* = 213]

61. Hollander PA, Blonde L, Rowe R et al. Efficacy and safety of inhaled insulin (exubera) compared with subcutaneous insulin therapy in patients with type 2 diabetes: Results of a 6-month, randomized, comparative trial. *Diabetes Care* 2004; 27(10): 2356–62. [RCT, *n* = 299]

62. Walkinshaw SA. Very tight versus tight control for diabetes in pregnancy. *Cochrane Database of Syst Rev* 2007; 2. [Meta-analysis; 2 RCTs, *n* = 182]

63. Middleton P, Crowther CA, Simmonds L. Different intensities of glycaemic control for pregnant women with pre-existing diabetes. *Cochrane Database Syst Rev* 2012; 8: CD008540. doi:10.1002/14651858 .CD008540.pub3. [Meta-analysis, 3 RCTs, *n* = 233]

64. Carroll MA, Yeomans ER. Diabetic ketoacidosis in pregnancy. *Crit Care Med* 2005; 33(10 Suppl.): S347–53. [Review]

65. ACOG practice bulletin. Pregestational diabetes mellitus. *Obstet Gynecol* 2005; 105: 675–84. [Review, guideline]

66. Boulvain M, Stan C, Irion O. Elective delivery in diabetic pregnant women. *Cochrane Database Syst Rev* 2001; 2(2). [Meta-analysis, 1 RCT, *n* = 200]

67. Kjos SL, Henry OA, Montoro M, Buchanan TA, Mestman JH. Insulin-requiring diabetes in pregnancy: A randomized trial of active induction of labor and expectant management. *Am J Obstet Gynecol* 1993; 169: 611–5. [RCT, *n* = 200]

68. Sanchez-Ramos L, Bernstein S, Kaunitz AM. Expectant management versus labor induction for suspected fetal macrosomia: A systematic review. *Obstet Gynecol* 2002; 100(5[1]): 997–1102. [Meta-analysis, 9 observational studies, 2 RCTs, 3751 subjects]

69. ACOG Practice Bulletin No. 22 (Replaces Technical Bulletin Number 159, September 1991). *Fetal macrosomia*. 2000. November. [Review]

70. Cordua S, Secher AL, Ringholm L, Damm P, Mathiesen ER. Real-time continuous glucose monitoring during labour and delivery in women with type 1 diabetes—Observations from a randomized controlled trial. *Diabet Med* 2013; 30(11): 1374–81. [Observational]

5

Gestational diabetes

A. Dhanya Mackeen and Melisa Lott

KEY POINTS

- **Poorly controlled** gestational diabetes (GDM) in pregnancy is associated with **increased risks of** fetal death, preterm birth, preeclampsia, polyhydramnios, macrosomia, operative (both vaginal and cesarean) delivery and birth injury (including brachial plexus), delayed lung maturity, respiratory distress syndrome, jaundice, hypoglycemia, hypocalcemia, and perinatal mortality.
- Prevention of GDM can be achieved with optimization of maternal health and body mass index prior to pregnancy, which often involves weight loss by proper diet and exercise.
- **Optimization of blood glucose control with diet and insulin to achieve fasting glucose ≤95 mg/dL and two-hour postprandial ≤120 mg/dL (or one-hour postprandial ≤140 mg/dL) is associated with reduced macrosomia, perinatal morbidity, and maternal comorbidities, including preeclampsia and depression.**
- **Insulin is superior to glyburide as it results in less fetal macrosomia and less neonatal hypoglycemia.** Compared to glyburide, **metformin is preferred given lower maternal weight gain and neonatal birth weight**.
- In GDM, **exercise** is associated with a similar rate of macrosomia as compared to insulin, improvement in glycemic control when done in combination with diet as compared to diet alone, and improvement in cardiovascular fitness.
- Women with GDM should be **screened for diabetes six to eight weeks postpartum.**

SCREENING/DIAGNOSIS

The term "gestational" before "diabetes" means that the **hyperglycemia is first recognized or diagnosed during pregnancy** [1]. If hyperglycemia is detected before 20 weeks, pregestational diabetes is probably present. The importance of screening for GDM and treatment to optimize glycemic control to reduce hyperglycemia-associated complications has been established [2–7]. Who, when, and how to screen, and the diagnostic glucose cutoffs to establish the diagnosis of GDM are controversial.

Who to Screen

The population that should be offered screening has not been uniformly identified. Low-risk women in whom screening may not be necessary (selective screening) must meet **all** of the following criteria: age <25 years; ethnic origin of low risk (not Hispanic, African, native American, south or east Asian, or Pacific Islander); BMI <25; no previous personal or family history of impaired glucose tolerance; no previous history of adverse obstetric outcomes associated with GDM [1–6,8].

However, **universal screening is most commonly adopted** and is endorsed by USPSTF [9]. The risk of developing GDM is directly associated with prepregnancy BMI [10].

When to Screen

To balance sensitivity and specificity with adequate treatment duration, screen women at **24 to 28 weeks**. However, the incidence of GDM (related to placental mass and hormone production) increases with gestational age. **Women with risk factors** (Table 5.1) **should be screened preconception or at first prenatal visit.** About 5% to 10% of women with these risk factors will have early GDM, and these represent 40% of all GDM diagnosed later at 24 to 28 weeks [11]. **If the early screen is negative, a repeat screen should be performed at 24 to 28 weeks gestation**. Typically, if a patient fails the early one-hour glucose screen and passes the early three-hour glucose tolerance test, the three-hour test should be repeated at 24–28 weeks.

How to Screen

Screening for GDM is somewhat controversial and can be performed either with a one-step or two-step process. One large trial has shown that **two-step screening is more cost-effective** than the one-step screening [12,13].

One-Step Process

The International Association of Diabetes and Pregnancy Study Groups (IADPSG), recommends using the **75-gram, one step** screening test at 24–28 weeks gestation for all women not known to have diabetes. The finding of one abnormal value is diagnostic of GDM: fasting ≥**92 mg/dL** (5.1 mmol/L), one hour ≥**180 mg/dL** (10.0 mmol/L) or two hour ≥**153 mg/dL** (8.5 mmol/L). [5]. This approach diagnoses twice as many women as having GDM than the two-step process generally employed in North America [14,15].

These recommendations were based on the finding of a multicenter study of 23,316 women that revealed an increased incidence of large for gestational age (LGA) infants, premature delivery, shoulder dystocia/birth injury, NICU admission, hyperbilirubinemia, and preeclampsia in women with glucose levels >75 mg/dL (fasting), 133 mg/dL (one hour), or 109 mg/dL (two hours) [16]. On the basis of the HAPO study [16], the IADPSG developed diagnostic cutoffs for the 75 g glucose load at the level shown to increase the odds of adverse outcomes by at least 1.75 as compared to the women with mean glucose measurements, i.e., fasting, 1 and 2 hour postprandials greater than or equal to 92, 180 and 153 mg/dL respectively. However, these have not been systematically reviewed [5,17]. **No trial has evaluated the efficacy of any therapy based on these new values**, and so they cannot be used yet for clinical care.

Table 5.1   Risk Factors for GDM

- Prior unexplained stillbirth
- Prior infant with congenital anomaly (if not screened in that pregnancy)
- Prior macrosomic infant
- History of gestational diabetes
- Family history of diabetes
- Obesity
- Chronic use of steroids
- Age >35 years
- Glycosuria
- Known impaired glucose metabolism

Two-Step Process

The first (screening) step involves a **50-g, one-hour oral glucose load** (*glucose challenge test*), applied in the nonfasting state [18] with a venous glucose value obtained one hour after consumption. Glucose polymer solutions are better tolerated than monomeric solutions [19]. Jelly beans have not been sufficiently tested to be a valid alternative [20]. Candy twists have recently been studied and may prove to be an option; however, data is currently insufficient to support its use [21]. Although studies have compared different GDM screening approaches including glucose polymer, glucose monomer, candy bars, and food, there is insufficient evidence to compare the effects of these different ways to glucose load and the subsequent management of GDM thereafter [12].

A positive result on the first part of the screening test is defined as 130, 135, or 140 mg/dL. The lower threshold identifies 90% of gestational diabetics but subjects 20% to 25% of those screened to the second diagnostic test. In contrast, the higher value has a lower sensitivity of 80%, but subjects fewer women, 14% to 18%, to further testing. ACOG recommends choosing 135 mg/dL or 140 mg/dL as the cutoff [1]. More than 80% of women with values ≥200 mg/dL will fail the three-hour glucose tolerance test (GTT), so many use this cutoff as meeting the diagnosis of GDM [22].

Definitive diagnosis of GDM is then made on the basis of the results of a **100-g, three-hour oral GTT** (administered after an overnight fast [8–14 hours], ideally following three days of unrestricted diet [including carbohydrate loading] and activity) while the patient remains seated and refrains from smoking.

Unfortunately, the criteria to establish diagnosis by this test are not universally accepted. The two competing criteria and their diagnostic levels are listed in Table 5.2. Two or more abnormal values on these tests establish the diagnosis of GDM. The Carpenter–Coustan stricter criteria increase by about 50% the number of women with a diagnosis of GDM compared to the NDDG criteria, and these pregnancies have elevated incidences of macrosomia and neonatal insulinemia [23]. Therefore, we **suggest using Carpenter–Coustan criteria**

Table 5.2   Criteria for Standard 100-g Glucose Load to Diagnose Gestational Diabetes

	National Diabetes Data Group		Carpenter–Coustan Criteria	
	mg/dL	mmol/L	mg/dL	mmol/L
Fasting	105	5.8	95	5.3
1 hour	190	10.6	180	10.0
2 hours	165	9.2	155	8.6
3 hours	145	8.0	140	7.8

as opposed to those of NDDG. In fact, there is evidence to suggest that hyperglycemia below the cutoff of even the Carpenter–Coustan criteria result in poor outcomes [16,24].

If **GDM is diagnosed <20 weeks, counseling and management should be as for pregestational diabetes.** The presence or absence of fasting hyperglycemia further subdivides this category.

If **one abnormal value** in the three-hour GTT is present, the patient should be counseled to avoid excess glucose consumption. Studies have shown that in these women better **glycemic control, achieved with either diet + insulin** or even just nutritional counseling, was associated with fewer neonatal complications and decreased incidence of LGA and cesarean when compared with no such therapies [25–29].

INCIDENCE

There is an overall **7%** incidence of GDM [30] using two-step screening and Carper–Coustan criteria in the United States, representing one of the most common medical complications facing obstetricians. Of cases of DM in pregnancy, 88% are GDM [1,31]. Incidence obviously depends on the screening strategy used with some suggesting that stricter criteria would result in 18% of pregnant women being diagnosed with GDM [16,17].

PATHOPHYSIOLOGY

The pathophysiology of GDM is insulin resistance caused by circulating hormonal factors: increased maternal and placental production of human placental lactogen, progesterone, growth hormone, cortisol, and prolactin. Increased body weight and caloric intake also contribute to the insulin resistance associated with pregnancy and may offset the normally increased insulin production in the pregnant woman [31]. Women with GDM have been found to have lower basal islet cell function in addition to insulin resistance when compared to a nondiabetic cohort. The combination of the two factors contributes to the development of GDM. This insulin resistance and decreased insulin production persists in the postpartum state and leads to the development of type II diabetes in this population. Low adiponectin levels may be a predictive biomarker for the development of GDM in obese women, but further studies are needed to ascertain the utility of this before clinical application [32]. Specific genes related to GDM and response to therapy are under investigation [33,34].

RISK FACTORS/ASSOCIATIONS

Pregnancy, obesity, hypertension, age greater than or equal to 35 years at delivery, metabolic syndrome, family history of type II DM, nonwhite ethnicity, previous macrosomia.

COMPLICATIONS

Incidence of complications is inversely proportional to glucose control. In poorly controlled DM, increased glucose in the mother causes abnormal metabolism while in the fetus it causes hyperinsulinemia and its consequences. However, treatment of even mild GDM reduced birth weight percentiles and neonatal fat mass [35]. Other complications are hypertensive disorders and preeclampsia, macrosomia, congenital malformations (OR 1.2–1.4) [36], operative delivery, and birth injury (confounded by maternal obesity; both related to macrosomia) [6,16,37]. Apart from transient neonatal hypoglycemia, no other metabolic derangement has been reported in the infant of the GDM mother. Long-term adult disorders, such as glucose intolerance and obesity, have been postulated to occur as frequently in these neonates as in neonates of women with pregestational diabetes, but this has not been verified by observational studies [38]. Elevated fasting glucose is associated with fetal macrosomia and with elevated C-peptide (which is correlated with increased fetal fat deposition) [39]. Approximately **50% of women identified as having GDM will develop frank diabetes within 10 years** if followed longitudinally [40].

PREVENTION

Low-glycemic diet [41], a diet with adequate (not excessive) caloric intake, and achieving and maintaining a normal BMI are probably beneficial, especially preconception, in preventing GDM, but have been insufficiently studied in RCTs so far. Structured moderate physical exercise programs during pregnancy decrease the risk of GDM and diminish maternal weight gain [42,43].

Myo-inositol has also been shown to be safe and effective in preventing GDM. **Myoinositol** (2 grams bid) improves insulin resistance [44] and reduces the incidence of GDM in nonobese Caucasian Italians [45], obese Italians [46], and in women with fasting glucose 92–126 mg/dL and BMI ≤35 [47]. Further studies are needed to determine safety regarding neonatal outcomes, efficacy in a diverse patient population, and whether there are increases in the diagnosis of GDM later in gestation.

TREATMENT OF GDM (TABLES 5.3 AND 5.4)

Treatment of GDM consists of **diet, exercise, and glucose monitoring**; medications, such as **oral hypoglycemic agents and/or insulin** are reserved for use when glycemic control is not achieved with diet and exercise.

Compared to usual prenatal care, treatment as described above is associated with significantly decreased incidences of **birth weight >4000 g, perinatal morbidity (death, shoulder dystocia, bone fracture, and nerve palsy), and preeclampsia in women with GDM** [3,48–50]. Incidence of CD is not significantly affected [3].

Diet

Dietary therapy consists of approximately 30 kcal/kg/day for the average patient and ±5 kcal/kg/day for underweight and overweight women, respectively [22]. Calories should be divided between three meals and three snacks: 45% carbohydrate, 20% protein, and 35% unsaturated fat. Because about 30% to 40% of gestational diabetics fail to achieve glucose control with diet alone, other interventions may be necessary. **If two glucose levels are >99 mg/dL (fasting) or ≥126 at ≤35 weeks or ≥144 after 35 weeks (two-hour postprandial) or ever ≥162 mg/dL (two-hour postprandial), despite diet and exercise, medical therapy should be considered** [6].

Dietary counseling has been shown to improve dietary intake in patients at risk for GDM [51] and may result in lower neonatal birth weight (133 g) and decreased incidence of LGA [52]. Although a diet with a low-glycemic index (e.g., decreased consumption of white bread, processed cereals, and potatoes) was felt to decrease the need for insulin in women with GDM [53], this recommendation was recently

Table 5.3 Management of the Gestational Diabetic Gravida

Preconception prevention
- Weight loss
- Exercise

Antepartum management
- Nutritional counseling for dietary control
- Finger stick blood sugar assessments: fasting values should be <95 mg/dL and two-hour postprandial values should be ≤120 mg/dL (or one-hour postprandial values should be ≤140 mg/dL)
- Exercise program
- Insulin or oral hypoglycemic agent if diet not sufficient to optimize blood sugars
- Fetal surveillance
  - Diet controlled: NSTs weekly (or twice weekly) after 40 weeks until delivery
  - Medication controlled: NSTs weekly (or twice weekly) from 32–36 weeks; twice weekly from 36 weeks until delivery

Intrapartum management (see Figure 4.1)
- Induction of labor
  - Diet controlled: at 41 weeks
  - Medication controlled: between 39 0/7 and 39 6/7 weeks
- Cesarean delivery if EFW ≥4500 g
- Frequent glucose assessment
  - Every one hour if required medication
  - Every four hours if diet controlled
- Target blood sugars 70–110 mg/dL
- IV insulin therapy if blood sugars greater than target blood sugars or with ketonuria
  - IV saline infusion at 125 cc/hour unless ketonuric, then add 5% dextrose solution at rate to keep blood sugar in target range

Postpartum management
- Standard 75-g glucose challenge test at 6 weeks postpartum visit (see Figure 5.3 and Table 4.1)

Abbreviations: EFW, estimated fetal weight; IV, intravenous; NSTs, nonstress tests.

challenged by a larger study which showed no benefit [54]. There is no difference in neonatal and adverse pregnancy outcomes for women on a low glycemic index diet versus a high fiber diet [55], and a low glycemic index diet compared to healthy eating did not show differences in birth weight, fetal percentile, or ponderal index [56]. A DASH diet has demonstrated improved glucose tolerance, lipid profiles, diastolic blood pressures, and serum insulin levels and decreased insulin requirement in small RCTs; however, large trials are needed to further assess effectiveness [57–59]. An oil-rich diet (45–50 g sunflower oil daily) versus a low-oil diet (20 g daily) did not have an effect on pregnancy outcomes [60].

Exercise

Exercising three times a week for 20 to 45 minutes is beneficial for women with GDM and those at risk for GDM [61]. In small RCTs, in women with GDM, exercise (as defined by 30 minutes of non-weight-bearing activity at 50% of aerobic capacity) has been associated with less gestational weight gain in obese gravida [62], a **similar rate of macrosomia compared to insulin** [63], **improvement in glycemic control when done in conjunction with diet compared to diet alone** [64,65], and **improvement in cardiovascular fitness** [66]. Although exercise later in pregnancy did not decrease the risk of developing GDM, it did reduce the GDM-related risk of neonatal macrosomia [61]. Improvement in maternal triglycerides [67,68], insulin sensitivity [67], and postprandial

Table 5.4 Randomized Controlled Trials of Medication for Treatment of Gestational Diabetes Mellitus

Study	Details	Testing	Intervention	Control	Outcomes
Casey [86]	n = 375 GA: 24–30	**Screening test:** 50 g 1-hour test ≥140 mg/dL **Diagnostic test:** 100 g 3-hour test with two or more abnormal values with cutoff fasting ≥105 mg/dL; 1-hour ≥190 mg/dL; 2-hour ≥165 mg/dL; 3-hour ≥145 mg/dL	(n = 189) Glyburide 2.5 mg daily titrated to a maximum dose of 20 mg daily Insulin initiated to achieve euglycemia if needed	(n = 186) Placebo All women with mild GDM received nutritional education and dietary counselling	**Primary:** 200-g birth weight decrement in neonates of mothers treated with glyburide was not found. **Secondary:** No difference in gestational hypertension, chorioamnionitis, shoulder dystocia, operative delivery, or third- or fourth-degree lacerations. Neonatal hyperbilirubinemia and hypoglycemia were uncommon. Glyburide in addition to diet improves glycemic control as compared to diet plus placebo.
Ibrahim [96]	n = 90 GA: 20–34	Included GDM and preexisting diabetes with insulin resistance (defined as poor glycemic control at a daily dose of 1.12 units/kg)	(n = 46) Oral metformin without increasing insulin dose If glycemic control not achieved then patient switched to conventional insulin dose-raising regimen	(n = 44) Oral metformin with increasing insulin dose	**Primary:** Those treated with insulin were more likely to achieve proper glycemic control. **Secondary:** As compared to increasing the insulin dose, the addition of metformin was associated with reductions in hospitalization rates, treatment cost, and frequency of maternal and neonatal hypoglycemia, NICU admission, and neonatal RDS. There were no differences in mode of delivery, fetal macrosomia, gestational age at delivery, or birth weight. Obesity negatively affected achievement of euglycemia with metformin.
Tertti [95]	n = 217 GA: 22–34	**Screening test:** none **Diagnostic test:** 75-g OGTT diagnostic cutoff values of plasma glucose up to December 2008 were the following: fasting ≥4.8 mmol/L, 1 h ≥10.0 mmol/L and 2 h ≥8.7 mmol/L, and thereafter ≥5.3, ≥10.0, and ≥8.6 mmol/L, respectively	(n = 111) Metformin 500 mg daily to maximum 1000 mg twice daily Insulin added if necessary for glycemic control	(n = 107) Insulin treatment was initiated using NPH insulin Protaphane®, and/or rapid-acting insulin lispro (Humalog®) or insulin aspart (Novorapid®)	**Primary:** No differences in birth weight. **Secondary:** No differences in macrosomia, LGA, or neonatal complications. Patients whose OGTT was performed earlier, who were older, and required oral medication earlier in pregnancy were more likely to need supplemental insulin in addition to metformin therapy.
Spaulonci [105]	n = 92 GA: any	**Screening test:** none **Diagnostic test:** 100-g or 75-g glucose with two or more abnormal values and cutoff: fasting ≥95 mg/dL, 1-h ≥180 mg/dL, 2-h ≥155 mg/dL, 3-h ≥140 mg/dL	(n = 46) Metformin Initial dose 1700 mg daily increased to 2550 mg daily Supplemental insulin added if needed for glycemic control All patients received nutritional counseling and daily caloric intake of 25–35 kcal/kg (based on BMI) was recommended	(n = 46) Insulin Human NPH insulin starting dose was 0.4 u/kg/day, with 1/2 dose before breakfast, 1/4 dose before lunch, and 1/4 dose at 10 p.m. Regular insulin was added for elevated postprandial values	**Primary:** Mean glucose levels were higher in the insulin group. **Secondary:** Patients in the metformin group gained less weight than those in the insulin group; there was no difference in frequency of preeclampsia, prematurity, or cesarean delivery; there was more neonatal hypoglycemia in those treated with insulin; no significant differences between the two groups were observed regarding neonatal outcomes, including gestational age at birth, Apgar scores, umbilical artery pH, or newborn weight. Supplemental insulin was required in 12 women (26%) in the metformin group.

(Continued)

Table 5.4 (Continued)   Randomized Controlled Trials of Medication for Treatment of Gestational Diabetes Mellitus

Study	Details	Testing	Intervention	Control	Outcomes
Tempe [85]	$n = 64$ GA: 0–28	**Screening test:** 50-g 1-hour test ≥130 mg/dL **Diagnostic test:** 100-g 3-hour with two or more abnormal values and cutoff: fasting ≥95 mg/dL, 1-h ≥180 mg/dL, 2-h ≥155 mg/dL, 3-h ≥140 mg/dL	($n = 32$) Glyburide 2.5 mg titrated to maximum dose 20 mg daily Switched to insulin if needed for glycemic control	($n = 32$) Insulin treatment 2/3 of the total dose administered in the morning and 1/3 at night; Lente and plain insulin were administered at a ratio of 2:1 in the morning and 2:1 or 1:1 at night	**Primary:** No difference in glycemic control. **Secondary:** No difference in maternal or neonatal complications.
Waheed [106]	$n = 68$ GA: >14	**Screening test:** none **Diagnostic test:** Fasting blood sugar >100 mg and random blood sugar >140 mg	($n = 34$) Metformin 500 mg daily up to 1500 mg maximum daily dose	($n = 34$) Insulin (dosage and insulin type not specified)	**Primary:** No differences in glycemic control
Hickman [91]	$n = 28$ GA: <20	**Screening:** not applicable **Inclusion:** pregestational diabetes mellitus type 2 on an oral hypoglycemic agent or GDMA2 diagnosed prior to 20 weeks	($n = 14$) Metformin 500 mg once or twice per day Insulin initiated to achieve euglycemia if needed after maximum dose of metformin (2500 mg) attained	($n = 14$) Weight-based insulin (0.7 U/kg/d) using NPH regular insulin Nutrition counseling and diabetes education was provided to all participants in both groups	**Primary:** No difference in average fasting glucose levels between groups. **Secondary:** Women managed with metformin required less insulin for euglycemia and had less hypoglycemic events; metformin was preferred by participants; there were no complications of shoulder dystocia, postpartum hemorrhage, stillbirths, or major congenital malformations. Supplemental insulin was required in six women (43%) in the metformin group.
Niromanesh [107]	$n = 160$ GA: 20–34	**Screening test:** 50-g 1-hour test ≥130 mg/dL **Diagnostic test:** 100-g 3-hour with two or more abnormal values and cutoff: fasting ≥95 mg/dL, 1-h ≥180 mg/dL, 2-h ≥155 mg/dL, 3-h ≥140 mg/dL	($n = 80$) Metformin 500 mg twice daily increased by 500–1000 mg one or two weeks to a maximum daily dose of 2500 mg, divided with each meal Insulin was needed if glycemic control was not achieved despite maximum metformin dose	($n = 80$) Insulin. NPH insulin with regular insulin as needed for elevated postprandial levels titrated to individual need All women were given counseling on diet and regular physical exercise.	**Primary:** No differences in maternal glycemic control; neonates born to mothers in the metformin group had lower birth weight than those in the insulin group. **Secondary:** Neonates from the metformin group had significantly lower anthropometric measurements (including head, arm, and chest circumference) and less LGA as compared to insulin group; there was no difference in incidence of birth defects, neonatal hypoglycemia, hyperbilirubinemia, or need for phototherapy; metformin was associated with less maternal weight gain compared to insulin. Supplemental insulin was required in 11 women (14%) in the metformin group.

(Continued)

Table 5.4 (Continued) Randomized Controlled Trials of Medication for Treatment of Gestational Diabetes Mellitus

Study	Details	Testing	Intervention	Control	Outcomes
Balaji [108]	n = 320 GA: 12–28	**Screening test:** 75 g OGTT with diagnosis when 2-hour glucose ≥140 mg/dL **Diagnostic test:** Inability to maintain euglycemia 2 weeks after medical nutritional therapy	(n = 163) BIAsp 30 six units before breakfast and adjusted as needed Biphasic insulin aspart (BIAsp) 30 contains 30% rapid-acting insulin aspart with 70% protamine crystallized insulin aspart to be used up to three times daily	(n = 157) BHI30 six units before breakfast and adjusted as needed Biphasic human insulin (BHI) 30 contains 30% short-acting and 70% intermediate acting neutral protamine hagedorn (NPH), to be used up to twice daily	**Primary:** No differences in LGA **Secondary:** No differences in overall glycemic control between groups (fasting and 2-hour postprandial, hgb A1c). The final mean insulin dose was significantly lower for BIAsp30 than BHI30.
Ijas [94]	n = 97 GA: 12–34	**Diagnostic test:** 75-g OGTT with one or more abnormal and cutoff values fasting 5.3 mmol/L, 11.0 mmol/L; 9.6 mmol/L	(n = 47) Metformin 750 mg once daily for first week, twice daily for second week, and three times daily from third week onward. Discontinued if significant side effect such as diarrhea. Supplemental insulin added if needed.	(n = 50) Insulin with long-acting insulin (Protophan) and rapid-acting (Humalog)	**Primary:** No differences in macrosomia or LGA. **Secondary:** No differences in NICU admissions, neonatal hypoglycemia, phototherapy treatment, or birth injuries; mean maternal weight gain, preeclampsia, and preterm delivery were not different between groups. In the metformin group, there was a higher incidence of vacuum extraction and cesarean deliveries as compared to the insulin group. Women that required additional insulin had higher BMI, higher fasting glucose, and required medication earlier in gestation than those controlled with metformin alone. Supplemental insulin was required in 15 women (32%) in the metformin group.
Moore [109]	n = 149 GA: 11–33	**Screening test:** 50-g 1-hour test ≥130 mg/dL **Diagnostic test:** 100 g 3-hour test with cutoff of fasting ≥95 mg/dL, 1-h ≥180 mg/dL, 2-h ≥155 mg/dL, 3-h ≥140 mg/dL with two or more abnormal values	(n = 74) Glyburide 2.5 mg twice daily initial dose titrated to maximum 20 mg daily dose Daily caloric intake of 25 to 30 kcal/kg (depending on BMI) was recommended.	(n = 75) Metformin 500 mg per day in divided doses to maximum dose of 2000 mg per day If failure to control glucose in either group, oral medication was discontinued and insulin was initiated.	**Primary:** Metformin had a failure rate 2.1 times higher than glyburide. **Secondary:** No differences in macrosomia, NICU admission, birth trauma, five minute Apgar score, preeclampsia, maternal or neonatal hypoglycemia, and route of delivery. Mean birth weight was lower in those treated with metformin as compared to glyburide. Metformin was associated with a higher rate of cesarean delivery compared to glyburide.
Rowan [110]	n = 733 GA: 20–33	Diagnosis of gestational diabetes mellitus according to the criteria of the Australasian Diabetes in Pregnancy Society (ADIPS)	(n = 363) Metformin ± insulin Metformin 500 mg once or twice daily with food and titrated to maximum dose 2500 mg. If blood glucose not controlled insulin was added	(n = 370) Insulin	**Primary:** No difference in composite neonatal complications **Secondary:** Neonatal anthropometric measures and umbilical-cord serum insulin concentrations were not different between the groups. Severe neonatal hypoglycemia occurred less often in the metformin group, although the rates of neonatal hypoglycemia were similar. Preterm birth was more common in the metformin group. Metformin was preferred by the participants. Supplemental insulin was required in 168 women (46%) in the metformin group.

(Continued)

Table 5.4 (Continued) Randomized Controlled Trials of Medication for Treatment of Gestational Diabetes Mellitus

Study	Details	Testing	Intervention	Control	Outcomes
Di Cianni [111]	$n = 96$ GA: not specified	**Screening test:** unclear **Diagnostic test:** 100-g glucose tolerance test with two or more abnormal values with cutoff: fasting ≥95 mg/dL, 1-h ≥180 mg/dL, 2-h ≥155 mg/dL, 3-h ≥140 mg/dL	Insulin aspart (ASP) $n = 31$ Insulin lispro (LIS) $n = 33$	Human regular insulin (HI) $n = 32$ Bedtime NPH insulin added if elevated fasting glucose values	**Primary:** Short-acting insulin may be associated with better glycemic control and newborn anthropometric measures than regular insulin. **Secondary:** There were no hypoglycemic episodes in any of the groups; there were no differences in insulin dose, duration of insulin therapy, fasting glucose, hgb A1c or maternal weight gain. Higher one-hour postprandial glucose levels were noted in HI group compared to ASP and LIS groups after patients were provided a standardized breakfast. LIS and ASP patients had lower birth weights compared to HI. The rates of macrosomia were not different between the two groups. Anthropometric measurements to evaluate for disproportionate growth were lower in the HI group.
Langer [84]	$n = 404$ GA: 11–33	**Screening test:** 50-g 1-hour test ≥130 mg/dL **Diagnostic test:** 100-g 3-hour with cutoff of 2 or more abnormal values: fasting ≥95 mg/dL, 1-h ≥180 mg/dL, 2-h ≥155 mg/dL, 3-h ≥140 mg/dL	($n = 201$) Glyburide 2.5 mg titrated to maximum 20 mg daily dose	($n = 203$) Insulin starting dose 0.7 unit/kg of actual body weight and increased as necessary	**Primary:** No difference in glycemic control **Secondary:** No differences in perinatal outcomes including LGA, fetal macrosomia, neonatal respiratory distress, hyperbilirubinemia, hypocalcemia, hypoglycemia, or need for IV glucose therapy. Cord serum analysis did not demonstrate the presence of glyburide in any of the infants' samples.

Abbreviations: BMI, body mass index; GA, gestational age (weeks); GDM, gestational diabetes mellitus; GDMA2, gestational diabetes mellitus – medication controlled; IUGR, intrauterine growth restriction; IV, intravenous; LGA, large for gestational age; n, sample size; NICU, neonatal intensive care unit; NPH, neutral protamine Hagedorn; OGTT, oral glucose tolerance test; RDS, respiratory distress syndrome.

glucose [68] have been demonstrated with exercise in pregnancy. Diet or exercise, or both, during pregnancy can reduce the risk of excessive gestational weight gain and decreases maternal hypertension [69]. The combined interventions have been shown to decrease neonatal respiratory morbidity. The amount and safety of exercise requires further research for the creation of safe guidelines [69]. If an exercise program is to be prescribed, early counseling regarding frequency and healthy practices is important to combat declining physical activity as pregnancy progresses [70–72]. Due to low compliance with exercise programs [73,74], the evidence supporting the beneficial effects of exercise in women with GDM with regards to maternal and neonatal outcome varies [4]. However, data seems to show that overall **exercise is beneficial** in this population although the frequency and intensity of the regimen must be individualized, taking into consideration the patient's comorbidities.

Glucose Monitoring

With a glucometer, **fasting and two-hour (or one-hour) postprandial glucose levels should be followed daily.** Although not in widespread use, studies have shown that continuous glucose monitoring may reveal more postprandial hyperglycemia than is detected by checking two-hour postprandial values [75,76]. Compared to preprandial monitoring, **postprandial monitoring is associated with improvement in glycosylated hemoglobin, less CD for dystocia, smaller birth weights, and less neonatal hypoglycemia** [77]. Because the risk of macrosomia appears to be linked with postprandial hyperglycemia, following these values appears to be reasonable and is what trials have tested [6,25,78,79]. Target goals (euglycemia) are **fasting glucose between 60 and 95 mg/dL and two-hour postprandial ≤120 mg/dL (or one-hour postprandial ≤140 mg/dL).** Fasting glucose ≤90 mg/dL in the third trimester may be associated with a lower risk of macrosomia, but trials were overall not high quality [80]. Achieving euglycemia decreases neonatal complications. If all values are within normal limits for extended periods, less frequent monitoring can be considered. Electronically reminding patients to transmit their blood glucose log data to their physicians did not influence maternal glucose values or infant birth weight, but did increase maternal reporting of blood sugars; however, sample size may have been too small to truly determine efficacy of these reminders [81].

Oral Hypoglycemic Agents

Oral hypoglycemic agents are safe in pregnancy. The second-generation sulfonylurea agents have been demonstrated to have low transplacental passage in both in vitro and in vivo models although glyburide has been detected in cord blood [82].

Glyburide

Although glyburide used to be considered equally efficacious to insulin with regards to pregnancy outcomes [83–86], recent evidence suggests that **insulin is superior to glyburide with a lower neonatal birth weight (109 g), less fetal macrosomia (RR 0.38), and less neonatal hypoglycemia (RR 0.49)** [87,88]. Approximately 10% to 20% of women on this regimen do not achieve euglycemia, especially women with a BMI >30. Obese women with GDM requiring medication to achieve euglycemia should probably be treated with insulin rather than with

oral agents [89]. If an oral hypoglycemic agent is chosen, metformin is preferred to glyburide [87]. If used, glyburide is started at 2.5 mg orally in the morning with a maximum dose of 20 mg daily.

Metformin

Metformin (Glucophage) is commonly used in women with polycystic ovarian syndrome to treat infertility related to anovulation. The incidence of miscarriage is decreased in women who are continued on this therapy throughout pregnancy [90], and there is evidence to suggest a decreased risk of GDM when metformin is continued [90]; however, this outcome is misleading as the medication may be masking the disease. No attributable birth defects or adverse outcomes in this patient population have been reported [1].

Compared to insulin therapy, metformin (± insulin if necessary) is associated with less maternal hypoglycemia [91], more preterm births (RR 1.5), less gestational hypertension (RR 0.53), less severe neonatal hypoglycemia (RR 0.62), and nonclinically significant differences of less maternal weight gain (1 kg) and lower gestational age at delivery (0.16 weeks) [87,92]. About one-third of patients failed metformin treatment. Metformin has no added benefit for postpartum weight loss [93]. Women with GDM who are obese, have a high fasting glucose, or need pharmacologic therapy early (e.g., <24 weeks) in pregnancy may be more suitable for insulin therapy or may require insulin as an adjunct to metformin therapy [94,95]. In women whose total insulin dose is ≥1.12 IU/kg, the addition of metformin has been shown to improve glycemic control, decrease maternal hypoglycemia, reduce neonatal hypoglycemia and decrease NICU admission [96]. Vitamin B12 stores are not affected by metformin [97].

Compared to glyburide, those treated with metformin had less maternal weight gain (2 kg), lower neonatal birth weights (206 g), less macrosomia, and fewer LGA infants [87].

In summary, **insulin is overall superior to oral glycemic agents for prevention of the complications of GDM.** If an oral hypoglycemic agent is chosen, it appears that **metformin may be preferred over glyburide.** Additionally, consideration can be given to the addition of metformin to an insulin regimen rather than continued increase of insulin dose.

Insulin

Useful sample calculations for the total daily insulin requirement and insulin regimen are in Table 5.5 [98–100] and Figures 5.1 and 5.2.

As with pregestational DM, insulin glargine, neutral protamine Hagedorn (NPH), and insulin lispro can be used

Table 5.5 Total Insulin Requirements

Trimester	Units/kg/day
1	0.7–0.8
2	0.8–1.0
3	0.9–1.2

Sources: Summaries for patients. Screening for gestational diabetes mellitus: U.S. preventive services task force recommendation statement. *Ann Intern Med*, 160, 6, 2014; Grant SM, Wolever TM, O'Connor DL, Nisenbaum R, Josse RG. *Diabetes Res Clin Pract*, 91, 1, 15–22, 2010; Wang H, Jiang H, Yang L, Zhang M. *Asia Pac J Clin Nutr*, 24, 1, 58–64, 2015.

Note: Patients with multifetal gestations or who have received steroids or betamimetics often require higher doses.

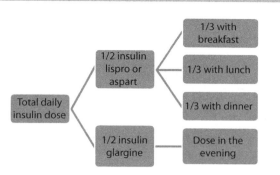

Figure 5.1. Distribution of insulin dose throughout the day if using insulin glargine and insulin lispro/aspart.

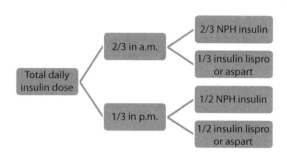

Figure 5.2 Distribution of insulin dose throughout the day if using NPH and insulin lispro/aspart.

for glucose control. Compared to regular insulin, insulin lispro is associated with a lower incidence of maternal hypoglycemic episodes in women with GDM [101]. Although early studies did not demonstrate benefit [102], it has been clearly established that in women with GDM, compared to no treatment or diet only, **diet and glucose monitoring with insulin**, if needed, are associated with **reduced macrosomia** [103] **and shoulder dystocia**; similar incidences of cesarean, NICU admission, and neonatal hypoglycemia [104]; and **no birth trauma** (bone fracture, nerve palsy) (vs. 1%) or **perinatal death** (vs. 1%) [3,6]. **Mood and quality of life are improved**, and the incidence of **depression decreases** with the above interventions and the optimization of glycemic control [6].

Table 5.5 shows characteristics of randomized trials comparing treatment of GDM with metformin, glyburide, and insulin.

Nutritional Supplementation

Calcium with vitamin D may have beneficial effects on glucose metabolism, lipid profiles [112,113], and biomarkers of oxidative stress [112], although the effect on blood glucose levels has been disputed [114]. Probiotic treatment (capsules or yogurt) [59,115,116] and DHEA supplementation [117,118] have not been shown to be beneficial.

Antepartum Testing

Antepartum fetal testing and ultrasound evaluations have not been standardly applied to the management of gestational diabetics as there is no clear literature to provide direction.

- *Euglycemia with diet only*: Although there is limited data, no testing seems to be necessary. Consider weekly or twice weekly nonstress tests (NSTs) starting at 40 weeks.
- *Hyperglycemia or medication necessary*: Consider management similar to pregestational diabetics: weekly or twice weekly NSTs from 32 to 35 6/7 weeks, then twice weekly NSTs from 36 weeks until delivery, which is usually accomplished between 39 and 40 weeks (see Chapter 4).

Ultrasound assessment of fetal weight is commonly employed, but because of the inherent inaccuracy of predicting macrosomia, it has not been supported by any studies, despite application of customized or normalized population growth curves [119].

Delivery

Timing, Mode, and Lung Maturity
There is insufficient evidence to assess the timing and mode of delivery in gestational diabetics. Compared to expectant management until 41–42 weeks, induction of labor at 38 weeks in women with insulin-dependent diabetes (of which >90% were gestational) is associated with reduced incidences of macrosomia [2,120]. However, the sample size was too small to evaluate the impact on perinatal mortality, which is a concern in women with diabetes who are delivered prior to 39 weeks [2]. **A secondary analysis of an RCT on those with mild gestational diabetes supports IOL prior to EDC as it reduces the risk of CD** [121].

In women requiring medication, management is usually similar to that of the pregestational diabetic, and delivery is advocated at around 39 0/7–39 6/7 weeks. In general, indicated delivery before 39 weeks, if truly indicated, should not require assessment of fetal maturity. If assessment of fetal lung maturity is done, laboratory tests are interpreted as in nondiabetic patients with phosphatidylglycerol ≥3% accepted by most authorities as the lab value indicating the least risk for fetal respiratory insufficiency in diabetic women; patients should be cautioned that a positive test does not preclude infant morbidities (see Chapter 57). While recognizing that macrosomia remains a difficult antenatal diagnosis both clinically and by ultrasound, delivery via cesarean is suggested for fetuses estimated to be ≥4500 g [1] (see Chapter 45). Operative deliveries should be avoided in women with fetuses estimated to be >4000 g and prolonged second stage of labor.

Intrapartum Glucose Management
Intrapartum management requires frequent assessment of blood glucose levels during labor (see Figure 4.1). For patients who have required insulin therapy, perform hourly assessments of blood sugars to maintain them between 70 and 120 mg/dL. Intravenous insulin may be necessary to maintain the above glucose levels, but is seldom required in these patients. Patients managed with diet alone may not need as frequent evaluations during labor and can have assessments every four hours.

Anesthesia

No specific adjustments necessary unless woman is obese.

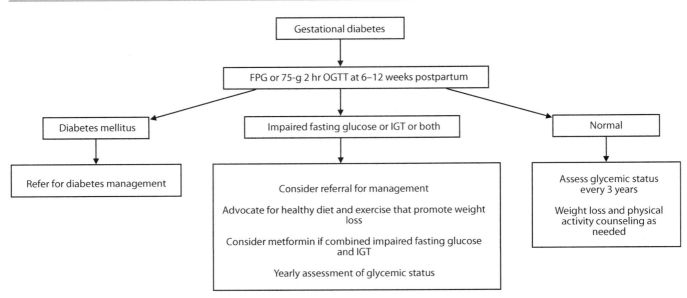

Figure 5.3 Postpartum screening of patients who had GDM. *Abbreviations*: FPG, fasting plasma glucose; IGT, impaired glucose tolerance; OGTT, oral glucose tolerance test. (Adapted from American College of Obstetricians and Gynecologists. *Obstet. Gynecol* 2013; 122: 406–16.)

Postpartum/Breast-Feeding

In the postpartum period, women with GDM do not, in general, require medication to control their blood sugars. Checking a fasting and postprandial value prior to discharge can be employed, especially if pregestational diabetes is suspected. Because these women have an increased risk of developing frank diabetes, **screening with a 75-g glucose challenge or other nonpregnant tests** (see Table 4.1) is advocated when the woman is **six to eight weeks postpartum** (Figure 5.3) [1] **and every two to three years thereafter** [40,122–124]. This can be accomplished by either the obstetrician with referral if values are abnormal or by referral for the screening to a medicine specialist. Breast-feeding, diet, and exercise should be encouraged in these women, particularly if they are obese. All forms of contraception are available to diabetics, providing they have no contraindications, such as hypertension or vascular disease.

Patients should be informed that they are at increased risk for developing diabetes during their lifetime, up to 50% over the next 10 years [40]. Women who are obese, diagnosed with GDM early in gestation, and have significantly abnormal screening results during and after pregnancy have the highest chance of adult onset diabetes. Prepregnancy obesity and fasting glucose >100 mg/dL (from 100-g glucose tolerance test) are associated with increased risks of development of metabolic syndrome [125]. Some suggest that women with an abnormal one-hour result are also at increased risk of metabolic derangements later in life despite a normal three-hour GTT [126]. Counseling regarding diet and exercise, maintenance of normal BMI, and surveillance with periodic screening are indicated. Cesarean delivery and gestational weight gain were associated with increases in depressive symptoms at six weeks postpartum [127].

REFERENCES

1. American College of Obstetricians and Gynecologists. Gestational diabetes. Practice bulletin no. 137. *Obstet Gynecol* 2013; 122: 406–16. [Review]
2. Boulvain M, Stan C, Irion O. Elective delivery in diabetic pregnant women. *Cochrane Database Syst Rev* 2001; 2(2). [Meta-analysis, 1 RCT, n = 200]
3. Alwan N, Tuffnell DJ, West J. Treatments for gestational diabetes. *Cochrane Database Syst Rev* 2009; 3(3): CD003395. [Meta-analysis, 8 RCTs, n = 1418]
4. Ceysens G, Rouiller D, Boulvain M. Exercise for diabetic pregnant women. *Cochrane Database Syst Rev* 2006; 3: CD004225. [Meta-analysis, 4 RCTs, n = 114]
5. American Diabetes Association. Diagnosis and classification of diabetes mellitus. *Diabetes Care* 2011; 34(Suppl. 1): S62–9. [Review, guideline]
6. Crowther CA, Hiller JE, Moss JR et al. Effect of treatment of gestational diabetes mellitus on pregnancy outcomes. *N Engl J Med* 2005; 352(24): 2477–86. [RCT, n = 1000. Impaired glucose tolerance (defined following 75 gm OGTT as fasting <7.0 mmol/L, two-hour between 7.8 mmol/L and 11.0 mmol/L). Diet, glucose monitoring, and insulin as needed vs. routine care]
7. Bancroft K, Tuffnell DJ, Mason GC, Rogerson LJ, Mansfield M. A randomised controlled pilot study of the management of gestational impaired glucose tolerance. *BJOG* 2000; 107(8): 959–63. [RCT, n = 68. Impaired glucose tolerance (defined following 75-gm OGTT as fasting 7.0 mmol/L in one week), serial ultrasound for growth and amniotic fluid, Doppler studies, CTG monitoring, unmonitored group received dietary advice, HbA1c monthly but no capillary glucose measurements]
8. Metzger BE, Buchanan TA, Coustan DR et al. Summary and recommendations of the fifth international workshop-conference on gestational diabetes mellitus. *Diabetes Care* 2007; 30(Suppl. 2): S251–60. [Review]
9. Summaries for patients. Screening for gestational diabetes mellitus: U.S. preventive services task force recommendation statement. *Ann Intern Med* 2014; 160(6). [Guideline]
10. Torloni MR, Betran AP, Horta BL et al. Prepregnancy BMI and the risk of gestational diabetes: A systematic review of the literature with meta-analysis. *Obes Rev* 2009; 10(2): 194–203. [Meta-analysis of 59 cohorts and 11 case controls with 671,945 women]

11. Meyer WJ, Carbone J, Gauthier DW, Gottmann DA. Early gestational glucose screening and gestational diabetes. *J Reprod Med* 1996; 41: 675–9. [II-3]

12. Tieu J, McPhee AJ, Crowther CA, Middleton P. Screening and subsequent management for gestational diabetes for improving maternal and infant health. *Cochrane Database Syst Rev* 2014; (2): CD007222. [Meta-analysis of 3 RCTs and 1 quasi-RCT, *n* = 3972]

13. Meltzer SJ, Snyder J, Penrod JR, Nudi M, Morin L. Gestational diabetes mellitus screening and diagnosis: A prospective randomised controlled trial comparing costs of one-step and two-step methods. *BJOG* 2010; 117(4): 407–15. [RCT, *n* = 1500]

14. Brody SC, Harris R, Lohr K. Screening for gestational diabetes: A summary of the evidence for the U.S. preventative services task force. *Obstet Gynecol* 2003; 101: 380–92. [Review]

15. Yeral MI, Ozgu-Erdinc AS, Uygur D, Seckin KD, Karsli MF, Danisman AN. Prediction of gestational diabetes mellitus in the first trimester, comparison of fasting plasma glucose, two-step and one-step methods: A prospective randomized controlled trial. *Endocrine* 2014; 46(3): 512–8. [RCT, *n* = 486]

16. HAPO Study Cooperative Research Group, Metzger BE, Lowe LP et al. Hyperglycemia and adverse pregnancy outcomes. *N Engl J Med* 2008; 358(19): 1991–2002. [Prospective, *n* = 25,505]

17. Coustan DR, Lowe LP, Metzger BE, Dyer AR. International Association of Diabetes and Pregnancy Study Groups. The hyperglycemia and adverse pregnancy outcome (HAPO) study: Paving the way for new diagnostic criteria for gestational diabetes mellitus. *Am J Obstet Gynecol* 2010; 202(6): 654. e1–6. [III]

18. Coustan DR, Widness JA, Carpenter MW, Rotondo L, Pratt DC, Oh W. Should the 50-gram, one hour plasma glucose screening test for gestational diabetes be administered in the fasting or fed state? *Am J Obstet Gynecol* 1986; 154: 1031–5. [II-2, *n* = 72]

19. Murphy NJ, Meyer BA, O'Kell RT, Hogard ME. Carbohydrate sources for gestational diabetes mellitus screening. A comparison. *J Reprod Med* 1994; 39(12): 977–81. [RCT, *n* = 108]

20. Lamar ME, Kuehl TJ, Cooney AT, Gayle LJ, Holleman S, Allen SR. Jelly beans as an alternative to a fifty gram glucose beverage for gestational diabetes screening. *Am J Obstet Gynecol* 1999; 181: 1154–7. [RCT, *n* = 160]

21. Racusin DA, Antony K, Showalter L, Sharma S, Haymond M, Aagaard KM. Candy twists as an alternative to the glucola beverage in gestational diabetes mellitus screening. *Am J Obstet Gynecol* 2015; 212(4): 522.e1–5. [RCT, *n* = 20]

22. Gabbe SG, Graves CR. Management of diabetes mellitus complicating pregnancy. *Obstet Gynecol* 2003; 102(4): 857–68. [III]

23. Magee MS, Walden CE, Benedetti TJ, Knopp RH. Influence of diagnostic criteria on the incidence of gestational diabetes and perinatal morbidity. *JAMA* 1993; 269(5): 609–15. [Observational study, *n* = 2,015]

24. Sevket O, Ates S, Uysal O, Molla T, Dansuk R, Kelekci S. To evaluate the prevalence and clinical outcomes using a one-step method versus a two-step method to screen gestational diabetes mellitus. *J Matern Fetal Neonat Med* 2014; 27(1): 36–41. [RCT, *n* = 786]

25. Langer O, Anyaegbunan A, Brustman L, Divon M. Management of women with one abnormal oral glucose tolerance test value reduces adverse outcome in pregnancy. *Am J Obstet Gynecol* 1989; 161: 593–9. [RCT, *n* = 272]

26. Deveer R, Deveer M, Akbaba E et al. The effect of diet on pregnancy outcomes among pregnant with abnormal glucose challenge test. *Eur Rev Med Pharmacol Sci* 2013; 17(9): 1258–61. [RCT, *n* = 100]

27. Kokanali MK, Tokmak A, Kaymak O, Cavkaytar S, Bilge U. The effect of treatment on pregnancy outcomes in women with one elevated oral glucose tolerance test value. *Ginekol Pol* 2014; 85(10): 748–53. [RCT, *n* = 411]

28. Grant SM, Wolever TM, O'Connor DL, Nisenbaum R, Josse RG. Effect of a low glycaemic index diet on blood glucose in women with gestational hyperglycaemia. *Diabetes Res Clin Pract* 2010; 91(1): 15–22. [RCT, *n* = 38]

29. Berggren EK, Mele L, Landon MB et al. Perinatal outcomes in Hispanic and non-Hispanic white women with mild gestational diabetes. *Obstet Gynecol* 2012; 120(5): 1099–104. [Secondary analysis, RCT, *n* = 1535]

30. American Diabetes Association. Diagnosis and classification of diabetes mellitus. *Diabetes Care* 2014; 37(Suppl. 1): S81–90. [Guideline]

31. American Diabetes Association. Gestational diabetes mellitus. *Diabetes Care* 2004; (Suppl. 1): S88–90. [Review]

32. Maitland RA, Seed PT, Briley AL et al. Prediction of gestational diabetes in obese pregnant women from the UK pregnancies better eating and activity (UPBEAT) pilot trial. *Diabet Med* 2014; 31(8): 963–70. [RCT, *n* = 106]

33. Bo S, Gambino R, Menato G et al. Isoleucine-to-methionine substitution at residue 148 variant of PNPLA3 gene and metabolic outcomes in gestational diabetes. *Am J Clin Nutr* 2015; 101(2): 310–8. [RCT, *n* = 200]

34. Wojcik M, Zieleniak A, Mac-Marcjanek K, Wozniak LA, Cypryk K. The elevated gene expression level of the A(2B) adenosine receptor is associated with hyperglycemia in women with gestational diabetes mellitus. *Diabetes/Metabolism Res Rev* 2014; 30(1): 42–53. [Prospective, *n* = 117]

35. Bahado-Singh RO, Mele L, Landon MB et al. Fetal male gender and the benefits of treatment of mild gestational diabetes mellitus. *Am J Obstet Gynecol* 2012; 206(5): 422.e1–5. [Secondary analysis, RCT, *n* = 932]

36. Balsells M, Garcia-Patterson A, Gich I, Corcoy R. Major congenital malformations in women with gestational diabetes mellitus: A systematic review and meta-analysis. *Diabetes/Metabolism Res Rev* 2012; 28(3): 252–7. [Meta-analysis, 17 RCTs, *n* > 500,000]

37. Landon MB, Spong CY, Thom E et al. A multicenter, randomized trial of treatment for mild gestational diabetes. *N Engl J Med* 2009; 361(14): 1339–48. [RCT, *n* = 958]

38. Kim SY, England JL, Sharma JA, Njoroge T. Gestational diabetes mellitus and risk of childhood overweight and obesity in offspring: A systematic review. *Exp Diabetes Res* 2011; 541308. [Meta-analysis, 12 Studies, *n* > 2900]

39. Durnwald CP, Mele L, Spong CY et al. Glycemic characteristics and neonatal outcomes of women treated for mild gestational diabetes. *Obstet Gynecol* 2011; 117(4): 819–27. [Secondary analysis, RCT, *n* = 460]

40. Kim C, Newton KM, Knopp RH. Gestational diabetes and the incidence of type 2 diabetes: A systematic review. *Diabetes Care* 2002; 25(10): 1862–8. [Review]

41. Tieu J, Crowther CA, Middleton P. Dietary advice in pregnancy for preventing gestational diabetes mellitus. *Cochrane Database Syst Rev* 2008; 2(2): CD006674. [Meta-analysis, 2 RCTs, *n* = 82]

42. Sanabria-Martinez G, Garcia-Hermoso A, Poyatos-Leon R, Alvarez-Bueno C, Sanchez-Lopez M, Martinez-Vizcaino V. Effectiveness of physical activity interventions on preventing gestational diabetes mellitus and excessive maternal weight gain: A meta-analysis. *BJOG* 2015; 122(9): 1167–74. [Meta-analysis, 13 RCTs, *n* = 2873]

43. Russo LM, Nobles C, Ertel KA, Chasan-Taber L, Whitcomb BW. Physical activity interventions in pregnancy and risk of gestational diabetes mellitus: A systematic review and meta-analysis. *Obstet Gynecol* 2015; 125(3): 576–82. doi:10.1097 /AOG.0000000000000691. [Meta-analysis; 10 RCTs, *n* = 3401]

44. Corrado F, D'Anna R, Di Vieste G et al. The effect of myoinositol supplementation on insulin resistance in patients with gestational diabetes. *Diabetic Med* 2011; 28(8): 972–5. [RCT, *n* = 69]

45. D'Anna R, Scilipoti A, Giordano D et al. Myo-inositol supplementation and onset of gestational diabetes mellitus in pregnant women with a family history of type 2 diabetes: A prospective, randomized, placebo-controlled study. *Diabetes Care* 2013; 36(4): 854–7. [RCT, *n* = 220]

46. D'Anna R, Di Benedetto A, Scilipoti A et al. Myo-inositol supplementation for prevention of gestational diabetes in obese pregnant women: A randomized controlled trial. *Obstet Gynecol* 2015; 126(2): 310–5. [RCT, *n* = 220]

47. Matarrelli B, Vitacolonna E, D'Angelo M et al. Effect of dietary myo-inositol supplementation in pregnancy on the incidence of maternal gestational diabetes mellitus and fetal outcomes: A randomized controlled trial. *J Matern Fetal Neonat Med* 2013; 26(10): 967–72. [RCT, *n* = 73]

48. Horvath K, Koch K, Jeitler K et al. Effects of treatment in women with gestational diabetes mellitus: Systematic review and meta-analysis. *BMJ* 2010; 340: c1395. [Meta-analysis, 5 RCTs, *n* = 2999]

49. Landon MB, Spong CY, Thom E et al. A multicenter, randomized trial of treatment for mild gestational diabetes. *N Engl J Med* 2009; 361(14): 1339–48. [RCT, *n* = 958]

50. Crowther CA, Hiller JE, Moss JR, McPhee AJ, Jeffries WS, Robinson JF et al. Effect of treatment of gestational diabetes mellitus on pregnancy outcomes. *NEJM* 2005; 352: 2477–86. [RCT, *n* = 1000. Impaired glucose tolerance (defined following 75 gm OGTT as fasting <7.0 mmol/L, two-hour between 7.8 mmol/L and 11.0 mmol/L). **Diet**, glucose monitoring, and **insulin** as needed vs. routine care]

51. Kinnunen TI, Puhkala J, Raitanen J et al. Effects of dietary counseling on food habits and dietary intake of Finnish pregnant women at increased risk for gestational diabetes—A secondary analysis of a cluster-randomized controlled trial. *Matern Child Nutrition* 2014; 10(2): 184–97. [Secondary analysis, RCT, *n* = 399]

52. Luoto R, Kinnunen TI, Aittasalo M et al. Primary prevention of gestational diabetes mellitus and large-for-gestational-age newborns by lifestyle counseling: A cluster-randomized controlled trial. *PLoS Med* 2011; 8(5): e1001036. [RCT, *n* = 399]

53. Moses RG, Barker M, Winter M, Petocz P, Brand-Miller JC. Can a low-glycemic index diet reduce the need for insulin in gestational diabetes mellitus? A randomized trial. *Diabetes Care* 2009; 32(6): 996–1000. [RCT, *n* = 63]

54. Moreno-Castilla C, Hernandez M, Bergua M et al. Low-carbohydrate diet for the treatment of gestational diabetes mellitus: A randomized controlled trial. *Diabetes Care* 2013; 36(8): 2233–8. [RCT, *n* = 152]

55. Louie JC, Markovic TP, Perera N et al. A randomized controlled trial investigating the effects of a low-glycemic index diet on pregnancy outcomes in gestational diabetes mellitus. *Diabetes Care* 2011; 34(11): 2341–6. [RCT, *n* = 99]

56. Moses RG, Casey SA, Quinn EG et al. Pregnancy and glycemic index outcomes study: Effects of low glycemic index compared with conventional dietary advice on selected pregnancy outcomes. *Am J Clin Nutr* 2014; 99(3): 517–23. [RCT, *n* = 576]

57. Asemi Z, Tabassi Z, Samimi M, Fahiminejad T, Esmaillzadeh A. Favourable effects of the dietary approaches to stop hypertension diet on glucose tolerance and lipid profiles in gestational diabetes: A randomised clinical trial. *Br J Nutr* 2013; 109(11): 2024–30. [RCT, *n* = 34]

58. Asemi Z, Samimi M, Tabassi Z, Esmaillzadeh A. The effect of DASH diet on pregnancy outcomes in gestational diabetes: A randomized controlled clinical trial. *Eur J Clin Nutr* 2014; 68(4): 490–5. [RCT, *n* = 52]

59. Asemi Z, Samimi M, Tabassi Z et al. Effect of daily consumption of probiotic yoghurt on insulin resistance in pregnant women: A randomized controlled trial. *Eur J Clin Nutr* 2013; 67(1): 71–4. [RCT, *n* = 70]

60. Wang H, Jiang H, Yang L, Zhang M. Impacts of dietary fat changes on pregnant women with gestational diabetes mellitus: A randomized controlled study. *Asia Pac J Clin Nutr* 2015; 24(1): 58–64. [RCT, *n* = 84]

61. Barakat R, Pelaez M, Lopez C, Lucia A, Ruiz JR. Exercise during pregnancy and gestational diabetes-related adverse effects: A randomised controlled trial. *Br J Sports Med* 2013; 47(10): 630–6. [RCT, *n* = 420]

62. Vinter CA, Jorgensen JS, Ovesen P, Beck-Nielsen H, Skytthe A, Jensen DM. Metabolic effects of lifestyle intervention in obese pregnant women. Results from the randomized controlled trial "lifestyle in pregnancy" (LiP). *Diabet Med* 2014; 31(11): 1323–30. [RCT, *n* = 304]

63. Bung P, Bung C, Artal R, Khodiguian N, Fallenstein F, Spatling L. Therapeutic exercise for insulin-requiring gestational diabetics: Effects on fetus–results of a randomized prospective longitudinal study. *J Perinat Med* 1993; 21: 125–37. [RCT]

64. Jovanovic-Peterson L, Durak EP, Peterson CM. Randomized trial of diet versus diet plus cardiovascular conditioning on glucose levels in gestational diabetes mellitus. *Am J Obstet Gynecol* 1989; 161(2): 415–9. [RCT, *n* = 33]

65. Ruchat SM, Davenport MH, Giroux I et al. Effect of exercise intensity and duration on capillary glucose responses in pregnant women at low and high risk for gestational diabetes. *Diabetes/Metabolism Res Rev* 2012; 28(8): 669–78. [RCT, *n* = 46]

66. Avery MD, Leon AS, Kopher RA. Effects of a partially home-based exercise program for women with gestational diabetes. *Obstet Gynecol* 1997; 89: 10–5. [RCT, *n* = 33]

67. van Poppel MN, Oostdam N, Eekhoff ME, Wouters MG, van Mechelen W, Catalano PM. Longitudinal relationship of physical activity with insulin sensitivity in overweight and obese pregnant women. *J Clin Endocrinol Metab* 2013; 98(7): 2929–35. [Prospective, longitudinal, *n* = 24]

68. Bo S, Rosato R, Ciccone G et al. Simple lifestyle recommendations and the outcomes of gestational diabetes. A 2 x 2 factorial randomized trial. *Diabetes Obes Metab* 2014; 16(10): 1032–35. [RCT, *n* = 400]

69. Muktabhant B, Lawrie TA, Lumbiganon P, Laopaiboon M. Diet or exercise, or both, for preventing excessive weight gain in pregnancy. *Cochrane Database Syst Rev* 2015; 6. [Meta-analysis, 49 RCTs, *n* = 11,444]

70. Korpi-Hyovalti E, Heinonen S, Schwab U, Laaksonen DE, Niskanen L. Effect of intensive counseling on physical activity in pregnant women at high risk for gestational diabetes mellitus. A clinical study in primary care. *Prim Care Diabetes* 2012; 6(4): 261–8. [RCT, *n* = 54]

71. Harrison CL, Lombard CB, Strauss BJ, Teede HJ. Optimizing healthy gestational weight gain in women at high risk of gestational diabetes: A randomized controlled trial. *Obesity (Silver Spring)* 2013; 21(5): 904–9. [RCT, *n* = 203]

72. Aittasalo M, Raitanen J, Kinnunen TI, Ojala K, Kolu P, Luoto R. Is intensive counseling in maternity care feasible and effective in promoting physical activity among women at risk for gestational diabetes? Secondary analysis of a cluster randomized NELLI study in Finland. *Int J Behav Nutr Physical Activity* 2012; 9: 104. [Secondary analysis, RCT, *n* = 399]

73. Oostdam N, van Poppel MN, Wouters MG et al. No effect of the FitFor2 exercise programme on blood glucose, insulin sensitivity, and birth weight in pregnant women who were overweight and at risk for gestational diabetes: Results of a randomised controlled trial. *BJOG* 2012; 119(9): 1098–107. [RCT, *n* = 121]

74. Stafne SN, Salvesen KA, Romundstad PR, Eggebo TM, Carlsen SM, Morkved S. Regular exercise during pregnancy to prevent gestational diabetes: A randomized controlled trial. *Obstet Gynecol* 2012; 119(1): 29–36. [RCT, *n* = 702]

75. Kestila KK, Ekblad UU, Ronnemaa T. Continuous glucose monitoring versus self-monitoring of blood glucose in the treatment of gestational diabetes mellitus. *Diabetes Res Clin Pract* 2007; 77(2): 174–9. [RCT, *n* = 71]

76. McLachlan K, Jenkins A, O'Neal D. The role of continuous glucose monitoring in clinical decision-making in diabetes in pregnancy. *Aust N Z J Obstet Gynaecol* 2007; 47(3): 186–90. [Descriptive study, *n* = 68]

77. De Veciana M, Major CA, Morgan MA, Asrat T, Tooney JS, Lien JM, Evans AT. Postprandial versus preprandial blood glucose monitoring in women with gestational diabetes mellitus requiring insulin therapy. *NEJM* 1995; 333: 1237–41. [RCT, *n* = 66]

78. Bancroft K, Tuffnell DJ, Mason GC, Rogerson LJ, Mansfield M. A randomised controlled pilot study of the management of gestational impaired glucose tolerance. *BJOG* 2000; 107(8): 959–63. [RCT, *n* = 68. Impaired glucose tolerance (defined following 75 gm OGTT as fasting <7.0 mmol/L, two-hour between 7.8 mmol/L and 11.0 mmol/L-same as Crowther). Monitored

group was given standard dietary advice, glucose metabolism was **monitored by capillary glucose** series five days a week, HbA1c was measured monthly (**insulin** was introduced if five or more capillary measurements >7.0 mmol/L in one week), serial ultrasound for growth and amniotic fluid, Doppler studies, CTG monitoring. Unmonitored group received dietary advice, HbA1c monthly but no capillary glucose measurements]

79. Ford FA, Bruce CB, Fraser RB. Preliminary report of a randomised trial of dietary advice in women with mild abnormalities of glucose tolerance in pregnancy. Personal communication 1997. [RCT, $n = 29$. Impaired glucose tolerance (defined following a 75-g OGTT as two-hour plasma glucose level between 8 mmol/L and 11 mmol/L-similar to Crowther. **Dietary** treatment group was given specific "diabetic type" advice (i.e., "high fiber, high carbohydrate, low fat, and appropriate energy"). No mention of insulin therapy. The control group received no specific dietary advice. Both groups attended clinic weekly and performed plasma glucose profiles]

80. Prutsky GJ, Domecq JP, Wang Z et al. Glucose targets in pregnant women with diabetes: A systematic review and meta-analysis. *J Clin Endocrinol Metab* 2013; 98(11): 4319–24. [Meta-analysis, 34 RCTs, $n = 9433$]

81. Homko CJ, Deeb LC, Rohrbacher K et al. Impact of a telemedicine system with automated reminders on outcomes in women with gestational diabetes mellitus. *Diabetes Tech Therapeut* 2012; 14(7): 624–9. [RCT, $n = 80$]

82. Hebert MF, Ma X, Naraharisetti SB et al. Are we optimizing gestational diabetes treatment with glyburide? The pharmacologic basis for better clinical practice. *Clin Pharmacol Ther* 2009; 85(6): 607–14. [Assessed steady-state PK of glyburide, insulin sensitivity, and β-cell responsivity after a mixed-meal tolerance test in women with GDM ($n = 40$), healthy pregnant women ($n = 40$), and nonpregnant women with DM ($n = 26$)]

83. Lain KY, Garabedian MJ, Daftary A, Jeyabalan A. Neonatal adiposity following maternal treatment of gestational diabetes with glyburide compared with insulin. *Am J Obstet Gyn* 2009; 200: 501.e1–6. [RCT of 83 neonates]

84. Langer O, Conway DL, Berkus MD, Xenakis EM, Gonzales O. A comparison of glyburide and insulin in women with gestational diabetes mellitus. *N Engl J Med* 2000; 343(16): 1134–8. [RCT, $n = 404$]

85. Tempe A, Mayanglambam RD. Glyburide as treatment option for gestational diabetes mellitus. *J Obstet Gynaecol Res* 2013; 39(6): 1147–52. [RCT, $n = 64$]

86. Casey BM, Duryea EL, Abbassi-Ghanavati M et al. Glyburide in women with mild gestational diabetes: A randomized controlled trial. *Obstet Gynecol* 2015; 126(2): 303–9. [RCT, $n = 375$]

87. Balsells M, Garcia-Patterson A, Sola I, Roque M, Gich I, Corcoy R. Glibenclamide, metformin, and insulin for the treatment of gestational diabetes: A systematic review and meta-analysis. *BMJ* 2015; 350: h102. [Meta-analysis, 15 RCTs, $n = 2509$]

88. Zeng YC, Li MJ, Chen Y et al. The use of glyburide in the management of gestational diabetes mellitus: A meta-analysis. *Adv Med Sci* 2014; 59(1): 95–101. [Meta-analysis, 5 RCTs, $n = 674$]

89. Langer O, Yogev Y, Xenakis EMJ, Brustman L. Overweight and obese in gestational diabetes: The impact on pregnancy outcomes. *Am J Obstet Gynecol* 2005; 192: 1768–76. [II-2]

90. De Leo V, Musacchio MC. The administration of metformin during pregnancy reduces polycystic ovary syndrome related gestational complications. *Eur J Obstet, Gynecol Reprod Biol* 2011; 157: 63–6. [Prospective cohort, $n = 208$]

91. Hickman MA, McBride R, Boggess KA, Strauss R. Metformin compared with insulin in the treatment of pregnant women with overt diabetes: A randomized controlled trial. *Am J Perinatol* 2013; 30(6): 483–90. [RCT, $n = 28$]

92. Gui J, Liu Q, Feng L. Metformin vs. insulin in the management of gestational diabetes: A meta-analysis. *PLoS One* 2013; 8(5): e64585. [Meta-analysis, 5 RCT, $n = 1270$]

93. Refuerzo JS, Viteri OA, Hutchinson M et al. The effects of metformin on weight loss in women with gestational diabetes: A pilot randomized, placebo-controlled trial. *Am J Obstet Gynecol* 2015; 212(3): 389.e1–9. [RCT, $n = 79$]

94. Ijas H, Vaarasmaki M, Morin-Papunen L et al. Metformin should be considered in the treatment of gestational diabetes: A prospective randomized trial. *BJOG* 2011; 118(7): 880–5. [RCT, $n = 100$]

95. Tertti K, Ekblad U, Koskinen P, Vahlberg T, Ronnemaa T. Metformin vs. insulin in gestational diabetes. A randomized study characterizing metformin patients needing additional insulin. *Diabetes Obes Metab* 2013; 15(3): 246–51. [RCT, $n = 217$]

96. Ibrahim MI, Hamdy A, Shafik A, Taha S, Anwar M, Faris M. The role of adding metformin in insulin-resistant diabetic pregnant women: A randomized controlled trial. *Arch Gynecol & Obstet* 2014; 289(5): 959–65. [RCT, $n = 90$]

97. Gatford KL, Houda CM, Lu ZX et al. Vitamin B12 and homocysteine status during pregnancy in the metformin in gestational diabetes trial: Responses to maternal metformin compared with insulin treatment. *Diabetes Obes Metab* 2013; 15(7): 660–7. [RCT, $n = 180$]

98. ACOG practice bulletin. Pregestational diabetes mellitus. *Obstet Gynecol* 2005; 105: 675–84. [Review, guideline]

99. Jovanovic L, Druzin M, Peterson CM. Effect of euglycemia on the outcome of pregnancy in insulin-dependent diabetic women as compared with normal control subjects. *Am J Med* 1981; 71(6): 921–7. [Level II-2]

100. Langer O, Anyaegbunam A, Brustman L, Guidetti D, Levy J, Mazze R. Pregestational diabetes: Insulin requirements throughout pregnancy. *Am J Obstet Gynecol* 1988; 159(3): 616–21. [II-2]

101. Jovanovic L, Ilic S, Pettitt DJ et al. Metabolism and immunologic effects of insulin lispro in gestational diabetes. *Diabetes Care* 1999; 22: 1422–7. [RCT, $n = 42$]

102. Garner P, Okun N, Keeley E et al. A randomized controlled trial of strict glycemia control and tertiary level obstetric care versus routine obstetric care in the management of gestational diabetes: A pilot study. *Am J Obstet Gynecol* 1997; 177(1): 190–5. [RCT, $n = 300$]

103. Thompson DJ, Porter KB, Gunnells DJ, Wagner PC, Spinnato JA. Prophylactic insulin in the management of gestational diabetes. *Obstet Gynecol* 1990; 7(6): 960–4. [RCT, $n = 108$]

104. Gojnic M, Perovic M, Pervulov M, Ljubic A. The effects of adjuvant insulin therapy among pregnant women with IGT who failed to achieve the desired glycemia levels by diet and moderate physical activity. *J Matern Fetal Neonat Med* 2012; 25(10): 2028–34. [RCT, $n = 280$]

105. Spaulonci CP, Bernardes LS, Trindade TC, Zugaib M, Francisco RP. Randomized trial of metformin vs. insulin in the management of gestational diabetes. *Am J Obstet Gynecol* 2013; 209(1): 34.e1–7. [RCT, $n = 92$]

106. Waheed S, Malik FP, Mazhar SB. Efficacy of metformin versus insulin in the management of pregnancy with diabetes. *J Coll Phys Surg–Pakistan* 2013; 23(12): 866–9. [RCT, $n = 68$]

107. Niromanesh S, Alavi A, Sharbaf FR, Amjadi N, Moosavi S, Akbari S. Metformin compared with insulin in the management of gestational diabetes mellitus: A randomized clinical trial. *Diabetic Res Clin Prac* 2012; 98(3): 422–9. [RCT, $n = 160$]

108. Balaji V, Balaji MS, Alexander C et al. Premixed insulin aspart 30 (BIAsp 30) versus premixed human insulin 30 (BHI 30) in gestational diabetes mellitus: A randomized open-label controlled study. *Gynecol Endocrin* 2012; 28(7): 529–32. [RCT, $n = 320$]

109. Moore LE, Clokey D, Rappaport VJ, Curet LB. Metformin compared with glyburide in gestational diabetes: A randomized controlled trial. *Obstet Gynecol* 2010; 115(1): 55–9. [RCT, $n = 149$]

110. Rowan JA, Hague WM, Gao W, Battin MR, Moore MP, MiG Trial Investigators. Metformin versus insulin for the treatment of gestational diabetes. *N Engl J Med* 2008; 358(19): 2003–15. [RCT, $n = 751$]

111. Di Cianni G, Volpe L, Ghio A et al. Maternal metabolic control and perinatal outcome in women with gestational diabetes mellitus treated with lispro or aspart insulin: Comparison with regular insulin. *Diabetes Care* 2007; 30(4): e11. [RCT, *n* = 96]

112. Asemi Z, Karamali M, Esmaillzadeh A. Effects of calcium-vitamin D co-supplementation on glycaemic control, inflammation and oxidative stress in gestational diabetes: A randomised placebo-controlled trial. *Diabetologia* 2014; 57(9): 1798–806. [RCT, *n* = 54]

113. Asemi Z, Hashemi T, Karamali M, Samimi M, Esmaillzadeh A. Effects of vitamin D supplementation on glucose metabolism, lipid concentrations, inflammation, and oxidative stress in gestational diabetes: A double-blind randomized controlled clinical trial. *Am J Clin Nutr* 2013; 98(6): 1425–1432. [RCT, *n* = 54]

114. Yap C, Cheung NW, Gunton JE et al. Vitamin D supplementation and the effects on glucose metabolism during pregnancy: A randomized controlled trial. *Diabetes Care* 2014; 37(7): 1837–44. [RCT, *n* = 158]

115. Lindsay KL, Brennan L, Kennelly MA et al. Impact of probiotics in women with gestational diabetes mellitus on metabolic health: A randomized controlled trial. *Am J Obstet Gynecol* 2015; 212(4): 496.e1–11. [RCT, *n* = 100]

116. Lindsay KL, Kennelly M, Culliton M et al. Probiotics in obese pregnancy do not reduce maternal fasting glucose: A double-blind, placebo-controlled, randomized trial (probiotics in pregnancy study). *Am J Clin Nutr* 2014; 99(6): 1432–39. [RCT, *n* = 138]

117. Zhou SJ, Yelland L, McPhee AJ, Quinlivan J, Gibson RA, Makrides M. Fish-oil supplementation in pregnancy does not reduce the risk of gestational diabetes or preeclampsia. *Am J Clin Nutr* 2012; 95(6): 1378–84. [RCT, *n* = 2399]

118. Min Y, Djahanbakhch O, Hutchinson J et al. Effect of docosahexaenoic acid-enriched fish oil supplementation in pregnant women with type 2 diabetes on membrane fatty acids and fetal body composition—Double-blinded randomized placebo-controlled trial. *Diabet Med* 2014; 31(11): 1331–40. [RCT, *n* = 117]

119. Costantine MM, Mele L, Landon MB et al. Customized versus population approach for evaluation of fetal overgrowth. *Am J Perinatol* 2013; 30(7): 565–72. [RCT, *n* = 491]

120. Kjos SL, Henry OA, Montoro M, Buchanan TA, Mestman JH. Insulin-requiring diabetes in pregnancy: A randomized trial of active induction of labor and expectant management. *Am J Obstet Gynecol* 1993; 169: 611–5. [RCT, *n* = 200]

121. Sutton AL, Mele L, Landon MB et al. Delivery timing and cesarean delivery risk in women with mild gestational diabetes mellitus. *Am J Obstet Gynecol* 2014; 211(3): 244.e1–7. [Secondary analysis, RCT, *n* = 679]

122. Bellamy L, Casas JP, Hingorani AD, Williams D. Type 2 diabetes mellitus after gestational diabetes: A systematic review and meta-analysis. *Lancet* 2009; 373(9677): 1773–9. [20 cohort studies (retrospective and prospective), *n* = 675,455]

123. Expert Committee on the Diagnosis and Classification of Diabetes Mellitus. Report of the expert committee on the diagnosis and classification of diabetes mellitus. *Diabetes Care* 2003; 26(Suppl. 1): S5–20. [Review, guideline]

124. The Royal Australian and New Zealand College of Obstetricians and Gynaecologists. College statement. Diagnosis of gestational diabetes mellitus. Melbourne: RANZCOG, 2008. [III]

125. Akinci B, Celtik A, Yener S, Yesil S. Prediction of developing metabolic syndrome after gestational diabetes mellitus. *Fertil Steril* 2010; 93(4): 1248–54. [Prospective, *n* = 164]

126. Retnakaran R, Qi Y, Sermer M, Connelly PW, Hanley AJ, Zinman B. An abnormal screening glucose challenge test in pregnancy predicts postpartum metabolic dysfunction, even when the antepartum oral glucose tolerance test is normal. *Clin Endocrinol (Oxf)* 2009; 71(2): 208–14. [Observational study, *n* = 259]

127. Nicklas JM, Miller LJ, Zera CA, Davis RB, Levkoff SE, Seely EW. Factors associated with depressive symptoms in the early postpartum period among women with recent gestational diabetes mellitus. *Maternal & Child Health Journal*. 2013; 17(9): 1665–72. [RCT, *n* = 71]

6

Hypothyroidism

Sushma Jwala

KEY POINTS

- **Hypothyroidism** is characterized by inadequate thyroid hormone production and usually requires for diagnosis **elevated thyroid-stimulating hormone (TSH) and low free thyroxine (FT4)** (or free triiodothyronine [FT3]).
- **Subclinical hypothyroidism** requires for diagnosis an **elevated TSH but normal FT4**.
- **Hashimoto's thyroiditis** is the most common cause of hypothyroidism in pregnancy with thyroid peroxidase antibodies in >90% of these women.
- Untreated or partially treated hypothyroidism is associated with increased risk of **preeclampsia, abruption, preterm birth, low birth weight, fetal death, and long-term impaired psychomotor function.**
- All physiologic changes and placental transfer should be known by the physician caring for thyroid disease in pregnancy (Table 6.1).
- **Women at high risk for hypothyroidism** (Table 6.3) should be **screened** with **TSH** and **FT4**.
- **Goal of** levothyroxine treatment in pregnancy is **maternal serum TSH 0.5 to 2.0 mµ/L**, and FT4 in upper third of normal range. **Most women with hypothyroidism need an increase in thyroxine replacement dose.**
- In women with overt hypothyroidism, **TSH and FT4 levels** should be checked **preconceptionally, at first prenatal visit in the first trimester,** four weeks after altering the doses (therefore, **every four weeks until TSH is normal**, especially in the first 20 weeks), **and at least every trimester in pregnancy.**
- **Iodine supplementation** in a population with high levels of endemic cretinism results in a reduction in deaths during infancy and early childhood with decreased endemic cretinism at four years of age and better psychomotor development scores between four and 25 months of age.
- There is **no evidence that screening and treatment of subclinical hypothyroidism during pregnancy improves maternal or fetal outcomes.**
- Screening and treating for hypothyroxinemia is also unnecessary as it is not associated with any maternal or child benefits.
- Every woman with a thyroid nodule should have fine-needle aspiration and TSH checked.

CLINICAL HYPOTHYROIDISM
Definitions (Figure 6.1)

- *Clinical (or overt) hypothyroidism*: Inadequate thyroid hormone production of any cause. Usually requires **elevated TSH and low FT4 (or FT3).**
- *Subclinical hypothyroidism*: Elevated TSH and normal FT4. Elevated TSH reflects the sensitivity of the hypothalamic-pituitary axis to small decreases in thyroid hormone; as the thyroid gland fails, the TSH level may rise above the upper limit of normal while the FT4 is still within the normal range.
- *Hypothyroxinemia*: Normal TSH and low FT4.
- TSH is also called thyrotropin, T4 is also called thyroxine, T3 is also called triiodothyronine; FT4 stands for free T4 and FT3 stands for free T3.

Incidence

1% in general population; about **0.3% in pregnant women** [1,2]. General screening of obstetric patients reveals an incidence of 2.5% of elevated serum TSH [2]. There is an increased incidence with concurrent autoimmune disease, that is, **5% to 8% incidence in patients with type I diabetes** [3]. Up to 25% of patients with type I diabetes develop postpartum thyroid dysfunction [3]. In the United States, 10% to 15% of pregnant women are iodine deficient (urinary iodine concentration <5 µg/dL) [4].

Signs/Symptoms

Thyroid disease may be masked by a hypermetabolic state of pregnancy. The most common signs include dry skin, weakness, facial puffiness, and mild-to-moderate weight gain [5]. Fatigue, constipation, cold intolerance, muscle cramps, insomnia, hair loss, goiter, prolonged relaxation phase of deep tendon reflexes, carpal tunnel syndrome, intellectual slowness, voice changes, myxedema, and (extremely rarely) coma are less common.

Pathophysiology

The thyroid maintains the metabolism in cells by stimulating transcription and translation. It also stimulates oxygen consumption and regulates lipid and carbohydrate metabolism and is necessary for normal growth and maturation. The thyroid is under the control of TSH from the anterior pituitary. TSH induces thyroid growth, differentiation, and iodine metabolism.

A majority (>99%) of cases of hypothyroidism are due to primary thyroid abnormality. Secondary hypothyroidism is pituitary in origin following irradiation or hypophysectomy or Sheehan's syndrome (postpartum pituitary necrosis). Tertiary hypothyroidism (hypothalamic) is rare.

Hashimoto's thyroiditis is the **most common cause of hypothyroidism in pregnancy**. It is a chronic autoimmune lymphocytic thyroiditis, characterized by antithyroid antibodies (**thyroid peroxidase [TPO] antibodies 90%**, thyroglobulin antibodies 20%–50%), and usually firm, painless goiter as a presenting symptom [6]. TPO antibodies are present in 6% of the general population. Less common causes are subacute viral thyroiditis; iodine deficiency (median urinary

Table 6.1 Thyroid Physiology Changes in Pregnancy and Transplacental Passage

	Change in Pregnancy	Placental Transfer
Thyroid-binding globulin (TBG)	↑	+
Total thyroxine (TT4)	↑	− (minimal)
Total triiodothyronine (TT3)	↑	−
Resin triiodothyronine uptake (RT3U)	↓	−
Thyroid-stimulating hormone (TSH)	−	−
Free thyroxine (FT4)	−	++
Free triiodothyronine (FT3)	−	++
TRH	−	− (<1%)
Iodide	↓	++
Thyroid-stimulating immunoglobulin (TSI)	−	++
Antithyroid peroxidase antibody	↓	++
Levothyroxine replacement	NA	− (minimal)
Thioamide (PTU or methimazole) therapy	NA	++
Free thyroxine index (FTI)	−	NA

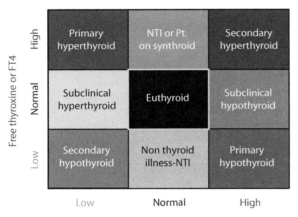

Figure 6.1 Basic thyroid evaluation.

iodine level <100 μg/L); "burned-out" Graves' disease, after radioiodine therapy, thyroidectomy, or antithyroid drugs; other head and neck surgery; other radiation therapy to the head, neck, or chest area; medications—lithium, iodine, amiodarone; rarely hypothalamic dysfunction, that is, Sheehan's syndrome.

Complications

Untreated or partially treated clinical hypothyroidism is associated with increased risk of **infertility, miscarriage, preeclampsia** (44%), **abruption** (19%), **preterm birth, low birth weight** (31%), or **fetal death** (12%) [7–9]. Fetal goiter does not develop in women with hypothyroidism unless they had previous hyperthyroidism and thyroid-stimulating immunoglobulins (TSIs) are still >200%. Infants whose mothers had serum FT4 below the 10th percentile may have a high incidence of **impaired psychomotor function** [10].

Management
Prevention
Recently, trace element **selenium** has been shown to reduce the incidence of hypothyroidism during pregnancy and postpartum periods [11]. Selenoproteins act as antioxidants and decrease thyroid inflammation in autoimmune thyroiditis by reducing TPO antibody titers. Up to 30% of women with TPO antibodies develop permanent hypothyroidism following postpartum thyroid dysfunction [12]. This may suggest a preventive role of selenomethionine supplementation in autoimmune thyroid dysfunction.

Preconception
In a small RCT, it was shown that preconception adjustment with increased dosage of levothyroxine supplementation in hypothyroid women of reproductive age results in better control by TSH and FT4 at first prenatal visit [13].

Pregnancy Considerations
Anatomy/Radiology
In pregnancy, moderate glandular hyperplasia and increased vascularity in the thyroid are physiologic. Thyroid volume by ultrasound increases a mean of 18% during pregnancy and returns to normal size in the postpartum period [4,14]. **Any significant goiter should be worked up**.

Maternal physiology
Several changes occur as shown in Table 6.1 (Chapter 3 of *Obstetric Evidence Based Guidelines*). **Thyroid-binding globulin** (TBG) increases about 200% secondary to estrogen-stimulated hepatocyte production and altered glycosylation, which inhibits degradation. **High levels of HCG**, which peak at 10 to 12 weeks, have some TSH-like activity and stimulate thyroid hormone secretion, which in turn **suppresses TSH**. Normal TSH levels in pregnancy are shown in Table 6.2. TSH suppression is even more marked for twins [15]. Peripheral metabolism of thyroid hormones is also altered by placental deiodinases, more in the second half of pregnancy [16].

Throughout pregnancy, there is an approximately 30% to 50% increase in T4 requirement [17,18]. Plasma iodide levels decrease during pregnancy because of fetal use of iodide and increased maternal renal clearance of iodide [19]. Pregnancy does not appear to alter the course of thyroid cancer [20].

Fetal Thyroid Physiology
In the fetus, the small amount of thyroxine that crosses the placenta provides all the thyroid hormone until 10 to 12 weeks. **Before 12 weeks** (time period for initiation of fetal brain development), **the fetus is entirely dependent on maternal transfer of thyroid hormones**. Upon beginning of activation of the fetal hypothalamic/pituitary–thyroid axis at this gestational age, the fetal thyroid begins to concentrate iodine and synthesize iodothyronines. At 18 to 20 weeks, the fetal thyroid is controlled by fetal pituitary TSH and mature hormone synthesis begins. TSH, T4, and T3 all begin to increase throughout gestation as there seems to be minimal negative feedback mechanism [19].

Placenta Physiology
It is important to be aware of which molecules cross the placenta and can affect the fetus. **FT4, FT3, thyrotropin-releasing**

Table 6.2 Thyroid-Stimulating Hormone Percentiles According to Gestational Age in Singleton Pregnancies

Gestational Age (Weeks)	2.5th Percentile	50th Percentile	97.5th Percentile
6	0.23	1.36	4.94
7	0.14	1.21	5.09
8	0.09	1.01	4.93
9	0.03	0.84	4.04
10	0.02	0.74	3.12
11	0.01	0.76	3.65
12	0.01	0.79	3.32
13	0.01	0.78	4.05
14	0.01	0.85	3.33
15	0.02	0.92	3.40
16	0.04	0.92	2.74
17	0.02	0.98	3.32
18	0.17	1.07	3.48
19	0.22	1.07	3.03
20	0.25	1.11	3.20
21	0.28	1.21	3.04
22	0.26	1.15	4.09
23	0.25	1.08	3.02
24	0.34	1.13	2.99
25	0.30	1.11	2.82
26	0.20	1.07	2.89
27	0.36	1.11	2.84
28	0.30	1.03	2.78
29	0.31	1.07	3.14
30	0.20	1.07	3.27
31	0.23	1.06	2.81
32	0.31	1.07	2.98
33	0.31	1.20	5.25
34	0.20	1.18	3.18
35	0.30	1.20	3.41
36	0.33	1.31	4.59
37	0.37	1.35	6.40
38	0.23	1.16	4.33
39	0.57	1.59	5.14
≥40	0.38	1.68	5.43

Source: Dashe JS, Casey BM, Wells CE, McIntire DD, Byrd EW, Leveno KJ et al. *Obstet Gynecol*, 106, 4, 753–7, 2005.

hormone, iodine, TSI, and anti-TPO cross placenta [21] (Table 6.1). **TSH does not cross.** The placenta rapidly deiodinases maternal T4 and T3 to the inactive reverse-T3.

Screening/Diagnosis

Universal screening for maternal hypothyroidism is not usually recommended [22–26]. **Women at high risk for hypothyroidism** should be **screened** (Table 6.3) [27]. Tests used for screening and diagnosis include **TSH** (most sensitive)

Table 6.3 Screening for Hypothyroidism in Pregnancy

Symptomatic (see signs/symptoms)
Previous therapy for hyperthyroidism
History of high-dose neck irradiation
Goiter/palpable thyroid nodules
Family history of thyroid disease
Suspected hypopituitarism
Type I DM [3]
Hyperlipidemia
Medications (iodine, amiodarone, lithium, dilantin, rifampin)

Source: Weetman AP, McGregor AM. *Endocr Rev*, 5, 2, 309–55, 1984.

Table 6.4 Primary vs. Secondary Hypothyroidism

Primary hypothyroidism	
TSH	↑
FT4	↓
Antithyroglobulin	+/−
Antithyroid peroxidase	+/−
Secondary hypothyroidism	
TSH	↓
FT4	↓

Abbreviations: FT4, free thyroxine; TSH, thyroid-stimulating hormone.

[28,29] and **FT4**. Elevated TSH and either low FT4 or low FT3 are consistent with clinical hypothyroidism (Table 6.4; Figure 6.1). In the first trimester, even a TSH level >2.5 is abnormal. Hypothyroidism in pregnancy is mainly (>99%) primary. Elevated TSH and normal FT4 are consistent with **subclinical hypothyroidism** (see below).

TPO antibody is present in not only 90% women with Hashimoto's thyroiditis, but also 10% of women with euthyroid at 12 weeks. It crosses the placenta, may increase incidence of spontaneous abortion [30], and increases the incidence of postpartum thyroid dysfunction [31]. TPO antibody levels >50 IU/mL have been shown to be associated with increased risk of abruption [32]. Measuring TPO or thyroglobulin antibodies is important for diagnosis, but serial levels are usually not indicated because treatment does not alter them. At present, routine testing of TPO antibodies during pregnancy is not recommended (see below).

Treatment

Goal

Maternal serum TSH 0.5 to 2.0 mµ/L, and FT4 in upper third of normal range. Interestingly, there are really no RCTs on treatment of overt hypothyroidism in pregnancy. Two trials of 30 and 48 hypothyroid women, respectively, compared levothyroxine doses, but both trials reported only biochemical outcomes [33].

Thyroxine Replacement: Dose

Preexisting hypothyroidism. Approximately **45% to 85% of hypothyroid women need** up to 45% **increase in thyroxine replacement dose** during pregnancy because of increased metabolism of thyroxine, weight gain, increased T4 pool, high serum TBG, placental deiodinase activity, and transfer of T4 to fetus [34,35]. Some advocate increasing replacement by 30% as soon as pregnancy is confirmed, but outcome data are not available [17].

New diagnosis. **Levothyroxine can be started at 0.1 to 0.15 mg/day** and adjusted by monitoring TSH levels. Thyroxine replacement will need to be increased as in preexisting disease.

Ferrous sulfate and calcium carbonate interfere with T4 absorption and should be taken at a different time of day from thyroxine therapy [36]. Therefore, **pregnant women should space their levothyroxine and prenatal vitamins by at least two to three hours.** Carbamazepine, phenytoin, and rifampin can increase the clearance of T4. **It takes approximately four weeks for thyroxine therapy to alter TSH level.** Not only under-replacement (see above) but also over-replacement (pregnancy loss, low birth weight) should be avoided [37].

Thyroxine Replacement: Type

Levothyroxine. Levothyroxine is the recommended thyroid replacement. Desiccated thyroid preparation, such as Armour Thyroid, at 30 mg/day initial dose, then increased incrementally by 15 mg every two to three weeks until maintenance dose of 60 to 120 mg/day, is an alternative if levothyroxine is unavailable.

Iodine supplement. **Iodine supplementation in a population with high levels of endemic cretinism results in a reduction of the condition** with no apparent adverse effects [38]. Iodine supplementation is associated with **a reduction in deaths during infancy and early childhood with decreased endemic cretinism at four years of age and better psychomotor development scores between four and 25 months of age.** About 10% to 15% of the U.S. population has iodine deficiency, which can manifest as subclinical hypothyroidism or with normal TSH and low T4. A daily dose of **250 μg of iodine is recommended during pregnancy and breast-feeding** [39].

Antepartum Management

- **TSH and FT4 levels** should be checked **preconception, at first prenatal visit in first trimester, four weeks after altering the doses (therefore, every four weeks until TSH is normal, especially in first 20 weeks), and at least every trimester in pregnancy.**
- Fetal heart rate should be assessed at each visit by doptone to rule out fetal bradycardia <120.
- Antepartum testing is not recommended if euthyroid; weekly nonstress tests beginning at about 32 weeks can be considered for clinically hypothyroid patients.
- Ultrasound is not recommended if euthyroid; monthly ultrasound can be considered for fetal growth, thyroid circumference [40], and fetal heart rate if clinically hypothyroid.
- Important to inform pediatrician at time of delivery.

Postpartum

Immediately post-delivery, the dosage of levothyroxine should be reduced to the prepregnancy dose, and TSH levels should be measured six to eight weeks postpartum with follow-up with medical doctor/endocrinologist.

Neonatal

The incidence of iodine-deficient **congenital hypothyroidism** is **1/4000 births,** 5% identified at birth by clinical symptoms, others by **newborn screening.** The United States screens all newborns. If discovered and treated in first few weeks of life, near-normal growth and intelligence are expected [41,42]. The majority of cases are due to agenesis/dysgenesis of fetal thyroid, dyshormonogenesis, or iodine deficiency. Fetuses are protected in utero by a small quantity of maternal T4 that crosses the placenta. Neonatal issues include neuropsychological abnormalities, deafness, respiratory difficulties, growth failure, lethargy, and hypotonia and myxedema of the larynx and epiglottis.

SUBCLINICAL HYPOTHYROIDISM
Incidence
2%–5% [43–45].

Diagnosis
Elevated TSH and normal FT4.

Screening and Management

Routine screening for subclinical hypothyroidism is currently not recommended because treatment of subclinical hypothyroidism has not been demonstrated to improve maternal or fetal outcomes [26]. Previously some observational studies have shown that subclinical hypothyroidism can be associated with impaired neurodevelopment in offspring [10] as well as increased incidences of preterm birth, abruption, severe pre-eclampsia, gestational diabetes, respiratory distress syndrome, and admission to intensive care nursery [43,46,47] but not consistently shown by other studies [44,48]. In a large randomized controlled trial (RCT), **levothyroxine supplementation given to asymptomatic women screened and identified to have a TSH ≥97.5th percentile was associated with a similar IQ and cognitive outcomes in their children at three years of age, compared to placebo** [26]. In another large RCT, **levothyroxine supplementation given to asymptomatic women screened and identified to have a TSH ≥4 mμ/L, and a normal free T4 (0.86–1.9 ng/dL) was associated with a similar IQ and cognitive outcomes in their children at five years of age compared to placebo** [49]. Therefore, **currently, there is no evidence that screening and treatment of subclinical hypothyroidism during pregnancy improves maternal or fetal outcomes** [22,26,49].

Women with subclinical hypothyroidism and thyroid antibodies (e.g., TPO) frequently progress to overt hypothyroidism and may develop hyperlipidemia and atherosclerotic heart disease [50].

HYPOTHYROXINEMIA
Incidence
1.3% [48].

Diagnosis
Normal TSH and low FT4.

Screening and Management

There are at least two large RCTs showing no benefit from screening and treating hypothyroxinemia. In a RCT, **levothyroxine supplementation given to asymptomatic women screened and identified to have a free T4 below the 2.5th percentile was associated with a similar IQ and cognitive outcomes in their children at three years of age compared to placebo** [26]. In another RCT, **levothyroxine supplementation given to asymptomatic women screened and identified to have a normal TSH (0.08–3.99 mμ/L) and a low free T4 (<0.86 ng/dL) was associated with a similar IQ and cognitive outcomes in their children at five years of age compared to placebo** [49]. Because isolated maternal hypothyroxinemia is not associated with adverse effects on perinatal outcome [48], there is no need to screen or treat for this condition. Therefore, there is evidence that **screening and treating for hypothyroxinemia is unnecessary** as it is not associated with any maternal or child benefits.

TPO-ANTIBODIES ONLY

Some women are euthyroid but have been identified to have TPO antibodies. In a RCT of euthyroid pregnant women with thyroid peroxidase antibodies, levothyroxine therapy significantly reduced the rate of PTB by 72% compared to placebo (RR 0.28; 95% CI 0.10–0.80), and the incidence of preeclampsia was similar (RR 0.61; 95% CI 0.11 to 3.48) [33,51]. **Routine thyroid screening and/or treatment for TPO in asymptomatic euthyroid women is not suggested** as a possible intervention for PTB prevention in absence of a clinical thyroid disease until further confirmed additional studies.

A trial of 169 TOP-positive, euthyroid women compared the trace element selenomethionine (selenium) with placebo and no significant differences were seen for either preeclampsia (RR 1.44; 95% CI 0.25 to 8.38) or preterm birth (RR 0.96; 95% CI 0.20 to 4.61) [33], but there was an improvement (decrease) in postpartum thyroiditis [11].

THYROID NODULE
Incidence
5% to 10% of thyroid tumors are neoplastic. Thyroid cancer occurs in 1/1000 pregnant women with palpable thyroid nodule.

Diagnosis
Ultrasound to define dominant nodule, followed by fine-needle aspiration for nodules >1 cm, which has a 95% diagnostic accuracy in pregnancy [52]. Radioisotope scanning is contraindicated in pregnancy. Serum TSH and FT4 should be checked.

Thyroid Surgery
For malignancy diagnosed on fine-needle aspiration, neck exploration should be performed ideally either in the second trimester or postpartum [52]. Neck irradiation for malignancy should be deferred until after pregnancy.

POSTPARTUM THYROIDITIS
Definition
Autoimmune inflammation of the thyroid gland that presents as new-onset painless hypothyroidism, transient thyrotoxicosis, or thyrotoxicosis followed by hypothyroidism **within one year postpartum**.

Incidence
Occurs in 5% of women in United States who do not have a history of thyroid disease [53] and may occur after delivery or pregnancy loss.

Risk Factors
Postpartum depression, high serum TPO antibody concentration, history of Graves's disease, or type I diabetes.

Etiology
Subacute lymphocytic thyroiditis or postpartum exacerbation of chronic lymphocytic thyroiditis.

Diagnosis
Documentation of new-onset abnormal levels of TSH and/or FT4 within the first postpartum year. All women with symptoms of thyroid dysfunction or who develop a goiter postpartum should be evaluated with TSH, FT4. If the diagnosis is unclear, an anti-TPO antibody level should be measured. Women with highest levels of TSH and anti-TPO antibodies have the highest risk for developing permanent hypothyroidism [54].

Three Clinical Presentations
1. Transient hyperthyroidism followed by recovery: 28%
2. Transient hyperthyroidism, followed by transient or rarely permanent hypothyroidism: 28%
3. Transient or permanent hypothyroidism: 44%

Management
Most women do not require treatment. Treatment is based on symptoms.

If symptomatic, thyrotoxicosis should be treated with a beta-adrenergic antagonist drug. Transient hypothyroidism is treated with thyroxine (25–75 mcg/day) for 6–12 months [22].

Recurrence Risk
Risk of recurrence is 70% [55].

Risk of developing permanent primary hypothyroidism in the five- to 10-year period following an episode of postpartum thyroiditis is markedly increased. Annual TSH level should be performed in them [56].

REFERENCES
1. Montoro MN. Management of hypothyroidism during pregnancy. *Clin Obstet Gynecol* 1997; 40(1): 65–80. [II-2]
2. Klein RZ, Haddow JE, Faix JD, Brown RS, Hermos RJ, Pulkkinen A et al. Prevalence of thyroid deficiency in pregnant women. *Clin Endocrinol (Oxf)* 1991; 35(1): 41–6. [II-2]
3. Alvarez-Marfany M, Roman SH, Drexler AJ, Robertson C, Stagnaro-Green A. Long-term prospective study of postpartum thyroid dysfunction in women with insulin dependent diabetes mellitus. *J Clin Endocrinol Metab* 1994; 79(1): 10–6. [II-2]
4. Hollowell JG, Staehling NW, Hannon WH, Flanders DW, Gunter EW, Maberly GF et al. Iodine nutrition in the United States. Trends and public health implications: Iodine excretion data from National Health and Nutrition Examination Surveys I and III (1971–1974 and 1988–1994). *J Clin Endocrinol Metab* 1998; 83(10): 3401–8. [II-2]
5. Rakel RE. *Textbook of Family Practice.* 6th ed. Philadelphia: WB Saunders; 2002. [Review]
6. Weetman AP, McGregor AM. Autoimmune thyroid disease: Developments in our understanding. *Endocr Rev* 1984; 5(2): 309–55. [III]
7. Reid SM, Middleton P, Cossich MC, Crowther CA. Interventions for clinical and subclinical hypothyroidism in pregnancy. *Cochrane Database Syst Rev* 2010; 7(7): CD007752. [Review]
8. Leung AS, Millar LK, Koonings PP, Montoro M, Mestman JH. Perinatal outcome in hypothyroid pregnancies. *Obstet Gynecol* 1993; 81(3): 349–53. [II-2]
9. Davis LE, Leveno KJ, Cunningham FG. Hypothyroidism complicating pregnancy. *Obstet Gynecol* 1988; 72(1): 108–12. [II-3]
10. Pop VJ, Kuijpens JL, van Baar AL, Verkerk G, van Son MM, de Vijlder JJ et al. Low maternal free thyroxine concentrations during early pregnancy are associated with impaired psychomotor development in infancy. *Clin Endocrinol (Oxf)* 1999; 50(2): 149–55. [II-2]

11. Negro R, Greco G, Mangieri T, Pezzarossa A, Dazzi D, Hassan H. The influence of selenium supplementation on postpartum thyroid status in pregnant women with thyroid peroxidase auto-antibodies. *J Clin Endocrinol Metab* 2007; 92(4): 1263–8. [RCT, *n* = 169]

12. Premawardhana LD, Parkes AB, Ammari F, John R, Darke C, Adams H et al. Postpartum thyroiditis and long-term thyroid status: Prognostic influence of thyroid peroxidase antibodies and ultrasound echogenicity. *J Clin Endocrinol Metab* 2000; 85(1): 71–5. [II-2]

13. Rotondi M, Mazziotti G, Sorvillo F, Piscopo M, Cioffi M, Amato G et al. Effects of increased thyroxine dosage pre-conception on thyroid function during early pregnancy. *Eur J Endocrinol* 2004; 151(6): 695–700. [RCT, *n* = 25]

14. Rasmussen NG, Hornnes PJ, Hegedus L. Ultrasonographically determined thyroid size in pregnancy and post partum: The goitrogenic effect of pregnancy. *Am J Obstet Gynecol* 1989; 160(5 Pt. 1): 1216–20. [II-3]

15. Dashe JS, Casey BM, Wells CE, McIntire DD, Byrd EW, Leveno KJ et al. Thyroid-stimulating hormone in singleton and twin pregnancy: Importance of gestational age-specific reference ranges. *Obstet Gynecol* 2005; 106(4): 753–7. [II-3]

16. Glinoer D, de Nayer P, Bourdoux P, Lemone M, Robyn C, van Steirteghem A et al. Regulation of maternal thyroid during pregnancy. *J Clin Endocrinol Metab* 1990; 71(2): 276–87. [II-3]

17. Alexander EK, Marqusee E, Lawrence J, Jarolim P, Fischer GA, Larsen PR. Timing and magnitude of increases in levothyroxine requirements during pregnancy in women with hypothyroidism. *N Engl J Med* 2004; 351(3): 241–9. [II-2]

18. Glinoer D. The regulation of thyroid function in pregnancy: Pathways of endocrine adaptation from physiology to pathology. *Endocr Rev* 1997; 18(3): 404–33. [III]

19. Burrow GN, Fisher DA, Larsen PR. Maternal and fetal thyroid function. *N Engl J Med* 1994; 331(16): 1072–8. [III]

20. Moosa M, Mazzaferri EL. Outcome of differentiated thyroid cancer diagnosed in pregnant women. *J Clin Endocrinol Metab* 1997; 82(9): 2862–6. [II-2]

21. Bajoria R, Fisk NM. Permeability of human placenta and fetal membranes to thyrotropin-stimulating hormone in vitro. *Pediatr Res* 1998; 43(5): 621–8. [II-3]

22. American College of Obstetricians and Gynecologists. Practice Bulletin No. 148: Thyroid disease in pregnancy. *Obstet Gynecol* 2015; 125(4): 996–1005. [Review]

23. Stagnaro-Green A, Abalovich M, Alexander E, Azizi F, Mestman J, Negro R et al. Guidelines of the American Thyroid Association for the diagnosis and management of thyroid disease during pregnancy and postpartum. *Thyroid* 2011; 21(10): 1081–125. [Review, guideline]

24. De Groot L, Abalovich M, Alexander EK, Amino N, Barbour L, Cobin RH et al. Management of thyroid dysfunction during pregnancy and postpartum: An Endocrine Society clinical practice guideline. *J Clin Endocrinol Metab* 2012; 97(8): 2543–65. [Review, guideline]

25. Negro R, Schwartz A, Gismondi R, Tinelli A, Mangieri T, Stagnaro-Green A. Universal screening versus case finding for detection and treatment of thyroid hormonal dysfunction during pregnancy. *J Clin Endocrinol Metab* 2010; 95(4): 1699–707. [II-2]

26. Lazarus JH, Bestwick JP, Channon S, Paradice R, Maina A, Rees R et al. Antenatal thyroid screening and childhood cognitive function. *N Engl J Med* 2012; 366(6): 493–501. [RCT, *n* = 794]

27. Gharib H, Cobin RH, Dickey RA. Subclinical hypothyroidism during pregnancy: Position statement from the American Association of Clinical Endocrinologists. *Endocr Pract* 1999; 5(6): 367–8. [Review, guideline]

28. American Association of Clinical Endocrinologists, editor. *AACE clinical practice guidelines for evaluation and treatment of hyperthyroidism and hypothyroidism.* American Association of Clinical Endocrinologists. Jackonville, FL: American Association of Clinical Endocrinologists; 1996. [Review, guideline]

29. Ladenson PW, Singer PA, Ain KB, Bagchi N, Bigos ST, Levy EG et al. American Thyroid Association guidelines for detection of thyroid dysfunction. *Arch Intern Med* 2000; 160(11): 1573–5. [Review, guideline]

30. Stagnaro-Green A, Roman SH, Cobin RH, el-Harazy E, Alvarez-Marfany M, Davies TF. Detection of at-risk pregnancy by means of highly sensitive assays for thyroid autoantibodies. *JAMA* 1990; 264(11): 1422–5. [II-3]

31. Kuijpens JL, Pop VJ, Vader HL, Drexhage HA, Wiersinga WM. Prediction of post partum thyroid dysfunction: Can it be improved? *Eur J Endocrinol* 1998; 139(1): 36–43. [II-2]

32. Haddow JE, McClain MR, Palomaki GE, Neveux LM, Lambert-Messerlian G, Canick JA et al. Thyroperoxidase and thyroglobulin antibodies in early pregnancy and placental abruption. *Obstet Gynecol* 2011; 117(2 Pt. 1): 287–92. [II-2]

33. Reid SM, Middleton P, Cossich MC, Crowther CA, Bain E. Interventions for clinical and subclinical hypothyroidism pre-pregnancy and during pregnancy. *Cochrane Database Syst Rev* 2013; 5: CD007752. [Meta-analysis; 4 heterogeneous RCTs]

34. Mandel SJ, Larsen PR, Seely EW, Brent GA. Increased need for thyroxine during pregnancy in women with primary hypothyroidism. *N Engl J Med* 1990; 323(2): 91–6. [II-2]

35. Kaplan MM. Management of thyroxine therapy during pregnancy. *Endocr Pract* 1996; 2(4): 281–6. [III]

36. Brent GA. Maternal hypothyroidism: Recognition and management. *Thyroid* 1999; 9(7): 661–5. [III]

37. Anselmo J, Cao D, Karrison T, Weiss RE, Refetoff S. Fetal loss associated with excess thyroid hormone exposure. *JAMA* 2004; 292(6): 691–5. [II-3]

38. Mahomed K, Gulmezoglu AM. Maternal iodine supplements in areas of deficiency. *Cochrane Database Syst Rev* 2007; 3(3): CD000135. [Meta-analysis: 3 RCTs, *n* = 1551]

39. WHO Secretariat, Andersson M, de Benoist B, Delange F, Zupan J. Prevention and control of iodine deficiency in pregnant and lactating women and in children less than 2 years old: Conclusions and recommendations of the Technical Consultation. *Public Health Nutr* 2007; 10(12A): 1606–11. [Review]

40. Ranzini AC, Ananth CV, Smulian JC, Kung M, Limbachia A, Vintzileos AM. Ultrasonography of the fetal thyroid: Nomograms based on biparietal diameter and gestational age. *J Ultrasound Med* 2001; 20(6): 613–7. [II-2]

41. Glorieux J, Dussault J, Van Vliet G. Intellectual development at age 12 years of children with congenital hypothyroidism diagnosed by neonatal screening. *J Pediatr* 1992; 121(4): 581–4. [II-2]

42. Rovet JF, Ehrlich RM, Sorbara DL. Neurodevelopment in infants and preschool children with congenital hypothyroidism: Etiological and treatment factors affecting outcome. *J Pediatr Psychol* 1992; 17(2): 187–213. [II-2]

43. Casey BM, Dashe JS, Wells CE, McIntire DD, Byrd W, Leveno KJ et al. Subclinical hypothyroidism and pregnancy outcomes. *Obstet Gynecol* 2005; 105(2): 239–45. [II-2]

44. Cleary-Goldman J, Malone FD, Lambert-Messerlian G, Sullivan L, Canick J, Porter TF et al. Maternal thyroid hypofunction and pregnancy outcome. *Obstet Gynecol* 2008; 112(1): 85–92. [II-1]

45. Fitzpatrick DL, Russell MA. Diagnosis and management of thyroid disease in pregnancy. *Obstet Gynecol Clin North Am* 2010; 37(2): 173–93. [III]

46. Tudela CM, Casey BM, McIntire DD, Cunningham FG. Relationship of subclinical thyroid disease to the incidence of gestational diabetes. *Obstet Gynecol* 2012; 119(5): 983–8. [II-2]

47. Wilson KL, Casey BM, McIntire DD, Halvorson LM, Cunningham FG. Subclinical thyroid disease and the incidence of hypertension in pregnancy. *Obstet Gynecol* 2012; 119(2 Pt. 1): 315–20. [II-3]

48. Casey BM, Dashe JS, Spong CY, McIntire DD, Leveno KJ, Cunningham GF. Perinatal significance of isolated maternal hypothyroxinemia identified in the first half of pregnancy. *Obstet Gynecol* 2007; 109(5): 1129–35. [II-2]

49. Casey B. Effect of maternal subclinical hypothyroidism or hypothyroxemia on IQ in offspring. *AJOG* 2016; 214(1 Suppl.): S2. [RCT, *n* = 677 for subclinical hypothyroidism; *n* = 526 for hypothyroxinemia]

50. Pearce EN, Farwell AP, Braverman LE. Thyroiditis. *N Engl J Med* 2003; 348(26): 2646–55. [III]

51. Negro R, Formoso G, Mangieri T, Pezzarossa A, Dazzi D, Hassan H. Levothyroxine treatment in euthyroid pregnant women with autoimmune thyroid disease: Effects on obstetrical complications. *J Clin Endocrinol Metab* 2006; 91(7): 2587–91. [RCT, *n* = 115]

52. Tan GH, Gharib H, Goellner JR, van Heerden JA, Bahn RS. Management of thyroid nodules in pregnancy. *Arch Intern Med* 1996; 156(20): 2317–20. [II-2]

53. Gerstein HC. How common is postpartum thyroiditis? A methodologic overview of the literature. *Arch Intern Med* 1990; 150(7): 1397–400. [III]

54. Lucas A, Pizarro E, Granada ML, Salinas I, Foz M, Sanmarti A. Postpartum thyroiditis: Epidemiology and clinical evolution in a nonselected population. *Thyroid* 2000;10(1): 71–7. [II-2]

55. Lazarus JH, Ammari F, Oretti R, Parkes AB, Richards CJ, Harris B. Clinical aspects of recurrent postpartum thyroiditis. *Br J Gen Pract* 1997; 47(418): 305–8. [II-3]

56. Azizi F. The occurrence of permanent thyroid failure in patients with subclinical postpartum thyroiditis. *Eur J Endocrinol* 2005; 153(3): 367–71. [II-2]

7

Hyperthyroidism

Sushma Jwala

KEY POINTS
- Hyperthyroidism occurs in 0.1% to 0.4% of pregnancies.
- Graves' disease accounts for 95% of women with hyperthyroidism.
- Untreated hyperthyroidism is associated with increased risks of **spontaneous pregnancy loss, preterm birth, preeclampsia, fetal death, abruption, fetal growth restriction (FGR), and neonatal Graves' disease as well as** maternal congestive heart failure and **thyroid storm.**
- **Hyperemesis gravidarum (HG)** can be associated with **gestational transient biochemical thyrotoxicosis** (low, usually undetectable thyroid-stimulating hormone [TSH], and/or elevated T4), but this biochemical change always resolves spontaneously. Therefore, there should be **no testing, follow-up, or treatment for biochemical thyrotoxicosis in women with HG**.
- Clinical hyperthyroidism is **diagnosed** by **suppressed TSH** and **elevated serum** free thyroxine (**FT4**). Thyroid-stimulating immunoglobulin (TSI) can be obtained as positive TSI is consistent with Graves' disease, and values >200% to 500% indicate higher risk for fetal/neonatal hyperthyroidism.
- Goal of treatment is to keep FT4 in high normal range. **Measure TSH and FT4** every four weeks until FT4 is consistently in the high normal range and then every trimester.
- Main treatment is with **either propylthiouracil (PTU) or methimazole**. Because of the very rare teratogenic effects of methimazole and the hepatotoxicity of PTU, **PTU can be used during the first trimester followed by switching over to methimazole in the second trimester and continuing it for the rest of the pregnancy.**
- Radioiodine is absolutely contraindicated in pregnancy.
- **Thyroid storm** is initially diagnosed clinically and treated aggressively with PTU, saturated solution of potassium iodide (SSKI), dexamethasone, and propranolol.

DEFINITIONS
Hyperthyroidism
Hyperfunctioning thyroid gland resulting in thyrotoxicosis. It usually implies low TSH and high FT4 (or FT3).

Graves' Disease
An autoimmune disease causing hyperthyroidism, characterized by production of **thyroid-stimulating immunoglobulins (TSIs)** or **thyroid-stimulating hormone-binding inhibitory immunoglobulins (TBIIs)**. TSIs coexist with TBIIs 30% of the time [1]. TSIs stimulate thyrotropin receptors. Instead, TBIIs can stimulate or inhibit TSH receptors [2].

TBIIs are seen in 30% of patients with Graves' disease and in 10% of patients with autoimmune Hashimoto's thyroiditis. TBIIs disappear, and patients achieve euthyroidism in 40% of the cases. Therefore, TBII assays have not been developed for clinical use because of higher costs involved in developing TBII assays as compared to the number of patients who would benefit from them.

TRAbs (TSH receptor antibodies) is a broader term used to include both TSIs and TBIIs. TRAb assays, in general, measure TSIs as TBII assays have not been established so far [3].

Thyrotoxicosis
Clinical and biochemical state that results from an excess production or exposure to thyroid hormone from any etiology.

Gestational Thyrotoxicosis
Biochemical tests consistent with hyperthyroidism during pregnancy but not a disease.

Thyroid Storm
Severe, acute, life-threatening exacerbation of the signs/symptoms of hyperthyroidism.

Subclinical Hyperthyroidism
Sustained TSH <0.1 mU/L with normal FT4 and free triiodothyronine (FT3) in the absence of nonthyroidal illness.

SIGNS/SYMPTOMS
Symptoms (may mimic hypermetabolic state of pregnancy): nervousness, tremor, frequent stools, excessive sweating, heat intolerance, insomnia, palpitations, decreased appetite, pruritus, decreased exercise tolerance, shortness of breath, eye symptoms of frequent lacrimation, double vision, and retro-orbital pain.

Physical Examination
Hypertension, goiter, tachycardia (>100 bpm, which does not decrease with Valsalva), wide pulse pressure, weight loss, ophthalmopathy (lid lag, lid retraction), and dermopathy (localized, pretibial myxedema). Goiter occurs only with iodine deficiency or thyroid disease and must be considered pathological.

INCIDENCE
0.1% to 0.4% of pregnancies [4,5].

ETIOLOGY

Graves' disease accounts for 95% of women with hyperthyroidism. It can be associated with diffuse thyromegaly or infiltrative ophthalmopathy. Non-Graves' hyperthyroidism accounts for 5% of women with hyperthyroidism and can be associated with gestational trophoblastic neoplasia [4,6], toxic nodular and multinodular goiter [5], hyperfunctioning thyroid adenoma, subacute thyroiditis, extra thyroid source of thyroid hormone (e.g., struma ovarii), iodine-induced hyperthyroidism, thyrotropin receptor activation [7], or viral thyroiditis.

Of women with hydatidiform mole or choriocarcinoma, 50% to 60% may have severe hyperthyroidism, which is primarily treated with evacuation of the mole or therapy directed against the choriocarcinoma.

BASIC PHYSIOLOGY/PATHOPHYSIOLOGY

See also hypothyroid guideline (see Chapter 6). **Ninety-five percent of cases are due to TSIs** [7] stimulating excess thyroid hormone production from the thyroid gland (**Graves' disease**). These IgG antibodies bind to and activate the G-protein-coupled thyrotropin receptor, which then stimulates follicular hypertrophy and hyperplasia as well as increases thyroid hormone production, T3 more than T4 [2]. Of women with Graves' disease, 40% to 50% have remission of the disease in 12 to 18 months [8].

COMPLICATIONS

Untreated hyperthyroidism preconception or in pregnancy is associated with increased risks of **spontaneous pregnancy loss, preterm birth, preeclampsia, abruption, fetal death, FGR, low birth weight,** maternal **congestive heart failure,** and **thyroid storm** [4,5,7,9–13]. **Neonatal Graves' disease** can affect neonates of women with Graves' disease. Fetal thyrotoxicosis is a possibility in women with Graves' disease. Long-term uncontrolled hyperthyroidism, even subclinical, is associated with increased maternal risk for atrial fibrillation, dementia, Alzheimer's, and hip fractures.

MANAGEMENT
Pregnancy Considerations

See also hypothyroid guideline in Chapter 6, including tables. **High levels of HCG,** which peak at 10 to 12 weeks, have some TSH-like activity and stimulate thyroid hormone secretion, which, in turn, **suppresses TSH.** Normal TSH levels in pregnancy are shown in Table 6.2. TSH suppression is even more marked for twins. Because of pregnancy physiologic changes, **hyperthyroidism typically ameliorates during the third trimester but may worsen postpartum.**

Hyperemesis gravidarum (HG) is diagnosed by severe nausea and vomiting associated with ketonuria and 5% weight loss (see Chapter 9). **Gestational transient biochemical thyrotoxicosis** (low, usually undetectable TSH, and/or elevated T4) may be related to high serum HCG and can occur in 3% to 11% of normal pregnancies especially during the period of highest serum HCG concentrations (10–12 weeks) [14]. Therefore, **no testing, follow-up, or treatment for thyroid disease in women with HG should be initiated** because there is no true thyroid disease, and the biochemical hyperthyroidism always spontaneously resolves [9]. Women with

signs or symptoms of hyperthyroidism from before pregnancy can be tested regardless of HG.

Women of childbearing age should have an average iodine intake of 150 µg/day. During pregnancy and breastfeeding, women should increase their daily iodine intake to 250 µg on average [15–17]. Most prenatal vitamins have at least 200 µg in them. In the United States, 10% to 15% of pregnant women are iodine deficient.

SCREENING/DIAGNOSIS

Women with signs/symptoms consistent with hyperthyroidism should be screened with serum **TSH and FT4** [18,19]. **Clinical hyperthyroidism is diagnosed by suppressed TSH and elevated serum FT4.** FT3 is measured in thyrotoxic patients with suppressed TSH but normal FT4 measurements (5% of hyperthyroid women). FT3 elevation indicates T3 thyrotoxicosis.

TSI can be obtained in women with clinical hyperthyroidism at the first visit and/or at 28 to 30 weeks [15–21]. A positive TSI is consistent with Graves' disease. **Values ≥200% to 500% indicate higher risk for fetal/neonatal hyperthyroidism and can help fetal and neonatal management.** Unfortunately, there is no standard test for TSI, often making comparisons between different laboratories or studies impossible. Presence of TSI differentiates Graves' disease from gestational thyrotoxicosis (biochemical tests consistent with hyperthyroidism during pregnancy, but no disease) and HG [5,10,12,22–24]. In patients with HG, routine measurements of thyroid function are **not** recommended unless other overt signs of hyperthyroidism are evident (see Chapter 9).

Women with thyroid surgery/ablation in the past who continue to produce antibodies (i.e., TSI) warrant assessment of maternal TSI level as these antibodies are associated with fetal/neonatal Graves' disease [20].

TREATMENT

There are no randomized controlled trials (RCTs) regarding management of hyperthyroidism in pregnancy [25]. The goal is to control symptoms of hyperthyroidism without causing fetal hypothyroidism, keeping **FT4 in the high normal range** and TSH in the low normal range with the lowest possible dose of thionamide. Propylthiouracil (PTU) >200 mg/day may result in fetal goiter [26], and keeping the FT4 in the upper nonpregnant reference range [27,28] minimizes the risk of fetal hypothyroidism. **It may be helpful to measure TSH and FT4 every four weeks until FT4 is consistently in the high normal range.** Then measurements every trimester may be obtained. Dosing may need to be decreased as pregnancy advances, and about 30% can discontinue antithyroid therapy and still remain euthyroid.

Pregnancy outcomes have not been shown to improve with treatment of maternal subclinical hyperthyroidism and may result in unnecessary exposure of the fetus to antithyroid drugs [4,22,29]. Identification and treatment of subclinical hyperthyroidism during pregnancy are unwarranted [29].

Thionamides
Propylthiouracil

PTU can be started at 100 mg every eight hours, and dose adjusted according to laboratory values and symptoms. It might take six to eight weeks to get adequate effect with initial clinical response in as little as two to three weeks. Usual doses are 50 to 150 mg every eight hours with requirements usually inversely proportional to gestational age (decrease as pregnancy advances) [30].

Methimazole

Can be started at 20 mg once a day and modified as needed according to laboratory values and symptoms. It is an acceptable alternative as it is equally effective. In fact, **in nonpregnant women, methimazole is often preferred to PTU as the longer half-life often allows once-daily dosing (compared to three times a day for PTU).** Efficacy of methimazole may be superior to PTU with fewer side effects [2]. The teratologic risks of aplasia cutis and esophageal and choanal atresia (nine cases in literature) are extremely rare [4,8,31–36]. There is no significant difference between PTU and methimazole in normalizing maternal TSH or on neonatal thyroid function, which might imply that transplacental transfer is similar [32]. Because of the very rare teratogenic effects of methimazole and the dual mechanism of action of PTU, some authors have recommended PTU as the thionamide of choice in pregnancy [8]. There is no trial comparing the two in pregnancy, and methimazole may be preferred because of once-daily dosing. Methimazole is a very reasonable alternative and can also be used when there is an allergic reaction to PTU. In 2009, the U.S. FDA had issued a safety alert on hepatotoxicity associated with PTU. Therefore, in order to balance methimazole embryopathy with PTU-induced hepatotoxicity, societies have recommended that **PTU be used during the first trimester followed by switching over to methimazole in the second trimester** [30,37] **for the rest of the pregnancy.**

Mode of Action

Both PTU and methimazole compete for peroxidase, blocking organification of iodide and so decreasing thyroid hormone synthesis. PTU also inhibits peripheral T4 to T3 conversion and is therefore thought to work faster with less transplacental crossing than methimazole [2].

Side Effects

Maternal. **Agranulocytosis** (granulocytes <250/mL) is the most serious side effect and occurs in 0.1% to 0.4% of cases. Risk factors are older gravidas and higher doses. It presents with fever, sore throat, malaise, and gingivitis. If hyperthyroid women treated with thionamides present with sore throat and fever, discontinue therapy and check a white blood count [8]. Other side effects (all with incidence of <5%) are thrombocytopenia, hepatitis, lupus-like syndrome, vasculitis, rash, hives, pruritus, nausea, vomiting, arthritis, anorexia, drug fever, and loss of taste or smell [8,38].

Fetal/neonatal. As PTU and methimazole both cross the placenta, they may cause **fetal hypothyroidism.** Transient hypothyroidism may cause goiter secondary to suppression of fetal pituitary–thyroid axis. This, however, rarely requires therapy. IQ scores of children exposed to thionamide in utero are normal compared to nonexposed siblings [39,40].

Radioiodine

Radioiodine therapy is often used in the United States as the first- or second-line (after thionamides) therapy. The goal of radioiodine therapy is induced hypothyroidism in order to prevent a recurrence of Graves' disease. This goal is achieved in about 80% of patients [2]. All women of reproductive age should have a pregnancy test immediately before this treatment. It is generally recommended that women do not attempt conception for 6 to 12 months after radioiodine treatment [2]. As the half-life for radioiodine is eight days, reassurance can be provided to women who present with conception more than four weeks from therapy.

This therapy is **absolutely contraindicated** in pregnancy. Fetal thyroid tissue will be ablated after 10 weeks. If given after 10 weeks, termination should be presented as an option. If given prior to 10 weeks, radioiodine does not appear to cause congenital hypothyroidism [41–43]. Breastfeeding should be avoided for 120 days after this therapy.

Beta-Blocker

Propranolol 20 to 40 mg orally every eight to 12 hours or atenolol 50 to 100 mg orally once a day are useful for rapid control of adrenergic symptoms of thyrothoxicosis until thionamide takes effect (four to six weeks). This therapy does not alter synthesis or secretion of the thyroid hormone. The goal is to keep the maternal heart rate at 80 to 90 bpm without palpitations. Prolonged therapy can lead to fetal side effects, such as FGR, fetal bradycardia, hypoglycemia, and subnormal response to hypoxemic stress.

Surgery

This is the least-often used treatment. Thyroidectomy may be indicated for women who [1] cannot tolerate thionamide, [2] need persistently high doses of antithyroid drugs, [3] are noncompliant with antithyroid drugs, [4] have goiter resulting in compressive symptoms, or [5] have other indications similar to nonpregnant women. The second trimester is the optimal time for surgery [44–46].

Iodine

Short-term use is safe for symptomatic relief [47]; however, use for longer than two weeks may cause fetal goiter [48].

ANTEPARTUM TESTING

- The **fetal heart rate** can be assessed for at least one minute at each visit by doptone to rule out fetal tachycardia >180.
- Thyroid function testing with **TSH and FT4** should be performed at least every trimester.
- Weekly **NSTs** can begin at 32 to 34 weeks, especially in women with uncontrolled hyperthyroidism or elevated TSIs.
- **Ultrasound** can assess fetal heart rate, thyroid (for goiter), and growth. If clinically hyperthyroid, ultrasounds every four weeks for growth may be indicated. If FGR or fetal tachycardia is present, fetal thyroid circumference can be assessed [49]. The sensitivity and specificity of fetal thyroid ultrasound at 32 weeks are 92% and 100%, respectively, for the diagnosis of clinically relevant fetal thyroid dysfunction [50].
- The fetus is at risk from either hypothyroidism from transplacental passage of antithyroid drugs or from hyperthyroidism from TSI. The presence of a fetal goiter

would point to fetal thyroid dysfunction but not distinguish between these two possibilities. **Fetal blood sampling** is rarely indicated but can be considered if high maternal TSI (200%–500% normal), and there are fetal signs suggestive of severe thyroid disease, that is, fetal hydrops, goiter, tachycardia, cardiomegaly, FGR, or history of prior fetus with hyperthyroidism [51,52]. Fetal hyperthyroidism should not be feared or tested for if TSIs are <130% (normal range). If the fetus is hypothyroid, injection of thyroxine in amniotic fluid is a possible intervention [53]. If fetus is hyperthyroid, maternal treatment with thionamide to prevent fetal effects may be indicated even if maternal T4 is low or normal [54].

- It is important to **inform pediatrician** at time of delivery of maternal diagnosis and drug therapy.

NEONATE

Neonates born to mothers with Graves' disease should be followed closely by a pediatrician for the possibility of transient neonatal hyperthyroidism [50,55,56]. **Neonatal Graves' disease** can affect 2% to 5% neonates of women with Graves' unrelated to maternal thyroid function and secondary to transplacental transfer of TSI or TBII. The risk is high if the TSI index is ≥5 or ≥200% to 500% [57]. Signs are tachycardia (>160 bpm), goiter, FGR, advanced bone age, craniosynostosis, hydrops, later motor difficulties, hyperactivity, or failure to thrive [57]. Neonates of women who have been treated surgically or with radioactive iodine before pregnancy and still gave TSI are at highest risk for neonatal Graves' disease because thionamide therapy is not present to counteract this effect. On the other hand, fetal and neonatal complications can also arise from thionamide treatment of the disease as, when this is excessive, signs of hypothyroidism can occur.

POSTPARTUM

Both PTU and methimazole are considered safe [58]. Only small amounts of PTU cross into breast milk although higher amounts of methimazole are present in breast milk [37,59]. Of pregnant patients in remission from Graves' disease, 75% will either relapse postpartum or develop postpartum thyroiditis [8].

TSH should be performed three and six months postpartum in women known to have thyroid peroxidase antibodies (TPO-Ab) [60,61]. Annual TSH level should be performed in women with a history of postpartum thyroiditis as they have a markedly increased risk of developing permanent primary hypothyroidism in the next five- to 10-year period following the episode of postpartum thyroiditis [62–65].

THYROID NODULE

Incidence of thyroid nodules in reproductive-aged women in 1%–2% [66]. Evaluation of thyroid nodule in pregnancy includes obtaining complete history and physical, TSH and neck ultrasound. If there is sonographic evidence of hypoechoic pattern, irregular margins, or micro calcifications, malignancy should be suspected [67]. If there is suspicion for malignancy, fine-needle aspiration and histologic evaluation for malignancy should be performed [68]. For thyroid cancer in pregnancy, see Chapter 42.

THYROID STORM
Incidence
Rare hypermetabolic, acute life-threatening condition in pregnancy, which occurs in 1% of hyperthyroid women.

Precipitating Factors
Labor, infection, preeclampsia, severe anemia, surgery.

Signs/Symptoms
Fever, tachycardia disproportionate to fever, mental status change, vomiting, diarrhea, dehydration, cardiac arrhythmia, congestive heart failure [5,69], and rarely seizures, shock, stupor, and coma.

Diagnosis
It initially should be made clinically with a combination of signs and symptoms. Confirmatory labs include increased FT4 (or increased FT3) and very low TSH.

Treatment
PTU, SSKI, dexamethasone, and propranolol should be given as shown in Table 7.1 [37]. The saturated solution of potassium iodide and sodium iodide block the release of thyroid hormone from the gland. Dexamethasone decreases thyroid hormone release and peripheral conversion of T4 to T3. Propranolol inhibits the adrenergic effects of excessive thyroid hormone. Supportive measures include IV fluids with glucose, acetaminophen (as antipyretic), and oxygen as needed. Fetal monitoring and maternal cardiac monitoring are recommended [21]. Delivery in the presence of thyroid storm should be avoided if possible, with maternal treatment leading to in utero fetal resuscitation. The underlying cause, for example, infection, should be treated.

Table 7.1 Suggested Possible Treatment of Thyroid Storm in Pregnant Women

1. Propylthiouracil (PTU), 600–800 mg orally, immediately, even before laboratory tests are back; then 150–200 mg orally every four to six hours. If oral administration is not possible, use methimazole rectal suppositories.
2. Starting one to two hours after PTU administration, saturated solution of potassium iodide (SSKI), two to five drops orally every eight hours; sodium iodide, 0.5–1.0 g intravenously every eight hours; Lugol's solution, eight drops every six hours; or lithium carbonate, 300 mg orally every six hours.
3. Consider dexamethasone, 2 mg intravenously or intramuscularly every six hours for four doses.
4. Propranolol, 20–80 mg orally every four to six hours or propranolol, 1–2 mg intravenously every five minutes for a total of 6 mg, then 1–10 mg intravenously every four hours.
5. If the patient has a history of severe bronchospasm, consider the following:
   Reserpine, 1–5 mg intramuscularly every four to six hours
   Guanethidine, 1 mg/kg orally every 12 hours
   Diltiazem, 60 mg orally every six to eight hours
6. Phenobarbital, 30–60 mg orally every six to eight hours as needed for extreme restlessness.

Source: American College of Obstetricians and Gynecologists. Practice Bulletin No. 148: Thyroid disease in pregnancy. *Obstet Gynecol*, 125, 4, 996–1005, 2015.

RESOURCES

- National Graves' Disease Foundation: http://www.ngdf.org
- American Thyroid Association Alliance for Patient Education: http://www.thyroid.org/patients/patients.html
- Thyroid Foundation of Canada: http://www.thyroid.ca

REFERENCES

1. Amino N, Izumi Y, Hidaka Y, Takeoka K, Nakata Y, Tatsumi KI et al. No increase of blocking type anti-thyrotropin receptor antibodies during pregnancy in patients with Graves' disease. *J Clin Endocrinol Metab* 2003; 88(12): 5871–4. [II-3]
2. Brent GA. Clinical practice. Graves disease. *N Engl J Med* 2008; 358(24): 2594–605. [III]
3. Zophel K, Roggenbuck D, Schott M. Clinical review about TRAb assay's history. *Autoimmun Rev* 2010; 9(10): 695–700. [III, Review]
4. Abalovich M, Amino N, Barbour LA, Cobin RH, De Groot LJ, Glinoer D et al. Management of thyroid dysfunction during pregnancy and postpartum: An Endocrine Society Clinical Practice Guideline. *J Clin Endocrinol Metab* 2007; 92(8 Suppl.): S1–47. [Review]
5. Mestman JH. Hyperthyroidism in pregnancy. *Best Pract Res Clin Endocrinol Metab* 2004; 18(2): 267–88. [Review]
6. Palmieri C, Fisher RA, Sebire NJ, Smith JR, Newlands ES. Placental-site trophoblastic tumour: An unusual presentation with bilateral ovarian involvement. *Lancet Oncol* 2005; 6(1): 59–61. [III]
7. Marx H, Amin P, Lazarus JH. Hyperthyroidism and pregnancy. *BMJ* 2008; 336(7645): 663–7. [Review]
8. Cooper DS. Antithyroid drugs. *N Engl J Med* 2005; 352(9): 905–17. [III, Review]
9. LeBeau SO, Mandel SJ. Thyroid disorders during pregnancy. *Endocrinol Metab Clin North Am* 2006; 35(1): 117–36, vii. [Review]
10. Davis LE, Lucas MJ, Hankins GD, Roark ML, Cunningham FG. Thyrotoxicosis complicating pregnancy. *Am J Obstet Gynecol* 1989; 160(1): 63–70. [II-2]
11. Mestman JH. Diagnosis and management of maternal and fetal thyroid disorders. *Curr Opin Obstet Gynecol* 1999; 11(2): 167–75. [III, Review]
12. Millar LK, Wing DA, Leung AS, Koonings PP, Montoro MN, Mestman JH. Low birth weight and preeclampsia in pregnancies complicated by hyperthyroidism. *Obstet Gynecol* 1994; 84(6): 946–9. [II-2]
13. Phoojaroenchanachai M, Sriussadaporn S, Peerapatdit T, Vannasaeng S, Nitiyanant W, Boonnamsiri V et al. Effect of maternal hyperthyroidism during late pregnancy on the risk of neonatal low birth weight. *Clin Endocrinol (Oxf)* 2001; 54(3): 365–70. [II-3]
14. Yeo CP, Khoo DH, Eng PH, Tan HK, Yo SL, Jacob E. Prevalence of gestational thyrotoxicosis in Asian women evaluated in the 8th to 14th weeks of pregnancy: Correlations with total and free beta human chorionic gonadotrophin. *Clin Endocrinol (Oxf)* 2001; 55(3): 391–8. [II-2]
15. Glinoer D. Pregnancy and iodine. *Thyroid* 2001; 11(5): 471–81. [Review]
16. Glinoer D. Feto-maternal repercussions of iodine deficiency during pregnancy. An update. *Ann Endocrinol (Paris)* 2003; 64(1): 37–44. [Review]
17. Hollowell JG, Staehling NW, Hannon WH, Flanders DW, Gunter EW, Maberly GF et al. Iodine nutrition in the United States. Trends and public health implications: Iodine excretion data from National Health and Nutrition Examination Surveys I and III (1971–1974 and 1988–1994). *J Clin Endocrinol Metab* 1998; 83(10): 3401–8. [II-2]
18. American Association of Clinical Endocrinologists. *AACE clinical practice guidelines for evaluation and treatment of hyperthyroidism and hypothyroidism.* Jacksonville, FL; 1996. [Review]
19. Ladenson PW, Singer PA, Ain KB, Bagchi N, Bigos ST, Levy EG et al. American Thyroid Association guidelines for detection of thyroid dysfunction. *Arch Intern Med* 2000; 160(11): 1573–5. [III]
20. Weetman AP. Graves' disease. *N Engl J Med* 2000; 343(17): 1236–48. [III, Review]
21. Ecker JL. Thyroid function and disease in pregnancy. *Curr Probl Obstet Gynecol Fertil* 2000; (23): 109–22. [III]
22. Tan JY, Loh KC, Yeo GS, Chee YC. Transient hyperthyroidism of hyperemesis gravidarum. *BJOG* 2002; 109(6): 683–8. [III]
23. Goodwin TM, Montoro M, Mestman JH. Transient hyperthyroidism and hyperemesis gravidarum: Clinical aspects. *Am J Obstet Gynecol* 1992; 167(3): 648–52. [III]
24. Goodwin TM, Montoro M, Mestman JH, Pekary AE, Hershman JM. The role of chorionic gonadotropin in transient hyperthyroidism of hyperemesis gravidarum. *J Clin Endocrinol Metab* 1992; 75(5): 1333–7. [II-2]
25. Earl R, Crowther CA, Middleton P. Interventions for hyperthyroidism pre-pregnancy and during pregnancy. *Cochrane Database Syst Rev* 2013; 11: CD008633. [Meta-analysis; 0 RCTs]
26. Hamburger JI. Thyroid nodules in pregnancy. *Thyroid* 1992; 2(2): 165–8. [III]
27. Momotani N, Noh J, Oyanagi H, Ishikawa N, Ito K. Antithyroid drug therapy for Graves' disease during pregnancy. Optimal regimen for fetal thyroid status. *N Engl J Med* 1986; 315(1): 24–8. [II-2]
28. Mortimer RH, Tyack SA, Galligan JP, Perry-Keene DA, Tan YM. Graves' disease in pregnancy: TSH receptor binding inhibiting immunoglobulins and maternal and neonatal thyroid function. *Clin Endocrinol (Oxf)* 1990; 32(2): 141–52. [II-3]
29. Casey BM, Dashe JS, Wells CE, McIntire DD, Leveno KJ, Cunningham FG. Subclinical hyperthyroidism and pregnancy outcomes. *Obstet Gynecol* 2006; 107(2 Pt. 1): 337–41. [II-2]
30. Bahn RS, Burch HB, Cooper DS, Garber JR, Greenlee MC, Klein I et al. Hyperthyroidism and other causes of thyrotoxicosis: Management guidelines of the American Thyroid Association and American Association of Clinical Endocrinologists. *Endocr Pract* 2011; 17(3): 456–520. [III]
31. Wing DA, Millar LK, Koonings PP, Montoro MN, Mestman JH. A comparison of propylthiouracil versus methimazole in the treatment of hyperthyroidism in pregnancy. *Am J Obstet Gynecol* 1994; 170(1 Pt. 1): 90–5. [II-2]
32. Momotani N, Noh JY, Ishikawa N, Ito K. Effects of propylthiouracil and methimazole on fetal thyroid status in mothers with Graves' hyperthyroidism. *J Clin Endocrinol Metab* 1997; 82(11): 3633–6. [II-2]
33. Clementi M, Di Gianantonio E, Pelo E, Mammi I, Basile RT, Tenconi R. Methimazole embryopathy: Delineation of the phenotype. *Am J Med Genet* 1999; 83(1): 43–6. [III]
34. Di Gianantonio E, Schaefer C, Mastroiacovo PP, Cournot MP, Benedicenti F, Reuvers M et al. Adverse effects of prenatal methimazole exposure. *Teratology* 2001; 64(5): 262–6. [II-2]
35. Yoshihara A, Noh J, Yamaguchi T, Ohye H, Sato S, Sekiya K et al. Treatment of Graves' disease with antithyroid drugs in the first trimester of pregnancy and the prevalence of congenital malformation. *J Clin Endocrinol Metab* 2012; 97(7): 2396–403. [II-3]
36. Laurberg P, Andersen SL. Antithyroid drug use in pregnancy and birth defects: Why some studies find clear associations, and some studies report none? *Thyroid* 2015; 25(11): 1185–90. [III]
37. American College of Obstetricians and Gynecologists. Practice Bulletin No. 148: Thyroid disease in pregnancy. *Obstet Gynecol* 2015; 125(4): 996–1005. [Review]
38. Abraham P, Avenell A, Watson WA, Park CM, Bevan JS. Antithyroid drug regimen for treating Graves' hyperthyroidism. *Cochrane Database Syst Rev* 2005; 2(2): CD003420. [Meta-analysis, Review]
39. Burrow GN, Klatskin EH, Genel M. Intellectual development in children whose mothers received propylthiouracil during pregnancy. *Yale J Biol Med* 1978; 51(2): 151–6. [II-2]
40. Eisenstein Z, Weiss M, Katz Y, Bank H. Intellectual capacity of subjects exposed to methimazole or propylthiouracil in utero. *Eur J Pediatr* 1992; 151(8): 558–9. [II-2]

41. Berg GE, Nystrom EH, Jacobsson L, Lindberg S, Lindstedt RG, Mattsson S et al. Radioiodine treatment of hyperthyroidism in a pregnant women. *J Nucl Med* 1998; 39(2): 357–61. [II-3]

42. Evans PM, Webster J, Evans WD, Bevan JS, Scanlon MF. Radioiodine treatment in unsuspected pregnancy. *Clin Endocrinol (Oxf)* 1998; 48(3): 281–3. [II-3]

43. Stagnaro-Green A, Abalovich M, Alexander E, Azizi F, Mestman J, Negro R et al. Guidelines of the American Thyroid Association for the diagnosis and management of thyroid disease during pregnancy and postpartum. *Thyroid* 2011; 21(10): 1081–125. [III]

44. Stice RC, Grant CS, Gharib H, van Heerden JA. The management of Graves' disease during pregnancy. *Surg Gynecol Obstet* 1984; 158(2): 157–60. [II-3]

45. Burrow GN. The management of thyrotoxicosis in pregnancy. *N Engl J Med* 1985; 313(9): 562–5. [Review]

46. Brodsky JB, Cohen EN, Brown BW Jr, Wu ML, Whitcher C. Surgery during pregnancy and fetal outcome. *Am J Obstet Gynecol* 1980; 138(8): 1165–7. [II-2]

47. Nohr SB, Jorgensen A, Pedersen KM, Laurberg P. Postpartum thyroid dysfunction in pregnant thyroid peroxidase antibody-positive women living in an area with mild to moderate iodine deficiency: Is iodine supplementation safe? *J Clin Endocrinol Metab* 2000; 85(9): 3191–8. [II-2]

48. Momotani N, Hisaoka T, Noh J, Ishikawa N, Ito K. Effects of iodine on thyroid status of fetus versus mother in treatment of Graves' disease complicated by pregnancy. *J Clin Endocrinol Metab* 1992; 75(3): 738–44. [II-2]

49. Ranzini AC, Ananth CV, Smulian JC, Kung M, Limbachia A, Vintzileos AM. Ultrasonography of the fetal thyroid: Nomograms based on biparietal diameter and gestational age. *J Ultrasound Med* 2001; 20(6): 613–7. [II-2]

50. Luton D, Le Gac I, Vuillard E, Castanet M, Guibourdenche J, Noel M et al. Management of Graves' disease during pregnancy: The key role of fetal thyroid gland monitoring. *J Clin Endocrinol Metab* 2005; 90(11): 6093–8. [II-3]

51. Nachum Z, Rakover Y, Weiner E, Shalev E. Graves' disease in pregnancy: Prospective evaluation of a selective invasive treatment protocol. *Am J Obstet Gynecol* 2003; 189(1): 159–65. [II-2]

52. Kilpatrick S. Umbilical blood sampling in women with thyroid disease in pregnancy: Is it necessary? *Am J Obstet Gynecol* 2003; 189(1): 1–2. [III]

53. Hanono A, Shah B, David R, Buterman I, Roshan D, Shah S et al. Antenatal treatment of fetal goiter: A therapeutic challenge. *J Matern Fetal Neonatal Med* 2009; 22(1): 76–80. [II-3]

54. Peleg D, Cada S, Peleg A, Ben-Ami M. The relationship between maternal serum thyroid-stimulating immunoglobulin and fetal and neonatal thyrotoxicosis. *Obstet Gynecol* 2002; 99(6): 1040–3. [II-2]

55. McKenzie JM, Zakarija M. Fetal and neonatal hyperthyroidism and hypothyroidism due to maternal TSH receptor antibodies. *Thyroid* 1992; 2(2): 155–9. [Review]

56. Mitsuda N, Tamaki H, Amino N, Hosono T, Miyai K, Tanizawa O. Risk factors for developmental disorders in infants born to women with Graves disease. *Obstet Gynecol* 1992; 80(3 Pt. 1): 359–64. [III]

57. Becks GP, Burrow GN. Thyroid disease and pregnancy. *Med Clin North Am* 1991; 75(1): 121–50. [III, Review]

58. American Academy of Pediatrics Committee on Drugs. Transfer of drugs and other chemicals into human milk. *Pediatrics* 2001; 108(3): 776–89. [Review]

59. Briggs GG, Freeman RK, Yaffe SJ, eds. *Drugs in Pregnancy and Lactation: A Reference Guide to Fetal and Neonatal Risk.* 6th ed.: Lippincott Williams & Wilkins; 2001. [II-2]

60. Premawardhana LD, Parkes AB, John R, Harris B, Lazarus JH. Thyroid peroxidase antibodies in early pregnancy: Utility for prediction of postpartum thyroid dysfunction and implications for screening. *Thyroid* 2004; 14(8): 610–5. [II-2]

61. Stagnaro-Green A. Clinical review 152: Postpartum thyroiditis. *J Clin Endocrinol Metab* 2002; 87(9): 4042–7. [Review]

62. Azizi F. The occurrence of permanent thyroid failure in patients with subclinical postpartum thyroiditis. *Eur J Endocrinol* 2005; 153(3): 367–71. [II-3]

63. Premawardhana LD, Parkes AB, Ammari F, John R, Darke C, Adams H et al. Postpartum thyroiditis and long-term thyroid status: Prognostic influence of thyroid peroxidase antibodies and ultrasound echogenicity. *J Clin Endocrinol Metab* 2000; 85(1): 71–5. [II-1]

64. Othman S, Phillips DI, Parkes AB, Richards CJ, Harris B, Fung H et al. A long-term follow-up of postpartum thyroiditis. *Clin Endocrinol (Oxf)* 1990; 32(5): 559–64. [II-2]

65. Tachi J, Amino N, Tamaki H, Aozasa M, Iwatani Y, Miyai K. Long term follow-up and HLA association in patients with postpartum hypothyroidism. *J Clin Endocrinol Metab* 1988; 66(3): 480–4. [II-2]

66. Fitzpatrick DL, Russell MA. Diagnosis and management of thyroid disease in pregnancy. *Obstet Gynecol Clin North Am* 2010; 37(2): 173–93. [III]

67. Gharib H, Papini E, Paschke R, Duick DS, Valcavi R, Hegedus L et al. American Association of Clinical Endocrinologists, Associazione Medici Endocrinologi, and European Thyroid Association medical guidelines for clinical practice for the diagnosis and management of thyroid nodules: Executive Summary of recommendations. *J Endocrinol Invest* 2010; 33(5): 287–91. [III]

68. Bartolazzi A, Gasbarri A, Papotti M, Bussolati G, Lucante T, Khan A et al. Application of an immunodiagnostic method for improving preoperative diagnosis of nodular thyroid lesions. *Lancet* 2001; 357(9269): 1644–50. [II-3]

69. Sheffield JS, Cunningham FG. Thyrotoxicosis and heart failure that complicate pregnancy. *Am J Obstet Gynecol* 2004; 190(1): 211–7. [III]

8

Prolactinoma

Katherine Husk

KEY POINTS

- **Diagnosis: elevated prolactin and MRI-proven pituitary adenoma.**
- **Preconception: treat with dopamine agonist** (bromocriptine or cabergoline) aiming to normalize prolactin and decrease size of adenoma, continuing therapy up to positive pregnancy test. Discourage pregnancy until those aims have been achieved and any neurologic or visual symptoms or suprasellar involvement have been resolved.
- **Maternal risk is adenoma enlargement**; this occurs in pregnancy in 1% to 5% of microadenomas and about 15% to 36% of macroadenomas.
- **Bromocriptine** and **cabergoline** have been shown to be safe for the fetus.
- Compared to cabergoline, bromocriptine has the following advantages: cheaper, more pregnancy safety data, no association with cardiac valve disease, but its disadvantages include twice daily (versus twice weekly) dosing and more side effects.
- **Management depends on the size of adenoma:**
  - **Microadenoma (<1 cm):** Consider stopping dopamine agonist in pregnancy, especially if normal prepregnancy prolactin and stable microadenoma >2 years. During the pregnancy, the woman should **be asked about headaches and changes in vision at each visit (at least every three months). The decision to treat with dopamine agonist is based on symptoms (e.g., headache) and signs (e.g., abnormal visual field examination) only.** Prolactin levels should not be checked because they physiologically (tenfold) increase in pregnancy.
  - **Macroadenoma (>1 cm): Dopamine agonist should be continued.** Monitoring as per microadenoma, plus **formal visual field testing every three months**. Transsphenoidal surgery is suggested usually only if maximal dopamine agonist therapy is ineffective.
  - **Postpartum:** Continue dopamine agonist therapy in those with macroadenomas. A prolactin level and MRI six to eight weeks postpartum can be performed to assess for regression/remission although prolactin levels may not normalize until six months postpartum. Continue dopamine agonist in women with microadenomas and elevated prolactin. Consider stopping therapy in women with microadenomas, stable >2 years, normal prolactin, and on low-dose therapy. If on dopamine agonist therapy, women should be advised against breast-feeding.

DIAGNOSIS/DEFINITION

Pituitary adenomas producing prolactin (prolactinomas or lactotroph adenomas) are diagnosed by sustained nonpregnant **elevation of serum prolactin** (usually >40 μg/L × 2; normal prolactin nonpregnant: <20 μg/L) *and* radiographic (best is MRI) evidence of pituitary adenoma. Rule out other causes of prolactinemia [1].

SYMPTOMS

Before pregnancy, galactorrhea in 80% of women and irregular menses (e.g., oligomenorrhea).

EPIDEMIOLOGY/INCIDENCE

Prolactinomas account for about 40% of pituitary tumors. They are the most common type of secretory pituitary tumor.

ETIOLOGY/BASIC PATHOPHYSIOLOGY

These adenomas produce prolactin. Outside of pregnancy, prolactin levels parallel tumor size fairly closely. Increased prolactin usually causes **infertility** because of the inhibitory effect of prolactin on secretion of GNRH, which in turn inhibits the release of LH and FSH, thus impairing gonadal steroidogenesis and ovulation and thereby conception. Sometimes the mass effect of a macroadenoma can also lead to infertility. Prolactinomas are usually benign and nonhereditary.

CLASSIFICATION

Microadenoma: <10 mm; macroadenoma: ≥10 mm.

COMPLICATIONS

Mother

The principal risk is the **increase in adenoma size** sufficient to cause neurologic symptoms, most importantly **visual impairment** or also headaches. In women with lactotroph adenomas who become pregnant, the hyperestrogenemia of pregnancy may increase the size of the adenoma. This should be distinguished from increase in pituitary (overall) size, which is physiologic in pregnancy. **The risk that the adenoma increase will be clinically important depends on the size of the adenoma before pregnancy.** The risk of a clinically important increase in the size of a lactotroph microadenoma during pregnancy is small. Because of enlargement, about 1% to 5% of pregnant women with **microadenomas** develop neurologic symptoms, such as headaches and/or a visual field abnormality and about 1% diabetes insipidus. With **macroadenomas**, neurologic symptoms occur in about 15% to 36% or higher of pregnant women and diabetes insipidus in about 1% to 2% [2–4]. Long-term hyperprolactinemia may lead to decrease in bone density, which again increases (not back to normal levels) after normal prolactin levels are reestablished [1].

Fetus

The main potential risk to the fetus is from dopamine agonist treatment of hyperprolactinemia. As dopaminergic neurons form early in fetal development, dopamine represents a key component of motor and cognitive development, and both bromocriptine and cabergoline cross the placenta [5,6]. Administration of bromocriptine during the first months of pregnancy does not harm the fetus (more than 6000 pregnancies reported) [7–9]. Data available about the use of bromocriptine later in pregnancy are less, but no adverse events have been reported. Cabergoline use in pregnancy is probably safe as well (more than 900 pregnancies reported), but less experience is reported in comparison to bromocriptine [5,6,9–13]. Because of the long half-life of cabergoline, concerns were raised about use in pregnancy induction (i.e., achieving pregnancy in a previously infertile woman) [5]; however, use of cabergoline in early pregnancy has not been associated with negative outcomes and thus far there is no evidence to suggest an increased risk of major malformations beyond the baseline risk [5,6,9,12,13]. There are, however, limited data available about use of cabergoline throughout pregnancy [5].

PREGNANCY CONSIDERATIONS

The ability to treat prolactinomas successfully with dopamine agonists in >90% of patients allows most women with this disorder to become pregnant. The theoretical basis for an **increase in size of the pituitary** during pregnancy is that hyperestrogenemia causes lactotroph hyperplasia. Secondary to estrogen causing lactotroph hyperplasia, there is a progressive increase in pituitary size throughout pregnancy, as assessed by MR imaging, so that the volume during the third trimester is more than double of that in nonpregnant women [14].

PREGNANCY-RELATED MANAGEMENT
Principles
Effect of Pregnancy on Disease
The whole pituitary enlarges in pregnancy, and the prolactinoma itself can enlarge. **Prolactin levels are physiologically elevated in pregnancy and cannot be used for management.** Serum levels of prolactin in nonpregnant patients with prolactinomas are usually proportional to the tumor mass, but this relationship is lost in pregnancy, particularly if dopamine agonists are discontinued early in pregnancy [9,15]. Prolactin levels do not correlate well with symptoms in both nonpregnant and pregnant patients with prolactinomas [16].

Effect of Disease on Pregnancy
No obstetrical effects unless major surgery is needed.

Workup
In Pregnancy (Figure 8.1)
- **Prolactin** levels are not helpful in pregnancy.
- **MRI** is more effective in revealing small tumors and the extension of large tumors compared to CT scan [1].
- **Visual field testing** is indicated in women with **macroadenomas**.

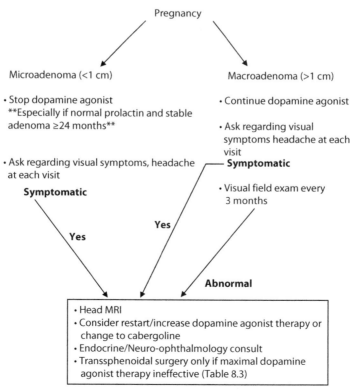

Figure 8.1 Management of prolactinoma in pregnancy (see also Table 8.2).

Table 8.1 Dose and Side Effect Profiles for Dopamine Agonists Approved for Use in the United States

Medication	Dose	Side Effects of Both Drugs[a]
Bromocriptine	Initial: 0.625–1.25 mg daily; usual range for maintenance dose: 2.5–10.0 mg daily	Nausea, headaches, dizziness (postural hypotension), nasal congestion, constipation. Infrequent: fatigue, anxiety, depression, alcohol intolerance. Rare: cold-sensitive vasospasm, psychosis
Cabergoline	Initial: 0.25–0.5 mg weekly; usual range for maintenance dose: 0.25–3.0 mg weekly	Possible: cardiac valve abnormalities (reported with cabergoline)

Source: Modified from Klibanski A. *N Engl J Med*, 362, 1219–26, 2010.
[a]More common with bromocriptine.

In Nonpregnant Women

If an elevated prolactin is detected, this should be repeated. If still elevated, then a head MRI is performed even in cases of mild hyperprolactinemia. At initial diagnosis, thyroid-stimulating hormone and free T4, renal and hepatic function should be assessed [16].

Treatment (Figure 8.1; Tables 8.1 and 8.2)

The primary therapy for all prolactinomas is a dopamine agonist. The dopamine agonists approved in the United States are bromocriptine and cabergoline. Dose recommendations and side effects are listed in Table 8.1 [16].

Bromocriptine (Parlodel)

Dose: Started at 0.625 mg po qhs with a snack for one week. Then add 1.25 mg qam for one week and increase by 1.25 mg. So at four weeks, a total of 5 mg total dose (split **2.5 mg ql2h**) is reached and prolactin rechecked. Usually a total of 5 to 7.5 mg (split ql2h) total dose is required. It can also be used intravaginally (same dose, less side effects, minimal vaginal irritation).

Mechanism of Action: Dopamine agonist (dopamine inhibits lactotroph receptors, so less prolactin is produced, and the size of tumors is decreased); ergot derivative.

Evidence for effectiveness: See below.

Safety in pregnancy: Safe (FDA category B); breast-feeding is contraindicated.

Side effects: Nausea, hypotension, and depression (less if therapy initiated at night).

Cabergoline (Dostinex)

Dose: Start at 0.25 mg twice weekly and increase monthly to normal prolactin. Usual required dose is 0.25 to 0.5 mg twice weekly; maximum dose should be 1 mg twice weekly.

Mechanism of action: Dopamine agonist (see above), non-ergot, high affinity for lactotroph dopamine receptors.

Table 8.2 Indications for Therapy in Patients with Prolactinomas

Main indication in pregnancy
Macroadenoma
Pregnant and nonpregnant
Enlarging microadenoma
Bothersome galactorrhea
Gynecomastia
Acne and hirsutism
Nonpregnant
Infertility
Oligomenorrhea or amenorrhea

Source: Modified from Klibanski A. *N Engl J Med*, 362, 1219–26, 2010.

Evidence for effectiveness: See below.

Safety in pregnancy: Safe (FDA category B); breast-feeding is contraindicated.

Side effects: Associated with heart valve disease in very high doses.

Preconception Counseling

Treatment of women with lactotroph adenomas outside of pregnancy is based on the size of the tumor, presence or absence of gonadal dysfunction, and the woman's desire regarding fertility [1]. Indications for therapy in patients with prolactinomas are listed in Table 8.2 [16].

Treatment should begin before conception with advice to the woman and her partner about the risks of pregnancy to her and the fetus. When a **dopamine agonist** is needed to lower the serum prolactin concentration to permit ovulation, counseling should include the fact that **bromocriptine** has larger safety data although **cabergoline** (Dostinex) has less data in pregnancy (although all reassuring thus far). Bromocriptine normalizes prolactin levels in >80% of women with microadenomas, restoring menses and fertility in >90%. **Compared to cabergoline, bromocriptine** has the following advantages: it is cheaper, there are more pregnancy safety data, and there is no association with heart valve disease, but its disadvantages include twice daily (vs. twice weekly) dosing, it is less effective at normalizing prolactin levels, and has more side effects [16]. If a woman cannot tolerate bromocriptine, cabergoline should be recommended; 70% of patients who do not have a response to bromocriptine respond to cabergoline. Overall, cabergoline is effective in inducing pregnancy at a high rate even in cases that have been traditionally considered difficult to treat, such as those with large tumor size, bromocriptine resistance, or bromocriptine intolerance [17]. There are, however, substantial numbers of women (approximately 18%), who are resistant to cabergoline and will require higher doses to achieve normalization of prolactin levels and to ovulate [9]. Quinagolide (Pergolide) should not be recommended because it is not FDA approved to treat hyperprolactinemia, has not been well studied during pregnancy, and has been associated with cardiac valvular defects [18]. In nonpregnant adults with prolactinomas, prolactin levels and MRI should be checked after diagnosis and stabilization once a year for three years and then about every two years if the patient's condition is stable. In patients with normal prolactin for ≥2 years on low-dose therapy, some consider stopping the dopamine agonist therapy. The risk of enlargement over time in untreated patients is about 20% [16].

Microadenomas

A woman who has a lactotroph microadenoma should be told that the risk of clinically important enlargement of her adenoma during pregnancy is very small (1%–5%) and that it **should not be a deterrent to becoming pregnant**. She should also be told that bromocriptine or cabergoline will likely be effective if symptoms do occur. If she is willing to take this small risk of enlargement, she should be **given bromocriptine or cabergoline before pregnancy in whatever dosage is necessary to lower her serum prolactin concentration to normal**. Bromocriptine is the drug associated with the greater experience. When the serum prolactin concentration is normal and menses have occurred regularly for a few months, the woman can attempt to become pregnant. Before pregnancy, the dopamine agonist should be tapered to the lowest effective dose and can be discontinued before pregnancy if used for >24 months with normal prolactin levels as about 25% of patients maintain normal levels even off of medication although most need to restart it.

Macroadenomas

A woman who has a lactotroph macroadenoma should be advised of the relatively higher risk of clinically important tumor enlargement during pregnancy [2–4]. A macroadenoma is an **absolute indication for therapy** (dopamine agonist, followed together with an endocrinologist) **in nonpregnant or pregnant women**. Doses of dopamine agonists sufficient to control the macroadenoma are usually higher (bromocriptine 7.5–10 mg/daily; cabergoline 0.5–1 mg twice weekly) than with microadenomas. The goals of treatment are to decrease prolactin levels and symptoms, to decrease and stabilize the tumor mass, and to prevent headaches and cranial nerve compression [16]. Before pregnancy, the dopamine agonist should be carefully tapered to lowest effective dose. This may take weeks to years. Advice and monitoring depend on the size of the adenoma.

- If the macroadenoma does not elevate the optic chiasm or extend behind the sella, treatment with bromocriptine or cabergoline for a sufficient period to shrink it substantially should reduce the chance of clinically important enlargement during pregnancy [2,19]. As with treatment with dopamine agonists, this risk is likely only somewhat increased compared with microadenomas [9]. Once sufficient decrease in size has occurred, the woman can attempt to become pregnant.

- If the adenoma is very large or elevates the optic chiasm, pregnancy should be strongly discouraged until the adenoma has been adequately treated. Despite ongoing treatment with dopamine agonists, large macroadenomas, particularly those with extension beyond the sella, have a 23% risk of undergoing a clinically significant increase in size during pregnancy [9]. If the macroadenoma extends behind the sella, the woman should undergo visual field examination and testing of anterior pituitary function. Transsphenoidal surgery may be necessary and perhaps postoperative radiation. Postoperative treatment with bromocriptine or cabergoline may also be helpful in reducing adenoma size further and lowering the serum prolactin concentration to normal. Such a regimen reduces the chance that symptomatic expansion will occur during pregnancy [2,3], but it may still occur. New evidence suggests that cabergoline has the potential for use as the primary therapeutic agent for macroadenomas, even those that extend beyond the sella, and may prevent the need for

traditional combination therapy with surgery, radiotherapy, and bromocriptine, but further studies are warranted [17].

- **Pregnancy should be discouraged in a woman whose macroadenoma is unresponsive to bromocriptine and cabergoline** even if it is not elevating the optic chiasm until the size has been greatly reduced by transsphenoidal surgery because medical treatment would not likely be effective if the adenoma enlarges during pregnancy.

PRENATAL CARE

See also section titled "Preconception Counseling."

Microadenoma

Bromocriptine and probably cabergoline are safe in pregnancy. They can be discontinued as soon as pregnancy has been confirmed if the patient who has a normal prolactin and a recent reassuring (adenoma <1 cm) MRI so desires. The risk of clinically significant tumor enlargement during pregnancy is about 3% for microprolactinomas [16].

During the pregnancy, the woman should be asked about headaches and changes in vision at each visit (or at least every three months). A formal visual field test every three months can be performed but is not absolutely necessary. **The decision to treat with a dopamine agonist is based on symptoms (e.g., headache) and signs (e.g., abnormal visual filed examination) only.** It should not be based on prolactin levels. In fact, **prolactin levels should not be checked** because they physiologically increase (about tenfold) in pregnancy. If no symptoms occur, serum prolactin can be measured about two months after delivery or cessation of nursing, and if it is similar to the pretreatment value, the drug can be resumed.

Macroadenoma

The **dopamine agonist should be continued during pregnancy** in most cases. In these patients, discontinuation of the drug usually leads to expansion of the adenoma [1]. Monitoring during pregnancy should be similar to that described above for women with microadenomas except for the fact that **formal visual field testing every three months should be performed**. The risk of clinically significant tumor enlargement during pregnancy is about 30% for macroprolactinomas [16].

A perceived change in vision should be assessed by a neuro-ophthalmologist, and an MRI (gadolinium-enhanced; more effective than CT scan) [1] should be performed if an abnormality consistent with a pituitary adenoma is confirmed. If the adenoma has enlarged to a degree that could account for the symptoms, the woman should be treated with higher doses of bromocriptine throughout the remainder of the pregnancy, which will usually decrease the size of the adenoma and alleviate the symptoms [20,21]. If the adenoma does not respond to bromocriptine, cabergoline may be successful [22]. If cabergoline is not successful, transsphenoidal surgery could be considered in the second trimester if vision is severely compromised; in comparison, surgery for persistent visual symptoms in the third trimester should be deferred until delivery if possible. Surgery is recommended only if medical therapy is ineffective. Indication for neurosurgery in patients with prolactinomas are listed in Table 8.3 [16].

Table 8.3   Indication for Neurosurgery in Patients with Prolactinomas

Pregnant or nonpregnant

Increasing tumor size despite optimal medical therapy
Dopamine agonist-resistant macroadenoma
Pituitary apoplexy
Inability to tolerate necessary dopamine agonist therapy
Persistent chiasmal compression despite optimal medical
   therapy
Medically unresponsive cystic prolactinoma
Cerebrospinal fluid leak during administration of dopamine
   agonist
Macroadenoma in a patient with a psychiatric condition for which
   dopamine agonists are contraindicated

Infertility patient

Dopamine agonist-resistant microadenoma if ovulation induction
   is not appropriate
Macroadenoma in proximity to optic chiasm despite optimal
   medical therapy (prepregnancy debulking recommended)

Source: Modified from Klibanski A. *N Engl J Med*, 362, 1219–26, 2010.

Surgical cure rates are <50% with macroadenomas with up to 80% of these patients experiencing recurrent hyperprolactinemia [16].

ANTEPARTUM TESTING

None needed (except if other indications present).

DELIVERY

No special precautions.

ANESTHESIA

No special precautions.

POSTPARTUM

A prolactin level and a gadolinium-enhanced MRI can be performed six to eight weeks postpartum. Prolactin levels may not normalize until six months postpartum [16]. Those with smaller adenoma size initially and/or normalization of pituitary MRI following pregnancy have a higher chance of remission [12]. The mechanisms of tumor regression/remission are unknown, but proposed mechanisms include changes in estrogen and/or dopamine status following pregnancy or autoinfarction of the tumor [6,17]. All women with macroadenomas and those with microadenomas and elevated prolactin should be continued/started on dopamine agonist therapy with endocrine follow-up. In women stable for more than two years with microadenoma with normal prolactin and low dose of therapy, consideration can be given to stopping therapy [16]. If therapy is stopped, close follow-up is necessary as even in stable patients with normal prolactin, recurrence of hyperprolactinemia is >30% for microprolactinomas and >50% for macroprolactinomas [16]. Other methods of contraception can be used, but oral estrogen-containing pills are also probably safe [16].

BREAST-FEEDING

A microadenoma is not a contraindication to nursing. If the woman has no neurologic symptoms at the time of delivery, nursing should not be of substantial risk, as breast-feeding does not appear to increase the risk of tumor enlargement and hyperprolactinemia recurrence [6]. If she does have neurologic symptoms at the time of delivery or if they develop during nursing, she should be treated with a dopamine agonist. Because dopamine agonists suppress lactation, the women on these drugs should be advised against breast-feeding.

REFERENCES

1. Schlechte JA. Prolactinoma. *N Engl J Med* 2003; 349: 2035–41. [III; review]
2. Gemzell C, Wang CF. Outcome of pregnancy in women with pituitary adenoma. *Fertil Steril* 1979; 31: 363. [A survey of 25 physicians in 1979 revealed that they had seen a total of 91 pregnancies in 85 women with lactotroph microadenomas and 46 women with lactotroph macroadenomas were followed during 56 pregnancies]
3. Molitch ME. Management of prolactinomas during pregnancy. *J Reprod Med* 1999; 44: 1121. [III; review]
4. Kupersmith MJ, Rosenberg C, Kleinberg D. Visual loss in pregnant women with pituitary adenomas. *Ann Intern Med* 1994; 121: 473. [II-3]
5. Glezer A, Bronstein MD. Prolactinomas, cabergoline, and pregnancy. *Endocrine* 2014; 47: 64–9. [III; review]
6. Auriemma RS, Perone Y, Di Sarno A, Grasso LF, Guerra E, Gasperi M, Pivonello R, Colao A. Results of a single-center 10-year observational survey study on recurrence of hyperprolactinemia after pregnancy and lactation. *J Clin Endocrinol Metab* 2013; 98: 372–9. [II-3; *n* = 143 pregnancies, 91 patients]
7. Turkalj I, Braun P, Krupp P. Surveillance of bromocriptine in pregnancy. *JAMA* 1982; 247: 1589. [The manufacturer of bromocriptine surveyed physicians known to prescribe bromocriptine. The survey evaluated 1410 pregnancies in 1335 women who took the drug during pregnancy, primarily during the first month [5]. The incidence of spontaneous abortions (11.1%) and major (1%) and minor (2.5%) congenital malformations was similar to that in the general population. Only eight women had taken bromocriptine after the second month of pregnancy]
8. Molitch ME. Pregnancy and the hyperprolactinemic woman. *N Engl J Med* 1985; 23: 1364–70. [II-c; safety of bromocriptine]
9. Molitch ME. Management of the pregnant patient with a prolactinoma. *Eur J Endocrinol* 2015; 172(5): R205–13. [III; review]
10. Robert E, Musatti L, Piscitelli G et al. Pregnancy outcome after treatment with the ergot derivative, cabergoline. *Reprod Toxicol* 1996; 10: 333. [II-3; *n* = 226]
11. Ricci E, Parazzini F, Motta T et al. Pregnancy outcome after cabergoline treatment in early weeks of gestation. *Reprod Toxicol* 2002; 16: 791–3. [II-3; cabergoline safety proven in 61 pregnancies]
12. Domingue M-E, Devuyst F, Alexopoulou O, Corvilain B, Maiter D. Outcome of prolactinoma after pregnancy and lactation: A study on 73 patients. *Clin Endocrinol* 2014; 80: 642–8. [II-3; *n* = 73]
13. Lebbe M, Hubinont C, Bernard P, Maiter D. Outcome of 100 pregnancies initiated under treatment with cabergoline in hyperprolactinaemic women. *Clin Endocrinol* 2010; 73: 236–42. [II-3; cabergoline safety proven in 100 pregnancies]
14. Gonzalez JG, Elizondo G, Saldivar D et al. Pituitary gland growth during normal pregnancy: An in vivo study using magnetic resonance imaging. *Am J Med* 1988; 85: 217. [II-3]
15. Melmed S, Casanueva FF, Hoffman AR, Kleinberg DL, Montori VM, Schlechte JA, Wass JAH. Diagnosis and treatment of hyperprolactinoemia: An Endocrine Society clinical practice guideline. *J Clin Endocrinol Metab* 2011; 96(2): 273–88. [III]
16. Klibanski A. Prolactinomas. *N Engl J Med* 2010; 362: 1219–26. [III]
17. Ono M, Miki N, Amano K et al. Individualized high-dose cabergoline therapy for hyperprolactinemic infertility in women with micro- and macroprolactinomas. *J Clin Endocrinol Metab* 2010; 95(6): 2672–9. [II-2]

18. Flowers CM, Racoosin JA, Lu SL et al. The US Food and Drug Administration's registry of patients with Pergolide-associated valvular heart disease. *Mayo Clin Proc* 2003; 78: 730. [II-3]

19. Ahmed M, Al-Dossary E, Woodhouse NJY. Macroprolactinomas with suprasellar extension: Effect of bromocriptine withdrawal during one or more pregnancies. *Fertil Steril* 1992; 58: 492. [II-2]

20. Konopka P, Raymond JP, Merceron RE et al. Continuous administration of bromocriptine in the prevention of neurological complications in pregnant women with prolactinomas. *Am J Obstet Gynecol* 1983; 146: 935. [II-3]

21. Van Roon E, van der Vijver JC, Gerretsen G et al. Rapid regression of a suprasellar extending prolactinoma after bromocriptine treatment during pregnancy. *Fertil Steril* 1981; 36: 173. [II-3]

22. Liu C, Tyrrell JB. Successful treatment of a large macroprolactinoma with cabergoline during pregnancy. *Pituitary* 2001; 4: 179. [II-3]

9

Nausea/vomiting of pregnancy and hyperemesis gravidarum

Rupsa C. Boelig

KEY POINTS

- **Diagnosis of hyperemesis gravidarum is nausea and vomiting ≥3 times a day** with **large ketones in urine** or acetone in blood (dehydration, fluid, and electrolyte changes) *and* **weight loss of >3 kg or >5% prepregnancy weight,** having excluded other diagnoses.
- Do not test for thyroid-stimulating hormone (TSH) in women with nausea/vomiting or hyperemesis gravidarum unless they have preexisting history/symptoms of hyperthyroidism.
- **For prevention, start prenatal vitamins before conception.**
- Start treating nausea and vomiting early to prevent hyperemesis gravidarum.
- **Therapies proven to improve nausea and vomiting of pregnancy and/or hyperemesis gravidarum are the following** (in approximate order of increasing risk/invasiveness/potency) (Figure 9.1):
  - Acupressure
  - **Ginger capsules**
  - **Vitamin B$_6$ with doxylamine**
  - Metoclopramide
  - **Ondansetron**
  - **Promethazine**

DIAGNOSIS/DEFINITION

Nausea and vomiting of pregnancy (NVP) can be quite variable, and symptoms can range from mild to severe (hyperemesis gravidarum, HG). Mild symptoms include intermittent nausea, odor and food aversion, retching, and vomiting.

Hyperemesis gravidarum (HG) or severe nausea/vomiting is generally defined as **intractable n/v ≥3 times a day** with signs of **dehydration** (large ketonuria, high urine specific gravity, or electrolyte imbalance) *and* **weight loss** of >3 kg or >5% prepregnancy weight, having excluded other diagnoses (Table 9.1).

EPIDEMIOLOGY/INCIDENCE

Nausea and vomiting are common in early pregnancy; approximately 50%–80% will experience nausea and 50% vomiting. HG, in contrast, affects only 0.3%–1% of pregnancies [1–3]. The onset is about four to six weeks, peak eight to 12 weeks, resolution <20 weeks. HG is the most common indication for hospital admission in the first trimester of pregnancy and second to preterm labor throughout the entire pregnancy. Of the cases, 60% resolve by the end of the first trimester, and 91% have complete resolution by 20 weeks [3]. For symptoms presenting after nine weeks, alternative diagnoses should be carefully considered (Table 9.1) [4].

GENETICS

More common in first-degree relatives (daughters, sisters, monozygotic more than dizygotic twins). Daughters born to mothers with HG have a three times higher risk of future development [5].

ETIOLOGY

Hypotheses:

1. Gastrointestinal (GI) motility decreases in pregnancy because of increasing levels of progesterone (but not particularly in HG; probably secondary phenomenon).
2. Hormones (hCG, thyroxine, cortisol, etc.) trigger the chemo-receptor trigger zone (CTZ) in the brainstem-vomiting center.
3. CTZ more sensitive to hormones.
4. Abnormalities in vestibulo-ocular reflex pathway [6].
5. N/v correlates with the rise and fall of hCG. It has been theorized that hCG stimulates the ovary to produce more estrogen, which is known to increase n/v [3].
6. Helicobacter pylori (IgG 90.5% in HG patients, 47.5% in controls [7]; no randomized controlled trials (RCTs) exist for treatment of H. pylori in HG) [2,7].
7. Possible psychologic predisposition, associated with unwanted, unplanned pregnancies or excessive life stressors (and conversion disorder) [4,8]. Of women with HG report, 85% have poor support by partner.
8. Some have also postulated that n/v is evolutionary to protect the fetus from teratogenic exposures because the time frame correlates with the period of organogenesis [4].
9. There is likely a strong genetic component involved in HG as the recurrence risk is significantly greater in women with a history of HG; however, the influence of paternity remains controversial [9–11].

CLASSIFICATION

A pregnancy-unique quantification of emesis/nausea (PUQE) index has been proposed, validated, and recently slightly modified, but it is seldom used clinically [12–14]. Management is based on clinical severity as well as a woman's perception of severity and desire for treatment.

RISK FACTORS/ASSOCIATIONS

Risk factors include young maternal age, nulliparity, prior HG (recurrence in about 67%), prior molar pregnancy, obesity, African-American race, female fetus, history of motion sickness, migraines, or psychiatric illness; preexisting

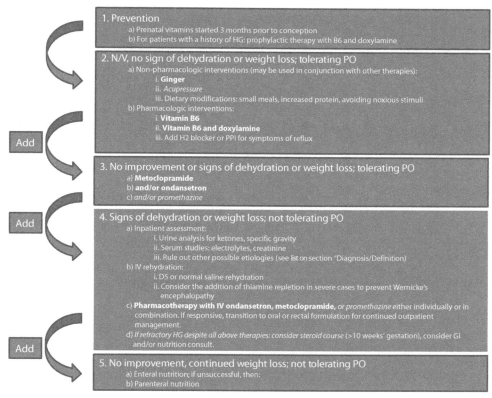

Figure 9.1 Management of Nausea and Vomiting of Pregnancy and Hyperemesis Gravidarum. Proceed through steps in a progressive, additive fashion. Therapies in bold have consistently demonstrated efficacy in randomized controlled trials for treatment of NVP and/or HG. Therapies in italics have been studied in RCTs with mixed results. *Abbreviations:* HG, hyperemesis gravidarum; H2 blocker, Histamine-2 receptor blockers; IV, intravenous; NVP, nausea and vomiting of pregnancy; N/V, nausea and/or vomiting; PO, per os/by mouth; PPI, proton pump inhibitor.

hyperthyroidism, diabetes, GI disorders, or asthma; conditions associated with high hCG levels (larger placental mass as in multiple pregnancy, molar pregnancy, Trisomy 21); and high estradiol levels. Women who experienced n/v related to estrogen exposure (i.e., oral contraceptive pill) outside pregnancy were more likely to experience NVP [4]. Smoking has been associated with a lower incidence of HG, possibly because it is associated with lower levels of hCG and estradiol [4,15,16].

A related condition symptomatically is **ptyalism**, defined by sialorrhea or excessive salivation although little is known about this condition. Diagnosis: salivation >1900 mL/day. Etiologic hypothesis: stimulation by starch (possibly pica). It is characterized by an inability to swallow rather than excessive production of saliva. No therapy (gum, lozenges, small meals, anticholinergics, ganglion-blocking agents, oxyphenonium bromide, etc.) has been studied appropriately or shown to be efficacious in pregnancy. Check hydration, nutrition, psychologic status, and other issues as per NVP [17].

COMPLICATIONS
Maternal
Mild cases are not associated with significant complications. For moderate-to-severe cases or HG, some women may experience significant psychosocial morbidity resulting in depression or decision to terminate (2.9% incidence of termination with HG in Sweden) [4,15,18]. Moderate-to-severe cases are also

associated with higher health care costs and economic burden from time lost from work and need for hospitalization [4]. Rare complications include Wernicke's encephalopathy (vitamin B_1 deficiency; permanent neurologic disability, or maternal death), peripheral neuropathies (vitamin B_6 and B_{12} deficiency), central pontine myelinolysis, splenic avulsion, esophageal rupture, pneumothorax, or acute tubular necrosis. In extreme and very rare cases of HG, maternal death can occur [4].

Fetal/Neonatal
Minimal complications (e.g., no increase in FGR) are found in NVP [4]. HG, however, is associated with a higher incidence of fetal growth restriction (especially if severe HG), low birth weight, small for gestational age, gestational hypertension, and preterm delivery [16,19]. HG is not associated with an increased risk of congenital malformation, and fetal death is very rare [4,19].

NVP and HG are also associated with lower incidence of pregnancy loss thought to be secondary to robust placental synthesis.

PREGNANCY MANAGEMENT
Principles
Prevention is better than treatment; that is, **intervening early in nausea/vomiting is helpful in preventing worsening symptoms** [20]. HG is a diagnosis of exclusion: see Table 9.1

Table 9.1   Differential Diagnosis of Nausea and Vomiting of Pregnancy

Gastrointestinal conditions
- Gastroparesis/Ileus
- Gastroenteritis
- Cyclic vomiting syndrome
- Achalasia
- Biliary tract disease
- Hepatitis
- Intestinal obstruction
- Peptic ulcer disease/H. pylori
- Pancreatitis
- Appendicitis
- Inflammatory bowel disease

Genitourinary tract conditions
- Pyelonephritis
- Uremia
- Ovarian torsion
- Kidney stones
- Degenerating uterine fibroids

Metabolic diseases
- Diabetic ketoacidosis
- Porphyria
- Addison's disease
- Hyperthyroidism
- Hyperparathyroidism

Neurologic disorders
- Pseudotumor cerebri
- Vestibular lesions
- Migraines
- Tumors of the central nervous system
- Lymphocytic hypophysitis

Miscellaneous
- Drug toxicity or intolerance
- Psychologic

Pregnancy-related conditions
- Acute fatty livery of pregnancy
- Preeclampsia
- Trophoblastic disease

Source: Adapted from American College of Obstetrics and Gynecology. *Obstet Gynecol* 2015; 126(3): e12–24.

for differential diagnosis. N/v tends to be undertreated by both some physicians and some patients although safe and effective therapies exist. Approximately 10% of patients with n/v during pregnancy will require medication [3].

Workup

Differential diagnostic possibilities should be ruled out, especially prior to the diagnosis of HG: see Table 9.1 [4].

History and Review of Systems
Special attention to severity of n/v, weight loss, prior GI diagnosis, and stressors—dietary, physical, and psychologic. Abdominal pain, fever, headache/migraine are atypical complaints of a patient with n/v of pregnancy.

Physical Exam
Special attention to vital signs, signs of dehydration, goiter, and abdominal and neurologic examinations.

Labs
- *Serum* (especially for severe cases): Electrolytes, BUN, creatinine, glucose, LFTs, amylase, lipase, acetone (quantitative hCG not helpful in management)
- *Urine*: ketones, specific gravity

- *Thyroid-stimulating hormone (TSH)*: **No need to send TSH** (60%–70% of HG have "transient biochemical hyperthyroidism of pregnancy" with decreased TSH and increased free thyroid index; this is secondary to hCG-stimulating thyroxine synthesis from pituitary; always resolves spontaneously in 1 to 10 weeks [21,22]; only test if pregnant woman has a history of thyroid disease or goiter).

Radiologic
Fetal ultrasound (to assess for molar pregnancy, multiple gestation, etc.).

Treatment
Figure 9.1 illustrates a suggested stepwise approach to the management of NVP and HG. Several interventions are available for treatment of n/v and HG [1,2] (Table 9.2). It is suggested to intervene early on n/v. A combination of interventions is often necessary. **For HG, consider starting at least at step 3**, but still consider implementing steps 1 and 2 as appropriate. Any underlining/concomitant GI disorder (reflux, ulcer, anorexia, etc.) should be treated appropriately.

Consults
For refractory cases consider nutrition, gastroenterology, and/or psychiatry consultation depending on history.

TREATMENT
Suggested Stepwise Therapeutic Approach (Figure 9.1).

Step 1: Prevention
Prenatal Multivitamin (MVI) before/at Conception
Vitamin B6 found in MVI has been shown to reduce the incidence of n/v [23], and the early use (prior to six weeks) of prenatal vitamin was associated with a decreased rate of vomiting [24].

Doxylamine/Vitamin B_6
One randomized controlled trial (RCT) found that in women with a history of HG, preemptive therapy with 10 mg **doxylamine with** 10 mg **pyridoxine** (Diclectin, delayed release) up to four tabs daily resulted in a significant **decrease in recurrence of HG** [25].

Step 2a: Nonpharmacologic Interventions
Lifestyle/Dietary Changes
Avoid odor/food triggers. Stop medications (e.g., iron, large vitamins) producing n/v. Counsel regarding safety and efficacy of treatment; provide reassurance regarding outcomes (see above). There is no evidence that rest improves n/v. Diet includes frequent, small meals: eat only one spoonful, wait, eat again, and so on; avoid an empty stomach; eat crackers in the morning upon waking; avoid fatty, greasy, spicy foods; ginger ale; prefer protein. One small nonrandomized prospective study found that protein-predominant meals produced decreased nausea compared to carbohydrate or fat predominant meals [26] but a prolonged high-protein diet is associated with higher incidences of preterm birth and fetal death.

Acupressure Wrist Bands
In the treatment of NVP, acupressure at the P6 "Neiguan" point [27–34] (Brands: Seaband, Bioband) has been associated with

Table 9.2 Selected Pharmacologic Treatment of NVP and HG

Agent	Dose	Side Effects	FDA Category	Comments
Ginger extract	125–250 mg tid/qid, po	Reflux, heartburn	C	Step 2a; OTC availability, food supplement
Vitamin B₆ (pyridoxine)	10–25 mg q8h po, do not exceed 100 mg qd		A	Step 2b; recommended as first-line pharmacologic intervention
Vitamin B₆–doxylamine	Pyridoxine, 10–25 mg q8h, po; doxylamine, 25 mg qhs, 12.5 mg bid prn, po; Diclegis (10 mg/10 mg) start 2–4 tabs qd-tid	Sedation	A	Step 1, 2b; Recommended as first line pharmacologic intervention. May be taken prophylactically if history of HG
Other Antihistamines (H₁-receptor antagonists)		Sedation, dizziness, drowsiness, anticholinergic effects		
• Diphenhydramine (Benadryl)	25–50 mg q4–6h prn; po, IV, IM Maximum: 100 mg/dose, 400 mg/day		B	May be helpful for relief of vestibular-type symptoms
• Meclizine (Bonine, Antivert)	25–50 mg q6h, po; maximum: 100 mg/24 hr		B	
• *Hydroxyzine (Atarax, Vistaril)*	25–100 mg q6–8h prn, po/IM; maximum: 600 mg/24 h		C	
• *Dimenhydrinate (Dramamine)*	50–100 mg q4–6h, po/pr/IM or 50 mg (in 50 cc saline over 20 min) q4–6h IV (not to exceed 400 mg/day, or 200 mg/day if also doxylamine		B	
H₂ receptor antagonists				
• Cimetidine (Tagamet)	1600 mg qd divided bid/qid		B	Step 2b; for patients with reflux, *H. pylori*
• Famotidine (Pepcid)	20–40 mg bid, po/IV			
• Ranitidine (Zantac)	75–150 mg prn, po (maximum 2 tabs/24 hr); 50 mg q6h IM/IV			
Proton pump inhibitors (PPIs)				Step 2b; Second line for reflux symptoms
• Omeprazole (Prilosec)	20–40 mg qd, po (maximum 80 mg/day)		B	
• Pantoprazole (Protonix)	40 mg bid, po			
• Esomeprazole (Nexium)	20–40 mg qd, po/NG/IV (maximum: 80 mg/day)			
• Lansoprazole (Prevacid)	15–30 mg qd, po			
Dopamine₂ antagonists		Sedation, anticholinergic effects		Step 3
• **Metoclopramide (Reglan)**	10–20 mg q6–8 h, po/IM/IV; 1–2 mg/kg IV	Tardive dyskinesia with increased duration of use (>12 week) and high total cumulative dose	B	Step 3. Also available as subcutaneous pump therapy, benefit of pump therapy is questionable
• Trimethobenzamide (Tigan)	300 mg tid/qid; po; 200 mg tid/qid, IM		C	Dopamine antagonist directly to emetic center CTZ
• Droperidol (Inapsine)	0.625–2.5 mg over 15 min, then 1.25 or 2.5 mg IM q3–4h prn, IM or continuous IV at 1–1.25 mg/hr (maximum: 2.5 mg/dose, slow push over 2–5 min, repeat doses with caution	Black box warning of torsades	C	Give with benadryl to prevent extrapyramidal symptoms
5-HT3 (Seratonin) receptor antagonist		Constipation, diarrhea, headache, fatigue, mild sedation		Step 3
• **Odansetron (Zofran)**	4–8 mg tid/qid po; 4–8 mg over 15 min q6–8h IV; or 1 mg/hr continuous for 24 h		B	Also available as an oral dissolving tablet and as a subcutaneous pump; benefit of pump therapy is questionable

(Continued)

Table 9.2 (Continued)   Selected Pharmacologic Treatment of NVP and HG

Agent	Dose	Side Effects	FDA Category	Comments
Phenothiazines (D$_2$ receptor antagonists)		Sedation; ↓BP if given too quickly, Parkinson's tremors, rash, anticholinergic side effects, tardive dyskinesia		Step 3
• *Promethazine (Phenergan)*	12.5–25 mg q4–6h, po/pr/IM/IV (maximum: 50 mg/dose po/IM; 25 mg/dose IV)	Severe tissue injury with undiluted IV use	C	May have similar or reduced efficacy with more side effects compared to ondansetron and metoclopramide
• Prochlorperazine maleate (Compazine; Bukatel)	5–10 mg q4–6h; po/IM/IV/ buccal, 10–25 mg q6h pr (maximum: 10 mg/dose, 40 mg/day)	D/c if unexplained decrease in WBCs	C	
Glucocorticoids		Increased risk of cleft lip if used before 10 weeks gestation	C	Step 4: for HG refractory to other medications. RCTs with mixed data on benefit. May be useful in refractory cases and decrease rate of readmission. Initial therapy for three days; if successful, may be tapered over one to two weeks, or for recurrent symptoms continued for maximum of six weeks for maximum duration with tapered dose if possible. If no improvement after 72 hours, discontinue.
• *Methylprednisolone*	• 16 mg PO TID			
• *Prednisolone*	• 5–20 mg PO qd-TID PO			
• *Methylprednisolone*	• 125 mg IV x 1 followed by oral taper			
• *Hydrocortisone*	• 300 mg IV qd			

Notes: Bold: therapies consistently demonstrating efficacy in RCTs in pregnancy; italics: therapies with efficacy demonstrated in at least one RCT in pregnancy although results may be mixed. Therapies listed without bold or italics have no RCTs proving efficacy in pregnancy. Food and Drug Administration (FDA) categories are as follows: A, controlled studies show no risk; B, no evidence of risk in humans; C, risk cannot be ruled out; D, positive evidence of risk; and X, contraindicated in pregnancy (http://www.fda.gov/).

Abbreviations: bid, twice a day; BP, blood pressure; CTZ, chemoreceptor trigger zone; d/c, discontinue; GI, gastrointestinal; HG, hyperemesis gravidarum; IM, intramuscular; IV, intravenous; min, minute; NG, nasogastric; NVP, nausea and vomiting of pregnancy; OTC, over the counter medication; PO, per os; PR, per rectum; prn, pro re nata or take as needed; qd, once daily; qhs, quaque hora somni or given at bedtime; qid, four times a day; q'X'h, given every 'X' hours; RTC, randomized controlled trial; SubQ, subcutaneous; tid, three times a day; WBCs, white blood cells.

improved nausea or symptom relief in one RCT and with no improvement in others when compared to placebo [1]. An RCT showed no significant difference between P6 acupressure versus vitamin B_6 therapy in nausea/vomiting of pregnancy [35].

In the treatment of HG, there are three RCTs, one with crossover design, comparing **acupressure** versus placebo. The results could not be combined for meta-analysis; however, the individual studies **demonstrated improved nausea and decreased number of anitemetics required** [2,36–39]. There are no pregnancy safety or breast-feeding concerns [2]. This intervention therefore can be considered either prior to (in mild cases) or as an adjunct to pharmaceutical interventions.

Acustimulation Wrist Bands
Acustimulation at the P6 Neiguan point [40,41] (Brand: Relief Band Device, Woodside Biomedical—http://www.reliefband.com). This device for noninvasive nerve electric stimulation was associated with less n/v and higher weight gain compared to placebo [40,41], but in the largest RCT, the assessment of the outcomes was not blinded, and the study was industry-sponsored by the makers of the device [41]. There are limited pregnancy safety or breast-feeding concerns.

Auricular Acupressure
One randomized controlled trial on the use of auricular acupressure found no significant benefit in either symptom improvement or number of antiemetic drugs needed as compared to controls [42]. There are no pregnancy safety or breast-feeding concerns.

Acupuncture
In the treatment of NVP, one trial found acupuncture to be equivalent to a sham procedure in the treatment of nausea of pregnancy [43]. Another trial found benefit of acupuncture compared to control in improvement of nausea but not vomiting although the sham procedure had some beneficial effect as well [44]. In the condition of HG, acupuncture was found to be as similar to metoclopramide in the reduction of nausea and vomiting [45]. **There does not appear to be a benefit with the use of acupuncture in the treatment of NVP or HG in pregnancy** [1,2].

Ginger
Ginger use has been suggested as early therapy in outpatients [4,46]. Side effects include reflux and heartburn. There have been several RCTs examining ginger for the treatment of NVP. A *Cochrane* review demonstrated **benefit of ginger compared to placebo** [1]. Although individual studies have demonstrated benefit in nausea reduction compared to vitamin B_6, a meta-analysis found no significant difference in symptom relief [1,47–50]. One RCT examined ginger versus doxylamine plus B_6 and found no difference in perceived severity of nausea and vomiting [51].

Regarding HG, one RCT found benefit with the use of ginger in HG; however, it was small (30 women) and crossover design [52].

Comparing it to other individual therapies, there was not found to be a significant difference in benefit with ginger vs. chamomile, dimenhydrate, or metoclopramide [1,47,53,54].

Other Nonpharmacologic Interventions
Regarding other nonpharmacologic interventions for n/v, there were two studies on oils versus placebo in NVP. One study on mint oil found no significant difference in severity of nausea and vomiting, and one study on lemon oil found no

difference in overall PUQE score but did show a significant reduction of symptoms from baseline to day three [55,56]. One study on **chamomile** found that it **improved symptoms** after one week [47].

In the setting of HG, **progressive muscle relaxation** with pharmacotherapy versus pharmacotherapy alone had better global improvement scores [57]. **Midwife-led outpatient care** had similar clinical outcomes but with decreased hours of hospital admission [58]. A holistic care plan versus standard medical therapy alone had a shorter length of hospital stay but no significant improvement in quality of life measures, nausea and vomiting severity, or cost [59].

There are no RCTs on hypnosis although there are case reports of some benefit [4,60]. There is insufficient evidence of benefit to suggest this as a therapy for NVP or HG.

In summary, ginger may be considered as an effective nonpharmacologic intervention in the setting of mild nausea and vomiting. Acupressure (by wristband and other means) **may also be a beneficial adjunct.** Intensive outpatient care may reduce inpatient hospitalization time. Acupuncture does not appear to be beneficial, and there is limited data to support the use of other nonpharmacologic interventions, such as nerve stimulation, muscle relaxation, hypnotherapy, and other dietary supplements.

Step 2b: Pharmacologic Interventions
Vitamin B_6
In the treatment of NVP, B_6 has been associated with a decrease in nausea, not in vomiting [1,61,62]. However, when used in women hospitalized for HG, it does not seem to affect n/v by itself [63].

Doxylamine and Vitamin B_6
Doxylamine is an antihistamine that has been studied in combination with vitamin B_6. This combination (formerly known as Bendectin and now available as Diclegis in the United States, Diclectin in Canada, and Debendox in the United Kingdom) is safe with no evidence of teratogenicity (proven with more than 200,000 exposures, by far the most for any other drug in pregnancy), and effective (>70% decrease in n/v) [3,4]. **Doxylamine and vitamin B_6 are associated with decrease in both n/v when used together** compared to no therapy or placebo [64–67]. A double-blind RCT showed Diclectin (a doxylamine–pyridoxine delayed-release preparation available) to significantly improve n/v and quality of life compared to placebo [67].

Other Antihistamines (Histamine-1 Receptor Antagonists)
Other antihistamines are generally safe and used mostly for the relief of vestibular-like symptoms. There may be an increased relative risk, but small absolute risk, of septal defects [68–70]. These include diphenhydramine, meclizine, hydroxyzine, and dimenhydrinate. An RCT showed that **dimenhydrinate** is as effective as ginger in the treatment of n/v with fewer side effects [53], and another demonstrated the benefit of **hydroxyzine** over placebo for nausea relief [71]. No RCTs exist for the other histamine-1 receptor antagonists (H_1RAs) to assess their effectiveness for n/v in pregnancy or HG.

Histamine-2 Receptor Antagonists
Cimetidine, famotidine, ranitidine, and nizatidine are approved for use in pregnancy to treat symptoms of heartburn, acid reflux, and *H. pylori*, which can exacerbate n/v. They may be added if symptoms are present. No RCTs exist

regarding their effectiveness for NVP or HG. A meta-analysis showed no increased risk of congenital malformations, risk of spontaneous abortions, or preterm delivery compared to controls [72]. In intractable cases of n/v with positive *H. pylori* serology, a nonrandomized study suggested benefit with triple therapy with ranitidine/flagyl/ampicillin [73].

Proton-Pump Inhibitor
Common proton-pump inhibitors (PPIs) used in pregnancy are omeprazole, pantoprazole, eso-meprazole, and lansoprazole. These can be used in conjunction with or separately from histamine-2 receptor antagonists (H₂RAs) for heartburn and reflux and *H. pylori* infections. A recent review [74], a meta-analysis [75], and a cohort study [76] showed that there is no evidence to suggest that the use of PPIs anytime during pregnancy increases the overall risk of birth defects, preterm delivery, or spontaneous abortion. There are no RCTs on this intervention for NVP or HG.

In summary, given its well-demonstrated safety and efficacy, vitamin B₆ with doxylamine should be considered first-line pharmacotherapy for the treatment of NVP [4,46]. If symptoms of reflux, heartburn, or *H. pylori* are present, H₂RAs and PPIs can also be considered.

Step 3: Antiemetic Therapy

Of the three commonly prescribed antiemetics, metoclopramide, promethazine, and ondansetron, only **metoclopramide** was studied in a placebo-controlled RCT; the remainder were studied in RCTs comparing one therapy with another. Less commonly used and much less studied, thiethylperazine and fluphenazine–pyridoxine were also studied in placebo-controlled trials [1,2].

Metoclopramide (Dopamine-2 Antagonist)
Metoclopramide (*Reglan*) is safe in pregnancy without increased risk of teratogenicity, preterm birth, low birth weight, or perinatal mortality [77–79]. In the setting of NVP, an RCT comparing metoclopramide to placebo found **improved n/v** [54]. An RCT showed that metoclopramide (with one IM shot of 50 mg of pyridoxine) is superior in decreasing vomiting and subjective improvement compared to monotherapy with either prochlorperazine or promethazine [80]. Compared with ondansetron, there was similar improvement in nausea but worse with vomiting [81].

Two recent RCTs compared metoclopramide and ondansetron in the setting of HG, and one found similar improvement in symptoms but did find that there was an **increased rate of drowsiness and dry mouth in the metoclopramide group**; the other found **improved vomiting with ondansetron** [82,83]. A recent RCT of inpatient HG patients showed that metoclopramide 10 mg IV q8h had similar efficacy and decreased drowsiness, dizziness, and dystonia when compared to IV promethazine [84].

A subcutaneous Reglan pump is an alternative mode of administering the drug, not yet tested in any pregnancy RCT. It is not necessarily cost-effective compared to inpatient management or home care and may have significant side effects, and thus it is not recommended for routine use in the management of NVP or HG [4,85,86].

Ondansetron (5-HT3 Receptor Antagonist)
Ondansetron (*Zofran*) is a serotonin 5-hydroxytryptamine-3 receptor antagonist. Although one study found an association

between first trimester ondansetron use and cardiac anomalies, especially septal defects, and another with cleft palate, the absolute risk was still quite low; other much larger studies have demonstrated its safety in pregnancy [87–90]. It must be prescribed with care as there is a risk of QT prolongation that could lead to potentially fatal arrhythmias. As such, the FDA has recommended it not be prescribed in IV doses >16 mg, and care should be taken to avoid other QT prolonging medications [4].

In the treatment of NVP, women treated with ondansetron **versus metoclopramide had similar levels of nausea but had reduced vomiting** [81]. Ondansetron was found to be **superior to pyridoxine and doxylamine** in improvement of n/v [91].

In the setting of HG, there was no significant difference when compared with promethazine in reduction of nausea or in adverse effects [92]. There are two RCTs **comparing ondansetron and metoclopramide** in the setting of HG. One study found similar efficacy in control of nausea with improved vomiting with ondansetron [83]; the other found **similar effects on n/v but with reduced side effects with ondansetron** [82]. There is limited evidence to support the use of a subcutaneous pump of ondansetron. There are no RCTs comparing subcutaneous with oral or IV administration. Although there may be some symptom improvement with a subcutaneous pump, a significant number of women experience complications with 25% stopping treatment related to complications [85,86]. Given the limited data on benefit and the significant side effects, the use of subcutaneous pumps is not recommended [4].

Promethazine (Phenothiazines)
Phenothiazines [prochlorperazine (Compazine), promethazine (Phenergan)] appear to be safe in pregnancy. A case-control study of promethazine showed no evidence of increase risk or rate of congenital anomalies in humans [89,93]. Phenothiazines are often used in addition to or instead of antihistamines. The level 1 evidence for effectiveness is limited. As said above, **metoclopramide** (with one IM shot of 50 mg of pyridoxine) **is superior in decreasing vomiting and subjective improvement** compared to monotherapy with either prochlorperazine or promethazine in NVP [80] and had similar efficacy with reduced side effects in HG [84]. Compared to ondansetron, there was no difference in severity of nausea in the setting of HG [92]. Two studies compared promethazine and corticosteroids in patients with HG. One study [94] found a decreased rate of hospital readmission with corticosteroids; the other study [95] found increased n/v at 48 hours but not after 17 days with prednisolone [2].

Other phenothiazines have been studied in the setting of NVP although they are not commonly used and their safety is not established. Thiethylperazine demonstrated improved symptoms compared to placebo, and fluphenzine-pyridoxine was not statistically significantly better than placebo in another [1,96,97].

In summary, if n/v persists despite steps 1 to 2, consider adding metoclopramide or ondansetron. Phenothiazine (promethazine) therapy may be added as well although it may not be as effective and has more side effects.

Step 4: Inpatient Assessment and Treatment
Inpatient Management
Admit if HG diagnosis is confirmed, woman is not tolerating oral intake, and failed outpatient management. Some

suggest just brief ER visits for severe cases needing emergent hydration. Home infusion services should be used as much as safely possible. Admission by itself does not improve HG, and should be limited. Other etiologies of n/v should be ruled out (Table 9.1), and work up should be initiated as described in "Pregnancy Management" above.

Intravenous Fluid (IVF) Hydration

IVF can be used if dehydration is present. Volume should be adequate to replenish loss and ongoing loss through vomiting. IV rehydration may be done with normal saline, lactated ringers, or dextrose normal saline along with electrolytes as needed. In severe cases, thiamine should be repleted to prevent the development of Wernicke's encephalopathy. Add thiamine 100 mg qd for two to three days, then multivitamins to IV fluids. Hypertonic solutions should be avoided; rapid overcorrection of hyponatremia may cause central pontine myelinolysis.

One RCT compared dextrose saline with normal saline and found that although there was improved nausea at hours 8 and 16 after treatment with dextrose saline, by 24 hours there was no difference in nausea score, quality of life, or length of hospital stay [98].

Additional Pharmacologic Therapy

Corticosteroids. Safety data on corticosteroids include possible increased incidence of oral cleft if used <10 weeks [4].

RCTs on the use of corticosteroids in the treatment of HG have had mixed results. A meta-analysis on this was limited by the difference in inclusion criteria and definition of HG. **Compared with placebo, the addition of corticosteroids to other antiemetic therapy does not appear to improve symptoms, but may reduce hospital readmission rate** [2]. One small RCT found decreased episodes of emesis compared to metoclopramide [99]. Two RCTs compared steroids with promethazine and one found increased side effects and delayed response compared to promethazine [95], and the other found decreased readmission associated with corticosteroids [94]. Adrenocorticoticotropic hormone (ACTH) is not beneficial [100]. **Corticosteroids are not recommended for the treatment of NVP but may be considered for a short course (up to three days) in refractory cases of HG after 10 weeks gestation.** Usual dosing is methylprednisolone 16 mg po/IV tid, prednisolone 20 mg po bid, or hydrocortisone 300 mg IV qd. For patients who do respond, this three-day course may be followed with a one to two week taper. ACOG suggests that patients who initially responded and then develop recurrent vomiting after the taper may be continued on an effective dose for up to 6 weeks although this is not based on any specific trial data [4].

Benzodiazepines

Do *not* use diazepam, a category D drug, because of possible fetal effects, despite one trial on its efficacy [101].

Clonidine

Clonidine is a centrally acting alpha-2 adrenergic agonist commonly used as an antihypertensive agent. It has been studied in the prevention of postoperative nausea and vomiting. One small crossover design RCT ($n = 12$) evaluated transdermal clonidine in addition to other antiemetic therapy for the treatment of refractory HG and found subjective and objective improvement in measures of nausea and vomiting; of note, this small study also reported one patient whose pregnancy course was complicated by central venous catheter associated sepsis [102]. Given this small limited study,

there is **insufficient data** on safety or efficacy to recommend clonidine for the treatment of NVP or HG.

In summary, for patients with dehydration, weight loss, and inability to tolerate PO, consider admission for IV rehydration, beginning treatment with the IV formulation of the antiemetics in step 3. Multiple combinations and dosing can be used. In the rare cases in which these are not successful, one may proceed with a short course of corticosteroids. Benzodiazepines are not recommended because of adverse fetal effects and limited data on benefit. Clonidine may be effective but is not recommended given the limited data on its benefits and safety.

Step 5: Nutritional Supplementation

If persistent weight loss or dehydration (e.g., more than five to seven days despite aggressive inpatient therapy), consider consulting gastroenterology and possibly psychiatry as well. In addition, supplement with either enteral (EN) or parenteral nutrition (PN) in conjunction with a nutrition consult.

Enteral Nutrition

Enteral nutrition requires a nasogastric (NG) tube. There are several types (e.g., 8 French Dobbhoff) of NG tubes with insufficient evidence to assess effectiveness of one versus the other. This intervention is best used for persistent n/v with no response to antiemetic therapy. There are no RCTs comparing NG tube or PN. One large retrospective cohort study compared EN with IVF and PN. They found the EN resulted in similar weight gain and pregnancy outcomes despite the fact that they had significantly greater weight loss on admission [103]. Because PN is associated with several possible complications, an NG tube should be tried first as tolerated [4]. A small case series of three patients demonstrated the feasibility and safety of endoscopically placed jejunosotomy tubes in the setting of refractory HG, and this may be an area for further study [104]. Enteral nutrition may be poorly tolerated and complicated by tube dislodgement requiring replacement.

Nutritional goals should be developed in conjunction with a nutrition consult. Specific nutritional requirement will depend on individual factors, such as degree of weight loss and severity of nausea and vomiting. In general, the Harris–Benedict equation for women may be used to calculate basal energy expenditure with an additional 300 calories added to meet the additional demands in pregnancy [105]. The weight used in the calculation may be current weight or prepregnancy weight depending on the degree of weight loss.

Nutrition (Harris–Benedict Equation)

- Basal Metabolic Rate = 655.1 + (9.56 × wt[kg]) + (1.85 × ht[cm]) − (4.68 × age[yr])
- Activity Factor: 1.2 to 1.9 (for sedentary activity level to extremely demanding activity level)
- (Basal Metabolic Rate × Activity Factor) + 300 = Daily caloric requirement in pregnancy
- Start at 25 mL/hr, increase by 25 mL/hr until goal. Then consolidate to give over eight to 12 hours overnight rather than continuously over 24 hours.

Parenteral Nutrition

Several catheters and regimens are possible (peripherally inserted central catheter [PICC], midline IV, etc.). As with EN, PN should be managed in conjunction with a nutrition consult. Generally PN is associated with **high incidence of** catheter complications, for example, infection, leading to sepsis (about 25%), thrombosis/occlusion, and dislodgement/mechanical failure with mixed reports on maternal or neonatal benefit and no RCTs assessing its efficacy [106–110]. Peripheral catheters have high morbidity and central catheters have central access complications. Other complications include pneumothorax, cholestasis, preterm birth, and fetal death. This is an expensive therapy to be used only when HG is refractory to treatment with significant weight loss (>5%) and failure of enteral nutrition.

In summary, for patients that are admitted with HG refractory to steps 1–4, order a nutrition consult and consider enteral over parenteral nutrition.

OTHER ISSUES

If persistent weight loss or dehydration (e.g., over five to seven days despite aggressive inpatient therapy), consider consulting **gastroenterology** and either enteral or parenteral nutrition. **Consider a psychiatric consult** in severe, refractory-to-therapy cases. Psychotherapy has not been evaluated in any trial. Woman can be **discharged home** on IV fluids and/or parenteral nutrition (PN) as long as stable, not losing weight, or other factors.

POSTPARTUM

The risk of recurrence of HG [2,4,9] is about 15% (vs. 0.7% in controls without prior HG). The risk may be reduced by change in paternity [9].

REFERENCES

1. Matthews A, Haas DM, Omathuna DP, Dowswell T. Interventions for nausea and vomiting in early pregnancy. *Cochrane Database Syst Rev* 2015 Sep; 8: 9. [Review]
2. Boelig RC, Barton SJ, Saccone G et al. Interventions for treating hyperemesis gravidarum. *Cochrane Database Syst Rev* 2016; *In Press.* [Review]
3. Niebyl JR. Nausea and vomiting in pregnancy. *N Engl J Med* 2010; 363: 1544–50. [Review]
4. American College of Obstetrics and Gynecology. Nausea and vomiting of pregnancy. ACOG Practice Bulletin No. 153. *Obstet Gynecol* 2015; 126(3): e12–24. [III]
5. Vikanes A, Skjaerven R, Grijbovski AM et al. Recurrence of hyperemesis gravidarum across generations: A population based cohort study. *BMJ* 2010; 340: c2050. [II-2]
6. Goodwin TM, Nwankwo OA, O'Leary LD et al. The first demonstration that a subset of women with hyperemesis gravidarum has abnormalities in the vestibuloocular reflex pathway. *Am J Obstet Gynecol* 2008; 199: 417.el–117.e9. [II-3]
7. Sandven I, Abdelnoor M, Nesheim BI et al. *Helicobacter pylori* infection and hyperemesis gravidarum: A systematic review and meta-analysis of case-control studies. *Acta Obstet Gynecol Scand* 2009; 88: 1190–200. [Meta-analysis, 25 case-control studies, 3425 pts total, 1970 controls]
8. El-Mallakh RS, Liebowitz NR, Hale MS. Hypermesesis gravidarum as conversion disorder. *J Nerv Ment Dis* 1990; 178(10): 655–9. [II-3]
9. Trogstad LI, Stoltenberg C, Magnus P et al. Recurrence risk in hyperemesis gravidarum. *BJOG* 2005; 112(12): 1641–5. [II-3]
10. Einsarson TR, Navioz Y, Maltepe C et al. Existance and severity of nausea and vomiting in pregnancy (NVP) with different partners. *J Obstet Gynaecol* 2007; 27(4): 360–2. [II-3]
11. Fejzo MS, Ching CY, Schoenberg FP et al. Change in paternity and recurrence of hyperemesis gravidarum. *JMFNM* 2011; 25(8): 1241–5. [II-2]
12. Koren G, Boskovic R, Hard M et al. Motherisk-PUQE (pregnancy-unique quantification of emesis and nausea) scoring system for nausea and vomiting of pregnancy. *Am J Obstet Gynecol* 2002; 186(5 Suppl.): s228–31. [II-3]
13. Lacasse A, Rey E, Ferreira E et al. Validity of a modified pregnancy-unique quantification of emesis and nausea (PUQE) scoring index to assess severity of nausea and vomiting of pregnancy. *Am J Obstet Gynecol* 2008; 198(l): 71.el–7. [II-3]
14. Ebrahimi N, Maltepe C, Bournissen G et al. Nausea and vomiting of pregnancy, using the 24-hour pregnancy-unique quantification of emesis (PUQE-24) Scale. *J Obstet Gynaecol Can* 2009; 31(9): 803–7. [II-3]
15. Fell DB, Dodds L, Joseph KS et al. Risk factors for hyperemesis gravidarum requiring hospital admission during pregnancy. *Obstet Gynecol* 2006; 107(2 Pt. l): 277–84. [II-2]
16. Temming L, Franco A, Istwan N et al. Adverse pregnancy outcomes in women with nausea and vomiting of pregnancy. *J Matern Fetal Neonatal Med* 2014; 27(1): 84–8. [II-2]
17. Van Dinter MC. Ptyalism in pregnant women. *J Obstet Gynecol Neonatal Nurs* 1991; 20: 206–9. [Review]
18. Poursharif B, Korst LM, Macqibbon KW. Elective pregnancy termination in a large cohort of women with hyperemesis gravidarum. *Contraception* 2007; 76(6): 451–5. [II-3]
19. Veenendaal MV, van Abeelen AF, Painter RC et al. Consequences of hyperemesis gravidarum for offspring: A systematic review and meta-analysis. *BJOG* 2011; 118(11): 1302–13. [Meta-analysis: 24 studies (cohort, case control, and cross-sectional)]
20. Brent R. Medical, social, and legal implications of treating nausea and vomiting of pregnancy. *Am J Obstet Gynecol* 2002; 186: s262–6. [Review]
21. Goodwin TM, Montoro M, Mestman JH. Transient hyperthyroidism and hyperemesis gravidarum: Clinical aspects. *Am J Obstet Gynecol* 1992; 167: 648–52. [II-3]
22. Goodwin TM, Mestman J. Transient hyperthyroidism of hyperemesis gravidarum. *Contemp Obstet Gynecol* 1996; 6: 65–78. [II-3, and review]
23. Czeizel AE, Dudas I, Fritz G et al. The effect of periconceptional multivitamin-mineral supplementation on vertigo, nausea and vomiting. *Arch Gynecol Obstet* 1992; 251: 181–5. [RCT, n = 48]
24. Emelianova S, Mazzotta P, Einarson A, Koren G. Prevalence and severity of nausea and vomiting of pregnancy and effect of vitamin supplementation. *Clin Invest Med* 1999 Jun; 22(3): 106–10. [II-2]
25. Maltepe C, Koren G. Preemptive treatment of nausea and vomiting of pregnancy: Results of a randomized controlled trial. *Obstet Gynecol Int* 2013; 2013: 809787. [RCT, n = 59]
26. Jednak MA, Shadigian EM, Kim MS, Woods ML et al. Protein meals reduce nausea and gastric slow wave dysrhythmic activity in first trimester pregnancy. *Am J Physiol* 1999 Oct; 277(4 Pt. 1): G855–61. [II-3]
27. Murphy PA. Alternative therapies for nausea and vomiting of pregnancy. *Obstet Gynecol* 1998; 91: 149–55. [Meta-analysis; 10 RCTs; 7 RCTs on acupressure]
28. Dundee JW, Sourial FB, Ghaly RG et al. P6 acupressure reduces morning sickness. *J Royal Soc Med* 1988; 81(8): 456–7. [RCT]
29. Hyde E. Acupressure therapy for morning sickness. A controlled clinical trial. *J Nurse Midwifery* 1989; 34(4): 171–8. [RCT]
30. de Aloysio D, Penacchioni P. Morning sickness control in early pregnancy by Neiguan point acupressure. *Obstet Gynecol* 1992; 80(5): 852–4. [RCT]
31. Bayreuther J, Lewith GT, Pickering R. A double-blind cross-over study to evaluate the effectiveness of acupressure at pericardium 6 (P6) in the treatment of early morning sickness (EMS). *Complem Ther Med* 1994; 2: 70–6. [RCT, n = 23]
32. Belluomini J, Litt RC, Lee KA et al. Acupressure for nausea and vomiting of pregnancy: A randomized, blinded study. *Obstet Gynecol* 1994; 84(2): 245–8. [RCT]
33. O'Brien B, Relyea MJ, Taerum T. Efficacy of P6 acupressure in the treatment of nausea and vomiting during pregnancy. *Am J Obstet Gynecol* 1996; 174: 708–15. [RCT]

34. Werntoft E, Dykes AK. Effect of acupressure on nausea and vomiting during pregnancy. *J Reprod Med* 2001; 46: 835–9. [RCT, *n* = 60]

35. Jamigorn M, Phupong V. Acupressure and vitamin B6 to relieve nausea and vomiting in pregnancy: A randomized study. *Archives Gynecol Obstet* 2007; 276(3): 245–9. [RCT, *n* = 66]

36. Shin HS, Song YA, Seo S. Effect of Neiguan point (P6) acupressure on ketonuria, nausea, and vomiting in women with hyperemesis gravidarum. *J Adv Nurs* 2007; 59: 510–9. [RCT, *n* = 66]

37. Habek D, Barbir A, Habek JC, Janculiak D et al. Success of acupuncture and acupressure of the pc6 acupoint in the treatment of hyperemesis gravidarum. *Forschende Komplementarmedizin und Klassische Naturheilkunde* 2004; 11(1): 20–3. [RCT, *n* = 36]

38. Mamo J, Mamo D, Pace M, Felice D. Evaluation of sea-band acupressure device for early pregnancy nausea and vomiting. 27th British Congress of Obstetrics and Gynaecology; 1995 July 4–7; Dublin, Ireland. 1995: 283. [RCT, *n* = 38]

39. Heazell A, Thornaycroft J, Walton V et al. Acupressure for the inpatient treatment of nausea and vomiting in early pregnancy: A randomized controlled trial. *Am J Obstet Gynecol* 2006; 194: 815–20. [RCT, *n* = 80]

40. Evans AT, Samuels SN, Marshall C et al. Suppression of pregnancy-induced nausea and vomiting with sensory afferent stimulation. *J Repro Med* 1993; 38: 603–6. [RCT, *n* = 23]

41. Rosen T, de Veciana M, Miller HS et al. A randomized controlled trial of nerve stimulation for relief of nausea and vomiting in pregnancy. *Obstet Gynecol* 2003; 102: 129–35. [RCT, *n* = 230]

42. Puangsricharern A, Mahasukhon S. Effectiveness of auricular acupressure in the treatment of nausea and vomiting in early pregnancy. *J Med Assoc Thai* 2008; 91(11): 1633–8. [RCT, *n* = 98]

43. Knight B, Mudge C, Openshaw S et al. Effect of acupuncture on nausea of pregnancy: A randomized, controlled trial. *Obstet Gynecol* 2001; 97: 184–8. [RCT, *n* = 55]

44. Smith C, Crowther C, Beilby J. Acupuncture to treat nausea and vomiting in early pregnancy: A randomized controlled trial. *Birth* 2002; 29: 1–9. [RCT, *n* = 593]

45. Neri I, Allais G, Schiapparelli P, Blasi I et al. Acupuncture versus pharmacological approach to reduce hyperemesis gravidarum discomfort. *Minerva Ginecol* 2005; 57(4): 471–5. [RCT, *n* = 88]

46. Arsenault MY, Lane CA, MacKinnon CJ, Bartellas E et al. The management of nausea and vomiting of pregnancy. *J Obstet Gynaecol Can* 2002; 24(10): 817–31. [III]

47. Modares M, Besharat S, Rahimi K, Besharat S et al. Effect of ginger and chamomile capsules on nausea and vomiting in pregnancy. *J Gorgan University of Medical Sciences.* 2012; 14(1): 46–51. [RCT, *n* = 70]

48. Chittumma P, Kaewkiattikun K, Wiriyasiriwach B. Comparison of the effectiveness of ginger and vitamin B6 for treatment of nausea and vomiting in early pregnancy: A randomized double-blind controlled trial. *J Med Assoc Thai* 2007; 90(l): 15–20. [RCT, *n* = 126]

49. Sripramote M, Lekhyananda N. A randomized comparison of ginger and vitamin B6 in the treatment of nausea and vomiting in pregnancy. *J Med Assoc Thai* 2003; 86: 846–53. [RCT, *n* = 128]

50. Smith C, Crowther C, Willson K et al. A randomized controlled trial of ginger to treat nausea and vomiting in pregnancy. *Obstet Gynecol* 2004; 103: 639–45. [RCT, *n* = 291]

51. Biswas SC, Bal R, Kamilya GS, Mukherjee J et al. A single-masked, randomized, controlled trial of ginger extract in the treatment of nausea and vomiting of pregnancy [abstract]. 49th All India Congress of Obstetrics and Gynaecology; 2006 Jan 6–9; Cochin, Kerala State, India. 2006: 53. [RCT, *n* = 63]

52. Fischer-Rasmussen W, Kjaer SK, Dahl C, Asping U. Ginger treatment of hyperemesis gravidarum. *Eur J Obstet Gynecol Reprod Biol* 1991 Jan 4; 38(1): 19–24. [RCT, *n* = 30, crossover design]

53. Pongrojpaw D, Somprasit C, Chanthasenanont A. A randomized comparison of ginger and dimenhydrate in the treatment of nausea and vomiting in pregnancy. *J Med Assoc Thai* 2007; 90(9): 1703–9. [RCT, *n* = 170]

54. Mohammadbeigi R, Shahgeibi S, Soufizadeh N, Reaiie M et al. Comparing the effects of ginger and metoclopramide on the treatment of pregnancy nausea. *Pak J Biol Sci* 2011; 14(16): 817–20. [RCT, *n* = 68]

55. Pasha H, Behmanesh F, Mohsenzadeh F, Hajahmadi M et al. Study of the effect of mint oil on nausea and vomiting during pregnancy. *Iran Red Crescent Med J* 2012; 14(11): 727–30. [RCT]

56. Kia PY, Safajou F, Shahnazi M, Nazemiyeh H. The effect of lemon inhalation aromatherapy on nausea and vomiting of pregnancy: A double-blind randomised controlled clinical trial. Unpublished data, reported in Matthew 2014 (ref 1). [RCT, *n* = 100]

57. Gawande S, Vaidya M, Tadke R, Kirpekar V. Progressive muscle relaxation in hyperemesis gravidarum. *Journal of SAFOG* 2011; 3(1): 28–32. [RCT, *n* = 30]

58. McParlin C, Carrick-Sen D, Steen IN, Taylor P et al. Hyperemesis in pregnancy study: A randomised controlled trial of midwife-led "outpatient" care. *Arch Disease in Childhood. Fetal and Neonatal Edition* 2008; 93 (Suppl. 1): Fa9. [RCT, *n* = 53]

59. Fletcher SJ, Waterman H, Nelson I, Carter LA et al. The effectiveness and cost-effectiveness of a holistic assessment and individualised package of care of women with hyperemesis gravidarum: Randomised controlled trial. *BJOG* 2013; 120(Suppl. s1): 552–3. [RCT, *n* = 273]

60. McCormack D. Hypnosis for hyperemesis gravidarum. *J Obstet Gynaecol* 2010; 30(7): 647–53. [III, systematic review]

61. Sahakian V, Rouse D, Sipes S et al. Vitamin B6 is effective therapy for nausea and vomiting of pregnancy: A randomized double-blind placebo-controlled study. *Obstet Gynecol* 1991; 78: 33. [RCT, *n* = 59; vitamin B6 25 mg orally q8h × 72 hours versus placebo]

62. Vutyavanich T, Wongtrangan S, Ruangsri RA. Pyridoxine for nausea and vomiting of pregnancy: A randomized, double-blind, placebo-controlled trial. *Am J Obstet Gynecol* 1995; 173: 881–4. [RCT, *n* = 342; vitamin B$_6$ 30 mg orally q8h versus placebo]

63. Tan PC, Yow CM, Omar ST. A placebo-controlled trial of oral pyridoxine in hyperemesis gravidarum. *Gynecol Obstet Invest* 2009; 77: 151–7. [RCT, *n* = 92]

64. Geiger CJ, Fahrenbach DM, Healey FJ. Bendectin in the treatment of nausea and vomiting in pregnancy. *Obstet Gynecol* 1959; 14: 688–90. [RCT, *n* = 110]

65. McGuiness BW, Binns DT. "Debendox" in pregnancy sickness. *J R Coll Gen Pract* 1971; 21: 500–3. [RCT, *n* = 81]

66. Wheatley D. Treatment of pregnancy sickness. *Br J Obstet Gynecol* 1977; 84: 444–7. [RCT, *n* = 56]

67. Koren G, Clark S, Hankins GDV et al. Effectiveness of delayed-release doxylamine and pyridoxine for nausea and vomiting of pregnancy: A randomized placebo controlled trial. *Am J Obstet Gynecol* 2010; 203: 571.el–7. [RCT, *n* = 256]

68. Seto A, Einarson T, Koren G. Pregnancy outcome following first trimester exposure to antihistamines: Meta-analysis. *Am J Perinatol* 1997 Mar; 14(3): 119–24. [Meta-analysis, 24 controlled studies, >20,000 patients]

69. Smedts HP, de Jonge L, Bandola SJ, Baardman ME, Bakker MK, Stricker BH et al. Early pregnancy exposure to antihistamines and risk of congenital heart defects: Results of two case-control studies. *Eur J Epidemiol* 2014 Sep; 29(9): 653–61. [II-2, 2 case-control studies]

70. Gilboa SM, Ailes EC, Rai RP, Anderson JA, Honein MA. Antihistamines and birth defects: A systematic review of the literature. *Expert Opin Drug Saf* 2014 Dec; 13(12): 1667–98. [Review, III]

71. Erez S, Schifrin BS, Dirim O. Double-blind evaluation of hydroxyzine as an antiemetic in pregnancy. *J Reprod Med* 1971; 7(1): 35–7. [RCT, *n* = 150]

72. Gill SK, O'Brien L, Koren G. The safety of histamine 2 (H2) blockers in pregnancy: A meta-analysis. *Dig Dis Sci* 2009; 54(9): 1835–8. [II-3, *n* = 2398 patients]

73. Mansour GM, Nashaat EH. Role of *Helicobacter pylori* in the pathogenesis of hyperemesis gravidarum. *Arch Gynecol Obstet* 2010. doi:10.1007/s00404-010-1759-8. [II-1, *n* = 160]

74. Majithia R, Johnson DA. Are proton pump inhibitors safe during pregnancy and lactation? Evidence to date. *Drugs* 2012 Jan 22; 72(2): 171–9. [Review]

75. Gill SK, O'Brien L, Einarson TR et al. The safety of proton pump inhibitors (PPIs) in pregnancy: A meta-analysis. *Am J Gastroenterol* 2009; 104: 1541–5. [Meta-analysis]

76. Pasternak B, Hviid A. The use of proton-pump inhibitors in early pregnancy and the risk of birth defects. *N Engl J Med* 2010; 363: 2114–23. [II-2]

77. Matok I, Gorodischer R, Karen G et al. The safety of metoclopramide use in the first trimester of pregnancy. *N Engl J Med* 2009; 360: 2528–35. [II-2, *n* = 3458]

78. Berkovitch M, Mazzota P, Greenberg R et al. Metoclopramide for nausea and vomiting of pregnancy: A prospective multicenter international study. *Am J Perinatol* 2002; 19: 311–6. [II-2, *n* = 175 neonates exposed in first trimester to metoclopramide]

79. Pasternak B, Svanstrom H, Molgaard-Nielsen D, Melbye M, Hviid A. Metoclopramide in pregnancy and risk of major congenital malformations and fetal death. *JAMA* 2013 Oct 16; 310(15): 1601–11. [II-2, case-control, 28,486 cases versus 113,698 control]

80. Bsat F, Hoffman DE, Seubert DE. Comparison of three outpatient regimens in the management of nausea and vomiting in pregnancy. *J Perinatol* 2003; 23: 531–5. [RCT, *n* = 169]

81. Ghahiri AA, Abdi F, Mastoo R, Ghasemi M. The effect of ondansetron and metoclopramide in nausea and vomiting of pregnancy. *Journal of Isfahan Medical School* 2011; 29(131). [RCT, *n* = 70]

82. Abas MN, Tan PC, Azmi N, Omar SZ. Ondansetron compared with metoclopramide for hyperemesis gravidarum: A randomized controlled trial. *Obstet Gynecol* 2014; 123(6): 1272–9. [RCT, *n* = 160]

83. Kashifard M, Basirat Z, Kashifard M, Golsorkhtabar-Amiri M et al. Ondansetron or metoclopramide? Which is more effective in severe nausea and vomiting of pregnancy? A randomized trial double blind study. *Clin Exp Obstet Gynecol* 2013; 40(1): 127–30. [RCT, *n* = 83]

84. Tan PC, Khine PP, Vallikkannu N et al. Promethazine compared with metoclopramide for hyperemesis gravidarum: A randomized control trial. *Obstet Gynecol* 2010; 115: 975–81. [RCT, *n* = 149]

85. Reichmann JP, Kirkbride MS. Reviewing the evidence for using continuous subcutaneous metoclopramide and ondansetron to treat nausea & vomiting during pregnancy. *Manag Care* 2012 May; 21(5): 44–7. [Review]

86. Klauser CK, Fox NS, Istwan N, Rhea D, Rebarber A, Desch C et al. Treatment of severe nausea and vomiting of pregnancy with subcutaneous medications. *Am J Perinatol* 2011 Oct; 28(9): 715–21. [II-3]

87. Einarson A, Maltepe C, Navioz Y et al. The safety of ondansetron for nausea and vomiting of pregnancy: A prospective comparative study. *BJOG* 2004; 111: 940–3. [II-2, *n* = 176 women with ondansetron exposure]

88. Danielsson B, Wikner BN, Kallen B. Use of ondansestron during pregnancy and congential malformations in the infant. *Reprod Toxicol* 2014; 50: 134–7. [II-2, *n* = 1349 infants with exposure]

89. Anderka M, Mitchell AA, Louik C, Werler MM, Hernandez-Diaz S, Rasmussen SA et al. Medications used to treat nausea and vomiting of pregnancy and the risk of selected birth defects. *Birth Defects Res A Clin Mol Teratol* 2012 Jan; 94(1): 22–30. [II-3]

90. Pasternak B, Svanstrom H, Hviid A. Ondansetron in pregnancy and risk of adverse fetal outcomes. *N Engl J Med* 2013 Feb 28; 368(9): 814–23. [II-2, 1848 exposed women, 7396 control]

91. Oliveira LG, Capp SM, You WB, Riffenburgh RH, Carstairs SD. Ondansetron compared with doxylamine and pyridoxine for treatment of nausea in pregnancy: A randomized controlled trial. *Obstet Gynecol* 2014 Oct; 124(4): 735–42. [RCT, *n* = 36; ondansetron 4 m PO versus 25 mg pyridoxine plus 12.5 mg doxylamine]

92. Sullivan CA, Johnson CA, Roach H et al. A pilot study of intravenous ondansetron for hyperemesis gravidarum. *Am J Obstet Gynecol* 1996; 174: 1565–8. [RCT, *n* = 30; ondansetron 10 mg IV versus promethazine 50 mg IV, both q8h]

93. Bartfai Z, Kocsis J, Puno EH et al. A population based case-control teratologic study of promethazine use during pregnancy. *Reprod Toxicol* 2008; 25: 276–85. [II-3]

94. Safari HR, Fassett MJ, Souter IC et al. The efficacy of methylprednisolone in the treatment of hyperemesis gravidarum: A randomized, double-blind, controlled study. *Am J Obstet Gynecol* 1998; 179: 921–4. [RCT, *n* = 40]

95. Ziaei S, Hosseiney FS, Faghihzadeh S. The efficacy of low dose prednisolone in the treatment of hyperemesis gravidarum. *Acta Obstet Gynecol Scand* 2004; 83: 272–5. [RCT, *n* = 80]

96. Newlinds JS. Nausea and vomiting in pregnancy: A trial of thiethylperzine. *Med J Aust* 1964; 15(1): 234–6. [RCT, *n* = 164]

97. Price JJ, Barry MC. A double blind study of fluphenazine with pyridoxine. *Pa Med J* 1964; 67: 37–40. [RCT, *n* = 78]

98. Tan PC, Norazilah MF, Omar SZ. Dextrose saline compared with normal saline rehydration of hyperemesis gravidarum: A randomized controlled trial. *Obstet Gynecol* 2013; 121(2 Pt. 1): 291–8. [RCT, *n* = 202]

99. Bondok RS, El Sharnouby NM, Eid HE et al. Pulsed steroid therapy is an effective treatment for intractable hyperemesis gravidarum. *Crit Care Med* 2006; 34: 2781–3. [RCT, *n* = 40]

100. Ylikorkala O, Kauppila A, Ollanketo ML. Intramuscular ACTH or placebo in the treatment of hyperemesis gravidarum. *Acta Obstet Gynecol Scand* 1979; 58(5): 453–5. [RCT, *n* = 32]

101. Ditto A, Morgante G, la Marca A et al. Evaluation of treatment of hyperemesis gravidarum using parenteral fluid with or without diazepam. A randomized study. *Gynecol Obstet Invest* 1999; 48: 232–6. [RCT, *n* = 50]

102. Maina A, Arrotta M, Cicogna L, Donvito V, Mischinelli M, Todros T et al. Transdermal clonidine in the treatment of severe hyperemesis. A pilot randomised control trial: CLONEMESI. *BJOG* 2014 Nov; 121(12): 1556–62. [RCT, *n* = 12]

103. Stokke G, Gjelsvik BL, Flaatten KT, Birkeland E, Flaatten H, Trovik J. Hyperemesis gravidarum, nutritional treatment by nasogastric tube feeding: A 10-year retrospective cohort study. *Acta Obstet Gynecol Scand* 2015 Apr; 94(4): 359–67. [II-3, *n* = 107 eneteral nutrition, *n* = 10 parenteral nutrition, *n* = 273 intravenous fluids]

104. Garg S, Contag S, Dutta S. Emerging role of endoscopically placed jejunostomy tubes in the management of severe hyperemesis gravidarum: A case series. *Gastrointest Endosc* 2014 Apr; 79(4): 685–8. [II-3]

105. Hsu JJ, Clark-Glena R, Nelson DK et al. Nasogastric enteral feeding in the management of hyperemesis gravidarum. *Obstet Gynecol* 1996; 88: 343–6. [II-3]

106. Russo-Stieglitz KE, Levine AB, Wagner BA et al. Pregnancy outcome in patients requiring parenteral nutrition. *J Matern Fetal Med* 1999; 8: 164–7. [II-2]

107. Folk JJ, Leslie-Brown HF, Nosovitch JT et al. Hyperemesis gravidarum: Outcomes and complications with and without total parenteral nutrition. *J Reprod Med* 2004; 49: 497–502. [II-2, *n* = 166]

108. Holmgren C, Aagaard-Tillery KM, Silver RM et al. Hyperemesis in pregnancy: An evaluation of treatment strategies with maternal and neonatal outcomes. *Am J Obstet Gynecol* 2008; 198(1): 56. [II-2]

109. Nuthalapaty FS, Beck MM, Mabie WC. Complications of central venous catheters during pregnancy and postpartum: A case series. *Am J Obstet Gynecol* 2009; 201: 311.el–5. [II-3]

110. Peled Y, Melamed N, Hiersch L, Pardo J, Wiznitzer A, Yogev Y. The impact of total parenteral nutrition support on pregnancy outcome in women with hyperemesis gravidarum. *J Matern Fetal Neonatal Med* 2014 Jul; 27(11): 1146–50. [II-2, *n* = 122 cases of HG with TPN, *n* = 1797 controls without HG]

10

Intrahepatic cholestasis of pregnancy

Giuliana Simonazzi and Steven K. Herrine

KEY POINTS

- The diagnosis of intrahepatic cholestasis of pregnancy (ICP) is defined as **first onset of pruritus in the second or third trimester, elevated serum bile acids >10 µmol/L, and spontaneous relief of signs and symptoms within four weeks after delivery**.
- ICP is diagnosed once all other forms of liver disease and cholestasis have been excluded.
- A total bile acid level of **>40 µmol/L** represents **severe** ICP.
- **Complications** of untreated, usually severe ICP, include spontaneous preterm birth, meconium, nonreassuring fetal heart tracing, fetal death, neonatal death, and postpartum hemorrhage. Fetal deaths occur mostly ≥37 weeks, and no increased perinatal deaths have occurred in recent series with ursodeoxycholic acid (UDCA) treatment and delivery by 37 to 38 weeks.
- **UDCA is the current treatment of choice** for ICP as it is associated with improvements in maternal pruritus, bile acids, and transaminases. UDCA treatment should be recommended for women with ICP and also to improve some fetal outcomes.
- Vitamin K 10 mg by mouth once a day at onset of ICP or 34 weeks has been suggested for prevention of postpartum hemorrhage, but there is insufficient evidence for a strong recommendation.
- There are several reports of sudden fetal death within 24 hours of a reactive nonstress test (NST) and insufficient evidence for a recommended fetal testing protocol.
- **Especially in severe cases, delivery should occur at about 37 0/7 to 37 6/7 weeks**.

HISTORIC NOTES

Old names such as "benign jaundice of pregnancy" or "idiopathic jaundice of pregnancy" should no longer be used.

DIAGNOSIS/DEFINITION

Intrahepatic cholestasis of pregnancy (ICP) is diagnosed when otherwise unexplained pruritus occurs in pregnancy with elevated bile acids >10 µmol/L (≥14 µmol/L) in >90%, often with elevations in serum alkaline phosphatase and aminotransferases, which all resolve after delivery [1]. In the setting of normal bile acids, some accept the diagnosis of pruritus and abnormal transaminases [14]. Other names used in the literature are gestational cholestasis or obstetric cholestasis. Other causes of pruritus and liver dysfunction should be excluded. Differential diagnosis may include hepatitis A, B, and C; Epstein–Barr and cytomegalovirus; autoimmune liver disease; gall bladder stones; tumors of the hepatobiliary tract; and a number of causes with elevated hepatic enzymes specified to pregnancy (e.g., preeclampsia, HELLP syndrome, and acute fatty liver) [2–5] (Figure 10.1, Table 10.1). Women with

persistent unexplained pruritus and normal biochemical tests should have liver function tests repeated every one to two weeks [1].

SYMPTOMS

ICP is characterized by mild to severe pruritus usually starting after 30 weeks, which often resolves within 48 hours following delivery [2]. The pruritus of ICP is typically **worse at night**, is often **widespread** throughout the whole body, and may be most severe in the **palms** of the hands and/or **soles** of the feet [1,6]. Mild jaundice, if present (incidence of 14%–25%), typically develops one to four weeks after onset of pruritis with mildly elevated serum levels of conjugated bilirubin. Insomnia, fatigue, anorexia, malaise, weight loss, epigastric discomfort, steatorrhea, gallstones, cholecystitis, vitamin K deficiency, and dark urine are other signs and symptoms associated with ICP [2].

INCIDENCE/EPIDEMIOLOGY

Incidence of ICP varies geographically with 0.01% to 0.5% in the United States; 0.5%–1.5% in Europe [7]; 5% Hispanics; 9.2% to 15.6% in South America [8]; and 2.3%–6.0% in China [9]. It commonly occurs in the late second and third trimesters, rapidly resolves within four weeks after delivery, and is associated with adverse pregnancy outcomes [1,8].

GENETICS

About 15% to 30% of women presenting with ICP have a family history of intrahepatic cholestasis (IC), but most cases are not related to known mutations of familial IC. Genetic predisposition is shown in high-prevalence regions, such as Chile and Scandinavia. Family clustering, prevalence of ethnic and geographic variations, and recently demonstrated mutations in gene coding for hepatobiliary transport proteins further indicate a genetic predisposition in ICP. There are many genetic variations described, which occur at different chromosomal locations, ATP8B1 at 18q 21-22, ABCB4 at 7q21, ABCB11 at 2q24 [10]. Genetic predisposition may lead to altered cell membrane composition of bile ducts and hepatocytes as well as the subsequent dysfunction of biliary canalicular transporters. Mutations in the hepatic phospholipid transporter (MDR3/ABCB4), amniophospholipid transporter (ATP8B1/FIC1), and bile salt export pump (BSEP/ABCB11) have been found in patients with ICP [2,6,8]. These genetic mutations are more frequent in women who developed severe ICP [6,8].

ETIOLOGY/BASIC PATHOPHYSIOLOGY

ICP is associated with a rise in conjungated bile salts, particularly the tauroconjugates of cholic and chenodeoxycholic

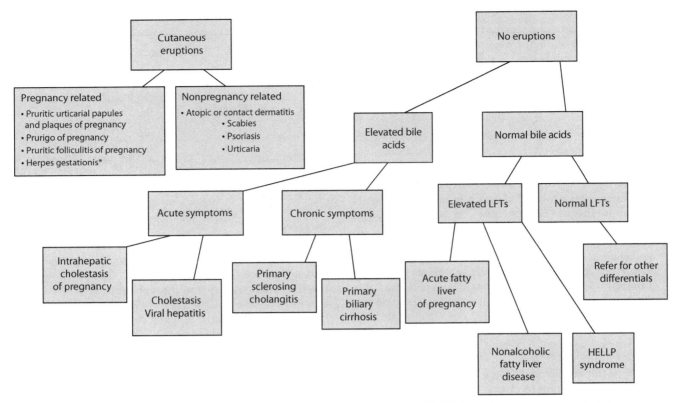

Figure 10.1 Pruritus during pregnancy. *Abbreviations*: LFT, liver function tests; HELLP, hemolytic anemia, elevated liver enzymes, and low platelet count. *See Chapter 43.

acid. Bile acids are the end products of hepatic cholesterol metabolism. The metabolic demands of pregnancy increase the demand for and exceed hepatic capacity for cholesterol metabolism in susceptible individuals. Bile acids, such as glycocholic and taurocholic acid, increase in serum and cause itching [6]. Bile acids are inherently cytotoxic, and thus their metabolism is tightly regulated. In ICP, the transport of bile salts from the liver to the gallbladder and intestine is disrupted, leading to compensatory transport of bile salts from hepatocytes into the blood [11].

The underlying mechanisms of obstetric complication (preterm delivery, meconium passage, fetal distress, and fetal death) are poorly understood [12]. First, research in animals has shown a detrimental effect of high bile acid levels on cardiomyocytes, which cause arrhythmias [13]. Such potentially lethal arrhythmias in the fetus could explain the increased incidence of stillbirth. Second, a vasoconstrictive effect of bile acids on human placental chorionic veins has been shown, possibly explaining the occurrence of fetal distress, asphyxia, and death [14]. Finally, several studies have shown bile acid to increase the sensitivity and expression of oxytocin receptors in the human myometrium, possibly clarifying the mechanism behind spontaneous preterm labor in pregnancies that are complicated by ICP [15,16].

CLASSIFICATION

A bile acid level of ≥40 µmol represents severe disease. Severe disease represents about 20% of cases of ICP. Complications occur mainly with severe ICP [17,18].

RISK FACTORS/ASSOCIATIONS

There is a higher incidence of ICP in women with multiple pregnancies, in women who have conceived after in vitro fertilization (2.7% compared with 2%), and in women older than 35 years of age. Multiparity, family clustering, ICP in previous pregnancy, and a history of oral contraceptive use are also associated with an increased incidence of ICP. Recurrence of ICP has been reported to occur between 40% and 60% with varying intensity in subsequent pregnancies in a random manner. Several environmental factors have been reported to play a role in the etiology of ICP in genetically susceptible individuals: high maternal serum copper and low maternal serum selenium and zinc. Interestingly, ICP is more common in some countries during the winter, when natural selenium levels are lower. Deficiency of vitamin D has been also reported in women with ICP [2,11].

COMPLICATIONS (WITHOUT TREATMENT)

Complications of untreated ICP include preterm birth (PTB) (15%–44%), passage of meconium (25% to 45%), nonreassuring fetal heart testing (NRFHT) 5% to 15%, fetal death (2% to 10%), neonatal death (1% to 2%), and postpartum hemorrhage (20% to 22%) [2]. Spontaneous PTB (SPTB) occurs mostly at 32 to 36 weeks as for other causes of SPTB. Fetal deaths occur mostly ≥37 weeks [3]. The etiology of fetal deaths is unclear. A relationship between bile acid levels and fetal death is suspected and remains the focus of much research. For example, a large study demonstrated that fetal compromise increased by 1%–2% for each additional µmol/L of bile acid concentration;

Table 10.1   Selected Differential Diagnoses of Pregnant Women with Pruritus

	Intrahepatic Cholestasis of Pregnancy	Viral Hepatitis	Primary Sclerosing Cholangitis	Primary Biliary Cirrhosis	Acute Fatty Liver of Pregnancy
Common trimester presentation	Third	Any	Any	Any	Second, third
Clinical features	Severe pruritis, jaundice	Nausea, vomiting, jaundice, prolonged abdominal pain and fluctuating jaundice and pruritis	Insidious and intermittent jaundice, fatigue, pruritis, abdominal pain	Fatigue, intermittent pruritis, RUQ pain, anorexia, and jaundice	Nausea, vomiting, abdominal pain, jaundice mental status changes, +/−preeclampsia, +/− HTN
Laboratory findings	Alkpho nl or elevated Trans elevated, sometimes to 1000 U/L Bilirubin: mildly elevated	Alkpho nl Trans 1000 to 2000 U/L; ALT > AST Bilirubin: nl or mildly elevated	Alkpho 3–5 × nl Trans 4–5 × nl Bilirubin: nl or mildly elevated	Alkpho 3–4 × nl Trans <3 × nl Bilirubin: early stage: nl, then increases slowly, may exceed >20 mg/dL	Alkpho nl Trans nl or moderately elevated Bilirubin: elevated
Pathology	Mutation in multidrug resistance-3 gene; environmental factors Bx: Bland changes typical of cholestasis of liver biopsy	Viral infection; sequalae from acute hepatitis can lead to cholestasis Bx: Marked inflammation	Idiopathic, associated with IBS; cholangiographic findings of multifocal structuring an ectasia of biliary tree Bx: thickened, fibrotic duct wall	Autoimmune inflammatory destruction of intralobular bile ducts Bx: Ductopenia: absence of interlobular bile ducts >50% portal tracts	Often idiopathic, some patients with inherited LCHAD deficiency; most common in primiparous and multiple gestations Bx: Microvesicular fatty liver disease
Treatments with reported benefit on symptoms	Ursodeoxycholic acid (first-line therapy); SAMe	Supportive measures	Ursodeoxycholic acid, treat underlying, liver transplant	Ursodeoxycholic acid, steroids	Delivery

Sources: Adapted from Kaaja RJ, Kontula KK, Raiha A et al. *Scand J Gastroenterol*, 29, 2, 178–81, 1994; Heinonen S, Kirkinen P. *Obstet Gynecol*, 94, 189–93, 1999; Alsulyman O, Ouzounian J, Ames-Castro M. *Am J Obstet Gynecol*, 175, 957–60, 1996.

Abbreviations: Alkpho, alkaline phosphatase; Bx, biopsy; HTN, hypertension; LCHAD, Long-chain 3-hydroxyacyl CoA dehydrogenase; nl, normal; RUQ, right upper quadrant; SAMe, S-adenosylmethionine; Trans, transaminases.

further statistical analysis suggested that, compared with control pregnancies, these rates increased significantly at bile acid level ≥40 micromoles/L [19]. In a recent multicenter retrospective cohort study, bile acids ≥40 μmol/L were associated with increased risk of meconium-stained amniotic fluid, and bile acids ≥100 μmol/L were associated with increased risk of stillbirth [20]. **No increase in perinatal deaths has occurred in recent series with treatment and delivery by 37 to 38 weeks** [13,21]. Subclinical steatorrhea may occur along with fat malabsorption. This condition may lead to vitamin K deficiency, resulting in a prolonged prothrombin time and postpartum hemorrhage [8].

PREGNANCY CONSIDERATIONS

Up to 50% of women recall pruritus during pregnancy, but few have elevated bile acids. Bile acids may initially be normal, later increasing at an average of three weeks after symptoms of pruritus. Of ICP diagnoses, 80% to 86% are made after 30 weeks.

PREGNANCY MANAGEMENT/EVALUATION
Principles

Usually only severe ICP is associated with perinatal complications so that the largest series has proposed no intervention for milder cases (i.e., bile acids <40 μmol) [18].

Workup

Laboratory evaluation includes **bile acids** (with serial measurement if initially negative and high clinical suspicion)

and **transaminases**, such as AST and ALT (which are elevated in approximately 60% of cases). GGT is not necessary but is elevated in 30% of cases. Serum bilirubin is elevated in about 25% of cases of ICP, rarely exceeding 6 mg/dL [2]. Hepatitis C antibody can be checked, especially in the presence of risk factors for the infection, as ICP is more common in these women. In the appropriate clinical setting, right upper quadrant ultrasound can be used to investigate the possibility of biliary obstruction (10% have cholelithiasis) (Figure 10.1, Table 10.1) [2–5]. Postnatal resolution of symptoms and biochemical abnormalities is required to confirm the diagnosis [1].

MANAGEMENT (FIGURE 10.2)
Prevention

No preventive measures have been proposed.

Therapy

Ursodeoxycholic Acid (Ursodiol)
　　Mechanism of action: Ursodiol is a hydrophilic bile acid that inhibits intestinal absorption of other bile acids, enhances excretory hepatocyte function and choleretic activity, stabilizes hepatocyte cell membranes and dilutes toxic bile acids in the enterohepatic circulation [13]. Ursodiol may also allow for transport of bile acids out of the fetal compartment.
　　Safety: FDA pregnancy category B.
　　Dose: 10 to 25 mg/kg orally divided into two doses daily. The standard starting dose is 300 mg to 500 mg orally twice a day.

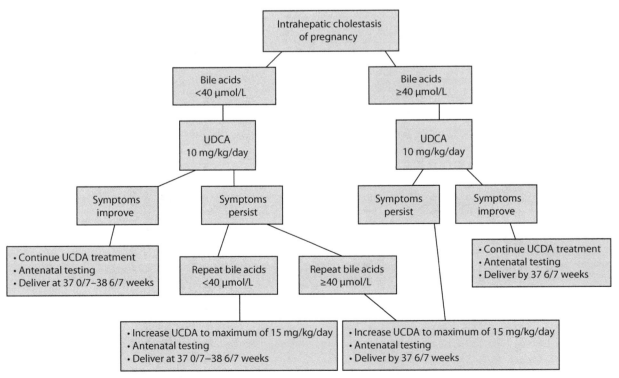

Figure 10.2 Treatment algorithm. *Abbreviations*: UDCA, ursodeoxycholic acid; SAMe, *S*-adenosylmethionine. (Adapted from Cappell M. *Med Clin North Am*, 92, 4, 739–60, 2008; Cappell M. *Med Clin North Am*, 92, 4, 717–37, 2008; Saleh M, Abdo K. *J Womens Health*, 16, 6, 833–41, 2007.)

Side effects: Headache, diarrhea, and constipation, all reported in less than 25% of patients. UDCA is generally well tolerated by pregnant women [22].

Effectiveness: Compared to placebo, **UDCA is associated with decreased pruritus, a significantly greater reduction in bile acids and transaminases, and lower incidence of preterm birth** [23–26]. When compared to other interventions, UDCA has been shown to have a **significant beneficial effect in decreasing pruritus, bile acids, and liver function tests** [27–29]. The outcome of fetal death is generally uncommon, but indirect evidence correlates lower bile acids with fewer fetal deaths and other complications. There is insufficient data concerning protection against stillbirth and safety to the fetus or neonate [1]. However, some studies suggested that UDCA therapy might also benefit fetal outcomes [22,30,31]. In a meta-analysis, including both non-RCTs and RCTs, the use of UDCA in the management of ICP was associated with improvement in some maternal outcomes (liver function tests, pruritus) and some fetal and neonatal outcomes (SPTB, neonatal intensive care unit admission). There were also a trend toward increased birth weight and decreased meconium staining associated with use of UDCA [32]. A Cochrane meta-analysis concluded that UDCA improves maternal pruritus in ICP, but cited insufficient evidence to recommend UDCA to improve fetal outcome. The analysis also reported an apparent decrease in fetal/neonatal morbidity associated with UDCA, including lower rates of meconium passage and higher mean gestational age at birth [27].

S-Adenosylmethionine

S-adenosylmethionine (SAMe) is a methyl donor that is thought to improve bile flow and biliary lipid metabolism. The dose should be 500 mg orally twice a day or 800 to 900 mg IV infusion once a day. Compared to placebo, one trial showed significantly **greater improvements in pruritus, bile salts, and liver enzymes** with SAMe [25,26,29,33–35]. **Compared to UDCA, SAMe is less effective at improving pruritus, bile acids, transaminases, and bilirubin** [25,36–39]. SAMe is not commonly used by itself given the tolerability and therapeutic superiority of UDCA.

UDCA and SAMe

Compared to placebo, **UDCA and SAMe resulted in greater improvements in pruritus, bile salts, and selected liver function assays**; however, combined UDCA and SAMe were no more effective than UDCA alone in regard to improvement in pruritus [26,27,39].

Other Therapies

Dexamethasone. Compared to dexamethasone, UDCA is associated with a greater reduction in bile acids and liver enzymes with improved pruritus only in women with severe ICP [27]. Dexamethasone should not be the first-line therapy for treatment of ICP, nor should it be used outside of a randomized controlled trial without a thorough consultation with the woman [1].

Cholestyramine. Cholestyramine is an anion exchange resin that binds to bile acids and decreases their absorption in the ileum. Cholestyramine should not be taken with other medications because of potential interference with their absorption. Safety: FDA pregnancy category C. Dose: 8 g

orally once a day. Significant side effects include a decrease in intestinal absorption of fat-soluble vitamins A, D, E, and K, increased intestinal gas, diarrhea, and poor palatability. No studies support the use of vitamin K supplementation to decrease risks associated with deficiency. Compared with UDCA, no significant differences were observed in pruritus, bile salts, or fetal/neonatal outcomes [28].

Guar gum. Guar gum is a type of dietary fiber that decreases the bile acid pool by binding to bile acids in the intestinal lumen [6] Safety: FDA pregnancy category B. Compared to placebo, there are no differences in pruritus, bile salts, or fetal/neonatal outcomes observed in a very small RCT [40].

Activated charcoal. Activated charcoal is a porous substance shown to adsorb bile salts, decrease bilirubin levels, and inhibit bile acid absorption [5]. Safety: FDA class C. Compared to no treatment, the reduction in bile salts was greater with charcoal, but there was no difference in pruritus or fetal/neonatal outcomes in a very small RCT [41].

Hydroxyzine. Hydroxyzine antagonizes central and peripheral histamine-1 receptors. Safety: FDA pregnancy category C; dose: 25 to 100 mg as needed every six hours orally. Hydroxyzine might improve tolerance to persistent itching, but this is not based on RCT data [8]. Antihistamines may provide some sedation at night but do not have a significant impact on pruritus.

Vitamin K. Vitamin K (FDA pregnancy category C) 10 mg once a day at onset of ICP or 34 weeks has been suggested for prevention of postpartum hemorrhage, but there is insufficient evidence for a strong recommendation [5]. Women should be advised that when prothrombin time is prolonged, the use of water-soluble vitamin K (for example, menadiol sodium phosphate) in a dose of 5–10 mg daily may be indicated [2].

Conclusion

UDCA monotherapy is the current treatment of choice and should be used as the first-line therapy for ICP. UDCA has been demonstrated to be equal or superior in safety, efficacy, cost-effectiveness, and convenience compared to other therapies. There is insufficient evidence to recommend SAMe, guar gum, activated charcoal, dexamethasone, cholestyramine alone or in combination in the management of women with ICP [27,39].

ANTEPARTUM TESTING

No RCT specifically addresses fetal surveillance and its frequency in ICP. No specific method of antenatal fetal monitoring for the prediction of fetal death can be recommended. Even if maternal detection of movements is simple, its role in monitoring pregnancy complicated by ICP has not been assessed. Ultrasound and cardiotocography are not reliable methods for preventing fetal death in ICP. Daily kick counts and nonstress tests (NSTs) once per week starting at diagnosis (usually on or after 32 weeks) have been proposed, but there are **several reports of fetal death after reactive NST** [42,43]. Despite this, expert opinion suggests that continuous fetal monitoring in labor should be offered [1].

DELIVERY

Stillbirths in ICP have been reported across all gestations, but the majority of unexplained fetal deaths occur after

37 weeks [6]. As gestation advances, the risk of delivery (prematurity, respiratory distress) versus the uncertain fetal risk of continuing the pregnancy (stillbirth) may justify offering women **induction of labor at 37 0/7–37 6/7 weeks, especially in severe cases (bile acid level of ≥40 µmol)** [6,13,26]. The decision should be made after careful counseling.

REFERENCES

1. Royal College of Obstetricians and Gynaecologists. *Obstetric cholestasis*. Green-top Guideline No. 43; April 2011. [Guideline; III]
2. Ozkan S, Ceylan Y, Ozkan OV, Yildirim S. Review of a challenging clinical issue: Intrahepatic cholestasis of pregnancy. *World J Gastroenterol* 2015; 21(23): 7134–41. [Review; III]
3. Cappell M. Hepatic disorders severely affected by pregnancy: Medical and obstetric management. *Med Clin North Am* 2008; 92(4): 739–60. [II-2]
4. Cappell M. Hepatic disorders mildly to moderately affected by pregnancy: Medical and obstetric management. *Med Clin North Am* 2008; 92(4): 717–37. [II-2]
5. Feldman M, Friedman L, Brandt L. *Gastrointestinal and Liver Disease*. 9th ed. Philadelphia, PA: Saunders, 2010. [Review]
6. Pathak B, Sheibani L, Lee R. Cholestasis of pregnancy. *Obstet Gynecol Clin North Am* 2010; 37(2): 269–82. [II-3]
7. Arrese M, Reyes H. Intrahepatic cholestasis of pregnancy: A past and present riddle. *Ann Hepatol* 2006; 5: 202–5. [Review; III]
8. Saleh M, Abdo K. Intrahepatic cholestasis of pregnancy: Review of the literature and evaluation of current evidence. *J Womens Health* 2007; 16(6): 833–41. [II-3]
9. Qi HB, Shao Y, Wu WX et al. Grading of intrahepatic cholestasis of pregnancy. *Zhonghua Fu Chan Ke Za Zhi* 2004; 39: 14–7. [II-3]
10. Floreani A, Gervasi MT. New insights on intrahepatic cholestasis of pregnancy. *Clin Liver Dis* 2016 Feb; 20(1): 177–89. [Review; III]
11. Williamson C, Geenes V. Intrahepatic cholestasis of pregnancy. *Obstet Gynecol* 2014 Jul; 124(1): 120–33. [Review; III]
12. Brouwers L, Koster MP, Page-Christiaens GC et al. Intrahepatic cholestasis of pregnancy: Maternal and fetal outcomes associated with elevated bile acid levels. *Am J Obstet Gynecol* 2015 Jan; 212(1): 100.e1–7. [II-2]
13. Gorelik J, Shevchuk A, de Swiet M et al. Comparison of the arrhythmogenic effects of tauro- and glycoconjugates of cholic acid in an in vitro study of rat cardiomyocytes. *BJOG* 2004; 111(8): 867–70. [II-2]
14. Sepulveda WH, Gonzalez C, Cruz MA, Rudolph MI. Vasoconstrictive effect of bile acids on isolated human placental chorionic veins. *Eur J Obstet Gynecol Reprod Biol* 1991; 42: 211–5. [II-3]
15. Israel EJ, Guzman ML, Campos GA. Maximal response to oxytocin of the isolated myometrium from pregnant patients with intrahepatic cholestasis. *Acta Obstet Gynecol Scand* 1986; 65: 581–2. [II-3]
16. German AM, Kato S, Carvajal JA et al. Bile acids increase response and expression of human myometrial oxytocin receptor. *Am J Obstet Gynecol* 2003; 189: 577–82. [II-3]
17. Sentilhes L, Bacq Y. The intrahepatic cholestasis of pregnancy. *J Obstet Gynecol Reprod Biol* 2008; 37(2): 118–26. [II-3]
18. Trauner M, Meier PJ, Boyer JL. Molecular pathogenesis of cholestasis. *N Engl J Med* 1998; 339(17): 1217–27. [Review; nonpregnant]
19. Glantz A, Marschall HU, Mattsson LA. Intrahepatic cholestasis of pregnancy: Relationships between bile acid levels and fetal complication rates. *Hepatology* 2004; 40(2): 467–74. [II-3; n = 693, largest series]
20. Kawakita T, Parikh LI, Ramsey PS et al. Predictors of adverse neonatal outcomes in intrahepatic cholestasis of pregnancy. *Am J Obstet Gynecol* 2015 Oct; 213(4): 570.e1–8. [Multicenter retrospective study, n = 233; II-2]
21. Kenyon AP, Percy CN, Girling J et al. Obstetric cholestasis, outcome with active management: A series of 70 cases. *BJOG* 2002; 109(3): 282–8. [II-3]
22. Joutsiniemi T, Timonen S, Leino R et al. Ursodeoxycholic acid in the treatment of intrahepatic cholestasis of pregnancy: A randomized controlled trial. *Arch Gynecol Obstet* 2014 Mar; 289(3): 541–7. [RCT, n = 20; I]
23. Roncaglia N, Locatelli A, Arreghini A et al. A randomized controlled trial of ursodeoxycholic acid and S-adenosyl-L-methionine in the treatment of gestational cholestasis. *BJOG* 2004; 111: 17–21. [RCT, n = 46]
24. Diaferia A, Nicastri PL, Tartagni M et al. Ursodeoxycholic acid therapy in pregnant women with cholestasis. *Int J Gynaecol Obstet* 1996; 52(2): 133–40. [RCT, n = 16]
25. Palma J, Reyes H, Ribalta J et al. Ursodeoxycholic acid in the treatment of cholestasis of pregnancy: A randomized, double-blind study controlled with placebo. *J Hepatol* 2000; 27(6): 1022–8. [RCT, n = 15]
26. Nicastri PL, Diaferia A, Tartagni M et al. A randomised placebo-controlled trial of ursodeoxycholic acid and S-adenosylmethionine in the treatment of intrahepatic cholestasis of pregnancy. *BJOG* 1998; 105(11): 1205–7. [RCT; UDCA = 8; SAMe = 8; both = 8; placebo = 8; RCT, n = 32; I]
27. Gurung V, Stokes M, Middleton P et al. Interventions for treating cholestasis in pregnancy. *The Cochrane Collaboration* 2014. [Meta-analysis; 21 RCT, n = 1197; I]
28. Glantz A, Marschall HU, Lammert F et al. Intrahepatic cholestasis of pregnancy: A randomized controlled trial comparing dexamethasone and ursodeoxycholic acid. *Hepatology* 2005; 2(6): 1399–405. [RCT, n = 130]
29. Binder T, Salaj P, Zima T et al. Randomized prospective comparative study of ursodeoxycholic acid and S-adenosyl-L-methionine in the treatment of intrahepatic cholestasis of pregnancy. *J Perinat Med* 2006; 34(5): 383–91. [RCT, n = 78]
30. Bacq Y, Sentilhes L, Reyes HB et al. Efficacy of ursodeoxycholic acid in treating intrahepatic cholestasis of pregnancy: A meta-analysis. *Gastroenterology* 2012 Dec; 143(6): 1492–501 [Meta-analysis of 9 RCT, n = 454; I]
31. Chappel LC, Gurung V, Seed PT et al. Ursodeoxycholic acid versus placebo, and early term delivery versus expectant management, in women with intrahepatic cholestasis of pregnancy: Semifactorial randomised clinical trial. *BMJ* 2012 Jun 13; 344: e3799 [Semifactorial RCT, n = 125; I]
32. Grand'Maison S, Durand M, Mahone M. The effects of ursodeoxycholic acid treatment for intrahepatic cholestasis of pregnancy on maternal and fetal outcomes: A meta-analysis including non-randomized studies. *J Obstet Gynaecol Can* 2014 Jul; 36(7): 632–41. [Meta-analysis; 11 RCTs and 6 non-RCTs, n = 836; I]
33. Kondrackiene J, Beuers U, Kupcinskas L. Efficacy and safety of ursodeoxycholic acid versus cholestyramine in intrahepatic cholestasis of pregnancy. *Gastroenterology* 2005; 129: 894–901. [RCT, n = 84]
34. Frezza M, Pozzato G, Chiesa L et al. Reversal of intrahepatic cholestasis of pregnancy in women after high dose S-adenosyl-L-methionine administration. *Hepatology* 1984; 4(2): 274–8. [RCT, n = 18]
35. Frezza M, Centini G, Cammareri G et al. S-Adenosylmethionine for the treatment of intrahepatic cholestasis of pregnancy. Results of a controlled clinical trial. *Hepatogastroenterology* 1990; 37(Suppl. 2): 122–5. [RCT, n = 30]
36. Ribalta J, Reyes H, Gonzalez MC et al. S-Adenosyl-L-methionine in the treatment of patients with intrahepatic cholestasis of pregnancy: A randomized, double-blind, placebo-controlled study with negative results. *Hepatology* 1991; 13(6): 1084–9. [RCT, n = 18]
37. Floreani A, Paternoster D, Melis A et al. S-Adenosylmethionine versus ursodeoxycholic acid in the treatment of intrahepatic cholestasis of pregnancy: Preliminary results of a controlled trial. *Eur J Obstet Gynecol Reprod Biol* 1996; 67(2): 109–13. [RCT, n = 20]

38. Roncaglia N, Locatelli A, Arreghini A et al. A randomized controlled trial of ursodeoxycholic acid and S-adenosyl-L-methionine in the treatment of gestational cholestasis. *BJOG* 2004; 111: 17–21. [RCT, *n* = 66]

39. Zhan L, Liu XH, Qi HB et al. Ursodeoxycholic acid and S-adenosylmethionine in the treatment of intrahepatic cholestasis of pregnancy: A multi-centered randomized controlled trial. *Eur Rev Med Pharmacol Sci* 2015 Oct; 19(19): 3770–6. [RCT, *n* = 135; I]

40. Riikonen S, Savonius H, Gylling H et al. Oral guar gum, a gel-forming dietary fiber relieves pruritus in intrahepatic cholestasis of pregnancy. *Acta Obstet Gynecol Scand* 2000; 79(4): 260–4. [RCT, *n* = 39]

41. Kaaja RJ, Kontula KK, Raiha A et al. Treatment of cholestasis of pregnancy with peroral activated charcoal. A preliminary study. *Scand J Gastroenterol* 1994; 29(2): 178–81. [RCT, *n* = 19]

42. Heinonen S, Kirkinen P. Pregnancy outcome with intrahepatic cholestasis. *Obstet Gynecol* 1999; 94: 189–93. [II-2]

43. Alsulyman O, Ouzounian J, Ames-Castro M. Intrahepatic cholestasis of pregnancy: Perinatal outcome associated with expectant management. *Am J Obstet Gynecol* 1996; 175: 957–60. [II-2]

11

Inflammatory bowel disease

Priyadarshini Koduri

KEY POINTS

- Inflammatory bowel disease (IBD) refers to Crohn's disease (CD) and ulcerative colitis (UC).
- Pathogenesis of IBD is not well known although both environmental and genetic factors play a role.
- If one parent has UC, the risk of the offspring developing UC is 1.6%; if one parent has CD, risk goes up to as high as 5.2%. With both parents having IBD, the offspring's risk goes up to 36%.
- Complications from IBD can be from intestinal or extraintestinal manifestations.
- **Women with IBD should be encouraged to plan conception when the disease is in remission and when their nutritional status is optimized**.
- Smoking cessation is an extremely important factor in keeping women with CD quiescent.
- CD has been associated with first-trimester miscarriage, preterm birth <37 weeks, and low birth weight. It may be associated with stillbirth and SGA infants.
- UC is associated with preterm birth <37 weeks. It may be associated with an increased risk of congenital anomalies, SGA, and stillbirth.
- Even if disease is well controlled, women with IBD remain at risk for adverse pregnancy outcomes.
- **The risk of a flare of IBD during pregnancy (33%) is similar to when they are not pregnant**.
- **Multiple medications are available for management of IBD. Most are considered safe for use in pregnancy and breast-feeding except for methotrexate and thalidomide. Aminosalicylates, such as sulfasalazine or mesalamine, are usually considered first-line therapies**.
- Surgical management for UC during pregnancy is only indicated in cases of massive hemorrhage, fulminant colitis unresponsive to medical management, perforation, or strongly suspected/known carcinoma. Colectomy in pregnancy is historically associated with high perinatal mortality.
- Ileal pouch–anal anastomosis does not confer additional maternal or fetal morbidity. Long-term pouch function is not affected by pregnancy or mode of delivery.
- **Mode of delivery in IBD remains controversial with no randomized controlled trials available to provide guidance. Limited evidence suggests that in women with IBD, vaginal delivery is appropriate in quiescent or absent perianal disease (abscess/fistula). A cesarean delivery may be performed for women with active perianal disease, such as perianal abscess or fistula**.
- **Mode of delivery does not impact development of IBD in children**.
- Thromboprophylaxis postpartum may be considered, particularly post cesarean section.
- Pregnancy and breast-feeding may have a mitigating effect on the course of IBD in the years following delivery.

BACKGROUND

Inflammatory bowel disease (IBD) refers to Crohn's disease (CD) and ulcerative colitis (UC). Both are chronic systemic diseases that affect women of reproductive age. They have a protracted relapsing and remitting course that extends over years. Although they share several common features, there are distinct differences between the two conditions summarized in Table 11.1. Differentiating between UC and CD, however, may be impossible in 15% of patients [1].

CROHN'S DISEASE
Definition
CD is a systemic inflammatory disease that mainly manifests as chronic, transmural, granulomatous inflammation of the gastrointestinal system. Any part of the GI tract can be affected. Although it commonly involves the colon and terminal ileum, the rectum may be involved in up to 50% of patients [1].

Diagnosis
Diagnosis is based on history, physical examination, laboratory evaluation and a combination of endoscopic, radiographic, and pathologic findings documenting the focal, asymmetric, and transmural features of the disease (Table 11.1). A diagnosis of CD is rarely made for the first time during pregnancy [2].

Signs/Symptoms
Manifestations of CD in pregnancy are similar to those in the nonpregnant state. Typical symptoms include chronic or intermittent diarrhea, abdominal pain, weight loss, fever, and rectal bleeding. Acute ileitis may mimic appendicitis. Additional clinical features include pallor, anorexia, palpable abdominal mass/tenderness, perianal fissures, fistula, or abscess. **Perianal manifestations are unique to CD. Extraintestinal symptoms are not uncommon and may involve a variety of organ systems (Table 11.2)**. Many of these manifestations are also seen in UC.

Epidemiology/Incidence
The incidence of CD varies by geographical region, but has been rising over the past decade. The incidence of CD in developed Western countries, including the United States, is estimated at seven per 100,000 population [3]. Disease frequency is two to four times higher in Jewish populations. The peak age of onset is in the second and third decades of life. Smoking is associated with a twofold increased risk of CD [1].

Table 11.1 Comparison of Ulcerative Colitis and Crohn's Disease

Feature	Ulcerative Colitis	Crohn's Disease
Extent of inflammation	Limited to mucosa	Involves all layers (transmural)
Intestine involved	Colon only	All segments of the gastrointestinal tract; terminal ileum most common
Rectal involvement	Always	Sometimes
Pattern of spread	Contiguous	Patchy, skip lesions
Granulomas	No	Yes (sometimes)
Fistula	No	Yes
Strictures	No	Yes
Abscess	No	Yes
Perianal disease	No	Yes
Bloody diarrhea	Yes	Maybe
Ileal disease on computed tomography	No	Yes
Increased colon cancer risk	Yes	Maybe (if colonic involvement)
Cure with surgery	Yes	No
Percent of patients who will need surgery	20%	70%

Table 11.2 Extraintestinal Manifestations of IBD

Dermatologic	Erythema nodosum
	Pyoderma gangrenosum
	Aphthous stomatitis
	Pyostomatitis vegetans
	Sweet's syndrome
	Anal skin tags
Musculoskeletal	Osteopenia/osteoporosis
	Osteomalacia
	Increased risk of fractures in hips, wrist, spine, and ribs
	Peripheral arthritis
	Axial arthropathies
Ocular	Conjunctivitis
	Uveitis
	Scleritis/episcleritis
Genitourinary	Nephrolithiasis
	Ureteral obstruction
	Fistulas
Hepatobiliary/pancreatic	Primary sclerosing cholangitis
	Cholelithiasis
	Pancreatitis
Thromboembolic	Increased risk of venous and arterial thromboses
	Hyperhomocysteinemia
Hematologic	Anemia
Pulmonary/cardiovascular	Chronic bronchitis
	Bronchiectasis
	Endocarditis/myocarditis
	Pleuropericarditis
	Reactive amyloidosis

Abbreviation: IBD, inflammatory bowel disease.

Etiology/Basic Pathophysiology

Etiology remains unclear. Genome-wide studies have identified multiple susceptibility loci on numerous chromosomes. Familial clustering and genetic anticipation have been confirmed [4]. However, these loci only explain approximately 20% of the heritability of CD, emphasizing the importance of other factors. The current hypothesis is that IBD results from a response to environmental triggers (infection, smoking, drugs, or other agents) in genetically susceptible individuals, resulting in a chronic dysregulation of mucosal immune function [5].

Complications
Maternal

Complications from CD may include serosal adhesions, partial and complete small bowel obstruction, fistula formation, perforation with resulting peritonitis, abscess formation, malabsorption, and perianal disease. Also, complications may arise from any extraintestinal manifestations (Table 11.2).

Fetal

The evidence related to fetal and neonatal outcomes remains conflicting and limited to observational studies. Retrospective studies suggest there may be an increased risk of first trimester miscarriage in women with CD when compared to controls [6,7]. However, this association has not been consistently demonstrated in large population-based cohort studies [7–9]. Several population-based studies and two meta-analyses demonstrate an increased risk of preterm birth <37 weeks and low birth weight infants [10–15]. The association with congenital anomalies remains questionable [10,15]. The risk of preterm birth may be higher in women who require oral systemic steroids and they may also be at increased risk for severe preeclampsia [8]. The data regarding the risk of small for gestational age (SGA) infants and stillbirth are inconsistent, but the most recent meta-analysis suggests an increased risk [10,15,16].

Pregnancy Considerations
Effect of Pregnancy on CD

Pregnant women with CD are no more likely to flare compared to nonpregnant women with CD [17]. Pregnancy may in fact have positive effects on disease activity as lower rates of relapse are observed in the three years following pregnancy [18,19]. Lower rates of stenosis and/or resection have also been noted in women with CD who have been pregnant during their disease course [20].

Effect of CD on Pregnancy

Regardless of disease activity, women with CD are at risk for adverse pregnancy outcomes that have been previously outlined [21]. Large population-based studies including women with IBD suggest an increased risk of adverse pregnancy outcomes with increasing disease activity [8,22]. Women with CD are at increased risk of cesarean delivery [10].

Management
Principles

Treatment of CD during pregnancy is similar to therapy in a nonpregnant patient. A multidisciplinary approach by an obstetrician/perinatologist and gastroenterologist is recommended. Most medications used in the management of CD are considered safe for use in pregnancy and have not been shown to be teratogenic. Women maintained in remission should continue their prepregnancy medications throughout their pregnancy unless they are on clearly teratogenic agents. Termination of pregnancy is not a therapeutic option for CD as there is no evidence that termination results in improved disease activity [23].

Workup

When a woman presents with symptomatic colitis and relapse is suspected, it is important to rule out infectious causes, including *Clostridium difficile* colitis. *C. difficile* may have a more fulminant course in patients with IBD [24]. Although imaging and colonoscopy/sigmoidoscopy may be indicated in the initial diagnosis of CD, they are often not necessary for workup of a relapse. Colonoscopy and/or flexible sigmoidoscopy may be performed safely during pregnancy.

Differential Diagnosis

Infectious colitis (bacterial, fungal, viral, or protozoan), diverticulitis, ischemic colitis, solitary rectal ulcer syndrome, nonsteroidal anti-inflammatory drug (NSAID)-related colitis.

Preconception Counseling

- A woman with CD should have a detailed discussion with her primary care provider, gastroenterologist, and obstetrician about her illness. Because the clinical course of CD during pregnancy depends on CD activity at the time of conception, it is important to **make sure that the disease is in remission before pregnancy** is planned. Contraceptive options should be reviewed as part of this discussion. **Quiescent disease at the time of conception (either spontaneous or on therapy) typically remains quiescent in two thirds of patients during pregnancy, and active disease remains active in up to 70% of patients**. Improvement during pregnancy is only noted in 30% [25]. In a recent meta-analysis, 46% of patients with active disease at time of conception remained active, and only 23% of women who were in remission at the time of conception relapsed [26].
- **Women are therefore encouraged to enter pregnancy when the disease is in remission for at least six months and their nutritional status has been optimized. Clinical remission is defined as normal bowel form and number (presence of formed stool and absence of diarrhea) without bleeding or abdominal pain** [27].

- CBC, folate, vitamin B_{12}, and iron should be assessed and appropriate replacement initiated if indicated [27].
- Women on methotrexate (MTX) should be counseled to be off the medication at least three to six months before conceiving. Additionally, women on sulfasalazine should be on folic acid at least one month prior to conception [28].
- Counsel women on **avoidance of exacerbating factors, including smoking and NSAID use** [3].
- The likelihood of a child developing CD should be discussed with parents although pregnancy should never be discouraged due to this reason. **The risk is estimated at 5.2% if one parent has CD** and 36% if both have IBD [16,29].
- The risk of infertility in patients with CD who have not had surgery seems to be the same as that of the general population.
- Review of vaccination history is important. Women on immunosuppressants should be immunized against influenza and pneumococcal infections. Under appropriate circumstances, they should also receive tetanus and meningococcal vaccines [24].

Prenatal Care

Comanagement with a gastroenterologist is recommended to ensure medication safety and appropriate management of any flares. Early evaluation and treatment of anemia, if applicable, is useful. To ensure appropriate weight gain during pregnancy, a nutrition consult may also be helpful. Serial growth surveillance should be considered particularly if a woman has active disease. There is no evidence that antenatal surveillance reduces stillbirth risk but may be considered in women with active disease.

Therapy

Treatment of CD is based on disease location, severity, and extraintestinal complications. Pharmacologic therapy is the mainstay of treatment. The goal of therapy is to maintain stable disease activity. Table 11.3 summarizes the pregnancy

Table 11.3 Medications Used in IBD

Type of Medication	Drug	Pregnancy Category	Recommendations for Pregnancy	Breast-Feeding
5-Amniosalicylic acid drugs	Sulfasalazine	B	First-line therapy; low risk; women should take 2 mg folic acid daily	Likely safe
	Mesalamine	C	Low risk	Likely safe
	Olsalazine	C	Low risk	Likely safe
	Balsalazide	B	Limited information	Limited information
Immunosuppressive agents	Azathioprine/ 6-mercaptopurine	D	Continue in pregnancy if efficacious; low risk	Likely safe
	Cyclosporine	C	Moderate risk	Not recommended
	Methotrexate	X	Contraindicated; teratogenic	Contraindicated, teratogenic
Anti-TNF-alpha agents	Infliximab	B	Low risk	Likely safe
	Adalimumab	B	Limited data; low risk	Safety unknown
	Certolizumab	B	Safety unknown	Safety unknown
Corticosteroids	Prednisone	C	Low risk; possible risk of cleft palate. PPROM and GDM	Likely safe
Antibiotics	Metronidazole	B	Low risk	Likely safe
	Quinolones	C	Low risk; possible cartilage damage with first-trimester exposure	Likely safe
Miscellaneous	Thalidomide	X	Contraindicated; teratogenic	Contraindicated; teratogenic

Abbreviations: GDM, gestational diabetes mellitus; IBD, inflammatory bowel disease; PPROM, premature preterm rupture of membranes; TNF, tumor necrosis factor.

recommendations for commonly used drugs in the therapy of IBD.

Aminosalicylates. **Sulfasalazine, mesalamine**, balsalazide, and olsalazine are in this category. These are usually considered the **first-line therapies**, both in nonpregnant and pregnant women. Drugs in this category have limited placental transfer and are generally considered safe for use in pregnancy and in breast-feeding. Aminosalicylates have not been shown to be teratogenic in humans [30–34]. They have not been shown to be associated with stillbirth, spontaneous abortion, preterm delivery, or low birth weight [30].

Because of the possible antifolate effects of sulfasalazine, women on sulfasalazine are recommended to take **2 mg folic acid/day in the prenatal period** and throughout the pregnancy [16,27].

Corticosteroids

Prednisone is generally safe in pregnancy and breast-feeding [23]. Although it does not cross the human placenta, animal studies report an increased risk of cleft palate in the offspring. Women on high doses should avoid breast-feeding within four hours of taking their dose to minimize possible neonatal effects. High-dose prednisone confers risk of diabetes (early glucola is warranted) and PPROM. A steroid taper is recommended when used for more than one week. Stress dose steroids are indicated only in special circumstances (see Chapter 25).

Antibiotics

Metronidazole and quinolones have been used in the management of IBD. Metronidazole is considered safe for use in pregnancy and breast-feeding. Quinolones have a high affinity for bone tissue and cartilage. Animal studies show cartilage damage in weight-bearing joints after quinolone exposure. Although risk with exposure is minimal, alternative therapies should be used in pregnancy when available [16]. Augmentin, another antibiotic used commonly in the management of both perianal and luminal CD, can be used safely during pregnancy. Rifamixin is a relatively new antibiotic, pregnancy category C, used in management of CD.

Immunomodulators/Immunosuppressants

Azathioprine/6-mercaptopurine. Mercaptopurine and azathioprine are often used to maintain remission in steroid-dependent patients with IBD [35,36]. Multiple case series and cohort studies have not demonstrated an increased risk of congenital anomalies, suggesting that these drugs are safe for use in pregnancy [36–43]. However, a recent meta-analysis demonstrated an increased risk of congenital anomalies in neonates born to women using thiopurines [44]. Nonetheless, **women who conceive on these medications should be allowed to remain on them through the pregnancy**. They should be counseled not to stop 6-mercaptopurine before conceiving as that may actually increase the risk of fetal loss [45]. Azathioprine and 6-mercaptopurine should ideally not be started for the first time in pregnancy due to response time and the small risk of severe side effects [27]. Several series suggest that breast-feeding on azathioprine/6-mercaptopurine may be safe [46–48].

Methotrexate. MTX is clearly teratogenic and use is **contraindicated in pregnancy** and in women considering pregnancy. Use in pregnancy or during organogenesis (six to eight weeks after conception) is associated with methotrexate embryopathy. Exposure later in pregnancy may be associated

with fetal toxicity and/or mortality. Women considering pregnancy should discontinue MTX three to six months before attempting conception [16]. MTX is contraindicated in breast-feeding.

Cyclosporine. This drug is typically used in patients with UC who are refractory to steroids. It should be used at the lowest effective dose. Cyclosporine has not been found to be teratogenic in humans [49–51]. It is associated with SGA infants and preterm birth [51]. Hypertension and seizures have also been reported with cyclosporine use. It should preferably not be initiated during pregnancy [38,39]. Breast-feeding is not recommended because of potential neonatal nephrotoxicity and immunosuppression [52,53].

Infliximab. Infliximab is a tumor necrosis factor (TNF)-alpha inhibitor used in patients with IBD [54–56]. Several studies and a meta-analysis have documented the **safety of infliximab in pregnancy and have shown no increased risk of congenital anomalies or other adverse pregnancy outcomes** [57–61]. Nonetheless, there are concerns regarding increased drug transfer across the placenta in the third trimester and newborn drug levels [62,63]. Newborn drug levels may in theory increase the risk of infectious complications in a neonate. This concern has led to a recommendation to avoid live vaccines for the first six months of life [61]. As such, current recommendations suggest that pregnant women should avoid treatment after 30 weeks gestation, and if necessary, the mother can be bridged with steroids to control the disease activity until delivery [63–65]. The final decision whether to discontinue medication should be made in partnership with a gastroenterologist. A neonatology or pediatric consultation can be offered to address vaccination concerns. The safety of infliximab in breast-feeding remains unknown although case reports of women on infliximab suggest it is safe [59,66].

Adalimumab. Adalimumab is an anti-TNF-alpha agent used in the management of CD. Human data on adalimumab use during pregnancy in IBD patients are limited. Case reports and a recent meta-analysis do not show an increased risk of congenital anomalies or other adverse pregnancy outcomes [61,67,68]. Similar to Infliximab, concerns regarding third-trimester use and newborn drug levels exist. There is limited data regarding the safety of Adalimumab in nursing but due to the miniscule amounts found in breast milk it is likely compatible.

Certolizumab. Certolizumab is a relatively new drug with decreased placental transfer compared to infliximab and adalimumab. It has not been associated with congenital anomalies or other adverse outcomes [61]. It has not been detected in breast milk, but data regarding safety of use in pregnancy or breast-feeding remains limited.

Miscellaneous Agents

Natalizumab. This is a humanized IgG4 monoclonal antibody more commonly used in multiple sclerosis patients although it has also been approved for treatment of CD. Data from the Natalizumab Pregnancy Exposure Registry do not show an association with adverse pregnancy outcomes [69]. It does cross the placenta during the third trimester of pregnancy. It is a pregnancy category C drug.

Thalidomide. Thalidomide has been successfully used in the treatment of some patients with CD [70]. Use in pregnancy and while breast-feeding is unequivocally contraindicated because of its well-known teratogenic effects.

Naltrexone. This is an opioid antagonist typically used in low doses to induce remission. There is insufficient evidence to deterime safety or efficacy in the nonpregnant population and no data yet on use in pregnant women [71].

Antepartum Testing

There is no literature to support the use of routine antenatal testing in patients with CD. However, it may be considered in women with active disease.

Delivery

No randomized controlled trials exist to determine the best form of delivery for women with CD. By current practice, **the method of delivery should be dictated by obstetric indication**. Vaginal delivery is acceptable for women with quiescent or absent perianal disease, and **cesarean delivery should be performed in those women with active perianal disease defined as perianal abscess or fistula** [72]. Episiotomy should be avoided as it places women with CD at risk for perineal disease peridelivery [73]. Mode of delivery does not appear to influence the development of IBD in offspring [74].

Women with IBD are considered "intermediate" risk for venous thromboembolism. Thromboprophylaxis (e.g., with low-molecular-weight heparin) should be considered for women postpartum (e.g., up to seven days), particularly for those women undergoing a cesarean delivery [75]. The first dose should be administered no sooner than four hours postoperatively and no later than 24 hours postoperatively.

Postpartum/Breast-Feeding

Breast-feeding is not associated with an increased risk of disease flare and may even be protective against a flare in the year following delivery [76,77].

ULCERATIVE COLITIS
Definition

UC is a chronic idiopathic systemic disease characterized by mucosal inflammation that usually involves the rectum and extends proximally to involve all or part of the colon. Disease is limited to the rectum and rectosigmoid in 40% to 50% of patients, and 30% to 40% have disease extending beyond the sigmoid but not involving the whole colon. In 20% of patients, the entire colon is involved [1].

Diagnosis

A diagnosis of UC is typically suspected on clinical grounds. It is confirmed by proctosigmoidoscopy or colonoscopy, histology of biopsy specimens, and by a negative stool exam ruling out infectious causes including *C. difficile* [24]. Alternative causes of diarrhea (infectious and noninfectious) should be ruled out before a definitive diagnosis can be made. Table 11.4 outlines criteria used to determine disease severity.

Signs/Symptoms

The manifestations of UC are similar in pregnant and nonpregnant women. The disease course is characterized by periods of remission and relapse. Extension of colonic disease can occur with time. Typical symptoms include diarrhea (often nocturnal), rectal bleeding, tenesmus, passage of mucus, and crampy abdominal pain. In severe disease, liquid

Table 11.4   Montreal Classification of Extent and Severity of Ulcerative Colitis

E1 (proctitis)	Inflammation limited to the rectum
E2 (left-sided; distal)	Inflammation limited to the splenic flexure
E3 (pancolitis)	Inflammation extends to the proximal splenic flexure
S0 (remission)	No symptoms
S1 (mild)	Four or less stools per day (with or without blood), absence of systemic symptoms, normal inflammatory markers
S2 (moderate)	Five stools per day, minimum signs of systemic symptoms
S3 (severe)	Six or more bloods per day, pulse rate ≥90 beats per min, Temperature ≥37.5°C, Hemoglobin concentration <105 g/L, ESR ≥30 mm/h

stool with blood, pus, and fecal matter may be experienced. Generalized symptoms may include anorexia, nausea, vomiting, fever, and weight loss. On physical examination, a tender anal canal and blood in the rectum may suggest proctitis. Severe pain and bleeding suggests toxic colitis, and tympany on abdominal exam suggests megacolon. Signs of peritonitis may suggest perforation [1]. Similar to CD, extraintestinal manifestations are not uncommon (Table 11.2).

Epidemiology/Incidence

The incidence of UC varies by geographical location. It is most common in Western nations and incidence in the United States is estimated at 8–12/100,000 population per year [24]. Ulcerative colitis has a bimodal pattern of incidence with the main peak at 15–30 years of age and a second peak at 50–70 years of age [78]. Unlike CD, the incidence of UC has remained stable over the past several decades [24]. Smoking and even a history of smoking increases the risk of UC. Former smokers have a 1.7-fold increased risk of developing UC compared to nonsmokers [1].

Etiology/Basic Pathophysiology

The etiology of UC remains unknown. The pathogenesis is currently thought to be similar to CD (see section titled "Etiology/Basic Pathophysiology" described earlier for CD).

Complications
Maternal

Massive hemorrhage typically from erosions in the colon (1%), toxic megacolon (5%), perforation (rare but fatal in 15% of cases), and strictures (5%–10%) [1]. The risk of colon cancer is related to the duration and extent of the disease. After 10 years, the colon cancer risk is estimated at 0.5% to 1% per year, necessitating annual or biannual colonoscopic surveillance [24]. Complications may also arise from any existing extraintestinal manifestations (Table 11.2).

In women with an ileal pouch–anal anastomosis (IPAA), pregnancy is considered safe and is not associated with an increased frequency of maternal morbidity or pouch complications [79]. Pouch complications reported in pregnancy include small bowel obstruction (2.8% antenatally, 6.8% postpartum), pouchitis (1.8%), and perianal abscess (0.4%) [80].

Fetal

UC is associated with preterm birth <37 weeks [10,15,81]. The risk of preterm birth may be higher in women who require systemic steroids and they may also be at increased risk for severe preeclampsia [8]. Evidence regarding other adverse pregnancy outcomes remains inconsistent. Several studies suggest that UC is not associated with low birth weight, intrauterine growth restriction, SGA infants, or stillbirth [7,10,82,83]. However, a recent meta-analysis shows an increased risk of SGA and stillbirth in patients with IBD [15]. Although some population-based studies and a meta-analysis suggest that UC may be associated with congenital anomalies, specifically limb deficiencies, obstructive urinary abnormalities, and multiple anomalies, these findings have not been replicated in other studies [8,10,82,84]. Similar to Crohn's disease, increased disease activity in pregnancy may be associated with worse pregnancy outcomes [8,22]. The presence of an IPAA does not confer additional fetal morbidity or mortality [79].

Pregnancy Considerations

Effect of Pregnancy on UC

Pregnant women with UC are just as likely to flare as non-pregnant women [85]. Pregnancy may result in fewer relapses in the years following delivery in women with UC [19,20].

In women with an IPAA, there may be transient worsening of pouch function during the pregnancy, but long-term function is preserved regardless of mode of delivery. Additionally, long-term pouch function in women who have had a vaginal delivery is similar to women who did not have a delivery following IPAA [79,86].

Effect of UC on Pregnancy

See section titled "Complications: Fetal."

Management

General Principles

Management of a pregnant woman with UC is best done in partnership with a gastroenterologist. The general principles for management of pregnant patients with UC are similar to management principles in women with CD.

Workup

See section titled "Workup" described earlier for CD.

Differential Diagnosis

Infectious diarrhea (bacterial, fungal, viral, or protozoan), diverticulitis, ischemic colitis, solitary rectal ulcer syndrome, NSAID-related colitis.

Preconception Counseling

- Women should be encouraged to optimize their medical management before conception and optimize nutritional status (see section titled "Crohn's Disease").
- Discontinue known teratogenic drugs. Women on methotrexate should wait three to six months after discontinuation before attempting pregnancy. Women on sulfasalazine should take 2 mg folic acid daily at least one month prior to conceiving and through the pregnancy.
- **Women should be up to date on relevant cancer screening as advised by their gastroenterologist.**

- CBC, folate, vitamin B_{12}, and iron should be assessed and appropriate replacement initiated if indicated [27].
- Counsel on the risk of inheritance of UC. The risk is estimated at 1.6% if the mother has UC and 36% if both have IBD [16].
- Review of vaccination history is important. Women on immunosuppressants should be immunized against influenza and pneumococcal infections. Under appropriate circumstances, they should also receive tetanus and meningococcal vaccines [24].

Prenatal Care

The pregnancy should be managed in partnership with a gastroenterologist. Although the data are conflicting regarding the increased risk of congenital anomalies, a careful anatomical survey is recommended. Serial growth surveillance can be considered, particularly in women with active disease. There is no evidence to support antenatal testing, but it may be considered in women with active disease.

Therapy

Treatment for ulcerative colitis is individualized based on disease severity and extent of colic involvement.

Pharmacological therapy. Many of the medications used to maintain remission or treat acute relapses are similar to the medications used in CD. See section titled "Therapy" (under CD) and Table 11.3. A meta-analysis showed Curcumin, an anti-inflammatory agent, to be successful in maintaining remission in nonpregnant patients with UC. Data regarding use and safety in pregnancy is lacking [87].

Surgery. Despite medical management, some women, particularly those with severe disease activity, may develop fulminant disease, necessitating operative intervention. The likelihood of colectomy depends on disease severity and presence of deep colonic ulcerations on admission [78]. Urgent or emergent surgery typically involves a subtotal colectomy with a temporary ileostomy without removal of the rectal stump. Subsequent IPAA and ileostomy closure is performed when the patient recovers. Proctocolectomy with IPAA is the standard of care for elective surgery [78]. Even when a surgical intervention for UC is performed in the third trimester, cesarean section should be reserved for obstetric indications [87].

Colectomy. Absolute indications for surgery are exsanguinating hemorrhage, perforation, and documented/strongly suspected carcinoma [4,24]. Other indications include severe fulminant colitis with or without toxic megacolon unresponsive to maximal medical therapy [24,78]. There are no prospective randomized trials comparing medical with surgical treatment efficacy for any indication in UC.

Historically, colectomy in pregnancy for fulminant UC has been associated with a high fetal mortality rate (49%) and concerning maternal mortality rate (22%) [88]. However, a more recent case series of women with fulminant UC undergoing total colectomy demonstrated no maternal or fetal mortality, which is consistent with other series published after 1987 [89].

Ileal Pouch–Anal Anastomosis

This is the most commonly performed procedure for UC. It involves resection of the large intestine and creation of an ileal J-pouch, which is attached to a rectal muscle cuff. It helps patients maintain their quality of life after colectomy because it maintains intestinal continuity and the function of defecation. IPAA is considered curative for UC.

However, recent data suggest that the risk of infertility in women with UC increases threefold after IPAA.

Antepartum Testing

There is no literature to base a recommendation for antenatal testing. However, antenatal testing may be considered in women with active disease.

Delivery

Similar to CD, mode of delivery should be dictated by obstetric indication. A vaginal delivery is considered safe for women with an IPAA [65,79]. As in the case of a woman with CD, thromboprophylaxis (e.g., with low-molecular-weight heparin) should be considered in women with UC.

Postpartum/Breast-Feeding

Breast-feeding may have a protective effect on the disease course of UC [64].

REFERENCES

1. Friedman S, Blumberg RS. Inflammatory bowel disease. In: Fauci AS, Braunwald E, Kasper DL et al. *Harrison's Principles of Internal Medicine*. 17th ed. Available at http://www.access medicine.com/content.aspx?aID=2883197. [Review]
2. Hill I, Clark A, Scott NA. Surgical treatment of acute manifestations of Crohn's disease during pregnancy. *J R Soc Med* 1997; 90: 64–6. [II-3]
3. Lichtenstein GR, Hanauer SB, Sandborn MD, and the Practice Parameters Committee of the American College of Gastroenterology. Management of Crohn's disease in adults. *Am J Gastroenterol* 2009; 104(2): 465–83. [III]
4. Baumgart DC, Sandborn W. Crohn's disease. *Lancet* 2012; 380: 1590–605. [III]
5. Carter MJ, Lobo AJ, Travis SPL, on behalf of the IBS Section of the British Society of Gastroenterology. Guidelines for the management of inflammatory bowel disease in adults. *Gut* 2004; 53(suppl. V): v1–16. doi:10.1136/gut.2004.043372. [III]
6. Mayberry JF, Weterman IT. European survey of fertility and pregnancy in women with Crohn's disease: A case control study by European Collaborative Group. *Gut* 1986; 27: 821–5. [II-2]
7. Mahadevan U, Sandborn WJ, Li DK et al. Pregnancy outcomes in women with inflammatory bowel disease: A large community-based study from Northern California. *Gastroenterology* 2007; 133(4): 1106–12. [II-2]
8. Boyd HA, Basit S, Harpsøe et al. Inflammatory bowel disease and risk of adverse pregnancy outcomes. *PLoS One* 2015 Jun 17; 10(6): e0129567. doi:10.1371/journal.pone.0129567. [II-2]
9. Bortoli A, Pedersen N, Duricova D et al. Pregnancy outcome in inflammatory bowel disease: Prospective European case-control ECCO–EpiCom study, 2003–2006. *Aliment Phrmacol Ther* 2011; 34: 724–34. [II-2]
10. Cornish J, Tan E, Teare J et al. A meta-analysis on the influence of inflammatory bowel disease on pregnancy. *Gut* 2007; 56: 830–7. doi:10.1136/gut.2006.108324. [II-2]
11. Fonager K, Sorenson HT, Olsen J et al. Pregnancy outcome for women with Crohn's disease: A follow-up study based on linkage between national registries. *Am J Gastroenterol* 1998; 93(12): 2426–30. [II-2]
12. Kornfeld D, Cnattingius S, Ekbom A. Pregnancy outcomes in women with inflammatory bowel disease—A population-based cohort study. *Am J Obstet Gynecol* 1997; 177(4): 942–6. [II-2]
13. Baird DD, Narendranathan M, Sandler RS. Increased risk of preterm birth for women with inflammatory bowel disease. *Gastroenterology* 1990; 99: 987–94. [II-2]
14. Reddy D, Murphy SJ, Kane SV et al. Relapses of inflammatory bowel disease during pregnancy: In hospital management and birth outcomes. *Am J Gastroenterol* 2008; 103: 1203–9. [II-2]
15. O'Toole A, Nwanne O, Tomlinson T. Inflammatory bowel disease increases risk of adverse pregnancy outcomes: A meta-analysis. *Dig Dis Sci* 2015; 60: 2750–61. [I]
16. Mahadevan U. Pregnancy and inflammatory bowel disease. *Med Clin North Am* 2010; 94: 53–73. [III]
17. Nielsen OH, Andreasson B, Bondesen S et al. Pregnancy in Crohn's disease. *Scand J Gastroenterol* 1984; 19(6): 724–32. [II-2]
18. Agret F, Cosnes J, Hassani Z et al. Impact of pregnancy on the clinical activity of Crohn's disease. *Aliment Pharmacol Ther* 2005; 21(5): 509–13. [II-3]
19. Castlglione F, Pignata S, Morace F et al. Effect of pregnancy on the clinical course of a cohort of women with inflammatory bowel disease. *Ital J Gastroenterol* 1996; 28(4): 199–204. [II-2]
20. Riis L, Vind I, Politi P et al. Does pregnancy change the disease course? A study in a European cohort of patients with inflammatory bowel disease. *Am J Gastroenterol* 2006; 101(7): 1539–45. [II-2]
21. Dubinsky M, Abraham B, Mahadevan U. Management of the pregnant IBD patient. *Inflamm Bowel Dis* 2008; 14(12): 1736–50. [III]
22. Bröms G, Granath F, Linder M et al. Birth outcomes in women with inflammatory bowel disease: Effects of disease activity and drug exposure. *Inflamm Bowel Dis* 2014; 20: 1091–8. [II-2]
23. Mottet C, Luillerat, Gonvers J et al. Pregnancy and Crohn's disease. *Digestion* 2005; 71: 54–61. [III]
24. Kornbluth A, Sachar DB, and The Practice Parameters Committee of the American College of Gastroenterology. Ulcerative colitis practice guidelines in adults: American College of Gastroenterology, Practice Parameters Committee. *Am J Gastroenterol* 2010; 105(3): 501–23. doi:10.1038/ajg.2009.727; published online January 12, 2010. [III]
25. Rogers RG, Katz VL. Course of Crohn's disease during pregnancy and its effect on pregnancy outcome: A retrospective review. *Am J Perinatol* 1995; 12: 262–4. [II-3]
26. Abhyankar A, Ham M, Moss AC. Meta-analysis: The impact of disease activity at conception on disease activity during pregnancy in patients with inflammatory bowel disease. *Aliment Pharmacol Ther* 2013; 38(5): 460–6. [I]
27. Mahadevan U, Matro R. Care of the pregnant patient with inflammatory bowel disease. *Obstet Gynecol* 2015; 126: 401–12. [III]
28. Faculty of Sexual and Reproductive Healthcare Clinical Guidance. *Sexual and reproductive health for individuals with inflammatory bowel disease: Clinical effectiveness unit*, June 2009. [III]
29. National Association for Colitis and Crohn's Disease. *Pregnancy and IBD* (NACC Information Sheet). 2008. Available at http://nacc.org.uk/downloads/factsheets/Pregnancy.pdf. Accessed March 2, 2009. [III]
30. Rahimi R, Nikfar S, Rezaie A et al. Pregnancy outcome in women with inflammatory bowel disease following exposure to 5-aminosalicylic acid drugs: A meta-analysis. *Reprod Toxicol* 2008; 25: 271–5. [II-l]
31. Mogadam M, Dobbin WO III, Korelitz BI et al. Pregnancy in inflammatory bowel disease: Effect of sulfasalazine and corticosteroids on fetal outcome. *Gastroenterology* 1981; 80(l): 72–6. [II-3]
32. Norgard B, Czeizel AE, Rockenbauer M et al. Population-based case control study of the safety of sulfasalazine use during pregnancy. *Aliment Pharmacol Ther* 2001; 15(4): 483–6. [II-2]
33. Diav-Citrin O, Park YH, Veerasuntharam G et al. The safety of mesalamine in human pregnancy: A prospective controlled cohort study. *Gastroenterology* 1998; 114: 23–8. [II-2]
34. Martineau P, Tennenbaum R, Elefant E et al. Foetal outcome in women with inflammatory bowel disease treated during pregnancy with oral mesalamine microgranules. *Aliment Pharmacol Ther* 1998; 12(11): 1101–8. [II-3]

35. Pearson DC, May GR, Fick G et al. Azathioprine for maintaining remission of Crohn's disease. *Cochrane Database Syst Rev* 2000: CD000067. [I]

36. Gisbert JP, Linares PM, McNicholl AG et al. Meta-analysis: The efficacy of azathioprine and mercaptopurine in ulcerative colitis. *Aliment Pharmcol Ther* 2009; 30: 126–37. [II-I]

37. Present DH, Meltzer SJ, Krumholz MP et al. 6-Mercaptopurine in the management of inflammatory bowel disease: short- and long-term toxicity. *Ann Intern Med* 1989; 111: 641–9. [II-3]

38. Alstead EM. Fertility and pregnancy in inflammatory bowel syndrome. *World J Gastroenterol* 2001; 7: 455–9. [III]

39. Alstead EM. Inflammatory bowel disease in pregnancy. *Postgrad Med I* 2002; 78: 23–6. [III]

40. Francella A, Dyan A, Dosian C et al. The safety of 6-mercaptopurine for childbearing patients with inflammatory bowel disease: A retrospective cohort study. *Gastroenterology* 2003; 124: 9–17. [II-2]

41. Moskovitz DN, Bodian C, Chapman ML et al. The effect on the fetus of medications used to treat inflammatory bowel disease patients. *Am J Gastroenterol* 2004; 99: 656–61. [II-3]

42. Polifka JE, Friedman JM. Teratogen update: Azathioprine and 6-mercaptopurine. *Teratology* 2002; 65: 240–61. [III]

43. Langagergaard V, Pedersen L, Gislum M et al. Birth outcome in women treated with azathioprine or mercaptopurine during pregnancy: A Danish nationwide cohort study. *Aliment Pharmacol Ther* 2007; 25: 73–81. [II-2]

44. Mozaffari S, Abdolghaffari, NS et al. Pregnancy outcomes in women with inflammatory bowel disease following exposure to thiopurines and anti-tumor necrosis factor drugs: A systematic review with meta-analysis. *Hum Exp Toxicol* 2015; 34(5): 445–59. [I]

45. Zlatanic J, Korelitz BI, Rajapakse R et al. Complications of pregnancy and child development after cessation of treatment with 6-mercaptopurinefor inflammatory bowel disease. *J Clin Gastroenterol* 2003; 36(4): 303–9. [II-3]

46. Moretti ME, Verjee Z, Ito S et al. Breast feeding during maternal use of azathioprine. *Ann Pharmcother* 2006; 40: 2269–72. [II-3]

47. Sau A, Clarke S, Bass J et al. Azathioprine and breastfeeding: Is it safe? *BJOG* 2007; 114: 498–501. [II-3]

48. Christensen LA, Dahlerup JF, Nielsen MJ et al. Azathioprine treatment during lactation. *Aliment Pharmacol Ther* 2008; 28: 1209–13. [II-3]

49. Armenti VT, Ahlswede KM, Ahlswede BA et al. National Transplant Pregnancy Registry—Outcomes of 154 pregnancies in cyclosporine-treated female kidney transplant recipients. *Transplantation* 1994; 57: 502–6. [II-3]

50. Armenti VT, Radomski JS, Moritz MJ et al. Report from the National Transplantation Pregnancy Registry (NTPR): Outcomes of pregnancy after transplantation. *Clin Transpl* 2005; 69–83. [II-3]

51. Bar Oz B, Hackman R, Einarson T et al. Pregnancy outcome after cyclosporine therapy during pregnancy: A meta-analysis. *Transplantation* 2001; 71: 1051–5. [II-I]

52. American Academy of Pediatrics Committee on Drugs. Transfer of drugs and other chemicals into human milk. *Pediatrics* 2001; 108: 776–89. [III]

53. Sifontis NM, Coscia LA, Constatinescu S et al. Pregnancy outcomes in solid organ transplant recipients with exposure to mycophenolate mofetil or sirolimus. *Transplantation* 2006; 82: 1698–702. [II-3]

54. Hanauer SB, Feagan BG, Lichtenstein GR et al. Maintenance infliximab for Crohn's disease: The ACCENT I randomized trial. *Lancet* 2002; 359: 1541–9. [I]

55. Rutgeerts P, Sandborn WJ, Feagan BG et al. Infliximab for induction and maintenance therapy for ulcerative colitis. *N Engl J Med* 2005; 353: 2462–76. [II-I]

56. Gisbert JP, Gonzalez-Lama J, Mate J. Infliximab therapy in ulcerative colitis: Systematic review and meta-analysis. *Aliment Pharmacol Ther* 2007; 25: 19–37. [II-I]

57. O'Donnell S, O'Morain C. Review article: Use of antitumour necrosis factor therapy in inflammatory bowel disease during pregnancy and conception. *Aliment Pharmacol Ther* 2008; 27: 885–94. [III]

58. Lichtenstein GR, Feagan BG, Cohen RD et al. Serious infections and mortality in association with therapies for Crohn's disease: TREAT registry. *Clin Gastroenterol Hepatol* 2006; 4: 621–30. [II-3]

59. Mahadevan U, Kane SV, Sandborn WJ et al. Intentional infliximab use during pregnancy for induction or maintenance of remission in Crohn's disease. *Aliment Pharmacol Ther* 2005; 21: 733–8. [II-3]

60. Katz JA, Antoni C, Keenan GF et al. Outcome of pregnancy in women receiving infliximab for the treatment of Crohn's disease and rheumatoid arthritis. *Am J Gastroenterol* 2004; 99: 2385–92. [II-2]

61. Narula N, Raed A, Dhillon A et al. Anti-TNFa therapies are safe during pregnancy in women with inflammatory bowel disease: A systematic review and meta-analysis. *Inflamm Bowel Dis* 2014; 20: 1862–9. [I]

62. Zelinkova Z, de Haar C, de Ridder L et al. High intrauterine exposure to infliximab following maternal anti-TNF treatment during pregnancy. *Aliment Pharmacol Ther* 2011; 33(9): 1053–8. [II-3]

63. Vasiliauskas ED, Church JA, Silverman N et al. Case report: Evidence for transplacental transfer of maternally administered infliximab to the newborn. *Clin Gastroenterol Hepatol* 2006; 4(10): 1255–8. [II-3]

64. Friedman S, Regueiro MD. Pregnancy and nursing in inflammatory bowel disease. *Gastroenterol Clin North Am* 2002; 31(1): 265–73, xii. [III]

65. Hou JK, Mahadevan U. A 24-year-old woman with inflammatory bowel disease. *Clin Gastroenterol Herpatol* 2009; 7: 944–7. [II-3]

66. Mahadevan U. Fertility and pregnancy in the patient with inflammatory bowel disease. *Gut* 2006; 55: 1198–206. [III]

67. Vesga L, Terdiman JP, Mahadevan U. Adalimumab use in pregnancy. *Gut* 2005; 54: 890. [II-3]

68. Mishkin DS, Van Deinse W, Becker JM et al. Successful use of adalimumab (Humira) for Crohn's disease in pregnancy. *Inflamm Bowel Dis* 2006; 12(8): 827–8. [II-3]

69. Cristiano L, Friend S, Bozie C et al. Evaluation of pregnancy outcomes from the Tysabri (natalizumab) Pregnancy Exposure Registry [abstract]. *Neurology* 2013; 80: P02.127. [III]

70. Ehrenpreis ED, Kane SV, Cohen LB et al. Thalidomide therapy for patients with refractory Crohn's disease: An open label trial. *Gastroenterology* 1999; 117(6): 1271–7. [II-3]

71. Segal D, MacDonald JK, Chande N. Low dose Naltrexone for induction of remission in Crohn's disease. *Cochrane Database Syst Rev* 2014 Feb 21; 2: CD010410. doi:10.1002/14651858.CD010410.pub2. [I]

72. Ilnyckyji A, Blanchard JF, Rawsthrone P et al. Perianal Crohn's disease and pregnancy: Role of mode of delivery. *Am J Gastroenterol* 1999; 94(ll): 3274–8. [II-2]

73. Brandt LJ, Estabrook SG, Reinus JF. Results of a survey to evaluate whether vaginal delivery and episiotomy lead to perineal involvement in women with Crohn's disease. *Am J Gastroenterol* 1995; 90: 1918–22. [II-3]

74. Bruce A, Black M, Bhattacharya S. Mode of delivery and risk of inflammatory bowel disease in the offspring: A systematic review and meta-analysis of observational studies. *Inflamm Bowel Dis* 2014; 20(7): 1217–26. [I]

75. Royal College of Obstetricians and Gynaecologists. *Reducing the risk of thrombosis and embolism during pregnancy and the puerperium.* Green-top Guideline No. 37, 2009. [III]

76. Moffatt DC, Ilnyckyj A, Bernstein CN. A population-based study of breastfeeding in inflammatory bowel disease: Initiation, duration, and effect on disease in the postpartum period. *Am J Gastroenterol* 2009; 104(10): 2517–23. [II-2]

77. Klement E, Cohen RV, Boxman J et al. Breastfeeding and risk of inflammatory bowel disease: A systematic review with meta-analysis. *Am J Clin Nutr* 2004; 80: 1342–52. [I]

78. Ordás I, Eckmann L, Talamini M et al. Ulcerative colitis. *Lancet* 2012; 380: 1606–19. [III]

79. McLeod RS. Ileal pouch anal anastomosis: Pregnancy—Before, during and after. *J Gastrointest Surg* 2008; 12(12): 2150–2. [III]

80. Seligman N, Sbar W, Berghella V. Pouch function and gastrointestinal complications during pregnancy after ileal pouch-anal anastomosis. *J Matern Fetal Neonatal Med* 2011; 24(3): 525–30. [II-3]

81. Norgard B, Fonager K, Sorenson HT et al. Birth outcomes of women with ulcerative colitis: A nationwide Danish cohort study. *Am J Gastroenterol* 2000; 95(11): 3165–70. [II-3]

82. Dominitz JA, Young JC, Boyko EJ. Outcomes of infants born to mothers with inflammatory bowel disease: A population-based cohort study. *Am J Gastroenterol* 2002; 97(3): 641–8. [II-2]

83. Molnar T, Farkas K, Nagy F et al. Pregnancy outcome in patients with inflammatory bowel disease according to the activity of the disease and the medical treatment: A case-control study. *Scand J Gastroenterol* 2010; 45(11): 1302–6. [II-2]

84. Norgard B, Puho E, Pedersen L et al. Risk of congenital abnormalities in children born to women with ulcerative colitis: A population-based, case-control study. *Am J Gastroenterol* 2003; 98(9): 2006–10. [II-2]

85. Nielson OH, Andreasson B, Bondeson S et al. Pregnancy in ulcerative colitis. *Scand J Gastroentol* 1983; 18(6): 735–42. [II-3]

86. Ravid A, Richard CS, Spencer LM et al. Pregnancy, delivery and pouch function after ileal pouch-anal anastomosis for ulcerative colitis. *Dis Colon Rectum* 2002; 45: 1283–8. [II-3]

87. Garg S, Ahuja V, Sankar JM et al. Curcumin for maintenance of remission in ulcerative colitis. *Cochrane Database Syst Rev* 2012 Oct 17; 10: CD008424. doi:10.1002/14651858.CD008424.pub2. [I]

88. Dozois EJ, Wolff BG, Tremaine WJ et al. Maternal and fetal outcome after colectomy for fulminant ulcerative colitis during pregnancy: Case series and literature review. *Dis Colon Rectum* 2005; 49: 64–73. [II-3]

89. Illnyckyj A. Surgical treatment of inflammatory bowel diseases and pregnancy. *Best Pract Res Clin Gastroenterol* 2007; 21(5): 819–34. [III]

12

Gallbladder disease

Priyadarshini Koduri

KEY POINTS

- Symptomatic gallstones are common in pregnant women, but acute cholecystitis is uncommon.
- **Pregnancy and the postpartum period increase the risk of gallstones and acute cholecystitis.**
- Biliary colic is the most common symptom associated with gallstones.
- Acute cholecystitis can be differentiated from biliary colic based on constant right upper quadrant or epigastric pain, Murphy's sign, and evidence of inflammation with systemic signs.
- Diagnosis of cholelithiasis or acute cholecystitis is based on characteristic signs, symptoms, and ultrasonographic findings.
- Acute cholecystitis is associated with significant maternal and fetal risks.
- In cases of biliary colic and acute cholecystitis failing a brief period (about 24 hours) of conservative management, laparoscopic surgery should not be delayed, following similar management to the nonpregnant adult.
- **Of women with acute cholecystitis, 27% fail conservative management and require a cholecystectomy.**
- **Cholecystectomy is unequivocally recommended in women with sepsis, ileus, or perforation.**
- **Endoscopic retrograde cholangiopancreatography (ERCP) and magnetic resonance cholangiopancreatography (MRCP) are considered safe in pregnancy.** Pregnancy is a risk factor for post-ERCP pancreatitis.
- Maternal and fetal outcomes are similar regardless of surgical approach to cholecystectomy. However, **the laparoscopic approach** has inherent surgical advantages, specifically shorter operative times, shorter hospital stays, and fewer operative complications. Surgery is best performed in the second trimester to minimize fetal risks.

CHOLELITHIASIS
Diagnosis/Definition

Presence of gallstones in the gallbladder. A diagnosis of cholelithiasis may be incidental or may be suspected on the basis of classic symptoms with confirmation on ultrasound.

Symptoms

Up to 50% of pregnant women with cholelithiasis are asymptomatic [1]. The most common symptom reported is biliary colic—**recurrent pain in the right upper quadrant or epigastrium** that is sudden in onset and may radiate to the interscapular area or right scapula. Biliary colic results from obstruction of the cystic or common bile duct. The resulting increased intraluminal pressure is unrelieved by repeated gallbladder contractions. Although nausea and vomiting often accompany biliary colic, the common triad of bloating, nausea, and heartburn is only weakly associated with the presence of gallstones [2].

Epidemiology/Incidence

Gallstones are fairly common and are found in up to 20% of women under age 40 in autopsy series [3]. Gallstones have been reported in 7% of nulliparous women and 20% of multiparous women [4]. Biliary sludge, which is a precursor to gallstones, is seen in up to 30% of pregnant women [2]. Gallbladder disease is the second most common indication for nonobstetrical surgery in pregnancy [5]. Increasing physical activity to moderate or vigorous levels did not decrease the incidence of sludge or gallstones in one trial [6].

Etiology/Pathophysiology

Gallstones form by concretion or accretion of normal or abnormal bile constituents. Increased biliary secretion of cholesterol and gallbladder hypomotility contributes to gallstone formation. There are three major types of gallstones: cholesterol, pigment, and mixed. Cholesterol and mixed stones constitute the majority of gallstones seen (80%), and pigment stones constitute the rest [3].

Risk Factors/Associations

Common risk factors for cholelithiasis are listed in Table 12.1. **Pregnancy is associated with an increased risk of cholelithiasis** likely due to decreased gallbladder motility and increased lithogenicity of bile [1,7]. Increased risk for cholelithiasis may remain up to five years postpartum [8]. Although the incidence of gallstones or sludge may increase with advancing gestation, regression in the postpartum period is not uncommon [9–13].

Differential Diagnosis

Acute cholecystitis (should be suspected if fever, chills, tachycardia, or other systemic signs accompany persistent right upper quadrant/epigastric pain), appendicitis, pancreatitis, peptic ulcer disease, pyelonephritis, HELLP syndrome, acute fatty liver disease, or hepatitis.

Complications
Maternal

Cholecystitis, cholangitis, choledocholithiasis, pancreatitis, or ileus.

Fetal

No reports suggest an increased fetal risk associated with biliary colic or the presence of gallstones.

Table 12.1   Risk Factors for Cholelithiasis

Cholesterol and mixed gallstones
    Race/Ethnicity: North American Indians, Hispanics
    Obesity
    Rapid weight loss (e.g., post gastric bypass)
    Female sex hormones (e.g., oral contraceptive pills)
    Ileal resection
    Advancing age
    Gallbladder hypomotility
    Diet: High calorie, high fat
Pigment stones
    Ethnicity: Asian
    Chronic hemolysis
    Alcoholic cirrhosis
    Chronic biliary tract infection, parasitic infection

Management

Principles
Conservative management may be an option at least initially in an attempt to avoid surgery. However, more recent evidence suggests having a **lower threshold for surgical intervention given the safety of the laparoscopic approach** and potentially improved fetal outcomes particularly in the second trimester [4,14,15]. Retrospective and survey-based studies suggest that conservative management of symptomatic cholelithiasis is associated with an increased symptom recurrence, hospitalizations, and emergency room visits [16–18].

Workup
Laboratory investigations. Blood count, transaminases, total bilirubin, serum amylase, and lipase.

    Imaging. **Ultrasound is the most useful and sensitive test** for detecting sludge and gallstones even as small as 2 mm [3,19]. Classic sonographic findings suggestive of gallstones include acoustic shadowing of opacities in the gallbladder lumen that change with the patient's position. The false negative and false positive rates for ultrasound in gallstone patients are estimated at 2% to 4% [3].

Therapy
All pregnant women with symptomatic cholelithiasis should be admitted to the hospital for observation. Although it is generally accepted that women without systemic symptoms should be conservatively managed initially in an effort to avoid surgery, this view was challenged in a retrospective review of 58 pregnant women with gallbladder disease, excluding those with acute cholecystitis [20]. **Compared to women surgically managed, women who were conservatively managed had twice the rate of obstetric complications.** However, this difference was not statistically significant and the obstetric complications were not directly linked to gallbladder disease.

    Conservative management should be attempted initially for about 24 hours. This typically includes bowel rest with NPO, intravenous hydration, and use of opioid analgesics. Surgical consultation should be obtained. **Indications for surgical management in symptomatic women without acute cholecystitis include worsening of symptoms, inability to tolerate oral intake, increasing abdominal tenderness, and patient preference.**

Pregnancy Considerations
Biliary colic alone does not appear to increase the risk of adverse obstetric outcome.

Labor and Delivery Issues
Mode of delivery is not impacted by the presence of gallstones. Cesarean section should be performed for obstetric indications.

ACUTE CHOLECYSTITIS
Diagnosis/Definition
Acute cholecystitis is inflammation of the gallbladder. A diagnosis of acute cholecystitis should be made on the basis of characteristic history and physical examination (Figure 12.1). Murphy's sign is a physical examination finding of increased abdominal rigidity on inspiration and right upper quadrant tenderness. This sign is pathognomonic for acute cholecystitis but may not always be present on exam, depending on gestational age and body habitus.

Classification
Table 12.2 summarizes criteria used to grade the severity of acute cholecystitis [21].

Persistent right upper quadrant pain

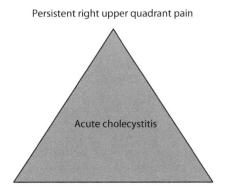

Right upper quadrant tenderness
(with or without Murphy's sign)

Inflammatory response
(indicated by symptoms and labs)

Figure 12.1   Diagnosing acute cholecystitis.

Table 12.2 Grading Severity of Acute Cholecystitis

Grade I (mild)
Acute cholecystitis in otherwise healthy patient with mild local inflammatory changes and without organ dysfunction
Criteria for Grade II or III not met

Grade II (moderate) – any one of the following characteristics
Leukocytosis (>18 cells per mm^3)
Palpable, tender mass in right upper quadrant
Symptom duration >72 hours
Marked local inflammation (gangrenous or emphysematous cholecystitis, pericholecystic or hepatic abscess, biliary peritonitis

Grade III (severe) – organ dysfunction in any one of the following systems
Cardiovascular: Hypotension requiring administration of ≥5 μg/kg/min of dopamine or any dose of norepinephrine
Neurologic: Decreased level of consciousness
Respiratory PaO$_2$:FiO$_2$ <300
Renal: Oliguria or Creatinine >2.0 mg/dL
Hepatic: INR >1.5
Hematologic: Platelet count <100,000/mm^3

Source: Adapted from Baron TH, Grimm IS, Swanstrom LL. *NEJM*, 373, 357–65, 2015.

Symptoms

Symptoms suggestive of acute cholecystitis are similar in the pregnant and nonpregnant state. **Common signs and symptoms include constant right upper quadrant pain or tenderness, fever, tachycardia, leukocytosis, anorexia, nausea, vomiting, and inability to tolerate oral intake.** Jaundice and signs consistent with peritonitis may also be present. In women with superimposed bacterial infection, sepsis may also be apparent.

Epidemiology/Incidence

Although cholelithiasis is fairly common in pregnancy, acute cholecystitis is relatively uncommon. It is estimated to complicate 0.1% of all pregnancies [22].

Risk Factors/Associations

See section titled "Cholelithiasis."

Complications

Maternal
Sepsis, cholangitis, pancreatitis, empyema of the gallbladder, gangrene and perforation, fistula formation, gallstone ileus, porcelain gallbladder with associated increased risk of gallbladder cancer.

Fetal
Fetal death (7% in women treated conservatively vs. 2% in women treated with laparoscopic cholecystectomy) [14], preterm delivery (3.5% in women treated conservatively vs. 6% in women treated surgically) [23], first-trimester miscarriage.

Etiology/Pathogenesis

The majority of cases of acute cholecystitis result from obstruction of the cystic duct by gallstones [2,24]. Inflammation of the gallbladder results from three factors: mechanical inflammation from increased intraluminal pressure, resulting in ischemia of the gallbladder wall and mucosa; chemical inflammation from release of tissue factors; and bacterial inflammation. Bacterial inflammation may play a role in 20% of all patients with acute cholecystitis [24]. Characteristic bacteria involved include *Escherichia coli*, *Klebsiella*, *Streptococcus faecalis*, *Staphylococcus*, and *Clostridium* [3,24].

Pregnancy Considerations

Principles
The appropriate and optimal management of pregnant women with acute cholecystitis remains controversial. Risks of conservative management include risk to the fetus from recurrent relapses, malnutrition, and other complications that may result from complicated gallbladder disease. However, surgery is not without maternal or fetal risk either. Management decisions for the pregnant woman with acute cholecystitis should be made in conjunction with a general surgeon to ensure optimal management for both mother and fetus.

Workup
Laboratory investigations. Complete blood count, transaminases, total bilirubin, alkaline phosphatase, serum amylase, and lipase.

Imaging. **Ultrasound is the image modality of choice in pregnancy for diagnosing cholecystitis.** Classic sonographic findings suggestive of acute cholecystitis are similar in pregnant and nonpregnant women. They include a thickened gallbladder wall (>3–5 mm), pericholecystic fluid, gallstones, and a sonographic Murphy's sign [2,21].

However, ultrasound is insensitive in diagnosing choledocholithiasis (presence of an obstructing gallstone in the common bile duct). If choledocholithiasis is suspected on the basis of a dilated biliary tree, abnormal liver tests or pancreatitis, further diagnostic modalities should be employed, namely MRCP or ERCP.

MRCP: Considering the safety of MRI in pregnancy, **MRCP is likely safe in pregnancy**. MRCP and ERCP have been shown to have similar diagnostic accuracy for choledocholithiasis in the nonpregnant population [25]. Nonetheless, there are no clear guidelines for use of MRCP in pregnancy. In doses several times the human dose, paramagnetic contrast agents have been associated with fetal abnormalities and increased risk of miscarriage in animals [26,27]. Safety of contrast agents during breast-feeding remains unknown.

ERCP: **ERCP followed by sphincterotomy and stone extraction is now the most common treatment modality for symptomatic choledocholithiasis.** In cases of acute cholecystitis, a cholecystectomy may be performed after an ERCP to prevent recurrence of obstruction. Several small retrospective studies support the **safety of ERCP** in pregnancy [28–35]. A large retrospective matched-cohort study showed that ERCP-associated complications of perforation, cholecystitis, and postsphincterotomy hemorrhage were rare in both pregnant and nonpregnant women [36]. However, pregnant women were found to have a significantly higher incidence of post-ERCP pancreatitis compared to nonpregnant women (12% vs. 5%, $P < 0.001$). Pregnancy complications were rare, and rates of maternal mortality, fetal distress, and fetal loss were comparable to national averages [36]. Interestingly, pregnant women post-ERCP had lower rates of preterm labor compared to the national average [36]. ERCP is best performed in the second trimester to minimize obstetric risks [29]. Fetal radiation exposure during an ERCP can vary depending on procedure time and fluoroscopy time. Although there is a correlation between fluoroscopy time and fetal radiation exposure, this relationship is not entirely linear [34]. In a series of 17 patients undergoing ERCP, fetal radiation doses were <200 mrad when fluoroscopy time was limited to less than one minute [34]. **Effort should be made to minimize fluoroscopy time, using shielding under the pelvis and over the lower part of the abdomen.** Modifying techniques to minimize fluoroscopy time have successfully been used to decrease fetal radiation exposure to negligible levels [37]. Nonradiation ERCP has been successfully performed during pregnancy without resultant adverse pregnancy outcomes [38–42]. However, the small number of reported procedures limits conclusions regarding safety of the procedure in pregnancy. Fetal monitoring before and after ERCP is recommended.

Management

All women with suspected acute cholecystitis should be **hospitalized** and a **surgical consultation** should be obtained. If acute cholecystitis is confirmed, conservative management for about 24 hours is a reasonable initial option to avoid surgery. **Conservative therapy typically includes NPO and bowel rest, intravenous hydration, and opioid analgesia.** Broad-spectrum antibiotics should be considered in women with systemic symptoms who do not improve in 12 to 24 hours [2].

The safety and possible efficacy of a short course of indomethacin in the second trimester to attempt to reverse the gallbladder inflammation has been reported [22]. Indomethacin use should be avoided after 32 weeks to avoid premature closure of the ductus arteriosus and oligohydramnios. Although ursodeoxycholic acid is used in nonpregnant women to dissolve gallstones, efficacy for use in pregnancy is uncertain [43].

A **majority of patients (40%–70%) who are treated conservatively relapse during the pregnancy** [4,14]. Approximately 27% of women will fail conservative management and require cholecystectomy [23]. **Definitive surgical therapy is required in pregnant women with sepsis, ileus, or perforation** [2]. Pregnant and nonpregnant women appear to have similar risk of major postoperative morbidity [44].

Laparoscopic vs. Open Cholecystectomy
A systematic review did not find any difference in maternal or fetal morbidity when the open laparoscopic approach was compared to the open approach [23]. A more recent study looking at 664 cholecystectomies performed during pregnancy found that the **laparoscopic approach** was associated with **shorter operative times, shorter length of stay, and fewer postoperative complications** [45]. The laparoscopic approach has been associated with a risk of bile duct injury, but such injury can be prevented by conversion to an open cholecystectomy if dissection is difficult or unsuccessful or the anatomy is difficult to ascertain [21]. The Society of American Gastrointestinal and Endoscopic Surgeons (SAGES) states that **laparoscopic cholecystectomy is the treatment of choice in the pregnant patient with gallbladder disease regardless of trimester** [46]. Ideally, surgery in pregnancy should be performed in the second trimester to minimize fetal risk. However, **laparoscopic cholecystectomy has been safely performed even in the third trimester** [47–50].

Regardless of mode of surgery, the pregnant patient should be placed in the left lateral position to avoid aortocaval compression. Perioperative monitoring should be performed. When the laparoscopic approach is used, care should be taken to avoid high intraperitoneal pressures, using the open technique for umbilical port insertion and using electrocautery away from the uterus. Steroids for fetal lung maturity should be considered between 23 and 33 6/7 weeks. Fetal monitoring before and after surgery is recommended.

Other surgical approaches have been described. There is a more recent technique, called NOTES (natural orifice translumenal endoscopic surgery), in which surgery is performed via a natural occurring orifice. There are no reports of a NOTES cholecystectomy performed during pregnancy. Percutaneous cholecystostomy is an older technique whereby the gallbladder is decompressed with a pigtail catheter placed under ultrasound guidance. It is a helpful management alternative in patients who cannot safely undergo surgery or who have contraindications to anesthesia. However, with the safety and acceptance of laparoscopic cholecystectomy, the role of percutaneous cholecystostomy is not well defined in pregnancy. A case series and observational study suggest that it can be performed safely in all trimesters [51,52]. Peroral endoscopic gallbladder drainage (transmural or transpapillary) has not been described in the pregnant population.

Labor and Delivery Considerations

Acute cholecystitis or history of cholecystectomy during the pregnancy should not impact mode of delivery. Cesarean section should be reserved for obstetric indications.

REFERENCES

1. Ramin KD, Ramsey PS. Disease of the gallbladder and pancreas in pregnancy. *Obstet Gynecol Clin North Am* 2001; 28: 571–80. [HI]
2. Gilo NB, Amini D, Landy HJ. Appendicitis and cholecystitis in pregnancy. *Clin Obstet Gynecol* 2009; 52(4): 586–96. [III]
3. Greenberger NJ, Paumgartner G. Diseases of the gallbladder and bile ducts. In: Fauci AS, Braunwald E, Kasper DL et al. eds. *Harrison's Principles of Internal Medicine.* 15th ed. New York: McGraw-Hill, 2001. [Review]
4. Swisher SG, Schmit PJ, Hunt KK et al. Biliary disease during pregnancy. *Am J Surg* 1994; 168: 576–9. [II-3]
5. Ellington SR, Flowers L, Legardy-Williams JK et al. Recent trends in hepatic diseases during pregnancy in the United States, 2002–2010. *Am J Obstet Gynecol* 2015; 212: 524.e1–7. [II-3]
6. Ko CW, Napolitano PG, Lee SP et al. Physical activity, maternal metabolic measures, and the incidence of gallbladder sludge or stones during pregnancy: A randomized trial. *Am J Perinatol* 2014; 31(1): 39–48. [I, RCT, n = 1196]
7. Everson GT. Gastrointestinal motility in pregnancy. *Gastroenterol Clin North Am* 1992; 21: 751–76. [III]
8. Thijs C, Knipschild P, Leffers P. Pregnancy and gallstone disease: An empiric demonstration of the importance of specification of risk periods. *Am J Epidemiol* 1991; 134: 186–95. [II-2]
9. Maringhini A, Marceno MP, Lanzarone F et al. Sludge and stones in gallbladder after pregnancy. Prevalence and risk factors. *J Hepatol* 1987; 5(2): 218–23. [II-3]
10. Tsimoyiannis EC, Antoniou NC, Tsaboulas C et al. Cholelithiasis during pregnancy and lactation. Prospective study. *Eur J Surg* 1994; 160(11): 627–31. [II-3]
11. Ko CW, Beresford SA, Schulte SJ et al. Incidence, natural history and risk factors for biliary sludge and stones during pregnancy. *Hepatology* 2005; 41: 359–65. [II-3]
12. Basso L, McCollum PT, Darling MR et al. A study of cholelithiasis during pregnancy and its relationship with age, parity, menarche, breastfeeding, dysmenorrhea, oral contraception and a maternal history of cholelithiasis. *Surg Gynecol Obstet* 1992; 175: 41–6. [II-2]

13. Valdivieso V, Covarrubias C, Siegel F et al. Pregnancy and cholelithiasis: Pathogenesis and natural course of gallstones diagnosed in early puerperium. *Hepatology* 1993; 17: 1. [II-3]

14. Jelin EB, Smink DS, Vernon AH et al. Management of biliary tract disease during pregnancy: A decision analysis. *Surg Endosc* 2008; 22: 54–60. [II-3]

15. Barone JE, Bears S, Chen S et al. Outcome study of cholecystectomy during pregnancy. *Am J Surg* 1999; 177(3): 232–6. [II-3]

16. Othman MO, Stone E, Hashimi M et al. Conservative management of cholelithiasis and its complications in pregnancy is associated with recurrent symptoms and more emergency department visits. *Gastrointest Endosc* 2012; 76(3): 564–9. [II-2]

17. Jorge AM, Keswani RN, Veerappan A et al. Non-operative management of symptomatic cholelithiasis in pregnancy is associated with frequent hospitalizations. *J Gastrointest Surg* 2015; 19(4): 598–603. [II-3]

18. Veerappan A, Gawron AJ, Soper NJ et al. Delaying cholecystectomy for complicated gallstone disease in pregnancy is associated with recurrent postpartum symptoms. *J Gastrointest Surg* 2013; 17(11): 1953–9. [II-3]

19. Shea JA, Berlin JA, Escarce JJ et al. Revised estimates of diagnostic test sensitivity and specificity in suspected biliary tract disease. *Arch Intern Med* 1994; 154: 2573–81. [II-3]

20. Dhupar R, Smaldone GM, Hamad GG. Is there a benefit to delaying cholecystectomy for symptomatic gallbladder disease during pregnancy? *Surg Endosc* 2010; 24(1): 108–12. [II-3]

21. Baron TH, Grimm IS, Swanstrom LL. Interventional approaches to gallbladder disease. *NEJM* 2015; 373: 357–65. [III]

22. Dietrich CS, Hill CC, Hueman M. Surgical disease presenting in pregnancy. *Surg Clin North Am* 2008; 88: 408–19. [III]

23. Date RS, Kaushal M, Ramesh A. A review of the management of gallstone disease and its complications in pregnancy. *Am J Surg* 2008; 196(4): 599–608. [III]

24. Indar AA, Beckingham IJ. Acute cholecystitis. *BMJ* 2002; 325: 639–43. [III]

25. Kaltenthaler EC, Walters SJ, Chilcott J et al. MRCP compared to diagnostic ERCP for diagnosis when biliary obstruction is suspected: A systematic review. *BMC Medical Imaging* 2006; 6: 9. [I]

26. American College of Obstetricians and Gynecologists. Guidelines for diagnostic imaging during pregnancy. ACOG Committee Opinion No. 299. *Obstet Gynecol* 2004; 104(3): 647–51. [III]

27. Kanal E, Borgstede JP, Barkovich AJ et al. American College of Radiology White Paper on MR safety: 2004 update and revisions. *Am J Roentgenol* 2004; 182(5): 1111–4. [III]

28. Chong VH, Jalihal A. Endoscopic management of biliary disorders during pregnancy. *Hepatobiliary Pancreat Dis Int* 2010; 9(2): 180–5. [II-3]

29. Al-Hashem H, Muralisharan V, Cohen H et al. Biliary disease in pregnancy with an emphasis on the role of ERCP. *J Clin Gastroenterol* 2009; 43(1): 58–62. [III]

30. Gupta R, Tandan M, Lakhtakia S et al. Safety of therapeutic ERCP in pregnancy—An Indian experience. *Indian J Gastroenterol* 2005; 24: 161–3. [II-3]

31. Jamidar PA, Beck GJ, Hoffman BJ et al. Endoscopic retrograde cholangiopancreatography in pregnancy. *Am J Gastroenterol* 1995; 90: 1263–7. [II-3]

32. Tham TC, Vandervoort J, Wong RC et al. Safety of ERCP during pregnancy. *Am J Gastroenterol* 2003; 98: 308–11. [II-3]

33. Tang SJ, Mayo MJ, Rodriguez-Frias E et al. Safety and utility of ERCP during pregnancy. *Gastrointest Endosc* 2009; 69: 453–61. [II-3]

34. Kahaleh M, Hartwell GD, Arseneau KO et al. Safety and efficacy of ERCP in pregnancy. *Gastrointest Endosc* 2004; 60: 287–92. [II-3]

35. Friedel D, Stavropoulos S, Iqbal S et al. Gastrointestinal endoscopy in the pregnant woman. *World J Gastrointest Endosc* 2014; 6: 156–67. [III]

36. Inamdar S, Berzin TM, Sejpal DV et al. Pregnancy is a risk factor for pancreatitis after endoscopic retrograde cholangiopancreatography in a national cohort study [published online ahead of print May 5, 2015]. *Clin Gastroenterol Hepatol*. doi:10.1016/j.cgh.2015.04.175. [II-2]

37. Smith I, Gaidhane M, Goode A et al. Safety of endoscopic retrograde cholangiopancreatography in pregnancy: Fluoroscopy time and fetal exposure, does it matter? *World J Gastrointest Endosc* 2013; 5(4): 148–53. [III]

38. Wu W, Faigel DO, Sun Gang et al. Non-radiation endoscopic retrograde cholangiopancreatography in the management of choledocholithiasis during pregnancy. *Dig Endosc* 2014; 26: 691–700. [III]

39. Uomo G, Manes G, Picciotto FP et al. Endoscopic treatment of acute biliary pancreatitis in pregnancy. *J Clin Gastroenterol* 1994; 18: 250–2. [II-3]

40. Simmons SC, Tarnasky PR, Rivera-Alsira ME et al. Endoscopic retrograde cholangiopancreatography (ERCP) in pregnancy without the use of radiation. *Am J Obstet Gynecol* 2004; 190: 1467–9. [II-3]

41. Sethi S, Thosani N, Banerjee S. Radiation-free ERCP in pregnancy: A "sound" approach to leaving no stone unturned. *Dig Dis Sci* 2015; 60: 2604–7. [III]

42. Ersoz G, Turan I, Tekin F et al. Nonradiation ERCP with endoscopic biliary sphincterotomy plus papillary balloon dilation for the treatment of choledocholithiasis during pregnancy [published online ahead of print April 4, 2015]. *Surg Endosc*. [III]

43. Ward A, Brogden R, Heel R et al. Ursodeoxycholic acid: A review of its pharmacologic properties and therapeutic efficacy. *Drugs* 1984; 27: 95–131. [III]

44. Silvestri MT, Pettker CM, Brousseau ED et al. Morbidity of appendectomy and cholecystectomy in pregnant and nonpregnant women. *Obstet Gynecol* 2011; 118(6): 1261–70. [II-2]

45. Cox TC, Huntington CR, Blair LJ et al. Laparoscopic appendectomy and cholecystectomy versus open: A study in 1999 pregnant patients [published online ahead of print June 20, 2015]. *Surg Endosc*. [II-2]

46. Pearl J, Price R, Richardson W, Fanelli R; Society of American Gastrointestinal Endoscopic Surgeons. Guidelines for diagnosis, treatment, and use of laparoscopy for surgical problems during pregnancy. *Surg Endosc* 2011; 11: 3479–92. [III]

47. Coelho JC, Vianna RM, da Costa MA et al. Laparoscopic cholecystectomy in the third trimester of pregnancy. *Arq Gastroenterol* 1999; 36: 90–3. [II-3]

48. Eichenberg BJ, Vanderlinden J, Miguel C et al. Laparoscopic cholecystectomy in the third trimester of pregnancy. *Am Surg* 1996; 62: 874–7. [II-3]

49. Sen G, Nagabhushan JS, Joypaul V. Laparoscopic cholecystectomy in the third trimester of pregnancy. *J Obstet Gynaecol* 2002; 22: 556–7. [II-3]

50. Pucci RO, Seed RW. Case report of laparoscopic cholecystetomy in the third trimester of pregnancy. *Am J Obstet Gynecol* 1991; 165: 401–2. [II-3]

51. Allmendinger N, Hallisey MJ, Ohki SK et al. Percutaneous cholecystostomy treatment of acute cholecystitis in pregnancy. *Obstet Gynecol* 1995; 86(4 Pt. 2): 653–4. [III]

52. Chiappetta Porras LT, Nápoli ED, Canullán CM et al. Minimally invasive management of acute biliary tract disease during pregnancy. *HPBSurgery* 2009: 829020. doi:10.1155/2009/829020. [III]

13

Pregnancy after liver and other transplantation

Ignazio R. Marino, Lucio Mandalà, and Augusto Lauro

KEY POINTS

- The best outcomes in pregnancy after liver transplant occur in patients with the following:
  - Good general health ≥1 year since transplant
  - Minimal or no proteinuria (<1 g/24 hours)
  - Creatinine <1.5 mg/dL
  - Well-controlled or no hypertension
  - No evidence of recent graft rejection
  - **Stable immunosuppressive regimen and liver function**
- Potential maternal and fetal complications include **preterm birth, preeclampsia, fetal growth restriction, and low birth weight**.
- Pregnancy in and of itself does not affect previously stable hepatic allograft function.
- The effect of **comorbid conditions (i.e., diabetes, hypertension)** should be considered and their **management optimized**.
- **Transplant recipients should have their baseline kidney function** (creatinine, 24-hour urine collection for total protein) **assessed**.
- Maintenance of current immunosuppression in pregnancy is usually recommended except for **mycophenolic acid products, for which fetal risks should be discussed and alternatives sought**.
- Summary of **management options in Table 13.4**.

PREGNANCY AFTER LIVER TRANSPLANTATION
Introduction and Historic Notes

Since the first human liver transplant performed in 1963 by Thomas Starzl (University of Colorado) [1], many advances in surgical techniques and immunosuppressive therapy have helped to increase the numbers of women who undergo allogenic organ transplantation each year. In 1978, Walcott [2] documented the first known pregnancy in a liver transplant recipient, which resulted in a successful delivery with both mother and infant in excellent health. Many times, a transplanted organ normalizes a woman's hormonal imbalance and restores fertility, thus offering the prospect of pregnancy and providing many women with end-stage organ disease a chance to conceive and bear children. As a result, among liver transplant recipients, a higher survival rate and a return to a good quality of life have been achieved. In 1991, the National Transplantation Pregnancy Registry (NTPR) was established at Thomas Jefferson University in Philadelphia, Pennsylvania, to analyze pregnancy outcomes in solid-organ transplant recipients [3].

Definition/Symptoms and Signs of ESLD

Liver transplantation (LTx): treatment of choice for all non-neoplastic end-stage liver diseases and for selected patients with nonresectable hepatic malignancies.

End-stage liver disease (ESLD): any hepatic disease that jeopardizes the survival or that seriously modifies the quality of life of the patient and for which the transplant is the only therapy because no other medical or surgical treatment exists that is able to provide a reasonable chance of recovery.

Before undergoing LTx, some patients remain in quite good clinical condition. There may be individual variations in terms of hospital care requirements. As the liver disease progresses, symptoms such as encephalopathy, weakness, and lethargy become more frequent. Intractable ascites, GI bleeding, peripheral edema, anorexia, jaundice, pruritus and cholestasis, peritonitis, and pneumonia may also develop. Often the patient is severely malnourished.

Indications

Although **chronic hepatitis C infection** (HCV) represents the leading indication for LTx in the United States, **autoimmune hepatitis** is probably the most frequent reason for transplantation among young female recipients who may become pregnant after transplant [4].

Epidemiology

Approximately one third of all patients who have undergone LTx are women, and about 75% of female recipients are of reproductive age [4]. The incidence indicates that more than 14,000 women of reproductive age are living in the United States after liver transplantation (LTx), and another 500 undergo LTx each year [5].

Pathophysiology

Women with decompensated liver disease commonly have menstrual dysfunction: Infertility is common in women with ESLD because of hypothalamic–pituitary–gonadal dysfunction, which decreased ovulation [6,7] and affects up to 50% of these patients. In fact, menstrual abnormalities may be the first signs of liver disease in females with chronic liver disease. In cirrhotic state, hypothalamic–pituitary dysfunction is associated with an inadequate response to the gonadotropin-releasing hormone agonists and clomiphene citrates as well as diminished gonadotrophin release relative to the reduced levels of circulating sex steroids [8]. Furthermore, serum levels of estradiol and testosterone are increased in patients with porto-systemic shunts. Thus pregnancy in decompensated cirrhosis is very uncommon. A successful transplant almost uniformly leads to a **prompt return to normal menstrual cycles and to reproductive functions** because of the recovery of the gonadotrophic function [8–11]. This is an important component of the restoration of normality of life for patients of childbearing age, and it is evidenced by the increasing number of post-transplantation pregnancies reported worldwide [12–24].

Preconception Counseling and Timing of Pregnancy

Pregnancy after liver transplant should be considered as a high-risk pregnancy and monitored closely by a team of transplant hepatologists and experts in obstetrics and maternal-fetal medicine. Female liver transplant recipients who are planning to become pregnant should be **counseled on contraception and optimal timing of pregnancy, proper vaccinations, and risks associated with immunosuppressive therapy**.

For this reason **an appropriate contraceptive plan should be recommended. Oral contraceptives are relatively contraindicated** in women with liver transplant because of many theoretical complications, such as the risk of thromboembolism, cholestasis, exacerbated hypertension, and interference in cyclosporin metabolism [7]. Although **intrauterine devices** may initially increase the risks of infection especially in immunocompromised women, their use is probably safe and **should be recommended**.

Many medications used for post-transplant immunosuppression have potential effects during pregnancy and breast-feeding. **The risks and benefits of each medication should be reviewed with patients contemplating pregnancy, and regimens should be tailored accordingly** [see below].

Ideally, **patients should be vaccinated prior to transplantation against influenza, pneumococcus, hepatitis B, and tetanus**. Alternatively, they should be vaccinated prepregnancy.

The optimal timing of conception post-transplant is controversial, but current recommendations suggest **waiting for at least one year after transplantation** based on rejection risks and to allow stabilization of allograft function and of immunosuppressive regimen [7–8,20] even though the shortest interval from OLTx to conception reported in the literature is three weeks [24]. Immunosuppressive agents are at their nadir one year post liver transplantation, and thus risk of allograft rejection is low at that time. Furthermore, renal and liver functions tend to stabilize during that period. Thus it is ideal to delay pregnancy until the patient is on a maintenance immunosuppression one to two years after transplantation to **minimize fetal exposure to high doses of immunosuppressants**. When choosing the timing of pregnancy after OLTx, **several factors should be considered**:

a. Good general health ≥1 year since transplant.
   1. Risk of acute graft rejection
   2. Risk of acute infection that might impact the fetus (cytomegalovirus [CMV] acute infection is most common within 6–12 months post-transplant)
b. Proteinuria and creatinine level.
   1. None or minimal proteinuria (<1 g/24 hours)
   2. Serum creatinine <1.5 mg/dL
c. Rejection and immunosuppression.
   1. No evidence of recent graft rejection (in the past year)
   2. Stable immunosuppression regimen (stable dosing)
d. Stable liver function.
   1. Patients with stable liver function generally have a low risk for opportunistic infections
e. Maternal age.
f. Medical noncompliance.

Comorbidity and Risk Factors

The outcome in liver transplant recipients from selected publications is shown in **Table 13.1**. The main comorbidity, risk factors about patient, graft, and fetus complications described in the English literature are also described below.

Hepatitis Virus Reactivation

Even if autoimmune hepatitis is the most frequent reason for transplantation among young female recipients who may become pregnant after transplant, a reactivation of viral hepatitis is considered one of the most serious risks for both mother and child.

For hepatitis B, for example, vertical transmission is reported between 10% and 20% of HBsAg-positive (HBeAg-negative) nontransplant mothers without immunoprophylaxis. It is recommended to vaccinate and give IVIg to all newborns born to HBsAg-positive women within 12 hours of birth as the hepatitis B virus (HBV) neonatal infection risks with these interventions decreases to less than 10% [25] (Chapter 30).

The rate of maternal-fetal HCV transmission in OLTx recipients is still unclear, requiring additional analysis. The vertical infection rate in pregnant HCV RNA-positive subjects is around 3% to 5% (in absence of other viral coinfections) [26]. A well-documented risk factor for HCV vertical transmission is maternal high viral load. Therefore, special attention should be given to patients with high viral load post-transplant (Chapter 31).

Hypertension and Renal Insufficiency

The immunosuppression regimen based on calcineurin inhibitors (cyclosporine and tacrolimus) is associated with an increased incidence of hypertension and renal insufficiency in the post-transplantation population. The pathogenesis is related to endothelial cell dysfunction and decreased endogenous nitric oxide production, causing renal dysfunction and hypertension: The side effect for the post-LTx pregnant women is an increased incidence of preeclampsia [6,21]. The same treatment with **calcium channel blockers** used in the nontransplant population is recommended [27].

Diabetes

The incidence of new-onset diabetes mellitus (NODM) is approximately **15%** among liver transplant recipients [28]. The immunosuppressive therapy plays an important role even if the impact of steroids is controversial. Most of the authors agree to **limit the use of steroids as much as possible and to reduce calcineurin inhibitors** at the minimum needed dose. The management of NODM is essentially similar to that of diabetes in the nontransplant population. NODM is associated with obesity, insulin resistance, insulin secretory defect, and subsequent development of type II diabetes in the offspring. Modern treatment protocols during pregnancy include **strict glycemic control** by a combination of diet and medications (Chapters 4 and 5). Traditionally, insulin therapy has been considered the gold standard for management of diabetes because of its efficacy in achieving better glucose control and the fact that it does not cross the placenta [29].

CMV Acute Infection

CMV infection represents one of the most common types of infection within six to 12 months in the post-transplant population, and it is very dangerous in early pregnancy because it is responsible for congenital malformation (microcephaly, cerebral palsy, sensorineural deafness) or congenital liver disease with an incidence of 10% to 15% of infected pregnancies. It is advisable to **screen all transplant recipients with CMV IgG and IgM**. If IgM positive, avidity testing should

Table 13.1   Fetal and Maternal Outcomes in Liver Transplant Recipients from Selected Studies

Author	No. of Pregnancies	Live Birth Rate (%)	Spontaneous Abortions (%)	Preterm (%)	Graft Dysfunction (%)	Cesarean Rate (%)	Birth Weight <2500 g (%)	Maternal Deaths (%)	Neonatal Deaths (%)
Alvaro E	30	66.6	26.6	NA	10	42	NA	0	6
Armenti VT	205	73	19	35	7	35	34	0	0
Dashpande NA	450	76.9	6.2	39.4	NA	44.6	NA	NA	NA
Christopher V	71	71	19	NA	17	40	20	4	NA
Coffin CS	20	70	5	27	5	38	NA	0	6
Dei Malatesta MF	285	78	NA	31	10	43	23	4	4
Jabiry-Zieniewicz Z	39	100	0	31	8	80	20	0	0
Jain AB	49	100	0	4	25	47	9	10	6
Nagy S	38	63	NA	29	17	46	17	17	0
Sibanda N	16	69	13	50	NA	62	57	NA	NA
Total	1203	76.7	7.95	30.8	12.37	47.76	25.7	4.3	3.1

Source: Adapted from Hammound GM, Almashhrawi AA, Ahmed KT et al. *World J Gastroenterol,* 19, 7647–51, 2013.

be performed (Chapter 47). The use of antiviral agents in the management of CMV infection during pregnancy remains controversial [8] (Chapter 47).

Acute Cellular Rejection

Acute cellular rejection (ACR) rate in the post-LTx pregnancies is reported **between 2% and 8%** [3,8,23] and **occurs during the earlier phases of pregnancy. Immunosuppression therapy should be maintained and monitored during pregnancy by serum levels** as a reduction or discontinuation may lead to rejection of the transplanted organ. **When acute rejection is suspected, an ultrasound-guided percutaneous liver graft biopsy is strongly recommended** and should be associated with a Doppler ultrasound study of the graft in order to exclude anatomic source of graft dysfunction. The ACR treatment includes adjustment of immunosuppressive medications and **use of steroids as antirejection therapy.**

Infrarenal Aortic Graft

One death due to aortic graft clotting by external compression from the gravid uterus has been reported [27]. For this reason, patients with infrarenal aortic graft should be monitored with color Doppler ultrasonography during pregnancy.

Pregnancy Complications (Table 13.1)

Preterm Birth and Low Birth Weight

The risk of prematurity is up to 50%, and the mean gestational age at delivery ranges between 36 and 37 weeks [3–5,20].

Intrauterine Growth Restriction

Intrauterine growth restriction (IUGR) is estimated to occur in about 20% of liver transplant recipients and is associated with perinatal morbidity and mortality (Chapter 45).

Table 13.2 FDA Classification of Risk of Immunosuppressive Drug in Pregnancy

Drugs	Pregnancy Category
Corticosteroids	B
Cyclosporin	C
Sirolimus	C
Tacrolimus	C
Azathioprine	D
Mycophenolate mofetil	D

Table 13.3 Selected Immunosuppressive Agents and Their Side Effects

Immunosuppressant	Side Effect
Prednisone[a]	Glucose intolerance
Azathioprine[a]	Leukopenia
Cyclosporine[a,b]	Hypertension, nephrotoxicity
Tacrolimus[a,b]	Hypertension, nephrotoxicity, neurotoxicity, glucose intolerance, myocardial hypertrophy
Mycophenolate Mofetil	GI disturbance
Sirolimus[a,b]	Leukopenia, thrombocytopenia, hyperlipidemia

[a]There have been no known teratogenic effects.
[b]Follow with blood levels.

Table 13.4 Pregnancy after Liver Transplantation: Management Options

Prepregnancy
- Patients should defer conception for at least one year after transplantation, with adequate contraception.
- Assessment of graft function (organ specific):
  - Recent liver biopsy
  - Proteinuria (24-hour collection for total protein)
  - Hepatitis B and C status (HBsAg; Hep. C Antibody)
  - *CMV, toxoplasmosis, herpes simplex status (IgG, IgM)*
- Maintenance immunosuppression options:
  - Azathioprine
  - Cyclosporine
  - Tacrolimus
  - Corticosteroids
  - *Mycophenolate mofetil (**avoid as feasible**)*
  - *Enteric-coated mycophenolate sodium (**avoid as feasible**)*
  - Sirolimus
- The effect of comorbid conditions, (i.e., diabetes, hypertension) should be considered and their management optimized.
- Vaccinations should be given if needed (i.e., rubella, etc.) (Chapter 38).
- Explore etiology of original disease.
- Discuss genetic issues if relevant.
- Discuss the effect of pregnancy on renal allograft function.
- Discuss the risks of intrauterine growth restriction, preterm birth, low birth weight, etc.

Prenatal
- Pregnancy in and of itself does not affect previously stable allograft function.
- Accurate early diagnosis and dating of pregnancy.
- Baseline laboratory tests should include:
  a. Liver enzymes (ALT and AST)
  b. Creatinine and bilirubin
  c. Immunosuppression medication (e.g., cyclosporine or tacrolimus) level
  d. 24-hour urinary protein and creatinine clearance
  e. Urine analysis and urine culture
  f. CMV, HSV, and Toxoplasma IgM and IgG
  g. HBsAg, HBsAb, HepCAb

Timing of repeat laboratory testing of at least tests a–e should be once every trimester until 32 weeks.
- Fetal surveillance.
- Monitor for hypertension and nephropathy.
- Careful surveillance for preeclampsia.
- Early screening for gestational diabetes.

Labor and delivery
- Vaginal delivery is optimal; cesarean delivery for obstetric reasons.

Post-natal
- Monitor immunosuppressive drug levels for at least one month postpartum, especially if dosages increased during pregnancy.
- Surveillance for rejection with biopsy if it is suspected.
- Breast-feeding discussion.
- Contraception counseling.

Preeclampsia

The incidence of hypertension and preeclampsia is approximately 20% in OLTx recipients and seems to occur mainly in patients taking **cyclosporine**, probably because of the related endothelial cell dysfunction, and less commonly with tacrolimus [3–6,23,27]. The management of preeclampsia is the same as in the nontransplant population (Chapter 1).

Abnormal Blood Chemistry and Liver Function Tests

In most series, **pruritus and cholestasis** seem to be the most frequent symptoms described in pregnancies after LTx. Differential diagnosis with ACR should be considered in all cases. HELLP syndrome and anemia have been reported [5].

Immunosuppression Therapy: Drugs and Their Side Effects

There is no consensus on the optimal maintenance regimen for transplant pregnant recipients. The use of immunosuppressive therapy after liver transplantation is unavoidable even taking into consideration the potential risks of the exposure of infants to immunosuppressive medications. **All immunosuppressive medications cross the placenta** and enter into fetal circulation and could potentially have effects in utero. Despite the fact that immunosuppressive agents such as Azathioprine, Cyclosporine, and Mycophenolic acid were teratogenic in animals, the risk of birth defects was not statistically different between those who received immunosuppressive medications and those who did not. Patients treated with either calcineurin inhibitors (**cyclosporine or tacrolimus**) **should have serial blood tests in pregnancy to follow medication levels** and to assess hepatic and renal function while avoiding unnecessary toxicity. Recent studies have reported an association between administration of **mycophenolic acid products (MPA) [myco-phenolate mofetil (MMF) and enteric-coated mycopheno-late sodium (EC-MPS)]** to transplant recipients and an increased risk of adverse outcomes in pregnancy-like specific pattern of **birth defects**. In 2007, the package inserts of MMF and EC-MPS included a change from pregnancy category C to **category D** [30–33]. The warning states that females of potential childbearing age must use contraception while taking MPA because its use during pregnancy is associated with increased rates of pregnancy loss and congenital malformations. Pregnancy outcomes with exposure to sirolimus remain limited: Reported to the NTPR are three liver recipients with three pregnancies (two live births, one spontaneous abortion) [3]. The Food and Drug Administration (FDA) classification of risk medication and their categories in pregnancy is reported in **Table 13.2**. Selected immunosuppressive drugs and their side effects are reported in **Table 13.3**.

Workup and Management

A summary of the suggested key points is in **Table 13.4**.

In case of elevations of liver function tests and/or bilirubin, an ACR should be ruled out. Evaluation of rejection includes liver ultrasound with Doppler to exclude anatomic sources of graft dysfunction. **Liver biopsy to diagnose rejection is *not* contraindicated in pregnancy.** Because of an increased risk of carbohydrate intolerance caused by the administration of prednisone or tacrolimus, **patients should be screened with glucose tolerance tests in the first trimester, followed by routine screening between 24 and 28 weeks.**

Antepartum Testing

A dating **ultrasound** should be performed in the first trimester. Ultrasound study should be performed every trimester with detailed fetus anatomy in the second trimester and serial assessment of fetal growth in the third trimester [3,19,34].

Weekly nonstress tests can begin at 32 weeks unless medical or obstetric complications indicate earlier testing.

Table 13.5   Pregnancy Outcomes among Solid-Organ Transplant Recipients

	Kidney[a]	Pancreas–Kidney	Liver	Heart	Lung
Maternal factors (n = pregnancies)	(987)	(75)	(287)	(103)	(30)
Mean transplant-to-conception interval (years)	3.6–6.1	3.0–5.5	5.7 ± 4.9	6.0 ± 4.7	3.6 ± 3.3
Hypertension during pregnancy	56%–65%	28%–95%	32%	39%	53%
Diabetes during pregnancy	4%–12%	0%–5%	7%	2%	23%
Infection during pregnancy	19%–23%	23%–62%	26%	13%	21%
Preeclampsia	30%–32%	27%–32%	22%	18%	17%
Rejection episode during pregnancy	1%–2%	0%–14%	7%	11%	6%
Graft loss within two years of delivery	8%–10%	18%–19%	7%	4%	14%
Outcomes (n)[b]	(1017)	(77)	(293)	(106)	(32)[c]
Therapeutic abortions	0.8%–8.4%	4%–5%	4%	5%	16%
Spontaneous abortions	12%–26%	9%–28%	18%	30%	28%
Ectopic	0.4%–1%	0%–3%	0.3%	2%	0
Stillborn	2%–3%	0	1.7%	1%	0
Live births	70.8%–76%	69%–86%	76%	62%	56%
Live births (n)	(762)	(58)	(221)	(66)	(18)
Mean gestational age (weeks)	35–35.8	34.2–34.8	36.4 ± 3.5	36.8 ± 2.6	33.9 ± 5.2
Preterm birth (<37 weeks)	52%–53%	65%–83%	42%	38%	61%
Mean birth weight (g)	2470–2547	1934–2263	2674 ± 796	2600 ± 568	2206 ± 936
Low birth weight (<2500 g)	42%–46%	50%–68%	34%	39%	61%
Cesarean section	43%–58%	61%–69%	41%	40%	31%
Neonatal deaths, % (n) (within 30 days of birth)	1%–2%	(1)	(1)	0	(2)[b]

Source: Adapted from Coscia LA, Constantinescu S, Moritz MJ et al. Report from the National Transplantation Pregnancy Registry (NTPR): Outcomes of pregnancy after transplantation. In: Cecka JM, Terasaki PI, eds. *Clinical Transplants* Los Angeles: UCLA Terasaki Foundation Laboratory. 65–85, 2011.

[a]Range of incidence due to different immunosuppressants.

[b]Includes twins, triplets, quadruplets.

[c]Includes one triplet pregnancy: one spontaneous abortion at 14 weeks and two born at 22 weeks and died within 24 hours of birth.

Labor and Delivery Issues

Patients who have received steroids during the antepartum period in the equivalent of more than 20 mg of prednisone for more than three weeks should receive "stress dose" steroids (i.e., hydrocortisone 100 mg IV every eight hours × 24 hours).

Cesarean delivery should be performed only for obstetric indications.

Breast-Feeding

Data collected from the NTPR [3] indicated no adverse outcomes in infants who were breast-fed during maternal cyclosporine use. Azathioprine seems also to be safe with breast-feeding. Nevertheless, mothers may be discouraged to breast-feed in the first few months post transplantation when immunosuppressive therapy is at high serum levels. The American Academy of Pediatrics advises that breast-feeding mothers can use prednisone and other glucocorticoids safely. Infant exposure to tacrolimus in milk is very low, and subsequently, **maternal tacrolimus therapy may be compatible with breast-feeding**.

PREGNANCY AFTER OTHER TRANSPLANTATIONS

For pregnancy after **renal transplantation**, please see Chapter 17.

Table 13.5 shows pregnancy **outcomes in kidney, kidney/pancreas, liver, heart, and lung recipients** for comparison [3]. Female heart transplant recipients are able to maintain pregnancy with the majority resulting in a live birth. Not all rejections are treated as some are low-grade. Maternal survival, independent of pregnancy-related events, should be considered as part of prepregnancy planning.

By comparison, lung recipients have a higher incidence of more significant rejection as well as graft loss in the peripartum period with smaller newborns. Successful pregnancy is possible post lung transplantation. Analyses of a larger number of cases may help to identify trends in pregnancy after lung transplantation. Whether long-term maternal survival is impacted by pregnancy warrants further study.

Intestinal transplantation has shown steady improvements in graft and patient survival over the past 20 years and is rapidly becoming more established worldwide [35]. The first pregnancy after intestinal transplant was described in 2006 [36], followed later by few other reports [37–40] with 100% success rate. Specific to this procedure, there are two factors affecting the transplant to be considered in case of pregnancy: higher need of immunosuppressants and absorptive function of transplanted bowel. Close monitoring of renal function and of the graft by endoscopies and biopsies must be performed during the pregnancy in order to prevent episodes of rejection or enteritis, preserving the fetus by temporary malnutrition.

ACKNOWLEDGMENT

We wish to thank **Ms. Claudia Cirillo** for her English language editing of our text.

REFERENCES

1. Starzl TE, Marchioro TL, Von Kaulla KN et al. Homotransplantation of the liver in humans. *Surg Gynecol Obstet* 1963; 117: 659–76. [III]
2. Walcott WO, Derick DE, Jolley JJ et al. Successful pregnancy in a liver transplant patient. *Am J Obstet Gynecol* 1978; 132: 340–1. [III]
3. Coscia LA, Constantinescu S, Moritz MJ et al. Report from the National Transplantation Pregnancy Registry (NTPR): Outcomes of pregnancy after transplantation. In: Cecka JM, Terasaki PI, eds. *Clinical Transplants 2010*. Los Angeles: UCLA Terasaki Foundation Laboratory. 2011: 65–85. [III]
4. Jabiry-Zieniewicz Z, Cyganek A, Luterek K et al. Pregnancy and delivery after liver transplantation. *Transplant Proc* 2005; 37: 1197–200. [III]
5. Deshpande NA, James NT, Kucirka LM et al. Pregnancy outcomes of liver transplant recipients: A systematic review and meta-analysis. *Liver Transp* 2012; 18: 621–9. [II-3]
6. Nagy S, Bush MC, Berkowitz R et al. Pregnancy outcome in liver transplant recipients. *Obstet Gynecol* 2003; 102(1): 121–8. [II-2, III]
7. McKay DB, Josephson MA, Armenti VT et al. Reproduction and transplantation: Report on the AST Consensus Conference on Reproductive Issues and Transplantation. *Am J Transplant* 2005; 5: 1592–9. [III]
8. Armenti VT, Herrine SK, Radomski JS et al. Pregnancy after liver transplantation. *Liver Transpl* 2000; 6: 671–85. [III]
9. Van Thiel DH, Lester R. The effect of chronic alcohol abuse on sexual function. *Clin Endocrinol Metab* 1979; 8: 499–510. [III]
10. Bonanno C, Dove L. Pregnancy after liver transplantation. *Semin Perinatol* 2007; 31: 348–53. [III]
11. Cundy TF, O'Grady JG, Williams R. Recovery of menstruation and pregnancy after liver transplantation. *Gut* 1990; 31: 337–8. [III]
12. Parolin MB, Rabinovitch I, Urbanetz AA et al. Impact of successful liver transplantation on reproductive function and sexuality in women with advanced liver disease. *Transplant Proc* 2004; 36: 943–4. [III]
13. Christopher V, Al-Chalabi T, Richardson PD et al. Pregnancy outcome after liver transplantation: A single-center experience of 71 pregnancies in 45 recipients. *Liver Transpl* 2006; 12: 1138–43. [II-3]
14. Hammound GM, Almashhrawi AA, Ahmed KT et al. Liver diseases in pregnancy: Liver transplantation in pregnancy. *World J Gastroenterol* 2013; 19: 7647–51. [III]
15. Dei Malatesta MF, Rossi M, Rocca B et al. Pregnancy after liver transplantation: Report of 8 new cases and review of the literature. *Transpl Immunol* 2006; 15: 297–302. [III]
16. Pan GD, Yan LN, Li B et al. A successful pregnancy following liver transplantation. *Hepatobiliary Pancreat Dis Int* 2007; 6: 98–100. [III]
17. Jankovic Z, Stamenkovic D, Duncan B et al. Successful outcome after technically challenging liver transplant during pregnancy. *Transplant Proc* 2007; 39: 1704–6. [III]
18. Jabiry-Zieniewicz Z, Bobrowska K, Pietrzak B. Mode of delivery in women after liver transplantation. *Transplant Proc* 2007; 39: 2796–9. [III]
19. Heneghan MA, Selzner M, Yoshida EM et al. Pregnancy and sexual function in liver transplantation. *J Hepatol* 2008; 49: 507–19. [III]
20. Surti B, Tan J, Saab S. Pregnancy and liver transplantation. *Liver Int* 2008; 28: 1200–6. [III]
21. Coffin CS, Shaheen AA, Burak KW et al. Pregnancy outcomes among liver transplant recipients in the United States: A nationwide case-control analysis. *Liver Transpl* 2010; 16: 56–63. [III]
22. Cash WJ, Knisely AS, Waterhouse C et al. Successful pregnancy after liver transplantation in progressive familial intrahepatic cholestasis, type 1. *Pediatr Transplant* 2010; 15: E174–6. [III]
23. Armenti VT, Constantinescu S, Moritz MJ et al. Pregnancy after transplantation. *Transplant Rev* 2008; 22: 223–40. [III]
24. Laifer SA, Darby MJ, Scantlebury VP et al. Pregnancy and liver transplantation. *Obstet Gynecol* 1990; 76: 1083–8. [III]
25. Lai CL, Ratziu V, Yuen MF et al. Viral hepatitis B. *Lancet* 2003; 362: 2089–94. [II-2]

26. Ferrero S, Lungaro P, Bruzzone BM et al. Prospective study of mother-to-infant transmission of hepatitis C virus: A 10-year survey (1990–2000). *Acta Obstet Gynecol Scand* 2003; 82: 229–34. [II-3]

27. Jain AB, Reyes J, Marcos A et al. Pregnancy after liver transplantation with tacrolimus immunosuppression: A single center's experience update at 13 years. *Transplantation* 2003; 76: 827–32. [III]

28. Marchetti P. New-onset diabetes after liver transplantation: From pathogenesis to management. *Liver Transpl* 2005; 11: 612–20. [III]

29. Homko CJ, Sivan E, Reece AE. Is there a role for oral antihyperglycemics in gestational diabetes and type 2 diabetes during pregnancy? *Treat Endocrinol* 2004; 3: 133–9. [III]

30. Anderka MT, Lin AE, Abuelo DN et al. Reviewing the evidence for mycophenolate mofetil as a new teratogen: Case report and review of the literature. *Am J Med Genet A* 2009; 149A: 1241–8. [III]

31. Sifontis NM, Coscia LA, Constantinescu S et al. Pregnancy outcomes in solid organ transplant recipients with exposure to mycophenolate mofetil or sirolimus. *Transplantation* 2006; 82: 1698–702. [III]

32. Roche Laboratories. Mycophenolate Mofetil Package Insert. Nutley, NJ: Roche Laboratories, 2009. [II-3]

33. Novartis Pharmaceuticals Corp. Mycophenolic acid package insert. East Hanover, NJ: Novartis Pharmaceuticals, 2009. [II-3]

34. Mastrobattista JM, Gomez-Lobo V, for the Society for Maternal-Fetal Medicine. Pregnancy after solid organ transplantation. *Obstet Gynecol* 2008; 112: 919–32. [III]

35. Abu-Elmagd K. The concept of gut rehabilitation and the future of visceral transplantation. *Nat Rev Gastroenterol Hepatol* 2015; 12: 108–20. [III]

36. Kosmach-Park B, Doshi B, Seward L et al. Successful pregnancy following intestine transplant in a long term survivor. *Am J Transplant* 2006; 6(Suppl. 2): 855 (World Transplant Congress, Boston 2006). [III]

37. Gomez-Lobo V, Landy HJ, Matsumoto C et al. Pregnancy in an intestinal transplant recipient. *Obstet Gynecol* 2012; 120: 497–500. [III]

38. Kosmach-Park B, Costa G, Mazariegos G. *Reproductive health and outcomes following intestine transplantation.* XIII ISBTS Annual Small Bowel Transplant Symposium, Oxford (UK) 2013. [III]

39. Srivastava R, Clarke S, Gupte GL et al. Successful pregnancy outcome following triple organ transplantation (small intestine, liver and pancreas). *Eur J Obstet Gynecol Reprod Biol* 2012; 163: 238–9. [III]

40. Marcus EA, Wozniak LJ, Venick RS et al. Successful term pregnancy in an intestine-pancreas transplant recipient with chronic graft dysfunction and parenteral nutrition dependence: A case report. *Transplant Proc 2015* 2015; 47: 863–7. [III]

14

Maternal anemia

Marcela C. Smid and Robert A. Strauss

KEY POINTS

- **Screening all pregnant women with Hgb** and mean corpuscular volume **(MCV)** for acquired and inherited anemias is recommended.
- Anemia in pregnancy is defined as a **hemoglobin (Hgb) <11 g/dL and hematocrit (Hct) <33% in the first or third trimesters and Hgb <10.5 g/dL and Hct <32% in the second trimester**. For African American women, recommend lowering cutoffs for Hgb and Hct by 0.8 g/dL and 2%, respectively.
- Key laboratory tests for the workup of anemia in pregnancy include a **complete blood count (CBC) with MCV**, red blood cell distribution width **(RDW)**, serum **ferritin** level, and **hemoglobin electrophoresis**. Workup of anemia in pregnancy is described in Figures 14.1 through 14.3.
- Individuals of African, Mediterranean, and Southeast Asian descent are at increased risk of hemoglobinopathies and/or inherited anemia. **All** women of **African ancestry** should have a **hemoglobin electrophoresis [1]. Women of Mediterranean and Southeast Asian descent** should be screened with CBC and MCV. If abnormal, further workup is recommended.
- The most **common cause of anemia in pregnancy** is **iron deficiency**. Iron deficiency anemia in pregnancy is defined as **serum ferritin <15 µg/L** with a Hgb <11 g/dL and Hct <33%.
- **Universal preventative oral iron supplementation during pregnancy**, with or without folate, is associated with a **reduced risk of maternal anemia and iron deficiency at term**.
- **Iron deficiency anemia is associated with adverse perinatal outcomes**, including preterm birth, low birth weight, and perinatal mortality although the evidence regarding the reduction of adverse outcomes with treatment of iron deficiency anemia in pregnancy are lacking.
- Treatment of iron deficiency anemia with oral iron treatment in pregnancy is associated with a **reduction in the number of women with hemoglobin <11 g/dL** and a **greater mean hemoglobin level**, but there are **insufficient data to conclude clear improvement in maternal or neonatal outcomes** (Figure 14.4).
- Parenteral iron may be considered in patients with severe iron deficiency anemia who cannot tolerate or will not take oral iron.
- Severe anemia from any etiology **(Hgb <4–6 mg/dL)** is associated with poor perinatal outcomes and increased perinatal and maternal mortality. Transfusion may be considered.

For sickle cell disease, see Chapter 15; for von Willebrand disease, see Chapter 16; for care of Jehovah's Witness pregnant women, see Chapter 9 in *Obstetric Evidence Based Guidelines*.

DEFINITION

Hemoglobin (Hgb) <11 g/dL and hematocrit (Hct) <33% in the first or third trimesters and <10.5 g/dL and Hct <32% in the second trimester [1,2]. For African American women, recommend lowering cutoffs for Hgb and Hct by 0.8 g/dL and 2%, respectively [3]. Iron deficiency anemia in pregnancy is defined as **serum ferritin <15 µg/L** with a Hgb <11 g/dL and Hct <33% [4,5].

SYMPTOMS

Usually asymptomatic unless hemoglobin <6 to 7 g/dL.

PREVALENCE

Worldwide, 38%–42% of pregnant women are anemic with estimates ranging from 22% in high resource areas to 56% in Africa [6,7]. In the United States, 5% of pregnant women are anemic; 18% are iron deficient with prevalence increasing from 7% in the first trimester to 28% in the third trimester. African American women (30%) and Mexican American women (24%) have a higher prevalence of iron deficiency anemia compared to European American (14%) [8].

GENETICS

Worldwide, 7% of the population are carriers for important hemoglobin disorders [9]. In the United States, approximately 1:12 African Americans have sickle cell trait, 1:300 have a form of sickle cell disease, and 1:600 have sickle cell anemia [10].

See Tables 14.1 through 14.3 for types of hemoglobins. Tables 14.4 and 14.5 describe the types of hemoglobinopathies and their clinical significance. *Cis*-α-thalassemia is common among women of Southeast Asian ancestry; β-thalassemia is common among women of Mediterranean, Asian, Middle Eastern, Hispanic, and West Indian ancestry. However, ethnicity is not a good predictor of risk as ethnic background is often mixed and many women partner outside their ethnic group [2].

ETIOLOGY/PATHOPHYSIOLOGY

Pregnant women undergo normal physiologic hemodynamic changes, which must be understood to correctly identify those who may benefit from additional testing and interventions. Total red blood cell (RBC) mass and plasma both increase; however, the plasma increase (40%–60%) is proportionally greater than the RBC increase (15%–30%), resulting in a lowering of the Hgb concentration compared to

Algorithms for diagnosing anemia generally fail in the presence of more than one cause.

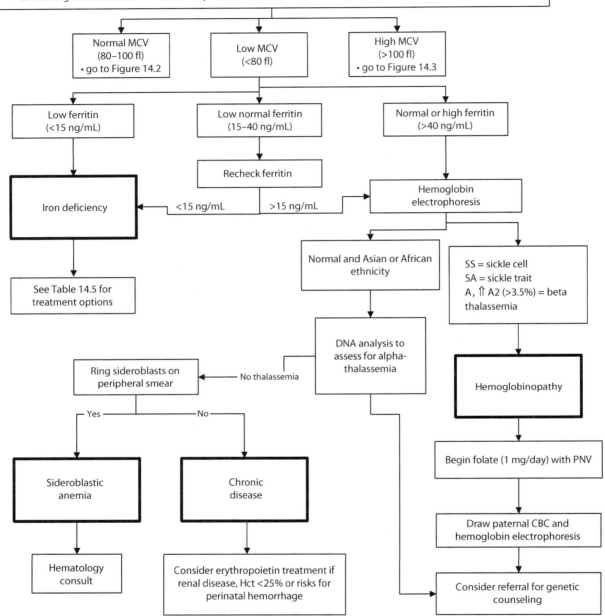

Figure 14.1   Evaluation of anemia in pregnancy. Algorithms for diagnosing anemia generally fail in the presence of more than one cause.

nonpregnant adults. Hgb 11–12 g/dL and Hct 33%–35% are normal pregnancy-related ranges.

Anemia may be inherited or acquired. Table 14.6 describes anemia by its pathophysiological mechanism. Anemia in pregnancy can be caused by decreased red blood cell production (nutritional deficiencies including iron, vitamin B_{12}, folate, decreased absorption, chronic disease, infection, bone marrow suppression, hormonal deficiencies),

increased red blood cell destruction (inherited hemolytic anemias, acquired hemolytic anemias), and blood loss.

Although this chapter focuses on anemia, the Centers for Disease Control notes that pregnant women with Hb concentration of greater than 15.0 g/dL or a Hct of greater than 45.0%, particularly in the second trimester, are at increased risk of poor perinatal outcomes (fetal growth restriction, preterm birth, fetal death) [2]. Increased Hb in the second or

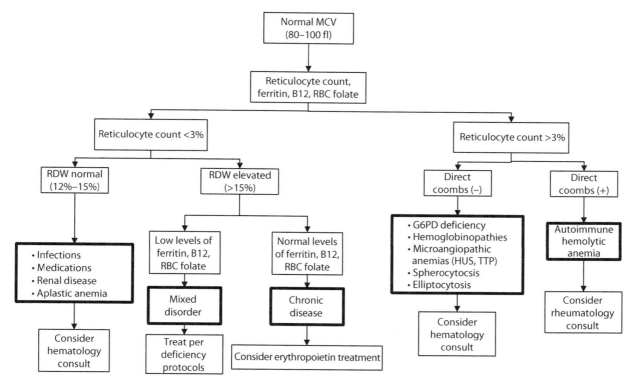

Figure 14.2 Normocytic anemia (MCV 80–100).

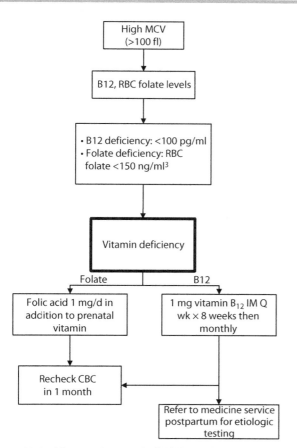

Figure 14.3 Macrocytic anemia (MCV >100).

Table 14.1 Types of Hemoglobins

Hemoglobin	α-Type Chains	β-Type Chains	Disease State
HgbA₁	2 α-chains	2 β-chains	Major adult hemoglobin
HgbA₂	2 α-chains	2 δ-chains	Minor adult hemoglobin
HgbF	2 α-chains	2 γ-chains	Fetal hemoglobin
HgbH	–	4 β-chains	α-Thalassemia major (–/–α)
Hgb Bart	–	4 γ-chains	Hydrops fetalis (–/–)
Hgb Gower	2 ε-chains	2 ς-chains	Embryonic hemoglobin

third trimester likely indicates poor blood volume expansion and should **not be considered an indication of adequate iron stores**.

Iron Deficiency Anemia

Iron deficiency anemia is the most common cause of anemia during pregnancy due to the nutrient demands required for the fetus and for maternal red blood cell mass expansion. Total iron loss associated with pregnancy and lactation is approximately 1 g. The typical diet in high-resource areas includes 15 mg of elemental iron per day. **The recommended daily intake of ferrous iron during pregnancy is 27 mg, which is present in most prenatal vitamins, and 10 mg during lactation** [11].

RISK FACTORS

Risk factors for iron deficiency or iron deficiency anemia include diet poor in iron-rich food, a diet poor in iron absorption enhancers (vitamin C–rich foods), a diet rich in foods that

Table 14.2 Types of α-Thalassemia

Clinical Nomenclature	Genotype	Disease
Silent carrier	−/α/α/α heterozygous α^+-thalassemia	Asymptomatic
α-Thalassemia trait	α −/α − (trans) Homozygous α^+-thalassemia Common among those with black African heritage or − −/α α (cis) Heterozygous α^0 thalassemia Common among those with Asian heritage	Mild anemia Similar to β-thalassemia minor
Hemoglobin H disease (α-Thalassemia major)	α −/− − α^+-thalassemia/ α^0-thalassemia	Severe HbH hemolytic anemia
Hydrops fetalis Bart's disease	− −/− − Homozygous α^0-thalassemia 80% Hb Bart/20% HbH	Lethal in utero without transfusions

Note: Because there are two α-chains on each chromosome 16, the possibility exists for four different disease states (unlike β-thalassemias, with which only two disease states are found).

Table 14.3 Types of β Thalassemia

β Thalassemia trait: one β chain affected β/β^0
Cooley anemia: both β chains affected β^0/β^0
β^0 absence of β chain production → causes more severe anemia
β^+ decrease in β chain production → causes milder anemia

diminish iron absorption (dairy, soy products, coffee, spinach), pica (eating nonfood substances, such as clay), gastrointestinal compromise affecting absorption (e.g., celiac disease, Crohn's disease, bariatric surgery, particularly restrictive surgeries), short pregnancy interval, parity ≥2, multiple gestation, low socioeconomic status, and history of blood loss (heavy menses, postpartum hemorrhage). Although iron deficiency anemia from ongoing blood loss from the gastrointestinal system is less common in women of reproductive age, when iron deficiency is recognized during pregnancy, all possible causes should be considered.

COMPLICATIONS

Observational studies suggest that maternal anemia and iron deficiency anemia are associated with poor perinatal outcomes, including increased risk of **low birth weight, preterm birth, and perinatal death** [12–19]. Maternal anemia in the first trimester is more consistently associated with adverse perinatal outcomes, compared to anemia diagnosed in the third trimester [17,20]. Severe maternal anemia is associated with abnormal fetal cerebral profusion and decreased amniotic fluid [21]. In low-resource areas, severe maternal anemia (Hgb <6–7 g/dL) is associated with **maternal cardiovascular compromise or death** [22,23]. Maternal anemia may also be associated with postpartum depression [24], impaired maternal postpartum cognition [25], poor mother–infant interaction, and infant cognitive function [26]. However, due to methodological inconsistencies among these studies, data to establish the association between maternal anemia and/or iron deficiency anemia and adverse maternal and perinatal outcomes remains insufficient [27].

DIAGNOSIS

An approach to determining the cause of maternal anemia is outlined in Figures 14.1 through 14.3. Anemia can be the result of more than one cause, and in such instances, **an algorithmic approach to the diagnosis may be incomplete**.

Workup

- Initial evaluation: **CBC with Hbg/Hct and MCV**. This initial anemia screening is recommended **for all pregnant women** [1] (Figure 14.1).
- All individuals of **African ancestry** should have a **hemoglobin electrophoresis**. See Tables 14.4 and 14.5. Solubility testing is inadequate for screening because it fails to identify other important hemoglobinopathies [2,28]. If documented results from a prior hemoglobin electrophoresis can be obtained, this test should not be repeated.

Microcytic Anemia

- Hgb <10.5–11 g/dL and **MCV <80 um³** represent a microcytic anemia (Figure 14.1).
- Obtain **ferritin** level, which has the highest sensitivity and specificity for diagnosing iron deficiency in anemic patients [29].
- Obtain **Hgb electrophoresis** to assess for a hemoglobinopathy (Table 14.4) [30].

Table 14.4 Hemoglobin Electrophoresis Patterns in Common Hemoglobinopathies

Condition	HbA	HbS	HbC	HbF	HbA2
Normal	95–98[a]	0	0	<1	2.5 ± 0.2
Beta thalassemia minor	90–95	0	0	1 to 3	>3.5
Sickle cell trait	50–60	35–45[a]	0	<2	<3.5
Sickle-beta(+) thalassemia	5–30	65–90	0	2 to 10	>3.5
Sickle-beta(0) thalassemia	0	80–92	0	2 to 15	>3.5
Sickle-HbC disease	0	45–50	45 to 50	1 to 8	<3.5
Homozygous sickle cell disease	0	85–95	0	2 to 15	<3.5

Source: Adapted from Schrier SL. Introduction to hemoglobin mutations. In: Post TW, ed. *UpToDate*, Waltham, MA.
[a]May be as low as 21 with sickle cell trait in presence of alpha thalassemia.
Abbreviation: Hb: hemoglobin.

Table 14.5 Hematological Studies and Clinical Severity of Thalassemias

Condition	Hb Level	HbA$_2$	HbF	Other Hb	Clinical Severity
Homozygotes					
α-Thalassemia	Severely low	0	0	80% Hb Bart, remainder HbH	Hydrops fetalis
β$^+$ Thalassemia	Very low	Variable	Variable	Some HbA	Moderately severe Cooley anemia
β^0 Thalassemia	Severely low	Variable	High	No HbA	Severe Cooley anemia
δβ^0 Thalassemia	Low	0	100%	No HbA	Thalassemia intermedia
Heterozygotes					
α-Thalassemia silent carrier	Normal	Normal	Normal	1%–2% Hb Bart at birth	Normal
α-Thalassemia trait	Low to normal	Normal	Normal	5% Hb Bart at birth	Very mild
HbH disease	Low	Normal	Normal	3%–30% HbH in adult; 35% HbH at birth	Thalassemia intermedia
β$^+$ Thalassemia	Mildly low to low	Elevated	Elevated	None	Mild
β^0 Thalassemia	Mildly low to low	Elevated	Very elevated	None	Mild

Table 14.6 Anemia Characterized by Mechanism

Dilutional (expansion of plasma volume)	Pregnancy Hyperglobinemia Massive splenomegaly
Decreased red blood cell production	Iron deficiency Vitamin B$_{12}$ deficiency Folic acid deficiency Bone marrow disorder or suppression Low levels of erythropoietin Hypothyroidism
Increased red blood cell destruction	Inherited: sickle cell, thalassemia major, hereditary spherocytosis Acquired: autoimmune hemolytic, thrombotic thrombocytopenia purpura, hemolytic uremic syndrome, malaria
Increased loss	Hemorrhage Gastrointestinal bleed

Table 14.7 Hematological Studies of Anemias

Marker	Anemia of Chronic Disease	Iron Deficiency Anemia	Thalassemia Alpha/Beta Trait or HbE
Hemoglobin	Normal to decreased	Normal to decreased	Normal to decreased
MCV	Normal to decreased	Decreased	Decreased can be <70
RDW	Normal to increased	Increased to >15	Normal
Transferrin saturation	Decreased	Decreased	Normal
Ferritin	No change to increased	Decreased	Normal

Normocytic Anemia

- If Hgb 10.5–11 g/dL and **MCV** ≥80–100 um^3, obtain reticulocyte count to determine if anemia is secondary to underproduction or hemolysis and obtain a history to identify any evidence of active bleeding, medication exposure, chronic disease, glucose-6-phosphate dehydrogenase (G6PD) deficiency, or a family history of RBC disorders (Figure 14.2).
- Obtain ferritin, vitamin B$_{12}$, and RBC folate.
- If high reticulocyte counts (≥3), then anemia may be secondary to hemolysis or blood loss. Consider 1) peripheral blood smear and haptoglobin (decreased), 2) direct coombs (suggests autoimmune hemolytic anemia), 3) Hgb electrophoresis to rule out SS or SC disease, and 4) hemoccult or other tests if other sources of blood loss are suggested by history.
- If low reticulocyte count (<3), then anemia is secondary to underproduction. Assess red cell distribution width (RDW) and follow algorithm.

Macrocytic Anemia

- If Hgb 10.5–11 g/dL and **MCV** >100 um^3, obtain vitamin B$_{12}$ and RBC folate level [29] (Figure 14.3).
- Anemia of chronic disease is usually associated with normocytic anemia (about 20% are associated

with microcytic anemia) (Table 14.7). Causes include chronic liver disease, thyroid disease, uremia, chronic infections, and malignancies. Workup may include liver function tests (LFTs), blood urea nitrogen (BUN) and creatinine, thyroid-stimulating hormone (TSH), and any tests for malignancy or chronic infection indicated by patient history and risk factors. Also check serum iron, serum B$_{12}$, and RBC folate to rule out combined deficiencies. Normal pregnancy-specific values can be found in Table 14.8.

- A **nutrition consult** should be obtained for patients with B$_{12}$, folate, and iron deficiencies.

Table 14.8 Trimester-Specific Pregnancy Reference Ranges (2.5th and 97.5th percentile)

	First Trimester	Second Trimester	Third Trimester
Serum ferritin level (ng/mL)	6–130	2–230	0–116
Total iron-binding capacity µg/dL	278–403	Not reported	359–609
Transferrin saturation (%)	Not reported	10–44	5–37
Plasma iron level (µg/dL)	72–113	44–178	30–193
Folate (RBC) (ng/mL)	137–589	94–828	109–663
Folate (serum) (ng/mL)	2.5–15.0	0.8–24.0	1.4–20.7
B$_{12}$ (cobalamin) pg/mL	118–438	130–656	99–526
MCV µm^3	81–96	82–97	81–99

Abbreviation: MCV, mean corpuscular volume.

- A **genetic consult** should be obtained for all patients with inherited disorders. Attempt to obtain a blood sample for hemoglobin electrophoresis from the father of the baby prior to the genetic consult. DNA testing for alpha-globin abnormalities is available.

PREVENTION

Daily and intermittent iron supplementation are associated with **prevention of low hemoglobin at term and at six weeks postpartum**. Insufficient evidence exists, however, that supplementation results in a significant reduction of **adverse perinatal outcomes**, including low birth weight, preterm birth, or infection [31,32]. Most of the RCTs provided very limited information about the clinical outcomes for women or their neonates. **Intermittent iron supplementation** appears to produce similar maternal and neonatal outcomes as daily supplementation with fewer side effects [31–33].

Except in women with hemochromatosis or other genetic disorders, there is little evidence of morbidity associated with iron supplementation. Common side effects of oral supplementation include constipation and gastrointestinal upset. **The recommended daily allowance of ferrous iron during pregnancy is 27 mg** as present in most prenatal vitamins [1]. Table 14.9 lists elemental iron content of available iron supplements.

Folate supplementation is associated with increased or maintained serum folate levels and red cell folate levels compared to placebo or no supplementation. Folate supplementation is associated with a **reduction in the proportion of women with megaloblastic anemia** but no difference in predelivery hemoglobin, serum folate, or RBC folate levels. Compared to placebo, folate supplementation is associated with **increase in mean birth weight** but **no difference in preterm birth or stillbirth/neonatal death**. Based on available data, there is **insufficient evidence** to conclude if folate supplementation has any substantial effect on maternal or neonatal outcomes [34].

THERAPY

There is a paucity of quality trials assessing the maternal and neonatal benefits of treatment of iron deficiency anemia in pregnancy [35]. Compared to placebo, **oral iron treatment** in pregnancy is associated with a reduction in the number of pregnant women with anemia in the second trimester and greater mean hemoglobin and ferritin levels (Figure 14.4). However, there is **insufficient evidence to assess change in clinical outcomes, including preterm birth, low birth weight, or maternal morbidity in treatment of anemia** [35]. Gastrointestinal side effects (e.g., constipation, nausea, and abdominal cramps) are common with oral iron treatments, and low-dose daily treatment may be effective in treating anemia with decreased side effects. Compared with standard

Table 14.9 Iron Supplements

Preparation	Elemental Iron Content
Ferrous fumarate	106 mg per 325 mg tablet
Ferrous sulfate	65 mg per 325 mg tablet
Ferrous gluconate	34 mg per 300 mg tablet
Iron dextran	50 mg/mL, IM or IV
Ferric gluconate	12.5 mg/mL IV
Iron sucrose	20 mg/mL IV
Ferric carboxymaltose	750 mg IV; 1500 mg maximum

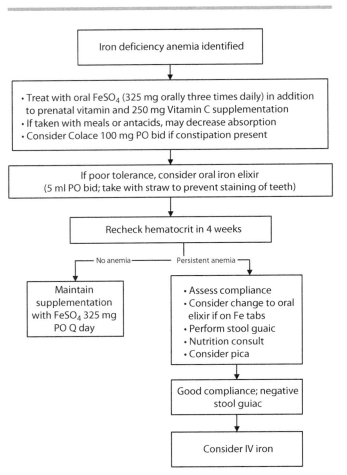

Figure 14.4 Treatment of iron deficiency anemia.

oral preparations, controlled release iron preparations are associated with a diminished frequency of constipation.

Compared to oral administration, **intravenous (IV) or intramuscular (IM) routes** of administration are associated with better hematologic indices, including higher mean Hgb and/or ferritin levels. Although serious adverse effects of parenteral iron appear uncommon, data are insufficient regarding effects such as venous thrombosis and severe allergic reaction [36–40]. When IV iron preparations are used, the safety profile of different preparations should be considered. Concern for anaphylactic reactions with high molecular weight IV dextran and long infusion times with iron polymaltose reduces their clinical use, particularly given limited information in pregnancy. Low molecular weight IV iron dextran offers an improved safety profile compared to high molecular weight IV iron dextran. IV sucrose has been shown to be well tolerated and increase hemoglobin and ferritin levels compared to oral iron in pregnant women [40]; however, this IV dosing requires six days of hospital administration. Ferric carboxymaltose offers an alternative. Although there are no RCTs, retrospective and prospective observational studies indicate that is associated with similar increases in mean Hgb and ferritin levels compared with IV iron sucrose and has a comparable safety profile while requiring only one infusion of up to 1000 mg of iron in 15 minutes [41].

There are insufficient data to assess the effects of other forms of prevention or therapy, including self-donation during pregnancy.

ANTEPARTUM TESTING

Consider growth ultrasound in the third trimester given association with anemia and low birth weight although there is limited evidence to support this practice.

DELIVERY AND ANESTHESIA

Prepare team regarding increased risk in the event of hemorrhage. Consider having blood available for possible transfusion in cases of severe anemia, for example, Hgb <8 g/dL.

POSTPARTUM/BREAST-FEEDING

There is **limited evidence** to assess different therapies for postpartum anemia. Outcome data on clinically relevant criteria are lacking. No effect on need for blood transfusions was apparent although the RCTs may have been of insufficient size to rule out important clinical differences. **Intravenous (IV) iron** was compared to oral iron in 10 studies [42]. In two studies, fatigue improved significantly in the IV group although there was no difference at six weeks postpartum. Gastrointestinal symptoms were reduced in the IV iron group compared to oral treatment in eight studies. Three allergic reactions were reported in the IV group, which was not statistically significant when compared to the oral treatment group. One study evaluated red blood cell **transfusion** versus nonintervention. General fatigue improved significantly more in the transfusion group at three days, but no difference between groups was seen at six weeks. Insufficient evidence exists to assess the safety profile of the IV route, including severe allergic reactions. In a recent RCT, IV ferrous sucrose for two days within 48 hours postpartum was not associated with significant benefits compared to placebo [43]. In two RCTs, ferric carboxymaltose compared to oral iron was associated with an earlier increase in hemoglobin postpartum [44,45]. Overall, **there is insufficient evidence to conclude that IV iron or blood transfusion significantly benefit women postpartum when compared to the risk of severe allergic reactions with IV iron preparations or maternal immunological sensitization with blood transfusion.**

Hematological indices (Hgb and Hct) show some improvement when **erythropoietin** was compared to iron only or iron and folate but not when compared with placebo [41]. When compared with oral iron therapy only, erythropoietin increases the likelihood of lactation at discharge from hospital in one very small trial.

Given that postpartum anemia is associated with several complications, including decreased ability to fully engage in child care, household tasks, and exercise as well as altered cognition, mood, and productivity, preventive measures for iron deficiency postpartum anemia may be considered although there is **insufficient evidence** to recommend this approach.

REFERENCES

1. American College of Obstetricians and Gynecologists. ACOG Practice Bulletin No. 95: Anemia in pregnancy. *Obstet Gynecol* 2008; 112(1): 201. [Review]
2. Yip R, Parvanta I, Cogswell ME, McDonnell SM, Bowman BA, Grummer-Strawn LM et al. Recommendations to prevent and control iron deficiency in the United States. *MMWR: Recommendations and Reports* 1998: i–29. [Review]
3. Institute of Medicine Committee on the Prevention, Management of Iron Deficiency Anemia Among USC, Women of Childbearing Age. In: Earl R, Woteki CE, editors. *Iron Deficiency Anemia: Recommended Guidelines for the Prevention, Detection, and Management Among US Children and Women of Childbearing Age.* Washington, DC: National Academies Press (US) Copyright 1993 by the National Academy of Sciences. All rights reserved; 1993. [Review]
4. Centers for Disease Control criteria for anemia in children and childbearing-aged women. *MMWR* 1989; 38(22): 400–4. [Review]
5. World Health Organization. *Iron deficiency anaemia: Assessment, prevention and control: A guide for programme managers.* 2001. [Review]
6. McLean E, Cogswell M, Egli I, Wojdyla D, De Benoist B. Worldwide prevalence of anaemia, WHO vitamin and mineral nutrition information system, 1993–2005. *Public Health Nutrition* 2009; 12(4): 444–54. [Review]
7. Stevens GA, Finucane MM, De-Regil LM, Paciorek CJ, Flaxman SR, Branca F et al. Global, regional, and national trends in haemoglobin concentration and prevalence of total and severe anaemia in children and pregnant and non-pregnant women for 1995–2011: A systematic analysis of population-representative data. *Lancet Global Health* 2013; 1(1): e16–25. [Systematic review; 107 countries]
8. Mei Z, Cogswell ME, Looker AC, Pfeiffer CM, Cusick SE, Lacher DA et al. Assessment of iron status in US pregnant women from the National Health and Nutrition Examination Survey (NHANES), 1999–2006. *Am J Clin Nutr* 2011; 93(6): 1312–20. [IIc]
9. Motulsky AG. Frequency of sickling disorders in U.S. blacks. *N Engl J Med* 1973; 288(1): 31–3. [IIc]
10. World Health Organization. *Genomics and world health: Report of the Advisory Committee on Health Research.* 2002. [Review]
11. Institute of Medicine. *Dietary Reference Intakes for Vitamin A, Vitamin K, Arsenic, Boron, Chromium, Copper, Iodine, Iron, Manganese, Molybdenum, Nickel, Silicon, Vanadium, and Zinc: A Report of the Panel on Micronutrients and of Interpretation and Uses of Dietary Reference Intakes, and the Standing Committee on the Scientific Evaluation of Dietary Reference Intakes.* National Academy Press; 2001. [Review]
12. Scholl TO, Hediger ML, Fischer RL, Shearer JW. Anemia vs iron deficiency: Increased risk of preterm delivery in a prospective study. *Am J Clin Nutr* 1992; 55(5): 985–8. [IIb]
13. Murphy JF, O'Riordan J, Newcombe RG, Coles EC, Pearson JF. Relation of haemoglobin levels in first and second trimesters to outcome of pregnancy. *Lancet* 1986; 1(8488): 992–5. [III]
14. Zhou LM, Yang WW, Hua JZ, Deng CQ, Tao X, Stoltzfus RJ. Relation of hemoglobin measured at different times in pregnancy to preterm birth and low birth weight in Shanghai, China. *Am J Epidemiol* 1998; 148(10): 998–1006. [III]
15. Klebanoff MA, Shiono PH, Selby JV, Trachtenberg AI, Graubard BI. Anemia and spontaneous preterm birth. *Am J Obstet Gynecol* 1991; 164(1 Pt. 1): 59–63. [IIb]
16. Singh K, Fong YF, Arulkumaran S. Anaemia in pregnancy—A cross-sectional study in Singapore. *Eur J Clin Nutr* 1998; 52(1): 65–70. [III]
17. Scholl TO, Hediger ML. Anemia and iron-deficiency anemia: Compilation of data on pregnancy outcome. *Am J Clin Nutr* 1994; 59(2 Suppl.): 492S–500S, discussion S–1S. [III]
18. Garn SM, Keating MT, Falkner F. Hematological status and pregnancy outcomes. *Am J Clin Nutr* 1981; 34(1): 115–7. [III]
19. Alwan NA, Cade JE, McArdle HJ, Greenwood DC, Hayes HE, Simpson NA. Maternal iron status in early pregnancy and birth outcomes: Insights from the baby's vascular health and iron in pregnancy study. *British J Nutr* 2015; 113(12): 1985–92. [IIb]
20. Haider BA, Olofin I, Wang M, Spiegelman D, Ezzati M, Fawzi WW. Anaemia, prenatal iron use, and risk of adverse pregnancy outcomes: Systematic review and meta-analysis. *BMJ (Clinical Research Ed)* 2013; 346: f3443. [Meta-analysis, 48 trials, n = 17,793]
21. Carles G, Tobal N, Raynal P, Herault S, Beucher G, Marret H et al. Doppler assessment of the fetal cerebral hemodynamic response to moderate or severe maternal anemia. *Am J Obstet Gynecol* 2003; 188(3): 794–9. [III]

22. Brabin BJ, Hakimi M, Pelletier D. An analysis of anemia and pregnancy-related maternal mortality. *J Nutrit* 2001; 131(2S–2): 604S–14S; discussion 14S–5S. [Systematic review; *n* > 10,000]

23. Geelhoed D, Agadzi F, Visser L, Ablordeppey E, Asare K, O'Rourke P et al. Maternal and fetal outcome after severe anemia in pregnancy in rural Ghana. *Acta Obstet Gynecol Scand* 2006; 85(1): 49–55. [IIb]

24. Corwin EJ, Murray-Kolb LE, Beard JL. Low hemoglobin level is a risk factor for postpartum depression. *J Nutrit* 2003; 133(12): 4139–42. [III]

25. Beard JL, Hendricks MK, Perez EM, Murray-Kolb LE, Berg A, Vernon-Feagans L et al. Maternal iron deficiency anemia affects postpartum emotions and cognition. *J Nutrit* 2005; 135(2): 267–72. [RCT, *n* = 81]

26. Perez EM, Hendricks MK, Beard JL, Murray-Kolb LE, Berg A, Tomlinson M et al. Mother-infant interactions and infant development are altered by maternal iron deficiency anemia. *J Nutrit* 2005; 135(4): 850–5. [RCT, *n* = 81]

27. Rasmussen K. Is there a causal relationship between iron deficiency or iron-deficiency anemia and weight at birth, length of gestation and perinatal mortality? *J Nutrit* 2001; 131(2s–2): 590S–601S; discussion S–3S. [Review]

28. American College of Obstetricians and Gynecologists. ACOG Practice Bulletin No. 78: Hemoglobinopathies in pregnancy. *Obstet Gynecol* 2007; 109: 229–37. [Review]

29. Ontario Association of Medical Laboratories. Guidelines for the use of serum test for iron deficiency. Guidelines for Clinical Laboratory Practice. 1995 Available at http://www.oaml.com/PDF/CLP002.pdf. Retrieved September 12, 2015. [Guideline]

30. Schrier SL. Introduction to hemoglobin mutations. In: Post TW, editor. *UpToDate*, Waltham, MA. [Review]

31. Pena-Rosas JP, De-Regil LM, Garcia-Casal MN, Dowswell T. Daily oral iron supplementation during pregnancy. *Cochrane Database Syst Rev* 2015; 7: Cd004736. [Meta-analysis; trials = 44, *n* = 43,274]

32. Cantor AG, Bougatsos C, Dana T, Blazina I, McDonagh M. Routine iron supplementation and screening for iron deficiency anemia in pregnancy: A systematic review for the U.S. Preventive Services Task Force. *Ann Int Med* 2015; 162(8): 566–76. [Meta-analysis, 11 trials, *n* > 2000]

33. Pena-Rosas JP, De-Regil LM, Dowswell T, Viteri FE. Intermittent oral iron supplementation during pregnancy. *Cochrane Database Syst Rev* 2012; 7: Cd009997. [Meta-analysis, 18 trials, *n* = 4071]

34. Lassi ZS, Salam RA, Haider BA, Bhutta ZA. Folic acid supplementation during pregnancy for maternal health and pregnancy outcomes. *Cochrane Database Syst Rev* 2013; 3: Cd006896. [Meta-analysis, 31 trials, *n* = 17,771]

35. Reveiz L, Gyte GM, Cuervo LG, Casasbuenas A. Treatments for iron-deficiency anaemia in pregnancy. *Cochrane Database Syst Rev* 2011; (10): Cd003094. [Meta-analysis, 23 trials, *n* = 3198]

36. Froessler B, Cocchiaro C, Saadat-Gilani K, Hodyl N, Dekker G. Intravenous iron sucrose versus oral iron ferrous sulfate for antenatal and postpartum iron deficiency anemia: A randomized trial. *J Matern Fetal Neonat Med* 2013; 26(7): 654–9. [II-b]

37. Kochhar PK, Kaundal A, Ghosh P. Intravenous iron sucrose versus oral iron in treatment of iron deficiency anemia in pregnancy: A randomized clinical trial. *J Obstet Gynaecol Res* 2013; 39(2): 504–10. [RCT, *n* = 100]

38. Khalafallah A, Dennis A, Bates J, Bates G, Robertson IK, Smith L et al. A prospective randomized, controlled trial of intravenous versus oral iron for moderate iron deficiency anaemia of pregnancy. *J Int Med* 2010; 268(3): 286–95. [RCT, *n* = 200]

39. Al RA, Unlubilgin E, Kandemir O, Yalvac S, Cakir L, Haberal A. Intravenous versus oral iron for treatment of anemia in pregnancy: A randomized trial. *Obstet Gynecol* 2005; 106(6): 1335–40. [RCT, *n* = 90]

40. Bayoumeu F, Subiran-Buisset C, Baka NE, Legagneur H, Monnier-Barbarino P, Laxenaire MC. Iron therapy in iron deficiency anemia in pregnancy: Intravenous route versus oral route. *Am J Obstet Gynecol* 2002; 186(3): 518–22. [RCT, *n* = 50]

41. Christoph P, Schuller C, Studer H, Irion O, De Tejada BM, Surbek D. Intravenous iron treatment in pregnancy: Comparison of high-dose ferric carboxymaltose vs. iron sucrose. *J Perinat Med* 2012; 40(5): 469–74. [II-2]

42. Markova V, Norgaard A, Jorgensen KJ, Langhoff-Roos J. Treatment for women with postpartum iron deficiency anaemia. *Cochrane Database Syst Rev* 2015; 8: Cd010861. [Meta-analysis, 22 trials, *n* = 2858]

43. Perello MF, Coloma JL, Masoller N et al. Intravenous ferrous sucrose versus placebo in addition to oral iron therapy for the treatment of severe postpartum anemia: A randomized controlled trial. *BJOG* 2014; 121: 706–13. [RCT, *n* = 72]

44. Van Wyck DB, Martens MG, Seid MH, Baker JB, Mangione A. Intravenous ferric carboxymaltose compared with oral iron in the treatment of postpartum anemia: A randomized controlled trial. *Obstet Gynecol* 2007; 110(2 Pt. 1): 267–78. [RCT, *n* = 352]

45. Seid, MH, Derman, RJ Baker, JB Banach W, Goldberg C, Rogers, R. Ferric carboxymaltose injection in the treatment of postpartum iron deficiency anemia: A randomized controlled clinical trial. *Am J Obstet Gynecol* 2008; 199(4): 435-e1. [RCT, *n* = 291]

15

Sickle cell disease

Mariam Naqvi and Jeffrey Ecker

KEY POINTS

- **Sickle cell disease is an autosomal recessive** disease resulting from an alteration in the structure of hemoglobin producing hemoglobin S (HbS). It is characterized by chronic hemolytic anemia and vaso-occlusive events.
- **Diagnosis is made by hemoglobin electrophoresis.**
- Severe complications during pregnancy and adverse pregnancy outcomes are most commonly experienced by women with **HbSS and HbSβ⁰ genotypes**, which result in **sickle cell anemia**.
- Complications may include pregnancy loss, fetal growth restriction, preterm birth, preeclampsia, placental abnormalities, anemia, painful crises, UTI and other infections, thromboembolic events, acute chest syndrome (ACS), alloimmunization, postpartum infections, and maternal mortality.
- Pneumococcal and influenza vaccines are important prevention interventions.
- Painful crises are managed with **narcotic** (preferably morphine) therapy and **IV fluids**. Antibiotics should be added if the woman is febrile, has an infection, or has ACS; **oxygen should be added if the woman has low oxygen saturation.**
- **Prophylactic blood transfusions are not beneficial** to improve maternal and perinatal outcomes. Blood transfusions are indicated for symptomatic or orthostatic anemia, hemoglobin <6 g/dL or hematocrit <25%, acute stroke, ACS, or multiple organ failure.
- In the 10% of patients with sickle cell disease who develop ACS, a chest X-ray is necessary. Antibiotics (usually cephalosporin and a macrolide) aimed at infectious pathogen(s) in pulmonary tree and bronchodilators are the mainstay of therapy.

HISTORIC NOTES

Sickle cell disease was first described in 1910 by Drs. Irons and Herrick. In 1949, Linus Pauling described the molecular structure of sickle cell hemoglobin by protein electrophoresis. In 1956, Ingram and Hunt discovered the single amino acid change in sickle cell hemoglobin [1]. In the 1960s, median survival age in the United States for those with sickle cell disease was estimated to be 42 years for men and 48 years for women [2]. During the past two decades, improvements in medical care and earlier detection (especially through newborn screening) have led to better survival rates (lifespan is still about two or three decades shorter), improved quality of life, and better pregnancy outcomes in women with sickle cell disease [3,4].

DEFINITION

Sickle cell disease is an inherited disorder resulting from an alteration in the structure of hemoglobin producing HbS. It is characterized by hemolysis and vaso-occlusive events. Sickle cell disease is associated with a mild to moderate chronic anemia. The term sickle cell disease **includes sickle cell anemia (HbSS)** (70% of cases), **hemoglobin S combined with hemoglobin C (HbSC)** (most of the remaining cases), **hemoglobin S combined with β-thalassemia (HbSβ⁺ or HbSβ⁰)**, and other double heterozygous conditions causing sickling and thus, clinical disease (e.g., hereditary persistence of fetal hemoglobin, HgS/HPHP), and hemoglobin E (HbS/HbE) [5]. The clinical manifestations vary among these genotypes with HbSβ⁰ usually with a similar severe phenotype as HbSS; HbSC associated with intermediate disease; and HbSβ⁺, HbSHPHP, and HbSE with mild or symptom-free disease [1,6]. The term **sickle cell anemia** includes HbSS and also HbSβ⁰ **(due to its similar phenotype)**.

DIAGNOSIS

The diagnosis is made by hemoglobin electrophoresis, according to the definition above. In all 50 U.S. states, newborns are screened for sickle cell disease at birth.

EPIDEMIOLOGY/INCIDENCE

Sickle cell disease occurs in about one in 600 African Americans and affects between 70,000 and 100,000 Americans. Sickle cell trait occurs in one in 12 African Americans, resulting in the birth of approximately 1100 infants with sickle cell disease annually in the United States. HbSS accounts for 60% to 70% of sickle cell disease in the United States. The prevalence of sickle cell disease and sickle cell trait is highest in West Africa (25% of the population have one mutation), the Mediterranean, Saudi Arabia, India, South and Central America, and Southeast Asia [1,6].

GENETICS/INHERITANCE

Sickle cell disease is an autosomal recessive disorder characterized by a mutation of a single nucleotide of the β-globin gene on chromosome 11p, changing the sixth amino acid in the β-globin chain from glutamic acid to valine. As noted above, other forms of sickle cell disease result from co-inheritance of HbS with other abnormal b-globin chain variants, the most common forms being sickle hemoglobin C disease (HbSC) and two types of sickle β-thalassemia (HbSβ⁺ thalassemia and HbSβ⁰ thalassemia). Inheriting one HbS gene results in sickle cell trait. Inheriting two HbS genes results in sickle cell disease. Concordant with an autosomal recessive pattern of inheritance, if both parents carry one HbS gene, the fetus has a 25% chance of having sickle cell disease, 50% chance of having sickle cell trait, and 25% chance of being unaffected [6].

PATHOPHYSIOLOGY

In most individuals without hemoglobinopathy, 96% to 97% of hemoglobin in humans is Hemoglobin A (which consists of two α- and two β-chains), with small portions of Hemoglobin A2 (two α- and two δ-chains), and at times Hemoglobin F (two α- and two γ-chains). Hemoglobin provides the oxygen carrying capacity of erythrocytes. HbS occurs because of a point mutation in which valine, a hydrophilic amino acid, is substituted for glutamic acid, a hydrophobic amino acid in the β-globin gene. This allows the sickle hemoglobin to polymerize when it is deoxygenated, triggering a cascade of repeated injury to the red cell membrane. As a consequence, these cells become very rigid, assume a characteristic sickle shape, hemolyze, and are unable to pass through small capillaries, leading to vessel occlusion and ischemia. This tissue ischemia leads to acute and chronic pain as well as to end-organ damage. As vaso-occlusion can occur in any vessel, this is a systemic disease that can affect multiple organs. The life span of a sickle cell is about 10 to 20 days compared to the 120-day life span of a normal red blood cell. This chronic hemolysis contributes to the anemia [1,6,7]. Dehydration, infection, decrease in oxygen tension, and acidosis are common triggers of cell sickling and sickle cell crisis. Sickle cell crisis is a term used to label several different and independent acute conditions occurring in patients with sickle cell disease (vaso-occlusive crisis, aplastic crisis, hemolytic crisis).

SYMPTOMS

1. **Chronic hemolytic anemia**
   - Fatigue, pallor, shortness of breath.
   - Aplastic crisis presents with severe anemia and reticulocytopenia. It is the most common hematologic crisis during pregnancy.
2. **Acute vaso-occlusive episodes**
   - Pain involving the chest, lower back, abdomen, head, and bones/extremities.
   - Dactylitis (inflammation of fingers and/or toes) often the first symptom of sickle cell disease.
   - Exacerbated by cold, infection, stress, dehydration, alcohol, and fatigue.
3. **Infections**
   - Urinary tract infections, pneumonia, osteomyelitis, endometritis.
   - Organisms include *Streptococcus pneumoniae*, *Hemophilus influenza*, *Staphylococcus*, Gram-negative organisms, *Salmonella*, and mycoplasma.
4. **Cardiac**
   - Systolic murmur, cardiomegaly, high output failure.
5. **Pulmonary**
   - ACS presents with chest pain, dyspnea, tachypnea, fever, cough, leukocytosis, and pulmonary infiltrates. It is usually a result of infection, vaso-occlusion, or bone marrow embolization.
6. **Gastrointestinal**
   - Right upper quadrant syndrome presents with abdominal pain, fever, hepatomegaly, hyperbilirubinemia, and increased liver function tests. Splenomegaly is common.
7. **Renal**
   - Hematuria, papillary necrosis, nephrotic syndrome, renal infarction, pyelonephritis, hyposthenuria, and renal medullary carcinoma.
8. **Neurologic**
   - Transient ischemic attacks, cerebrovascular accidents, seizures, coma, hemiparesis, hemianesthesia, visual field changes, and cranial nerve palsy.
   - Moyamoya disease is a progressive occlusive process of the cerebral vasculature that results in the formation of collateral vessels with the appearance of "puffs of smoke" ("Moyamoya" in Japanese) on angiography.
9. **Skeletal**
   - Avascular necrosis most often occurs in the humeral and femoral heads and is characterized by pain.

COMPLICATIONS

Pregnancy in women with sickle cell disease is complicated by both the underlying disease and the physiologic changes and adaptations of pregnancy, which may compound or exacerbate organ damage. Despite this, most women can achieve a successful pregnancy: The majority tend to deliver beyond 28 weeks gestation with a >80% live birth rate although 50% will require transfusion or medically indicated hospitalization, and 75% will have a pain crisis during the pregnancy [8].

Several complications have been reported: effects of sickle cell disease on pregnancy—Table 15.1 [8–12]; effects of pregnancy on sickle cell disease—Table 15.2 [8,11,12]. Stroke occurs in 24% of women with sickle cell disease by age 45. Venous thromboembolism in 25% of women with sickle cell disease by age 30 [9]. During pregnancy, of women with sickle cell disease, about 50%–70% require hospitalization and 30%–40% blood transfusion [10].

PREGNANCY MANAGEMENT
Principles

Multidisciplinary team approach, involving providers from hematology, blood bank, primary care, obstetrics and/or maternal fetal medicine, and any other involved specialists (e.g., providers from pulmonology, cardiology, pain management, and social services).

Workup

- *For diagnosis:* Hemoglobin electrophoresis
- *For a crisis:* Hemoglobin, hemoglobin electrophoresis, urine culture, and culture of any other possible infectious source; blood gas if hypoxia is present

Preventive Care

Pneumococcal and influenza vaccines. Avoid triggers (especially infections). Optimize hemoglobin status by educating on good nutrition and prescribe vitamins/folic acid/iron as needed; establish a plan for the home medication regimen, and educate on analgesia safety in pregnancy.

Preconception

Patients are no longer counseled to avoid pregnancy. Counseling should consist of a review of the effects of sickle cell disease on pregnancy, highlighting an increased risk for hospital admissions, pain crises, infections, severe anemia, maternal mortality, preeclampsia, and other maternal

Table 15.1 Complications: Effects of Sickle Cell Disease on Pregnancy

Complication	HBSS	HBSC	HBSβ⁰
Pregnancy loss (mostly first trimester)	7%–36% [8,11,12]	9% [12]	
Fetal death	No increase [8,11]	No increase [8,11]	
Fetal growth restriction (FGR)	45% [11]	21% [11]	
Small for gestational age (SGA)[a]	21% [13]		
Acute anemia	4% [13]		15% [13]
Painful crises[b]	20%–50% [8,11,13]	19%–26% [11,13]	
Urinary tract infections	15% [8]		
Preterm birth	45% [11,13][c]	22% [11]	
Preeclampsia	10% [11,14]	3%	
Alloimmunization[d]	24% [21]	6% [21]	4% [21]
Antepartum admissions[e]	62% [11]	26% 2.8 [11]	
Postpartum infections[f]	1.4 [14]		

Note: % is reported if available in the source study.

[a] Preeclampsia and acute anemia episodes are risk factors for SGA. High hemoglobin F levels are protective for fetal growth [13].

[b] There is no difference in the rate of painful episodes before, during, and after pregnancies [13].

[c] The mean gestational age at delivery is 34 to 37 weeks [11,13].

[d] Percentages reflect women who were not randomized to prophylactic transfusions; there were no differences in alloimmunization among women with HbSS that were randomized to prophylactic transfusions and controls (29% versus 21%). Any woman with sickle cell disease is at increased risk for Rh and other antibodies if she has had blood transfusions in the past.

[e] Because of all the above complications, in particular painful crises, and increased incidences of infections in general, women with sickle cell disease in pregnancy are at increased risk for hospitalization.

[f] More likely to have postpartum infections secondary to endometritis or pyelonephritis. The effect is listed as odds ratio compared to the African American population. No increase risk for postpartum hemorrhage [8,11].

Table 15.2 Complications: Effects of Pregnancy on Sickle Cell Disease

Complication	HBSS
Maternal mortality	0.5%–2.1% [8,13,14]
Acute chest syndrome	7%–20% [8,13]
Thromboembolic events	2.5 [14]
Cerebral vein thrombosis	4.9 [14]
Pyelonephritis	1.3 [14]
Pneumonia	9.8 [14]
Sepsis	6.8 [14]
SIRS	12.6 [14]
Pulmonary hypertension	6.3 [14]
No. of blood transfusions	22.5 [14]
Postpartum infection	1.4 [14]

Note: % is reported if available in the source study. Otherwise, the effect is listed as odds ratios or relative risks.

complications (Tables 15.1 and 15.2) [8,11–14]. The discussion should also entail the effects of sickle cell disease on the fetus, which include early pregnancy loss, growth restriction, and perinatal mortality as well as a risk for inherited hemoglobinopathies. Preventive care should be emphasized. Try to optimize hemoglobin status by prescribing up to **4 mg folic acid** and a prenatal vitamin [4,15]. Discuss medication use during pregnancy and change/stop teratogenic medications (ACE inhibitors, iron chelators, and possibly hydroxyurea). Hydroxyurea is strongly recommended for adults with three or more crises per year, pain or chronic anemia interfering with daily life, or severe or recurrent episodes of ACS. Vaccinate as needed (see above).

Genetic counseling for women with sickle cell disease with possible preimplantation genetic diagnosis for those at risk of having a baby with sickle cell anemia can be offered.

Allogenic hematopoietic stem cell transplantation has been done with some success, almost exclusively in children, with bone marrow cells from HLA-identical siblings and is associated with a 92%–94% survival and 82%–86% event-free survival [16]. Despite rare reports of successful pregnancies in these women, almost all become infertile after the chemotherapy.

Prenatal Care

1. Initial visit: medical (assess for chronic organ damage, especially pulmonary hypertension, renal disease, and congestive heart failure), obstetrical, transfusion, and social history; nutritional assessment; discuss precipitating factors for painful crises and prior successful pain management. Counseling regarding risks (Tables 15.1 and 15.2), nutrition, hydration, and preventative care. Low-dose aspirin may be considered as the U.S. Preventative Services Task Force recommends the use of aspirin 81 mg/day starting early in pregnancy, i.e., in the first trimester, in women who are at high risk for preeclampsia. There are no trials specifically on this preventive intervention in this population, and we do not routinely offer it. Maternal-fetal medicine and hematology consults can be considered.

2. Initial laboratory studies: CBC; reticulocyte count; Hb electrophoresis; ferritin; bilirubin; liver function tests; hepatitis A, B, and C; HIV; BUN; creatinine, urine protein (by protein/creatinine ratio or 24-hour urine); antibody screen; rubella antibody titer; VDRL; tuberculosis skin test; Pap smear as appropriate; and chlamydia and gonorrhea cultures.

3. Offer laboratory evaluation to the father of the baby (CBC, hemoglobin electrophoresis). Offer genetic counseling if the father is positive for HbS. If the father is positive for HbS, offer prenatal diagnosis via chorionic villous sampling or amniocentesis through direct DNA analysis (polymerase chain reaction). Interestingly, the vast majority of women at risk of an affected fetus decline prenatal diagnosis.

4. Serial urine cultures every four to eight weeks.
5. CBC every trimester.
6. **Folate supplementation up to 4 mg daily** plus prenatal vitamin [4,13]. Ferrous sulfate 325 mg only if iron studies suggestive of iron deficiency. Iron overload should be avoided (ferritin >1000 ng/mL suggestive of overload).
7. Pneumococcal, influenza, and meningococcal vaccines.
8. Recommend first-trimester ultrasound for more accurate dating, which will aid in screening for growth restriction later during pregnancy. Ultrasound at 18 to 20 weeks for a detailed anatomy scan and then growth scans starting at 28 to 32 weeks as clinically indicated.
9. Some recommend maternal echocardiogram, especially if signs of pulmonary hypertension [17].
10. For patients with multiple red cell alloantibodies and an anticipated need for a blood transfusion, consider to have phenotypically matched units of PRBC identified.
11. Rescreen for red cell alloantibodies in third trimester [18].

THERAPY

1. **Painful crisis** (diagnosis made by history, often no physical or laboratory finding).
   - **Narcotics**: Morphine or hydromorphone are the preferred agents. Consider using a patient-controlled analgesia (PCA) system for severe pain. Oral controlled-release morphine is as effective as intravenous morphine in nonpregnant adults. Ask women regarding which narcotic or other pain medication works best for them and implement as appropriate. After 28 to 32 weeks, avoid NSAIDs, which are safe and effective earlier in pregnancy. Prescribe stool softeners with narcotic use [19].
   - **Intravenous fluids**: Effective in nonpregnant adults. Adequate fluid intake is 60 mL/kg/24 hours in adults [19]. Consider running fluids at a rate of 150 cc/hour. Monitor fluid balance.
   - **Antibiotics**: Broad-spectrum antibiotics should be used if patient is febrile (T >38°C), or if there is evidence of infection. A third-generation cephalosporin is typically given with addition of a macrolide (e.g., azithromycin or erythromycin) if chest symptoms are present [19].
   - **Oxygen**: Use only for ACS or if O_2 saturation is less than patient's known state or <95% [4] (such treatment is ineffective in nonpregnant patients and may be so in pregnant women as well) [19].
   - **Incentive spirometry** should be used by women hospitalized for vaso-occlusive crises.
   - **Labor and delivery**: There is no need to alter general recommendations for labor and delivery in women in sickle cell crisis. A crisis is not an indication for cesarean delivery or other special intervention. Close monitoring of mother and fetus for adequate oxygenation is paramount. Pain during labor can be managed with narcotics, regional anesthesia, or local anesthesia via pudendal block [20]. Pediatricians should be aware of any chronic narcotic use in pregnancy as such is a risk for neonatal withdrawal.
2. **Anemia**
   - **Transfusions**: There is limited evidence to assess the efficacy of prophylactic blood transfusions for pregnant women with sickle cell disease. Compared to transfusion only for Hb <6 g/dL, transfusion (or exchange transfusion) with two units of red cells every week for three weeks or until hemoglobin level is 10 to 11 g/dL or HbS <35% is associated with no significant difference in perinatal outcome [21]. Prophylactic transfusions decreased the number of painful crisis (14% vs. 50%). Disadvantages of prophylactic transfusion include increase in costs, number of hospitalizations, and risk of alloimmunization [21]. Therefore, prophylactic blood transfusions are not indicated universally for pregnant women with sickle cell disease.

   Indications for transfusions are any woman who is symptomatic or orthostatic from anemia and/or with a hemoglobin <6 g/dL or hematocrit <25% or with acute stroke, chest syndrome, or multiple organ failure.

   Sickle cell crisis is not an absolute indication to transfusion. Persistent crises are an indication to transfusion to avoid recurrence. If blood transfusion is indicated, it should always be leukodepleted and matched for Rh and Kell antigens.

   Goal of transfusion is usually hematocrit >35%, HbA_1 >40%, and HbS <35%.

   There is insufficient evidence to compare exchange versus regular blood transfusions for sickle cell disease in pregnancy. For a hematocrit <15%, a direct transfusion is always preferable. For a hematocrit >15%, an exchange transfusion can be considered.

   A serum ferritin level of >1000 ng/mL is suggestive of iron overload and is a contraindication to iron supplementation.
   - **Iron, folic acid, and multivitamins**: Only prescribe iron if patient is deficient (avoid iron overload).
   - **Hydroxyurea** (hydroxycarbamide): In nonpregnant women, hydroxyurea has been shown to decrease the number and severity of painful crises and to improve overall survival [22]. Data in pregnancy is limited; however, available case reports do not appear to demonstrate an increased risk of congenital malformations [23–25]. **If felt to be beneficial for management, its use could be considered during pregnancy.**

ALLOIMMUNIZATION

If the antibody screen is positive as a result of sensitization from past transfusions, follow recommendations in Chapter 52. The antigen status of the father of the pregnancy should be tested as he often does not carry the offending antigen with the maternal antibody usually acquired by prior transfusions. Bilirubin level (Delta OD450) in amniotic fluid of women with sickle cell disease is unreliable for detecting fetal anemia as maternal hemolysis and hyperbilirubinemia increase fetal and AF bilirubin levels. Fetal anemia may be assessed by middle cerebral artery Doppler (see Chapter 52).

ANTENATAL TESTING

There are no prospective studies on the use of antepartum testing in sickle cell disease women [10]. Fetal monitoring can be started at 32 weeks with weekly nonstress tests (or biophysical profiles), especially if the fetus is growth restricted [6].

DELIVERY

It is safe for patients to deliver vaginally. Inductions and cesarean deliveries should be reserved for obstetrical indications [4]. Although some have proposed delivery around 37 weeks [10], there is no strong evidence for delivery before 39 0/7 and 39 6/7 weeks unless complications (e.g., preeclampsia) occur. There is one case report of a sickle cell crisis triggered by induction of labor with a prostaglandin [26]. Some recommend prophylactic transfusion before a cesarean delivery to avoid precipitating a crisis because of blood loss in patients with hemoglobin 7 to 8 g/dL or less [20].

ANESTHESIA

There are no contraindications to anesthesia (IV, regional, or general) [4].

POSTPARTUM

During the postpartum period, early ambulation and adequate hydration is encouraged. Compression boots and incentive spirometry should be used. Guidelines from the Royal College of Obstetricians and Gynecologists recommend administration of prophylactic LMWH for 10 days postpartum in all women with sickle cell disease [27]. Although U.S. guidelines are more lenient, the American College of Obstetricians and Gynecologists does recommend consideration of pharmacologic prophylaxis in women after cesarean birth if additional risk factors are present; thus, it seems prudent to consider postpartum prophylaxis with LMWH in women with sickle cell disease after cesarean birth or if additional risk factors are present [28]. Decision making regarding VTE prophylaxis in women after a vaginal birth should consider risk factors in addition to sickle cell disease (e.g., age, obesity); those with several risk factors may warrant chemoprophylaxis. Anemia should be assessed and transfusion only if indicated (see above). Breast-feeding is encouraged. About 5%–6% of neonates of mothers with sickle cell disease can have neonatal withdrawal syndrome due to maternal chronic opioid use [29].

CONTRACEPTION

Progestin-containing contraception agents are safe among women with sickle cell disease; these include depot medroxyprogesterone acetate (DMPA) etonogestrel implants and the levonorgestrel intrauterine device [30,31]. The copper intrauterine device system is a safe, effective, and excellent choice in these women. Although these women are at higher risk of VTE and anemia, estrogen-containing contraceptives can be considered if the advantages outweigh the risks for that individual [30].

ACUTE CHEST SYNDROME
Definition

New pulmonary infiltrate of at least one complete lung segment with alveolar consolidation and excluding atelectasis and presence of chest pain, temp T >38.5°C, tachypnea, wheezing, or cough. Hypoxia, decreasing hemoglobin levels, and progressive pneumonia are frequent. Mostly associated with pulmonary fat embolism and pulmonary infection with 3% to 10% chance of death related to pulmonary embolism and pneumonia.

Incidence

Acute chest syndrome develops in about 10% of women with sickle cell disease.

Pathophysiology

Cause of ACS remains mainly unknown. Infection leading to sickle crisis, anemia, hypoxia, and vaso-occlusion with ischemic damage are the most common associations.

Symptoms

Chest pain, pain in arms and legs, dypnea, fever, etc.

Complications

ACS is one of the most common causes of death (3%–10%) among those with sickle cell disease. Neurologic complications, probably secondary to CNS hypoxia, occur in about 20% of patients. Pulmonary emboli and infarction can also occur.

Workup

For ACS, chest X-ray, sputum culture, nasopharyngeal sample, and/or culture of bronchoscopy washings (*Chlamydia pneumoniae* and *Mycoplasma pneumoniae* are most common pathogens).

Therapy

Antibiotics (usually cephalosporin and a macrolide) aimed at infectious pathogen(s) in pulmonary tree, and bronchodilators (even if no evidence of reactive airway disease). Blood transfusions (especially in hypoxic and/or anemic women), oxygen (15% need mechanical ventilation), and pain control as needed [31].

SICKLE CELL TRAIT

Pregnant women with sickle cell trait should be screened with a hemoglobin electrophoresis if this has not been done before, and testing of the father and genetic counseling should be offered. They are at increased risk of **urinary tract infections** and therefore should have a urine culture at the first prenatal visit and in every trimester. Asymptomatic bacteriuria should be treated.

HBSC DISEASE

HbC is due to a single nucleotide substitution (A for G) in the sixth codon of the β-globin gene (making it a Hb C gene) in chromosome 11, leading to substitution of lysine for glutamic acid on the β-globin chain, resulting in β^c globin. Of African Americans, 1% are carriers (trait). Diagnosis is by electrophoresis. No disease with trait only.

HbSC occurs in about 1/833 African Americans. About 40% to 60% have same clinical course as HbSS disease, and others have milder disease. Preventive and prenatal management should be as for HbSS.

HBS-/βTHAL

There are two types of sickle cell-beta thalassemia, and they are classified according to the amounts of beta globin chain present. Women with HbSβ⁰ have complete absence of beta globin, and are clinically similar to HbSS (hemoglobin electrophoresis: absent HbA; elevated HbA2 and HbF). Women with HbSβ⁺ have reduced amounts of beta globin (hemoglobin electrophoresis: low HbA; elevated HbA2 and HbF) and are typically managed similar to women with HbSS but tend to have milder disease [32,33].

HEMOGLOBIN E

Prevalent in Southeast Asia. No increase in mortality; may have slight decrease in birth weight and increase in abruption.

REFERENCES

1. Rust OA, Perry KG. Pregnancy complicated by sickle hemoglobinopathy. *Clin Obstet Gynecol* 1995; 38(3): 472–84. [Review]
2. Serjeant GR, Higgs DR, Hambleton IR. Elderly survivors with homozygous sickle cell disease. *N Engl J Med* 2007; 356(6): 642–3. [III]
3. World Health Organization. *Sickle Cell Anaemia: Report by the Secretariat*. 59th World Health Assembly; 2006. [III]
4. ACOG Committee on Obstetrics. ACOG Practice Bulletin No. 78: Hemoglobinopathies in pregnancy. *Obstet Gynecol* 2007; 109(1): 229–37. [III]
5. Serjeant GR. The emerging understanding of sickle cell disease. *Br J Haematol* 2001; 112(1): 3–18. [Review]
6. Rappaport VJ, Velazquez M, Williams K. Hemoglobinopathies in pregnancy. *Obstet Gynecol Clin North Am* 2004; 31(2): 287–317, vi. [Review]
7. Stuart MJ, Nagel RL. Sickle-cell disease. *Lancet* 2004; 364(9442): 1343–60. [Review]
8. Serjeant GR, Loy LL, Crowther M, Hambleton IR, Thame M. Outcome of pregnancy in homozygous sickle cell disease. *Obstet Gynecol* 2004; 103(6): 1278–85. [II-2]
9. Naik RP, Streiff MB, Haywood C, Nelson JA, Lanzkron S. Venous thromboembolism in adults with sickle cell disease: A serious and under-recognized complication. *Am J Med* 2013; 126(5): 443–9. [II-2]
10. Ngô C, Kayem G, Habibi A, Benachi A, Goffinet F, Galactéros F et al. Pregnancy in sickle cell disease: Maternal and fetal outcomes in a population receiving prophylactic partial exchange transfusions. *Eur J Obstet Gynecol Reprod Biol* 2010; 152(2): 138–42. [II-3]
11. Sun PM, Wilburn W, Raynor BD, Jamieson D. Sickle cell disease in pregnancy: Twenty years of experience at Grady Memorial Hospital, Atlanta, Georgia. *Am J Obstet Gynecol* 2001; 184(6): 1127–30. [II-2]
12. Milner PF, Jones BR, Döbler J. Outcome of pregnancy in sickle cell anemia and sickle cell-hemoglobin C disease. An analysis of 181 pregnancies in 98 patients, and a review of the literature. *Am J Obstet Gynecol* 1980; 138(3): 239–45. [II-3]
13. Smith JA, Espeland M, Bellevue R, Bonds D, Brown AK, Koshy M. Pregnancy in sickle cell disease: Experience of the Cooperative Study of Sickle Cell Disease. *Obstet Gynecol* 1996; 87(2): 199–204. [II-2]
14. Villers MS, Jamison MG, De Castro LM, James AH. Morbidity associated with sickle cell disease in pregnancy. *Am J Obstet Gynecol* 2008; 199(2): 125.e1–5. [III]
15. Bennett L, Chapman C, Davis B et al. Pregnancy, contraception and fertility. In: *Standards for the Clinical Care of Adults with Sickle Cell Disease in the UK London: Sickle Cell Society*. 2008. [III]
16. Yawn BP, Buchanan GR, Afenyi-Annan AN, Ballas SK, Hassell KL, James AH et al. Management of sickle cell disease: Summary of the 2014 evidence-based report by expert panel members. *JAMA* 2014; 312(10): 1033–48. [III]
17. Klings ES, Machado RF, Barst RJ, Morris CR, Mubarak KK, Gordeuk VR et al. An official American Thoracic Society clinical practice guideline: Diagnosis, risk stratification, and management of pulmonary hypertension of sickle cell disease. *Am J Respir Crit Care Med* 2014; 189(6): 727–40. [III]
18. Okusanya BO, Oladapo OT. Prophylactic versus selective blood transfusion for sickle cell disease in pregnancy. *Cochrane Database Syst Rev* 2013; 12: CD010378. [I]
19. Rees DC, Olujohungbe AD, Parker NE, Stephens AD, Telfer P, Wright J et al. Guidelines for the management of the acute painful crisis in sickle cell disease. *Br J Haematol* 2003; 120(5): 744–52. [II-3]
20. Firth PG, Head CA. Sickle cell disease and anesthesia. *Anesthesiology* 2004; 101(3): 766–85. [Review]
21. Koshy M, Burd L, Wallace D, Moawad A, Baron J. Prophylactic red-cell transfusions in pregnant patients with sickle cell disease. A randomized cooperative study. *N Engl J Med* 1988; 319(22): 1447–52. [RCT, *n* = 72]
22. Rees DC, Williams TN, Gladwin MT. Sickle-cell disease. *Lancet* 2010; 376(9757): 2018–31. [Review]
23. Ballas SK, McCarthy WF, Guo N, DeCastro L, Bellevue R, Barton BA et al. Exposure to hydroxyurea and pregnancy outcomes in patients with sickle cell anemia. *J Natl Med Assoc* 2009; 101(10): 1046–51. [II-2]
24. Jackson N, Shukri A, Ali K. Hydroxyurea treatment for chronic myeloid leukaemia during pregnancy. *Br J Haematol* 1993; 85(1): 203–4. [II-2]
25. Liebelt EL, Balk SJ, Faber W, Fisher JW, Hughes CL, Lanzkron SM et al. NTP-CERHR expert panel report on the reproductive and developmental toxicity of hydroxyurea. *Birth Defects Res B Dev Reprod Toxicol* 2007; 80(4): 259–366. [III]
26. Faron G, Corbisier C, Tecco L, Vokaer A. First sickle cell crisis triggered by induction of labor in a primigravida. *Eur J Obstet Gynecol Reprod Biol*. 2001 Feb; 94(2):304–6. [II-3]
27. *Green-top Guideline No. 37a: Reducing the Risk of Venous Thromboembolism during Pregnancy and the Puerperium*. 2015. [III]
28. James A, Committee on Practice Bulletins—Obstetrics. Practice bulletin no. 123: Thromboembolism in pregnancy. *Obstet Gynecol* 2011; 118(3): 718–29. [III]
29. Kellogg A, Rose CH, Harms RH, Watson WJ. Current trends in narcotic use in pregnancy and neonatal outcomes. *Am J Obstet Gynecol* 2011; 204(3): 259.e1–4. [II-3]
30. *WHO Medical eligibility criteria for contraceptive use*. Fourth edition, 2009. http://whqlibdoc.who.int/publications/2010/9789241563888_eng.pdf. [III]
31. Manchikanti A, Grimes DA, Lopez LM, Schulz KF. Steroid hormones for contraception in women with sickle cell disease. *Cochrane Database Syst Rev* 2007; (2): CD006261. [I]
32. Platt OS, Thorington BD, Brambilla DJ, Milner PF, Rosse WF, Vichinsky E et al. Pain in sickle cell disease. Rates and risk factors. *N Engl J Med* 1991; 325(1): 11–6. [II-3]
33. Castro O, Brambilla DJ, Thorington B, Reindorf CA, Scott RB, Gillette P et al. The acute chest syndrome in sickle cell disease: Incidence and risk factors. The Cooperative Study of Sickle Cell Disease. *Blood* 1994; 84(2): 643–9. [II-3]

von Willebrand disease

Dawnette Lewis and Srikanth Nagalla

KEY POINTS

- It is difficult to establish a diagnosis of type I von Willebrand disease (vWD) in pregnant women. The diagnostic workup includes 1) prolonged bleeding time, 2) low levels of factor VIII, 3) decreased von Willebrand Factor (vWF) antigen (Ag), and 4) decreased ristocetin cofactor activity. Be aware of **physiologic increase of factor VIII and vWF levels in pregnancy.**
- Workup therefore includes these key **labs: factor VIII, vWFAg, ristocetin cofactor activity, bleeding time.**
- **DDAVP responsiveness** should be tested preconception or in the second or third trimester.
- **Prophylactic therapy for most common type (type I) of vWD if factor VIII <50% of normal is DDAVP.**
- **Prophylactic therapies for other types of vWD are according to type and include DDAVP, vWF concentrates (Humate P, Alphanate SD/HT), and/or adjuvant therapy (antifibrinolytic amino acids [amniocaproic acid and tranexamic acid], used in conjunction with desmopressin and plasma concentrates).**
- If possible, avoid pudendal blocks and operative vaginal deliveries as well as scalp lead and scalp pH given the usually 50% chance of the fetus being affected.

HISTORIC NOTES

von Willebrand disease (vWD) was first described in 1926 by a Finnish pediatrician, Erik von Willebrand. He also reported that the condition was inherited in an autosomal dominant fashion and improved with blood transfusions.

DIAGNOSIS/DEFINITION

Diagnosis of vWD is complex (Table 16.1) [1–7]. vWD is usually associated with prolonged bleeding time with aPT and aPTT frequently normal (aPTT is only prolonged in patients with severe vWD due to decreased Factor VIII level). For type I, the most important laboratory tests are the following:

- **Ristocetin cofactor activity** [binding of vWF:Ag to the platelet membrane glycoprotein Iba, mediated by the antibiotic ristocetin] (*decreased*) or **von Willebrand activity** (this test uses a monoclonal antibody against the GPIb binding site of vWF) (*decreased*).
- **vWF:Ag** [von Willebrand factor antigen; an immunoreactive protein] (*decreased*)
- **Factor VIII** (*decreased*)

As a patient progresses through pregnancy, many of the values for diagnosis are normal due to the hormonal effects on the vWF levels, and diagnosis cannot be made reliably. For distinguishing types (Table 16.1), also send multimeric analysis and factor VIII binding assay. Factor VIII levels are best (but not that good) at predicting surgical/soft-tissue bleeding.

SYMPTOMS

Abnormal bleeding symptoms include **epistaxis, bleeding from the gums and with dental surgery, ecchymoses, prolonged bleeding after minor cuts, menorrhagia, postpartum hemorrhage, delayed postpartum hemorrhage, and postoperative bleeding.** Ask for a detailed personal history (menstruation, injuries, surgeries, etc.) and family history.

EPIDEMIOLOGY/INCIDENCE

Incidence is about 1%–2% in the general population; it is the most common congenital hemorrhagic disease affecting males and females and all ethnic groups.

GENETICS

Usually autosomal dominant (Table 16.2). vWF is a large multimeric glycoprotein encoded on chromosome 12 and is synthesized and released from endothelium and megakaryocytes. There are more than 250 mutations of all types known.

ETIOLOGY/BASIC PATHOPHYSIOLOGY

Decrease (quantitative: types I and III) in von Willebrand factor (vWF; also known as factor VIII cofactor) or (qualitative: type II) its function. This cofactor is critical for normal platelet adhesion at site of vascular injury (Figure 16.1) [1–7].

CLASSIFICATION: TYPES

1. **(60%–85%) Autosomal Dominant.** Partial quantitative decrease of vWF. **Mild-moderate decrease in vWF.** Also **decreased factor VIII** 5–30 (nl 50–150 IU/dL); **decreased vWF:Ag, decreased** vWF:Ac (tinty)-measured by **ristocetin-induced cofactor** assay.
2. (10%–30%) Autosomal dominant. Qualitative defect of vWF. **Normal vWF but dysfunction:**
   A. Decreased vWF function due to decrease in large multimers
   B. Gain of function mutation causing increased binding of vWF to platelets and resulting in moderate thrombocytopenia.
   M and N types are uncommon.
3. (1%–5%) Autosomal recessive. Quantitative decrease. **No vWF** and very low factor VIII. Severe symptoms **do not respond to DDAVP.**

   Acquired – during certain disease states.

Table 16.1 Common Laboratory Findings in von Willebrand Disease

Subtype[a]	von Willebrand Factor Antigen	von Willebrand Factor Ristocetin Cofactor Activity	von Willebrand Factor Ristocetin Cofactor Activity/von Willebrand Factor Antigen (ratio)	Factor VIII	Low Dose Ristocetin-Induced Platelet Aggregation	Multimer Assay
Type 1	Low	Low	>0.5–0.7	Low or normal	No reaction	Normal
Type 2A	Low	Low	<0.5–0.7	Low or normal	No reaction	Decrease in large multimers
Type 2B	Low	Low	<0.5–0.7	Low or normal	Positive	Decrease in large multimers
Type 2M	Low	Low	<0.5–0.7	Low or normal	No reaction	Normal
Type 2N	Normal to low	Normal to low	>0.5–0.7	Low	No reaction	Normal
Type 3	Absent	Absent		Low	No reaction	Absent

Source: Adapted from Pacheco LD, Constantine MM, Saade GR, Mucowski S, Hankins GDV, Sciscione AC. *Am J Obstet Gynecol*, 203, 194–200, 2010.

Table 16.2 Mechanism, Inheritance, and Treatment for the Different Types of von Willebrand Disease

Type	Mechanism	Inheritance	Treatment	Second-Line Therapy
1	Quantitative (partial) decrease vWF	Autosomal dominant	DDAVP	Factor VIII/vWF concentrates
2	Qualitative/functional defect vWF	Autosomal dominant		
A	Platelet-dependent vWF— absence of large or intermediate size multimers	Autosomal dominant	Factor VIII/vWF concentrates	DDAVP
B	Large multimers absent (increase in binding with platelets and vWF)	Autosomal dominant	None	
M		Autosomal dominant	Factor VIII/vWF concentrates	DDAVP
N	Defect in binding of vWF with platelets	Autosomal dominant	Factor VIIII/vWF concentrates	DDAVP
3	Severe or absent vWF and Factor VIII deficiency	Autosomal recessive	Factor VIII/vWF concentrates (without alloantibodies) Recombinant factor VIII (with alloantibodies)	
Acquired	Occurs in disease states, such as cancer, valvular heart disease (AS), thrombocythemia, autoimmune diseases	Increased clearance of vWF from plasma	Treatment of underlying condition	Desmopressin, plasma concentrates, IVIg

Abbreviations: DDAVP, 1-deamino-8-D-arginine vasopressin; vWF, von Willebrand factor.

COMPLICATIONS

Intra- and postpartum hemorrhage. Postpartum hemorrhage occurs in 16%–29% of women within 24 hours and delayed (after 24 hours, usually within 2 weeks) in 20%–29% of women. Does not impair fertility or increase pregnancy loss.

PREGNANCY CONSIDERATIONS

Factor VIII and vWF levels rise in pregnancy, so they might be normal at term even with vWD.

PREGNANCY MANAGEMENT

Principles

Treat as you would in nonpregnant adult.

Workup (labs)

See "Diagnosis" above (Tables 16.1 and 16.2).

Management

Preconception counseling: Obtain history, type of vWD, records, etc.; hematology and genetic counseling consult as necessary; baseline laboratory tests (see workup above); hepatitis B vaccine. If vWD type I with factor VIII levels <50 IU/dL, type II or III, or history of severe bleeding, consider care in a high-risk center with close collaboration with hematologist.

    Prenatal care: First trimester: See "Preconception counseling" if not done yet. Prenatal diagnosis, including CVS, is possible (give DDAVP or other prophylaxis as appropriate per type—see below); Second/third trimester: Anesthesia consult; test response to DAVVP. Third trimester: monitor laboratory tests; birth plan (anesthesia, DDAVP, etc.). Aim to achieve factor VIII levels of ≥50 mu/dL, associated with very low risk of any bleeding complications [2,6,7].

    Therapy: See Table 16.2 and Figure 16.2.

TYPE I

DDAVP (desmopressin, i.e., 1-deamino-8-D-arginine vasopressin; synthetic vasopressin [AntiDiureticHormone] analog)

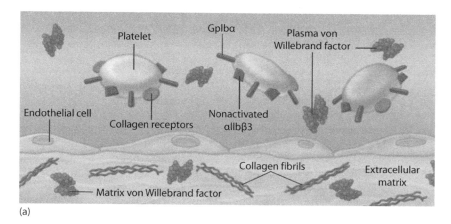

(a)

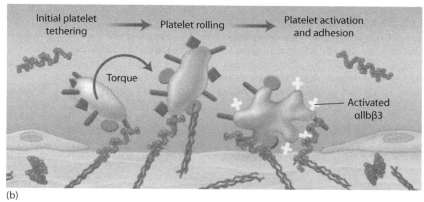

(b)

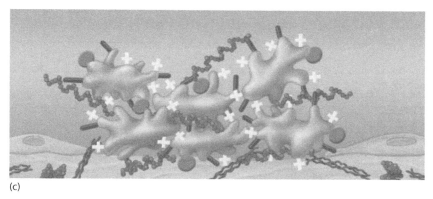

(c)

Figure 16.1 Platelet adhesion at site of vascular injury. (a) In the intact vessel wall, endothelial cells hamper the interactions of circulating platelets and their membrane glycoproteins Ibα (GpIbα), nonactivated IIb–IIIa (αIIbβ3), and collagen receptors GpVI and α2β1 with von Willebrand factor and collagen fibrils localized in the subendothelial extracellular matrix. When the vessel wall is intact and blood flow is normal, plasma von Willebrand factor that is present in a coiled structure and platelets coexist in circulating blood with minimal interactions. (b) In the damaged vessel wall, collagen and von Willebrand factor of the subendothelial matrix become exposed to flowing blood and shear forces. Plasma von Willebrand factor efficiently binds to exposed collagen and uncoils its structure, supporting the adhesion of circulating platelets in synergy with collagen. Bound von Willebrand factor interacts, at first, only with the platelet receptor GpIbα and platelet tethering occurs. This interaction has a fast dissociation rate, and platelets tethered to the vessel wall still move in the direction of flow (rolling). In this interaction, collagen receptors GpVI and α2β1 bind to collagen and promote platelet adhesion and activation in synergy with the von Willebrand factor–GpIbα interactions. (b and c) Once platelets are activated (represented by irregular margins), a conformational change of αIIbβ3 enhances its affinity for the ligand von Willebrand factor (receptors are shown as crosses). This event, together with the rolling of platelets due to the von Willebrand factor–GpIbα interaction, allows αIIbβ3 to bind platelets to the vessel wall (c) αIIbβ3 is also responsible for platelet-to-platelet interactions that eventually lead to platelet-plug formation mediated by von Willebrand factor and, at slow flow conditions, by fibrinogen (not shown). (From Mannucci P. *NEJM*, 351, 683–94, 2004. Reprinted with permission.)

0.3 mcg/kg IV over 30 minutes (maximum dose: 25–30 mcg). Works within one hour (peak occurs in 30–90 minutes after the infusion). Also available SQ (0.3 mcg/kg) or nasal inhalation (300 mcg in adults). Mechanism of action is promoting release of vWF and factor VIII from endothelial cells. So increases ristocetin cofactor activity and increases x 3 vWF:Ag level, factor VIII procoagulant level (FVIII:C). Can give test dose and then **check Factor VIII** and ristocetin cofactor activity at peak—one hour—and clearance—four hours. It lasts up to 10 hours, so repeat every 12 hours, maximum two to four doses. **DDAVP is first-line therapy for type I; second line for IIa; and contraindicated for type IIb.**

Safe in pregnancy for mother and fetus (does not cross placenta) [2] and during breast-feeding (Category B).

If not responsive to DDAVP: **alphanate** (factor VIII and vWF mixed). This is better than cryoprecipitate because there are no infectious disease issues. Otherwise use **humate-P** (purified Factor VIII). Usual loading dose for these 2 vWF concentrates is 40–60 IU/kg. Alternatives, especially more for treatment of hemorrhage more than prophylaxis, are **cryoprecipitate** (fibrinogen and vWF), **FFP** (watch volume overload), **cryoprecipitate** (fibrinogen and vWF), or **FFP**

(watch volume overload). Applies to all above: Safety: limited data, but probably safe. Counsel regarding blood product precautions.

Type IIa

Preferred therapy is Factor VIII/vWF concentrates (as alphanate, humate-P, etc.).

Type IIb

No specific treatment is available, but can treat as per Figure 16.2.

Type III

Without alloantibodies: factor VIII/vWF concentrates; with alloantibodies: recombinant factor VIII.

Antepartum Testing

Not indicated unless other complications present (no known direct fetal risks).

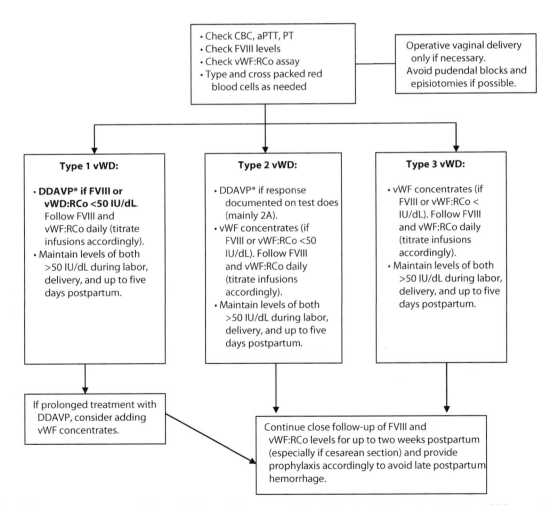

Figure 16.2 Peripartum management of von Willebrand disease. aPTT, activated partial thromboplastin time; CBC, complete blood count; DDAVP, 1-deamino-8-D-arginine vasopressin; vWF, von Willebrand factor; vWF:RCo, von Willebrand factor ristocetin cofactor activity. *Avoid hypotonic solutions at time of delivery if using DDAVP in order to prevent hyponatremia. (Adapted from Pacheco LD, Constantine MM, Saade GR, Mucowski S, Hankins GDV, Sciscione AC. *Am J Obstet Gynecol*, 203, 194–200, 2010.)

Delivery (Figure 16.2)

Types I and II: Measure 1) bleeding time, 2) **factor VIII**, 3) vWFAg, and 4) ristocetin cofactor activity. **If vWF activity levels are ≥50 mu/dL, there is very low risk of bleeding with vaginal or cesarean delivery. If lower, prophylactically administer DDAVP (if DDAVP responder) or concentrates/ blood products** (see above, according to type) *at time of delivery (if possible one hour before)* **and 12 hours thereafter** (then as needed).

Type III: Do not measure vWF activity as always low. Treat daily as above starting before delivery.

Oxytocin dose should be carefully monitored because fluid retention can be a side effect of both oxytocin and DDAVP and lead to life-threatening hyponatremia. As fetus has a 50% chance of having von Willebrand disease, scalp lead, scalp pH, and operative vaginal delivery should be avoided.

Anesthesia

Regional anesthesia is safe if normal PTT, factor VIII levels of ≥50 mu/dL and normal ristocetin cofactor activity.

Postpartum/Breast-Feeding

Measure factor VIII one to two weeks postpartum because increased level during pregnancy will again physiologically decrease in vWD disease. Risk of postpartum bleeding in fact continues for about two to four weeks, so that additional doses of DDAVP and close monitoring are required. As the neonate has a 50% chance of having von Willebrand disease, circumcision may need to be delayed until after testing.

FUTURE

vWF produced by recombinant DNA techniques; gene therapy.

RARE/RELATED

Glanzman disease (congenital thromboasthenia): congenital bleeding disorder defined by defective or quantitatively abnormal glycoprotein (GP) IIb/IIIa receptors (Figure 16.1). Diagnosis: bleeding and abnormal platelet aggregation in response to stimuli, prolonged bleeding times, normal platelet counts [3]. Four pregnancies in the world's literature up to 1978, very few if any after.

REFERENCES

1. Mannucci P. Treatment of von Willebrand disease. *NEJM* 2004; 351: 683–94. [Review]
2. James AH. Von Willebrand disease. *Obstet Gynecol Survey* 2006; 61: 136–45. [Review]
3. Newman PJ, Seligsohn U, Lyman S et al. The molecular genetic basis of Glanzmann thrombasthenia in the Iraqi-Jewish and Arab populations in Israel. *Proc Natl Acad Sci USA* 1991; 88: 3160–4. [II-3]
4. Pacheco LD, Constantine MM, Saade GR, Mucowski S, Hankins GDV, Sciscione AC. Von Willebrand disease and pregnancy: A practical approach for the diagnosis and treatment. *Am J Obstet Gynecol* 2010; (203): 194–200. [Review]
5. Kadir RA, Lee CA, Sabin CA, Pollard D, Economides DL. Pregnancy in women with von Willebrand's disease or factor XI deficiency. *BJOG* 1998; 105: 314–21. [II-3]
6. Lipe BC, Dumas MA, Ornstein DL. Von Willebrand disease in pregnancy. *Hematol Oncol Clin N Am* 2011; 25: 335–58. [Review]
7. Chi C, Kadir RA. Inherited bleeding disorders in pregnancy. *Best Pract Res Clin Obstet Gynaecol* 2012; 26: 103–17. [Review]

17

Renal disease

Rebekah McCurdy

KEY POINTS

- The frequency of complications in pregnancies with maternal renal disease is directly proportional to the severity of renal dysfunction, typically correlated with the initial creatinine level.
- Complications include **preterm birth, preeclampsia, fetal growth restriction, low birth weight, and perinatal mortality.** In women with **creatinine ≥1.4 mg/dL,** about 10% will have progressive **renal deterioration. Creatinine >2.3 mg/dL may be regarded as a contraindication to pregnancy.**
- **Workup** includes serum **creatinine, blood urea nitrogen, and electrolytes** as well as **24-hour urine collection for protein and creatinine clearance.**
- Hypertension is commonly associated with renal disease and should be treated to **keep diastolic <90 mmHg.**
- Women with end-stage renal disease (ESRD) on **dialysis** should be counseled **preconception** that they **should receive a renal transplant** and **then wait one to two years** before attempting pregnancy. Women on dialysis or with a recently transplanted kidney should be maintained on **effective contraception.** If pregnant, counseling should include review of the very **high rates** of the above **complications.**
- There is an overall **success** of pregnancy (live births) in women after **renal transplantation of >90%.**
- In women with **moderate-to-severe** renal insufficiency, **low-dose aspirin started in early pregnancy** may reduce the incidence of **preeclampsia.**
- **Pelvic floor exercises** during and after pregnancy **decrease the incidence of urinary incontinence in the third trimester and postpartum.**
- Asymptomatic bacteriuria should be assessed for at the first prenatal visit and treated promptly as 20%–40% of women will develop pyelonephritis if left untreated.

DIAGNOSES/DEFINITIONS

- *Chronic renal insufficiency (CRI)*: Synonymous with chronic renal failure (CRF). Includes five stages, the most severe of which are characterized by irreversible, progressive impaired kidney function (Table 17.1) [1,2], ultimately leading to end-stage renal disease. The most mild forms may be associated with little or no long-term adverse outcomes. Table 17.2 [3] details CRI staging from the National Institutes of Health.
- *End-stage renal disease (ESRD)*: Patients with ESRD (Stage 5 CRF) no longer have kidney function adequate to sustain life and **require dialysis or kidney transplantation.** Without proper treatment, ESRD is fatal.

SYMPTOMS

Include a frequent need to urinate and edema as well as possible anemia, fatigue, weakness, headaches, and loss of appetite. As renal disease progresses, other symptoms, such as nausea, vomiting, bad breath, and pruritus, may develop as toxic metabolites, normally filtered out of the blood by the kidneys, build up to harmful levels.

EPIDEMIOLOGY/INCIDENCE

The overall incidence of renal disease (excluding asymptomatic bacteriuria) in the general obstetric population is 0.03% to 0.2% [4–6].

PHYSIOLOGIC RENAL CHANGES IN PREGNANCY

Pregnancy is marked by vasodilation, occurring soon after conception. This results in a drop in blood pressure, an increase in cardiac output, and an increase in renal blood flow and glomerular filtration rate (GFR). These changes persist until late gestation. Likely causes include increased progesterone, nitric oxide, relaxin, and estrogen. Functionally, there is increased renal plasma flow (peaks 60%–80% in the second trimester, then falls to 50%–60% above baseline during the third trimester). GFR increases 30% during the first trimester and peaks at 50% above prepregnancy values in the second trimester. Creatinine and urea production remains unchanged, resulting in a drop in serum creatinine and urea levels to mean values of 0.6 and 9 mg/dL, respectively. Near term, a 15% to 20% decrease in GFR occurs [7,8] (Chapter 3 of *Obstetric Evidence Based Guidelines*). Ideally, evaluation of renal function in pregnancy should be based on GFR with creatinine clearance probably the best way to approximate GFR (normal values: Table 17.3) [9]. There is an increase in the size of the kidneys and urinary collecting system. Kidney length increases approximately 1 cm and volume increases 30% [10]. The entire collecting system becomes dilated, which may be confused with an obstructive uropathy. Mild hydronephrosis, particularly common on the right, may be present and physiologic in more than 90% of normal pregnancies [11].

CLASSIFICATION

See Tables 17.1 and 17.2 [1,2].

RISK FACTORS/PRECONCEPTION COUNSELING

As functional loss progresses, the risks to mother and fetus increase substantially [1,12]. The goal is to optimize prepregnancy health.

Table 17.1 Classification of Renal Insufficiency

Category	Serum Creatinine[a] (µmol/L [mg/dL])
Preserved	<100 (<1.1)
Mildly impaired renal function	100–124 (1.1–1.3)
Moderate renal insufficiency	125–250 (1.4–2.8)
Severe renal insufficiency	>250 (>2.8)

Sources: Adapted from Lindheimer MD, Davison JM, Katz AI. *Semin Nephrol*, 21, 2, 173–89, 2001; Modena A, Hoffman M, Tolosa JE. *Am J Obstet Gynecol*, 193, 6, S86, 2005.
[a]In early pregnancy.

Table 17.2 Stages of Chronic Kidney Disease[a]

Stage	Description	GFR
1	Normal kidney function but urine findings or structural abnormalities or genetic trait point to kidney disease	>90
2	Mildly reduced kidney function, and other findings point to kidney disease	60–89
3	Moderately reduced kidney function	30–59
4	Severely reduced kidney function	15–29
5	Very severe or end-stage kidney failure	<15 or on dialysis

Source: Modified from Levey AS, Coresh J, Balk E, Kausz AT, Levin A, Steffes MW et al. *Ann Intern Med*, 139, 2, 137–47, 2003.
[a]National Kidney Foundation 2002 (http://www2.kidney.org/professionals /KDOQI/guidelines_ckd/p4_class_g1.htm).

Table 17.3 Normal Ranges of Renal Functions during Pregnancy

	Nonpregnant Adult	First Trimester	Second Trimester	Third Trimester
Creatinine (mg/dL)	0.5–0.9	0.4–0.7	0.4–0.8	0.4–0.9
Glomerular filtration rate (ml/min)	106–132	131–166	135–170	117–182

Source: Modified from Abbassi-Ghanavati M, Greer LG, Cunningham FG. *Obstet Gynecol*, 114, 6, 1326–31, 2009.

Specific Diseases

- *Vasculopathy*: Patients with vasculopathy from scleroderma and polyarteritis nodosa should be discouraged from pregnancy because of high maternal and fetal morbidity and mortality [1,13,14].
- *Lupus nephritis*: Patients with lupus nephritis do well when the disease is in remission for six months prior to conception with a live birth rate up to 95% [15,16]. Rates of preterm delivery and preeclampsia are based on degree of renal insufficiency. Total live birth rate for all lupus patients is 58% to 95% [15,17]. Low complement levels at conception are predictive of adverse pregnancy outcomes (RR 19), and use of low-dose aspirin during pregnancy is associated with a decrease in adverse outcomes (RR 0.11) [16]. Presence of antiphospholipid antibodies is also associated with increased risk [18]. In addition, the risk of lupus flare is increased in patients with >1 g of proteinuria or GFR <60 mL/min [16] (see Chapter 25).
- *IgA nephropathy*: Women with biopsy-proven IgA nephropathy can be counseled that pregnancy does not appear to impact kidney function [19].
- *Mild renal insufficiency*: Typically successful pregnancy outcomes with no adverse effect on the course of their disease [20].
- *Moderate and severe renal insufficiency*: Prognosis is more guarded. Deterioration in renal function is seen in 43% of which 10% do not improve postpartum [21].

CHRONIC RENAL INSUFFICIENCY
Complications

Prognosis is directly related to the degree of renal insufficiency (Table 17.4) [14,22–26]. The best outcomes are in women with preconception serum creatinine levels below 2 mg/dL and diastolic blood pressure of 90 mmHg or less although women with only mild renal insufficiency may still be at increased risk for adverse outcomes [1,6,27]. Creatinine clearance below 70 mL/min prior to conception is associated with poor outcomes even when serum creatinine levels are in the minimal dysfunction category [28]. Needing more than one antihypertensive medication for optimal control is associated with a significant decrease in live birth rate [20]. Proteinuria (>1 g/24 hr) and reduced GFR (<40 mL/min) in combination are risk factors for progression of renal disease to end stage

Table 17.4 Rate of Complications According to Degree of Renal Insufficiency (%)

Creatinine	PTB	Preeclampsia	HTN	FGR	Perinatal Mortality	Live Birth	Decline in Renal Function
<1.4	20	11	25	24	9	>90	16
1.4–2.8	36–60	42	56	31–37	7	>90	50
>2.8	73–86	86	56	43–57	36	N/A	40
Dialysis	48–84	20	100	50–80	60	40–50	N/A
Renal transplant	52–75	23–37	47–63	20–66	7	74–80	14

Sources: Adapted from Jones DC. *Clin Perinatol*, 24, 2, 483–96, 1997; Airoldi J, Weinstein L. *Obstet Gynecol Surv*, 62, 2, 117–24, 2007; Hou SH. *Am J Kidney Dis*, 23, 1, 60–3, 1994; Armenti VT, Radomski JS, Moritz MJ, Gaughan WJ, Philips LZ, McGrory CH et al. *Clin Transpl*, 97–105, 2001; Luders C, Castro MC, Titan SM, De Castro I, Elias RM, Abensur H et al. *Am J Kidney Dis*, 56, 1, 77–85, 2010; Crowe AV, Rustom R, Gradden C, Sells RA, Bakran A, Bone JM et al. *QJM*, 92, 11, 631–5, 1999.
Abbreviations: FGR, fetal growth restriction; HTN, hypertension; N/A, not available; PTB, preterm birth.

and also predict a shorter time to dialysis therapy and lower birth weight [29].

- *Infertility*: Conception with GFR <25 mL/min is rare secondary to alterations in hypothalamic–pituitary–adrenal (HPA) axis [30].
- *Hypertension*: Incidence of hypertension increases from 28% at baseline to approximately 50% by the third trimester [21].
- *Proteinuria*: Urinary protein excretion >3 g in 24 hours increases from approximately 25% to 41% during pregnancy [21].
- *Preeclampsia*: Increased incidence. Diagnosis is difficult because of the high frequency of baseline hypertension and proteinuria.
- *Preterm labor*: Incidence as high as 85% [31].
- *Low birth weight*: 66% [31].
- *Perinatal mortality*: 10% to 20% [20,21].
- *Cost*: Women with chronic renal disease have increased median cost of pregnancy [4].

Pregnancy Considerations

Pregnancy does not appear to adversely affect the natural history of renal disease in women with mild dysfunction. However, 10% with moderate-to-severe disease will suffer irreversible deterioration during pregnancy [5,21,32]. Preconception assessment of renal function should be recommended to all patients with diabetes mellitus seeking pregnancy as adverse outcomes are more common with diabetic nephropathy [33]. Referral to a nephrologist should be considered for all diabetics with a creatinine >1.4 [34].

Workup

Serum creatinine, BUN, and electrolytes as well as **24-hour urine collection for protein and creatinine clearance**. A 24-hour urine >300 mg protein is considered abnormal and correlates roughly to 1+ proteinuria on a urine dipstick. Urine dipstick should not be the only testing for women with suspected renal disease as this can miss up to one in 11 hypertensive pregnant women with actual proteinuria [35]. A 24-hour urine collection has long been the gold standard although **a random protein-creatinine ratio has been shown to accurately predict baseline proteinuria in early pregnancy** [36,37]. Renal biopsy should be reserved for those whose diagnosis is in question, particularly in those with sudden deterioration in renal function for no known reason as it may change the management in up to 66% of cases [38]. It is generally recommended only before 32 weeks of pregnancy as delivery after 32 weeks may be accomplished with relatively good outcomes for the neonate after which the biopsy may be performed. Severe renal disease may increase the risk of complications from the renal biopsy. A skilled physician and ultrasound guidance should be used in the performance of a renal biopsy in a pregnant individual [10].

Prevention

Aim to preserve whatever renal function remains. Screen for diabetes and hypertension and arrange for appropriate consultation and treatment so as to prevent end-organ complications. In addition, dose medications appropriately for chronic renal disease so as to avoid acute or chronic kidney injury.

Management

Patients with moderate or severe renal insufficiency should be managed with a **multidisciplinary approach** in conjunction with a perinatologist, nephrologist, and neonatologist.

Prenatal Care

Prenatal Visits

Women may be seen every two to four weeks until 32 weeks gestation, after which they may need to be seen weekly because of the markedly increased risk for severe preeclampsia. Careful monitoring of blood pressure and proteinuria for early detection of hypertension and superimposed preeclampsia should be performed at every visit.

Laboratory Tests

Evaluation of renal function should include a **24-hour creatinine clearance and protein excretion** at least at the first visit in early pregnancy and, depending on severity of renal insufficiency, each trimester. Frequent **urine culture** should be done for early detection of asymptomatic bacteriuria or confirmation of urinary tract infection. Maternal anemia should be corrected with iron supplementation or erythropoietin if severe. Pregnant women may need higher doses of erythropoietin to maintain hematocrit >35% [39].

Antenatal Testing

- Frequent (e.g., monthly) ultrasound for fetal growth
- Biophysical assessment (e.g., nonstress tests, or biophysical profile scores) of fetal well-being beginning weekly at ≥32 weeks

Patient Education

The symptoms of preterm labor and preeclampsia should be reviewed with women who have chronic renal disease.

Therapy

Hypertension

Hypertension should be treated aggressively in obstetric patients with underlying renal dysfunction to preserve kidney function. The goal is to **keep diastolic blood pressure <90 mmHg**. Use of antihypertensive medication in pregnancy is discussed in Chapter 1.

Preeclampsia

Magnesium is not contraindicated but should be **used with extreme caution** begun at 1 to 2 g/hr, possibly without a bolus, or just giving boluses (no continuous infusion rate) as needed. Evaluation for side effects of magnesium should occur at least hourly, and magnesium levels should be checked often (e.g., every two to four hours) in labor to adjust the dose. Calcium gluconate should be available. An alternative is to use phenytoin 15 to 20 mg/kg IV. **Low-dose aspirin** should be started in the first trimester in women with moderate to severe CRI and in women with a history of lupus nephritis to reduce the incidence of preeclampsia and fetal growth restriction (FGR) [16,40,41].

Preterm Labor

Magnesium and indomethacin should be used with caution as they are renally excreted.

Delivery

Delivery should be performed at a tertiary care center. Mode of delivery should be for standard obstetric indications. Deliberate preterm birth may be necessary in the face of worsening maternal renal function, severe preeclampsia, or worsening fetal status.

Postpartum/Breast-Feeding

Little is known about the quantities of immunosuppressive agents in breast milk. Although small series have shown little toxicity, caution should be used when recommending breast-feeding to patients taking these agents [42].

Long-Term Renal Prognosis

When kidney dysfunction is mild, pregnancy does not appear to adversely alter the natural history with the possible exception of a few disorders [20]. **In women with moderate-to-severe renal insufficiency (maternal serum creatinine ≥1.4 mg/dL), 10% of patients will have progressive renal deterioration at 12 months postpartum [21].**

NEPHROTIC SYNDROME
Definition

Nephrotic syndrome (NS): Defined by >3.5 g of proteinuria in 24 hours in nonpregnant adults [43]. A condition caused by any disease that damages the kidneys' filtering system, the glomeruli. Because of the decrease in oncotic pressure in pregnant women, nephrotic syndrome is associated with hypoalbuminemia, edema, venous thromboembolism, and hypercholesterolemia.

General

The most common causes of adult nephrotic syndrome outside of pregnancy are focal glomerulosclerosis, membranous nephropathy, and minimal-change disease [44].

Epidemiology/Incidence

Nephrotic syndrome occurs in 0.012% to 0.025% of all pregnancies [43].

Workup

Newly diagnosed nephrotic syndrome in early pregnancy has been associated with hydatidiform molar pregnancies; therefore, this should be evaluated [37,44,45]. If the diagnosis is made prior to pregnancy, histologic diagnosis can help direct treatment. In most cases of stable disease, renal biopsy can be deferred until postpartum if histologic diagnosis is not already made. Renal biopsy in pregnancy is considered a safe option, especially if the results are expected to potentially change management [46,47]. The presence of proteinuria >1 g in combination with GFR <40 mL/min is predictive of worse prognosis in pregnancy [29]. For this reason, **patients with newly diagnosed proteinuria prior to 20 weeks gestation (1+ or greater on urine dipstick on two samples at least six hours but no more than seven days apart [8]) should have a 24-hour urine collection for both protein and creatinine clearance in order to estimate GFR [48]. Testing for proteinuria on urine dipstick is associated with a high false positive rate and contamination (blood, semen, detergents, etc.).**

Complications

Nephrotic syndrome rarely causes complications in pregnancy in the absence of hypertension and abnormal renal function. Most of the literature on nephrotic syndrome in pregnancy is based on case reports; therefore, the incidence of specific complications is unknown.

Specific Diseases

Membranous nephropathy is associated with increased fetal demise, preterm delivery (43%), hypertension, and a decline in maternal renal function [49].

Prenatal Care, Fetal Monitoring, and Labor Management

A similar approach to antepartum and intrapartum care can be used to that of patients with chronic renal insufficiency (see preceding section). Patients should be managed with a **multidisciplinary** approach, in conjunction with a perinatologist, nephrologist, and neonatologist.

Management

It may be necessary to treat nephrotic syndrome with steroids, which requires early and repeat screening for gestational diabetes (GDM). Thromboprophylaxis should be considered for women with proteinuria >5 g/day [34].

Long-Term Prognosis

Relates to the specific diagnosis. Most evidence suggests that pregnancy does not worsen or accelerate the overall disease process in women with primary glomerular disease, at least at five-year follow-up [50]. The exception to this appears to be women with membranous glomerulonephritis, who do worse after experiencing a pregnancy.

DIALYSIS
Principles/Counseling

Women with ESRD on dialysis have impaired fertility secondary to suppression of hypothalamic–pituitary–adrenal (HPA) axis function, leading to anovulation and amenorrhea. Fertility rates are improving with advances in dialysis, overall decreased serum creatinine levels, and improvement of azotemia. Published rates of fertility range from 1% to 7%. Dialysis-dependent patients with ESRD should be **offered contraception** [51].

Women on dialysis should be counseled preconception that they should receive a renal transplant and then wait for one to two years before attempting pregnancy [52]. For successful outcomes in pregnant women on dialysis, the key is **coordination of multidisciplinary care** to maintain blood pressure control, fluid balance, and adequate nutrition. There is an overall >70% likelihood of fetal survival [53]. Live births in women on dialysis during pregnancy has improved from 23% [54] to about 50% in 1994 [21] to 79% in 1998 [53] and to 92% in 2002 [51].

Of note, in dialysis patients, serum levels of B-human chorionic gonadotropin may be borderline elevated in women who are not pregnant; an ultrasound should be used to confirm the diagnosis of pregnancy [52].

Complications

Stillbirth (8%–50%), **neonatal death** (9%–25%), **preterm delivery** (48%–84%), **severe preeclampsia** (11%) [31,55], **polyhydramnios** (40%) [25], **FGR** (50%–80%), **hypertension** (100%), **anemia** (100%), and even **maternal death** despite recent improved overall outcomes [51]. Most of the neonatal morbidity occurs secondary to prematurity. The risk of congenital anomalies does not appear to be increased. Preeclampsia is a poor prognostic factor in these patients, associated with increased rates of stillbirth, low birth weight, and prematurity [25].

Pregnancy Management

- Counseling regarding complications should be reviewed. Because of the high incidence of complications, termination may be discussed as well as the possibility of a better outcome after renal transplant [51].
- Intensive hemodialysis (HD) for patients with ESRD **six to seven times a week** is recommended. There appears to be a trend toward better infant survival in women who received dialysis >20 hr/wk [31].
- Plasma urea level appears to be the most important factor influencing pregnancy outcome in dialysis patients. A predialysis urea of 30 to 50 mg/dL (5–8 mmol/L) is associated with improved outcomes [56].
- Prepregnancy dialysis regimen should be increased by approximately 50%.
- HD may be superior to peritoneal dialysis (PD), but this has not been studied in any trial in pregnancy. Older reports have demonstrated more successful pregnancies in women undergoing HD (79%) compared to PD (33%) [51]. Newer small series demonstrate comparable outcomes between HD and PD [57,58], but no clear benefit of PD over HD. For this reason, PD is not recommended in the general pregnant patient population. If patients are already established on PD, there is no compelling evidence to change to HD [31,55]. PD can be complicated by intra-abdominal infection, and this differential should be considered in pregnant patients using PD presenting with abdominal pain.
- Aggressively use HD to decrease azotemia for improving pregnancy outcomes. As a goal, predialysis urea level should be <100 mg/dL and BUN should be low (7–10 mg/dL), so that there is not osmotic diuresis in the fetus.
- Avoid maternal hypotension during HD. Keep BP 130–150/80–90.
- Avoid excessive fluid shifts. Ensure minimal fluctuations and limit volume changes.
- Alter heparin regimen near delivery if possible.
- Use maternal dry weight to base HD volume.
- There are no studies of fetal surveillance during HD.
- Altering HD rates to achieve maximal volume control may decrease incidence of polyhydramnios.
- Obtain a nutritional consult [52].
- Be aware of other metabolic changes:
  - Good general health ≥1 year since transplant.
  - Keep bicarbonate 22 to 26 mEq/L.
  - Keep hemoglobin 11 to 12 mg/dL with erythropoietin (can be given in pregnancy, does not cross the placenta). Because of resistance to erythropoietin in pregnancy, the dose must be increased by as much as 50% to maintain the target hemoglobin [56]. Anemia is associated with worse neonatal outcomes [25].
  - Replace calcium (>2 g/day), phosphorus.
  - Dialysate: may need more potassium, less calcium.
- Adequate calorie and protein supply needs to be assured.
- Ensure good blood pressure control.
- Maintain attention toward signs and symptoms of preterm labor.
- Maternal serum screening for aneuploidy is unreliable in this group of patients [51,59].
- Indocin may worsen kidney function. Magnesium should be avoided if possible or used cautiously with frequent levels.
- Close antepartum fetal surveillance is warranted because of risk of FGR and fetal heart rate abnormalities.
- Consider delivery at 34 to 36 weeks.
- There are insufficient data to assess the effects of antenatal steroids and the risk of gestational diabetes mellitus in HD patients.
- Neonatologists should be available to assess the neonate. Neonates are born with BUN and creatinine levels equal to the mother's and often experience osmotic diuresis, resulting in volume contraction and electrolyte abnormalities. Intrauterine hypercalcemia may result in postnatal hypocalcemia and tetany [60].
- Asymptomatic bacteriuria in dialysis and transplant patients should be treated for two weeks, and suppression may be given for the remainder of the pregnancy [52]. Antepartum care should otherwise be similar to those patients with chronic renal disease.

Postpartum

Most women return to prepregnancy dialysis regimens and have uncomplicated postpartum recoveries. Postpartum care must address contraception. A renal transplant should precede future pregnancies.

RENAL TRANSPLANTATION
Principles

Management should be at a center with a **transplant nephrologist** and requires attention toward **serial assessment of renal function, diagnosis and treatment of rejection, blood pressure control, and control of anemia**. There is an overall **success** of pregnancy (live births) in women after renal transplantation of >90% [61]. Fertility can normalize soon after transplantation, so patients should be maintained on contraception until ready to attempt a pregnancy. If graft function is adequate and stable, pregnancy does not cause accelerated graft demise [62]. However, one case-control study suggested that graft function is adversely affected by pregnancy [63]. At 10-year follow-up, graft survival was 69% in pregnant patients and 100% in nonpregnant controls.

Complications

Slightly increased incidences of fetal growth restriction, premature rupture of membranes, preterm delivery, and preeclampsia.

Preconception Counseling

Ideal candidate for pregnancy is a woman with the following:

1. Good general health for at least one year post-transplant before attempting conception.
2. Minimal (ideally <300 mg or at least <1000 mg/24 hr) proteinuria.

3. Absence (ideal) or at least good control of hypertension.
4. No evidence of graft rejection.
5. Absence of pelvicaliceal distention on intravenous pyelogram.
6. Stable renal function (maternal serum creatinine <1.4 mg/dL or ideally <1.1 mg/dL). Fetal survival improves from 75% with creatinine >1.4% to 95% with normal creatinine. **Creatinine >2.3 mg/dL may be regarded as a contraindication to pregnancy** as all transplant patients with a creatinine >2.3 mg/dL experienced progression of renal failure requiring retransplant or dialysis within two years of pregnancy [26].
7. Stable immunosuppressive regimen.
8. If possible, drug therapy should be reduced to maintenance levels: prednisone <15 mg/day, azathioprine <2 mg/kg/day, cyclosporine <5 mg/kg/day [52].
9. Preconception recommendations: discontinue ACE inhibitors and determine immune status for hepatitis B, herpes simplex, CMV, and toxoplasmosis [52].

Prenatal Care

Attempt to obtain operative records from transplant surgery to identify location of kidney. Be aware of side effects of immunosuppressive agents (Table 17.5) [64]. A common immunosuppressive drug is currently tacrolimus (Prograf). It crosses the placenta but has not been associated with an increase in congenital anomalies. Avoid nephrotoxic drugs. Be aware of significant drug interactions with cyclosporine (Table 17.6) [65].

- *Antenatal visits*: should be every two to four weeks up to 32 weeks and weekly thereafter.
- *Lab work*: includes monthly assessment of *CBC, BUN, serum creatinine, electrolytes, serum urate, 24-hour creatinine clearance and protein* levels, and urine specimen for *culture*. Initial labs should also include serum serologies for *cytomegalovirus, toxoplasmosis,* and *herpes simplex virus* (IgM and IgG for each) and *LFTs. Levels of immunosuppressive agent* (tacrolimus, cyclosporine, etc.) should

Table 17.5 Immunosuppressive Agents Commonly Used and Their Side Effects

Agent → Side effect

- Prednisone[a] → glucose intolerance, neonatal adrenal insufficiency, thymic hypoplasia
- Azathioprine[a] → leukopenia (maintain maternal white blood count >7500 pL)
- Cyclosporine[a,b] → hypertension, nephrotoxicity (watch for drug interactions—see Table 17.4), intrauterine growth retardation
- Tacrolimus[a,b] → hypertension, nephrotoxicity, neurotoxicity, glucose intolerance, myocardial hypertrophy, hyperkalemia, neonatal anuria
- Sirolimus[b] → GI disturbance, weakness; animal studies raise concern regarding potential for human fetotoxicity although no teratogenesis is evident.
- Mycophenolate mofetil → GI disturbance; animal studies raise concern regarding potential for human teratogenicity. At least 12 cases of human deformity associated with mycophenolate mofetil, including microtia (11), auditory canal atresia (8), cleft lip and palate (6), and micrognathia (4).

Sources: Adapted from Hou S. *Am J Kidney Dis*, 33, 2, 235–52, 1999; Merlob P, Stahl B, Klinger G. *Reprod Toxicol*, 28, 1, 105–8, 2009.
[a]These have no known teratogenic effects.
[b]Follow with blood levels.

Table 17.6 Drug Interactions with Cyclosporine

Drugs that exhibit nephrotoxic synergy

Gentamicin	Cimetidine
Tobramycin	Ranitidine
Vancomycin	Diclofenac
Amphotericin B	Trimethoprim with sulfamethoxazole
Ketoconazole	Azapropazon
Melphalan	

Careful monitoring of renal function should be practiced when Sandimmun® (cyclosporine) is used with nephrotoxic drugs.

Drugs that alter cyclosporine levels

Cyclosporine is extensively metabolized by the liver. Therefore, circulating cyclosporine levels may be influenced by drugs that affect hepatic microsomal enzymes, particularly the cytochrome P-450 system. Substances known to inhibit these enzymes will decrease hepatic metabolism and increase cyclosporine levels. Substances that are inducers of cytochrome P-450 activity will increase hepatic metabolism and decrease cyclosporine levels. Monitoring of circulating cyclosporine levels and appropriate cyclosporine dosage adjustment are essential when these drugs are used concomitantly.

Drugs that increase cyclosporine levels

Diltiazem	Danazol
Nicardipine	Bromocriptine
Verapamil	Metoclopramide
Ketoconazole	Erythromycin
Fluconazole	Methylprednisone
Intracondazole	

Drugs that decrease cyclosporine levels

Rifampin	Phenobarbital
Phenytoin	Carbamazepine

Other drug interactions

Reduced clearance of prednisolone, digoxin, and lovastatin has been observed when these drugs are administered with Sandimmun (cyclosporine). In addition, a decrease in the apparent volume of distribution of digoxin has been reported after cyclosporine administration. Severe digitalis toxicity has been seen within days of starting cyclosporine in several patients taking digoxin. Cyclosporine should not be used with potassium-sparing diuretics because hyperkalemia can occur. During treatment with cyclosporine, vaccination may be less effective: and the use of live vaccines should be avoided. Myositis has occurred with concomitant lovastatin, frequent gingival hyperplasia with nifedipine, and convulsions with high dose methylprednisolone. Further information on drugs that have been reported to interact with cyclosporine is available from Sandoz Pharmaceuticals Corporation (New Jersey, U.S.).

Source: Adapted from *Physician's Desk Reference*. 52nd ed. Montvale, NJ: Thompson PDR; 1998.

be obtained at least every trimester. If the patient is on prednisone or tacrolimus, obtain a fasting and two-hour postprandial blood sugar upon presentation. If these values are normal, perform a glucose challenge test at 24 weeks. Renal transplant patients are at considerable risk for urinary tract infections (up to 40%) and should be screened regularly [26].
- *Fetal surveillance*: should follow the recommendations for chronic renal disease.

Labor Management

Labor management should include careful monitoring of maternal fluid balance, cardiovascular status, and temperature.

Cesarean delivery should be for obstetric indications only. Women who have received steroids for long periods during the antepartum period, i.e., 20 mg or more of prednisone or equivalent for more than 3 weeks, should receive "stress dose" steroids. Notification of the use of immunosuppressants to the pediatrician is important for proper follow-up of the neonate.

Renal Graft Rejection

Occurs in 4% to 9% pregnant allograft recipients and is difficult to diagnose. Factors that increase risk include increased number of episodes of rejection during the year prior to conception, maternal serum creatinine >2 mg/dL, proteinuria >500 mg/dL, and graft dysfunction during pregnancy [45]. Clinical hallmarks include fever, oliguria, deteriorating renal function, renal enlargement, and tenderness. **Renal ultrasound** and **biopsy** for diagnosis is necessary before aggressive antirejection therapy is begun.

Postpartum/Breast-Feeding

In general, not enough data are available to make a formal recommendation. However, breast-feeding is contraindicated in patients on cyclosporine.

Resources

Gift of Life Institute National Transplant Pregnancy Registry: http://ntpr.giftoflifeinstitute.org/, toll-free phone 1-877-955-6877.

URINARY TRACT INFECTIONS
Screening

All pregnant women should be screened at the first prenatal visit for asymptomatic bacteriuria. The prevalence of asymptomatic bacteriuria in pregnancy is comparable to nonpregnant patients, between 2% and 10% [66]. If asymptomatic bacteriuria goes untreated in pregnancy, 20% to 40% of patients will develop pyelonephritis, compared to 3% of women who are treated [66,67]. Women with risk factors for urinary tract infections [UTIs] (DM, GDM, neurogenic bladder, prior frequent UTIs, sickle cell disease or trait) should be screened every trimester. Patients with sickle cell trait are at increased risk for pyelonephritis, but it has not been demonstrated that frequent screening reduces the risk [68].

Complications

Pregnant women with asymptomatic bacteriuria are at increased risk for symptomatic infection and **pyelonephritis**. There is also a positive relationship between untreated bacteriuria, **low birth weight**, and **preterm birth**. Other complications of UTIs or pyelonephritis include fetal mortality, possibly long-term mental retardation, and developmental delay [69], preeclampsia, anemia, and pulmonary and renal insufficiency. Treatment of asymptomatic bacteriuria helps prevent these complications (see Chapters 2 and 16 of *Obstetric Evidence Based Guidelines*).

Prevention

Daily intake of 10 to 16 oz. of **cranberry juice** decreases the incidence of recurrent *Escherichia coli* UTIs. *Lactobacillus GG* drink does not have any benefit [70].

Diagnosis

A threshold of ≥**100,000** colony-forming units (CFUs) of the same bacterial strain on two consecutive voided specimens is the indication for treatment. Additionally, asymptomatic bacteriuria may be defined as >100 colony-forming units per milliliter (CFU/ml) of a single recognized uropathogen when the specimen was obtained with a catheterized specimen [71].

Group B *Streptococcus* should be appropriately treated at any concentration (see Chapter 16 of *Obstetric Evidence Based Guidelines*). It is important to avoid contamination by cleansing the perineum and then collecting "midstream" urine.

Treatment

Check allergies and sensitivities. The most effective and safest antibiotic regimen for the initial treatment of asymptomatic bacteriuria in pregnancy is not known. If appropriate, **nitrofurantoin** 100 mg orally twice per day can be used for seven days. If not effective, oral alternatives are cephalexin 250 mg every six hours, amoxicillin 250 mg every eight hours, or trimethoprim-sulfamethoxazole 160/800 mg orally every 12 hours for 7 days [72]. Nitrofurantoin and sulphonamides should be avoided in the first trimester if other antiobiotic alternatives are available; however, if not, they can be used [73]. Given the lack of conclusive evidence, it may be useful for clinicians to consider factors such as cost, local availability, and side effects [74].

Follow-Up

A **test of cure** is necessary [75]. If positive, give another antibiotic regimen (consider different, sensitive regimen) and assess compliance. Intramuscular treatment can be given if compliance remains an issue. Suppressive therapy (once a day of nitrofurantoin 50 mg, amoxicillin 250 mg, or cephalexin 250 mg) is indicated after two UTIs or one episode of pyelonephritis.

PYELONEPHRITIS
Incidence
1% to 2% [76].

Diagnosis

Urinary tract infection with costovertebral angle tenderness, usually accompanied by systemic symptoms such as fever and chills. Positive urine culture is necessary for diagnosis.

Management

- **Urine culture sensitivity is crucial to assure adequate antibiotic coverage.**
- Workup should include CBC, electrolytes, creatinine, and liver function tests. Intravenous fluids. Approximately 15%–20% of pyelonephritis is complicated by bacteremia; however, more research is needed to recommend routine collection of blood cultures [77].
- Usually inpatient treatment. Outpatient therapy can be considered for uncomplicated compliant women with pyelonephritis after IV ceftriaxone [78,79].
- **Intravenous antibiotics** for 24 to 48 hours or at least >24 hours afebrile:
  - Drug of choice:
    - **Ceftriaxone 1 to 2 g every 24 hours** [80,81]

- Alternatives:
  - Ancef 1 to 2 g every six to eight hours [79]
  - Ampicillin 1 to 2 g every six hours with gentamicin 1.5 mg/kg every eight hours
  - Trimethoprim-sulfamethoxazole 160/800 mg every 12 hours
- If not afebrile within 48 hours with appropriate regimen or if recurrent pyelonephritis, consider renal ultrasound to rule out renal abscess.
- Once IV therapy completed, oral therapy for 10 to 14 days, followed by suppression and frequent urine cultures (see above) [82,83].

URINARY NEPHROLITHIASIS
Incidence
At least 1/1500 but may occur more commonly [84,85]. Up to 12% of the general population has had a urinary stone during their lifetime with recurrence rates approaching 50% [84]. Nephrolithiasis is also called renal calculi or stones. Given the low incidence, it is unclear if the occurrence of nephrolithiasis is or is not increased in pregnancy with some authors reporting an incidence as high as 1/200.

Risk Factors
More common in Caucasians, second and third trimester, right side [86], recurrent UTIs, gout, prior renal stones or renal disease, family history.

Complications
Possibly increased preterm birth and pyelonephritis [87].

Diagnosis
A typical presentation for renal colic includes nausea, vomiting, hematuria, and flank or abdominal pain. Urinalysis may reveal hematuria, as well as pyuria in up to 42% of patients [88,89]. The best imaging technique in the nonpregnant adult is unenhanced helical CT scan of the abdomen and pelvis, which has 96% sensitivity and 100% specificity [84]. If CT is unavailable, plain abdominal X-ray should be performed because 75% to 90% of urinary stones are radiopaque. **Ultrasonography** has a sensitivity of only 11% to 24% with >90% specificity in nonpregnant adults, but because of a **sensitivity of about** 67% in pregnancy, it is **currently the first-line screening test in pregnancy.** Doppler ultrasound has been shown to be somewhat useful in distinguishing ureteral obstruction from physiologic hydronephrosis. A difference of >0.04 in the resistive indices of the obstructed and normal kidneys can be used to predict obstruction. In addition, comparison of bilateral ureteral jets on ultrasound can be helpful [90]. **If initially the ultrasound is negative, an MRU (magnetic resonance urography)** [91] should be considered **or, if unavailable, X-ray** second and CT third. Renal stones are poorly visualized by MRI alone. It is important to know that mild-to-moderate hydronephrosis is physiologic in pregnancy and is usually worse on the right kidney.

Management
Composition, location, and size of stone should be assessed. Up to 64% to 70% of women can pass stones spontaneously during pregnancy and an additional 50% of the remaining pass the stones in the postpartum period [89]. Most patients with stones will not require intervention; therefore, conservative management with **hydration and pain control is the typical first-line management.** There are no trials in pregnancy or even in nonpregnant adults. Ketorolac and diclofenac appear to be as effective as narcotics. All can be used acutely intravenously.

Usually **increases in fluids and movement** are used as initial interventions in pregnancy as well as nonpregnant adults. **More than 70% of stones in pregnancy resolve with conservative management.** A urinary stone seen by ultrasound (or CT) but not X-ray is probably a uric acid stone; 20 mmol of potassium citrate orally two to three times daily (aim to alkalinize urine to pH 6.5–7.0) can be effective medical therapy for dissolution of this type of stone. **Urgent intervention is indicated with** obstruction, infected upper urinary tract, impending renal deterioration, intractable pain or vomiting, anuria, or high-grade obstruction of a solitary or transplanted kidney.

If conservative therapy fails, insertion of **stents** is a safe intervention in pregnancy. Double pigtail stent insertion may be more effective (100%) and have a lower failure rate than conservative management (80% success) but a higher discomfort rate [11]. Fetal risk is low for stent placement. **Percutaneous nephrostomy** is needed only rarely but is safe in pregnancy. Ureteroscopy has also been shown to be safe and effective in pregnancy with complication rates similar to the nonpregnant patient [84,85]. **Shock wave lithotripsy** is considered first-line therapy for proximal ureteral stones <1 cm in nonpregnant adults but is seldom used in pregnancy. Even if inadvertent lithotripsy is performed in pregnancy, it is not a cause for concern [89,92].

PREVENTION OF URINARY INCONTINENCE
Incidence
Urinary incontinence has been reported to occur in 5% to 40% of pregnant and postpartum women.

Prevention
Pelvic floor exercises *during pregnancy* **decrease the incidence of urinary incontinence in the third trimester and postpartum** up to six months after birth [93–95]. Pelvic floor muscle strength is also significantly higher. Group training with a physiotherapist for 60 minutes once per week and twice daily at home for a period of 12 weeks between 20 and 36 weeks holding the pelvic floor muscle contraction six to eight seconds each time (for ~10 times) with rest periods of six seconds is one accepted and effective intervention [95].

Pelvic floor muscle training *after childbirth* is **effective in prevention and treatment of urinary incontinence** [96–100].

POSTPARTUM URINARY RETENTION
Definition
Absence of spontaneous micturition six hours post vaginal delivery or six hours after catheter removal (after cesarean delivery). A residual <50 mL is normal and >200 mL is abnormal [101].

Incidence
0.2% to 3% [102].

Risk Factors

Nulliparity, prolonged stages of labor, epidural anesthesia, operative or cesarean delivery.

Management

There are no trials to assess any intervention. Oral analgesia, standing and walking, warm bath, and/or immersing hands in cold water may help. If bladder volume by ultrasound <400 mL, wait; if >400 mL, **intermittent catheterization every four to six hours until the woman is able to void and then the first residual volume is <150 mL** is usually recommended and preferable to indwelling catheterization. Pharmacologic treatment should be avoided. If the woman still has retention upon discharge and/or after 48 hours, self-catheterization should be taught. Prophylactic antibiotics are indicated in women who require catheterization. There are no clear long-term sequelae of postpartum urinary retention. Complete resolution of voiding dysfunction is expected within 28 days with no increased risk for long-term voiding abnormalities. Higher post-void residual volumes at 72 hours after delivery are predictive of a longer time to full recovery [102].

MICROSCOPIC HEMATURIA IN PREGNANCY
Definition

Microscopic hematuria: 5–10 red blood cells per high power field in a spun catheterized specimen.

Incidence

3% during pregnancy, 2%–16% in nonpregnant population [103]

Differential Diagnosis

Pseudohematuria may be present from excessive consumption of beets, berries, rhubarb, or food coloring as well as certain laxatives and medications.

- *Acute Renal Disease*: Hematuria may be sole presentation; differential diagnosis includes HELLP syndrome, hemolytic uremic syndrome, thrombotic thrombocytopenic purpura, preeclampsia with severe features, renal cortical necrosis, acute pyelonephritis, acute fatty liver of pregnancy, or urinary tract obstruction [103].
- *Chronic renal disease*: As discussed earlier.
- *Infectious renal disease*: Pyelonephritis, cystitis, urethritis.
- *Trauma in Pregnancy*: Hematuria may be the presenting sign in a pregnant patient who is a victim of domestic violence.
- *Placental Pathology*: If the placenta invades the bladder (placenta percreta), hematuria may result.
- *Uncommon causes* of hematuria in pregnancy: Youssef syndrome (vesicouterine fistula), hydatidiform mole (either with malignancy or renal failure), hemangiomas, arteriovenous malformations, renal vein thrombosis, nutcracker syndrome (compression of left renal vein leading to increased pressure gradient and hematuria).

Risk Factors for Significant Disease [101]

- Age >40 years
- Smoking history
- History of gross hematuria
- Occupational exposure to chemicals or dyes (benzenes or aromatic amines)
- Previous urologic disease (e.g., chronic cystitis or bacterial infections)
- History of irritative voiding symptoms
- Analgesic abuse
- History of pelvic irradiation
- Cyclophosphamide exposure

Management

- Repeat dipstick; if negative, no need for further workup.
- Evaluate for vaginal bleeding possibly contaminating urine specimen.
- Send for microscopy; if abnormal casts or dysmorphic RBCs, consider nephrology consultation for glomerular etiology.
- Urine culture; if positive, treat with appropriate antibiotics.
- Urine cytology; if positive, cystoscopy and referral.
- Obtain renal ultrasound to look for pathological basis for hematuria.
- Renal biopsy reserved for sudden deterioration of renal function, relatively safe in pregnancy.

REFERENCES

1. Lindheimer MD, Davison JM, Katz AI. The kidney and hypertension in pregnancy: Twenty exciting years. *Semin Nephrol* 2001; 21(2): 173–89. [Review]
2. Modena A, Hoffman M, Tolosa JE. Chronic renal disease in pregnancy: A modern approach to predicting outcome. *Am J Obstet Gynecol* 2005; 193(6): S86. [Abstract II-2]
3. Levey AS, Coresh J, Balk E, Kausz AT, Levin A, Steffes MW et al. National Kidney Foundation practice guidelines for chronic kidney disease: Evaluation, classification, and stratification. *Ann Intern Med* 2003; 139(2): 137–47. [Systematic Review]
4. Fink JC, Schwartz SM, Benedetti TJ, Stehman-Breen CO. Increased risk of adverse maternal and infant outcomes among women with renal disease. *Paediatr Perinat Epidemiol* 1998; 12(3): 277–87. [II-2]
5. Bar J, Ben-Rafael Z, Padoa A, Orvieto R, Boner G, Hod M. Prediction of pregnancy outcome in subgroups of women with renal disease. *Clin Nephrol* 2000; 53(6): 437–44. [II-1]
6. Fischer MJ, Lehnerz SD, Hebert JR, Parikh CR. Kidney disease is an independent risk factor for adverse fetal and maternal outcomes in pregnancy. *Am J Kidney Dis* 2004; 43(3): 415–23. [II-3]
7. Milne JE, Lindheimer MD, Davison JM. Glomerular heteroporous membrane modeling in third trimester and postpartum before and during amino acid infusion. *Am J Physiol Renal Physiol* 2002; 282(1): F170–5. [II-2]
8. Vidaeff AC, Yeomans ER, Ramin SM. Pregnancy in women with renal disease. Part I: General principles. *Am J Perinatol* 2008; 25(7): 385–97. [Review]
9. Abbassi-Ghanavati M, Greer LG, Cunningham FG. Pregnancy and laboratory studies: A reference table for clinicians. *Obstet Gynecol* 2009; 114(6): 1326–31. [Systematic Review]
10. Wide-Swensson D, Strevens H, Willner J. Antepartum percutaneous renal biopsy. *Int J Gynaecol Obstet* 2007; 98(2): 88–92. [II-2]
11. Tsai YL, Seow KM, Yieh CH, Chong KM, Hwang JL, Lin YH et al. Comparative study of conservative and surgical management for symptomatic moderate and severe hydronephrosis in pregnancy: A prospective randomized study. *Acta Obstet Gynecol Scand* 2007; 86(9): 1047–50. [I]
12. Nevis IF, Reitsma A, Dominic A, McDonald S, Thabane L, Akl EA et al. Pregnancy outcomes in women with chronic kidney disease: A systematic review. *Clin J Am Soc Nephrol* 2011; 6(11): 2587–98. [Systematic Review]

13. Jungers P, Houillier P, Forget D, Henry-Amar M. Specific controversies concerning the natural history of renal disease in pregnancy. *Am J Kidney Dis* 1991; 17(2): 116–22. [III]

14. Jones DC. Pregnancy complicated by chronic renal disease. *Clin Perinatol* 1997; 24(2): 483–96. [II-2]

15. Huong DL, Wechsler B, Vauthier-Brouzes D, Beaufils H, Lefebvre G, Piette JC. Pregnancy in past or present lupus nephritis: A study of 32 pregnancies from a single centre. *Ann Rheum Dis* 2001; 60(6): 599–604. [II-2]

16. Imbasciati E, Tincani A, Gregorini G, Doria A, Moroni G, Cabiddu G et al. Pregnancy in women with pre-existing lupus nephritis: Predictors of fetal and maternal outcome. *Nephrol Dial Transplant* 2009; 24(2): 519–25. [II-3]

17. Hayslett JP. The effect of systemic lupus erythematosus on pregnancy and pregnancy outcome. *Am J Reprod Immunol* 1992; 28(3–4): 199–204. [II-2]

18. Smyth A, Oliveira GH, Lahr BD, Bailey KR, Norby SM, Garovic VD. A systematic review and meta-analysis of pregnancy outcomes in patients with systemic lupus erythematosus and lupus nephritis. *Clin J Am Soc Nephrol* 2010; 5(11): 2060–8. [Systematic Review]

19. Limardo M, Imbasciati E, Ravani P, Surian M, Torres D, Gregorini G et al. Pregnancy and progression of IgA nephropathy: Results of an Italian multicenter study. *Am J Kidney Dis* 2010; 56(3): 506–12. [II-2]

20. Jungers P, Chauveau D, Choukroun G, Moynot A, Skhiri H, Houillier P et al. Pregnancy in women with impaired renal function. *Clin Nephrol* 1997; 47(5): 281–8. [II-2]

21. Jones DC, Hayslett JP. Outcome of pregnancy in women with moderate or severe renal insufficiency. *N Engl J Med* 1996; 335(4): 226–32. [II-2]

22. Airoldi J, Weinstein L. Clinical significance of proteinuria in pregnancy. *Obstet Gynecol Surv* 2007; 62(2): 117–24. [III]

23. Hou SH. Frequency and outcome of pregnancy in women on dialysis. *Am J Kidney Dis* 1994; 23(1): 60–3. [II-3]

24. Armenti VT, Radomski JS, Moritz MJ, Gaughan WJ, Philips LZ, McGrory CH et al. Report from the national transplantation pregnancy registry (NTPR): Outcomes of pregnancy after transplantation. *Clin Transpl* 2001: 97–105. [II-2]

25. Luders C, Castro MC, Titan SM, De Castro I, Elias RM, Abensur H et al. Obstetric outcome in pregnant women on long-term dialysis: A case series. *Am J Kidney Dis* 2010; 56(1): 77–85. [II-3]

26. Crowe AV, Rustom R, Gradden C, Sells RA, Bakran A, Bone JM et al. Pregnancy does not adversely affect renal transplant function. *QJM* 1999; 92(11): 631–5. [II-3]

27. Bramham K, Briley AL, Seed PT, Poston L, Shennan AH, Chappell LC. Pregnancy outcome in women with chronic kidney disease: A prospective cohort study. *Reprod Sci* 2011; 18(7): 623–30. [II-2]

28. Abe S. An overview of pregnancy in women with underlying renal disease. *Am J Kidney Dis* 1991; 17(2): 112–5. [II-3]

29. Imbasciati E, Gregorini G, Cabiddu G, Gammaro L, Ambroso G, Del Giudice A et al. Pregnancy in CKD stages 3 to 5: Fetal and maternal outcomes. *Am J Kidney Dis* 2007; 49(6): 753–62. [II-3]

30. Holley JL, Bernardini J, Quadri KH, Greenberg A, Laifer SA. Pregnancy outcomes in a prospective matched control study of pregnancy and renal disease. *Clin Nephrol* 1996; 45(2): 77–82. [II-2]

31. Okundaye I, Abrinko P, Hou S. Registry of pregnancy in dialysis patients. *Am J Kidney Dis* 1998; 31(5): 766–73. [II-2]

32. Cunningham FG, Cox SM, Harstad TW, Mason RA, Pritchard JA. Chronic renal disease and pregnancy outcome. *Am J Obstet Gynecol* 1990; 163(2): 453–9. [II-2]

33. Piccoli GB, Clari R, Ghiotto S, Castelluccia N, Colombi N, Mauro G et al. Type 1 diabetes, diabetic nephropathy, and pregnancy: A systematic review and meta-study. *Rev Diabet Stud* 2013; 10(1): 6–26. [Systematic Review]

34. National Collaborating Centre for Women's and Children's Health (UK). *Diabetes in pregnancy: Management of diabetes and its complications from preconception to the postnatal period. NICE Guideline.* 2015 Feb. [Systematic Review]

35. Phelan LK, Brown MA, Davis GK, Mangos G. A prospective study of the impact of automated dipstick urinalysis on the diagnosis of preeclampsia. *Hypertens Pregnancy* 2004; 23(2): 135–42. [II-2]

36. Hirshberg A, Draper J, Curley C, Sammel MD, Schwartz N. A random protein-creatinine ratio accurately predicts baseline proteinuria in early pregnancy. *J Matern Fetal Neonatal Med* 2014; 27(18): 1834–8. [II-2]

37. Cote AM, Brown MA, Lam E, von Dadelszen P, Firoz T, Liston RM et al. Diagnostic accuracy of urinary spot protein: Creatinine ratio for proteinuria in hypertensive pregnant women: Systematic review. *BMJ* 2008; 336(7651): 1003–6. [Review]

38. Piccoli GB, Daidola G, Attini R, Parisi S, Fassio F, Naretto C et al. Kidney biopsy in pregnancy: Evidence for counselling? A systematic narrative review. *BJOG* 2013;120(4): 412–27. [Systematic Review]

39. Sienas L, Wong T, Collins R, Smith J. Contemporary uses of erythropoietin in pregnancy: A literature review. *Obstet Gynecol Surv* 2013; 68(8): 594–602. [Review]

40. National Collaborating Centre for Women's and Children's Health (UK). *Hypertension in Pregnancy. NICE Clinical Guideline.* 2010 Aug. [Systematic Review]

41. Bujold E, Roberge S, Lacasse Y, Bureau M, Audibert F, Marcoux S et al. Prevention of preeclampsia and intrauterine growth restriction with aspirin started in early pregnancy: A meta-analysis. *Obstet Gynecol* 2010; 116(2 Pt. 1): 402–14. [Meta-Analysis of RCTs]

42. Nyberg G, Haljamae U, Frisenette-Fich C, Wennergren M, Kjellmer I. Breast-feeding during treatment with cyclosporine. *Transplantation* 1998; 65(2): 253–5. [II-3]

43. Cohen AW, Burton HG. Nephrotic syndrome due to preeclamptic nephropathy in a hydatidiform mole and coexistent fetus. *Obstet Gynecol* 1979; 53(1): 130–4. [II-3]

44. Alvarez L, Ortega E, Rocamora N, Tormo A, Gil CM, Trigueros M et al. An unusual cause of nephrotic syndrome and hypertension in a young woman. *Nephrol Dial Transplant* 2002; 17(11): 2026–9. [II-3]

45. Komatsuda A, Nakamoto Y, Asakura K, Yasuda T, Imai H, Miura AB. Case report: Nephrotic syndrome associated with a total hydatidiform mole. *Am J Med Sci* 1992; 303(5): 309–12. [II-3]

46. Packham DK, North RA, Fairley KF, Whitworth JA, Kincaid-Smith P. Membranous glomerulonephritis and pregnancy. *Clin Nephrol* 1987; 28(2): 56–64. [II-3]

47. Day C, Hewins P, Hildebrand S, Sheikh L, Taylor G, Kilby M et al. The role of renal biopsy in women with kidney disease identified in pregnancy. *Nephrol Dial Transplant* 2008; 23(1): 201–6. [II-2]

48. American College of Obstetricians and Gynecologists, Task Force on Hypertension in Pregnancy. Hypertension in pregnancy. Report of the American College of Obstetricians and Gynecologists' Task Force on Hypertension in Pregnancy. *Obstet Gynecol* 2013; 122(5): 1122–31. [Review]

49. Packham D, Fairley KF. Renal biopsy: Indications and complications in pregnancy. *Br J Obstet Gynaecol* 1987; 94(10): 935–9. [II-3]

50. Barcelo P, Lopez-Lillo J, Cabero L, Del Rio G. Successful pregnancy in primary glomerular disease. *Kidney Int* 1986; 30(6): 914–9. [II-3]

51. Chao AS, Huang JY, Lien R, Kung FT, Chen PJ, Hsieh PC. Pregnancy in women who undergo long-term hemodialysis. *Am J Obstet Gynecol* 2002; 187(1): 152–6. [II-3]

52. Hou S. Pregnancy in chronic renal insufficiency and end-stage renal disease. *Am J Kidney Dis* 1999; 33(2): 235–52. [II-3]

53. Romao JE Jr, Luders C, Kahhale S, Pascoal IJ, Abensur H, Sabbaga E et al. Pregnancy in women on chronic dialysis. A single-center experience with 17 cases. *Nephron* 1998; 78(4): 416–22. [II-3]

54. Successful pregnancies in women treated by dialysis and kidney transplantation. Report from the Registration Committee of the European Dialysis and Transplant Association. *Br J Obstet Gynaecol* 1980; 87(10): 839–45. [II-3]

55. Chan WS, Okun N, Kjellstrand CM. Pregnancy in chronic dialysis: A review and analysis of the literature. *Int J Artif Organs* 1998; 21(5): 259–68. [II-3]

56. Asamiya Y, Otsubo S, Matsuda Y, Kimata N, Kikuchi K, Miwa N et al. The importance of low blood urea nitrogen levels in pregnant patients undergoing hemodialysis to optimize birth weight and gestational age. *Kidney Int* 2009; 75(11): 1217–22. [II-2]

57. Jefferys A, Wyburn K, Chow J, Cleland B, Hennessy A. Peritoneal dialysis in pregnancy: A case series. *Nephrology (Carlton)* 2008; 13(5): 380–3. [II-3]

58. Chou CY, Ting IW, Lin TH, Lee CN. Pregnancy in patients on chronic dialysis: A single center experience and combined analysis of reported results. *Eur J Obstet Gynecol Reprod Biol* 2008; 136(2): 165–70. [II-2]

59. Cheng PJ, Liu CM, Chang SD, Lin YT, Soong YK. Elevated second-trimester maternal serum hCG in patients undergoing haemodialysis. *Prenat Diagn* 1999; 19(10): 955–8. [II-3]

60. Blowey DL, Warady BA. Neonatal outcome in pregnancies associated with renal replacement therapy. *Adv Ren Replace Ther* 1998; 5(1): 45–52. [Review]

61. Armenti VT, Radomski JS, Moritz MJ, Gaughan WJ, Philips LZ, McGrory CH et al. Report from the National Transplantation Pregnancy Registry (NTPR): Outcomes of pregnancy after transplantation. *Clin Transpl* 2002: 121–30. [II-2]

62. Armenti VT, McGrory CH, Cater JR, Radomski JS, Moritz MJ. Pregnancy outcomes in female renal transplant recipients. *Transplant Proc* 1998; 30(5): 1732–4. [II-2]

63. Salmela KT, Kyllonen LE, Holmberg C, Gronhagen-Riska C. Impaired renal function after pregnancy in renal transplant recipients. *Transplantation* 1993; 56(6): 1372–5. [II-2]

64. Merlob P, Stahl B, Klinger G. Tetrada of the possible mycophenolate mofetil embryopathy: A review. *Reprod Toxicol* 2009; 28(1): 105–8. [Review]

65. *Physician's Desk Reference*. 52nd ed. Montvale, NJ: Thompson PDR; 1998. [III]

66. Smaill FM, Vazquez JC. Antibiotics for asymptomatic bacteriuria in pregnancy. *Cochrane Database of Syst Reviews* 2015; (8). [Systematic Review]

67. Gilstrap LC 3rd, Ramin SM. Urinary tract infections during pregnancy. *Obstet Gynecol Clin North Am* 2001; 28(3): 581–91. [Review]

68. Thurman AR, Steed LL, Hulsey T, Soper DE. Bacteriuria in pregnant women with sickle cell trait. *Am J Obstet Gynecol* 2006; 194(5): 1366–70. [II-2]

69. McDermott S, Callaghan W, Szwejbka L, Mann H, Daguise V. Urinary tract infections during pregnancy and mental retardation and developmental delay. *Obstet Gynecol* 2000; 96(1): 113–9. [II-2]

70. Kontiokari T, Sundqvist K, Nuutinen M, Pokka T, Koskela M, Uhari M. Randomised trial of cranberry-lingonberry juice and Lactobacillus GG drink for the prevention of urinary tract infections in women. *BMJ* 2001; 322(7302): 1571. [I-RCT, n = 150]

71. Nicolle LE, Bradley S, Colgan R, Rice JC, Schaeffer A, Hooton TM et al. Infectious Diseases Society of America guidelines for the diagnosis and treatment of asymptomatic bacteriuria in adults. *Clin Infect Dis* 2005; 40(5): 643–54. [Review]

72. Widmer M, Gulmezoglu AM, Mignini L, Roganti A. Duration of treatment for asymptomatic bacteriuria during pregnancy. *Cochrane Database Syst Rev* 2011; (12): CD000491. doi(12):CD000491. [Systematic Review]

73. American College of Obstetricians and Gynecologists Committee on Obstetric Practice. ACOG Committee Opinion No. 494: Sulfonamides, nitrofurantoin, and risk of birth defects. *Obstet Gynecol* 2011; 117(6): 1484–5. [III]

74. Guinto VT, De Guia B, Festin MR, Dowswell T. Different antibiotic regimens for treating asymptomatic bacteriuria in pregnancy. *Cochrane Database Syst Rev* 2010; (9): CD007855. doi(9):CD007855. [Systematic Review]

75. Ennis M, Callaway L, Lust K. Adherence to evidence-based guidelines for the management of pyelonephritis in pregnancy. *Aust N Z J Obstet Gynaecol* 2011; 51(6): 505–9. [II-2]

76. Hill JB, Sheffield JS, McIntire DD, Wendel GD Jr. Acute pyelonephritis in pregnancy. *Obstet Gynecol* 2005; 105(1): 18–23. [II-3]

77. Gomi H, Goto Y, Laopaiboon M, Usui R, Mori R. Routine blood cultures in the management of pyelonephritis in pregnancy for improving outcomes. *Cochrane Database Syst Rev* 2015; 2: CD009216. [Systematic Review]

78. Millar LK, Wing DA, Paul RH, Grimes DA. Outpatient treatment of pyelonephritis in pregnancy: A randomized controlled trial. *Obstet Gynecol* 1995; 86(4 Pt. 1): 560–4. [I-RCT, n = 120]

79. Wing DA, Hendershott CM, Debuque L, Millar LK. Outpatient treatment of acute pyelonephritis in pregnancy after 24 weeks. *Obstet Gynecol* 1999; 94(5 Pt. 1):683–8. [I-RCT, n = 92]

80. Sharma P, Thapa L. Acute pyelonephritis in pregnancy: A retrospective study. *Aust N Z J Obstet Gynaecol* 2007; 47(4): 313–5. [II-2]

81. Sanchez-Ramos L, McAlpine KJ, Adair CD, Kaunitz AM, Delke I, Briones DK. Pyelonephritis in pregnancy: Once-a-day ceftriaxone versus multiple doses of cefazolin. A randomized, double-blind trial. *Am J Obstet Gynecol* 1995; 172(1 Pt. 1): 129–33. [I-RCT, n = 178]

82. Lenke RR, VanDorsten JP, Schifrin BS. Pyelonephritis in pregnancy. A prospective randomized trial to prevent recurrent disease evaluating suppressive therapy with nitrofurantoin and close surveillance. *Am J Obstet Gynecol* 1983; 146(8): 953–7. [I-RCT, n = 200]

83. Brost BC, Campbell B, Stramm S, Eller D, Newman RB. Randomized clinical trial of antibiotic therapy for antenatal pyelonephritis. *Infect Dis Obstet Gynecol* 1996; 4(5): 294–7. [I-RCT, n = 67]

84. Teichman JM. Clinical practice. Acute renal colic from ureteral calculus. *N Engl J Med* 2004; 350(7): 684–93. [Review]

85. Semins MJ, Trock BJ, Matlaga BR. The safety of ureteroscopy during pregnancy: A systematic review and meta-analysis. *J Urol* 2009; 181(1): 139–43. [Systematic Review]

86. Lewis DF, Robichaux AG 3rd, Jaekle RK, Marcum NG, Stedman CM. Urolithiasis in pregnancy. Diagnosis, management and pregnancy outcome. *J Reprod Med* 2003; 48(1): 28–32. [II-3]

87. Swartz MA, Lydon-Rochelle MT, Simon D, Wright JL, Porter MP. Admission for nephrolithiasis in pregnancy and risk of adverse birth outcomes. *Obstet Gynecol* 2007; 109(5): 1099–104. [II-2]

88. Thomas AA, Thomas AZ, Campbell SC, Palmer JS. Urologic emergencies in pregnancy. *Urology* 2010; 76(2): 453–60. [Review]

89. Stothers L, Lee LM. Renal colic in pregnancy. *J Urol* 1992; 148(5): 1383–7. [II-2]

90. Shokeir AA, Mahran MR, Abdulmaaboud M. Renal colic in pregnant women: Role of renal resistive index. *Urology* 2000; 55(3): 344–7. [II-2]

91. Spencer JA, Chahal R, Kelly A, Taylor K, Eardley I, Lloyd SN. Evaluation of painful hydronephrosis in pregnancy: Magnetic resonance urographic patterns in physiological dilatation versus calculous obstruction. *J Urol* 2004; 171(1): 256–60. [II-3]

92. Asgari MA, Safarinejad MR, Hosseini SY, Dadkhah F. Extracorporeal shock wave lithotripsy of renal calculi during early pregnancy. *BJU Int* 1999; 84(6): 615–7. [II-3]

93. Sampselle CM, Miller JM, Mims BL, Delancey JO, Ashton-Miller JA, Antonakos CL. Effect of pelvic muscle exercise on transient incontinence during pregnancy and after birth. *Obstet Gynecol* 1998; 91(3): 406–12. [I-RCT, n = 46]

94. Reilly ET, Freeman RM, Waterfield MR, Waterfield AE, Steggles P, Pedlar F. Prevention of postpartum stress incontinence in primigravidae with increased bladder neck mobility: A randomised controlled trial of antenatal pelvic floor exercises. *BJOG* 2014; 121 (Suppl. 7): 58–66. [1-RCT, n = 268]

95. Morkved S, Bo K, Schei B, Salvesen KA. Pelvic floor muscle training during pregnancy to prevent urinary incontinence: A single-blind randomized controlled trial. *Obstet Gynecol* 2003; 101(2): 313–9. [I-RCT, n = 301]

96. Morkved S, Bo K. The effect of postpartum pelvic floor muscle exercise in the prevention and treatment of urinary incontinence. *Int Urogynecol J Pelvic Floor Dysfunct* 1997; 8(4): 217–22. [I-RCT, *n* = 198]

97. Morkved S, Bo K. Effect of postpartum pelvic floor muscle training in prevention and treatment of urinary incontinence: A one-year follow up. *BJOG* 2000; 107(8): 1022–8. [RCT follow-up]

98. Wilson PD, Herbison GP. A randomized controlled trial of pelvic floor muscle exercises to treat postnatal urinary incontinence. *Int Urogynecol J Pelvic Floor Dysfunct* 1998; 9(5): 257–64. [1-RCT, *n* = 230]

99. Chiarelli P, Cockburn J. Promoting urinary continence in women after delivery: Randomised controlled trial. *BMJ* 2002; 324(7348): 1241. [1-RCT, *n* = 676]

100. Glazener CM, Herbison GP, Wilson PD, MacArthur C, Lang GD, Gee H et al. Conservative management of persistent postnatal urinary and faecal incontinence: Randomised controlled trial. *BMJ* 2001; 323(7313): 593–6. [I-RCT, *n* = 747]

101. Yip SK, Sahota D, Pang MW, Day L. Postpartum urinary retention. *Obstet Gynecol* 2005; 106(3): 602–6. [Review]

102. Groutz A, Levin I, Gold R, Pauzner D, Lessing JB, Gordon D. Protracted postpartum urinary retention: The importance of early diagnosis and timely intervention. *Neurourol Urodyn* 2011; 30(1): 83–6. [II-2]

103. Sandhu KS, LaCombe JA, Fleischmann N, Greston WM, Lazarou G, Mikhail MS. Gross and microscopic hematuria: Guidelines for obstetricians and gynecologists. *Obstet Gynecol Surv* 2009; 64(1): 39–49. [III]

18

Headache

Stephen Silberstein and Shuhan Zhu

KEY POINTS

- **Most causes of headache in pregnancy** are not due to ominous causes but to migraine or tension-type headache.
- **Migraines affect up to 18% of pregnant women; this condition frequently is diagnosed before pregnancy.**
- **New-onset headache in pregnancy** requires a **thorough neurological evaluation that** may include **neuroradio-graphic studies and/or cerebrospinal fluid (CSF) analysis**.
- Some worrisome disorders that cause headache occur more commonly in pregnant women. These include subarachnoid hemorrhage, stroke, pituitary tumor or apoplexy, and cerebral venous thrombosis.
- **Education about avoiding specific foods, caffeine, and alcohol triggers** for migraine may reduce the need for both preventive and acute medications. Pregnant patients with headache should **avoid skipping meals, optimize sleep and exercise habits, and consider yoga, meditation, or biofeedback** as an adjunctive migraine preventive modality.
- **Certain acute and preventive medication can be used** with caution in pregnancy; most are not absolutely contraindicated.
- **Most** patients with migraine without aura and many with migraine with aura **improve during pregnancy**, particularly during the second and third trimesters.
- Patients who are unknowingly pregnant and who have taken medications in the nonsteroidal anti-inflammatory class or the triptan class early in pregnancy can be reassured that drugs of these classes have not been shown to increase the incidence of teratogenicity.
- For **acute treatment** of primary headache, **acetaminophen alone (preferably) or with codeine (for refractory headache)** should be the first choice during all trimesters. **Naproxen and ibuprofen** are safe and well tolerated in pregnancy but should be **avoided after 28 weeks**. Severe unrelenting migraine responds well to parenteral antiemetics, such as metaclopramide and prochlorperazine. **Propranolol or metoprolol can be considered as a prophylactic medication** for the pregnant patient whose headache frequency requires daily preventive medication, and for whom nonpharmacologic approaches to headache prophylaxis have failed.

BACKGROUND/EPIDEMIOLOGY

The relationship between headache and pregnancy is of concern for two reasons: First, primary headache disorders (migraine or tension-type headaches) are far more common in women than men, and the impact of headache in women is directly affected by reproductive life events. One-year migraine prevalence is 18% in women in the United States.

It has a peak incidence following menarche in young girls, is most prevalent in the reproductive age of 20 to 50, is commonly exacerbated by menses, influenced by hormonal contraception and replacement therapy, and is often improved following menopause. Migraine, particularly migraine without aura, generally improves with pregnancy and worsens in the postpartum period.

Pregnancy has been a common exclusion criterion for controlled clinical trials. Therefore, data on the safety of drugs used for primary headache types in pregnant women, such as migraine and tension-type headache, are scant. Yet, in a survey of drug utilization by the World Health Organization, 68% of pregnant women took some form of medication.

Clinicians should be particularly vigilant regarding secondary headaches associated with pregnancy, such as stroke, cerebral venous thrombosis, pituitary apoplexy, and posterior reversible encephalopathy associated with eclampsia [1].

DIAGNOSIS

Diagnostic criteria as per the International Headache Society are shown in Table 18.1 [2].

Diagnostic Considerations for Headache in Pregnancy

Some secondary causes of headache (because of another, often ominous, disorder):

- Cortical venous thrombosis or cranial sinus thrombosis
- Subarachnoid hemorrhage
- Preeclampsia or eclampsia associated with elevated blood pressure (associated with reversible cerebral vasoconstriction syndrome [RCVS])
- Stroke
- Idiopathic intracranial hypertension (pseudotumor cerebri)
- Pituitary tumor and pituitary apoplexy
- Headache associated with trauma to the head or neck or to infection or disease of the meninges, sinuses, eyes, or ears

Some primary causes of headache:

- Migraine with and without aura
- Tension-type headache
- Trigeminal autonomic cephalgias (cluster headache)
- Cough headache

Red flags suggesting a secondary (ominous) headache:

- Sudden-onset (thunderclap) headache
- Secondary risk factors (HIV, systemic cancer)
- Headache associated with systemic symptoms (fever, weight loss, meningeal signs, papilledema) or focal

Table 18.1 International Headache Society Criteria for the Diagnosis of Migraine

Migraine without Aura
A. At least five attacks fulfilling criteria B–D
B. Headache duration of 4–72 hours (untreated or unsuccessfully treated)
C. Headache with at least two of the following:
   a. Unilateral location
   b. Pulsating quality
   c. Moderate or severe pain intensity
   d. Aggravation by routine physical activity
D. During headache at least one of the following:
   a. Nausea and/or vomiting
   b. Photophobia and phonophobia
E. Not better accounted for by another diagnosis

Migraine with Aura
A. At least two attacks fulfilling criteria B and C
B. One or more of the following fully reversible aura symptoms:
   1. Visual
   2. Sensory
   3. Speech and/or language
   4. Motor
   5. Brainstem
   6. Retinal
C. At least two of the following four characteristics:
   1. At least one aura symptom spreads gradually over ≥5 minutes and/or two or more symptoms occur in succession
   2. Each individual aura symptom lasts 5–60 minutes
   3. At least one aura symptom is unilateral
   4. The aura is accompanied or followed within 60 minutes, by headache
D. Not better accounted for by another diagnosis, and transient ischemic attack has been excluded

Tension-type headache
A. At least 10 episodes occurring on <1 day/month on average and fulfilling criteria B–D
B. Headache lasting from 30 minutes to 7 days
C. Headache that has at least two of the following characteristics:
   1. Bilateral location
   2. Pressing/tightening (nonpulsatile) quality
   3. Mild or moderate intensity
   4. Not aggravated by routine physical activity
D. Both of the following:
   1. No nausea or vomiting
   2. No more than one of photophobia or phonophobia
E. Not better accounted for by another diagnosis

Source: Adapted from International Headache Society. *Cephalalgia*, 33, 9, 629–808, 2013.

neurologic signs (confusion, impaired alertness, or incoordination)
- New, different, or progressively worsening headache
- Positional headache that occurs only in the upright posture and is relieved with recumbency (CSF leak)

EPIDEMIOLOGY/PATHOPHYSIOLOGY

In the past year, 18% of women and 6% of men had a **migraine** headache, but nearly half of these patients remain undiagnosed. It is estimated that an even greater number of women (approximately 40%) suffer from episodic or chronic tension-type headache. Migraine usually improves during pregnancy, but a first migraine can occur, typically in the

first trimester. The elevated and sustained levels of plasma estrogens are felt to be protective during pregnancy and the fall in estrogen at the onset of menses is a factor in menstrually associated migraine. Estrogens are known to increase pain thresholds in animal studies [3] and endogenous opioids also increase as pregnancy progresses. Migraine often recurs postpartum, usually within three to six days.

The meninges, proximal cerebral blood vessels, and venous sinuses are pain sensitive. Therefore, it is not surprising that subarachnoid hemorrhage from a ruptured aneurysm or vessel distension from a venous thrombosis would produce head pain. Pus and subarachnoid blood act as irritants, setting up an inflammatory reaction and potentially interfering with CSF reabsorption, causing hydrocephalus.

The pathophysiology of migraine is complex. Even less is known about the genesis of tension-type headache. The migraine aura is probably due to cortical spreading depression (CSD). CSD is a spreading decrease in electrical activity that moves across the cerebral cortex at 2 to 3 mm/min. It is characterized by shifts in cortical steady-state potential, transient increases in potassium, nitric oxide, and glutamate and transient increases in CBF, followed by sustained decreases. Functional MRI studies of patients with migraine show that a period of hyperemia precedes the oligemia present during the migraine aura and the headache itself can begin before hyperemia while blood flow in the cerebral cortex is still reduced. Headache probably results from activation of meningeal and blood vessel nociceptors combined with a change in central pain modulation. Headache and its associated neurovascular changes are subserved by the trigeminal system. Stimulation results in the release of substance P and calcitonin gene-related peptide (CGRP) from sensory C-fiber terminals and neurogenic inflammation [4]. Neurogenic inflammation sensitizes nerve fibers (peripheral sensitization), which now respond to previously innocuous stimuli, such as blood vessel pulsations, partly causing the pain of migraine. Central sensitization of trigeminal nucleus caudalis neurons can also occur. Central sensitization may play a key role in maintaining the headache. The migraine aura can trigger headache: CSD activates trigeminovascular afferents. This replaces the older theories of migraine pathophysiology of aura caused by vasoconstriction and headache caused by vasodilation.

GENETICS

Migraine is a group of familial disorders with a genetic component. Familial hemiplegic migraine (FHM) is a group of autosomal dominant disorders associated with attacks of migraine, with and without aura, and hemiparesis [5]. FHM1 accounts for approximately two thirds of cases and is due to at least 10 different missense mutations in the CACNA1A gene, which codes for the α_1-subunit of a voltage dependent P/Q Ca^{2+} channel. FHM2 results from a new mutation in the α_2-subunit of the Na/K pump. FHM3 is due to a missense mutation in gene SCN1A (Glnl489Lys), which encodes an α_1-subunit of a neuronal voltage-gated Na+ channel (Na_vl.l).

PREGNANCY CONSIDERATIONS
Effect of Pregnancy on the Disorder

Several retrospective studies of the course of migraine in pregnancy have been performed [6]. Most women with migraine improve during pregnancy, women without aura more commonly than women with aura, generally by the second and third trimesters. Women whose migraines began during the menarche and **those with menstruation-associated migraine are more likely to have headaches recede during pregnancy** [1]. Large prospective trials are now available. The MIGRA study prospectively reviewed headache and migraine during pregnancy and puerperium. More than 2000 pregnant women with headache participated, with 208 fulfilling IHS criteria for a diagnosis of migraine. There was a **significant decrease in the frequency of migraine during pregnancy, specifically during the second and third trimesters** [7].

Effect of the Disorder on Pregnancy

Patients with migraine were not believed to have an increased incidence of teratogenicity, toxemia, stillbirths, or miscarriage compared with controls [8]. A recent study from Taiwan found that, compared with unaffected mothers, women with migraines were at increased risk of having low-birth-weight preterm babies, preeclampsia, and delivery by caesarean [9]. A prospective cohort study in Italy found that migraine was a risk factor for subsequent development of hypertensive disorders during pregnancy although there were no significant associations with low birth weight, fetal loss, or premature delivery [10].

MANAGEMENT
Evaluation of Headache in Pregnancy

Headache in pregnancy should be evaluated in the same manner as any other time with the awareness of specific disorders that are more frequent or only occur with pregnancy. The clinician should be alert to the warning signs of ominous headache. Certain conditions that cause worrisome headache are more common in pregnancy. Headache that presents in a sudden (thunderclap) fashion may indicate subarachnoid hemorrhage, particularly if associated with a change in consciousness or focal neurologic signs. Sudden headache can also accompany preeclampsia (consider RCVS) or pituitary apoplexy. Venous or sinus thrombosis, associated with the puerperium, can present with seizure, precipitous headache, vomiting or focal signs, and, if intracranial pressure is elevated, papilledema.

Whether or not to obtain a CT or an MRI as part of the evaluation of headache in pregnancy depends on the degree of suspicion for an ominous cause of headache. Generally speaking, **head CT and MRI are safe in pregnancy** although the decision to obtain the study should be based on the risk of missing a structural or serious cause of headache without the study. **Gadolinium**, used as a contrast agent for MRI scanning, does cross the placenta [11]. However, if an intracerebral bleed, mass lesion, or meningitis is suspected, the benefit of CT, MRI, or MRA far outweighs the potential risks, including the risk of gadolinium. Gadolinium was deemed **safe** by the European Society of Radiology as after gadolinium contrast media no effect on the fetus has been reported in the literature [12]. Lumbar puncture to diagnose meningitis or hemorrhage may be delayed until CT of the brain without contrast is obtained to avoid the risk of herniation if a mass or cerebral edema is suspected.

Acute Therapy for Headache

Acute migraine treatments in nonpregnant women include, among others, simple analgesics (acetominophen, aspirin), nonsteroidal anti-inflammatory drugs (NSAIDs), opioids, ergot alkaloids, isometheptene caffeine-barbiturate combinations, and triptans (Table 18.2).

Migraine typically improves as pregnancy progresses. However, in the first trimester, when headache often worsens, concern arises as to the potential effect of acute medication on embryogenesis. The situation is particularly poignant as many women, unknowingly pregnant, will have used acute medications to treat migraine or tension-type headache in the very early days or weeks after conception.

Acetaminophen is the drug most commonly taken during pregnancy. There is no evidence of any teratogenic effect (FDA B). Concerns regarding the safety of aspirin arose from early data when used at therapeutic doses for analgesic or antipyretic purposes. These concerns do not appear to apply to low-dose (60–100 mg/day) aspirin (FDA C; D if third trimester). Although aspirin is labeled category C, aspirin is unique in that there are clinical trials that studied aspirin during pregnancy for conditions other than headache, for example, in patients with antiphospholipid antibody

Table 18.2   Proposed Management of Primary Headache in Pregnancy

Nonpharmacologic methods: Optimize sleep, nutrition, exercise. Education, counseling, reassurance		Recommended for all pregnant women Ideally should be discussed as preconception planning	
Analgesic	**FDA Cat[a]**	**Before 28 Weeks**	**After 28 Weeks**
Acetaminophen	B	First line	First line
Ibuprofen	B	Ibuprofen used more commonly,	NOT RECOMMENDED, all NSAIDs are
Naproxen	B	naproxen also consider low risk	FDA category D in third trimester
Antiemetic			
Metoclopramide	B	Antiemetic class generally safe, effective for nausea and migraine pain, can be given	
Promethazine	C	intravenously and in combination with an appropriate analgesic	
Prochlorperazine	C		
Opioid			
Meperidine	B	Recommend short opiate courses to	Limit opioids during late pregnancy to
Codeine	C	prevent medication over use headache	reduce neonatal withdrawal
Morphine	C		
Others			
Caffeine	C	May be combined appropriate analgesic	
Prednisone	C	Recommend short courses of steroids, limit to three- to six-day courses to reduce	
Dexamethasone	C	risk of fetal side effects	

[a]US Food and Drug Administration Pregnancy Category.

syndrome [13]. Recommended dosing of aspirin is high, at 500 to 1000 mg per attack [8]. Other category B drugs (no evidence of risk in humans but without controlled human studies) include **ibuprofen and naproxen in the first two trimesters only; NSAIDs are considered category D during the last trimester due to risk of premature ductus arteriosus closure and neonatal pulmonary hypertension** [14]. **Caffeine** is a category C drug and may be used alone or in combination with NSAID or acetaminophen, depending on the gestational age. The caffeine content of one cup of drip coffee is approximately 100 mg [15]; consumption of up to 200 mg of caffeine a day is generally considered low risk during pregnancy [16,17].

Meperidine (FDA B), **codeine** (FDA C), **and morphine** (FDA C) may be used with the caveat that chronic use, particularly during late pregnancy, can result in neonatal withdrawal syndromes [1]. Prednisone or dexamethasone may be used for intractable migraine although chronic exposure can result in fetal adrenal suppression and other complications [1].

Ergotamine and dihydroergotamine are category X and should be avoided in pregnant women. Ergots are abortifacients and have been shown to cause fetal distress and birth defects.

Antiemetic medicines, such as **metoclopramide (FDA B), promethazine (FDA C), and prochlorperazine (FDA C)**, are effective parenterally for the head pain itself in addition to the nausea and vomiting that can accompany migraine. These are generally considered safe for use during pregnancy. Intravenous or intramuscular antiemetics, with fluid replacement, are effective in aborting status migrainosus or severe headache in the emergency room or urgent care center.

The triptans are 5-HT IB/ID receptor agonists effective in treating migraine headache and the accompanying symptoms of photosensitivity, nausea, and vomiting. The data obtained from 12 years of prospective monitoring of pregnancies exposed to sumatriptan and naratriptan failed to show a signal for a substantial increase in the risk of all major birth defects. However, the size of the registry is currently insufficient to evaluate the risk of specific defects or to permit definitive conclusions of the risks associated with sumatriptan or naratriptan [18]. The triptan class is category C and is not recommended for pregnant migraineurs. Nevertheless, on the basis of the pregnancy registry, if a patient has unwittingly taken **sumatriptan** prior to knowledge of her pregnancy, **reassurance is appropriate given the lack of teratogenicity of this drug**. It is not known whether this positive outcome may also be extrapolated to other medications in the triptan class.

Headache Prophylaxis in Pregnancy

Clinicians should be encouraged to treat headaches in early pregnancy with acute medications such as acetaminophen or low doses of codeine. **Preventive therapy should be reserved for women whose headaches continue to worsen throughout pregnancy.** There are no prospective randomized clinical trials of migraine prophylactic drugs in pregnant women.

Nonpharmacologic therapies should be initiated first. **Relaxation training and thermal biofeedback,** combined with relaxation techniques and **cognitive behavioral therapies,** have been subjected to rigorous, well-designed, randomized clinical trials and show efficacy in migraine prevention [19]. In contradistinction, evidence based therapy recommendations for acupuncture, hypnosis, and chiropractic manipulation for headache prevention are not yet available.

Whenever a second comorbid condition exists with migraine, it is advisable to use one drug to treat both conditions. Examples include migraine and epilepsy, wherein an anticonvulsant may be effective to treat both conditions, and migraine and depression, for which a selective serotonin reuptake inhibitor (SSRI), such as fluoxetine (category B), may similarly permit monotherapy.

Propranolol or **metoprolol** are the drugs of choice as headache preventive during pregnancy [1]. Verapamil (calcium channel blocker) may also be beneficial [20]. Valproic acid should be avoided for headache prophylaxis because of its potential for causing neural tube defects. The use of topiramate and gaba-pentin should be restricted for headache prophylaxis in view of their potential association with fetal defects although these drugs can be very effective for nonpregnant migraineurs.

Education about avoiding specific foods, caffeine, and alcohol triggers for migraine may reduce reliance on both preventive and acute medications. Pregnant patients with headache should **avoid skipping meals, optimize sleep and exercise habits, and consider meditation or yoga.**

REFERENCES

1. MacGregor E. Headache in pregnancy. *Continuum (Minneap Minn)* 2014; 20(1): 128–47. [Review]
2. International Headache Society. The international classification of headache disorders. 3rd ed (beta version). *Cephalalgia* 2013; 33(9): 629–808. [Review]
3. Dawson-Basoa M, Gintzler A. 17-Beta-estradiol and progesterone modulate an intrinsic opioid analgesic system. *Brain Res* 1993; 601(1–2): 241–5. [II-3]
4. Dimitriadou V, Buzzi M, Theoharides T, Moskowitz M. Ultrastructural evidence for neurogenically mediated changes in blood vessels of the rat aura mater and tongue following antidromic trigeminal stimulation. *Neuroscience* 1992; 48(1): 187–203. [II-2]
5. Silberstein S, Dodick D. Migraine genetics: Part II. *Headache* 2013; 53(8): 1218–29. [Review]
6. Loder E, Silberstein S. Headaches in woman. In: Silberstein SD, Lipton RB, Dodick DW, eds. *Wolff's Headache and Other Head Pain.* 8th ed. New York: Oxford University Press, 2008: 691–710. [Review]
7. Kvisvik E, Stovner L, Helde G, Bovim G, Linde M. Headache and migraine during pregnancy and puerperium: The MIGRA-study. *J Headache Pain* 2011; 12(4): 443–51. [II-2]
8. Wainscott G, Sullivan F, Volans G, Wilkinson M. The outcome of pregnancy in women suffering from migraine. *Postgrad Med J* 1978; 54(628): 98–102. [II-2]
9. Chen H, Chen S, Chen Y, Lin H. Increased risk of adverse pregnancy outcomes for woman with migraines: A nationwide population-based study. *Cephalalgia* 2010; 30(4): 443–8. [II-2]
10. Facchinetti F, Allais G, Nappi R, D'Amico R, Marozio L, Bertozzi L et al. Migraine is a risk factor for hypertensive disorders in pregnancy: A prospective cohort study. *Cephalalgia* 2009; 29(3): 286–92. [II-3]
11. Schwartz R. Neurodiagnostic imaging of the pregnant patient. In: Deinsky O, Feldmann E, Hainline B, eds. *Neurologic Complications of Pregnancy.* New York: Raven Press, 1994: 243–8. [Review]
12. Webb J, Thomsen H, Morcos S. The use of iodinated and gadolinium contrast media during pregnancy and lactation. *Eur Radiol* 2005; 15(6): 1234–40. [Review]
13. Vainio M, Kujansuu E, Iso-Mustajärvi M, Mäenpää J. Low dose acetylsalicylic acid in prevention of pregnancy-induced hypertension and intrauterine growth retardation in women with bilateral uterine artery notches. *BJOG* 2002; 109(2): 161–7. [II-2]

14. Morris J, Rosen D, Rosen K. Nonsteroidal anti-inflammatory agents in neonates. *Paediatr Drugs* 2003; 5(6): 385–405. [Review]

15. United States Department of Agriculture Agricultural Research Service. *National Nutrient Database for Standard Reference Release 28.* In: usda.gov (online). Available at: http://ndb.nal.usda.gov/ndb/foods/show/4277?fgcd=&manu=&lfacet=&format=&count=&max=35&offset=&sort=&qlookup=14209. Accessed January 12, 2016. [Review]

16. Jahanfar S, Jaafar SH. Effects of restricted caffeine intake by mother on fetal, neonatal and pregnancy outcomes. *Cochrane Database Syst Rev* 2015; 9(6): CD006965. [Review]

17. Maslova E, Bhattacharya S, Lin SW, Michels KB. Caffeine consumption during pregnancy and risk of preterm birth: A meta-analysis. *Am J Clin Nutr* 2010; 92(5): 1120–32. [Review]

18. Cunnington M, Ephross S, Churchill P. The safety of sumatriptan and naratriptan in pregnancy: What have we learned? *Headache* 2009; 49(10): 1414–22. [Review]

19. Campbell JK, Penzien DB, Wall EM, and the US Headache Consortium. *Evidence-based guidelines for migraine headache: Behavioral and physical treatments.* In: AOA.net (online). Available at: http://tools.aan.com/professionals/practice/pdfs/gl0089.pdf. Accessed January 2, 2016. [Review]

20. Silberstein S, Freitag F, Bigal M. Migraine treatment. In: Silberstein SD, Lipton RB, Dodick DW, eds. *Wolff's Headache and Other Head Pain.* 8th ed. New York: Oxford University Press, 2008: 177–292. [Review]

19

Seizures

Sally Mathias and Meriem K. Bensalem-Owen

KEY POINTS

- **Epilepsy** is a chronic neurological condition characterized by **recurrent unprovoked seizures**. The most important diagnostic tool is the history.
- Approximately 0.3% to 0.5% of all pregnancies are among women with epilepsy.
- For the majority of the patients, seizure frequency remains unchanged during pregnancy. Status epilepticus is rare during pregnancy.
- **Fetal loss, perinatal death, congenital anomalies** (4%–8% or about twice the baseline risk), **low birth weight, prematurity, induction, developmental delay**, and **childhood epilepsy** have been reported in the past to be more frequent, but more recent data do not confirm an increase in these complications.
- **Supplemental folic acid** (0.4 up to 4 mg daily, usually 2–4 mg) may be given to all women of childbearing age taking **antiepileptic drugs** (AEDs) prior to conception and continued during pregnancy. There is **insufficient published information** to address the **dosing of folic acid**.
- **Counsel** women with seizures or epilepsy about the risk of AED-*associated* teratogenicity and neurodevelopmental delay, folic acid supplementation, possible changes in seizure frequency during pregnancy, importance of medication compliance and AED level monitoring, inheritance risks for seizures, and breast-feeding. **Encourage enrollment in a pregnancy registry.**
- In general, the best choice for therapy is the AED that best controls the seizures. **Monotherapy at the lowest possible dose of the AED most efficient in controlling seizures** should be **the goal**. All treatment decisions involve a discussion of benefits and harms of treatment options.
- **Carbamazepine, phenobarbital, primidone, phenytoin, valproate, and topiramate** are FDA category D drugs and should be avoided if possible.
- **Optimize AED therapy and complete AED changes** if possible **at least six months before planned conception.**
- **Seizure freedom for at least nine months prior to pregnancy is probably associated with a high likelihood of remaining seizure-free during pregnancy.**
- **Stopping or changing an AED during pregnancy for the sole purpose of reducing teratogenicity is not advised.**
- **Prenatal testing** should include first-trimester ultrasound, **alpha-fetoprotein (AFP) levels, anatomy, and echocardiographic ultrasounds** and, if needed, amniocentesis for amniotic fluid AFP and acetylcholinesterase.
- As pregnancy progresses, **both total and nonprotein-bound plasma concentrations of some AEDs may decline.**
- Monitor AED levels through the eighth postpartum week.
- There is **insufficient evidence to support or refute a benefit of prenatal vitamin K supplementation for reducing the risk of hemorrhagic complications in the newborns** of women with epilepsy.
- There is possibly a substantial **increased risk of preterm birth for women with epilepsy who smoke**.
- **Encourage breast-feeding** and monitor for sedation or feeding difficulties, which can be caused by certain AEDs, usually those with low protein binding.
- Emphasize that **>90% of women with epilepsy have successful pregnancies and deliver healthy babies.**

BACKGROUND

Recommendations and guidelines presented in this chapter are in large part based on the updated three companion Practice Parameters of the Quality Standards Subcommittee and Therapeutics and Technology Assessment Subcommittee of the American Academy of Neurology, American Epilepsy Society, and the updated Epilepsy Quality Measurement Set [1–4].

DIAGNOSES/DEFINITIONS

Seizures result from an abnormal paroxysmal discharge of a group of cerebral neurons. **Epilepsy** is a **chronic neurological condition**. Epilepsy is defined as **at least two unprovoked (or reflex) seizures occurring greater than 24 hours apart** or **one unprovoked (or reflex) seizure and a probability of further seizures similar to the general recurrence risk after two unprovoked seizures, occurring over the next 10 years** [5]. The most important diagnostic tool is the **history**. The examination is very often normal unless the patient has a structural brain lesion. The history should include the following information:

- The presence or absence of an aura, which is a recurrent stereotypic abnormal sensation or experience. The aura is a simple partial seizure or focal seizure without impairment of consciousness or awareness according to the newly proposed classification of seizures and epilepsies [6].
- Seizure description by an eyewitness, including duration.
- Postictal phase, description, and duration.
- Exacerbating factors.
- Birth history, especially when the seizure onset is in the neonatal period or early childhood.
- History of febrile convulsions, central nervous system infections, head trauma with loss of consciousness or known structural lesion in the brain.
- Family history.

Ancillary tests include **EEG**, laboratory tests as indicated by the history, and imaging of the brain. **MRI of the head is** more sensitive than CT scan for detecting subtle lesions. EEG poses no risk to the fetus, so workup for diagnosis should proceed in pregnancy just as in nonpregnant adults.

SYMPTOMS

In partial onset or focal seizures, some patients may experience a subjective feeling, called an aura. The particular site of the brain affected determines usually the symptomatology and/or the clinical expression of the seizure.

EPIDEMIOLOGY/INCIDENCE

Epilepsy occurs in 0.5% to 0.8% of the general population, with 5% of people reporting a seizure at some time in their life. Approximately one in 26 people will develop epilepsy at some point in their lives [7]. The prevalence of epilepsy in the United States indicates that approximately one half million women with epilepsy are of childbearing age. Approximately **0.3% to 0.5% of all pregnancies are among women with epilepsy** [8].

ETIOLOGY/BASIC PATHOPHYSIOLOGY

Paroxysmal discharges of neurons occur when the threshold for firing of neuronal membranes is reduced. The pathophysiology of epileptic disorders is not very well understood. Structural abnormalities of neuronal transmitter receptors, channelopathies, excessive excitatory activity, cortical remodeling, and loss of inhibitory neuronal activity have all been implicated as possible mechanisms.

CLASSIFICATION

The International League Against Epilepsy (ILAE) proposed a new classification for seizures and epilepsies in 2010 [6]. Depending on their onset, seizures are classified as **focal, generalized, or unknown**. Focal seizures can be further subdivided into seizures with or without impairment of consciousness also known as **simple partial** or **complex partial** seizures (CPS). When awareness is preserved, the patient may either experience focal motor manifestations or experience a subjective feeling, called an aura. The prototype for generalized seizures is the generalized tonic clonic (GTC) seizure.

Auras can be olfactory, gustatory, sensory, auditory, visual, vertiginous sensations, or psychic experiences (such as "deja vu"). Focal seizures with impairment of consciousness can evolve into bilateral convulsive seizure (also known as secondarily generalized seizure).

RISK FACTORS/ASSOCIATIONS

Risk factors for seizures are numerous and could include malformations of cortical development, head trauma, central nervous system infections, family history, complicated febrile convulsions, and possibly history of difficult birth (anoxia or trauma) or complicated (fetal infections and/or preterm birth) pregnancy.

COMPLICATIONS

Epileptic women of childbearing age should be informed of the risks associated with antiepileptic drug (AED) use prior to

conception [3] and that seizures may be harmful to mother and fetus [4]. A recently published retrospective cohort study evaluated the effect of pregnancy planning in women with epilepsy on seizure control during pregnancy and on maternal and neonatal outcomes. Planned pregnancies had a significantly greater portion of patients receiving AED monotherapy and of not using valproic acid. This group also had a lower frequency of seizures during pregnancy as well as a significantly lower likelihood of altering their AED regimen during pregnancy [9].

Maternal Complications

The American Academy of Neurology (AAN) reviewed the scientific literature and published practice parameters in 2009, which stated that probably no substantially increased risk exists of cesarean delivery, late pregnancy bleeding, or preterm labor and delivery in women with epilepsy who are taking antiepileptic drugs [1–3]. There is insufficient evidence to support or refute an increased risk of preeclampsia, gestational hypertension, spontaneous abortion, a change in seizure frequency or an increased risk of status epilepticus in pregnant women with epilepsy. Only class IV studies could be found on this subject. On the basis of class II studies, seizure freedom for at least nine months prior to pregnancy is probably associated with a high likelihood (84%–92%) of remaining seizure-free during pregnancy. Women can injure themselves during convulsive seizures.

Fetal Complications

GTC seizures increase the risk of hypoxia and acidosis as well as injury from blunt trauma. Generalized seizures but not partial seizures occurring during labor can affect fetal heart rate. According to a recent study, women with epilepsy on AED therapy and experiencing more than one GTC seizure during pregnancy had an overall five times higher preterm birth risk, a shorter gestational age, and a reduced birth weight in boys [10]. **Fetal loss** (1.3%–14%) and **perinatal death** (1.3%–7.8%), **congenital malformation anomalies** (4%–8%, or about twice the baseline risk), **low birth weight** (7%–10%), **preterm birth** (4%–11%), **induction, developmental delay**, and childhood epilepsy can be associated with in utero exposure to AEDs. There is insufficient evidence to determine whether the risk of neonatal hemorrhagic complications in the newborns of women with epilepsy taking AEDs is substantially increased. **Evidence is inadequate to determine whether prenatal vitamin K in women with epilepsy reduces the risk of hemorrhagic complications in the newborns.**

Congenital malformations are more common among offspring of women on AEDs (5%) than among offspring of untreated patients (3%). Major congenital malformations include neural tube defects (NTDs), congenital heart disease, cleft lip/palate, and urogenital defects. Minor congenital malformations include coarse hair, epicanthal folds, small nail beds, and skin tags. Most common congenital malformations, which differ for different AEDs, are cardiac, neural tube, craniofacial, and involving the fingers.

Epilepsy and pregnancy registries have been operational for approximately 15 years and were developed in order to better understand the risks of birth defects associated with AED treatment, and more importantly, to systematically study the range of birth defects resulting from use of each AED [11]. Two class I studies, including one from the U.K. Epilepsy and Pregnancy Registry, revealed that exposure during the first trimester to valproic acid monotherapy is associated with a greater risk for major congenital malformations than carbamazepine monotherapy [12,13]. Valproic acid as part of polytherapy was associated with greater risk than polytherapy without valproic acid [12].

Data from the North American Antiepileptic Drug (NAAED) Pregnancy Registry indicate that **the rate of major malformations is 9% with valproate** [14], **6% with phenobarbital, 2% with lamotrigine, 2.2% with levetiracetam, 4.5% with topiramate, and 3.1% with carbamazepine**. Valproic acid is associated with neural tube defects, oral clefts, hypospadias, poor cognitive outcome, and cardiac malformations. Exposure to phenytoin, carbamazepine, topiramte, and lamotrigine was associated with oral clefts. Avoidance of phenobarbital may reduce the risk of cardiac malformations.

MANAGEMENT
Principles

Effect of pregnancy on disease: Increase in hepatic cytochrome P450 enzyme activity and renal clearance causes the concentration of some AEDs to fall. Decreased protein binding results **in higher levels of unbound biologically active AEDs** and may cause toxicity (Table 19.1). On the basis of current studies, there is insufficient evidence to support or refute an increased risk of a change in seizure frequency or status epilepticus during pregnancy.

Preconception Counseling
Also include in first prenatal visit the following:

a. Conception should be deferred until seizures are **well controlled on a minimum dose of medication.**
b. **Monotherapy is preferable.** Good compliance with AEDs is essential to avoid any seizures.
c. Inform women with epilepsy that infants exposed in utero to AED have a **4% to 8% risk of congenital malformation**, most notably neural tube defects, cardiac, and craniofacial defects, compared to 2% to 3% for the general population. Epilepsy pregnancy registries have been operational for more than 15 years and have collected an

Table 19.1 Pharmacokinetic Profile and Adverse Effects of the Most Commonly Used AEDs

	Mechanism	Pregnancy Category	Protein Binding (%)
First-generation AEDs			
Phenytoin (Dilantin)	Na	D	90
Carbamazepine (Tegretol)	Ca, GABA	D	75
Valproic acid (Depakote, Depakene)	Na, GABA	D	85–95
Ethosuximide	T-type Ca	C	0
Second- and third-generation AEDs			
Gabapentin (Neurontin)	Ca	C	0
Pregabalin (Lyrica)	Ca	C	0
Lamotrigine (Lamotrigine)	Na, Glutamate	C	55
Levetiracetam (Keppra)	SV2a	C	0
Oxcarbazepine (Oxcarbamazepine)	Na, Ca	C	40
Tiagabine (Gabatril)	GABA reuptake	C	96
Topiramate (Topiramate)	Multiple	D	10
Zonisamide (Zonegran)	Na, T-Ca	C	40–60
Lacosamide (Vimpat)	Na (slow inactivation)	C	15
Rufinamide (Banzel)	Na	C	34
Vigabatrin (Sabril)	GABA	C	0
Eslicarbazepine (Aptiom)	Na	C	<40

	Adverse Effects
First-generation AEDs	
Phenytoin (Dilantin)	Rash, ataxia, hirsutism, gingival hypertrophy, osteoporosis
Carbamazepine (Tegretol)	Rash, diplopia, sexual dysfunction, osteoporosis
Valproic acid (Depakote, Depakene)	Weight gain, tremor, hair loss, encephalopathy, hepatotoxicity, pancreatitis, polycystic ovaries
Ethosuximide	Nausea, vomiting, anorexia, rash
Second- and third-generation AEDs	
Gabapentin (Neurontin)	Weight gain, edema, myoclonus
Pregabalin (Lyrica)	Increased appetite, confusion, somnolence
Lamotrigine (Lamotrigine)	Rash, aseptic meningitis
Levetiracetam (Keppra)	Behavioral changes, asthenia
Oxcarbazepine (Oxcarbamazepine)	Hyponatremia, diplopia, rash
Tiagabine (Gabatril)	Encephalopathy, status epilepticus
Topiramate (Topiramate)	Renal stones, speech difficulties, paresthesias, weight loss, acidosis, closed-angle glaucoma
Zonisamide (Zonegran)	Renal stones, weight loss, paresthesias, contraindicated if history of allergy to sulfa drugs
Lacosamide (Vimpat)	Dizziness, nausea, vomiting, double vision
Rufinamide (Banzel)	Headaches, drowsiness, dizziness, vomiting
Vigabatrin (Sabril)	Visual field loss, somnolence, headaches, dizziness
Eslicarbazepine (Aptiom)	Dizziness, disturbance in gait and coordination

impressive amount of data. **Carbamazepine, phenobarbital, primidone, phenytoin, valproate, and topiramate** are FDA category D drugs and **should be avoided** if possible at least in the first trimester. Recent pregnancy databases have suggested that valproate is significantly more teratogenic than carbamazepine, and the combination of valproate with lamotrigine and valproate with carbamazepine is particularly teratogenic [15]. If valproate is used, high plasma levels (>70 µg/mL) should be avoided unless necessary to control seizures, and the drug should be given in divided doses three or four times daily. To date, the most comprehensive prospective study of cognitive development reported IQ in children exposed to low dose of valproate comparable to IQ in children exposed to other antiepileptic drugs [16]. Lamotrigine has been associated with facial clefts; however, the lowest rates of MCMs were seen when lamotrigine dose was <300 mg/day [17].

d. Seizure freedom for at least nine months prior to pregnancy is probably associated with a high likelihood of remaining seizure-free during pregnancy.

e. Consider **neurological consultation** regarding the possibility of tapering off and stopping anticonvulsant medications if the patient has been seizure-free for greater than two years and has a normal EEG. The patient should be observed for six to 12 months off AED before attempting conception.

f. Preconception folic acid supplementation (usually 2–4 mg) may be considered to reduce the risk of major congenital malformations.

g. Driving privileges should be suspended for several months after a seizure; the exact length varies depending on the state [18].

h. Home/work: Avoid baths, take showers instead. Avoid manipulation of heavy machinery or working at heights [18].

i. Enzyme-inducing AEDs (Table 19.1) enhance the metabolism of oral contraceptives, therefore decreasing their efficacy. Pregnancies should be planned.

j. **Emphasize that 90% of women with epilepsy have successful pregnancies and deliver healthy babies** [19].

Prenatal Counseling

At the first prenatal visit and during pregnancy as necessary, counsel women with seizures or epilepsy regarding all of the above preconception issues. In addition, discuss the following:

- There is a possible change in seizure frequency during pregnancy. A recent prospective study found, however, that pregnancy does not appear to affect seizure frequency in women with epilepsy [20].
- **Although no AED is specifically indicated for use in pregnant women, the AED that renders the patient seizure-free and side effect-free should be the drug of choice during pregnancy.**
- The risk-to-benefit ratio must be considered when selecting a drug.
- There is a risk of AED-associated teratogenicity and neurodevelopment delay.
- **Importance of medication compliance and AED level monitoring during pregnancy.** AED levels decline due to enhanced AED hepatic metabolism, changes in

volume distribution, and increase in glomerular filtration rate, which leads to increased renal clearance and decreased protein binding. Therefore, levels should be measured on highly protein bound AEDs (Table 19.1).

- In a retrospective population-based study, a tenfold increase in mortality was noted in pregnancy in women with epilepsy compared to women without epilepsy. Etiology for mortality was not found, thus leaving many questions answered. Most of these deaths were Sudden Unexpected Death in Epilepsy (SUDEP) demonstrating the importance of complete seizure control and a heightened clinical attention for these pregnancies [21,22].
- Breast-feeding issues (see below).
- Inheritance risks for seizures.
- Child care issues [23].
- **Educate patients about various pregnancy registries and encourage enrollment in a registry.** The goal of any registry is to gather and publish information on the rate of major malformations in infants whose mothers had taken AEDs during pregnancy and to determine the safety of seizure medications. The North American Anti-Epileptic Drug Pregnancy Registry enrolls pregnant women with epilepsy from the United States and Canada (http://www.aedpregnancyregistry.org). Likewise, every region has its own pregnancy registry, and newer AED manufacturers have a registry of their own.

Prenatal Care

- Supplemental **folic acid** (usually 2–4 mg/day) in women with epilepsy before they become pregnant is generally recommended to reduce the risk of major congenital malformations.
- A first-trimester ultrasound is indicated for exact dating.
- Anatomic ultrasound at 11 to 13 weeks can identify most severe defects, such as anencephaly.
- Prenatal testing for neural tube defects with **alpha-fetoprotein** levels at 15 to 18 weeks gestation (up to 21 weeks).
- If appropriate, amniocentesis for amniotic fluid alpha-fetoprotein and acetylcholinesterase levels.
- **Ultrasound at 16 to 20 weeks** gestation can assess anatomic anomalies, such as orofacial clefts, heart defects, and caudal neural tube defects.
- Fetal **echocardiogram** at about 22 weeks.
- An ultrasound for growth at >32 weeks is not mandatory.
- Neonates should receive vitamin K, 1 mg IM at birth. The benefit of prenatal maternal vitamin K therapy is unknown with no trial available for assessment.

THERAPY (TABLE 19.1)

- **Multidisciplinary** communication between the primary care provider, obstetrician, geneticist, and neurologist/epileptologist for counseling and management of seizures and epilepsy during pregnancy is crucial.
- **There is no trial that indicates which AED is safest during pregnancy.** The best choice is the AED that best controls the seizures. **All the AEDs are FDA category C except for the following AEDs that are category D: carbamazepine, phenobarbital, primidone, phenytoin, valproate, and**

topiramate (Table 19.1). **These six AEDs should therefore be avoided if possible** by using a different therapy beginning in the preconception period. Switching and abruptly stopping of AEDs are to be avoided.

- Regarding AED therapy, at the beginning of pregnancy it is recommended that the patient is on **monotherapy** with the AED of choice for the seizure type, achieving optimal seizure control at the lowest effective dose.
- **Monitoring the serum levels** of **lamotrigine, carbamazepine, and phenytoin** during pregnancy should be considered, and monitoring of levetiracetam and oxcarbazepine (as monohydroxy derivative) levels may be considered. Free levels (serum or saliva) are available for carbamazepine, valproic acid, phenobarbital, and phenytoin. Avoid high peak levels by spreading out the total daily dose into multiple smaller doses. Studies provide some evidence supporting active monitoring of AED levels during pregnancy, particularly of lamotrigine, as changes in lamotrigine levels were associated with increased seizure frequency [24]. **It seems reasonable to individualize this monitoring for each patient with the aim of maintaining a level close to preconception level, presumably the one at which the woman with epilepsy was doing well with seizure control.** One study showed that during pregnancy the clearance of lamotrigine increases with a peak of 94% in the third trimester; hence, frequent adjustments of the dose are required during pregnancy [19].
- AEDs have effects on sodium, potassium, or calcium channels. They also can affect neurotransmitters enhancing the inhibitory neurotransmitter, GABA, or inhibiting the excitatory glutamate.
- AED Pregnancy Registry: Phone number 1-888-233-2334. http://www.aedpregnancyregistry.org.

DELIVERY

AED medication should be continued in labor and in the immediate postpartum period. Women should be encouraged to bring their own AEDs to the delivery, and medications should be taken at their usual times during labor [25]. Consider intravenous formulations of AEDs if these cannot be taken orally. A recent study found that women with epilepsy on polytherapy versus monotherapy had an increased risk of cesarean section [26]. **There is possibly a substantial increased risk of preterm birth or women with epilepsy who smoke [27].**

POSTPARTUM/BREAST-FEEDING

Breast-feeding is not contraindicated. The greater the protein binding of the AED (Table 19.1), the lower is its concentration in breast milk. Breast-feeding is not contraindicated in patients on anticonvulsant medications unless excess neonatal sedation occurs. **Monitor newborns** or infants for sedation when breast-feeding mothers with seizures take low-protein-bound AEDs. The AED concentration profiled in breast milk follows the plasma concentration curve. The total amount of drug transferred to infants via breast milk is usually much smaller than the amount transferred via the placenta during pregnancy. However, as drug elimination mechanisms are not fully developed in early infancy, repeated administration of a drug via breast milk may lead to accumulation in the infant. Extended release formulations of AEDs should be avoided. It appears that there are no adverse effects of AED exposure via breast milk on cognition and development observed at three years and six years [28].

Valproic acid, phenobarbital, phenytoin, and carbamazepine may be considered as not transferring into breast milk to as great an extent as, for example, levetiracetam, gabapentin, lamotrigine, and topiramate.

For most AEDs, the pharmacokinetics in the mother will return to prepregnancy levels within 10 to 14 days after delivery. Monitor AED levels through the eighth postpartum week and adjust doses accordingly to avoid toxicity. **Sleep deprivation may exacerbate seizures**, and should therefore be avoided. Women with epilepsy should not bathe their child while they are alone at home and should avoid stair climbing while carrying the baby; a portable changing pad placed on the floor should be used. New mothers should avoid using a carrier in front or on their back. A portable carrier with handles is a safer alternative in the event of a seizure and subsequent fall [23]. Because enzyme-inducing AEDs (Table 19.1) lower estrogen concentrations by 40% to 50%, thereby compromising contraceptive effectiveness, hormonal contraceptives prescribed to women with epilepsy on these AEDs should contain ≥50 µg of ethinyl estradiol [29]. Oral contraceptives induce lamotrigine metabolism, requiring adjustment of its dose [30].

REFERENCES

1. Harden CL, Pennell PB, Koppel BS et al. Practice parameter update: Management issues for women with epilepsy—Focus on pregnancy (an evidence-based review): III. Vitamin K, folic acid, blood levels, and breastfeeding: Report of the Quality Standards Subcommittee and Therapeutics and Technology Assessment Subcommittee of the American Academy of Neurology and American Epilepsy Society. *Neurology* 2009; 73(2): 142–9. [Guideline; III]
2. Harden CL, Hopp J, Ting TY et al. Practice parameter update: Management issues for women with epilepsy—Focus on pregnancy (an evidence-based review): I. Obstetrical complications and change in seizure frequency: Report of the Quality Standards Subcommittee and Therapeutics and Technology Assessment Subcommittee of the American Academy of Neurology and American Epilepsy Society. *Neurology* 2009; 73: 126–32. [Guideline; III]
3. Harden CL, Meador KJ, Pennell PB et al. Practice parameter update: Management issues for women with epilepsy—Focus on pregnancy (an evidence-based review): II. Teratogenesis and perinatal outcomes: Report of the Quality Standards Subcommittee and Therapeutics and Technology Assessment Subcommittee of the American Academy of Neurology and American Epilepsy Society. *Neurology* 2009; 73: 133–41. [Guideline; III]
4. Fountain NB, Van Ness PC, Bennett A et al. Quality improvement in neurology: Epilepsy update quality measurement set. *Neurology* 2015; 84(14): 1483–7. [Guideline; III]
5. Fisher R, Acevedo C, Arzimanoglou A et al. A practical clinical definition of epilepsy. *Epilepsia* 2014; 55: 475–82. [Review]
6. Berg AT, Berkovic SF, Brodie MJ et al. Revised terminology and concepts for organization of seizures and epilepsies: Report of the ILAE Commission on Classification and Terminology, 2005–2009. *Epilepsia* 2010; 51: 676–85. [Guideline; III]
7. England MJ, Liverman CT, Schultz AM, Strawbridge LM. Institute of Medicine Committee on the Public Health Dimensions of the Epilepsies. *Epilepsy Behav* 2012 Oct; 25(2): 266–76. [Review]
8. Hirtz D, Thurman DJ, Gwinn-Hardy K et al. How common are the "common" neurologic disorders? *Neurology* 2007; 68(5): 326–37. [II-3]

9. Abe K, Hamada H, Yamada T et al. Impact of planning of pregnancy in women with epilepsy on seizure control during pregnancy and on maternal and neonatal outcomes. *Seizure* 2014; 23: 112–6. [II-3]

10. Rauchenzauner M, Ehrensberger M, Rieschi M et al. Generalized tonic-clonic seizures and antiepileptic drugs during pregnancy—A matter of importance for the baby? *J Neurol* 2013; 260: 484–8. [II-3]

11. Meador KJ, Pennell PB, Harden CL et al. Pregnancy registries in epilepsy: A consensus statement on health outcomes. *Neurology* 2008; 71: 1109–17. [II-3]

12. Morrow J, Russell A, Guthrie E et al. Malformation risks of antiepileptic drugs in pregnancy: A prospective study from the UK Epilepsy and Pregnancy Register. *J Neurol Neurosurg Psychiatry* 2006; 77(2): 193–8. [II-2]

13. Wide K, Winbladh B, Kallen B. Major malformations in infants exposed to antiepileptic drugs in utero, with emphasis on carbamazepine and valproic acid: A nation-wide, population-based register study. *Acta Paediatr* 2004; 93(2): 174–6. [II-2]

14. Wyszynski DF, Nambisan M, Surve T et al., for the Antiepileptic Drug Pregnancy Registry. Increased rate of major malformations in offspring exposed to valproate during pregnancy. *Neurology* 2005; 64(6): 961–5. [II-3]

15. Tomson T, Battino D, Craig J et al., ILAE Commission on therapeutic strategies. Pregnancy registries: Differences, similarities, and possible harmonization. *Epilepsia* 2010; 51(5): 909–15. [III]

16. Meador KJ, Baker GA, Browning N et al., NEAD Study Group. Fetal antiepileptic drug exposure and cognitive outcomes at age 6 years (NEAD study): A prospective observational study. *Lancet Neurol* 2013; 12(3): 244–52. [II-3]

17. Holmes LB, Baldwin EJ, Smith CR et al. Increased frequency of isolated cleft palate in infants exposed to lamotrigine during pregnancy. *Neurology* 2008; 70(22 Pt. 2): 2152–8. [II-2]

18. Dean P. Safety issues for women with epilepsy. In: Morrell MJ, Flynn K, eds. *Women with Epilepsy*. 1st ed. Cambridge: University Press, 2005: 263–8. [II-3]

19. McAuley JW, Anderson GD. Treatment of epilepsy in women of reproductive age: Pharmacokinetic considerations. *Clin Pharmacokinet* 2002; 41: 559–79. [II-3]

20. La Neve A, Boero G, Francavilla T, Plantamura M, De Agazio G, Specchio L. Prospective, case–control study on the effect of pregnancy on seizure frequency in women with epilepsy. *Neurol Sci* 2015; 36: 79–83. [II-1]

21. Edey S, Moran N, Nashef L. SUDEP and epilepsy-related mortality in pregnancy. *Epilepsia* 2014; 55(7): e72–74. [II-2]

22. MacDonald SC, Bateman BT, McElrath TF, Hernández-Díaz S. Mortality and morbidity during delivery hospitalization among pregnant women with epilepsy in the United States. *JAMA Neurol* 2015; 72(9): 981–8. [II-3]

23. Callanan M. Parenting for women with epilepsy. In: Morrell MJ, Flynn K eds. *Women with Epilepsy*. 1st ed. Cambridge: University Press, 2005: 228–34. [III]

24. Pennell PB, Peng L, Newport DJ et al. Lamotrigine in pregnancy: Clearance, therapeutic drug monitoring, and seizure frequency. *Neurology* 2008; 70: 2130–6. [II-3]

25. Thomas SV, Syam U, Devi SJ. Predictors of seizures during pregnancy in women with epilepsy. *Epilepsia* 2012; 53(5): e85–8. [II-2]

26. Viale L, Allotey J, Cheong-See F et al. for EBMCONNECT Collaboration. Epilepsy in pregnancy and reproductive outcomes: A systematic review and meta-analysis. *Lancet* 2015; published online Aug 26. http://dx.doi.org/10.1016/S0140-6736(15)00045-8. [Review; II-1]

27. Hvas CL, Henriksen TB, Ostergaard JR et al. Epilepsy and pregnancy: effect of antiepileptic drugs and lifestyle on birth weight. *BJOG* 2000; 107: 896–902. [II-3]

28. Meador KJ, Baker GA, Browning N et al., for the Neurodevelopmental Effects of Antiepileptic Drugs (NEAD) Study Group. Breastfeeding in children of women taking antiepileptic drugs: Cognitive outcomes at age 6 years. *JAMA Pediatric* 2014; 168: 729–36. [II-2]

29. Harden CL, Leppik I. Optimizing therapy of seizures in women who use oral contraceptives. *Neurology* 2006; 67: S56–8. [II-3]

30. Christensen J, Petrenaite V, Atterman J et al. Oral contraceptives induce lamotrigine metabolism: Evidence from a double-blind, placebo-controlled trial. *Epilepsia* 2007; 48: 484–9. [RCT]

20

Spinal cord injury

Megan Gooding and Leonardo Pereira

KEY POINTS

- Spinal cord injury (SCI) in pregnant women is associated with increased risks of urinary tract infections, preterm birth, and anemia. **The most worrisome, potentially fatal** complication is **autonomic dysreflexia (ADR)**.
- Antenatal management of women with preexisting SCI includes **frequent urinary cultures** *or* **antibiotic suppression (self, intermittent catheterization** is preferred), **stool softeners** and a **high-fiber diet**, routine **skin exams**, and **frequent position changes**. In women with lesions above the level of T5, baseline and serial pulmonary function tests can be used to assess vital capacity. There is insufficient data at this time to recommend universal thromboprophylaxis.
- ADR affects up to **85% of women with lesions at or above the level of T6**. The most common sign of ADR is **systemic hypertension**. Symptoms are synchronous with uterine contractions. Prevention involves avoidance of triggers (constipation, cathetherization, exams, etc.) and **early epidural anesthesia**. Antihypertensive therapy for ADR includes **nitroprusside, amyl nitrate, trimethaphan**, and **hydralazine**.
- Several **prophylactic procedures** are necessary for **labor and delivery** in the SCI woman. Among these, **continuous hemodynamic monitoring during labor by maternal electrocardiogram, pulse oximetry, and arterial line** should be performed in patients with **baseline pulmonary insufficiency**.

DIAGNOSIS/DEFINITION

Spinal cord injury (SCI) is diagnosed neurologically. It can occur following trauma to the spinal cord and also because of a variety of pathologies (e.g., neural tube defect, congenital, transverse myelitis, etc.).

EPIDEMIOLOGY/INCIDENCE

About 12,000 new spinal cord injuries per year occur in women of childbearing age in the United States, and each year, about 2000 women with SCI will become pregnant [1]. SCI diagnosed during pregnancy is rare. SCI preexisting pregnancy is relatively more common.

CLASSIFICATION

SCI is classified by its etiology and, especially, by the level of the lesion. The higher the functional level of the lesion, the worse the disease and prognosis.

Complications (for women with preexisting SCI): **Asymptomatic bacteriuria, lower urinary tract infections** (up to 35% incidence) [2], and **pyelonephritis** are common. The risk of preterm birth is between 8% and 13% [2–5].

Anemia can occur in 12% of women with SCI, especially with history of chronic pyelonephritis, decubitus, and/or renal failure. The most worrisome, potential fatal complication is autonomic dysreflexia (ADR).

PREGNANCY MANAGEMENT
Preconception Counseling

Women with preexisting SCI who are contemplating pregnancy should be referred for preconception counseling. If the spinal cord lesion is congenital or hereditary in origin then genetic counseling is warranted. Women with congenital spinal lesions, such as meningomyelocele, should be made aware of the increased risk of spinal cord lesions to their offspring and placed on 4 mg/day of folic acid [6]. All other SCI women should take at least 400 mg of folic acid preconception. Women with Klippel–Trenaunay or von Hippel–Lindau syndromes are at risk for epidural or subdural hemangiomas and should undergo MRI to determine the safety of neuraxial anesthesia [7].

Patients with preexisting SCI are probably at no greater risk than the general obstetric population for either congenital malformations or fetal death [8]. In contrast to patients with SCI antecedent to pregnancy, patients who suffer traumatic SCI during pregnancy may be at risk for **spontaneous abortion, fetal malformation, abruptio placentae, or direct fetal injury** [9]. A fetal malformation rate of 11% has been reported in 45 patients who suffered spinal cord injuries during pregnancy [8].

Prenatal Care
Acute SCI during Pregnancy

Acutely, SCI results in neurogenic shock or "spinal shock" because of the loss of sympathetic innervation. This typically presents with hypotension, bradycardia, and hypothermia because of parasympathetic effects. Adequate volume resuscitation and pressor support should be administered. Direct measurements of pulmonary capillary wedge pressure with a pulmonary artery catheter will assist clinical management. Internal hemorrhage should be identified and treated with the aid of a trauma surgeon if possible.

In the setting of acute SCI, initial stabilization of the neck and spinal column should occur immediately and airway patency secured. This may require a jaw thrust maneuver, nasal trumpet, or nasal intubation. Administration of methyl-prednisolone within eight hours of SCI may improve neurologic recovery in select cases [10]. The risk of deep venous thrombosis and pulmonary embolism is greatest within eight weeks of traumatic SCI [11]. Prophylactic anticoagulation should be considered during this period.

In rare cases, acute SCI may result from acute hemorrhage, malignancy, or aggressive hemangiomas. In those cases, embolization or decompressive surgery may be necessary during pregnancy [7,12].

Antenatal Management of Preexisting SCI

Urinary. Recurrent UTIs and or sepsis are common complications of SCI. **Frequent urinary cultures or antibiotic suppression with nitrofurantoin should be considered** [13–15] although there is a paucity of data to guide optimal genitourinary care in pregnancy [16]. Continuous indwelling catheterization appears to have a near 100% incidence of UTI in SCI patients, so self, **intermittent catheterization** every four to six hours may be preferable.

Gastrointestinal. **Stool softeners** and a **high-fiber diet** to prevent constipation.

Dermatology. Routine **skin exams** for any evidence of decubitus ulcers at each visit and **frequent position changes**. Wheelchairs may need to be resized or fitted with extra padding. Supplemental Vitamin D (2000 IU daily) is recommended [17].

Pulmonary. In patients with high thoracic or cervical spine lesions, usually above the level of T5, baseline and serial **pulmonary function tests** to assess vital capacity (VC), and especially if VC <13 mL/kg, **possible need for ventilatory assistance** in labor are recommended [13,15]. Supine tilted positioning is suggested for labor.

Thromboembolic. Despite an incidence of venous thromboembolism reported as high as 8% [18], there are **insufficient data at this time to recommend universal administration of heparin** during pregnancy. However, range of motion exercises and thrombolytic stockings should be considered for all women, and heparin prophylaxis should be administered to women with additional risk factors (prior VTE or known thrombophilia) [19]. Each case should be addressed individually. Women suffering acute SCI during pregnancy should receive thromboprophylaxis for at least eight weeks post trauma on the basis of the high rate of deep venous thromboses reported in nonpregnant patients during this time period [11].

Hematology. Screen for and treat anemia aggressively.

General support. Spasticity and muscle contractions frequently complicate SCI. A regular program of range of motion exercises in lower extremities, leg elevation, and exercises to increase upper body strength is recommended, as are social support services [14,20].

Autonomic dysreflexia. ADR is the most serious complication impacting obstetric management, affecting **about 90% of patients with lesions at or above the level of T6** [3,21] (above sympathetic outflow and above the upper level of greater splanchnic flow). It is potentially fatal. It is attributed to loss of hypothalamic control over sympathetic spinal reflexes of somatic or visceral sensory impulses still active distal to the level of the lesion [22]. **The most common sign of ADR is systemic hypertension** (vasoconstriction),

which is often severe. Maternal clinical manifestations include hyperthermia, piloerection, diaphoresis, increased extremity spasticity, pupil dilation, nasal congestion, respiratory distress, bradycardia (most common) or tachycardia or cardiac arrhythmia, extreme fear and anxiety, headache, loss of consciousness, intracranial bleed, convulsions, and even death. **Symptoms are synchronous with uterine contractions**. BP rises with contractions, then normalizes in between.

ADR may be mistaken for preeclampsia, but several findings may help differentiate the two conditions (Table 20.1).

Triggers: Afferent stimuli (usually distension) from hollow viscus (bladder, bowel, uterus) or skin (irritation or temp change) below level of the spinal cord lesion. These include uterine contractions, cervical manipulation/pelvic examinations, cold stirrups, insertion of speculum, manipulation of urinary catheters, catheter obstruction, constipation, and decubitus ulcers.

Preventive management of ADR in susceptible patients:

1. Routine bladder catheterization with topical anesthetic.
2. Avoidance of constipation with bowel regimen.
3. Pelvic exams: consider pudendal block or topical anesthetic (lidocaine) prior to exams. Avoid cold stirrups or speculums if possible.
4. Prophylactic **antihypertensive therapy** (as necessary to prevent recurrent ADR) with oral nifedipine (10–20 mg), terazosin (1–10 mg qhs), or clonidine.
5. **Epidural anesthesia** at the onset of labor.

Treatment of ADR:

1. Remove offending stimulus. Expedite delivery if in second stage with forceps or vacuum or perform cesarean delivery (discuss this with patient prior to labor).
2. Positioning: tilt head upward, loosen tight clothing around neck.
3. Antihypertensive therapy—rapid onset [21].
   - **Nitroprusside** (0.5 ug/kg/min intravenously, titrate to BP) or sublingual sodium nitroglycerin (0.3–0.6 mL)
   - **Amyl nitrate** (one capsule crushed for inhalation)
   - Ganglionic blocking agent: **trimethaphan** (Arfonad), 1 ampule in 500 mL D5W at 3 to 4 mg/min continuous intravenously
   - Prazosin, α–adrenergic blocker: 0.5–1.0 mg PO bid or TID
   - Direct vasodilator: **hydralazine**, 10 mg orally, or nifedipine bite and swallow tablet 10 to 20 mg
4. Anesthesia—**regional** (preferred) or general anesthesia can treat ADR.

Antepartum testing. No specific testing is recommended.

Ascertainment and preparation for (preterm or term) labor. Women with spinal cord transection above T10, especially

Table 20.1 Differentiating ADR from Preeclampsia

Disease	Symptoms	Hematologic	Hepatic Function	Urinalysis	Treatment
Preeclampsia	Independent of uterine contractions	Decreased platelets	Elevated uric acid and/or liver function tests	Proteinuria	Intravenous MgSO$_4$ (most commonly)
ADR	Synchronous with uterine contractions	Normal	Normal	Norepinephrine	Remove stimulus; antihypertensive therapy

Abbreviations: ADR, autonomic dysreflexia; MgSO$_4$, magnesium sulfate.

above T6, may have **painless labor** and are at risk for unattended delivery. Even with lower levels, if transection is complete, patients may not feel contractions. Symptoms that are related through the sympathetic nervous system may alert patients to labor. These should be reviewed with patients as they near term: abdominal or leg spasms, shortness of breath, or increased spasticity. **Uterine palpation techniques** should be reviewed with patients. Consider inpatient hospitalization, especially if patients dilated and have (>T6) high lesions (because of possible unattended delivery with ADR).

Psychological challenges. Successful pregnancy outcome in women with SCI relies on multidisciplinary team coordination with providers from high-risk obstetrics, anesthesiology, and spinal cord injury service when possible [14,23]. Women with SCI should have an anesthesia consult with a plan for epidural at onset of labor. Professional support from a multidisciplinary team that focuses on patient empowerment and the degree of controllability can make the pregnancy experience a positive one for women with SCI [24]. Depression is commonly associated with SCI and treatment options include cognitive behavioral therapy, acupuncture, and selected antidepressants (some increase spasticity while others have fetal effects) [25].

DELIVERY

Patients with spinal cord transection above the level of T10 are at risk for unattended delivery secondary to unrecognized contractions. About 20% of women with SCI will deliver preterm; surveillance with cervical checks can be considered starting at 28 weeks [4]. Consider inpatient hospitalization for patients with advanced cervical dilation because of the risk of unattended delivery or for women with spinal cord lesions above the level of T6 because of the high risk of ADR [2,15].

Labor is the period during which ADR is most likely to arise. Therefore, there should be a plan for delivery in a unit capable of invasive hemodynamic monitoring. **Appropriate antihypertensive therapy should be available at the patient's bedside during labor.** If induction is necessary, women with cervical ripening should have continuous blood pressure monitoring and possibly an epidural. **Continuous hemodynamic monitoring during labor by maternal electrocardiogram, pulse oximetry, and arterial line** should be performed in patients with **baseline pulmonary insufficiency** [15]. Body temperature should be closely monitored, without assuming that temperature increases are due to intra-amniotic infection (may be caused by underlying thermodisregulation). A Foley catheter may be placed during labor to avoid bladder distension or repeated catheterizations. Patients should change position and have a skin examination every two hours to prevent decubitus ulcer formation. Episiotomy should be avoided, not only because it is not beneficial in general, but also because it is a possible trigger for ADR.

The rate of spontaneous vaginal delivery and need for assisted vaginal delivery depends on the level of the spinal cord lesion. Approximately 30% of SCI patients will be delivered by cesarean [2,3,5,12,14,23] (Table 20.2).

ANESTHESIA

Epidural anesthesia should be administered early in labor [21,26]. This is to prevent ADR, with a goal for T10 level.

Table 20.2 Mode of Delivery Stratified by Level of SCI

Delivery Mode	≥T6 Level (%)	<T6 Level (%)	All SCI (%)
NSVD	15 (24)	18 (42)	33 (31)
AVD	22[a] (34)	7 (16)	29 (27)
CD	27 (42)	18 (42)	45 (42)
Total	64 (100)	43 (100)	107 (100)

Sources: Wanner MB, Rageth CJ, Zach GA. *Paraplegia*, 25, 482–90, 1987; Verduyn WH. *Paraplegia*, 24, 231–40, 1986; Hughes SJ, Short DJ, Usherwood MM et al. *BJOG*, 98, 513–8, 1991; Ouafae S, Jayi S, Alaoui FF, Bouguern H, Chaara H, Fikri G, Rachidi SA, Houssaini NS, Hlimmich M, Melhouf MA. *BioMed Central*, 8, 207, 2014; Skowronski E, Hartman K. *Roy Austral NZ Coll Obstet Gynaecol*, 48, 485–91, 2008; Engel S, Ferrara G. *International Spinal Cord Society*, 51, 170–1, 2012.
Abbreviations: AVD, assisted vaginal delivery; CD, cesarean delivery; NSVD, normal spontaneous vaginal delivery; SCI, spinal cord injury.
[a]Majority of assisted vaginal deliveries performed because of autonomic dysreflexia.

Prehydration is very important as these patients tend to be hypotensive.

POSTPARTUM CARE AND BREAST-FEEDING

The concept of women with SCI becoming parents frequently generates negative societal reactions; however, research has demonstrated that the children of women with SCI when compared with peers with able-bodied mothers have the same attitudes toward their parents, gender roles, and family functioning [27].

In the postpartum period, bladder distension and constipation should be avoided. The use of thromboprophylaxis of SCI patients during the puerperium is controversial. Breast-feeding should be encouraged. Oral contraceptive pills appear to be safe [3,28] although some authors discourage their use [29]. Progesterone-only pills, transdermal patches, intramuscular medroxyprogesterone injections, condoms and spermicide, and intrauterine devices are all acceptable alternatives.

GUILLAIN–BARRÉ SYNDROME

With many of the features of SCI in common, pregnant women with Guillain–Barré syndrome (GBS) face similar challenges [30]. The risk of UTI and DVT are both increased in this population, and extreme muscle weakness can lead to paralysis and the need for ventilatory support. The safety and effectiveness of **plasmaphoresis and IVIG** to treat GBS in pregnancy have been established and should be considered in cases involving severe or worsening weakness. Delivery can often be accomplished by regional anesthesia and passive or assisted second stage. The use of general anesthesia can be particularly dangerous in GBS patients, specifically in regards to the need for avoidance of succinylcholine, risk of hyperkalemima, autonomic instability, and the challenges of extubation in severely weakened patients. A multidisciplinary team approach is highly recommended.

RESOURCES

SCI patients and nonmedical personnel may be referred to the following website: http://www.spinalcord.org/resources posted by the National Spinal Cord Injury Association (NSCIA) for more information.

REFERENCES

1. National Spinal Cord Injury Statistics Center. *UAB Spinal Cord Injury Info Sheet #15*. Birmingham, AL: University of Alabama; 2009. Updated 2012. [Epidemiologic study]
2. Wanner MB, Rageth CJ, Zach GA. Pregnancy and autonomic hyperreflexia in patients with spinal cord lesions. *Paraplegia* 1987; 25: 482–90. [II–3]
3. Verduyn WH. Spinal cord injured women, pregnancy and delivery. *Paraplegia* 1986; 24: 231–40. [II–3]
4. Westgren N, Hultling C, Levi R et al. Pregnancy and delivery in women with a traumatic spinal cord injury in Sweden, 1980–1991. *Obstet Gynecol* 1993; 81: 926–30. [II–3]
5. Hughes SJ, Short DJ, Usherwood MM et al. Management of the pregnant woman with spinal cord injuries. *BJOG* 1991; 98: 513–8. [II–3]
6. Wilson RD, Johnson JA, Wyatt P et al. Pre-conceptional vitamin/folic acid supplementation 2007: The use of folic acid in combination with a multivitamin supplement for the prevention of neural tube defects and other congenital anomalies. *J Obstet Gynaecol Can* 2007; 12: 1003–26. [II–2]
7. Vercauteren M, Waets P, Pitkanen M, Forster J. Neuraxial techniques in patient with pre-existing back impairment or prior spine interventions: A topical review with special reference to obstetrics. *Int J Anesthesiol Intensive Care, Pain, Emergency Med* 2011; 55: 910–7. [Review; III]
8. Göller H, Paeslack V. Pregnancy damage and birth-complications in the children of paraplegic women. *Paraplegia* 1972; 10(3): 213–7. [II–3]
9. Atterbury JL, Groome LJ. Pregnancy in women with spinal cord injuries. *Nurs Clin North Am* 1998; 33(4): 603–13. [Review]
10. Gilson GJ, Miller AC, Clevenger FW et al. Acute spinal cord injury and neurogenic shock in pregnancy. *Obstet Gynecol Surv* 1995; 50(7): 556–60. [II–3]
11. Sugarman B. Medical complications of spinal cord injury. *Q J Med* 1985; 54:3–18.[II–3]
12. Ouafae S, Jayi S, Alaoui FF, Bouguern H, Chaara H, Fikri G, Rachidi SA, Houssaini NS, HIimmich M, Melhouf MA. An aggressive vertebral hemangioma in pregnancy: A case report. *BioMed Central* 2014; 8: 207. [II–3]
13. Obstetric management of patients with spinal cord injuries. ACOG Committee Opinion No. 275. American College of Obstetricians and Gynecologists. *Obstet Gynecol* 2002; 100: 625–7. [Review]
14. Skowronski E, Hartman K. Obstetric management following traumatic tetraplegia: Case series and literature review. *Roy Austral NZ Coll Obstet Gynaecol* 2008; 48: 485–91. [II–3; Review]
15. Greenspoon JS, Paul RH. Paraplegia and quadriplegia: Special considerations during pregnancy and labor and delivery. *Am J Obstet Gynecol* 1986; 155: 738–41. [III]
16. Pannek J, Bertschy S. Mission impossible? urological management of patients with spinal cord injury during pregnancy: A systematic review. *Spinal Cord* 2011; 49: 1028–32. [II–2; Review]
17. Dorner B, Posthauer ME. The role of nutrition in pressure ulcer prevention and treatment: NPUAP white paper. *Adv Skin Wound Care* 2009; 22: 212–26. [Review]
18. Ghidini A, Healey A, Andreani M, Simonson MR. Pregnancy and women with spinal cord injuries. *Acta Obstet Gynecol Scand* 2008; 87: 1006–10. [Review]
19. Baschat AA, Weiner CP. Chronic neurologic diseases and disabling conditions in pregnancy. Welner SL, Haseltine F, eds. *Welner's Guide to the Care of Women With Disabilities*. Philadelphia PA: Lippincott, Williams & Wilkins; 2004: 145–58. [Review]
20. Ditunno JF, Formal CS. Current concepts: Chronic spinal cord injury. *N Engl J Med* 1994; 330: 550–6. [Review]
21. Krassioukov A, Warburton DE, Teasell R, Eng J. Spinal Cord Injury Rehabilitation Evidence Research Team. A systematic review of the management of autonomic dysreflexia after spinal cord injury. *Arch Phys Med Rehabil* 2009 April; 90: 682–95. [Review]
22. Berghella V, Spector T, Trauffer P et al. Pregnancy in patients with preexisting transverse myelitis. *Obstet Gynecol* 1996; 87: 809–12. [III; two new case reports of transverse myelitis]
23. Engel S, Ferrara G. Obstetric outcomes in women who sustained a spinal cord injury during pregnancy. *International Spinal Cord Society* 2012; 51: 170–1. [II–2]
24. Tebbet M, Kennedy P. The experience of childbirth for women with spinal cord injuries: An interpretive phenomenology analysis study. *Disabil Rehabil* 2012: 34(9): 762–9. [II–2]
25. Olkin R. Disability and depression. Welner SL, Haseltime F, eds. *Welner's Guide to the Care of Women With Disabilities*. Philadelphia, PA: Lippincott, Williams & Wilkins; 2004: 279–99. [Review]
26. Baker ER, Cardenas DD. Pregnancy in spinal cord injured women. *Arch Phys Med Rehabil* 1996; 77(5): 501–7. [Review]
27. Signore C, Spong CY, Krotoski D, Shinowara NL, Blackwell SC. Pregnancy in women with physical disabilities. *Obstet Gynecol* 2011; 117: 935–47. [Review]
28. Jackson AB, Wadley V. A multicenter study of women's self-reported reproductive health after spinal cord injury. *Arch Phys Med Rehabil* 1999; 80: 1420–8. [II–2]
29. Sipski ML. The impact of spinal cord injury on female sexuality, menstruation and pregnancy: A review of the literature. *J Am Paraplegia Soc* 1991; 14(3): 122–6. [Review]
30. Chan LYS, Tsui MHY, Leung TN. Guillain–Barré syndrome in pregnancy. *Acta Obstet Gynecol Scand* 2004; 83: 319–25. [Review]

21

Mood disorders

Madeleine A. Becker, Tal E. Weinberger, Ann Chandy, Nazanin E. Silver, and Elisabeth J. S. Kunkel

KEY POINTS

- Depression is twice as common in women as in men, and rates are highest during the childbearing years.
- Depression is common in pregnancy. **Up to 70% of pregnant women report symptoms of depression**.
- Postpartum blues is a temporary, common condition, affecting up to 85% of new mothers.
- **Postpartum depression occurs in 5% to 20% of women.**
- **Postpartum psychosis affects about 0.1% to 0.2% of women**. There is a very high risk of postpartum psychosis in mothers with bipolar disorder.
- Pregnant women who discontinue their antidepressant medications during pregnancy demonstrate a high rate of relapse.
- Maternal depression has been associated with an increase in premature births, low birth weight, fetal growth restriction, and postnatal complications.
- **Untreated maternal depression has been associated with an increased risk of subsequent childhood psychopathology**.
- The **Edinburgh Postnatal Depression Scale** is a short and easy-to-administer screening tool to assess for postpartum depression.
- Bipolar depression is often misdiagnosed as a major depressive disorder.
- **The risk of postpartum affective episodes is very high among women with bipolar disorder** with the majority of women experiencing symptoms within the first three weeks of delivery.
- The incidence of infanticide in women with untreated postpartum psychosis may be as high as 4%.
- **Patients with mood disorders should be stabilized on the minimal number of medications at the lowest *effective* dose before pregnancy.**
- **Paroxetine has been associated with an increased risk in cardiac malformations and should generally be avoided during pregnancy if possible.**
- **Other selective serotonin reuptake inhibitors (SSRIs) are not considered teratogenic.**
- Individual decisions about medication management during pregnancy should take into account multiple factors, such as severity of maternal illness, frequency of mood episodes, efficacy of past medication trials, and strength of maternal support system.
- In neonates exposed to **lithium** during the first trimester, the risk of **Ebstein's anomaly** has been estimated to be between 0.05% and 0.1%.
- The risk for major congenital anomalies in infants exposed to **valproic acid** in utero is estimated to be between **6.2% and 13.3%**.
- There are still limited data regarding the safety of second-generation (atypical) antipsychotics during pregnancy.

- All psychotropic medications cross the placenta and can enter breast milk.
- Most SSRIs produce low infant levels and should be continued in breast-feeding mothers who need to take antidepressant medications.

MOOD DISORDERS IN PREGNANCY AND POSTPARTUM
Definitions and Epidemiology

Major depressive disorder (MDD) is a syndrome characterized by sustained depressed mood or loss of interest in daily activities along with "neurovegetative symptoms" of depression, which include a decrease or increase in appetite, insomnia or hypersomnia, psychomotor retardation or agitation, and decreased energy. Other symptoms of MDD include feelings of worthlessness or guilt, loss of interest in usually pleasurable activities (or anhedonia), difficulty concentrating, and recurrent thoughts of death or suicidal ideation [1]. Women have approximately twice the lifetime rate of depression as men [2]. In women, the highest rates of major depression occur during the childbearing years between the ages of 25 to 44. Depression is one of the most common complications during pregnancy and in the postpartum period [3]. **Up to 70% of pregnant women report symptoms of depression during their pregnancy** with 10% to 16% fulfilling the criteria for major depression [4,5]. There is a high rate of psychiatric illness in mothers after childbirth. This may be attributable to hormonal factors but also can be associated with psychological stress and prior psychiatric illness [6,7].

Postpartum blues is a common condition, affecting up to 85% of new mothers. It is characterized by tearfulness, mood lability, irritability, and anxiety. Symptoms are typically mild and begin around postpartum day 2 to 4 and resolve spontaneously, usually in about two weeks [8]. Women with postpartum blues may be at increased risk for the subsequent development of postpartum depression [9] and warrant close follow-up after delivery.

Postpartum depression occurs in 5% to 20% of women [10]. Symptoms of postpartum depression are the same as for major depressive disorder and include depressed mood, insomnia, anhedonia, suicidal ideation, guilt, worthlessness, fatigue, impaired concentration, change in appetite, and change in motor activity. The *DSM-5* categorizes "peripartum onset" as a specifier of MDD, applied to the first four weeks after childbirth (ICD-10 coding permits classifications of postpartum mental disorders up to six weeks after childbirth) [1]. In practice, many clinicians would contemplate depressive symptoms to be considered "postpartum depression" for a much longer period than this, generally for up to one year after childbirth [11].

Postpartum psychosis is much less common than postpartum depression, affecting about **0.1% to 0.2%** of all women [12]. It is characterized by mood lability, agitation, confusion, thought disorganization, hallucinations, and disturbed sleep. Postpartum psychosis has been associated with an increased risk of suicide, infant neglect, and infanticide [13,14], and is considered a psychiatric emergency. Although relatively rare in the general population, the risk of postpartum psychosis is significantly increased in mothers with a history of previous inpatient psychiatric hospitalization [15,16]. **There is a very high risk of postpartum psychosis in mothers with bipolar depression, reportedly as high as 46% [4,6,7].** Additionally, women who have had an episode of postpartum psychosis are at increased risk for subsequently developing bipolar affective disorder, leading many researchers to speculate that postpartum psychosis is really an episode of bipolar disorder [17].

RISK FACTORS

The strongest risk factor for depression during pregnancy is a history of major depressive disorder [18]. Women with a history of anxiety disorder, depression, postpartum depression, or other previous psychiatric disorders are also at an increased risk for postpartum depression [10,13,19,20]. Social isolation, poor social support, high parity, unintended pregnancy, younger age, and exposure to trauma, domestic violence, and birth complications are also factors that are associated with postpartum depression [8,21–24]. **Women who discontinue antidepressant medications during pregnancy are also at risk for relapse. One study of pregnant women with a history of moderate to severe recurrent depression, who discontinued their antidepressant medication during pregnancy, showed a 68% rate of relapse during pregnancy.** This was compared to a 25% relapse rate for those women who continued antidepressants throughout their pregnancies [19].

Hormonal factors also have been implicated as risk factors for depression. Rapid changes in estradiol and progesterone levels have been associated with postpartum depression. Women with thyroid autoantibodies also appear to be at higher risk for postpartum depression [17].

The U.S. Preventative Services Task Force (USPSTF) and American College of Obstetricians and Gynecologists (ACOG) recommends screening for depression in pregnant and postpartum women. Screening should be implemented with adequate systems in place to ensure accurate diagnosis, effective treatment, and appropriate follow-up [3,25].

COMPLICATIONS

Untreated maternal depression is associated with multiple problems, both during pregnancy and postpartum, and can negatively affect mother–child interactions. **Maternal depression has been associated with an increase in premature births [26,27], low birth weight, fetal growth restriction, and postnatal complications** [4,27,28].

Untreated maternal depression during pregnancy may result in poor compliance with prenatal care and increased exposure risk to illicit drugs, herbal remedies, alcohol, and tobacco [4]. Infants of mothers with untreated depression have been shown to cry more, are more difficult to console, more irritable, less active, and less attentive. They also display fewer facial expressions [29,30]. Women who have depression, anxiety, or stress while being pregnant are at an increased risk for their child having impaired cognitive development,

emotional problems, or symptoms of attention deficit hyperactivity disorder [31]. **Maternal depression has been associated with an increased risk of subsequent childhood psychopathology**, including behavioral problems, anxiety disorders, and depression [32–36]. Correspondingly, remission of maternal depression positively affects both mother and child, resulting in a significantly lower rate of childhood psychiatric symptoms and diagnoses [37].

Studies also show that mothers with depression have a poor pattern of infant health care utilization, including increased use of acute care and emergency room visits as well as decreased utilization of preventative services, including well-care visits and up-to-date vaccinations [38]. Depressed mothers are also less likely to continue to breastfeed [39].

Screening

The **Edinburgh Postnatal Depression Scale (EPDS)** is recommended for screening in women at risk for postpartum depression. This screening tool is short and easy to administer. It is a self-administered scale, consisting of 10 questions assessing emotional symptoms experienced by the mother over the seven days prior to evaluation. The EPDS can be completed in about five minutes [40]. Scores on the EPDS range from 0 to 30, and a **score of 9 or greater should prompt further clinical evaluation**. No scale is a substitute for clinical judgment, and in any situation in which there is significant clinical concern for postpartum depression, the patient should be evaluated thoroughly and if warranted referral should be made and treatment initiated [3].

An initial validation study revealed a sensitivity of 86% and a specificity of 78% of the EPDS [40]. However, a more recent review of multiple studies validating the EPDS demonstrated heterogeneity of sensitivity and specificity across different studies. This suggests that the **EPDS may not be equally valid in different settings** [41] (Figure 21.1).

Thyroid function tests and a complete blood count are useful for identifying other medical conditions that can present with symptoms of depression. Prompt psychiatric consultation should be obtained when depression is suspected, especially when symptoms are severe or when psychotic or suicidal features are present. The presence of psychosis or suicidal or homicidal ideation or intent should be considered an emergency.

BIPOLAR DISORDER IN PREGNANCY AND POSTPARTUM
Definitions and Epidemiology

Bipolar disorder is a psychiatric illness characterized by episodes of depression alternating with sustained episodes of elevated mood and/or irritability, which are classified as either "mania" or "hypomania." Hypomania is an attenuated form of mania with no associated functional impairment. Both mania and hypomania are associated with increased energy, decreased need for sleep, rapid speech and/or thoughts, distractibility, impulsivity, mood lability, and grandiosity. "Mood swings" are not adequate for a diagnosis of bipolar disorder; rather, a patient must have a syndrome characterized by *sustained* symptoms lasting for days to weeks.

Bipolar disorder, type I (BAD I) is a severe form of bipolar disorder defined by at least one lifetime manic or

Name: _____

Address: _____

Baby's Age: _____

As you have recently had a baby, we would like to know how you are feeling.
Please UNDERLINE the answer which comes closest to how you have felt IN THE
PAST 7 DAYS, not just how you feel today.

1. I have been able to laugh and see the funny side of things.

   As much as I always could
   Not quite so much now
   Definitely not so much now
   Not at all

2. I have looked forward with enjoyment to things.

   As much as I ever did
   Rather less than I used to
   Definitely less than I used to
   Hardly at all

3. * I have blamed myself unnecessarily when things went wrong.

   Yes, most of the time
   Yes, some of the time
   Not very often
   No, never

4. I have been anxious or worried for no good reason.

   No, not at all
   Hardly ever
   Yes, sometimes
   Yes, very often

5. * I have felt scared or panicky for not very good reason.

   Yes, quite a lot
   Yes, sometimes
   No, not much
   No, not at all

6. * Things have been getting on top of me.

   Yes, most of the time I haven't been able to cope at all
   Yes, sometimes I haven't been coping as well as usual

   No, most of the time I have coped quite well
   No, I have been coping as well as ever

7. * I have been so unhappy that I have had difficulty sleeping.

   Yes, most of the time
   Yes, sometimes
   Not very often
   No, not at all

8. * I have felt sad or miserable.

   Yes, most of the time
   Yes, quite often
   Not very often
   No, not at all

9. * I have been so unhappy that I have been crying.

   Yes, most of the time
   Yes, quite often
   Only occasionally
   No, never

10. * The thought of harming myself has occurred to me.

   Yes, quite often
   Sometimes
   Hardly ever
   Never

Figure 21.1 Edinburgh Postnatal Depression Scale (EPDS). Response categories are scored 0, 1, 2, and 3 according to increased severity of the symptoms. Items marked with an asterisk are reverse scored (i.e., 3, 2, 1, and 0). The total score is calculated by adding together the scores for each of the ten items. (Adapted from Cox JL, Holden JM, Sagovsky R. *Br J Psychiatry*, 150, 782–6, 1987.)

mixed episode. Mixed episodes are characterized by simultaneous manic and depressive symptoms. The lifetime prevalence estimate is 1% for BAD I [42]. Men and women are affected at equal rates. **Bipolar disorder, type II** (BAD II) is characterized by episodes of depression and hypomania. The lifetime prevalence estimate is 1.1% for BAD II. Women with BAD II outnumber men by a ratio of approximately 2:1 [43]. The average age of onset of bipolar disorder is in the late teens to early 20s, placing affected women at high risk for mood episodes during their reproductive years.

Risk Factors

Extremely high susceptibility to postpartum episodes is a unique feature of bipolar disorder, as opposed to other mood or psychotic disorders [44] with a 67% risk of postpartum depression reported in one study [43]. Between 25% and 50% of women with BAD will have an episode of postpartum mania; a **family history** of postpartum psychosis further increases the risk of a postpartum psychotic episode [43].

Women with a **previous history of postpartum psychosis** are at extremely high risk in subsequent pregnancies [45].

A strong association between **primiparity** and risk of postpartum psychosis has been identified; this may be related to prophylactic strategies being implemented faster and more aggressively in women who have had previous deliveries affected by postpartum psychosis [46]. As opposed to nonpsychotic postpartum depression, studies have consistently found no association between stressful life events and onset of postpartum psychosis [44]. Immunological dysregulation has also been implicated and requires further study [47].

Postpartum women have nearly seven times the risk of a psychiatric hospital admission for a first affective episode and two times the risk of a recurrent affective episode compared with pregnant and nonpregnant women [48]. Onset of symptoms is often sudden. **The peak prevalence of symptom onset is between postpartum days 1 to 3 with the majority of women experiencing symptoms within three weeks after delivery** [43]. Approximately 50% of episodes of postpartum psychosis are the first manifestation of mental illness with sudden onset and precipitous worsening of symptoms [44].

Women with a **history of bipolar disorder or postpartum psychosis** have a very high risk of relapse postpartum; a clinical dilemma that commonly arises in this setting is whether medication should be continued during pregnancy or started immediately after delivery. A recent small study demonstrated that women with a history of episodes restricted to the postpartum period were not at high risk during pregnancy; postpartum prophylaxis was highly effective in this group. However, those with episodes occurring outside the postpartum period were at high risk during pregnancy as well; postpartum prophylaxis was much less effective in this setting [49].

Complications

Unplanned pregnancy and **voluntary termination** of pregnancy may occur more frequently in women with BAD [48]. Adverse neonatal outcomes, such as **preterm delivery, severe large for gestational age birth weight, neonatal morbidity (such as RDS, sepsis, and neonatal abstinence syndrome), congenital malformations, and neonatal hospital readmission,** have been found to be more common among women with a history of hospitalization for bipolar disorder. The cause of the higher percentage of adverse outcomes in this population is unknown; potential explanations include direct physiological effect of psychiatric illness, health care and lifestyle behaviors related to mood symptoms, or effects of psychiatric medication [50].

Exposure to bipolar disorder during pregnancy has been associated with **premature birth, low birth weight, and behavioral disturbances in the children of women with untreated illness** [51].

Pregnancy Considerations

Women who discontinue mood stabilizer treatment shortly before or after conception have twice the risk of recurrence and a fourfold shorter latency to a new affective episode as compared to women who continue their mood stabilizers [52]. Perinatal affective episodes are often depressive rather than manic or hypomanic and, after occurring in one pregnancy, tend to recur in subsequent pregnancies [4]. The proportion of women experiencing mood episodes during pregnancy was found to be approximately 22.7% in one large study and was similar for women with BAD I and BAD II [53]. Younger age at illness onset was found to be strongly associated with perinatal illness [53]. **Maintenance of mood stability during pregnancy is crucial** as recurrence of symptoms during this time strongly predicts the onset of postpartum episodes [54].

Screening

Misclassification of BAD as MDD is common in the general population. This can lead to inappropriate treatment and consequent lack of improvement or worsening of the patient's psychiatric condition. The use of selective serotonin reuptake inhibitors (SSRIs) in bipolar disorder is controversial but may be associated with treatment resistance or more frequent mood episodes in patients with the rapid-cycling form of the disorder [55]. Some markers of bipolar depression

(as opposed to unipolar or major depression) include atypical symptoms (i.e., increased sleep or appetite), psychotic depression, early age of symptom onset, treatment resistance to antidepressants, and a family history of bipolar disorder [54].

Misdiagnosis of BAD as MDD in the postpartum period also may occur. Hypomania often is overlooked in the general psychiatric population as patients often dismiss symptoms that do not disrupt (or even enhance) their functioning. Clinicians may not inquire about episodes of elevated mood. Hypomania after delivery may be misconstrued as normal joy related to the birth of a child [42].

There are no screening instruments specifically designed to detect mood episodes in patients with bipolar disorder before or after delivery. Commonly used screening instruments, such as the EPDS, have not been validated in postpartum women with BAD [42]. Of all the screening instruments for BAD used in the general population, the Mood Disorders Questionnaire (MDQ) has been most widely studied, both in psychiatric settings as well as primary care and community settings. In one study, the MDQ demonstrated excellent sensitivity and specificity in screening for BAD (with use of a modified scoring algorithm) during pregnancy and the postpartum period in women referred for psychiatric evaluation [56]. No measures demonstrate high sensitivity in a community sample, making a universal screening scale difficult to recommend. Women who present with depressive symptoms during the perinatal or postpartum period should be screened clinically for BAD, given the risk of inappropriate treatment associated with misdiagnosis [43].

No screening instrument is intended to replace a thorough clinical evaluation. Any patient who has a positive screen for symptoms of mood disorder should be referred in a timely fashion for mental health evaluation. Immediate screening by a mental health professional is warranted for suspected suicidal ideation or homicidal ideation toward the baby as well as for any concern regarding postpartum psychosis. **The incidence of infanticide in women with untreated postpartum psychosis has been estimated to be as high as 4%** [57]. Emergent intervention (such as psychiatric hospitalization) may be necessary to address immediate safety issues.

PHARMACOLOGIC MANAGEMENT OF MOOD DISORDERS

All psychotropic medications cross the placenta and can enter breast milk [4]. Risks of medication exposure to the fetus need to be weighed against the risks (to both mother and fetus) of untreated maternal illness. When a mood disorder is suspected, referral to a psychiatrist is recommended. Psychotherapy should always be considered as part of the treatment plan and can be effective in many cases. **Psychotherapy has been shown to be effective for some symptoms of depression in pregnancy** [58]. When symptoms are severe, or there is a high risk of relapse, medications can be helpful and/or necessary.

Fetal exposure to either maternal depression or antidepressants carries risk to the developing fetus [59]. Individual decisions about medication management during pregnancy should take into account multiple factors, such as severity of maternal illness, frequency of mood episodes, efficacy of past medication trials, and strength of maternal support system. In general, a single medication at a higher dose is preferable to multiple medications [4]. Multidisciplinary collaboration regarding psychotropic medication management during pregnancy should include the obstetrician, primary care doctor, psychiatrist, pediatrician, and patient's family. The risks of discontinuing medication versus any known risks of the prenatal exposure should be fully discussed with the patient, and this discussion should be documented.

During the postpartum period, in addition to concerns about medication passage into breast milk, important considerations include the impact of sleep disruption on maternal illness. Sleep deprivation can be extremely destabilizing in women with bipolar disorder. This is particularly concerning given the fact that the postpartum period is already a time of additional vulnerability in patients with mood disorders.

Antidepressants (Table 21.1)

Selective Serotonin Reuptake Inhibitors (SSRIs)
The most commonly prescribed medications for depression are the SSRIs. According to a *Cochrane* review, SSRIs are more effective for treating perinatal depression than placebo [60]. Compared to other classes of antidepressant medications, there are much more data available for the safety of these medications during pregnancy. The potential impact of maternal psychiatric depression on neonatal outcome has been difficult to evaluate independently of medication effects, resulting in some difficulty in clearly interpreting these data. The lowest effective dose of medication should be used during pregnancy to minimize exposure risk to the fetus. The need for using medications during pregnancy should always be weighed against any known risk of exposure of the fetus or nursing infant [8].

Teratogenicity
Several large reviews of the available data have shown **no specific pattern of major malformations in women exposed to SSRIs or other antidepressants in pregnancy** [61,62], and they are not considered to be teratogens [61,62]. The National Birth Defects Prevention study found that there was an increased risk of omphalocele, anencephaly, and craniosynostosis, but absolute risks were small [63]. These risks were found only after more than 40 statistical tests were performed and, thus, may be attributed to chance [4]. In the Sloane Epidemiology Center Birth Defects Study, no increased risk of omphalocele or craniosynostosis was found to be associated with SSRI use. Both of these studies were limited by the small number of exposures for each congenital malformation [4].

There have been some reports showing that women exposed to **paroxetine** in the first trimester are at higher risk (1.5- to twofold) for **cardiac malformations** [28,64–68], but there are also reports that do not support this association [61,64,68–71]. In light of these findings, the manufacturer reclassified paroxetine's pregnancy category to "D" [72], and so paroxetine should be avoided in pregnancy. If a patient were already taking paroxetine, one should attempt to switch to another antidepressant [4], preferably before pregnancy.

Although the data are conflicting, the majority of databases, including two recent, large, case-controlled studies, have found no significant increased rate of congenital heart defects with exposure to SSRIs other than paroxetine [4,28,54,62,63,71,73]. There are conflicting reports regarding the association of antidepressants and cardiovascular defects with a recent systematic review of the literature showing a recurrent pattern of heart defects [74]. A large multinational population study, however, found no substantial increase in prevalence of cardiovascular defects for either the SSRIs or for venlafaxine [63]. An increase in prevalence of septal and right ventricular outflow tract defects was present but was found to lack association with antidepressant exposure with further sibling-controlled analysis [62]. Another large recent meta-analysis found an increase in cardiac and septal heart defects, which although it reached statistical significance was not found to be clinically significant [75].

The use of antidepressants during pregnancy has been associated with reductions in birth weight [76] and infants who are small for gestational age [28,77]. Numerous studies show that SSRIs and TCAs (as well as the other antidepressants) are associated with preterm delivery (<37 weeks) [28,77,78]. These results are not consistent, and this association was not found in all studies. When effects were found, the differences in gestational age among exposed and non-exposed infants were typically modest (one week or less). As similar results were found among women using SSRIs and TCAs (which have different mechanisms of action), **maternal illness rather than medication effects may explain some of these findings** [68].

Neonatal Toxicity
Other risks concerning the use of SSRIs during pregnancy include reports of an increased risk of **persistent pulmonary hypertension of the newborn** (PPHN). PPHN involves right-to-left shunting of blood through the fetal ductus arteriosus and foramen ovale and results in neonatal hypoxia. If this is severe, it can result in right heart failure and is fatal in approximately 10% of cases. A meta-analysis has found an increased risk of PPHN among newborns whose mothers were exposed to SSRIs later in pregnancy (after 20 weeks gestation) [79]. PPHN was found to occur in about **three to six per 1000 exposed infants**. The baseline rate or occurrence of PPHN is between 0.5 and two per 1000 babies in the general population [28]. Two large, retrospective cohort studies [80,81] found no increased risk of PPHN in infants exposed to SSRIs. Four recent studies supported an association between SSRI use and PPHN with an adjusted odds ratio ranging from 3.44 to 6.1 [68,82–85]. The mechanism may be related to high circulating levels of serotonin in the fetal lungs [82]. Further research is needed to clarify this association.

Antidepressant exposure late in pregnancy has also been associated with transient neonatal complications. Symptoms may include jitteriness, tremor, tachypnea, hypoglycemia, temperature instability, weak cry, poor tone, and mild respiratory distress [4,86,87]. These symptoms are common and may occur in up to one third of infants exposed to antidepressants during the pregnancy [88]. Symptoms usually occur in the first neonatal days and generally resolve in a period of two weeks or less [28]. It is not clear whether the mechanism is a withdrawal syndrome or related to medication toxicity [61,87,89].

Neurodevelopmental Effects
Long-term neurodevolopmental effects after in utero SSRI exposure have been evaluated in a few small studies. Two studies found differences on some behavioral measures between exposed and unexposed children [90,91]. However, in two studies by Nulman et al., evaluating children exposed to fluoxetine and to various TCAs, no differences were found between exposed children and controls [92,93]. One study demonstrated that the effects of in utero SSRI exposure on children's motor functioning is transitory and a longitudinal

Table 21.1 Antidepressants in Pregnancy and Lactation

Class	Medication	FDA Risk Category	Teratogenicity	Late Pregnancy Exposure	Neonatal Toxicity	Breast-Feeding
Selective serotonin reuptake inhibitors	**Citalopram** (Celexa®)	C	Most studies have not identified an increased risk of major malformations [4,28,61–63]	Conflicting reports regarding risk of PPHN in infants exposed to SSRIs after 20 weeks' gestation [68,79,82–85]	• Conflicting results regarding risk of preterm birth, low birth weight, and small for gestational age in SSRI exposed pregnancies • Late pregnancy exposure associated with neonatal adaptation problems, NICU admission, low Apgar scores • All of these findings may be attributable to maternal illness rather than medication exposure [28,76–78]	RID: <1%–9% [10] Infant serum concentration low or undetectable in several studies [94,95] • One reported case of high infant serum levels [10,94,95]
	Fluoxetine (Prozac®, Prozac Weekly®, Sarafem®)	C	Most studies have not identified an increased risk of major malformations [4,28,61–63]	As above	As above	RID ≤10% Infant plasma concentration variable • Less favored because of long half-life and active metabolite • A few reports of adverse effects, but most studies with none in exposed infants [10,94,95]
	Sertraline (Zoloft®)	C	Most studies have not identified an increased risk of major malformations [4,28,61–63]	As above	As above	RID = 2% Infant serum concentration low to undetectable [10,94,95]
	Escitalopram (Lexapro®)	C	Very limited studies, but as escitalopram is the S-enantiomer of citalopram, it is likely comparable with this medication [4,28,61–63]	As above	As above	Limited data, but infant exposure thought to be similar to citalopram [10,94,95]
	Fluvoxamine (Luvox®, Luvox CR®)	C	No increased risk identified, but data are limited [4,28,61–63]	As above	As above	RID 1%–2% Limited data; infant plasma levels variable [10,94,95]
	Paroxetine (Paxil®, Paxil CR® Pexeva®)	D	Some data consistently supporting **increased risk of cardiac malformations** [28,64–71]	As above	As above	RID 1%–3% Infant serum concentration low to undetectable [10,94,95]

(Continued)

Table 21.1 (Continued)   Antidepressants in Pregnancy and Lactation

Class	Medication	FDA Risk Category	Teratogenicity	Late Pregnancy Exposure	Neonatal Toxicity	Breast-Feeding
Serotonin-norepinephrine reuptake inhibitors	**Venlafaxine** (Effexor®, Effexor XR®, Venlafaxine ER)	C	No increased risk identified, but data are limited [62,63]	As above	As above	Limited data, mean infant dose is 4.7%–9.2% of maternal levels; no adverse effects noted [10,96,97]
	Duloxetine (Cymbalta®)	C	Very limited data	As above	As above	Very limited data available
Other	**Mirtazapine** (Remeron®, Remeron SolTab®)	C	No increased risk identified, but data very limited [4,28,98–102]	As above	As above	Very limited data, low to undetectable infant levels; no adverse events noted [103–105]
	Bupropion (Budeprion SR, Budeprion XL, Buproban Wellbutrin®, Wellbutrin SR®, Wellbutrin XL®, Zyban ®)	C	Limited data, but most studies have not identified an increased risk of major malformations [4,28,98–102]		None reported	Limited data • One case report of a seizure in an exposed infant [106–108]

Note: RID, weight adjusted relative infant dose or % of weight adjusted maternal dose ingested by the infant.

pattern of poor developmental outcomes has not been established [109]. There is **limited information** available on the long-term effects of antidepressant exposure. Data on this topic must be interpreted carefully as the effects of maternal depression are also likely to have a significant impact on behavior and cognitive development [28].

Autism Spectrum Disorders
Findings from published studies regarding association of SSRIs with autism spectrum disorder are **inconsistent and not conclusive**. Multiple studies have found an association with first trimester exposure to SSRIs as well as maternal depression and an increased risk of autism spectrum disorders [110]. One study found that prenatal SSRI exposure was three times as likely in boys with autism spectrum disorder compared with children with typical development. This association was most strongly linked with first trimester exposure to the SSRIs [111]. Other studies have found only a small increase in risk [112]. A large study from Denmark did not find an association between antidepressant exposure and autism spectrum disorders when controlling for confounding factors [113]. It may be that depression itself may be attributable to some of these associations.

Tricyclic Antidepressants (TCAs)
TCAs have not been shown to be associated with a higher risk of congenital malformations when taken in the first trimester [28,70,114]. Complications for the newborn after tricyclic exposure during later pregnancy include tachycardia, irritability, jitteriness, hypertonia, convulsions, and anticholinergic symptoms, such as urinary retention [114].

Monoamine Oxidase Inhibitors (MAOIs)
Monoamine oxidase inhibitors are prescribed much less commonly because of multiple food and drug–drug interactions. There are much less data available for this class of medications. One small study shows an increased rate of congenital malformations [115]. Given the paucity of data on this class of medications, MAOIs should be avoided during pregnancy if possible [114].

Serotonin-Norepinephrine Reuptake Inhibitors (SNRIs)
and Other Classes
Commonly used medications in these classes include venlafaxine, duloxetine, mirtazapine, and bupropion. Overall, existing data suggest no significantly increased rate of congenital malformations with these antidepressants, but there are much less data available than for the SSRIs or TCAs [4,28,98,99]. In one study, the rate of preterm delivery with the serotonin-norepinephrine reuptake inhibitors (SNRIs) or norepinephrine reuptake inhibitors (NRIs) was significantly increased, and neonatal symptoms were similar to those symptoms seen in infants whose mothers were taking SSRIs during pregnancy [100]. In a recent population-based, case-control study, there was a small positive association with maternal bupropion use during pregnancy and left outflow tract heart defects [101]. However, other studies found no increased rate of major malformations [28,102,116].

Other Effects of Prenatal Exposure to Antidepressants
In some past studies, there was found to be increased risk of *spontaneous abortion (SAB)* that is associated with the use of several classes of antidepressants in pregnancy. Miscarriage rates were 12.4% in exposed women versus 8.7% in women who were not exposed to medications. There were no differences found between the different classes of antidepressants. The studies, however, were variable in controlling for confounding variables, such as health habits, smoking, and age [28,117–119]. Other more recent studies do not support this association [77,120,121] with incidence of SAB in women exposed to various SSRIs not exceeding the SAB rates in control groups [90].

Expert guidelines and algorithms to guide the physician on decision making for continuing and/or initiating medications for MDD during pregnancy have been published [28].

Mood Stabilizers (Table 21.2)
Lithium
Lithium is associated with an increased risk of Ebstein's anomaly, a cardiac defect characterized by congenital displacement of the tricuspid valve toward the apex of the right ventricle. In the general population, the risk of Ebstein's anomaly is 1:20,000. **In neonates exposed to lithium during the first trimester, the risk of Ebstein's anomaly is 1:1500, 0.05% to 0.1%** [122]. Thus, although the relative risk of Ebstein's anomaly is significantly higher with prenatal lithium exposure, the absolute risk still remains small [48]. A recent meta-analysis of trials evaluating lithium toxicity concluded that lithium's teratogenic risk has been overestimated [123].

In one trial, birth weight of lithium-exposed infants was found to be significantly higher than matched controls [124]. Individual cases of arrhythmia, nephrogenic diabetes insipidus, thyroid dysfunction, hypotonia, hypoglycemia, and hyperbilirubinemia have been reported. These problems are generally transient and have no long-term sequelae. Lithium-exposed infants may have poor respiratory effort and/or cyanosis at delivery. Neonatal hypotonicity, bradycardia, cyanosis, and hypoglycemia are preventable if lithium is discontinued immediately before delivery; however, given the high risk of postpartum mood episodes in these patients, lithium should be reinstated immediately afterward [125].

Lithium is distributed in total body fluid volume, and levels can be affected by vomiting and changes in sodium intake [48]. Thyroid function should be monitored during pregnancy because of the possibility of lithium-induced thyroid toxicity. In the last trimester, renal excretion of lithium increases by 30% to 50% [125], which may necessitate a dose increase at this time. Decreasing the dose of lithium at delivery may be necessary to avoid maternal lithium toxicity associated with the dramatic decrease in vascular volume occurring at delivery. Adequate hydration should be maintained during labor [48].

Many experts recommend continuing lithium during pregnancy in women with severe symptoms who have had a good response to lithium [122]. However, given the small absolute risk of Ebstein's anomaly, some patients with less frequent, less severe episodes may be able to discontinue lithium during pregnancy or at least during the first trimester. When the decision is made to discontinue lithium, the drug should be tapered slowly (over the course of >15 days) as rapid discontinuation of lithium is associated with higher frequency of, and reduced latency to recurrence of symptoms [52]. Prenatal screening, including high-resolution ultrasound and fetal echocardiography, should be conducted at 16 to 18 weeks' gestation in pregnant women with first-trimester lithium exposure [48].

Table 21.2 Mood Stabilizers in Pregnancy and Lactation

Medication	FDA Risk Category	Teratogenicity	Neonatal Toxicity	Breast-Feeding	Comments
Lithium (Eskalith®, Lithobid®)	D	• 20- to 40-fold increased risk of Ebstein's anomaly but absolute risk is small [122–124]	Cases of transient arrythmia, nephrogenic diabetes insipidus, thyroid dysfunction, hypotonia, hypoglycemia, and hyperbilirubinemia [125]. • Infants may have poor respiratory effort or cyanosis at delivery [125]	Variable infant serum levels [160]. Risk of toxicity in the newborn. Monitor lithium levels and CBC in breast-fed exposed infants [126–128]	Monitor serum levels and thyroid function frequently. Fluid shifts and changes in metabolism may necessitate dose adjustment [48,125]. • Infants may have poor respiratory effort or cyanosis at delivery [125]. High-resolution ultrasound and fetal echocardiography at 16 to 18 weeks gestation [48]
Valproic acid (Depakene®, Stavzor®)/Divalproex sodium (Depakote®, Depakote ER®, Depakote Sprinkles®)	D	• 6.2%–13.3% risk of major anomalies: NTDs, cardiovascular anomalies, limb defects, and hypospadias [130,132] • 1%–2% risk of NTDs [130,132] • Risk of facial dysmorphic features "antiepileptic drug syndrome" [132] • Risk of cognitive deficits and ASD [133]	None noted	Considered compatible with breast-feeding [129], low infant serum levels [129]	Teratogenicity and cognitive effects likely dose dependent [1], also polytherapy associated with greater risk [130,131] • Supplement with high-dose folic acid [132]
Carbamazepine (Carbatrol®, Equetro®, Tegretol®, Tegretol XR®)	D	• Risk of NTD 0.5%–1%; overall risk of major malformations 2.2%–5.4% [130] • Risk of facial dysmorphic features "antiepileptic drug syndrome" [48]	Risk of hemorrhagic disease in the newborn because of fetal vitamin K deficiency [48,131]	Considered compatible with breast-feeding [129] with variable infant serum levels; few reports of infant hepatotoxicity, monitor serum levels and LFTs in exposed infants [129,134–136]	Can cause fetal vitamin K deficiency, supplementation in last month of pregnancy recommended [129] • Supplement with high-dose folic acid [129]
Oxcarbazepine (Trileptal®)	C	Available teratogenic information is reassuring but database is too small to draw definitive conclusions [130]	None noted	Limited data	Levels may decrease during pregnancy [48]

(Continued)

Table 21.2 (Continued)   Mood Stabilizers in Pregnancy and Lactation

Medication	FDA Risk Category	Teratogenicity	Neonatal Toxicity	Breast-Feeding	Comments
Lamotrigine (Lamictal®, Lamictal XR®)	C	Conflicting results regarding risk of oral clefts [137–139]; if elevated, absolute risk is low • May be higher risk of malformations at higher doses [137]	None noted	High infant exposure, approximately 30% of maternal levels [129] Hypothetical risk of SJS in the newborn [141,142]	Changes in clearance during pregnancy and after delivery may necessitate dose adjustment [140]. • Safety data are reassuring compared to other treatment options [140] • Periconceptional folic acid supplementation [140]
Atypical antipsychotics Olanzapine (Zyprexa®, Zyprexa Zydis®) Risperidone (Risperdal®, Risperdal M-Tab®) Quetiapine (Seroquel®, Seroquel XR®) Aripiprazole (Ability®, Ability Discmelt®) Ziprasidone (Geodon®) Clozapine (Clozaril®, FazaClo®)	C: Olanzapine, risperidone, quetiapine, aripiprazole, ziprasidone. B: Clozapine	Limited data, but no evidence for increased risk with olanzapine, risperidone, clozapine, or quetiapine [143,144]. Very limited data with aripiprazole and ziprasidone	No reports of neonatal toxicity	Limited data. Low to undetectable levels in case reports with quetiapine, risperidone, olanzapine exposure [145,146]. Possibly some EPS with olanzapine exposure [146]. Very limited data for aripiprazole and ziprasidone [147–149] Clozapine: variable levels in infant serum. Hypothetical risk of agranulocytosis [146]	Can cause maternal weight gain and diabetes • Some evidence of association with LGA infants [143]

Abbreviations: ASD, autism spectrum disorder; EPS, extrapyramidal symptoms; LGA, large for gestational age; NTD, neural tube defects; SJS, Steven's–Johnson syndrome.

Valproic Acid

On the basis of data from several large antiepileptic pregnancy registries, **the risk for major congenital anomalies in infants exposed to valproic acid (VPA) in utero is estimated to be between 6.2% and 13.3%** [130]. Congenital anomalies seen with VPA include neural tube defects (NTDs), cardiovascular anomalies, limb defects, and hypospadias. About 1% to 2% of exposed infants present with NTDs [130,132]. Lumbosacral meningomyelocele is the most common NTD associated with VPA exposure, likely representing a drug effect on neural crest closure [48]. This defect occurs 10 to 20 times more frequently in VPA-exposed infants than in the general population [132].

A specific combination of facial dysmorphic features has been described in infants exposed to VPA in utero; this same syndrome was later described in children of women using other antiepileptic drugs (AEDs) (including carbamazepine) during pregnancy. This syndrome is known as the "antiepileptic drug syndrome" and is characterized by intrauterine growth retardation, long and thin upper lip, shallow philtrum, epicanthal folds, and midfacial hypoplasia with flat nasal bridge, small upturned nose, and down-turned angles of the mouth [132]. In infants exposed to VPA in utero, these features are often associated with other major anomalies and developmental delay. Cognitive deficits, attention deficit disorder, and learning difficulties have been repeatedly reported in children exposed to VPA in utero [130,132]. Perinatal valproate exposure also is associated with autism spectrum disorder [132].

Teratogenicity and cognitive effects related to prenatal VPA exposure are likely dose dependent with doses greater than 800 to 1000 mg associated with significantly greater risk [130,131]. Polytherapy with VPA and other anticonvulsants results in a higher rate of teratogenicity than monotherapy with VPA alone [132].

Valproic acid should not be used during pregnancy unless the benefits clearly outweigh the risks. Valproate is known to interfere with folic acid metabolism, so high-dose folate supplementation (4–5 mg/day) is currently recommended prior to conception and during the first trimester in women taking VPA (as well as with other anticonvulsants) during pregnancy. Folic acid supplementation decreases the incidence of NTDs, but the benefit of using high-dose folate for decreasing the rate of NTD in this population is unclear. As lamotrigine and carbamazepine interfere with folic acid absorption, supplementation is recommended in women taking these medications as well [132]. The UK and Ireland Epilepsy and Pregnancy Registers recently found that folate supplementation had no significant effect on pregnancy outcome in women exposed to carbamazepine, lamotrigine, and valproic acid [150].

Carbamazepine and Oxcarbazepine

Rates of malformations with carbamazepine exposure range from 2.2% to 5.4% in different large AED pregnancy registries. Carbamazepine is associated with a risk of NTDs of 0.5% to 1%. Recent data suggest that carbamazepine exposure may not cause cognitive impairment. Malformation rates are consistently higher with VPA than with carbamazepine [130]. Pregnancies exposed to high doses of carbamazepine (>1000 mg) resulted in a higher rate of malformations than lower doses (<400 mg) [150].

Carbamazepine can cause fetal vitamin K deficiency. Vitamin K is necessary for normal midfacial growth and for normal clotting factor function; thus, carbamazepine exposure during pregnancy may increase the risk of neonatal bleeding and midfacial abnormalities. Many experts recommend oral vitamin K in the last month of pregnancy [48]. There is currently insufficient evidence to determine whether vitamin K supplementation reduces the rate of neonatal hemorrhagic complications [131].

Data on malformation rates with oxcarbazepine exposure are still limited. A literature review on infants exposed to oxcarbazepine in utero, including data from the worldwide Novartis safety database and other pregnancy registries and study centers, revealed no increased risk of malformations. However, the number of exposed pregnancies was insufficient to draw definitive conclusions regarding safety of this medication [151]. Oxcarbazepine does not produce the same toxic epoxide metabolite as carbamazepine, and thus authors speculate that oxcarbazepine may be less harmful to the developing fetus [48]. Plasma concentrations of oxcarbazepine may decrease during pregnancy [152], which may necessitate dose adjustment.

Lamotrigine

The reproductive safety data regarding lamotrigine seems to be reassuring compared to other treatments for BAD. The North American AED Pregnancy Registry reported a 10.4-fold increased risk of cleft lip and/or cleft palate in infants exposed to lamotrigine in utero; the absolute risk of cleft lip and/or palate in the registry was 7.3:1000 [137]. Other large pregnancy registries did not substantiate this association [138,139]. One pregnancy registry reported a higher risk of major malformations with lamotrigine doses greater than 200 mg/day. No effects on cognition have been found, but data remain limited [130]. However, in another registry, the rate of congenital malformations with high-dose lamotrigine was still found to be lower than that with high dose valproate [150].

Lamotrigine clearance is increased during pregnancy, which may necessitate dose increases to maintain therapeutic effect. After delivery, lamotrigine clearance returns rapidly to baseline, requiring carefully monitoring and dose adjustment to avoid toxicity [140].

Antipsychotics

Data regarding the safety of second-generation (atypical) antipsychotics during pregnancy is still too limited to draw definitive conclusions regarding risk of structural teratogenicity [143]. A large cohort study of women exposed to both first- and second-generation antipsychotics has not revealed any substantial risk of teratogenicity [144]. Current available evidence regarding olanzapine, risperidone, quetiapine, and clozapine does not consistently reveal any increased risk for teratogenicity above that in the general population. In one study, quetiapine demonstrated the lowest amount of placental passage when compared to haloperidol, risperidone, and olanzapine [153]. Minimal information is available regarding ziprasidone and aripiprazole [143]. No information is available regarding paliperidone, iloperidone, asenapine, or lurasidone. The second-generation antipsychotics are known to cause maternal weight gain and diabetes, which are independently associated with pregnancy complications. Clozapine and olanzapine should be considered highest risk for metabolic complications in pregnancy in this class [143]. Some data indicate that second-generation antipsychotic exposure can result in a higher incidence of large-for-gestational-age infants [54]. One recent study demonstrated deficits in neuromotor performance in infants with prenatal antipsychotic exposure [154].

Data regarding exposure to haloperidol, a commonly used first-generation (typical) antipsychotic, are limited but generally are reassuring. An extrapyramidal syndrome has been reported in some cases of babies exposed to first-generation antipsychotics in utero [54].

NONPHARMACOLOGIC MANAGEMENT OF MOOD DISORDERS
Therapy

Empirically validated treatments exist for both depression during pregnancy and postpartum depression [155,156]. **Interpersonal psychotherapy** and **cognitive-behavioral therapy** are primary among these treatments and have been demonstrated to be effective for women with mild-to-severe depression. Interpersonal psychotherapy is a validated treatment for perinatal depression and should be a first-line treatment option [156–158]. Evidence from clinical trials indicates that interpersonal psychotherapy by itself or in combination with antidepressants may help speed time to recovery from postpartum depression and prolong the time spent in remission [158,159]. Randomized controlled trials are needed to further assess the efficacy of psychotherapy during pregnancy and postpartum [160,161].

According to a *Cochrane* review, pregnant women who receive psychological intervention for depression were significantly less likely to develop postnatal depression than were those who received standard care. Interventions included postpartum home visits, telephone support, and interpersonal psychotherapy [162].

Behavioral Educational Interventions

In an RCT of Black and Latina mothers just postpartum, behavioral educational intervention aimed to prepare and educate mothers about modifiable risk factors associated with symptoms of postpartum depression reduced positive depression screens [163]. Postpartum nurse home visits aimed at relationship-focused behavioral coaching (Communicating and Relating Effectively, CARE) are associated with significant increases in quality of mother–infant interaction and decreases in postpartum depression severity [164].

Electroconvulsive Therapy

In pregnant adults, electroconvulsive therapy (ECT) has well-proven efficacy in the treatment of MDD (complete response to treatment 84% and partial response 16%) and BAD (complete response to treatment 92% and partial response 8%) [165]. ECT is **not recommended as a first-line treatment but may be considered in patients who have demonstrated treatment resistance, when depression is life threatening, and when psychotic features are present** [166]. Side effects include transient memory loss, muscle soreness, and headache.

In pregnant women treated for depression, risks to the mother and child are low to moderate in all trimesters, possibly with more risk in the first trimester. The American Psychiatric Association (APA) recommends considering ECT as a primary treatment for MDD and bipolar disorder in pregnancy, consulting with an obstetrician before the pregnancy,

immediate access to obstetrical services during ECT treatments, fetal heart rate and ultrasound monitoring, and routine anesthetic measures with a consideration of intubation [167,168]. The most common complications of ECT in pregnant women are fetal bradyarrhythmias, uterine contractions, and induction of premature labor, which occurred at a rate of up to 29% with a child mortality rate of 7% (in a case series of 67 patients) [169]. Fetal bradyarrhythmias likely occur as a result of hypoxia. Positioning the woman with her right hip elevated will minimize the risk of hypoxia in the fetus. Induction of labor may be related to postictal elevations of oxytocin. Uterine activity can be monitored during ECT administration [165,170]. Fetal monitoring is suggested during ECT because of the potential for fetal sedation from general anesthesia. Methohexital sodium and propofol are the anesthetic agents most commonly used for ECT in the United States. Succinylcholine is generally used as a muscle relaxant as it does not cross the placenta at usual doses [168]. Neither ECT nor any of these agents have known teratogenicity [170,171]. ECT does not generate current through the uterus. One case of fetal death after status epilepticus was reported [170]. Limiting seizure duration during ECT in the general population is standard practice.

MANAGEMENT DURING LACTATION

All psychiatric medications are passed into breast milk. The American Academy of Pediatrics (AAP) has rated the compatibility of individual drugs with lactation. This rating is based on case reports found in the literature and is intended to assist the physician in counseling the mother regarding breast-feeding while taking medication [172]. Given the high rate of psychiatric illness during and after pregnancy, the health care practitioner should carefully evaluate the postpartum patient who is at risk for psychiatric illness to determine whether medication is necessary.

Antidepressants

The AAP Committee on Drugs rates antidepressant medications as "effects unknown, and may be of concern in breast-feeding" [172]. However, a pooled analysis of antidepressant levels in lactating mothers suggests that it is probably safe to use most antidepressants during lactation [94] and that antidepressant use is not considered to be a contraindication to **breast-feeding**. Antidepressant exposure in breast milk is five to 10 times lower than exposure in utero [10]. There are few reports of adverse effects in infants exposed to these medications. Most antidepressant drugs do not pose a risk to the nursing infant; however, consideration to the individual risk/benefit is necessary in each individual patient. This is especially true of drugs that have long half-lives and those that accumulate in breast milk and of vulnerable infants, such as those that are premature and those with immature organ function or underlying medical conditions [95].

Selective Serotonin Reuptake Inhibitors
The growing evidence is generally reassuring concerning the safety of the use of SSRIs in breast-feeding mothers. The excretion of SSRIs into breast milk is relatively low to undetectable [10]. Low infant plasma levels have been found with all the SSRIs, but higher concentrations have been reported for fluoxetine, citalopram, sertraline, and venlafaxine [95]. However, **if a woman has been stable on an antidepressant**

throughout her pregnancy, preference is usually to remain on that agent postpartum as evidence suggests that most infant SSRIs levels have been found to be quite low. Long-term effects of infant exposure to SSRIs through nursing have been less well studied.

Tricyclic Antidepressants

The AAP rates effects of TCAs during breast-feeding as "unknown but may be of concern." Infant plasma levels of TCAs were found to be <1% of maternal dose [173]. Most reports show no adverse effects in the nursing infant [4,10,173,174]. One exception is doxepin, with which there was one report of respiratory depression in an infant exposed through breast milk [4].

Monoamine Oxidase Inhibitors

No current data were found.

Venlafaxine

There are very few case reports published on the safety of venlafaxine in nursing. These show low-to-variable infant plasma levels in breast-fed infants. The mean infant dose or percentage of maternal intake ranged from 4.7% to 9.2% (mean of 6.4%), which is below the 10% estimated level of concern but still relatively high compared with data published for other antidepressants [96]. No adverse effects were found in exposed infants [10,96,97].

Duloxetine

At this time, there is an extremely limited amount of data available on effects on infants exposed to duloxetine while nursing.

Bupropion

There are no studies and only a few case reports on the safety of bupropion in breast-fed infants. Low infant serum levels were found [6,106], and no adverse effects were reported in two exposed infants [107]. One study reported a seizure in a six-month-old infant, which was possibly attributable to the use of bupropion during breast-feeding [108].

Trazodone

There are very little data on trazodone. In the few cases examined, levels in breast milk have been found to be low [175].

Mirtazapine

There are few published cases of infant exposure to mirtazapine. In these few cases, infant levels were low to undetectable. No adverse effects were seen in the exposed infants, including sedation or weight gain, which are common side effects of this medication [103–105].

Mood Stabilizers

Lithium

The AAP Committee on Drugs considers lithium to be associated "with significant effects on some nursing infants and should be given to nursing mothers with caution." Infant levels have been reported as variable but higher than those with many other medications, from one half to one third of maternal levels [176]. More recent studies found considerable variability (0%–30% of maternal dose) in infant serum levels of lithium as well as levels that were generally lower than previously thought [126,127]. In a few case reports,

adverse infant effects have included cyanosis, hypotonia, heart murmur, EKG changes, lethargy, and hypothermia [128,133]. Occasional and transient laboratory abnormalities, including elevated blood urea nitrogen (BUN), creatinine, and thyroid-stimulating hormone were observed in the sample of infants studied [126]. Infants may be more susceptible to both dehydration and lithium toxicity because of their immature kidney function and potential for rapid dehydration.

Valproic Acid

AAP Committee on Drugs considers valproic acid to be "compatible" with breast-feeding. Levels have been found to be very low in breast milk [129]. One adverse event of thrombocytopenia and anemia in an exposed infant was reported [177].

Carbamazepine

The AAP Committee on Drugs considers carbamazepine to be compatible with breast-feeding. Levels reported in infant serum were highly variable, but have not been found to penetrate breast milk in clinically significant amounts [129]. In two case reports, however, carbamazepine was associated with infant hepatotoxicity [134–136]. Exposed infants should be monitored by checking serum levels and liver function tests.

Lamotrigine

Effects of lamotrigine during breast-feeding are classified by the AAP as "unknown, but may be of concern." Lamotrigine is excreted in relatively high levels in breast milk. Infant serum levels were one third (about 30%) of maternal levels, likely because of a slow, immature elimination in infants. Most of the case reports found no adverse effects in infants [129] although there were some cases of mild thrombocytosis in one study [141]. There have been no reported cases of Stevens-Johnson syndrome in nursing infants to date, but because this may be a concern, infants should be closely monitored [142].

The Neurodevelopmental Effects of Antiepileptic Drugs Study is a prospective multicenter observational study examining cognitive outcomes in children at age 3 that were exposed to AEDs, both in utero and during breast-feeding. The study consisted of 199 children of mothers with epilepsy who were taking AEDs while pregnant. This study found no deleterious effects of AED therapy (valproate, carbamazepine, and lamotrigine) on cognitive outcomes of children that were exposed both in utero and while breast-feeding [178]. Although this study looked at effects on children of mothers with epilepsy rather than bipolar disorder, the effects of exposure would likely be applicable to either population.

Antipsychotics

The AAP Committee on Drugs rates the effects of haloperidol, chlorpromazine, thiothixene, mesoridazine, and trifluoperazine to be unknown and may be of concern to nursing infants. Haloperidol is excreted in relatively high amounts in breast milk but has not been associated with adverse effects on the infant [179,180]. Chlorpromazine exposure has been associated with drowsiness and lethargy in one infant [181]. In one study of seven infants with exposure to chlorpromazine through breast milk, there were no adverse effects reported at 16-month and five-year follow-up evaluations [182].

Atypical Antipsychotics
The atypical antipsychotics have not yet been rated by the AAP Committee on Drugs. There are only a few case reports published. Generally, risperidone, olanzapine, and quetiapine levels have been found to be low to undetectable in samples of nursing infants, and most infants showed no or few adverse effects from these medications [145,146]. There was one report of an infant with cardiomegaly, jaundice, and sedation after exposure to olanzapine [145]. There have also been a few cases of extrapyramidal reactions in infants exposed to olanzapine [146]. In a worldwide safety database maintained by the manufacturer of olanzapine, there were no adverse events reported in 82.3% of infants breast-feeding during olanzapine treatment. Most commonly reported adverse events in the remaining 15.6% of infants were somnolence, irritability, tremor, and insomnia [183]. The data for ziprasidone and aripiprazole are limited. In one case report, ziprasidone use in pregnancy and lactation did not result in any adverse outcomes for the infant, and in another case report, the concentration of ziprasidone in human milk was found to be low [147,148]. Likewise, in one case report, aripiprazole use during pregnancy and lactation did not result in any adverse outcomes, and there were no detectable levels of aripiprazole or its metabolite in the breast milk [149].

There are very few studies published on the safety of clozapine. The AAP rates effects as "unknown and of concern" in breast-feeding. In one case report, clozapine was shown to have a relatively high accumulation in breast milk [184]. In an infant exposed to clozapine both prenatally and during breast-feeding, delayed speech acquisition may have been attributable to clozapine [185]. Although no cases have been reported of agranulocytosis in nursing infants, it is a theoretical risk. Therefore, it is not recommended that clozapine be used during breast-feeding [10,146]. With limited data available, if women decide to breast-feed while taking an antipsychotic medication, infants should be monitored for possible adverse effects.

REFERENCES

1. American Psychiatric Association. *Diagnostic and Statistical Manual of Mental Disorders, 4th ed, Text Revision (DSM-IV-TR)*, Washington, DC: American Psychiatric Publishing, 2000. [III]
2. National Institute of Mental Health (US). *The numbers count: Mental disorders in America.* NIH Publication No. 06-4584. Bethesda (MD): NIMH, 2006. [III]
3. Committee on Obstetric Practice. The American College of Obstetricians and Gynecologists Committee Opinion no. 630. Screening for perinatal depression. *Obstet Gynecol* 2015 May; 125(5): 1268–71. [Report of expert committee, III]
4. ACOG Committee. Clinical Management Guidelines for Obstetrician–Gynecologists: Use of psychiatric medications during pregnancy and lactation. ACOG Practice Bulletin No. 92. *Obstet Gynecol* 2008; 111(4): 1001–20. [Review, III]
5. Gentile S. Use of contemporary antidepressants during breast-feeding: A proposal for a specific safety index. *Drug Saf* 2007; 30(2): 107–21. [Review, III]
6. Kendell RE, Chalmers JC, Platz C. Epidemiology of puerperal psychosis. *Br J Psychiatry* 1987; 150: 662–73. [II-3]
7. McNeil TF. A prospective study of postpartum psychoses in a high-risk group. 1. Clinical characteristics of the current postpartum episodes. *Acta Psychiatr Scand* 1986; 74(2): 205–16. [Prospective case-control study, II-1]
8. Howard, LM, Molyneux, E, Dennis, CL, Tamsen R, Stein A, Milgrom J. Non-psychotic mental disorders in the perinatal period. Perinatal mental health 1. *Lancet* 2014; 384: 1775–88. [Literature review of studies that included RCTs and observational studies, III]
9. Newport DJ, Hostetter A, Arnold A et al. The treatment of postpartum depression: Minimizing infant exposures. *J Clin Psychiatry* 2002; 63(Suppl. 7): 31–44. [Review, III]
10. Eberhard-Gran, Eskild A, Opjordsmoen S. Use of psychotropic medications in treating mood disorders during lactation: Practical recommendations. *CNS Drugs* 2006; 20(3): 187–98. [Review, III]
11. Cox J. Postnatal mental disorder: Towards ICD-11. *World Psychiatry* 2004; 3(2): 96–7. [Commentary, III]
12. Gentile S. Clinical utilization of atypical antipsychotics in pregnancy and lactation. *Ann Pharmacother* 2004; 38: 1265–71. [Review, III]
13. Hales RE, Yudofsky SC, eds. *American Psychiatric Publishing Textbook of Clinical Psychiatry. 4th ed.* Arlington, VA: American Psychiatric Publishing, 2005. [III]
14. Spinelli MG. A systematic investigation of 16 cases of neonaticide. *Am J Psychiatry* 2001; 158(5): 811–3. [Case series, II-3]
15. Nager A, Sundquist K, Ramirez-Leon V et al. Obstetric complications and postpartum psychosis: A follow-up study of 1.1 million first-time mothers between 1975 and 2003 in Sweden. *Acta Psychiatr Scand* 2008; 117(1): 12–9. [Retrospective cohort, n = 1413, II-2]
16. Harlow BL, Vitonis AF, Sparen P et al. Incidence of hospitalization for postpartum psychotic and bipolar episodes in women with and without prior prepregnancy or prenatal hospitalizations. *Arch Gen Psychiatry* 2007; 64(1): 42–8. [Retrospective cohort, n = 2259, II-2]
17. Stewart D, Vigod S, Stotland NL. Obstetrics and gynecology. In: Levenson JL, ed. *The American Psychiatric Publishing Textbook of Psychosomatic Medicine. Psychiatric Care of the Medically Ill.* Washington, DC: American Psychiatric Publishing, Inc., 2010: 797–826. [III]
18. Raisanen S, Lehto SM et al. Risk factors for perinatal outcomes of major depression during pregnancy: A population-based analysis during 2002–2010 in Finland. *BMJ Open* 2014; 4(11): e004883. [Cross-sectional study, II-3]
19. Cohen LS, Altshuler LL, Harlow BL et al. Relapse of major depression during pregnancy and in women who maintain or discontinue antidepressant treatment. *JAMA* 2006; 295(5): 499–507. [Prospective study, n = 201, II-2]
20. Bloch M, Rotenberg N, Koren D et al. Risk factors associated with the development of postpartum mood disorders. *J Affect Disord* 2005; 88(1): 9–18. [Prospective study, n = 1800, II-1]
21. Nielsen Forman D, Videbech P, Hedegaard M et al. Postpartum depression: Identification of women at risk. *BJOG* 2000; 107(10): 1210–7. [Prospective study, n = 5252, II-1]
22. Katon W, Russo J et al. Predictors of postpartum depression. *J Womens Health* 2014; 23(9): 753–9. [Prospective cohort, II-2]
23. Mercier RJ, Garrett J et al. Pregnancy intention and postpartum depression: Secondary data analysis from a prospective cohort. *BJOG* 2013: 120(9): 1116–22. [Prospective cohort, II-2]
24. Verreault N, Da Costa D. Rates and risk factors associated with depressive symptoms during pregnancy and with postpartum onset. *J Psychosom Obstet Gynaecol* 2014: 35(3): 84–91. [Prospective cohort, II-2]
25. USPSTF. Final Recommendation Statement; Depression in Adults: Screening. *JAMA* 2016; 315(4): 380–7. [Guideline]
26. Szegda K, Markenson G, Bertone-Johnson ER, Chasan-Taber L. Depression during pregnancy: A risk factor for adverse neonatal outcomes? A critical review of the literature. *J Matern Fetal Neonatal Med* 2014 Jun; 27(9): 960–7. [Data largely obtained from prospective cohort studies, II-2]
27. Grigoriadis S, VonderPorten EH, Mamisahvili L et al. The impact of maternal depression during pregnancy on perinatal outcomes: A systematic review and meta-analysis. *J Clin Psychiatry* 2013 Apr; 74(4): e321–41. [Cohort studies were analyzed, II-2]

28. Yonkers KA, Wisner KL, Stewart DE et al. The management of depression during pregnancy: A report from the American Psychiatric Association and the American College of Obstetricians and Gynecologists. *Gen Hosp Psychiatry* 2009; 31(5): 403–13. [Review, III]

29. Zuckerman B, Bauchner H, Parker S et al. Maternal depressive symptoms during pregnancy, and newborn irritability. *J Dev Behav Pediatr* 1990; 11(4): 190–4. [Prospective study, n = 1123, II-1]

30. Field T, Diego M, Hernandez-Reif M. Prenatal depression effects on the fetus and newborn: A review. *Infant Behav Dev* 2006; 29: 445–55. [Review, III]

31. Glover, V. Maternal depression, anxiety, and stress during pregnancy and child outcome: What needs to be done. *Best Practice Res Clin Obstet Gynecol* 2014: 28(1): 25–35. [Literature review and expert opinion, III]

32. Pilowsky DJ, Wickramaratne PJ, Rush AJ et al. Children of currently depressed mothers: A STAR*D ancillary study. *J Clin Psychiatry* 2006; 67(1): 126–36. [Cross-sectional cohort, n = 151, II-3]

33. Biederman J, Faraone SV, Hirshfel-Becker DR et al. Patterns of psychopathology and dysfunction in high-risk children of parents with panic disorder and major depression. *Am J Psychiatry* 2001; 158(1): 49–57. [Case-control, n = 380, II-1]

34. Brennan PA, Hammen C, Anderson MJ et al. Chronicity, severity, and timing of maternal depressive symptoms: Relationships with child outcomes at age 5. *Dev Psychol* 2000; 36(6): 759–66. [Prospective cohort, n = 4953, II-1]

35. Hammen C, Brennan PA. Severity, chronicity and timing of maternal depression and risk for adolescent offspring diagnosis in a community sample. *Arch Gen Psychiatry* 2003; 60(3): 253–8. [Cross-sectional cohort, n = 816, II-3]

36. Gao W, Paterson J, Abbott M et al. Maternal mental health and child behaviour problems at 2 years: Findings from the Pacific Islands Families Study. *Aust N Z J Psychiatry* 2007; 41(11): 885–95. [Prospective cohort, n = 1398, II-1]

37. Weissman MM, Pilowsky DJ, Wickramaratne PJ et al. Remissions in maternal depression and child psychopathology: A STAR*D-child report. *JAMA* 2006; 295(12): 1389–98. [Prospective cohort, n = 151, II-1]

38. Minkovitz CS, Strobino D, Scharfstein D et al. Maternal depressive symptoms and children's receipt of health care in the first 3 years of life. *Pediatrics* 2005; 115(2): 306–14. [Prospective cohort, n = 5565, II-1]

39. Hatton DC, Harrison–Hohner J, Coste S et al. Symptoms of postpartum depression and breastfeeding. *J Hum Lact* 2005; 21(44): 444–9. [Prospective cohort, n = 377, II-1]

40. Cox JL, Holden JM, Sagovsky R. Detection of postnatal depression. Development of the 10-item Edinburgh Postnatal Depression Scale. *Br J Psychiatry* 1987; 150: 782–6. [Case-controlled validation study, II-2]

41. Gibson J, McKenzie-McHarg L, Shakespeare J et al. A systematic review of studies validating the Edinburgh Postnatal Depression Scale in antepartum and postpartum women. *Acta Psychiatr Scand* 2009; 119(5): 350–64. [Meta-analysis and review, III]

42. Sharma V. Management of bipolar II disorder during pregnancy and the postpartum period. *Can J Clin Pharmacol* 2009; 16(1): e33–41. [Review, III]

43. Chessick CA, Dimidjian S. Screening for bipolar disorder during pregnancy and the postpartum period. *Arch Womens Ment Health* 2010; 13(3): 233–48. [Review, III]

44. Jones I, Chandra P, Dazzan P, Howard L. Bipolar disorder, affective psychosis, and schizophrenia in pregnancy and the postpartum period. *Lancet* 2014; 384: 1789–99. [Literature review and discussion of prospective cohort studies, III]

45. Robertson E, Jones I, Haque S. Risk of puerperal and non-puerperal recurrence of illness following bipolar affective puerperal (post-partum) psychosis. *Br J Psychiatry* 2005; 186: 158–9. [Prospective cohort study, II-2]

46. Di Florio A, Jones L, Forty L et al. Mood disorders and parity—A clue to the aetiology of the postpartum trigger. *J Affect Disord* 2013; 152–4: 334–9. [Case-control study, II-2]

47. Berginck V, Burgerhout KM, Weigelt K et al. Immune system dysregulation in first-onset postpartum psychosis. *Biol Psychiatry* 2013; 73(10): 1000–7. [Cohort study, II-2]

48. Yonkers KA, Wisner KL, Stowe Z et al. Management of bipolar disorder during pregnancy and the postpartum period. *Am J Psychiatry* 2004; 161: 608–20. [Review, III]

49. Berginck V, Bouvy PF, Vervoort JS et al. Prevention of postpartum psychosis and mania in women at high risk. *Am J Psychiatry* 2012; 169: 609–15. [Nonrandomized controlled study, II-1]

50. Mei-Dan E, Ray J, Vigod S. Perinatal outcomes among women with bipolar disorder: A population-based cohort sudy. *Am J Obstet Gynecol* 2015; 212: 367e1–8. [Cohort study, II-2]

51. Sharma V, Pope C. Pregnancy and bipolar disorder: A systematic review. *J Clin Psychiatry* 2012; 73(11): 1447–55. [Review of largely prospective observational data, II-2]

52. Viguera AC, Whitfield T, Baldessarini RJ et al. Risk of recurrence in women with bipolar disorder during pregnancy: Prospective study of mood stabilizer discontinuation. *Am J Psychiatry* 2007; 164(12): 1817–24. [Prospective cohort, n = 89, II-1]

53. Viguera AC, Tondo L, Koukopoulos AE. episodes of mood disorders in 2,252 pregnancies and postpartum periods. *Am J Psychiatry* 2011; 168: 1179–85. [Retrospective observational study, II-2]

54. Einarson A, Boskovic R. Use and safety of antipsychotic drugs during pregnancy. *J Psychiatr Pract* 2009; 15(3): 183–92. [Review, III]

55. Ghaemi SN. Why antidepressants are not antidepressants: STEP-BD, STAR*D, and the return of neurotic depression. *Bipolar Disord* 2008; 10(8): 957–68. [Review, III]

56. Frey B, Simpson W, Wright L, Steiner M. Sensitivity and specificity of the mood disorder questionnaire as a screening tool for bipolar disorder during pregnancy and the postpartum period. *J Clin Psychiatry* 2012; 73(11): 1456–61. [Cohort study, II-2]

57. Spinelli MG. Postpartum psychosis: Detection of risk and management. *Am J Psychiatry* 2009; 166: 405–8. [Case Report and Review, III]

58. Spinelli M, Endicott J. Controlled clinical trial of interpersonal psychotherapy versus parenting education program for depressed pregnant women. *Am J Psychiatry* 2003; 160(3): 555–62. [RCT, N = 38, I]

59. Suri R, Lin AS et al. Acute and long-term behavioral outcomes of infants and children exposed in utero to either maternal depression or antidepressants: A review of the literature. *J Clinical Psychiatry* 2014; 75(10): e1142–52. [Literature review, III]

60. Molyneaux E, Howard L, McGeown H, Karia AM, Trevillion K. Antidepressant treatment for postnatal depression. *Cochrane Database Syst Rev* 2014; 9: CD002018. [Cochrane Review of 6 RCTs with 596 participants, I]

61. Yonkers KA, Blackwell KA, Glover J, Forray A. Antidepressant use in pregnant and postpartum women. *Annu Rev Clinc Psychol* 2014; 10: 369–92. [Literature review of largely observational studies, including prospective cohort studies, II-2]

62. Furu K, Kieler H, Haglund B et al. Selective serotonin reuptake inhibitors and venlafaxine in early pregnancy and risk of birth defects: Population based cohort study and sibling design. *BMJ* 2015; 350: 1798.1-9. [Cohort study, II-2]

63. Alwan S, Reefhuis J, Rasmussen SA et al., for National Birth Defects Prevention Study. Use of selective serotonin-reuptake inhibitors in pregnancy and the risk of birth defects. *N Engl J Med* 2007; 356(26): 2684–92. [Cross-sectional study, n = 6582, II-3]

64. Wurst KE, Poole C, Ephross SA et al. First trimester paroxetine use and the prevalence of congenital, specifically cardiac, defects: A meta-analysis of epidemiological studies. *Birth Defects Res A Clin Mol Teratol* 2010; 88(3): 159–70. [Meta-analysis Review, III]

65. Bakker MK, Kerstjens-Fredierikse WS, Buys CH et al. First trimester use of paroxetine and congenital heart defects: A population-based case-control study. *Birth Defects Res A Clin Mol Teratol* 2010; 88(2): 94–100. [Retrospective case-controlled study, *n* = 1293, II-2]

66. Cole JA, Ephross SA, Cosmatos IS et al. Paroxetine in the first trimester and the prevalence of congenital malformations. *Pharmacoepidemiol Drug Saf* 2007; 16(10): 1075–85. [Retrospective cohort, II-3]

67. Kallen BA, Otterblad Olausson P. Maternal use of selective serotonin-reuptake inhibitors in early pregnancy and infant congenital malformations. *Birth Defects Res A Clin Mol Teratol* 2007; 79(4): 301–8. [Retrospective cohort, II-3]

68. Reis M, Kallen B. Delivery outcome after maternal use of antidepressant drugs in pregnancy: An update using Swedish data. *Psychol Med* 2010; 40(10): 1723–33. [Retrospective cohort, II-3]

69. Einarson A, Pistelli A, DeSantis M et al. Evaluation of the risk of congenital cardiovascular defects associated with the use of paroxetine during pregnancy. *Am J Psychiatry* 2008; 165(6): 749–52. [Epidemiologic study, *n* = 3285, II-2]

70. Davis RL, Rubanowice D, McPhillips H et al. Risk of congenital malformations and perinatal events among infants exposed to antidepressant medication during pregnancy. *Pharmacoepidemiol Drug Saf* 2007; 16(10): 186–94. [Retrospective cohort, II-3]

71. Huybrechts KF Palmesten K, Avorn et al. Antidepressant use in pregnancy and the risk of cardiac defects. *N Engl J Med* 2014 June; 370(25): 2397–407. [Cohort study of 949,504 women, II-2]

72. Available at: http://www.fda.gov/Drugs/DrugSafety/Postmarket DrugSafetyInformationforPatientsandProviders/Drug SafetyInformationforHealthcareProfessionals/PublicHealth Advisories/ucm051731.htm. [III]

73. Louik C, Lin A, Werler M et al. First-trimester use of selective serotonin-reuptake inhibitors and the risk of birth defects. *N Engl J Med* 2007; 356(26): 2675–83. [Retrospective observational case-controlled study, *n* = 9849, II-2]

74. Gentile S. Early pregnancy exposure to selective serotonin reuptake inhibitors, risks of major structural malformations, and hypothesized teratogenic mechanisms. *Expert Opin Drug Metab Toxicol* 2015 Jul 1; 1–13. [Expert opinion, III]

75. Grigoriadis S, VonderPorten EH, Mamishvili L et al. Antidepressant exposure during pregnancy and congenital malformations: Is there an association? A systemic review and meta-analysis of the best evidence. *J Clin Psychiatry* 2013 Apr; 7(4): e293–308. [Cohort and case-control studies reviewed, II-2]

76. Huang H, Coleman S, Bridge JA, Yonkers K, Katon W. A meta-analysis of the relationship between antidepressant use in pregnancy and the risk of preterm birth and low birth weight. *Gen Hosp Psychiatry* 2014; 36(1): 13–8. [Meta-analysis included prospective and retrospective observational studies, II-2]

77. Ross LE, Grigoriadis S, Mamisashvili L et al. Selected pregnancy and delivery outcomes after exposure to antidepressant medication: A systematic review and meta-analysis. *JAMA Psychiatry* 2013; 70(4): 436–43. [Studies reviewed are largely cohort studies, II-2]

78. Huybrechts KF, Sanghani RS, Avorn J, Urato AC. Preterm birth and antidepressant medication use during pregnancy: A systemic review and meta-analysis. *PLoS One* 2014; 9(3): e92778. [Analysis of largely prospective and retrospective cohort studies, II-2]

79. Grigoriadis S, Vonderporten EH, Mamisashvili L et al. Prenatal exposure to antidepressants and persistent pulmonary hypertension of the newborn: Systematic review and meta-analysis. *BMJ* 2014; 14348: f6932. [Analysis of cohort and case-control studies, II-2]

80. Andrade SE, McPhillips H, Loren D et al. Antidepressant medication use and risk of persistent pulmonary hypertension of the newborn. *Pharmacoepidemiol Drug Saf* 2009; 18: 246–52. [Retrospective cohort-control study, *n* = 1104 and 1104 controls, II-2]

81. Wichman CL, Moore KM, Lang TR et al. Congenital heart disease associated with selective serotonin reuptake inhibitor use during pregnancy. *Mayo Clin Proc* 2009; 84: 23–27. [Retrospective study, *n* = 808 and 24,406 controls, II-2]

82. Chambers et al. Selective serotonin reuptake inhibitors and the risk of persistent pulmonary hypertension of the newborn. *N Engl J Med* 2006; 354: 579–87. [Retrospective cohort-control, II-2]

83. Kallen B, Olausson PO. Maternal use of selective serotonin re-uptake inhibitors and persistent pulmonary hypertension of the newborn. *Pharmacoepidemiol Drug Saf* 2008; 17(8): 801–6. [Retrospective cohort, II-3]

84. Kieler H, Artama M et al. Selective serotonin reuptake inhibitors during pregnancy and the risk of persistant pulmonary hypertension in the newborn: Population based cohort study from the five Nordic countries. *BMJ* 2012; 344. [II-1]

85. Huybrechts KF, Bateman BT, Palmsten K et al. Antidepressant use later in pregnancy and the risk of persistent pulmonary hypertension of the newborn. *JAMA* 2015; 313(21): 2142–51. [Cohort study, II-2]

86. Moses-Kolko EL, Bogen D, Perel J et al. Neonatal signs after late in utero exposure to serotonin reuptake inhibitors: Literature review and implications for clinical applications. *JAMA* 2005; 293: 2372–83. [Review of cohort studies, case series and case controls, III]

87. Grigoradis S, VonderPorten EH, Mamisashvili L et al. The effect of prenatal exposure on neonatal adaptation: A systematic review and meta-analysis. *J Clin Psychiatry* 2013 Apr; 74(4): e309–20. [Review of cohort and case-control studies, II-2]

88. Chambers CD, Johnson KA, Kick LM, Feliz RJ, Jones KL. Birth outcomes in pregnant women taking fluoxetine. *N Engl J Med* 1996; 335(14): 1010–5. [Prospective cohort study, II-2]

89. Tuccori M et al. Safety concerns associated with the use of serotonin reuptake inhibitors and other serotonergic/noradrenergic antidepressants during pregnancy: A review. *Clin Ther* 2009; 31: 1426–53. [Review, III]

90. Casper RC, Fleisher BE, Lee-Ancajas JC et al. Follow-up of children of depressed mothers exposed or not exposed to antidepressant drugs during pregnancy. *J Pediatr* 2003; 142: 402–8. [Retrospective study, II-3]

91. Mortensen JT, Olsen J, Larsen H et al. Psychomotor development in children exposed in utero to benzodiazepines, antidepressants, neuroleptics, and antiepileptics. *Eur J Epidemiol* 2003; 18: 769–71. [Retrospective study, II-3]

92. Nulman I, Rovet J, Stewart DE et al. Neurodevelopment of children exposed in utero to antidepressant drugs. *N Engl J Med* 1997; 336: 258–62. [Retrospective study, II-3]

93. Nulman I, Rovet J, Stewart DE et al. Child development following exposure to tricyclic antidepressants or fluoxetine throughout fetal life: A prospective, controlled study. *Am J Psychiatry* 2002; 159(11): 1889–95. [II-1]

94. Weissman AM, Levy BT, Hartz AJ et al. Pooled analysis of antidepressant levels in lactating mothers, breast milk and nursing infants. *Am J Psychiatry* 2004; 161(6): 1066–78. [Meta-analysis, II-2]

95. Sachs HC; Committee on Drugs. The transfer of drugs and therapeutics into human milk: An update on selected topics. *Pediatrics* 2013; 132(3): e796–809. [Report of expert committee, III]

96. Ilett KF, Kristensen JH, Hackett LP et al. Distribution of venlafaxine and its O-desmethyl metabolite in human milk and their effects in breastfed infants. *Br J Clin Pharmacol* 2002; 53(1): 17–22. [II-3]

97. Newport DJ, Ritchie JC, Knight BT et al. Venlafaxine in human milk and nursing infant plasma: Determination of exposure. *J Clin Psychiatry* 2009; 70(9): 1304–10. [Uncontrolled investigational study, II-3]

98. Einarson TR, Einarson A. Newer antidepressants in pregnancy and rates of major malformations: A meta-analysis of prospective comparative studies. *Pharmacoepidemiol Drug Saf* 2005; 14(12): 823–7. [Meta-analysis and review, III]

99. Einarson A, Choi J, Einarson TR et al. Incidence of major malformations in infants following antidepressant exposure in pregnancy: Results of a large prospective cohort study. *Can J Psychiatry* 2009; 54(4): 242–6. [Prospective case-control, II-1]

100. Lennestal R, Kallen B. Delivery outcome in relation to maternal use of some recently introduced antidepressants. *J Clin Psychopharmacol* 2007; 27: 607–13. [Retrospective case-control, II-2]

101. Alwan S, Reefhuis J, Botto LD et al. Maternal use of bupropion and risk for congenital heart defects. *Am J Obstet Gynecol* 2010; 203(1): 52.e1–6. [Retrospective case-control, II-2]

102. Cole JA, Modell JG, Haight BR et al. Bupropion in pregnancy and the prevalence of congenital malformations. *Pharmacoepidemiol Drug Saf* 2007; 16(5): 474–84. [Retrospective study, II-3]

103. Kristenen JH, Ilett KF, Rampono J et al. Transfer of the antidepressant mirtazapine into breast milk. *Br J Clin Pharmacol* 2007; 63(3): 322–7. [II-3]

104. Klier CM, Mossaheb N, Lee A et al. Mirtazapine and breastfeeding: Maternal and infant plasma levels. *Am J Psychiatry* 2007; 164(2): 348–9. [II-3]

105. Aichhorn W, Whitworth AB, Weiss U et al. Mirtazapine and breastfeeding. *Am J Psychiatry* 2004; 161(12): 2325. [II-3]

106. Briggs GG, Samson JH, Ambrose PJ et al. Excretion of bupropion in breast milk. *Ann Pharmacother* 1993; 27(4): 431–3. [II-3]

107. Baab SW, Peindl KS, Piontek CM et al. Serum bupropion levels in 2 breastfeeding mother-infant pairs. *J Clin Psychiatry* 2002; 63(10): 910–1. [II-3]

108. Chaudron LH, Schoenecker CJ. Bupropion and breastfeeding: A case of a possible infant seizure. *J Clin Psychiatry* 2004; 65(6): 881–2. [II-3]

109. Santucci AK, Singer LT et al. Impact of prenatal exposure to serotonin reuptake inhibitors or maternal major depressive disorder on infant developmental outcomes. *J of Clinical Psychiatry* 2014; 75(10): 1088–95. [Prospective cohort, II-2]

110. Rai D, Lee BK, Dalman C, Golding J, Lewis G, Manusson C. Parental depression, maternal antidepressant use during pregnancy, and the risk of autism spectrum disorders: Population based case-control study. *BMJ* 2013; 346 f2059. [Case-control, II-2]

111. Harrington RA, Lee LC, Crum RM, Zimmerman AW, Hertz-Picciotto I. Prenatal SSRI use and offspring with autism spectrum disorder or developmental delay. *Pediatrics* 2014; 133(5): e1241–8. [Case-control, II-2]

112. Croen LA, Grether JK, Yoshida CK, Odouli R, Hendrick V. Antidepressant use during pregnancy and childhood autism spectrum disorders. *Arch Gen Psychiatry* 2011; 68(11): 1104–12. [Case-control, II-2]

113. Sorensen MJ, Gronborg TK, Christensen J, Parner ET, Vestergaard M, Schendel D, Pedersen LH. Antidepressant exposure in pregnancy and risk of autism spectrum disorders. *Clin Epidemiol* 2013; 5: 449–59. [Cohort study, II-2]

114. Altshuler LL, Cohen L, Szuba MP et al. Pharmacologic management of psychiatric illness during pregnancy: Dilemmas and guidelines. *Am J Psychiatry* 1996; 153: 592–606. [Meta-analysis and review, III]

115. Heinonen OP, Slone D, Shapiro S. *Birth defects and drugs in pregnancy.* Littleton, MA: Publishing Sciences Group, 1977. [III]

116. Chun-Fai-Chan, Koren G et al. Pregnancy outcome of women exposed to bupropion during pregnancy: A prospective comparative study. *Am J Obstet Gynecol* 2005; 192: 932–6. [Prospective case-control, II-1]

117. Einarson A, Choi J, Einarson TR et al. Rates of spontaneous and therapeutic abortions following the use of antidepressants in pregnancy: Results from a large prospective database. *J Obstet Gynaecol Can* 2009; 31(5): 452–6. [Prospective case-control, II-1]

118. Nakhai-Pour HR, Broy P, Berard A. Use of antidepressants during pregnancy and the risk of spontaneous abortion. *CMAJ* 2010; 182(10): 1031–7. [Retrospective study, II-3]

119. Djulus J, Koren G, Einarson TR et al. Exposure to mirtazapine during pregnancy: A prospective comparative study of birth outcomes. *J Clin Psychiatry* 2006; 67(8): 1280–4. [Prospective case-control, II-1]

120. Stephansson O, Kieler H, Haglund B et al. Selective serotonin reuptake inhibitors during pregnancy and the risk of stillbirth and infant mortality. *JAMA* 2013; 309: 48–54. [Cohort study, II-2]

121. Jimenez-Solem E, Andersen JT, Petersen M et al. SSRI use during pregnancy and risk of stillbirth and neonatal mortality. *Am J Psychiatry* 2013; 170: 299–304. [Cohort study, II-2]

122. Yacobi S, Ornoy A. Is lithium a real teratogen? What can we conclude from the prospective versus retrospective studies? A review. *Isr J Psychiatry Relat Sci* 2008; 45(2): 95–106. [Review, III]

123. McKnight RF, Adida M, Budge K et al. Lithium toxicity profile: A systematic review and meta-analysis. *Lancet* 2012; 379: 721–28. [Review and analysis of seven cohort studies, seven case-control studies, and 48 case reports, II-2]

124. Jacobson SJ, Jones K, Johnson K et al. Prospective multicentre study of pregnancy outcome after lithium exposure during first trimester. *Lancet* 1992; 339(8792): 530–3. [II-2]

125. Pinelli JM, Symington AJ, Cunningham KA et al. Case report and review of the perinatal implications of maternal lithium use. *Am J Obstet Gynecol* 2002; 187: 245–9. [Review, III]

126. Viguera AC, Newport DJ, Ritchie J et al. Lithium in breast milk and nursing infants: Clinical implications. *Am J Psychiatry* 2007; 164(2): 342–5. [II-3]

127. Moretti ME, Koren G, Verjee Z et al. Monitoring lithium in breast milk: An individualized approach for breast-feeding mothers. *Ther Drug Monit* 2003; 25(3): 364–6. [II-3]

128. Tunnessen WW Jr, Hertz CG. Toxic effects of lithium in newborn infants: A commentary. *J Pediatr* 1972; 81: 804–7. [III]

129. Chen L, Lui F, Yoshida S et al. Is breastfeeding of infants advisable for epileptic mothers taking antiepileptic drugs? *Psychiatry Clin Neurosci* 2010; 64(5): 460–8. [II-3]

130. Tomson T, Battino D. Teratogenic effects of antiepileptic medications. *Neurol Clin* 2009; 27: 993–1002. [Review, III]

131. Harden CL, Pennell PB, Koppel BS. Practice parameter update: Management issues for women with epilepsy—Focus on pregnancy (an evidence-based review). Vitamin K, folic acid, blood levels, and breastfeeding: Report of the Quality Standards Subcommittee and Therapeutics and Technology Assessment Subcommittee of the American Academy of Neurology and American Epilepsy Society. *Neurology* 2009; 73(142): 142–9. [III]

132. Ornoy A. Valproic acid in pregnancy: How much are we endangering the embryo and fetus? *Reprod Toxicol* 2009; 28: 1–10. [Review; III]

133. Woody JN, London WL, Wilbanks GD Jr. Lithium toxicity in a newborn. *Pediatrics* 1971; 47: 94–6. [Case report, III]

134. Merlob P, Mor N, Litwin A. Transient hepatic dysfunction in an infant of an epileptic mother treated with carbamazepine during pregnancy and breastfeeding. *Ann Pharmacother* 1992; 26(12): 1563–5. [II-3]

135. Frey B, Schubiger G, Musy JP. Transient cholestatic hepatitis in a neonate associated with carbamazepine exposure during pregnancy and breastfeeding. *Eur J Pediatr* 1990; 150(2): 136–8. [II-3]

136. Frey B, Braegger CP, Ghelfi D. Neonatal cholestatic hepatitis from carbamazepine exposure during pregnancy and breast feeding. *Ann Pharmacother* 2002; 36(4): 644–7. [II-3]

137. Holmes LB, Baldwin EJ, Smith CR et al. Increased frequency of isolated cleft palate in infants exposed to lamotrigine during pregnancy. *Neurology* 2008; 70: 2152–8. [Prospective cohort, II-2]

138. Dolk H, Jentink J, Loane M et al. Does lamotrigine use in pregnancy increase orofacial cleft risk relative to other malformations? *Neurology* 2008; 71: 714–22. [II-2]

139. Morrow J, Russell A, Guthrie E et al. Malformation risks of anti-epileptic drugs in pregnancy: A prospective study from the UK Epilepsy and Pregnancy Register. *J Neurol Neurosurg Psychiatry* 2006; 77: 193–8. [Prospective case-control, II-1]

140. de Haan GJ, Edelbroek P, Segers J et al. Gestation-induced changes in lamotrigine pharmacokinetics: A monotherapy study. *Neurology* 2004; 63: 571–3. [Case series, *n* = 12, II-3]

141. Newport DJ, Pennell PB, Calamaras MR et al. Lamotrigine in breast milk and nursing infants: Determination of exposure. *Pediatrics* 2008; 122(1): e223–31. [II-3]

142. Ohman I, Vitols S, Tomson T. Lamotrigine in pregnancy: Pharmacokinetics during delivery, in the neonate, and during lactation. *Epilepsia* 2000; 41(6): 709–13. [II-3]

143. Gentile S. Antipsychotic therapy during early and late pregnancy: A systematic review. *Schizophrenia Bulletin* 2010; 36(3): 518–44 [Largely nonrandomized prospective observational studies, II-2]

144. Habermann F, Fritzsche J, Fuhlbruck F et al. Atypical antipsychotic drugs and pregnancy outcome: A prospective cohort study. *J Clin Psychopharmacol* 2013; 33: 453–62. [Prospective cohort study, II-2]

145. Goldstein DJ, Corbin LA, Fung MC. Olanzapine-exposed pregnancies and lactation: Early experience. *J Clin Psychopharmacol* 2000; 20(4): 399–403. [Meta-analysis and review, III]

146. Gentile S. Infant safety with antipyschotic therapy in breast-feeding: A systematic review. *J Clin Psychiatry* 2008; 69(4): 633–4. [Systematic review]

147. Werremeyer A. Ziprasidone and citalopram use in pregnancy and lactation in a woman with psychotic depression. *Am J Psychiatry* 2009; 166(11): 1298. [II-3]

148. Schlotterbeck P, Saur R, Hiemke C et al. Low concentration of ziprasidone in human milk: A case report. *Int J Neuropsychopharmacol* 2009; 12(3): 437–8. [II-3]

149. Lutz UC, Hiemke C, Wiatr G et al. Aripiprazole in pregnancy and lactation: A case report. *J Clin Psychopharmacol* 2010; 30(2): 204–5. [II-3]

150. Campbell E, Kennedy F, Russell A et al. Malformation risks of antiepileptic drug monotherapies I pregnancy: Updated results from the UK and Ireland Epilepsy and Pregnancy Registers. *J Neurol Neurosurg Psychiatry* 2014; 85: 1029–34 [Prospective observational study, II-2]

151. Montouris G. Safety of the newer antiepileptic drug oxcarbazepine during pregnancy. *Curr Med Res Opin* 2005; 21(5): 693–701. [III]

152. Battino D, Tomson T. Management of epilepsy during pregnancy. *Drugs* 2007; 67(18): 2727–46. [Review, III]

153. Newport DJ. Atypical antipsychotic administration during late pregnancy: Placental passage and obstetrical outcomes. *Am J Psych* 2007; 164(8): 1214–20. [Prospective observational study, II-2]

154. Johnson KC, LaPrairie JL, Brennan PA. Prenatal antipsychotic exposure and neuromotor performance during infancy. *Arch Gen Psychiatry* 2012; 69(8): 787–94. [Prospective observational study, II-2]

155. Muldner-Nieckowski L, Cyranka K et al. Psychotherapy for pregnant women with psychiatric disorders. *Psychiatr Pol* 2015; 49(1): 49–56. [Review of literature, including *Cochrane* review of RCTs, III]

156. Stuart S, Koleva H. Psychological treatments for perinatal depression. *Best Pract Res Clin Obstet Gyn* 2014; 28(1): 61–70. [Review of literature, including *Cochrane* review of RCTs, III]

157. McGregor M, Coghlan M et al. The effect of physician-based cognitive behavioral therapy among pregnant women with depressive symptomatology: A pilot quasi-experimental trial. *Early Interv Psychiatry* 2014; 8(4): 348–57. [Nonrandomized controlled clinical trial, II-1]

158. Spinelli MG, Endicott J et al. A controlled clinical treatment trial of interpersonal psychotherapy for depressed pregnant women at 3 New York City Sites. *J Clin Psychiatry* 2013; 74(4): 393–9. [RCT, I]

159. Dimidjian S, Goodman SH et al. An open trial of mindfulness-based cognitive therapy for the prevention of perinatal depressive relapse/recurrence. *Arch Womens Ment Health* 2015; 18(1): 85–94. [Uncontrolled investigational study, II-3]

160. Miniati M, Callari A et al. Interpersonal psychotherapy for post-partum depression: A systemic review. *Arch Womens Mental Health* 2014; 17(4): 257–68. [Review included RCTs, I]

161. Nardi B, Laurenzi S et al. Is the cognitive-behavioral therapy an effective intervention to prevent postnatal depression? A critical review. *Int J Psychiatry Med* 2012; 43(3): 211–25. [Review of 8 RCTs, I]

162. Dennis C-L, Dowswell T. Psychosocial and psychological interventions for preventing postpartum depression. *Cochrane Database Syst Rev* 2013; 2: CD001134. [Review of RCTs, I]

163. Howell EA, Balbierz A, Wang J et al. Reducing postpartum depressive symptoms among Black and Latina mothers: A randomized controlled trial. *Obstet Gynecol* 2012; 119: 942–9. [RCT, *n* = 540]

164. Horowitz J, Murphy CA, Gregory K et al. Nurse home visits improve maternal/infant interaction and decrease severity of postpartum depression. *JOGNN* 2013; 42: 287–300. [RCT, *n* = 134]

165. Bulbul F, Copoglu US, Alpak G et al. Electroconvulsive therapy in pregnant patients. *Gen Hosp Psychiat* 2013; 35: 636–9. [Case series, III]

166. Marcus SM, Flynn HA, Tandon R et al. Treatment guidelines for depression in pregnancy. *Int J Gynecol Obstet* 2001; 72: 61–70. [Review, Expert opinion, III]

167. American Psychiatric Association Committee on Electroconvulsive Therapy. The practice of electroconvulsive therapy, recommendation for treatment, training, and privileging a task force report of the American Psychiatric Association. Washington, DC: American Psychiatric Association, 2001. [Organizational guidelines, Report of expert committee, III]

168. Rabheru K. The use of electroconvulsive therapy in special patient populations. *Can J Psychiat* 2001; 46: 710–9. [Review, Unable to access full article. Abstract says that review largely consists of case reports, case series, and a few controlled trials, III]

169. Leiknes KA, Cooke MJ, Jarosch-von Schweder L et al. Electroconvulsive therapy during pregnancy: A systematic review of case studies. *Arch Womens Ment Health* 2015; 18: 1–39. [Meta-analysis of case series, analysis of case studies, III]

170. Anderson EL, Reti IM. ECT in pregnancy: A review of the literature from 1941 to 2007. *Psychosom Med* 2009; 71(2): 235–42. [Review of articles, case reports, letters, chapters, and Web sites providing original contributions and/or summarizing prior data on ECT administration during pregnancy, III]

171. Saatcioglu O, Tomruk NB. The use of electroconvulsive therapy in pregnancy: A review. *Isr J Psychiat Relat Sci* 2011; 48: 6–11. [Review, Mostly case reports and case series reviewed, III]

172. American Academy of Pediatrics Committee on Drugs. Transfer of drugs and other chemicals into human milk. *Pediatrics* 2001; 108(3): 776–89. [III]

173. Yoshida K, Smith B, Craggs M et al. Investigation of pharmacokinetics and possible adverse effects in infants exposed to tricyclic antidepressants in breast-milk. *J Affect Disord* 1997; 43(3): 225–37. [II-3]

174. Wisner KL, Perel JM, Foglia JP. Serum clomipramine and metabolite levels in four nursing mother-infant pairs. *J Clin Psychiatry* 1995; 56(1): 17–20. [II-3]

175. Verbeeck RK, Ross SG, McKenna EA. Excretion of trazadone in breast milk. *Br J Clin Pharmacol* 1986; 22(3): 367–70. [II-3]

176. Schou M, Amdison A. Lithium and pregnancy. 3. Lithium ingestion by children breast-fed by women on lithium treatment. *Br Med J* 1973; 2(5859): 138. [II-3]

177. Stahl MM, Neiderud J, Vinge E. Thrombocytopenic purpura and anemia in a breast-fed infant whose mother was treated with valproic acid. *J Pediatr* 1997; 130(6): 1001–3. [II-3]

178. Meador KJ, Baker GA, Browning N et al. Effects of breastfeeding in children of women taking antiepileptic drugs. *Neurology* 2010; 75(22): 1954–60. [Prospective case-control study, II-2]

179. Whalley LJ, Blain PG, Prime JK. Haloperidol secreted in breast milk. *Br Med J (Clin Res Ed)* 1981; 282(6278): 1746–7. [Case report, II-3]

180. Yoshida K, Smith B, Craggs M et al. Neuroleptic drugs in breast-milk: A study of pharmacokinetics and of possible adverse effects in breast-fed infants. *Psychol Med* 1998; 28(1): 81–91. [Prospective case-control study, II-2]

181. Wiles DH, Orr MW, Kolakowska T. Chlorpromazine levels in plasma and milk of nursing mothers. *Br J Clin Pharmacol* 1978; 5(3): 272–3. [II-3]

182. Kris EB, Carmichael DM. Chlorpromazine maintenance therapy during pregnancy and confinement. *Psychiatr Q* 1957; 31: 690–5. [Case series, $n = 14$, II-3]

183. Brunner E, Falk DM, Jones M. Olanzapine in pregnancy and breastfeeding: A review of data from global safety surveillance. *BMC Pharmacol Toxicol* 2013; 14: 38 [Cohort study, II-2]

184. Barnas C, Bergant A, Hummer M et al. Clozapine concentrations in maternal and fetal plasma, amniotic fluid and breast milk. *Am J Psychiatry* 1994; 151(6): 945. [Case report, II-3]

185. Mendheker DN. Possible delayed speech acquisition with clozapine therapy during pregnancy and lactation. *J Neuropsychiatry Clin Neurosci* 2007; 19: 196–7. [Case report, II-3]

22

Smoking

Jorge E. Tolosa and David M. Stamilio

KEY POINTS

- **Smoking** is the most significant **preventable risk factor** associated with **low birth weight, preterm birth, perinatal death, and other maternal and perinatal complications.**
- Smoking cessation in pregnancy reduces the incidences of low birth weight, preterm birth, and perinatal death.
- Comprehensive screening for women who smoke in pregnancy is necessary by asking if she smokes; if no, need to ask if she smoked in the last year; if no, if she uses electronic cigarettes. If the answer to any of these three questions is yes, counseling and intervention are necessary.
- **Counseling** with behavioral and educational interventions is **associated with the highest cessation rates** (Tables 22.1 through 22.4).
- **Pharmacotherapies** are **either contraindicated or their safety and efficacy is insufficiently studied in pregnancy.**
- **Nicotine replacement therapies** are safe and effective in the general population, but there is **insufficient evidence** for recommending them in pregnant smokers.
- **Nicotine replacement therapy** is associated with known **adverse fetal effects.**
- The greatest risk of **relapse** occurs in the **postpartum period.**
- There is **insufficient evidence** to recommend specific **interventions to prevent relapse in pregnant and postpartum women.**

HISTORIC NOTES

The 20th century saw the rise of the manufactured cigarette and its popularity grew [1]. People continue to smoke despite known adverse effects [1].

DIAGNOSIS/DEFINITION

Tobacco dependence is a chronic addictive condition that requires repeated intervention for cessation.

EPIDEMIOLOGY/INCIDENCE

- Approximately 176 million adult women are daily smokers worldwide with the majority living in high-income countries. There is a very concerning trend toward increased rates of tobacco use, smoked and smokeless, in low- and middle-income countries [1,2].
- In 2012 in the United States, nearly 15 of every 100 adult women smoked [3].
- The incidence of smoking in pregnancy in the United States was 12.3% in 2010 (a significant reduction from 13.3% in 2000) [4]. Estimated smoking rates during pregnancy among reproductive-age women vary in different countries from 0.1% to 50% [5].
- By race, the highest prevalence of smoking occurs among those reporting multiple races and whites. The lowest prevalence occurs among Hispanics and Asian Pacific Islander women [6].
- **Women are more likely to stop smoking in pregnancy than in any other time in their lives** [7].
- Up to 46% of preconception smoking women stop smoking before their first antenatal visit or during pregnancy [8,9]. Pregnancy can help motivate women to quit smoking.
- **50% to 60% of those who quit smoking in pregnancy relapse within the first four months postpartum** [4,9].
- More than 300 million people around the world, the vast majority of whom live in South Asia, use smokeless tobacco products. Its use in high-income countries remains stable (not including use of vaporized nicotine delivery systems) [1]. Regional variations ranging from 6% (Congo) to 33.5% (Orissa, India) exist among low- and middle-income countries [10].
- Among high-income countries, both the United States and Sweden have seen increases in smokeless tobacco use that may offset decreases in cigarette consumption [11,12].

GENETICS

- Maternal genotype may affect the risk of low birth weight in cigarette smokers [13].
- The *CYP1A1*, *CYP2A6*, and *GSTT1* genes encode enzymes active in metabolism and elimination of toxic substances in cigarette smoke [13–15].
- In women who smoked, heterozygous variants of *CYP1A1* and absence of *GSTT1* genes resulted in significantly greater reductions in birth weight.

ETIOLOGY/BASIC PATHOLOGY

- Tobacco smoke has more than 7000 chemicals, hundreds of which are toxic and negatively affect almost all organ systems [1]. Nicotine and carbon monoxide are documented fetal neurotoxins and major compounds of tobacco smoke [16].
- Other toxic compounds include ammonia, polycyclic aromatic hydrocarbons, hydrogen cyanide, vinyl chloride, and nitrogen oxide.
- Smoking may result in damage to fetal genetic material [17].

Table 22.1 Multiple-Choice Questionnaire Improves Initial Disclosure Rates of Smoking/Tobacco Use

(A) I have **never** smoked or I have smoked less than 100 cigarettes in my lifetime.

(B) I stopped smoking **before** I found out I was pregnant, and I am not smoking now.

(C) I stopped smoking **after** I found out I was pregnant, and I am not smoking now.

(D) I smoke some now, but I **cut down** on the number of cigarettes I smoke since I found out I was pregnant.

(E) I smoke regularly now, about the **same** as before I found out I was pregnant.

(F) Do you use any other tobacco product? (If yes, inquire about details as above)

If the patient responds to B or C, reinforce her decision to quit, congratulate her on success of quitting, and encourage her to remain smoke free.

If the patient responds to D or E, she should be classified as a smoker. Document in the chart and proceed to the other 5As of the 5A framework: Ask, Advise, Assess, Assist, and Arrange.

Source: Adapted from Mullen PD, Carbonari JP, Tabak ER et al. *Am J Obstet Gynecol*, 165, 2, 409–13, 1991.

Table 22.2 "The 5 Rs" for Smokers Who Are Unwilling to Quit Smoking

1. ***Relevance:*** Motivational information to a patient is more effective if it is relevant to a patient's personal circumstances (i.e., smoking can cause adverse effects in pregnancy).
2. ***Risks:*** Stress the acute and long-term risks of smoking. Try to associate it with the patient's current health or illnesses.
3. ***Rewards:*** Ask the patient to identify potential benefits of smoking.
4. ***Roadblocks:*** Identify barriers or impediments to quitting and note treatment options that could address the barriers.
5. ***Repetition:*** Repeat the motivational intervention at each visit.

Table 22.3 "The 5 As" for Patients Who Are Willing to Quit Smoking

1. ***Ask:*** Tobacco status is inquired and documented. A multiple-choice question method (Table 22.1) improves disclosure.
2. ***Advise:*** Urge all tobacco users to quit in a clear, strong, personalized manner. Review risks associated with continued smoking.
3. ***Assess:*** Determine the patient's willingness to quit in the next 30 days. If unwilling, the provider should ask and advise at each subsequent office visit.
4. ***Assist:*** Provide smoking cessation materials and provide support. Help the patient develop a plan and provide practical counseling. Pharmacotherapy may be considered for the general population of smokers although there are insufficient data on safety and efficacy in pregnancy.
5. ***Arrange:*** Provide follow-up contact, either in person or by telephone, soon after the quit date and further follow-up encounters as needed. Congratulate success during each visit. Review circumstances if a relapse occurred and use it as a learning experience for the patient. Consider referral or more intensive treatment. Assess pharmacotherapy use and problems.

Table 22.4 Smoking Cessation Counseling (Skills Training and Problem Solving Techniques)

1. Identify activities that increase risk of smoking or relapse.
2. Explore coping skills and describe the time and nature of withdrawal.
3. Tell patients they may experience anxiety, frustration, depression, and intense cravings for cigarettes.
4. Withdrawal symptoms become manageable in a few weeks.
5. Make lifestyle changes to reduce stress and improve quality of life.
6. Minimize time spent in the company of smokers.
7. Provide as much information to the patient as possible: supplement discussions with pamphlets, booklets, videos, hotlines (1-800-QUIT-NOW), Internet, or support groups (http://www.smokefree.gov, http://www.smokefreefamilies.org).

Nicotine

- Crosses the placenta and can be detected in the fetal circulation at levels that exceed maternal circulation levels by 15% [18].
- **Amniotic fluid levels** are 88% **higher than maternal plasma levels** [18].
- Causes for impaired fetal oxygen delivery: vasoconstriction and changes in capillary volume and villous membrane contribute to abnormal gas exchange within the placenta [19].
- Fetal central nervous system effects: Abnormalities in cell proliferation and differentiation lead to decreased number of cells and eventually altered synaptic activity. Nicotine not only affects multiple transmitter pathways and influences the development of the fetal brain, but also affects eventual programming and synaptic competence [18].
- Studies have been focused on short-term developmental fetal effects, such as sympathetic activation, leading to increased fetal heart rate and reduction in fetal breathing movement. However, animal studies suggest that fetal exposure to nicotine alone impacts the incidence of late-onset diseases, including Type II diabetes, obesity, hypertension, neurobehavioral deficits, and respiratory dysfunction [20].

Carbon Monoxide

- Crosses the placenta rapidly and can be detected in the fetal circulation at **levels that exceed maternal circulation** levels by 15% [16,18].
- Exposure causes formation of carboxyhemoglobin. Carboxyhemoglobin is cleared slowly from the fetal circulation and diminishes tissue oxygenation via competitive inhibition with oxyhemoglobin. There is a left shift of the oxyhemoglobin dissociation curve, causing decreased availability of oxygen to the fetus [18].
- A 10% maternal carboxyhemoglobin concentration would result in a decrease of available oxygen supply to the fetus akin to a 60% reduction in blood flow.

Carcinogens

- More than 69 carcinogens have been identified in smoked tobacco products, compounds that are toxic to rapidly dividing cells.
- Levels of cyanide and at least one tobacco-specific carcinogen are higher in smokers [16,18].

RISK FACTORS

- Social disadvantage and lower education [6,21]
- High parity
- Low levels of social support and/or being without a partner
- Exposure to domestic violence
- Having a partner that smokes or exposure to second-hand smoke at home
- Depression, coexisting emotional/psychiatric problems, substance abuse
- Job strain
- Poor coping skills
- Younger age
- Fear of weight gain and dissatisfaction with female body image

Spontaneous quitters usually smoke less, are more likely to have stopped smoking before, are more likely to have a nonsmoker partner or have more support and encouragement at home for quitting, and have stronger beliefs about the dangers of smoking [7].

COMPLICATIONS Smoking is the **most modifiable risk factor associated with adverse pregnancy outcomes** [9,16,22–24].

- *Congenital anomalies*: There is sufficient evidence to infer a causal relationship between maternal smoking in early pregnancy and orofacial clefts and suggestive evidence of a possible association with clubfoot, gastroschisis, and atrial septal defects [25].
- *Low birth weight (LBW)*: Women who smoke are more likely to have a low-birth-weight baby (<2500 g) with relative risk (RR) of 1.3 to 10. The mean birth weight **deficit is 200 to 300 g** by term [3]. Up to 19% of term LBW has been attributed to smoking [26], including environmental tobacco smoke exposure in pregnancy [27]. Low birth weight causes a substantial economic burden [4].
- *Preterm birth*: Women who smoke are 1.3 to 2.5 times more likely to have a preterm delivery. It is estimated that up to 5%–8% of preterm births may be attributed to smoking [26].
- *Pregnancy loss*: Women who smoke are 1.2 to 3.4 times more likely to have an early pregnancy loss.
- *Premature rupture of membranes (PROM)*: Smoking increases PROM risk by at least twofold (RR of 1.9–4.2).
- *Preeclampsia*: Smoking in the second trimester of pregnancy is associated with a **reduced** incidence of preeclampsia. The mechanism for the risk reduction has not been elucidated [28].
- *Placental abruption*: Smoking increases the rate of abruption (RR of 1.4–2.5).
- *Placenta previa*: Smoking is associated with a higher rate of placenta previa (RR of 1.4–4.4).
- *Fetal death*: Large case-control and cohort studies suggest a fetal death RR of 1.2–1.4 associated with cigarette smoking.
- *Postnatal morbidities*: Increased risk of sudden infant death syndrome (SIDS), respiratory infections, reactive airway diseases, otitis media, bronchiolitis, short stature, hyperactivity, obesity, and decreased school performance. Up to 34% of cases of SIDS have been attributed to smoking [26].
- Health cost resulting from tobacco use includes annual expenditures for health and developmental problems of infants and children caused by mothers smoking or by being exposed to second-hand smoke during pregnancy or by kids being exposed to parents smoking after birth. Annual health expenditures solely from secondhand exposure amounted to $6.06 billion [29]. Also not included above are costs from smokeless chewing tobacco use, adult secondhand smoke exposure, or pipe/cigar smoking.
- *Maternal lifetime complications*: Atherosclerotic disease, lung cancer, chronic obstructive pulmonary disease, many forms of lung disease, increased risk of ectopic pregnancy, premature menopause, infertility and osteoporosis.

Smokeless Tobacco Complications

Study of adverse outcomes related to use of **smokeless tobacco** has been limited. One study of the Swedish Medical Birth Registry reports an increased risk of **stillbirth** with an adjusted odds ratio (OR) of 1.6 [CI 1.1–2.3] [30]. This finding had been previously reported in India [31].

Electronic Cigarettes (E-cigarettes) in Pregnancy

Although the prevalence of e-cigarette use has increased considerably since their U.S. market introduction in 2007, currently there are **very limited data on safety and efficacy of e-cigarettes to aid in achieving smoking cessation in pregnant patients.** In addition to nicotine, e-cigarettes contain nitrosamines, diethylene glycol, and variable amounts of trace metals, including arsenic, chromium, cadmium, nickel, and lead. Contents, including nicotine amount, of the e-cigarette vapor vary considerably among the multitude of products [32].

- Pregnancy and maternal affects of the non-nicotine vapor contents are unknown.
- Although e-cigarette nicotine pregnancy effects have not been studied, there is an abundance of animal research that provides evidence that prenatal nicotine exposure has deleterious effects to offspring, including lung disease, central nervous system abnormalities that produce adverse cognitive and neurologic outcomes, stress-induced cardiac defects, high blood pressure, and reduced fertility [32].
- In nonpregnant patients there are limited observational data that e-cigarettes may assist in reducing cravings and the number of cigarettes smoked per day, but efficacy has not been studied in pregnant patients [33–35].
- Misconceptions about e-cigarettes are common among pregnant women, including a belief (in 43%) that e-cigarettes are safer to the fetus than traditional cigarettes. These misconceptions could pose risks to both maternal and child health [36[.
- A survey indicates that misconceptions exist among obstetric providers with 29% responding that e-cigarettes are safer than traditional cigarettes and 14% reporting that e-cigarettes have no adverse health effects [37].

PREGNANCY CONSIDERATIONS

- Pregnancy is a **unique opportunity** for medical intervention and may be the only time women seek medical attention.

- Concerns over the dangers of smoking to the fetus may serve as a motivation for smoking cessation.
- Behavioral interventions, such as voucher based contingency management and other support/reward programs, have demonstrated efficacy in pregnancy [21,24,38].
- **The safety and efficacy of existing pharmacotherapies remain uncertain in pregnancy [7,8,24,25].**

PRINCIPLES

- Goal: Cessation of tobacco products use during pregnancy, postpartum, and for a lifetime.
- Tobacco-dependence treatments are clinically and economically effective relative to other medical disease prevention interventions [24].
- **Smoking cessation in pregnancy could prevent** 19% of low-birth-weight births, and 5%–8% of preterm deliveries [26]. Smoking in the third trimester has the greatest impact on birth weight [39,40].
- Women who quit smoking by the third trimester have birth weights similar to those of nonsmokers [39].

MANAGEMENT

- **Document smoking status at each initial prenatal visit** [41] (Table 22.1). **For tobacco users, document smoking status at each follow-up prenatal visit.**
- The patient should also be asked about the use of any other tobacco product.
- **Comprehensive screening for women who smoke in pregnancy is necessary by asking if she smokes; if no, need to ask if she smoked in the last year; if no, if she uses electronic cigarettes. If the answer to any of these three questions is yes, counseling and intervention are necessary.**
- Although most pregnant women do disclose their smoking, **urine cotinine testing** can aid in uncovering the few who do not disclose, which may help in managing smoking cessation [42]. Biochemical verification of smoking status is an important component to the research setting and may also help to guide intervention in the clinical setting.
- Smoking cessation programs are helpful compared to no intervention at all [7].
- Most smokers make many attempts to quit before success is achieved. First-time quitters need to be aware of this trend [24].
- Explore reasons for previous failures: assess for nonadherence to therapy and improper use of cessation aides in the past [24].
- Assess for psychosocial comorbidities that may affect smoking cessation [43].
- Address secondhand tobacco exposures.
- Comprehensive tobacco control programs, including **mass media campaigns**, are effective in changing smoking behavior in adults [44].
- Other political and social interventions, such as **smoking taxation, smoking bans in public and other places, bans on tobacco advertising and promotion, increases in retail prices, antismoking advocacy**, and other public policies, **are effective in smoking cessation** [45]. For example, smoke-free legislation, such as smoking bans

in workplaces, public places, or both, is associated with significant reductions in preterm births and child hospital admission for asthma [46].

THERAPY
Assessment for Intervention

- **Assess and document** tobacco use and status at every visit. This increases the likelihood of smoking-related discussions between patients and health care providers and increases cessation rates (Table 22.1). There is insufficient evidence (no RCTs) to assess the effect of an objective method to assess smoking status (e.g., a breath carbon monoxide monitor or cotinine measurement use systematically) in pregnant women.
- The five-step assessment (the 5Rs) can be used to address the patient who reports she is not willing to initiate smoking cessation (Table 22.2) [24].
- The **five-step intervention (the 5As)** is recommended in clinical practice to help pregnant women quit smoking if they verbalize a desire to quit in the next 30 days (Table 22.3) [24]. Use of the 5As is endorsed by The American College of Obstetricians and Gynecologists [9], the National Cancer Institute, and the British Thoracic Society.

Counseling

- Simple advice has a small but positive effect on cessation rates [47].
- All health care providers should give **clear, strong, and personalized advice** to every patient to quit smoking as evidence demonstrates that a **three-minute intervention** raises abstinence rates [24].
- Disclosure rates improve 40% if a **multiple-choice format for disclosure** is used rather than a yes/no format (Table 22.1) [41].
- **Oral and written advice at each prenatal visit** regarding the risk of smoking for mother and fetus and a plan to quit are effective (Table 22.4) [24].
- On the basis of >56 randomized controlled trials with >21,000 women participants, use of **support and reward techniques** to help quit smoking have been associated with a **23% decrease in continued smoking late in pregnancy** [48,49].
- **Voucher-based contingency management** is a promising mode of therapy as it has been associated with increased abstinence rates and improved neonatal birth weights [21,38]. **Financial incentives** significantly increase rates of smoking cessation [50]. For example, serial vouchers (£50–£400) provided for validated abstinence were associated with more smokers stopping smoking (22.5%) compared to controls (8.6%) [51]. In particular, reward-based programs (e.g., $800 for smoking cessation) are much more commonly accepted than deposit-based programs (e.g., refundable deposit of $150 plus $650 in reward payments), leading to higher rates of sustained abstinence from smoking. But smokers who were accepted to enroll were more likely to quit in the deposit-based program, e.g., if they stood to lose money if they failed [52].
- There is a strong dose–response relationship between the **duration and frequency of counseling** and its

effectiveness [24]. **Videos, self-help manuals, self-help guides, and telephone calls** are other examples of effective smoking cessation interventions [9].

- Women who received psychosocial interventions had an 18% reduction in preterm births and infants with low birth weight [8].
- **Telephone hotlines** (aka, QUITLINE; 1-800-QUIT-NOW) and **web information** (http://www.smokefree.gov; http://www. smokefreefamilies.org) sites are helpful and increase efficiency in implementing smoking cessation care in the clinical office. Patient uptake of QUITLINE assistance is improved with provider encouragement for its use and with proactive referral by the provider (with patient consent) rather than passively providing the phone number to a patient.
- Interventions to increase *smoking cessation among the partners* of pregnant women with the additional aim of facilitating cessation by the women themselves have been insufficiently studied [7]. Nonetheless, from studies including nonpregnant women, **partner smoking cessation counseling and intervention should be performed during pregnancy.**

Pharmacotherapies

Nicotine Replacement Therapy

- General
  - Nicotine replacement therapy (NRT) includes **patches, gums, inhalers, lozenges, and nasal spray.**
  - NRT is a part of an **effective strategy** to promote smoking cessation **in the general nonpregnant** population [53] (Table 22.5). All of the commercially available forms of NRT (gum, transdermal patch, nasal spray, inhaler, and sublingual tablets/lozenges) can help people who make a quit attempt to increase their chances of successfully stopping smoking. NRTs increase the rate of quitting by about 50% to 70%, regardless of setting. Quit rates are increased 43% with nicotine gum (4 mg more effective than 2 mg) and 66% with the patch. In fewer trials, nicotine inhaler, tablets/lozenges, and nasal spray are associated with 90% to 100% increase in quit rates. All of these effects were largely independent of the duration of therapy, the intensity of additional support provided, or the setting in which the NRT was offered [53].

- In pregnancy, NRT may help with nicotine withdrawal, has not yet been shown to have a significant advantage over other types of interventions, and has not been proven to effectively reduce smoking rates in pregnant smokers [54,55].
- In pregnancy, some studies show that NRT is associated with a trend for benefit [56–59], but safety/efficacy concerns remain [9,54].
- There is a risk of adverse effects of nicotine on the fetus through alterations in the uterine, placental, or cerebral blood flow [16–18,54].
- Animal studies suggest nicotine may be toxic to the developing central nervous system [16–18,54].
- The American College of Obstetricians and Gynecologists cautions that the use of NRT should only be undertaken with close supervision and after careful consideration and discussion with the patient of the known risk of continued smoking and the possible risks of NRT [9].
- There is **insufficient evidence to assure safety or efficacy of NRT in pregnancy with unclear ratio of risks and benefits** [7,9,54].
- Biomarkers such as plasma, urine, or salivary cotinine, thiocyanate, carboxyhemoglobin, or cotinine may be useful to monitor NRT use in pregnancy.
- Nicotine gum
  - FDA class C drug with known adverse effect on fetus in animal models.
  - Nicotine gum 2 mg was associated with a nonsignificant increase in smoking cessation from 10% to 13%, and significantly increased birth weights and gestational age at birth, compared to placebo [60].
- Nicotine patch
  - **Class D drugs with known human risk in pregnancies.**
  - Nicotine patches during pregnancy have been associated with nonsignificant effects on smoking cessation in pregnant smokers [58–61]. Multiple meta-analyses of studies on other nicotine replacement therapies in pregnancy indicate that there is insufficient evidence that NRT (mostly patch) is effective or safe in prenatal smoking cessation [54,62,63]. Myung et al. concluded that there is a mean 13% abstinence rate in their meta-analysis; they included seven studies of which one is a prospective study of bupropion, one is a quasi-RCT that studied use of a multimodal

Table 22.5 Nicotine Replacement Therapy

Only Recommended in the General Nonpregnant Population			
Nicotine Replacement	Dosing Regimen	Advantages	Disadvantages
Nicotine patch: Nicoderm CQ® or Nicotrol®	Nicoderm CQ®: 21 mg/day for 6 wk, then 14 mg/day for 2 wk, then 7 mg/day for 2 wk. Nicotrol: single dose patch for 16 hr/day for 6 wk (no tapering recommended)	Over-the-counter, easy dosing	Local skin irritation in up to 50% of users, insomnia with 24-hr dosing. 30–60 min required for maximal effect
Nicotine gum or lozenge	Start on quit date: 2 mg tab if <25 cigarettes per day or 4 mg tab if >25 cigarettes per day	Over-the-counter, satisfy oral behavior	Low nicotine levels, multiple dosing
Nicotine nasal spray	1–2 doses per hr × 3 mo. Most patients require from 7–40 sprays over 24 hr	Rapid and higher nicotine levels	Initial adverse effects may include throat and nasal irritation, discouraging use
Nicotine inhaler	10 mg cartridges used over 20 min. 6–16 cartridges per day	Substitutes for smoking behavior	Low nicotine levels

intervention, and the other five were RCTs of NRT that did not show an effect [63].

- No significant effect on birth weight or preterm birth were associated with nicotine patch use [56,58,61].
- Nicotine inhaler, tablets/lozenges, and nasal spray
  - Class D drugs with known human risk in pregnancies. There is insufficient evidence to assess the safety and effectiveness of nicotine inhaler, tablets/lozenges, and nasal spray, with no RCTs of pregnant smokers.
- Electronic cigarettes
  - There are insufficient data on the safety and smoking cessation efficacy of electronic cigarettes during pregnancy with no RCTs or well-designed observational studies in pregnant patients. Based on the lack of human data for safety and efficacy and potential for fetal harm from nicotine, electronic cigarettes are not recommended in pregnant or breast-feeding patients.

Bupropion HCl (Zyban®, Wellbutrin®)

- Class C drug in pregnancy with no known adverse fetal effects.
- There is an FDA black box warning relating to the risk of serious maternal neuropsychiatric events, including suicide.
- In controlled clinical trials, this antidepressant increased success for moderate to heavy smokers >15 cigarettes/day by 50% to 100% in the general population of nonpregnant smokers [7].
- **There are no published clinical trials to assess the safety and efficacy of bupropion as a smoking cessation intervention in pregnancy [7,55].**
- Dose: 300 mg/day (in two divided doses to minimize side effects). Start 2 weeks prior to anticipated quit date and continue up to 7 to 12 weeks.
- Advantages: in non-pregnant populations, non-nicotine may be used in combination with patch for greater efficacy, provides therapy for comorbid depression.
- Disadvantages: contraindicated if history of seizures, head trauma, alcohol abuse, or anorexia. Multiple-drug interactions with anti-HIV medications.

Varenicline (Chantix®)

- Class C drug in pregnancy with no adequate or well-controlled studies in pregnant women.
- There is an FDA black box warning relating to the risk of serious neuropsychiatric events, including suicide.
- Varenicline is a partial nicotine agonist sharing structural similarity with nicotine and competitively binds nicotine acetylcholine receptors.
- In nonpregnant populations, a meta-analysis of nine randomized trials shows that varenicline increased abstinence over placebo at six months or longer (RR 2.33 [CI 1.95–2.80]), over bupropion at one year (RR 1.52 [CI 1.22–1.88]), and over NRT at one year (RR 1.31 [CI 1.01–1.71]) [64].
- **There are no published clinical trials to assess the safety and efficacy of varenicline as a smoking cessation intervention in pregnancy [55].**
- As varenicline shares close structural similarity to nicotine and occupies identical receptor sites and safety data are nonexistent, it is not advisable to use varenicline during gestation and lactation.

- Disadvantages: risk of serious neuropsychiatric events; risk of angioedema and serious skin reactions; twofold increase in adverse effects of nausea, vomiting, vivid dreams, and constipation compared to placebo.

Combination Therapies

More studies are needed to determine whether combination therapy of NRT or other pharmaceutical in combination with behavioral modification, such as contingency management, increases efficacy or safety [2,59,64–66].

NOT Recommended

- *Clonidine*: Limited efficacy. Not superior to placebo. Side effects include drowsiness, fatigue, and dry mouth [67].
- *Nortriptyline (a tricyclic agent)*: Some benefit but not FDA approved. Class C drug. Unsafe in pregnancy [23,68].
- *Maclobemide (a monoamine oxidase inhibitor)*: Some benefit but not FDA approved. Class C drug. Uncertain safety in pregnancy [69].
- *Serotonin reuptake inhibitors*: Not effective [68].
- *Opioids*: Naloxone and naltrexone. Not effective [68].

Alternative Treatments

- *Acupuncture*: There is no clear evidence that acupuncture, acupressure, laser therapy, or electrostimulation are effective at smoking cessation [70].
- Hypnosis and meditation have been insufficiently studied in pregnant smokers to make a recommendation [9].
- *Stages of change* or *feedback* known as the transtheoretical model of behavior change assesses an individual's readiness to act on a new healthier behavior and provides strategies or processes of change to guide the individual through the stages of change to action and maintenance. It is composed of the following constructs: stages of change, processes of change, self-efficacy, decisional balance, and temptation; it has not shown benefit [7].

BREAST-FEEDING

- Abstinence increases breast-feeding initiation and duration [71–73].
- Breast-fed infants of smoking mothers have urinary cotinine levels 50 times higher than breast-fed infants of non-smoking mothers and levels are 10 times higher among bottle-fed infants of women who smoke [23]. Mothers unable to quit smoking in the postpartum period should still be encouraged to breast-feed. Mothers should be counseled to avoid smoking at home [72].
- Incentive-based programs for tobacco cessation may increase duration of breast-feeding [71].

POSTPARTUM

- **50% to 60% of those who quit smoking relapse in the first four months after delivery [4,9],** likely due to a period of great stress and emotional fluctuations.
- Risk factors for relapse include depression, family members who smoke, prepregnancy tobacco use, and low weight gain in pregnancy [73].

- Effective strategies for preventing relapse have not yet been identified [73,74], but smoking cessation interventions should be continued in collaboration with primary physicians and other health care personnel (Table 22.5).

PREVENTION
Relapse Prevention

- Insufficient evidence to support use of any specific interventions for helping smokers who have successfully quit for a short time and prevent relapse [73].
- It may be more efficient to focus efforts on initial cessation attempts [7,74].
- Biochemical markers may be used to monitor abstinence once cessation has occurred: carbon monoxide and urinary cotinine [23]. More research is needed to validate this method [7].

Reduce Initiation of Smoking

Prevent sale of tobacco to young people, prohibit smoking in public places, increase tobacco taxation, workplace smoking cessation programs, ban on tobacco sponsorship of sporting and cultural events [7,44,45,75].

Reduce Pregnancy Complications of Smoking

Vitamin C 1000 mg and vitamin E 400 IU supplementation has been associated with a reduction in placental abruption and preterm birth among smokers [76].

Reduce Consequences of Smoking in Newborn

Supplemental vitamin C 500 mg a day started before 22 weeks by smokers who decline to quit improves newborn pulmonary function tests and decreases wheezing through one year in the offspring [77].

FUTURE

- Development of clinical trials needed to determine safety and efficacy of pharmacologic therapies, such as nicotine replacement, bupropion, and varenicline [7–9,55].
- Clinical trials of alternative interventions, such as contingency management with use of incentives to reduce tobacco use in pregnancy.
- Evaluation of introduction and use of biochemical markers of exposure to tobacco in pregnancy and the postpartum period.
- Existing tobacco surveillance practices should be modified to include screening and intervention for use of smokeless tobacco and electronic cigarettes.
- Continued investigations should include an antinicotine vaccine—initial trials have not been successful—and new pharmaceutical approaches.

REFERENCES

1. Eriksen MP, Ross H et al. *The Tobacco Atlas*. 5th ed. Atlanta, GA: American Cancer Society, 2015. [Epidemiologic data]
2. Oncken CA, Dietz PM, Tong VT et al. Prenatal tobacco prevention and cessation interventions for women in low- and middle-income countries. *Acta Obstet Gynecol Scand* 2010; 89(4): 442–53. [Review; Tobacco prevention and intervention strategies for decreasing tobacco exposure and use in LMIC countries are reviewed. Recommendations of a working group of tobacco control and perinatal experts are reviewed. Key research priorities are identified, including evaluating the impact of tobacco control policy on tobacco use and SHS exposure among pregnant and reproductive-age women, development of culturally adapted interventions, exploring use of concurrent population level and clinical interventions for cessation among pregnant and reproductive-age women.]
3. Centers for Disease Control and Prevention. Current cigarette smoking among adults—United States, 2005–2014. *MMWR* 2015; 64(44): 1233–40. Accessed December 8, 2015.
4. Tong VT, Jones JR, Dietz PM et al. Trends in smoking before, during, and after pregnancy—Pregnancy Risk Assessment Monitoring System (PRAMS), United States, 40 sites, 2000–2010. *MMWR Surveill Summ* 2013; 62(SS06); 1–19. [Epidemiologic data]
5. WHO Report on the Global Tobacco Epidemic, 2009: Implementing smoke-free environments, World Health Organization, 2009. [III]
6. Centers for Disease Control and Prevention (CDC). Cigarette smoking among adults and trends in smoking cessation—United States, 2009. *MMWR* 2010; 59(35): 1135–40. [Epidemiologic data]
7. U.S. Department of Health and Human Services. *Women and smoking: A report of the Surgeon General*. Rockville: U.S. Department of Health and Human Services, Public Health Service, Office of the Surgeon General, 2001. [Epidemiologic data]
8. Chamberlain C, O'Mara-Eves A, Oliver S, Caird JR, Perlen SM, Eades SJ, Thomas J. Psychosocial interventions for supporting women to stop smoking in pregnancy. *Cochrane Database System Rev* 2013, 10: CD001055. doi:10.1002/14651858.CD001055.pub4. [77 trials > 29,000 women; Update of previous Cochrane Review on this topic. Seven new RCTs included and four cluster RCTs. Smoking cessation interventions significantly reduced low birth weight (RR 0.83; 0.73–0.95) and preterm birth (RR 0.86: 0.74–0.98) as well as smoking in pregnancy (RR 0.94: 0.93–0.96). Eight trials of smoking relapse prevention (n > 1000) showed no significant reduction in relapse rates.]
9. ACOG. Smoking cessation during pregnancy. ACOG Committee Opinion No. 471. *Obstet Gynecol* 2010; 116(5): 1241–4. [Guideline]
10. England LJ, Kim YS, Tomar SL et al. Non-cigarette tobacco use among women and adverse pregnancy outcomes. *Acta Obstet Gynecol* 2010; 89: 454–64. [Review]
11. Swedish National Board of Health and Welfare. Available at: http://www.socialstyrelsen.se/publikationer2008/2008-125-18. Accessed 2/16/2011. [II-2; Observational study spanning 2000–2006 of Swedish cigarette and other tobacco product use in pregnancy using national database.]
12. Connolly GN, Alpert HR. Trends in the use of cigarettes and other tobacco products, 2000–2007. *JAMA* 2008; 299: 2629–30. [II-3]
13. Wang X, Zuckerman B, Pearson C et al. Maternal cigarette smoking, metabolic gene polymorphism, and infant birth weight. *JAMA* 2002; 287: 195–202. [II-2, n = 741; Case-control study. Mothers of singleton live births were evaluated by PTB, LBW, and maternal smoking status in pregnancy. The maternal genotype of CYP1A1 and GSTT1 genotypes for each variable was assessed. The greatest reduction for birth weight was found in smoking mothers with CYP1A1 Aa/aa genotypes with absent GSTT1 (–1285 g, $p < 0.001$). LBW infants and PTB were also significantly more prevalent in pregnant smokers with CYP1A1 Aa/aa genotypes with absent GSTT1.]
14. Tyndale RF. Genetics of alcohol and tobacco use in humans. *Ann Med* 2003; 35: 94–121. [Review]
15. Aagaard-Tillery K, Spong KY, Thom E et al. Pharmacogenomics of maternal tobacco use: Metabolic gene polymorphisms and risk of adverse pregnancy outcomes. *Obstet Gynecol* 2010; 115: 568–77. [II-2, n = 1004; Case-control study of 502 smokers with

matched controls were evaluated for adverse pregnancy outcome on the basis of GSTT1 (del), CYP1A1, and CYP2A6 gene polymorphisms in mother and fetus. Fetal GSTT1(del) was significantly and specifically associated with low birth weight in pregnant smokers. Other adverse pregnancy outcomes were not associated with the gene polymorphisms studied.]

16. Dempsey DA, Benowitz NL. Risks and benefits of nicotine to aid smoking cessation in pregnancy. *Drug Safety* 2001; 24: 277–322. [Review]

17. Chica RA, Ribas I, Giraldo J et al. Chromosomal instability in amniocytes from fetuses of mothers who smoke. *JAMA* 2005; 293: 1212–22. [II-1]

18. Andres RL, Day MC. Perinatal complications associated with maternal tobacco use. *Semin Neonatol* 2000; 5: 231–41. [II-2]

19. Burton GJ, Palmer ME, Dalton KJ. Morphometric differences between the placental vasculature of non-smokers, smokers, and ex-smokers. *BJOG* 1989; 96(8): 907–15. [II-3]

20. Bruin JE, Hertzel CG, Holloway AC. Long-term consequences of fetal and neonatal nicotine exposure: A critical review. *Toxicol Sci* 2010; 116: 364–74. [Review; Landmark toxicology review with focus on long-term effects of developmental nicotine exposure using existing data from animal models. "The evidence provided in this review overwhelmingly indicates that nicotine should no longer be considered the 'safe' component of cigarette smoke. In fact, many of the adverse postnatal health outcomes associated with maternal smoking during pregnancy may be attributable, at least in part, to nicotine alone."]

21. Heil SH, Scott TL, Higgins ST. An overview of principles of effective treatment of substance use disorders and their potential application to pregnant cigarette smokers. *Drug Alcohol Depend* 2009; 104(Suppl. 1): S106–14. [Review; Novel interventions for tobacco cessation in pregnancy can be found from interventions for other substance use disorders. Promising modalities include contingency management using alternative reinforcers that accommodate deficits in D2 dopamine receptor density (voucher-based CM); medications modafinil and deprnyl; cotreatment of depression. "Certainly, pharmacotherapies offer a potentially important treatment strategy for improving outcomes with pregnant smokers." "The evidence that cessation medications increase abstinence rates in pregnant smokers is inconclusive."]

22. Castles A, Adams EK, Melvin CL et al. Effects of smoking during pregnancy: Five meta-analyses. *Am J Prev Med* 1999; 16(3): 208–15. [Meta-analyses, 34 articles; Meta-analyses of 34 articles culled from 124 evaluating relative risk and odds ratio for PPROM, preeclampsia, abruption, placenta previa, and ectopic pregnancy among smokers in pregnancy.]

23. *UpToDate: Smoking and Pregnancy*, 2011. Available at: http://www.uptodate.com. [Review]

24. Fiore MC, Jaen CR, Baker TB et al. *Treating Tobacco Use and Dependence: 2008 Update. Clinical Practice Guideline.* Rockville, MD: U.S. Department of Health and Human Services, Public Health Service, 2008. [Guideline]

25. U.S Department of Health and Human Services. *The Health Consequences of Smoking-50 Years of Progress.* A Report of the Surgeon General. Atlanta, GA: U.S. Department of Health and Human Services, Centers for Disease Control and Prevention, National Center for Chronic Disease Prevention and Health Promotion, Office of Smoking and Health, 2014. Printed with corrections, January 2014. [Review]

26. Dietz PM, England LJ, Shapiro-Mendoza CK et al. Infant morbidity and mortality attributable to prenatal smoking in the U.S. *Am J Prev Med* 2010; 39(1): 45–52. [II-2]

27. Heggard HK, Kjaergaad H, Moller LF et al. The effect of environmental tobacco smoke during pregnancy on birth weight. *Acta Obstet Gynecol Scand* 2006; 85(6): 675–81. [II-2]

28. Karumanchi SA, Levine RJ. How does smoking reduce the risk of preeclampsia? *Hypertension* 2010 May; 55(5): 1100–1. Published online 2010 Mar 15. doi:10.1161/HYPERTENSIONAHA.109.148973. PMCID: PMC2855389. [Review]

29. Health care costs updated to 2009 dollars, based on data in Behan, DF et al., *Economic Effects of Environmental Tobacco Smoke, Society of Actuaries*, March 31, 2005, https://www.soa.org/Research/Research-Projects/LifeInsurance/research-economic-effect.aspx. [Review]

30. Wikstrom AK, Cnattingius S, Stephansson O. Maternal use of Swedish snuff (snus) and risk of stillbirth. *Epidemiology* 2010; 21(6): 772–8. [II-2; Population-based cohort study of Swedish Medical Birth Register involving 7629 snuff users, 41,488 smokers of one to 10 daily cigarettes, and 17,014 smokers of greater than 10 cigarettes. Stillbirth rate was significantly elevated for snuff users [aOR 1.6 (1.1–2.3)], "light" smokers [aOR 1.4 (1.2–1.7)], and heavy smokers [aOR 2.4 (2.0–3.0)] when compared to 504,531 nonsmoking controls.]

31. Gupta PC, Subramoney S. Smokeless tobacco use and risk of stillbirth a cohort study in Mumbai, India. *Epidemiology* 2006; 17: 47–51. [II-1]

32. Suter MA, Mastrobattista J, Sachs M, Aagaard K. Is there evidence for potential harm of electronic cigarette use in pregnancy? Birth Defects Research (Part A) 2015; 103: 186–195. [II-3]

33. Siegel MB, Tanwar KL, Wood KS. 2011. Electronic cigarettes as a smoking-cessation: Tool results from an online survey. *Am J Prev Med* 40: 472–5. [II-3]

34. Polosa R, Caponnetto P, Morjaria JB et al. Effect of an electronic nicotine delivery device (e-Cigarette) on smoking reduction and cessation: A prospective 6-month pilot study. *BMC Public Health* 2011; 11: 786. [II-1]

35. Caponnetto P, Campagna D, Cibella F et al. EffiCiency and Safety of an electronic cigAreTte (ECLAT) as tobacco cigarettes substitute: A prospective 12-month randomized control design study. *PLoS One* 2013; 8: e66317. [RCT]

36. Mark KS, Farquhar B, Chisolm BM, Coleman-Cowger VH, Terplan M. Knowledge, attitudes, and practice of electronic cigarette use among pregnant women. *J Addict Med* 2015; 9: 266–72. [II-3]

37. England LJ, Anderson BL, Tong VTK et al. Screening practices and attitudes of obstetricians-gynecologists toward new and emerging tobacco products. *Am J Obstet Gynecol* 2014; 211: 695.e1–7. [II-3]

38. Heil SH, Higgins ST, Bernstein IM. Effects of voucher-based incentives on abstinence from cigarette smoking and fetal growth among pregnant women. *Addiction* 2008; 103(6): 1009–18. [I, $n = 82$ pregnant tobacco users; Participants were randomized to contingent or noncontingent voucher conditions. Vouchers could be exchanged for retail items during pregnancy and up to 12 weeks postpartum. Contingent vouchers were earned for biochemically verified abstinence. Participants in the contingent voucher system had significantly increased abstinence at delivery (41% vs. 10%; $p = 0.003$) and 12 weeks postpartum (24% vs. 3%; $p = 0.006$). Birth weight was significantly increased (3355 g vs. 3102 g, $p = 0.06$). Trend toward lower % LBW and % PTB was observed but not significant. Cost of incentive was $334 per participant.]

39. Lieberman E, Gremy I, Lang JM et al. Low birth weight at term and timing of fetal exposure to maternal smoking. *Am J Public Health* 1994; 84(7): 1127–31. [II-2]

40. McCowan LM, Dekker GA, Chan E et al. Spontaneous preterm birth and small for gestational age infants in women who stop smoking early in pregnancy: Prospective cohort study. *BMJ* 2009; 338: b1081. [II-2, $n = 2504$; Prospective cohort study. No differences noted in rate of PTB or SGA between nonsmokers and cessation in early pregnancy. Tobacco users screening positive at 14 to 16 wga had higher rates of spontaneous PTB (10% vs. 4%, $p = 0.006$) and SGA (17% vs. 10%, $p = 0.03$) than those who accomplished cessation in early pregnancy. Rates of adverse effects may be mitigated with cessation prior to 14 wga.]

41. Mullen PD, Carbonari JP, Tabak ER et al. Improving disclosure of smoking by pregnant women. *Am J Obstet Gynecol* 1991; 165(2): 409–13. [II-3]

42. Swamy GK, Reddick KL, Brouwer RJ et al. Smoking prevalence in early pregnancy: Comparison of self-report and anonymous urine cotinine testing. *J Matern Fetal Neonatal Med* 2011; 24(1): 86–90. [II-3]

43. Kleber HD, Weiss RD, Anton RF Jr et al. Treatment of patients with substance use disorders, second edition. American Psychiatric Association. *Am J Psychiatry* 2007; 164(4 Suppl.): 5–123. [Guideline]

44. Bala M, Strzeszynski L, Cahill K. Mass media interventions for smoking cessation in adults. *Cochrane Database Syst Rev* 2008; (1): CD004704. [Meta-analysis; 11 "campaigns"]

45. Ali MK, Koplan JP. Promoting health through tobacco taxation. *JAMA* 2010; 303(4): 357–8. [Review III]

46. Been JV, Nurmatov UB, Cox B et al. Effect of smoke-free legislation on perinatal and child health: A systematic review and meta-analysis. *Lancet* 2014; 383(9928): 1549–60. [Meta-analysis, 11 studies]

47. Lancaster T, Bergson G, Stead LF. Physician advice for smoking cessation. *Cochrane Database Syst Rev* 2008; (4): CD000165. [Meta-analysis; 41 trials, n = 31,000 nonpregnant participants; Brief advice versus no advice detected a significant increase in quitting (RR 1.66; 1.42–1.94, 17 trials). More intensive intervention increased estimated effect (RR 1.84; 1.60–2.13, 11 trials). A small benefit of more intensive intervention over brief advice was noted. Assuming an unassisted quit rate of 2% to 3%, quit rates may increase further 1% to 3%.]

48. Sexton M, Hebel JR. A clinical trial of change in maternal smoking and its effect on birth weight. *JAMA* 1984; 251(7): 911–5. [RCT]

49. Donatelle RJ, Prows SL, Champeau D et al. Randomised controlled trial using social support and financial incentives for high risk pregnant smokers: Significant Other Supporter (SOS) program. *Tob Control* 2000; 9(Suppl. 3): iii67–69. [RCT]

50. Volpp KG, Troxel AB, Pauly MV et al. A randomized, controlled trial of financial incentives for smoking cessation. *N Engl J Med* 2009; 360: 699–709. [RCT, n = 878 nonpregnant adults]

51. Tappin D, Bauld L, Purves D et al. Financial incentives for smoking cessation in pregnancy: Randomised controlled trial. *BMJ* 2015; 350: h134. [RCT, n = 612]

52. Halpern SD, French B, Small DS et al. Randomized trial of four financial-incentive programs for smoking cessation. *NEJM* 2015; 372: 2108–17. [RCT, 2538]

53. Stead LF, Perera R, Bullen C et al. Nicotine replacement therapy for smoking cessation. *Cochrane Database Syst Rev* 2008; (1): CD000146. [Meta-analysis; 111 trials, N > 40,000 nonpregnant adults; NRT of any type resulted in abstinence compared to control (RR 1.58; 1.50–1.66): Nicotine gum (RR 1.43; 1.33–1.53), nicotine patch (RR 1.66; 1.53–1.81), nicotine inhaler (RR 1.90; 1.36–2.67), lozenge (RR 1.2.00; 1.63–2.45), and nasal spray (RR 2.02; 1.49–3.73); 4 mg gum was associated with significant benefit when compared to 2 mg gum in heavy smokers. Quit rates were increased by 50% to 70% with the addition of an NRT.]

54. Lumley J, Chamberlain C, Dowswell T, Oliver S, Oakley L, Watson L. Interventions for promoting smoking cessation during pregnancy. *Cochrane Database System Rev* 2009; 3: CD001055. doi:10.1002/14651858.CD001055.pub3. [Meta-analysis; Seventy-two trials are included. Fifty-six randomized controlled trials (over 20,000 pregnant women) and nine cluster-randomized trials (over 5000 pregnant women) provided data on smoking cessation outcomes. There was a significant reduction in smoking in late pregnancy following interventions [risk ratio (RR) 0.94, 95% confidence interval (CI) 0.93 to 0.96]. Smoking cessation interventions reduced low birthweight (RR 0.83, 95% CI 0.73 to 0.95) and preterm birth (RR 0.86, 95% CI 0.74 to 0.98), and there was a 53.91g (95% CI 10.44 g to 95.38 g) increase in mean birthweight.]

55. Oncken CA, Kranzler HR. What do we know about the role of pharmacotherapy for smoking cessation before or during pregnancy? *Nicotine Tob Res* 2009; 11: 1265–73. [Review; NRT has not been demonstrated to have an advantage over placebo treatment. Studies are limited to small sample size and/or poor medication compliance. NRT use is associated with increased birth weight. Psychosocial interventions should be first treatment option for pregnant smokers.]

56. Pollack KJ, Oncken CA, Lipkus IM et al. Nicotine replacement and behavioral therapy for smoking cessation in pregnancy. *Am J Prev Med* 2007; 33: 297–305. [RCT, n = 181; Women were randomized to a self-selected NRT arm (patch, gum, lozenge, or no therapy arm) (N = 122) versus behavioral modification (N = 59). This trial was stopped by DSMB after an a priori criterion of a near-twofold increase in adverse pregnancy outcomes in the NRT arm (30% vs. 17%). Further analysis revealed that this effect was no longer present when controlling for history of preterm birth (32% vs. 12%, respectively).]

57. Wisborg K, Henriksen TB, Secher NJ. A prospective intervention study of stopping smoking in pregnancy in a routine antenatal care setting. *BJOG* 1998; 105(11): 1171–6. [RCT, n = 250]

58. Kapur B, Hackman R, Selby P et al. Randomized, double blind, placebo-controlled trial of nicotine replacement therapy in pregnancy. *Curr Ther Res* 2001; 62(4): 274. [RCT, n = 30]

59. Hegaard H, Hjaergaard H, Moller L et al. Multimodel intervention raises smoking cessation rate during pregnancy. *Acta Obstet Gynecol Scand* 2003; 82: 813–9. [RCT]

60. Oncken C, Dornelas E, Greene J et al. Nicotine gum for pregnant smokers: A randomized controlled trial. *Obstet Gynecol* 2008; 112: 859–67. [RCT, n = 194; RCT women randomized to 2 mg nicotine gum (N = 100) versus placebo (N = 94) for six weeks. NRT group was associated with higher birth weight, decreased LBW, and lower risk of delivery prior to 37 weeks' gestation. The mean gestational age at delivery was clinically significant (38.9 vs. 38 weeks, p < 0.014). The cessation rate was low (13% NRT vs. 9.6% on placebo) at six weeks. This trial remained underpowered and was suspended by the DSMB for poor cessation.]

61. Wisborg K, Henriksen TB, Jespersen LB et al. Nicotine patches for pregnant smokers: A randomized controlled study. *Obstet Gynecol* 2000; 96: 967–71. [RCT, n = 250; Behavior modification therapy combined with either 15-mg NRT patch for eight weeks followed by 10-mg NRT patch for three weeks (N = 120) or placebo (N = 122). No differences in birth weight, LBW, preterm birth with adequate power. Only 11% of those in the treatment group completed a full course of therapy.]

62. Coleman T, Chamberlain C, Cooper S, Leonardi-Bee J. Efficacy and safety of nicotine replacement therapy for smoking cessation in pregnancy: Systematic review and meta-analysis. *Addiction* 2011 Jan; 106(1): 52–61. doi:10.1111. [Meta-analysis]

63. Myung S, Ju W, Jung H, Park C, Oh S, Seo H, Kim H. Efficacy and safety of pharmacotherapy for smoking cessation among pregnant smokers: A meta-analysis. *BJOG* 2012; 119: 1029–39. [Meta-analysis]

64. Cahill K, Stead LF, Lancaster T. Nicotine receptor partial agonists for smoking cessation. *Cochrane Database Syst Rev* 2008; (3): CD006103. [Meta-analysis; nine RCTs, n = 7627; Meta-analysis of nine randomized trials of varenicline increased abstinence over placebo at six months or longer (RR 2.33; 1.95–2.80), over bupropion at one year (RR 1.52; 1.22–1.88), and over NRT at one year (RR 1.31; 1.01–1.71). There is a need for independent community-based trials of varenicline to test its efficacy and safety in smokers with varying comorbidities and risk patterns. There is a need for further trials of the efficacy of treatment extended beyond 12 weeks.]

65. Simon JA, Duncan C, Carmody TP et al. Bupropion for smoking cessation: A randomized trial. *Arch Intern Med* 2004; 164(16): 1797–803. [RCT]

66. Jorenby DE, Leischow SJ, Nides MA et al. A controlled trial of sustained-release bupropion, a nicotine patch, or both for smoking cessation. *N Engl J Med* 1999; 340(9): 685–91. [RCT]

67. Gourlay SG, Stead LF, Benowitz NL. Clonidine for smoking cessation. *Cochrane Database Syst Rev* 2004; (3): CD000058. [Meta-analysis]

69. Hughes JR, Stead LF, Lancaster T. Antidepressants for smoking cessation. *Cochrane Database Syst Rev* 2007; (1): CD000031. [Meta-analysis; 66 trials; Meta-analysis of 66 trials using antidepressants for smoking cessation. Bupropion (36 trials, n = 11,140,

RR 1.69; 1.53–1.85), nortryptilene (6 trials, $n = 975$, RR 2.03; 1.48–2.78); both increased long-term cessation. Insufficient evidence to demonstrate any additional benefit with the addition of NRT to these medications. There is no significant effect of SSRIs, MAOi, or venlafaxine.]

68. David S, Lancaster T, Stead LF. Opioid antagonists for smoking cessation. *Cochrane Database Syst Rev* 2001; (3): CD003086. [Meta-analysis; four trials; No significant differences in long-term (6 months) abstinence rates.]

70. White AR, Rampes H, Campbell JL. Acupuncture and related interventions for smoking cessation. *Cochrane Database Syst Rev* 2006; (1): CD000009. [Meta-analysis; 24 studies; No significant differences in short-or long-term abstinence rates.

71. Higgins TM, Higgins ST, Heil SH et al. Effects of cigarette smoking cessation on breastfeeding duration. *Nicotine Tob Res* 2010; 12(5): 483–88. [II-1, $n = 158$; RCT where first 32 participants were assigned (not randomized) to their treatment or control group for pilot study purposes. Participants received incentive-based intervention or routine administration of comparable vouchers (control). Women receiving incentive-based treatment have significantly higher breastfeeding duration 35% versus 17% at 12 weeks postpartum ($p = 0.002$) as well as abstinence 25% versus 3% ($p < 0.01$).]

72. Gartner L, Morton J, Lawrence RA et al. American Academy of Pediatrics policy statement: Breastfeeding and the use of human milk. *Pediatrics* 2005; 115(2): 496–506. [Guideline]

73. Soloman LJ, Higgins ST, Heil SH et al. Predictors of postpartum relapse to smoking. *Drug Alcohol Depend* 2007; 90(2–3): 224–7. [II-3, $n = 87$; Multivariate analyses of predictors of postpartum relapse of women who quit smoking in pregnancy. Relapse rate of 48% within 6 months postpartum. Friends/family members who smoke, heavy prepregnancy smoking, higher depression scores, and lower weight gain concerns were associated with increased risk of relapse. Interventions at targeting postpartum relapse include reducing postpartum depression.]

74. Hajek P, Stead LF, West R. Relapse prevention interventions for smoking cessation. *Cochrane Database Syst Rev* 2009; (1): CD003999. [Meta-analysis, 36 RCTs; There is insufficient evidence to support the use of any specific behavioral or pharmacologic intervention for helping smokers who have successfully quit for a short time and avoid relapse.]

75. Cahill K, Moher M, Lancaster T. Workplace interventions for smoking cessation 2008. *Cochrane Database Syst Rev* 2008; (4): CD003440. [51 studies]

76. Abramovici A, Gandley RE, Clifton RG, Leveno KJ, Myatt L, Wapner RJ, Thorp JM Jr, Mercer BM, Peaceman AM, Samuels P, Sciscione A, Harper M, Saade G, Sorokin Y, for the Eunice Kennedy Shriver National Institute of Child Health Human Development Maternal-Fetal Medicine Units Network. Prenatal vitamin C and E supplementation in smokers is associated with reduced placental abruption and preterm birth: A secondary analysis. *BJOG* 2015; 122: 1740–7. [Secondary analysis of RCT, $n = 9969$]

77. McEvoy CT, Schilling D, Clay N, Jackson K, Go MD, Spitale P, Bunten C, Leiva M et al. Vitamin C supplementation for pregnant smoking women and pulmonary function in the newborn infants. A randomized clinical trial. *JAMA* 2014; 311: 2074–82. [RCT, $n = 179$]

23

Drug abuse

Neil S. Seligman

KEY POINTS

- Estimates of the incidence of drug abuse during pregnancy, based on patient interview and toxicologic testing, vary from 0.4% to 27%. Polysubstance abuse (including tobacco and alcohol) is common.
- All pregnant women should be screened for illicit drug using tools such as the **4Ps** (Table 23.3).
- Treatment of substance-abusing pregnant women requires a multidisciplinary team.
- Promoting **preconception behavioral change** or, ideally, strategies to prevent initiation of substance use is preferred over drug abuse treatment during pregnancy.

Marijuana

- Marijuana is the most commonly used drug during pregnancy; approximately one in 20 pregnant women use marijuana.
- The effects of marijuana exposure are mild, limited to decreased length of gestation (0.8 weeks) and birth weight (172 g), and are likely the result of alterations in hemodynamics. Marijuana use during pregnancy may increase the risk of sudden infant death syndrome.
- Marijuana is believed to alter fetal brain development by binding to opioid receptors in the central nervous system, which are present as early as the 14th week of gestation.

Opioids

- Infections (including hepatitis, HIV, and others) account for the majority of complications related to parenteral opioid use.
- **Neonatal withdrawal from opioids occurs in 60% to 70% of exposed neonates.**
- **Oral replacement therapy is the standard treatment for opioid addiction**. Replacement therapy diminishes the risks of perinatal transmission of hepatitis C and HIV and increases utilization of prenatal care among other benefits. Higher recidivism rates and an increased rate of complications are seen with detoxification. **Methadone** (often preferred) **and buprenorphine are the most common options for replacement therapy**. Methadone is titrated to the effective dose that prevents withdrawal symptoms.
- Opioids decrease baseline fetal heart rate and variability. Optimal timing of a nonstress test or biophysical profile is at least four to six hours following the last dose of medication.

Cocaine

- Systemic effects of cocaine include hypertension, tachycardia, and mydriasis. Pregnancy is associated with increased sensitivity of the cardiovascular system to the harmful effects of cocaine, such as arrhythmias and myocardial infarction.
- Fetal and neonatal effects of cocaine include higher rates of congenital malformations, intrauterine growth restriction, low birth weight (<2500 g), small for gestational age, preterm premature rupture of membranes, preterm birth, abruption, stillbirth, and emergent delivery. Cocaine exposure also results in shorter gestation, smaller head circumference, decreased length, and neonatal withdrawal.
- Interventions for cocaine dependence primarily involve **psychosocial therapies**; currently, there are no Food and Drug Administration (FDA)-approved pharmacotherapies for treatment of cocaine dependence during pregnancy.

Others

- The incidence of amphetamine use during pregnancy varies from 0.1% to 1.0% whereas methamphetamine use may be up to 5.2% in some high prevalence areas. Ecstasy use among pregnant women varies from 0.6% to 8.8%.
- Amphetamine and methamphetamine use during pregnancy has been associated with an increased risk of preterm birth, alterations in fetal and neonatal size, neonatal withdrawal, and long-term developmental consequences. The complications of ecstasy use during pregnancy are not well characterized.
- Benzodiazepine exposure is associated with preterm birth, delivery by cesarean section, low birth weight, low Apgar score, and neonatal sedation and withdrawal.
- Phencyclidine does not appear to cause congenital malformations but is associated with a higher incidence of prematurity, intrauterine growth restriction, low birth weight, and small for gestational age infants. Developmental effects, including neurological effects, behavioral problems, and sleep disturbances, have been noted.
- An increased risk of limb reduction defects, central nervous system anomalies, and neural tube defects has been reported in association with lysergic acid diethylamide (LSD) use.

BACKGROUND

Drug abuse is a chronic medical illness. In general, continued use of harmful substances is not intended to harm the fetus

Table 23.1 Definitions

- ***Substance use disorder***: defined by the *DSM-V* as variable consumption resulting in significant impairment or distress including: 1) social or interpersonal consequences; 2) failure to fulfill obligations at work, school, or home; 3) physically hazardous situations; 4) tolerance; 5) withdrawal; 6) tolerance; 7) substance is taken in larger amounts and for longer than was expected; 8) persistent desire or unsuccessful efforts to cut down; 9) excessive time is spent in obtaining or using the substance; 10) important work, recreation, or social life activities are reduced or given up; 11) substance use is continued despite knowledge of the adverse consequences; 12) craving or strong desire or urge to use a specific substance.
  Mild: 2–3 of the above within a 12 month period; replaces "*abuse*."
  Moderate (4–5) or severe (≥6): of the above within a 12 month period; replaces "*substance dependence*."
- ***Physical dependence***: adaptation to use such that withdrawal symptoms manifest with abrupt discontinuation or tolerance.
- ***Addiction***: a primary chronic disease characterized by impaired control over behavior, drug craving, inability to consistently abstain from drug use, and diminished recognition of significant problems with behaviors and interpersonal relationships.

but rather a response to acute psychological or physical need [1]. In current terminology, the term "substance use disorder" has replaced "abuse" and "addiction" (Table 23.1). There is no safe pattern of illicit substance use.

INCIDENCE

Despite well-established risks, the prevalence of illicit substance use by reproductive-age women has steadily increased. Substance use by reproductive-age females represents possible teratogenic exposures. Estimates of use in the general population are available from the 2013 National Survey on Drug Use and Health (NSDUH) [2]:

- 24.6 million Americans (9.4%) aged 12 and older used drugs in the past month.
- 6.9 million were diagnosed with dependence or abuse of illicit drugs.
- Most commonly used illicit drugs were marijuana, nonmedical use of psychotherapeutics (narcotics, tranquilizers, stimulants, and sedatives), cocaine, and hallucinogens.
- Substance abuse is lower in females (7.3%) than in males (11.5%).

During pregnancy, substance use ranges from **0.4%** to **27%** depending on the population surveyed based on patient interviews and urine toxicology testing at the initial prenatal visit and delivery [3]. According to the 2013 NSDUH [2],

- **5.4% of pregnant women aged 15–44 reported current illicit drug use**, corresponding to >200,000 infants born annually exposed to illicit drugs in utero.
- Illicit drug use during pregnancy is more prevalent among younger women (15–17 years old: 14.6% vs. 18–25: 8.6% and 26–44: 3.2%).
- **Fewer** women reported current drug use **during the third trimester** compared to the first or second trimester (2.4% vs. 9.0% and 4.8%, respectively).

Estimates based on surveys may underestimate the rate of substance abuse by as much as 50% or more. In a study of universal screening for substance abuse in an inner city population, **19%** of women screened positive for one or more substances at the time of admission to labor and delivery, of which only 32.6% gave a history of drug use [4].

RISK FACTORS

Attributes common among pregnant substance-abusing women include a history of domestic violence, sexual assault, poverty, poor self-esteem, and difficulty with relationships. The use of multiple substances at the same time is common. Substance use increases the risk of sexually transmitted infections, including hepatitis C and HIV, endocarditis, and tuberculosis [5] through needle sharing, risky sexual behaviors (e.g., unprotected intercourse, sex with multiple partners, trading drugs for sex, and prostitution), and incarceration (resulting from the purchase and sale of illicit drugs, prostitution, or theft). Drug-dependent women have higher rates of psychopathology, which may impede optimal management. Factors that may heighten the suspicion of drug abuse are shown in Table 23.2.

WORKUP

Options for the evaluation of illicit substance use include interview, questionnaires, and chemical tests. Use of open-ended questions and motivational interviewing techniques may be helpful [6]. The **"4Ps"** is a frequently recommended screening tool for pregnant women (Table 23.3) [7]. T-ACE, TWEAK (both specifically designed for pregnant women), CAGE-AID, CRAFFT (for adolescents), and The Drug Abuse Screening Test (DAST) are other available options.

Table 23.2 Common Signs and Symptoms That Should Indicate a High Risk of Drug Use

- No prenatal care, limited prenatal care (three or fewer prenatal visits prior to 28 weeks gestation), or late prenatal care (initiation of prenatal care after the first trimester)
- Multiple missed prenatal care appointments
- Impaired school or work performance
- History of unexplained adverse obstetrical or neonatal outcomes (e.g., abruption)
- Children with neurodevelopmental problems
- Children not currently living in the home or involvement by child protective services
- Medical history of substance abuse or substance abuse-related problems
- Women on maintenance therapy with either methadone or buprenorphine
- Family history of substance abuse
- Frequent encounters with law enforcement
- Partners who have a history of substance abuse
- Homelessness
- Physical stigmata of substance use (track marks, related infections) or withdrawal
- History of physical or sexual abuse
- Sudden behavioral changes or inappropriate behavior, including disorientation, somnolence, loose associations, unfocused anger
- Signs or symptoms of preterm labor or abruption
- Severe hypertension (blood pressure >160/110 mmHg)
- Unexplained vaginal bleeding or fetal demise

Table 23.3   4Ps

1. **P**arents: Did any of your parents have a problem with alcohol or other drug use?
2. **P**artner: Does your partner have a problem with alcohol or drug use?
3. **P**ast: In the past, have you had difficulties in your life because of alcohol or other drugs, including prescription medications?
4. **P**resent: In the past month have you drank any alcohol or used other drugs?

Scoring: Any "yes" should trigger further questions.

Source: Adapted from ACOG CO 524 and Ewing H. A practical guide to intervention in health and social services with pregnant and post-partum addicts and alcoholics: *theoretical framework, brief screening tool, key interview questions, and strategies for referral to recovery resources.* In Martinez (CA): The Born Free Project, Contra Costa County Department of Health Services; 1990.

Chemical tests using samples of maternal blood, hair, saliva, sweat, or urine or fetal/neonatal specimens (amniotic fluid, cord blood, meconium, blood, hair, or urine) are available for most illicit substances. Verbal consent should be obtained before obtaining these tests. **Urinalysis** is the most commonly used laboratory screening for substance use. **Providers should be aware of the strengths and limitations of this test.** False negative test results can occur when drug ingestion occurred too recently for the substance to appear in the urine, when sufficient time has passed to allow complete drug clearance, or with dilute urine (Table 23.4). False positive results can be as high as 5% [8]. For example, labetalol may create a false positive result on urine drug screening for amphetamines [9]. Not all substances can be detected with a typical urine drug screen [8]. For example, more specific testing may be required when oxycodone use is suspected. Urine drug testing cannot diagnose a drug-use disorder or its severity, nor can it determine frequency, amount, or route of use [8]. The physician should also be aware of the limitations of neonatal testing. Drugs may be present in meconium for months, making it difficult to differentiate between the occasional user, continued substance use, and women on treatment (e.g., methadone maintenance therapy) with no recent substance use. Maternal self-report alone underestimates the prevalence of substance abuse; however, routine urine drug screening is not currently recommended.

When maternal history and/or laboratory tests are positive for illicit drug use, a complete drug history should be

Table 23.4   Length of Time Drugs Are Present in Urine

Opioids	
Codeine	2 days
Morphine	2 days
Heroin	1 day
Methadone	3 days
Cocaine	1–3 days
Amphetamines	2 days
Benzodiazepines	
Single use	3 days
Chronic use	6 weeks
Marijuana	
Single use	3 days
Chronic use	30 days

obtained for each substance. The acronym "DRUG" may be useful to remember the components of the drug history.

> **D**rug name
> **R**oute (e.g., intravenous, oral)
> **U**sed how much, how often
> **G**otten how (e.g., prostitution, theft)

The initial evaluation of substance-abusing pregnant women presenting to the labor and delivery unit for any reason should include a urine drug screen, ideally with consent.

MANAGEMENT

In general, pregnant women are highly motivated to decrease or stop using illicit substances to avoid potential negative consequences for the fetus. Women who acknowledge their use of illicit substances should be counseled and offered treatment as necessary [10,11]. Treatment of substance-abusing pregnant women requires a **multidisciplinary team**. Providers must be aware of the specific needs of the pregnant substance abuser. Management options include **psychosocial treatments** [3] **such as motivational interviewing** [6], **cognitive behavioral therapies, 12-step approaches, community/social network approaches contingency management, pharmacologic therapies, and inpatient treatment. Contingency management strategies (rewards for good behavior) are effective in improving retention of pregnant women in illicit drug treatment programs** [12].

PREVENTION

The prevention of drug abuse is paramount to drug abuse treatment. Prevention strategies are focused on **increasing public awareness of the harmful effects of drug use through advertising campaigns, school programs, and encouraging parents to educate their children. Physicians** should take an active role in drug abuse prevention by **routinely counseling their patients about the negative consequences of drug abuse.**

PRECONCEPTION COUNSELING

Substance use is an important component of the history in women seeking preconception counseling because fetal drug exposure is preventable. Women with a positive history and/or laboratory testing for substance abuse should be counseled about the reproductive effects of the specific substances along with the risks and benefits of pharmacological and nonpharmacologic treatment. Women should be encouraged to postpone conception until after initiating or completing drug treatment. Because of the reproductive risks of certain pharmacological treatments, reliable methods of contraception should be encouraged. Anovulatory cycles and infertility are more common in substance-abusing women, especially with opioid use; however, it should be stressed that pregnancy can definitely occur without adequate contraception. There is some evidence that **prepregnancy health promotion is associated with a positive effect on maternal behavior change (specifically binge drinking)** but more research is needed [13] (see Chapter 1 of *Obstetric Evidence Based Guidelines*).

PRENATAL CARE

All pregnant women should be screened for the use of illicit substances, tobacco, and alcohol [7,14,15]. In fact, all

Table 23.5 Elements of the Initial Evaluation

- History of drug sequelae (thrombophlebitis, bacterial endocarditis, hepatitis)
- Psychosocial history (abuse, domestic violence, depression/anxiety/bipolar, inpatient psych admission)
- Thorough drug history (what, how much, how often, how obtained, taken how)
- Observation for signs and symptoms of intoxication or withdrawal
- Assessment of nutritional status
- Physical exam (sequelae of drug use: track marks, skin lesions from intradermal injection aka "skin popping," abscess scars, dentition)
- Dating ultrasound
- Laboratory evaluation: CBC with differential, basic metabolic panel, liver function tests, hepatitis B and C antibody, RPR, blood type and antibody screen, HIV (with counseling), urinalysis and culture, urine drug screen, TB skin test, gonorrhea, chlamydia, wet mount (trichomonas)

women over 12 years old should be screened [16]. Obtaining a history of drug abuse may be facilitated by creating a private, safe, nonjudgmental atmosphere (see earlier section titled "Workup"). Women should be informed that screening is universal, the intent is to ensure appropriate prenatal care, and answers are confidential [7]. Maternal history alone may not be sufficient when there is a high suspicion of substance abuse. Reluctance to admit substance use may stem from fear of legal repercussions and involvement of child protective services. Providers should address misinformation and dispel any myths about the risks and ramifications of substance use. Eighteen states consider substance abuse during pregnancy a form of child endangerment and have laws requiring mandatory reporting of substance abuse during pregnancy [1]. **Criminalization of addiction in pregnancy is both ineffective and ethically inappropriate** [1].

Components of the history and physical exam and the recommended laboratory evaluation are shown in Table 23.5. Because of the frequent association with poor nutrition, these women may benefit from nutritional counseling. Continued positive drug screens may warrant ultrasound and nonstress test (NST) surveillance. Whether referral to a maternal-fetal medicine specialist is required depends on physician experience and the presence of other comorbidities. Regardless, pregnant women who abuse illicit drugs may benefit from **referral to specialized programs** integrating addiction treatment, obstetrical and medical care, social services, and psychiatric support where available [1,8].

MARIJUANA (CANNABIS) AND SYNTHETIC CANNABANOIDS
Historic Notes
Cannabis has been used for medicinal purposes for thousands of years and is among the earliest non-food-bearing plants cultivated by humans [17].

Diagnosis/Definition
More than 400 chemicals are found in *Cannabis sativa,* many of which are the same toxic substances found in cigarette smoke. The primary active chemical in marijuana is **tetrahydrocannabinol (THC)**, but marijuana contains more than 400 chemicals. Marinol (dronabinol), a synthetic preparation of

Δ^9-THC, is indicated for treatment of anorexia and weight loss in patients with AIDS and of nausea and vomiting associated with chemotherapy. Dried cannabis leaves contain up to 12% THC. Some common street names for marijuana include pot, grass, herb, weed, Mary Jane, reefer, skunk, boom, gangster, kif, chronic, and ganja. Marijuana is most commonly smoked but can also be taken orally. "Spice" or K2 refers to marijuana alternatives made from dried plant material mixed with synthetic cannabinoids [18].

Symptoms
The symptoms of marijuana intoxication include euphoria, tachycardia, conjunctival congestion, and anxiety [19].

Epidemiology/Incidence
Marijuana is the **most commonly used illicit drug** in the United States and the most commonly used illicit drug during pregnancy. Of women who use illicit drugs during pregnancy, 75% to 80% use marijuana [20]. The prevalence of marijuana use during pregnancy ranges from 2%–28% (typically 2%–5%) [21,22]. Additionally, continued marijuana use decreases across gestation; therefore, marijuana use at term most likely represents chronic use. Admission for treatment of marijuana use is increasing. Among pregnant women admitted for substance abuse treatment, marijuana was the primary drug in 6% of women in 1992 compared to 20% in 2012 [23]. Legalization and increased societal acceptance of marijuana is expected to result in increased marijuana use during pregnancy. Medicinal marijuana use should not be condoned during pregnancy [22].

Etiology/Basic Pathophysiology
THC crosses the placenta and can be detected in fetal tissues for several weeks after use [24]. Fetal plasma levels are approximately 10% of maternal levels, but greater exposure can result from repetitive use [22]. Chronic marijuana use alters uterine artery blood flow [25] and may **decrease uteroplacental perfusion** [26]. Compared to cigarettes, smoking marijuana is associated with fivefold higher levels of carbon monoxide [21]. When taken in combination, marijuana can potentiate the effects of other illicit drugs.

Risk Factors/Associations
Women who use marijuana during pregnancy are less likely to take folic acid and are more likely to be underweight, single, have lower levels of education and income, and be victims of intimate partner violence [22]. Alcohol and tobacco use is two to three times more likely among marijuana users [27].

Complications
Limitations of the current research on the effects of marijuana use during pregnancy include ascertainment (e.g., self-report), frequent use of other substances, (especially tobacco), sociodemographic differences, and recent increase in prevalence of prenatal marijuana use. Although it is difficult to separate the effects of marijuana from its contextual associations of use, subtle effects could have a large impact because exposure is so frequent [28]. Additionally, much of the research was performed during a period in which marijuana potency

was fourfold less than it is today. Overall, the risk of obstetrical and/or neonatal complications increases in relation to the amount of marijuana use and is greatest among frequent users (≥4–6 times per week) [29]. Infrequent use appears to pose limited risk. Little is known about the reproductive risks of synthetic cannabanoids.

- *Congenital anomalies*: Multiple large studies have shown no obvious pattern of malformations associated with prenatal marijuana use [22,30]. One study reported an increased incidence of anencephaly with first trimester marijuana use (OR 2.5, 95% CI 1.3–4.9), which may reflect less frequent use of supplemental folic acid [22].
- *Obstetrical complications*: Frequent marijuana use >5 times per week is associated with a 0.8-week **reduction in length of gestation** [31] but does not appear to be an independent risk factor for PTB. Likewise, marijuana exposure was not a predictor of other adverse outcomes [21,32]; however, NICU admission may be more likely (OR 1.54 95% CI 1.14–2.07). Reports of an increased risk of stillbirth are at least partially confounded by cigarette smoking [22,32].
- *Fetal/neonatal morphometrics*: Continued marijuana use was associated with a 172 g (95% CI –208 to –35 g) **reduction in mean birth weight** [33]. Marijuana use during the first 18 weeks was associated with a smaller, but still significant, reduction in weight (–95.4 g 95% CI –168 to –23 g). Heavy use (i.e., daily) was associated with the greatest reduction in weight. The effect, if any, on SGA (OR 1.3, 95% CI 1.03–1.62), length, and head circumference (approximately –0.5 cm) is small [20,22,32,34]. Additionally, there are mixed findings with respect to low birth weight (LBW) [22].
- *Neonatal withdrawal*: Examination of **neonates** of moderate to heavy marijuana smokers using the Brazelton Neonatal Assessment Scale demonstrated **altered responses to visual stimuli, increased tremulousness, and a high-pitched cry** [35]. These findings were no longer present by one month of age.
- *Long-term neonatal outcome*: Exposure to marijuana through second-hand smoke is a risk factor for **sudden infant death syndrome** [36,37]. Cannabinoid receptors in the fetal central nervous system, present as early as 14 weeks, play a role in normal brain development. Marijuana is believed to **alter fetal brain development** by binding these receptors leading to changes in synaptic structure and function and thus altered behavior, a predilection for adult neuropsychiatric disorders, and early onset marijuana use [22,37,38]. The main findings from longitudinal studies of perinatal marijuana exposure are: impaired mental development at nine months, increased aggression and inattention at 18 months (in girls), impaired memory and decreased verbal scores at 36–48 months, increased anxiety and depression, increased externalizing behavior (e.g., impulsivity, hyperactivity) at 6–10 years, impaired abstract and visual reasoning at 10 years, impaired visuoperceptual functioning at 9–12 years, and altered visuospatial memory at 18–22 years [39].

Therapy

Currently, there is no approved pharmacotherapy for marijuana abuse.

Antepartum Testing

The role of antepartum surveillance for marijuana exposure is insufficiently studied to make recommendations.

Anesthesia

Drugs affecting maternal heart rate and blood pressure should be used with caution. Adverse interactions have been reported between marijuana and drugs such as propranolol [40]. Likewise, during cesarean section under general anesthesia, the combination of marijuana and certain inhaled anesthetics can result in pronounced myocardial depression [40]. If general anesthesia is planned, the airway effects of chronic smoke inhalation should be considered [40]. Cross-tolerance to opioids and benzodiazepines may make dosing difficult [40].

Postpartum/Breast-Feeding

THC levels in breast milk are up to eight times higher than in maternal serum [37]. Reported effects of marijuana use during breast-feeding include sedation, lethargy, less frequent and shorter feedings, and delayed motor development at one year [41]. The AAP, ACOG, and ABM strongly advise that **women should not use marijuana while breast-feeding** as it may be hazardous to the infant and nursing mother [22,37,41,42].

OPIOIDS: HEROIN AND PRESCRIPTION OPIOID ANALGESICS
Historic Notes

Opioids are among the world's oldest known drugs. Opium is the dried "latex" of the opium poppy, which is grown mainly in Southeast Asia. Use of opium for its therapeutic benefits predates recorded history. Historically, opium has incited significant social, political, and economic strife. Opium contains morphine, codeine, and thebaine (converted chemically into oxycodone, oxymorphone, nalbuphine, naloxone, naltrexone, and buprenorphine). Opium can also be converted into heroin, a highly addictive and rapid acting opioid with a short half-life. Its origin dates back to 1874 when it was first introduced as a cure for morphine addiction [43]. Opioid maintenance therapy was adopted in the 1960s as a treatment for heroin addiction [1].

Diagnosis/Definition

Opioids are chemicals that bind to the opioid receptor. The term "opiate" refers to the naturally occurring alkaloids (morphine, codeine, heroin) found in opium. Street names for heroin in the United States include "big H," "black tar," "chiva," hell dust," "horse," "negra," and "smack." Opioids can be taken orally, sniffed, smoked, absorbed through the skin, or injected (most common route of administration for heroin). Heroin may be "cut" with adulterants, such as quinine, cornstarch, and baby formula powder.

Symptoms

Acute intoxication causes euphoria, altered pain sensation, and sedation; however, opioids can affect multiple organ systems (e.g., hypotension, constipation, urinary retention, sedation, miosis). **Withdrawal** presents as abdominal cramps, restlessness, insomnia, mydriasis, tachycardia, tachypnea, hypertension, lacrimation, rhinorrhea, yawning, piloerection, drug craving, irritability, and anxiety. Withdrawal symptoms **may start within four to six hours and last up to one week** (longer for methadone) [7]. Opioid **overdose**, the most serious complication, presents with respiratory depression, miotic pupils, pulmonary edema, obtundation, and/or coma. Overdose because of opioids is usually managed by securing an airway, supporting respiration, and administration of naloxone (Narcan).

Epidemiology/Incidence

Abuse of heroin and prescription opioids in the United States has **dramatically increased**. 1/1000 pregnant women reported heroin use during pregnancy, and an additional 5.6–12/1000 pregnant women reported misuse of prescription opioid analgesics [8,44]. However, estimates range **from <1% to as high as 21%** depending on the population [45]. Oxycodone and hydrocodone are the most commonly abused prescription opioid analgesics. Neonatal withdrawal from opioids, also called neonatal abstinence syndrome (NAS), tripled in the United States from 2004 to 2013, indicating a rise in opioid use during pregnancy [46].

Risk Factors/Associations

Many opioid-addicted pregnant women are unmarried (18%), poorly educated (20% finished high school), and prostitute themselves (22%) [43]. The percentage of women who do not receive prenatal care is as high as 80% [43]. Poverty, polysubstance abuse, concomitant mental illness, domestic violence, and a history of physical or sexual assault are common [1].

Complications

Maternal medical complications because of chronic parenteral opiate abuse (particularly needle sharing) account for much of the obstetrical issues in these women. Of greatest concern are infections, especially **hepatitis B, hepatitis C, and HIV**. However, other sequelae include, but are not limited to, **bacteremia/sepsis, cellulitis, endocarditis, tuberculosis/pneumonia, and sexually transmitted infections** [47]. Recent literature on obstetrical complications pertains mainly to women on methadone maintenance. For the purpose of this section, studies of methadone-maintained women were largely excluded. Few studies have independently evaluated nonsupervised or "street" methadone or misuse of prescription opioid analgesics. Complications related to illicit opioid use and prescribed opioids when used as directed use may not be comparable.

- *Congenital anomalies*: There is **no established increased risk of congenital anomalies** or pattern of malformations related to fetal opioid exposure [1]; however, a recent case-control study demonstrated an association between prescription opioid analgesics and certain birth defects—conoventricular septal defects (OR 2.7, 95% CI, 1.1–6.3), atrioventricular septal defects (OR 2.0, 95% CI, 1.2–3.6), hypoplastic left heart syndrome (OR 2.4, 95% CI, 1.4–4.1), spina bifida (OR 2.0, 95% CI, 1.3–3.2), or gastroschisis (OR 1.8, 95% CI, 1.1–2.9) [48]. This study was based on maternal recall and did not take into account dose [7]. Most prescription opioid analgesics are FDA pregnancy category B and C.

- *Obstetrical complications*: *Heroin* use is associated with a sixfold increase in obstetric complications [49]. The risk of **miscarriage** is increased. When the results of four observational studies are averaged, the **rate of preterm birth (PTB) is 28%** (range 17%–45% [50]) among women addicted to heroin [43]. The incidence of meconium staining ranges from 21% to 46% compared to 12% to 13.8% in drug-free controls [43]; however, some studies have reported no difference. Additionally, there are higher rates of **abruption and stillbirth** [7]. A retrospective cohort study examining the effect of the type of narcotic used demonstrated rates of "fetal distress" between 47% and 52% for women abusing unsupervised methadone, heroin, and polydrug abuse [51]. Respiratory distress may be less common because of fetal stress from repeated episodes of withdrawal.

- *Fetal/neonatal morphometrics*: Heroin use is associated with **decreased birth weight**. In a retrospective study, mean birth weight of infants exposed to heroin during pregnancy was lower than controls (2490 g vs. 3176 g) [52]. Combining the results of four controlled studies yielded similar results (mean 2553 g; −691 g compared to controls) [43]. It is **not clear whether this is entirely due to heroin or is secondary to other aspects related to heroin addiction (e.g., malnutrition and smoking)**. One theory is that heroin affects birth weight by lowering fetal plasma leptin levels. Likewise, intrauterine growth restriction (IUGR) and LBW are more common [7]. Averaging the results from controlled studies, the rate of LBW is 41% (vs. 26% in methadone, $p \leq 0.01$ and 19% in drug-free controls, $p \leq 0.0025$) [43], much of which is due to a higher incidence of IUGR (20% vs. 4%) [53], and small for gestational age (SGA) infants (18% vs. 12% in methadone and 5% in drug-free controls) [43].

- *Neonatal withdrawal*: The **incidence of NAS** is approximately **60%–70%** among opioid-exposed neonates. Symptoms typically appear within the first 72 hours after birth but can occur any time within the first two weeks [7]. NAS is characterized by central nervous system hyperirritability, gastrointestinal dysfunction, respiratory distress, and autonomic symptoms [47,54]. The most serious, life-threatening sequela of NAS is seizures. Up to 30% of opioid-exposed neonates will demonstrate abnormalities on electroencephalogram, and 2% to 11% will have overt seizures [55]. There are several scoring systems to measure the severity of NAS, the most common of which was proposed by Finnegan [56]. Neonates with high NAS scores (e.g., a cumulative Finnegan score of ≥24) may be candidates for replacement therapy (usually neonatal opium solution, morphine, clonidine, or phenobarbital, but buprenorphine has also been recently studied with promising results) [57]. In utero withdrawal is a largely hypothetical concept.

- *Long-term neonatal outcome*: With the exception of methadone, data on long-term outcome of infants exposed to opioids are limited [7]. In a study using videotaped interactions between drug-dependent women and their infants at four months, global ratings of interaction quality were lower compared to non–drug-exposed dyads [54]. Greater body tension and poorer coordination was also observed in the drug-exposed infants. Neurological impairment was also more common at 18 months and three years of age [58]. Other effects include increased temper, impulsivity, aggressiveness, poorer self-confidence, and impaired memory and perception [30,59].

Therapy

The incidence of obstetrical complications is lower among women undergoing treatment [47]. Oral replacement therapy is the standard treatment for opioid-use disorder with dependence. Randomized controlled trials (RCTs) demonstrate an approximately threefold reduction in heroin use and a threefold increase in retention in treatment relative to non-pharmacological treatment [3,60]. In pregnancy, the maternal and fetal benefits are extensive and, among others, include preventing complications of illicit drug use (e.g., acquiring and vertically transmitting hepatitis C and HIV), encouraging prenatal care and drug treatment, reducing criminal activity, and avoiding other risks associated with drug culture [7]. Long-term studies have shown that pregnant women enrolled in opioid maintenance therapy rarely resume illicit substance use and can maintain a relatively normal family life [1].

Two approaches to pharmacological treatment are maintenance and detoxification. The goal of maintenance therapy is to substitute heroin with another licit drug in quantities sufficient to prevent symptoms of withdrawal and drug craving. Detoxification, however, aims to replace heroin with progressively lower doses of a licit substance until treatment is no longer required. High rates of return to illicit opioid use has been observed with detoxification in pregnant women [61,62] and nonpregnant individuals [3,63,64]; however, these two approaches to therapy have not been compared in RCTs of pregnant women. Moreover, opiate detoxification in pregnancy requires significant time commitment and extended treatment, with one study reporting 56% success with inpatient detoxification [65]. Additionally, the safety of detoxification during pregnancy is not well studied. Detoxification has been associated with miscarriage, stillbirth, and alterations in fetal adrenal hormone levels [66,67], but larger, more recent studies have not confirmed these findings [68,69]. Medically supervised withdrawal is preferred to continued illicit substance use [7]. Pregnant women are given priority in opioid maintenance programs. A list of providers can be found at https://findtreatment.samhsa.gov/TreatmentLocator/faces/quickSearch.jspx. Opioid replacement is only one aspect of a comprehensive drug treatment program.

Methadone

Methadone (FDA category C), a long-acting synthetic μ receptor agonist, is the preferred treatment for opioid addiction during pregnancy. Four RCTs have shown that methadone maintenance decreases illicit opioid use, criminal activity, and mortality rates in nonpregnant heroin-addicted adults [70]. Typical initial stabilization doses range from 10 to 30 mg with the dose increased in 5- to 10-mg increments thereafter. The most appropriate methadone dose is controversial. Doses of at least 60 mg are more effective than lower doses [3,71]. We recommend titrating the daily methadone dose to achieve the dose that effectively prevents symptoms of withdrawal and drug cravings. In our experience the average maintenance dose of methadone is approximately 120 mg/day. As a result of the physiologic changes that occur during pregnancy

(decreased plasma levels and increased clearance), dose increases are often needed in the later part of pregnancy to prevent withdrawal. A methadone trough level may be useful in guiding dose adjustments as symptomatic women have significantly lower mean methadone levels than asymptomatic women (0.18 mg/L vs. 0.24 mg/L) [72]. Likewise, trough levels >0.3 mg/L in symptomatic women should be clinically correlated to urine drug screen results because of the possibility of withdrawal from other illicit substances. Rarely, split daily dosing may be required because of rapid metabolism [7]. Caution should be taken when prescribing other medications to women on methadone because of the potential for drug–drug interactions. For example, both methadone and the commonly prescribed antibiotic metronidazole increase the QTc interval, which can lead to potentially fatal ventricular arrhythmias.

Methadone maintenance is associated with improved obstetrical and neonatal outcome compared to illicit opioid abuse (more adequate prenatal care, longer gestation, increased birth weight and head circumference, etc.) but not to the level of drug-free controls. The rate of continued illicit substance abuse is 15%–36% in some studies, and this continued substance abuse may attenuate some of the beneficial effects of drug treatment programs [50,73].

The most common neonatal sequela of opioid exposure is neonatal withdrawal, also referred to as NAS. Rates of NAS reported in the literature range from 31% to 80% [72,74]. However, maternal methadone dose is not associated with either the incidence of NAS or the length of neonatal treatment [1,75–77]. Methadone has also been associated with decreased birth weight and head circumference [78], jaundice, and thrombocytosis. Less commonly recognized is the effect of methadone on the developing visual system. In a group of 20 exposed infants and children, ophthalmic abnormalities included decreased visual acuity (95%), nystagmus (70%), delayed visual maturation (50%), strabismus (30%), refractive errors (30%), and cerebral visual impairments (25%) [79]. Neither the long-term effects nor the independent effect of other illicit substances are clear.

Buprenorphine

Use of buprenorphine is increasing. Buprenorphine (Subutex, FDA category C) is a partial μ receptor agonist and κ receptor antagonist. Randomized trials demonstrate that buprenorphine increases treatment retention (RR 1.21–1.52) and decreases heroin use [3,60] in nonpregnant adults compared to methadone. Effectiveness during pregnancy is similar to methadone [8]. The main advantages of buprenorphine are lower risk of overdose ("ceiling effect") and respiratory depression, fewer drug interactions, and that it does not require supervised daily administration [7]. Buprenorphine can be prescribed by any physician with the appropriate credentialing, which improves accessibility and confidentiality and decreases the social stigma [1]. There is also evidence of less severe NAS. In a Cochrane systematic review of maintenance agonist treatments for opiate-dependent pregnant women, compared to methadone, buprenorphine was not associated with a difference in dropout (RR 1.00, 95% CI 0.41–2.44), continued illicit heroin use (RR 2.50, 95% CI 0.11–54.87), rate of neonatal treatment for NAS (RR 1.28, 95% CI 0.58–2.85), or length of neonatal treatment for NAS (RR 0.50, 95% CI –1.84–2.84) [49]. However, a recent randomized, placebo-controlled trial comparing methadone and buprenorphine for treatment of maternal opioid dependency found that buprenorphine was associated with significantly lower doses of morphine for treatment of NAS (mean total amount 1.1 vs. 10.4 mg), shorter duration of treatment for NAS (4.1 vs. 9.9 days), and shorter neonatal hospital stay (10.0 vs. 17.5 days) but no difference in continued illicit substance use (15% vs. 9%, $p = 0.27$) or the rate of neonatal treatment for NAS (57% vs. 47%, $p = 0.26$) [73]. This trial has yet to be included in the *Cochrane* systematic review. A limitation of the trial was a markedly higher attrition rate from the buprenorphine treatment arm than from the methadone arm (18% vs. 33%, $p = 0.02$). On the other hand, induction is more difficult, and some patients express dissatisfaction likely due to partial μ receptor agonist properties. **With informed consent, buprenorphine may be an appropriate first-line medication for women who are not yet on treatment** [7].

Suboxone is a combination of buprenorphine and naltrexone. The addition of naltrexone is meant to deter parenteral use and lowers the risk of diversion. In general, pregnant women taking Suboxone should be **switched to an equivalent dose of buprenorphine** (Subutex). As with methadone, dose increases during pregnancy are common.

Other Treatments
Other treatments for opioid-addicted pregnant women include oral slow-release morphine, heroin-assisted treatment, L-*A*-acetylmethadol (LAAM), and clonidine. In a small RCT, oral slow-release morphine was superior to methadone in abstinence from heroin, but there was no statistically significant difference in birth weight or duration of NAS [49,80]. There are two case reports of "heroin-assisted" treatment in a total of five pregnant women. Heroin-assisted treatment combines methadone and injectable heroin. The selection criteria for this program are a history of addiction for more than two years, failure of at least two alternative treatments, and risk of further physical or social decline. The authors observed a higher birth weight compared to women treated with methadone alone [81]. LAAM is a m receptor agonist with a longer half-life than methadone. LAAM was taken off of the market in 2003 because it prolongs the QT interval, leading to potentially life-threatening ventricular arrhythmias. Clonidine, an α-agonist antihypertensive medication, has been used alone or in addition to other medications for mild withdrawal. The blood pressure–lowering effect of clonidine is due to its α_2-agonist properties. Likewise, clonidine prevents withdrawal symptoms through the same mechanism. In summary, **treatments other than methadone or buprenorphine have limited evidence for safety and efficacy and therefore should be avoided.**

Antepartum Testing
Reports of an increased risk of intrauterine fetal demise (IUFD) associated with intravenous opiate abuse [47] have led some authors to suggest weekly fetal monitoring beginning at 32 weeks. However, **for women in a treatment program who have repetitively negative urine drug screens, antepartum testing should be reserved for standard obstetrical indications** (e.g., IUGR). Opiates are associated with decreases in baseline, variability, and accelerations. Ideally, to avoid misinterpretation, women on methadone or other prescribed narcotics should have nonstress test or biophysical profile scheduled before or at least four to six hours after a dose of methadone.

Delivery
As per common obstetric practices.

Anesthesia
Peripheral intravenous access can be difficult in chronic intravenous drug abusers. Dosing of other opioid analgesics for pain control during labor and postpartum can be challenging because of recent use or tolerance from chronic receptor stimulation [19] and hyperalgesia. In a retrospective study, **methadone-maintained women required 70% more oxycodone equivalents after cesarean section than controls** [82]. Opioid antagonists or agonist-antagonists can precipitate acute withdrawal [82]. Examples of these drugs are Nubain®, Talwin®, Stadol®, and Narcan®. If any of these drugs are accidentally given, withdrawal can also be reversed with any opioid [82].

Regional anesthesia is safe. However, hypotension may occur more frequently because of concomitant malnutrition and/or liver disease. If general anesthesia becomes necessary, poor dentition, airway burns, chronic lung disease, and decreased gastric emptying may result in airway compromise [8].

After delivery, fluid shifts may increase opioid levels. However, we have not observed any cases of oversedation or other complications postpartum. **Opioid replacement should be continued throughout labor and delivery** as it is not part of the labor analgesia. Similarly, complaints of pain should be taken seriously and not assumed to be drug-seeking behavior.

Postpartum/Breast-Feeding
Methadone or buprenorphine should be continued during the immediate peripartum period. Oversedation from methadone because of changes in volume of distribution and hepatic clearance is rare in practice [83]. Dose reductions should be based on clinical signs and symptoms rather than protocol.

The American Academy of Pediatrics (AAP) strongly advises that women should not use heroin while breast-feeding as it may be hazardous to the infant and nursing mother [42]. Tremors, restlessness, vomiting, and poor feeding have been reported in breast-fed infants of women using heroin [41]. Breast-feeding is not contraindicated in women taking opioids for acute (e.g., Percocet for postoperative pain) or chronic pain.

Women taking **methadone** should be **encouraged to breast-feed, irrespective of dose**, assuming the patient is enrolled in a treatment program and remains abstinent [7,37,41,42]. Potential benefits include **improved maternal-infant bonding and favorable effects on NAS** [37,83–87]. However, close observation is warranted because lethargy, respiratory difficulty, and poor weight have also been observed [41]. **Methadone levels in human milk are <3% of the maternal weight-adjusted dose, and infant plasma concentrations are <3% of the maternal trough concentration.** With such low exposure, it is not clear whether the favorable effects of breast-feeding on NAS are related to methadone in breast milk or the act of breast-feeding itself [88].

Likewise, women prescribed **buprenorphine** should also be **encouraged to breast-feed** [7]. Although this contradicts the package labeling, the amount of buprenorphine in breast milk is also low. Infant exposure is <2.4% of the maternal weight-adjusted dose [41], which is unlikely to have any negative effects on development [37]. Similar to methadone, buprenorphine also appears to have favorable effects on NAS [37].

COCAINE (BENZOYLMETHYLECOGNINE)
Historic Notes

The leaves of the South American erythroxylon coca plant have been consumed to increase energy and reduce fatigue and hunger since as early as 3000 BC [89]. Cocaine was purified in 1862 by Albert Neiman, and although Sigmund Freud first introduced cocaine into modern medicine in 1884 with his treatise *On Coca*, its use as a topical anesthetic (cocaine-saturated saliva) dates back thousands of years. Cocaine is still used in some ophthalmologic procedures. Coca-Cola® contained cocaine until 1903; today the soft drink still contains a non-narcotic extract prepared from the coca plant.

Diagnosis/Definition

As a hydrochloride, cocaine (also known as "snow") is sold in the form of a powder or as granules or crystals. Crack, also known as crack cocaine, rock, or freebase, is cocaine returned to its pure, alkalinized form by heating it with baking soda and water. The name "crack" comes from the characteristic sound made during the "cooking" process [89]. Cocaine can be injected, snorted, or smoked (in cigarettes or with marijuana). Inhalation is the preferred route of administration by crack users [90].

Symptoms, Signs, and Cardiopulmonary Complications

Cocaine produces a brief euphoria by interfering with presynaptic neurotransmitter uptake, thereby increasing sympathomimetic neurotransmitters (serotonin, norepinephri, serotonin, norepinephrine, and dopamine) [91]. Systemic effects include **hypertension** (mean rise 25 mmHg systolic and 6 mmHg diastolic), **tachycardia** (mean increase 20 beats per minute), and **dilated pupils** [89]. More severe consequences include arrhythmias, hypotension, myocardial infarction, seizures, stroke, gastrointestinal ischemia, thrombosis, hyperthermia, and sudden death. Pulmonary complications of smoking crack include interstitial pneumonitis, spontaneous pneumothorax, and "crack lung," which is characterized by acute dyspnea, hypoxia, fever, hemoptysis, and respiratory failure. The active metabolites may have delayed activity. The combination of cocaine and alcohol produces cocaethylene, which increases the risk of cardiac events 40-fold and sudden death 25-fold.

Pregnancy is associated with increased sensitivity of the cardiovascular system to cocaine [92,93]. Plasma cholinesterase activity, the enzyme responsible for metabolizing cocaine, is decreased during pregnancy, which prolongs the adverse effects of cocaine [94]. Additionally, other physiologic changes during pregnancy (increased oxygen demand and limited or decreased supply because of increases in heart rate, blood pressure, and left ventricular contractility) [91] increase the cardiopulmonary toxicity of cocaine [94,95].

Cocaine use may present as the constellation hypertension, proteinuria, and edema, and therefore may be confused for preeclampsia. Withdrawal symptoms from cocaine include drug craving, fatigue, and mental depression.

Epidemiology/Incidence

Cocaine use peaked in the 1980s (8%–17% in urban hospitals) [96] and has since declined. From 1993 to 1995, 9.1% of pregnant women used cocaine by self-report or positive meconium at four urban centers (3.4% history and positive meconium) [97]. According to another study, in the late 1990s, the prevalence of cocaine use by pregnant women was approximately **0.28% (1/10th of overall drug use during pregnancy)** [98]. More recently, between 2000 and 2001, at a public hospital in São Paulo, Brazil, the rate of cocaine use by pregnant teens 11 to 19 years old in the third trimester was 1.7% using hair analysis.

Etiology/Basic Pathophysiology

Cocaine readily crosses the placenta and can be detected in fetal blood and tissues [96]. The maternal and fetal sequelae of cocaine may be related to the effects of cocaine on the cardiovascular system [95,99]. Uterine artery vasospasm and vasoconstriction in response to cocaine-mediated increases in norepinephrine results in decreased uteroplacental blood flow and uteroplacental insufficiency, which can lead to fetal acidosis, hypoxia, and distress. Additionally, increased maternal plasma norepinephrine and the β-agonist properties of cocaine stimulate uterine contractions [98], an effect that has been reproduced in vitro [100]. Uterine contractions and acute vasoconstriction of vessels in the placental bed are thought to be the mechanisms of abruption related to cocaine use [94,101]. Cocaine has the ability to potentiate the effects of or be potentiated by other drugs. The combination of cocaine and ethanol produces cocaethylene, a biologically active substance with unknown reproductive effects [95]. Cocaine is metabolized through the liver; hence preexisting liver disease may potentiate its effects.

Risk Factors/Associations

As with other substances, women who use cocaine are more likely to use other illicit substances, tobacco, and/or alcohol. Cocaine use during pregnancy is more common among black women compared with the racial distribution of other substances. Pregnant women who use cocaine also tend to be older, have less than a high school education, have higher gravidity, and are more likely to have had a prior abortion [102]. Poverty, poor nutrition, depression, physical abuse, poor social support, and sexually transmitted infections have also been associated with cocaine use.

Maternal and Perinatal Complications

- *Congenital anomalies*: Cocaine use alone (RR 1.7, 95% CI 1.12–2.60) or in addition to other drugs (RR 2.10, 95% CI 1.42–3.09) during pregnancy is associated with a **higher rate of congenital malformations**, which is likely the effect of factors other than cocaine itself [97,103,104]. The overall rate of malformations is **10%** [89]. Vasoconstriction leads to disruption of the fetal bowel (atresia, infarction, perforation, necrotizing enterocolitis in the neonate), CNS (microcephaly in 16%, porencephaly), and/or limbs (reduction). Exposure to cocaine has been suggested in the etiology of hydranencephaly [95]. Neonates exposed to cocaine are at risk for structural and functional (arrhythmias, conduction abnormalities, etc.) congenital heart disease [105].

- *Obstetrical complications*: **Miscarriage, shorter gestation** (–1.47 weeks 95% CI –1.97 to –0.98), **PTB** (OR 3.38, 95% CI 2.72–4.21), **PPROM** (RR 1.85, 95% CI 1.35–2.52 cocaine alone; RR 3.18, 95% CI 1.61–6.29 cocaine with other drugs), **abruption** (RR 4.55, 95% CI 3.19–6.50 cocaine alone; RR 4.95, 95% CI 2.08–11.81 cocaine with other drugs), pre-eclampsia, **stillbirth** (18.2%) [106]; meconium staining of the amniotic fluid and fetal heart rate abnormalities are the most frequently cited obstetrical complications of cocaine use [19,95,96,104,107,108]. Women who use cocaine during pregnancy are four times more likely to require **emergent delivery**. Precipitous delivery is also common (13.4%) [109]. Women presenting with PPROM in association with cocaine exhibit more advanced cervical dilation and shorter latency [110,111]. Body packing, the ingestion of multiple packets of cocaine for the purpose of smuggling, can cause serious complications if a packet ruptures, and at least one case of perimortem cesarean section has been reported in this situation [112]. **Cocaine use increases vertical transmission of HIV fourfold** [113].
- *Fetal/neonatal morphometrics*: Cocaine use during pregnancy is associated with **decreased birth weight** (–492 g, 95% CI –562 to –421), **LBW** (OR 3.66, 95% CI 2.90–4.63), **IUGR, SGA infants** (OR 3.23, 95% CI 2.43–4.30), **decreased head circumference** (–1.21 to –1.72 cm), **and decreased length** (–2.17 to –2.57 cm) [104,107,114]. Poor placental perfusion and appetite suppression leading to poor maternal weight gain are hypothesized to cause the observed changes in growth.
- *Neonatal withdrawal*: Abrupt discontinuation of cocaine at birth results in a constellation of withdrawal symptoms, best described as "neonatal toxicity." These symptoms include **jitteriness/tremulousness** (OR 2.17, 95% CI 1.44–3.29), **high-pitched cry** (OR 2.44; 95% CI 1.06–5.66), **irritability** (OR 1.81, 95% CI 1.18–2.80), **excessive suck** (OR 3.58, 95% CI 1.63–7.88), **hyperalertness** (OR 7.78, 95% CI 1.72–35.06), and **autonomic instability** (OR 2.64, 95% CI 1.17–5.95) and typically occur in the first two to three days of life [97].
- *Long-term neonatal outcome*: Initial studies reported adverse neurological consequences of antenatal cocaine exposure (so-called "crack babies"); however, more recent studies have found that **much of the effect is related to co-occurring exposures**. Nonetheless, cocaine is not without consequence. Antenatal exposure to cocaine is associated with slower growth and higher rates of obesity and elevated blood pressure [103,115]. The mechanism that has been postulated to explain increased obesity is poor maternal nutrition and LBW, which has been linked to later obesity. Children followed up to 10 years demonstrate poorer adolescent functioning and perceptual reasoning, impaired perceptual learning, internalizing, externalizing, and total behavior problems, more symptoms of oppositional defiant disorder and attention deficit hyperactivity disorder (ADHD), impairment of executive function, adverse effects on short-term memory, and poorer language development, which is at least in part due to associated sociodemographic factors (e.g., poverty) [103]. Brain magnetic resonance imaging of these children shows lesser total gray matter especially in the prefrontal and frontal regions [116]. Cocaine also has **effects on the visual system**. Strabismus and refractive errors are more likely among children prenatally exposed to cocaine. Cases of permanent eyelid edema have also been reported.

Therapy

There are currently no FDA-approved pharmacologic therapies available for detoxification or maintenance of cocaine dependence. Interventions for cocaine dependence primarily involve **psychosocial therapies** (e.g., cognitive behavioral therapy, motivational interviewing). Very few interventions have been specifically studied in pregnancy. Treatment programs for cocaine have a favorable impact on pregnancy outcome; rates of PTB and LBW were decreased by 67% and 84% [99]. Motivational enhancement therapy was compared to "usual" counseling for pregnant women abusing cocaine in a randomized trial that found no difference in treatment utilization. The use of motivational incentives, also known as **voucher-based contingency management**, was studied in a small, randomized trial of pregnant women abusing cocaine. Treatment retention and abstinence from cocaine was high in both groups and there was a trend toward increased attendance at prenatal care visits ($p = 0.077$) [117]. In a separate study, **motivational interviewing** was associated with a significant reduction in neonatal intensive care unit admission and length of stay and cost savings amounted to $5000 per mother/infant pair above the cost of the program [118]. A recent pilot study demonstrated that progesterone may have some promise as a treatment for cocaine use disorder in postpartum women [119].

Withdrawal from cocaine is usually mild, if present, and not life threatening for the mother or fetus. Benzodiazepines can be given to relieve symptoms [98]. Rarely, psychotic symptoms during withdrawal may require treatment with antipsychotic medications.

Antepartum Testing

The role of antepartum testing (ultrasound and nonstress tests or biophysical profiles) for cocaine use is insufficiently studied to make recommendations. Based on expert opinion, weekly antenatal testing is recommended starting at 32 weeks [120].

Anesthesia

Regional anesthesia should be used with caution because of combative behavior, altered perception of pain, cocaine-induced thrombocytopenia, and ephedrine-resistant hypotension (usually responds to phenylephrine). Women may perceive pain despite adequate spinal/epidural anesthesia levels [105]. Hydralazine is the drug of choice for management of cocaine-induced hypertension, labetalol plus nitroglycerin may be a reasonable alternative [19]. Propranolol should be avoided because of the potential for unopposed α-adrenergic stimulation; however, labetalol is generally considered safe. The use of general anesthesia also presents challenges; all volatile anesthetics can cause arrhythmia and increased systemic vascular resistance [121].

Postpartum/Breast-Feeding

The AAP strongly advises that women **should not use cocaine while breast-feeding** as it may be hazardous to the infant and nursing mother [42]. Cocaine intoxication, seizures, irritability, vomiting, diarrhea, and tremulousness have been reported in breast-fed infants of women using cocaine [41].

AMPHETAMINES: AMPHETAMINE, METHAMPHETAMINE, 3,4-METHYLENEDIOXYMETHAMPHETAMINE (ECSTASY), SYNTHETIC CATHINONES ("BATH SALTS")
Historic Notes

Amphetamines were first synthesized in 1887 [122]. Amphetamine is FDA approved (schedule II) for the treatment of (ADHD) and narcolepsy. The more potent stimulant, methamphetamine (schedule II), is FDA approved for the treatment of ADHD and obesity. Methamphetamine is easily made from over-the-counter cold medications, and addiction can occur after as little as one use [123]. Ecstasy, which is chemically similar to methamphetamine, was patented in 1912 [124]. In the 1970s, psychotherapists used ecstasy to enhance "openness" with their patients [124]. Ecstasy was classified as a schedule I drug in 1985 [124]. Bath salts are a group of synthetic cathinones (naturally occurring alkaloids that are chemically similar to amphetamines) with amphetamine-like stimulant properties. "Bath salts," sometimes also sold as "jewelry cleaner," "phone screen cleaner," or "plant food," get their name from the resemblance of the crystalline powder to the real thing [125]. Bath salts are not detected on routine urine drug screens.

Diagnosis/Definition

Amphetamines are a group of synthetic stimulants that are structurally similar to norepinephrine [126]. Amphetamines increase levels of norepinephrine, serotonin, and dopamine by increasing release and blocking reuptake [127]. Street names for amphetamines include dexies, bennies, ice (methamphetamine), and crystal (methamphetamine). Amphetamines can be injected, snorted, smoked (78.3% for methamphetamines), or taken orally or anally [128]. Gamma-hydroxybutyrate (GHB) is sometimes referred to as "liquid ecstasy" but is chemically and pharmacologically unrelated to 3,4-methylenedioxymethamphetamine.

Symptoms, Signs, and Organ Toxicity

Symptoms of amphetamine use include alertness, decreased fatigue, sleeplessness, euphoria, exhilaration, emotional openness, reduction of negativity, and decreased inhibition [129]. Systemic effects include hypertension, dilated pupils, tremor, and hyperactivity [126]. Release of serotonin is responsible for some of the hallucinogenic effects of amphetamines [126]. Rarely, at high doses, toxicity mimicking cocaine toxicity can be seen, including hypertension, retinal damage, cardiac arrhythmia, hyperthermia, seizure, shock, stroke, and death [126]. Amphetamine use can damage brain structure including the gray matter, temporal lobe, and basal ganglia. Methamphetamine abuse can cause toxic hepatitis, which presents similarly to acute viral hepatitis. Consequences of long-term methamphetamine use include anxiety, confusion, insomnia, memory loss, weight loss, dental problems ("meth mouth"), depression, violence, paranoia, hallucinations, and formication [127]. Symptoms of amphetamine withdrawal are mild and not life threatening (e.g., depression, insomnia).

Ecstasy produces symptoms of euphoria, intimacy, and decreased anxiety. Methylenedioxyprolevone, a constituent of bath salts, can cause hypertension and acute neurological, cardiovascular, and psychiatric symptoms.

Epidemiology/Incidence

Amphetamines are the most abused prescription medication [130] and are overall the second most commonly abused drug worldwide. Despite similarity with cocaine, the greater popularity of amphetamines is likely related to longer half-life, greater sympathomimetic effects, lower cost, and greater accessibility [131]. Use of methamphetamine, the most commonly abused amphetamine, is an escalating problem in the United States and other parts of the world [124,127,132]. In recent years, hospitalization for amphetamine abuse by pregnant women has doubled [133]. The reported incidence of methamphetamine use during pregnancy is between **0.1% and 1.0% and up to 5.2% in the highest use areas** [134,135]. Methamphetamine use during pregnancy is significantly more common in cities and in the West, Midwest, and Southeast United States [128]. Methamphetamine accounts for nearly a quarter of drug treatment admissions during pregnancy [128]. The rate of ecstasy exposure during pregnancy is less clear. Ecstasy is one of the most widely used illicit drugs in the United Kingdom where the rate of self-reported use ranged from 0.6% to 8.8% in 2004 [124]. In the United States, ecstasy use peaked in 2001 and has since declined. There has been a recent epidemic of bath salt use.

Etiology/Basic Pathophysiology

Methamphetamine crosses the placenta and is detectable in fetal tissues. Studies of methamphetamine in pregnant sheep suggest that vasoconstriction may be the mechanism that leads to obstetrical and neonatal complications [136].

Risk Factors/Associations

Pregnant methamphetamine users are more likely to be young, white (although an increasing proportion of women are Hispanic), and unmarried [127]. Other characteristics of amphetamine-using mothers include late initiation of prenatal care, lower SES, less education, less likely to have private insurance, and less likely to have social support and are more likely to be homeless, victims of domestic violence, involved in criminal activity, have comorbid psychiatric conditions, and engage in risky sexual behavior [137]. Women who use ecstasy during pregnancy are more likely to be younger (mean 23.2 years vs. 31.2 years, $p < 0.0001$), report that the pregnancy was unplanned (84% vs. 54%, $p < 0.05$), use alcohol (66% vs. 31%, $p < 0.0001$), smoke cigarettes (54% vs. 20%, $p < 0.0001$), and use other illicit drugs during pregnancy compared to nonusers [137,138]. Similar patterns of polysubstance abuse are observed among women who abuse amphetamine and methamphetamine [128,139].

Complications

Given that amphetamines and cocaine have similar effects on the central nervous system, both agents produce similar effects during pregnancy and are often combined in studies. Amphetamines concentrate in the fetus at levels that eventually exceed those in the mother [140]. Proving an association between amphetamines and adverse outcomes is difficult because of multiple accompanying confounders.

- *Congenital anomalies*: Although central nervous system, cardiac, gastrointestinal, and limb malformations and cleft lip have been reported, the best available evidence suggests that **exposure to amphetamines, excluding** ecstasy, during pregnancy is unlikely to cause congenital anomalies [127,131]. Data from the United Kingdom National Teratology Information Service demonstrated a 15% rate of congenital anomalies after prenatal *ecstasy* exposure (expected 2%–3%). Among these malformations, talipes equinovarus occurred more frequently than expected (all three female, 38/1000 [95% CI 8.0–109.0] vs. expected 3:1 male predominance, 1/1000) [141]. There was also a trend toward higher-than-expected rates of congenital heart disease (26/1000 [95% CI 3.0–90.0] vs. expected 5–10/1000). Chemical additives used to expand drug volume (e.g., talc, inositol, methylsulfonylmethane) pose an unknown risk of congenital anomalies [127].

- *Obstetrical and neonatal complications*: Amphetamine use is associated with an increased risk of PTB (OR 4.11, 95% CI 3.05–5.55). An increased risk of abruption has also been reported, which is thought to be due to amphetamine-mediated platelet activation and uterine contractions [140]. In a retrospective study evaluating outcomes in pregnancies complicated specifically by methamphetamine use, complications that occurred significantly more frequently included **gestational hypertension** (OR 1.8, 95% CI 1.6–2.0), **preeclampsia** (OR 2.7, 95% CI 2.4–3.0), **IUFD** (OR 5.1, 95% CI 3.7–7.2), **abruption** (OR 5.5, 95% CI 4.9–6.3), **PTB** (OR 2.9, 95% CI 2.7–3.1), **neonatal death** (OR 3.1 95% CI 2.3–4.2), and **infant death** (OR 2.5, 95% CI 1.7–3.7) [131]. The obstetrical and neonatal complications of ecstasy use are insufficiently studied.
- *Fetal/neonatal morphometrics*: A systematic review of 10 studies demonstrated a 279 g **decrease in mean birth weight** (95% CI −485 to −74) and **increases in LBW** (OR 3.97, 95% CI 2.45–6.43), and **SGA** (OR 5.79, 95% CI 1.39–24.06) among *amphetamine*-addicted women [141]. Likewise, exposure to *methamphetamine* specifically has also been consistently associated with an increased risk of **IUGR**, SGA (OR 2.05–3.5), LBW (OR 2.0), and decreased birth weight, head circumference, and length [131,136,139,143,144].
- *Neonatal withdrawal*: Neonatal withdrawal from *amphetamines* is characterized by abnormal sleep, poor feeding, tremors, hypertonia, agitation, and tachypnea.
- *Long-term neurodevelopmental outcome*: In a longitudinal follow-up study of Swedish children exposed to *amphetamine* prenatally, the children demonstrated **deficits in behavior and school performance**, including language, mathematics, and physical fitness at age 14 years [145]. Earlier follow-up of these children showed increased **sleepiness, characteristics of autism, speech abnormalities, and stranger anxiety** by one year old, **lower IQ** at four years old, and **aggressive behavior and difficulty with peers** at eight years old [146]. This study included a relatively small sample and lacked a control group. The IDEAL study examined developmental outcomes of *methamphetamine-exposed* children vs. matched controls. These children were more likely to have behavioral problems, including emotional reactivity, anxiety/depression, externalizing behavior (i.e., "lashing out"), and ADHD at three to five years [146]. Further follow-up of these same children showed a much higher likelihood of cognitive problems (OR 2.8, 95% CI 1.2–6.5) at 7.5 years old [146], placing them at risk of poor academic achievement and behavioral problems. Magnetic resonance imaging studies of children up to 16 years old with prenatal exposure to *methamphetamine* showed smaller brain structures correlating with impairment in **executive functioning (e.g., attention deficit) and verbal memory** [147]. A cohort of infants followed up to 24 months demonstrated fine and gross motor deficits following in utero exposure to ecstasy [148] No long-term studies of prenatal *ecstasy* exposure are available [124].

Therapy

There are currently no FDA-approved medications available for detoxification or maintenance of amphetamine dependence. Nonetheless, these women should be referred for treatment because **psychosocial interventions** (e.g., cognitive behavioral therapy) can be beneficial; due to the intensive schedule, a residential center may be preferred.

Antepartum Testing

The role of antepartum surveillance for exposure to amphetamines is insufficiently studied to make recommendations. Based on expert opinion, weekly antenatal testing is recommended starting at 32 weeks [120].

Anesthesia

Sympathectomy caused by regional anesthesia can result in profound hypotension in women using amphetamines, and vasopressors should be used with caution [40]. Small doses of benzodiazepines may be useful for agitation. Dosing of general anesthetics may be altered by acute and chronic amphetamine use [40]. Potent inhalation anesthetics (e.g., halothane) sensitize the myocardium to the effect of catecholamines, which are increased by amphetamines, increasing the risk arrhythmia.

Postpartum/Breast-Feeding

The AAP and ACOG strongly advise that women **should not ingest amphetamines while breast-feeding** [42,127]. Amphetamines can decrease breast milk supply by inhibiting prolactin release [127]. Additionally, amphetamines **concentrate in breast milk**, resulting in levels 2.8–7.5 times higher than in maternal plasma [127]. Adverse effects on the neonate have been reported (irritability, poor sleep, hypertension, tachycardia, seizures) [41,42]. **Infant fatality from continued methamphetamine use during breast-feeding has been reported** [41. Like amphetamines, ecstasy is also concentrated in breast milk [41]. At prescription doses, methylphenidate levels in breast milk are very low (relative infant dose 0.7%; <10% is generally considered acceptable for breast-feeding) [149].

BENZODIAZEPINES
Historic Notes

Benzodiazepines have been studied as potential treatments for threatened abortion, preterm labor, preeclampsia, and as adjuncts for pain management in labor.

Diagnosis/Definition

Benzodiazepines are a group of compounds formed through the fusion of a benzene and a diazepine ring. They are categorized by half-life as short-, medium-, and long-acting. Street names for benzodiazepines include "benzos," "downers," "nerve pills," and "tranks." Benzodiazepines are usually taken orally.

Symptoms

Benzodiazepines are sedative drugs, used mainly for the treatment of anxiety, and have the potential for addiction. They act on the GABAa receptor inhibiting postsynaptic signaling.

Epidemiology/Incidence

Benzodiazepines were the most commonly prescribed drugs in pregnancy [150]. In the 1970s and 1980s, 1.6% to 2.2% of pregnant women in the United States and Europe used benzodiazepines during pregnancy; however, the exact incidence of benzodiazepine exposure is unclear with rates varying from <1% to 40% [151].

Etiology/Basic Pathophysiology

Benzodiazepines cross the placenta; fetal and neonatal concentration vary between benzodiazepines. Whereas diazepam levels in the neonate are one- to threefold higher than those of the mother, neonatal levels of midazolam are lower than those of the mother [150].

Risk Factors/Associations

Benzodiazepine exposure in Swedish women is associated with older age, higher incidence of smoking, less education, and use of other psychoactive drugs [151].

Complications

A clear understanding of the effects of benzodiazepines is limited by significant heterogeneity between studies: benzodiazepines studied as a class versus individual agents; effect of the underlying medical condition (e.g., epilepsy) or obstetrical complication (e.g., preeclampsia); prescribed use of therapeutic doses versus illicit use; concomitant use of other psychoactive drugs, illicit substances, tobacco, or alcohol.

- *Congenital anomalies*: Benzodiazepines do not carry a significant risk of teratogenesis [152,153]. In a meta-analysis of first trimester exposure to benzodiazepines there was **no increase in major malformations** (OR 1.06 95% CI 0.91–1.25) [154]. Although previous reports suggested an increased risk of cleft lip and palate, the absolute risk of oral cleft from prenatal benzodiazepine exposure was increased by only 0.01%, from six in 10,000 to seven in 10,000 [155]. Considering benzodiazepine individually rather than as a class, the OR for anal atresia was 6.15 (95% CI 2.44–15.74) following exposure to lorazepam [156].
- *Obstetrical and neonatal complications*: **PTB** (early exposure: aOR 1.48, 95% CI 1.26–1.75; late exposure aOR 2.57 95% CI 1.92–3.43), **LBW** (early exposure: aOR 1.30, 95% CI 1.06–1.59; late exposure: aOR 1.89, 95% CI 1.89–2.76), **low Apgar scores** <7 at five minutes (late exposure: aOR 2.02, 95% CI 1.13–3.65), all have been associated with benzodiazepine exposure [157]. After exclusion of women with reported use of antidepressants, there was no significant increased risk of PTB or low APGAR score <7 at five minutes. Benzodiazepine use immediately prior to delivery may result in delivery of a **sedated neonate**.
- *Neonatal withdrawal*: Neonatal withdrawal from benzodiazepines is characterized by **hypoventilation**, irritability, hypertonicity, and "floppy infant syndrome" (hypotonia, lethargy, poor respiratory effort, and feeding difficulties). Other withdrawal symptoms include irritability, sleep disturbance, **restlessness, hyperreflexia, tremulousness, jitteriness, and gastrointestinal symptoms** (diarrhea and vomiting) [152]. Symptoms of withdrawal may be delayed, not occurring until day 12 to 21, and may last for several months [152]. We recommend limiting as clinically feasible administration of benzodiazepines to pregnant women, especially those on methadone maintenance therapy. Benzodiazepine use by women on methadone maintenance therapy is associated with more severe neonatal NAS [55,70,77,158]. In a multivariate analysis, the mean length of treatment was two weeks longer among neonates exposed to methadone and benzodiazepines versus methadone alone [77].
- *Long-term neonatal outcome*: There is a paucity of long-term data; however, benzodiazepines have been available for >40 years, and there is **no significant evidence of a harmful effect on brain development** [152,153]. At 18 months, compared to children of women without psychiatric disorders, benzodiazepine (mainly diazepam-exposed children (n = 17) showed impaired fine motor skills and abnormal tone and patterns of movement (e.g., walking) [159]. However, in a study of children with prenatal exposure to chlordiazepoxide, there was no evidence of abnormal neurodevelopment (IQ or motor status) at eight months (n = 501 children) or four years (n = 435 children) [160].

Therapy

Abrupt discontinuation of benzodiazepines may cause **serious maternal withdrawal**. Mild symptoms include tremor, diaphoresis, tachycardia, and other vital sign changes. More serious symptoms include seizure, delirium, autonomic instability, and suicidal ideation. Benzodiazepine withdrawal is less likely if a woman has not taken therapeutic doses (i.e., three to four times per day) for ≥4 weeks. These women should be reassessed for benzodiazepine withdrawal if they have changes in vital signs (systolic blood pressure ≥150 mmHg, diastolic blood pressure ≥100 mmHg, pulse >110 beats/min, temperature >101°F, or SpO_2 <96%) or symptoms of anxiety or agitation. **Psychiatry consultation** is suggested **for women who are dependent on benzodiazepines** (i.e., use of benzodiazepine at therapeutic doses for ≥4 weeks). **Typically scheduled tapering is done with a longer-acting benzodiazepine (e.g., Klonopin) to reduce the risk of benzodiazepine withdrawal seizure.** Protocols based on objective measures (e.g., vital signs), symptoms, and subjective complaints, such as the Clinical Institute Withdrawal Assessment of Alcohol Scale, Revised, can be used instead of or in addition to tapering. There are no published guidelines for detoxification during pregnancy. Likewise, there are currently no FDA-approved medications available for maintenance of benzodiazepine dependence.

Antepartum Testing

The role of antepartum surveillance for benzodiazepine exposure is insufficiently studied to make a recommendation.

Postpartum/Breast-Feeding

Approximately 0.1% to 11% of the weight-adjusted maternal benzodiazepine dose is transferred to the breast milk and is drug-specific [141]. Nonetheless, most prescription benzodiazepines are "**moderately safe**" (lactation risk category L3) during breast-feeding and few adverse events are reported [161]. However, CNS depression, accumulation of metabolites, and prolonged half-life in the neonate have been noted [41]. Sedation may be more likely when multiple CNS depressant medications are taken together [152]. Women are strongly advised to refrain from nonmedical use of benzodiazepines while breast-feeding [42].

PHENCYCLIDINE
Historic Notes

Phencyclidine (PCP) was developed as an anesthetic agent and produced effective anesthesia and analgesia with minimal respiratory and cardiovascular depression but was removed from the market because of a high incidence of delirium, agitation, and violence [162]. The dissociative anesthetic ketamine is a derivative of PCP [162].

Diagnosis/Definition

The chemical name of PCP is 1-(1-phenylcyclohexyl) piperidine. Street names for PCP include angel dust, hog, ozone, rocket fuel, shermans, wack, crystal, and embalming fluid. PCP is most commonly smoked (73%) or snorted (13%) but can also be swallowed (12%) or injected (2%) [163,164].

Symptoms

Most women who abuse PCP do so only occasionally, and a typical dose is 5 mg. Chronic use may lead to habituation and the need for doses as high as 100 mg to achieve the same feeling [165]. Common symptoms of intoxication are nystagmus, hypertension, altered consciousness (e.g., depressed), mental status changes (e.g., disorientation and hallucinations), and bizarre behavior (e.g., agitation and violence) [162]. Although rare, acute psychosis and death have been reported [166].

Epidemiology/Incidence

Although popular in the 1970s, PCP abuse declined in the late 1980s and 1990s but has recently reemerged as a drug of abuse. In the early 1980s, PCP use by pregnant women in Cleveland ranged from **5.8%** (by testing) to **6.4%** (by history) [164,167].

Etiology/Basic Pathophysiology

The exact mechanism of action of PCP is unclear. PCP is an *N*-methyl D-aspartate (NMDA) receptor antagonist [168]. PCP crosses the placenta and can be detected in amniotic fluid, umbilical cord blood [169–171], and neonatal urine [172]. Concentrations in the fetus may exceed maternal levels [43,95,132].

Risk Factors/Associations

The rate of concomitant tobacco use ranges from 43% to 84% [173–175]. The majority of pregnant women who use PCP during pregnancy also abuse other illicit drugs (e.g., cocaine) and alcohol.

Pregnancy Complications

There is a **high rate of polysubstance abuse by women using PCP**, which limits the ability to tease out the obstetrical and neonatal effects of PCP abuse. The use of matched, non–drug-exposed controls was infrequent.

- *Congenital anomalies*: Although there were early case reports of infants exposed antenatally to PCP born with dysmorphic facial features [167,176], microcephaly [172], and cerebellar malformations, **no increased rate of congenital malformations** have been reported in a literature review totaling 206 neonates with prenatal PCP exposure [177].
- *Obstetrical complications*: The rate of **PTB** among PCP-exposed neonates was 20% to 22% [173,176].
- *Fetal/neonatal morphometrics*: Prenatal exposure to PCP has not been consistently shown to affect birth weight, length, or head circumference [164,174,175]. However, higher-than-expected rates of **IUGR** (32%) [173], **LBW** (30%) [176], and **SGA** (17%) [176] have been reported.
- *Neonatal withdrawal*: Neonatal withdrawal from PCP is characterized by neurological (e.g., tremor, abnormal tone, and hypertonic reflexes) and gastrointestinal (e.g., emesis and diarrhea) symptoms, irritability, exaggerated responses to auditory and tactile stimuli, lethargy and rapid shifts in consciousness [164,165,172,175,176,178]. Symptoms of withdrawal were reported in 55% of 22 infants with exposure to PCP alone [176]. Symptoms of withdrawal can be managed conservatively (e.g., swaddling), by acidification of the urine, or when medications are indicated, with phenobarbital, diazepam, or paregoric.
- *Long-term neonatal outcome*: Studies of long-term neurodevelopmental outcome are limited by small size and dropout rates of over 50%. Attachment disorder has been described during the first year of life [176]. At 12 to 18 months of age, exposed infants demonstrated **impaired fine motor skills** [178]. Caretakers reported **behavioral problems (e.g., temper tantrums and oppositional behaviors), inconsolability, and sleep disturbances** [176,178].

Therapy

Mild symptoms can be managed by placing the individual in a dark, quiet environment with as little stimulation as possible. Additional symptoms and their treatments are as follows: convulsions are treated with diazepam, hypertension with antihypertensives (e.g., hydralazine), fever with antipyretics, and severe rigidity and rhabdomyolysis with dantrolene [43,179]. There are currently no FDA-approved medications available for detoxification or maintenance of PCP dependence.

Antepartum Testing

The role of antepartum surveillance is insufficiently studied to make recommendations. However, hypertension in response to moderate to high doses of PCP may be an indication for nonstress testing and/or ultrasound to estimate fetal weight [43].

Postpartum/Breast-Feeding

PCP is present in breast milk [169,170] in sufficient quantities to cause intoxication [41]. The AAP advises that women should not use PCP while breast-feeding [41,42].

HALLUCINOGENS: LYSERGIC ACID DIETHYLAMIDE, PSILOCYBIN (MAGIC MUSHROOMS), PEYOTE (MESCALINE)
Historic Notes
Naturally occurring hallucinogens have been used for centuries as part of religious and cultural activities. LSD, the prototypical synthetic hallucinogen, was synthesized in 1938 by the chemist Albert Hofmann, who recognized its hallucinogenic capabilities when he was accidentally exposed.

Diagnosis/Definition
The active ingredients in psilocybin and peyote are psilocin (N, N-dimethyl-4-phosphoryloxytryptamine) and 3,4,5-trimethoxypheneylamine. LSD is an ergot (rye fungus) derivative. Street names are as follows:

- LSD: acid, trips, microdots, dots, blotters (or named by the design on the blotting paper), mellow, or tabs
- Psilocybin: magic mushrooms, shrooms, magics, blue meanies, liberty caps, golden tops, mushies
- Peyote: buttons, cactus, mesc

LSD can be taken orally as a tablet, capsule, or liquid applied to blotter paper, sniffed, injected, or smoked. Psilocybin and peyote are usually taken orally; peyote can also be smoked.

Symptoms
Hallucinogens principally alter sensory perceptions, mood, and thought patterns through alteration of serotonin pathways in the central nervous system [59]. Vital sign abnormalities are uncommon, but may include increased blood pressure and heart rate. Rare complications include hyperthermia and serotonin syndrome.

Epidemiology/Incidence
According to the National Household Survey on Drug Abuse, **0.2%** of reproductive age women aged 15 to 44 years reported hallucinogen use in the past month. Among pregnant women screened for inclusion in a study of prenatal methamphetamine exposure, <0.5% used hallucinogens. In Europe, the rate of LSD and hallucinogenic mushroom use is 0.4%–2.0% (7.5% in the United Kingdom) and 0.2%–12.8%, respectively [180].

Etiology/Basic Pathophysiology
Evidence that LSD causes DNA damage in vitro raises concerns about its potential as a teratogen [181].

Complications
The effects of hallucinogen exposure on obstetrical neonatal outcome are not well studied.

- *Congenital anomalies*: In a literature review including 162 pregnancies with parental LSD use before or during pregnancy, there were seven anomalies (4.3%) not attributable to other causes. **Limb reduction defects** accounted for five of the seven anomalies; a higher-than-expected incidence (1.78/1000) [182]. Another series of 148 pregnancies, including specimens from spontaneous and induced abortions with parental LSD use showed a 9.6% rate of major anomalies that were mainly **central nervous system** (hydrocephalus and arteriovenous malformations) and **neural tube defects.** Eye abnormalities have also been reported [59]. Because of lack of appropriate controls and confounding by use of other illicit substances, tobacco, and alcohol, **a cause-and-effect relationship cannot be established** [182,183]. There are no reports of human teratogenesis because of psilocybin or peyote [181].
- *Obstetrical and neonatal complications*: There is no evidence that LSD or other hallucinogens increased the risk of PTB or have an effect on birth weight.
- *Long-term neonatal outcome*: Follow-up of children whose parents used LSD to 2.5 years old showed no growth or developmental abnormalities [183].

Therapy
In most cases, supportive care is all that is necessary. Benzodiazepines are the first-line treatment for acute agitation. Rarely, severe hyperthermia may require medically induced paralysis. There are currently no FDA-approved medications available for detoxification or maintenance of hallucinogen dependence.

Antepartum Testing
The role of antepartum surveillance is insufficiently studied to make recommendations. However, hyperthermia and serotonin syndrome may be an indication for fetal monitoring.

REFERENCES
1. Kremer ME, Arora KS. Clinical, ethical, and legal considerations in pregnant women with opioid abuse. *Obstet Gynecol* 2015; 126(3): 474–8. [Review; III]
2. *Results from the 2013 National Survey on Drug Use & Health: Summary of National Findings*. Available at: http://www.samhsa.gov/data/sites/default/files/NSDUHresultsPDFWHTML2013/Web/NSDUHresults2013.pdf. Last accessed February 3, 2016. [Survey; level III]
3. Rayburn WF, Bogenschutz MP. Pharmacotherapy for pregnant women with addictions. *Am J Obstet Gynecol* 2004; 191(6): 1885–97. [Review; III]
4. Azadi A, Dildy GA 3rd. Universal screening for substance abuse at the time of parturition. *Am J Obstet Gynecol* 2008; 198(5): e30–2. [II-3]
5. Martin J, Payte JT, Zweben JE. Methadone maintenance treatment: A primer for physicians. *J Psychoactive Drugs* 1991; 23(2): 165–76. [Review; III]
6. ACOG. Motivational interviewing: A tool for behavioral change. ACOG Committee Opinion No. 423. *Obstet Gynecol* 2009; 113(1): 243–6. [III]
7. ACOG. Opioid abuse, dependence, and addiction in pregnancy. ACOG Committee Opinion No. 524. *Obstet Gynecol* 2012; 119(5): 1070–6. [III]
8. Jones HE, Deppen K, Hudak ML et al. Clinical care for opioid-using pregnant and postpartum women: The role of obstetric providers. *Am J Obstet Gynecol* 2014; 210(4): 302–10. [Review; III]
9. Oei, JL, Kingsbury A, Dhawan A et al. Amphetamines, the pregnant woman and her children: A review. *J Perinatol* 2012; 32(10): 737–47. [Review; III]
10. Kuczkowski KM. The effects of drug abuse on pregnancy. *Curr Opin Obstet Gynecol* 2007; 19(6): 578–85. [Review; III]
11. ACOG. Cocaine in pregnancy. ACOG Committee Opinion No. 114. *Int J Gynaecol Obstet* 1993; 41(1): 102–105. [III]

12. Terplan M, Lui S. Psychosocial interventions for pregnant women in outpatient illicit drug treatment programs compared to other interventions. *Cochrane Database Syst Rev* 2007; 17(4): CD006037. [Systematic Review; I]

13. Whitworth M, Dowswell T. Routine pre-pregnancy health promotion for improving pregnancy outcomes. *Cochrane Database Syst Rev* 2009; 7(4): CD007536. [Systematic Review; I]

14. ACOG. Substance abuse in pregnancy. ACOG Technical Bulletin No. 195. *Int J Gynaecol Obstet* 1994; 47(1): 73–80. [III]

15. ACOG. Alcohol abuse and other substance use disorders: Ethical issues in obstetric and gynecologic practice. ACOG Committee Opinion No. 633. *Obstet Gynecol* 2015; 125(6): 1529–37. [III]

16. National Institute on Drug. *Abuse screening for drug use in general medical settings.* Available at: https://d14rmgtrwzf5a.cloudfront.net/sites/default/files/resource_guide.pdf. Last accessed February 3, 2016. [III]

17. Childers SR, Breivogel CS. Cannabis and endogenous cannabinoid systems. *Drug Alcohol Depend* 1998; 51(1–2): 173–87. [Review; III]

18. *DrugsFacts: Synthetic Cannabinoids.* Available at: http://www.drugabuse.gov/publications/drugfacts/k2spice-synthetic-marijuana. Last accessed February 3, 2016. [III]

19. Kuczkowski KM. Marijuana in pregnancy. *Ann Acad Med Singapore* 2004; 33(3): 336–9. [III]

20. de Moraes Barros MC, Guinsburg R, de Arújo Peres C et al. Exposure to marijuana during pregnancy alters neurobehavior in the early neonatal period. *J Pediatr* 2006; 149(6): 781–7. [Review; III]

21. Conner SN, Carter EB, Tuuli MG et al. Maternal marijuana use and neonatal morbidity. *Am J Obstet Gynecol* 2015; 213(3): 422 e1–4. [II-2]

22. ACOG. Marijuana Use During Pregnancy and Lactation. ACOG Committee Opinion No. 637. *Obstet Gynecol* 2015; 126(1): 234–8. [III]

23. Maritn CE, Longinaker N, Mark K et al. Recent trends in treatment admissions for marijuana use during pregnancy. *J Addict Med* 2014; 00: 1–6. [II-3]

24. Kozer E, Koren G. Effects of prenatal exposure to marijuana. *Can Fam Physician* 2001; 47: 264. [III]

25. El Marroun H, Tiemeier H, Steegers EA et al. A prospective study on intrauterine cannabis exposure and fetal blood flow. *Early Hum Dev* 2010; 86(4): 231–6. [II-2]

26. Cornelius MD, Taylor PM, Geva D et al. Prenatal tobacco and marijuana use among adolescents: Effects on offspring gestational age, growth, and morphology. *Pediatrics* 1995; 95(5): 738–43. [II-2]

27. Ko JY, Farr SL, Tong VT et al. Prevalence and patterns of marijuana use among pregnant and nonpregnant women of reproductive age. *Am J Obstet Gynecol* 2015; 213: 201 e1–10. [II-2]

28. Jobe AH. Marijuana effects on neurobehavior of newborns. *J Pediatr* 2006; 149(6): a1. [III]

29. Linn S, Schoenbaum SC, Monson RR et al. The association of marijuana use with outcome of pregnancy. *Am J Public Health* 1983; 73(10): 1161–4. [II-2]

30. Viteri, OA, Soto EE, Bahado-Singh RO et al. Fetal anomalies and long-term effects associated with substance abuse in pregnancy: A literature review. *Am. J Obstet Gynecol* 2015; 32(5): 405–16. [III]

31. Fried PA, Watkinson B, Willan A. Marijuana use during pregnancy and decreased length of gestation. *Am J Obstet Gynecol* 1984; 150(1): 23–7. [II-2]

32. Warshak CR, Regan J, Moore B et al. Association between marijuana use and adverse obstetrical and neonatal outcomes. *J Perinatol* 2015; 35(12): 991–5. [II-2]

33. El Marroun HE, Tiemeier H, Steegers EAP et al. Intrauterine cannabis exposure affects fetal growth trajectories: The generation R study. *J Am Acad Child Adolesc Psychiatry* 2009; 48(12): 1173–81. [II-2]

34. Bada HS, Reynolds EW, Hansen WF. Marijuana use, adolescent pregnancy, and alteration in newborn behavior: How complex can it get? *J Pediatr* 2006; 149(6): 742–5. [Comment]

35. Fried PA. Prenatal exposure to tobacco and marijuana: Effect during pregnancy, infancy, and early childhood. *Clin Obstet Gynecol* 1993; 36(2): 319–37. [Review; III]

36. Scragg RK, Mitchell EA, Ford RP et al. Maternal cannabis use in the sudden death syndrome. *Acta Paediatr* 2001; 90(1): 57–60. [II-2]

37. Reece-Stremtan S, Marinelli KA. ABM clinical protocol #21: Guidelines for breastfeeding and substance use or substance use disorder, revised 2015. *Breastfeed Med* 2015; 10(3): 135–41. [III]

38. Day NL, Goldschmidt L, Day R et al. Prenatal marijuana exposure, age of marijuana initiation, and the development of psychotic symptoms in young adults. *Psychol Med* 2015; 45(8): 1779–87. [II-3]

39. Calvigioni DH, Hurd YL, Harkany T et al. Neuronal substrates and functional consequences of prenatal cannabis exposure. *Eur Child Adolesc Psychiatry* 2014; 23(10): 931–41. [Review; III]

40. Kuczkowski KM. Anesthetic implications of drug abuse in pregnancy. *J Clin Anesth* 2003; 15(5): 382–94. [Review; III]

41. Sachs HC, Frattarelli DA, Galinkin JL et al. The transfer of drugs and therapeutics into human breast milk: An update on selected topics. *Pediatrics* 2013; 132(3): e796–809. [III]

42. Eidelman AI, Schanler RJ, Johnston M et al. Breastfeeding and the use of human milk. *Pediatrics* 2012; 129(3): e827–41. [III]

43. Glantz CJ, Woods JR Jr. Cocaine, heroin, and phencyclidine: Obstetric perspective. *Clin Obstet Gynecol* 1993; 36(2): 279–301. [Review; III]

44. Wilbourne P, Wallerstedt C, Dorato V et al. Clinical management of methadone dependence during pregnancy. *J Perinat Neonatal Nurs* 2001; 14(4): 26–45. [Review; III]

45. Brown HL, Britton KA, Mahaffey D et al. Methadone maintenance in pregnancy: A reappraisal. *Am J Obstet Gynecol* 1998; 179(2): 459–63. [Review; III]

46. Tolia VN, Patrick SW, Bennett MM et al. Increasing incidence of the neonatal abstinence syndrome in US neonatal ICUs. *N Engl J Med* 2015; 372(22): 2118–26. [II-3]

47. Kaltenbach K, Berghella V, Finnegan L. Opioid dependence during pregnancy: Effects and management. *Obstet Gynecol Clin North Am* 1998; 25(1): 139–51. [Review; III]

48. Broussard CS, Rasmussen SA, Reefhuis J et al. for the National Birth Defects Prevention Study. Maternal treatment with opioid analgesics and risk for birth defects. *Am J Obstet Gynecol* 2011; 204(4): 314.e1–11. [II-2]

49. Minozzi S, Amato L, Vecchi S et al. Maintenance agonist treatments for opiate dependent pregnant women. *Cochrane Database Syst Rev* 2008; 16(2): CD006318. [Systematic Review; I]

50. Almario CV, Seligman NS, Dysart KC et al. Risk factors for preterm birth among opiate-addicted gravid women in a methadone treatment program. *Am J Obstet Gynecol* 2009; 201(3): 326. e1–6. [II-2]

51. Stimmel B, Goldberg J, Reisman A et al. Fetal outcome in narcotic-dependent women: The importance of the type of maternal narcotic used. *Am J Drug Alcohol Abuse* 1982; 9(4): 383–95. [II-2]

52. Kandall SR, Albin S, Lowinson J et al. Differential effects of maternal heroin and methadone use on birthweight. *Pediatrics* 1976; 58(5): 681–5. [II-2]

53. Doberczak TM, Thronton JC, Bernstein J et al. Impact of maternal drug dependency on birth weight and head circumference of offspring. *Am J Dis Child* 1987; 141(11): 1163–7. [II-2]

54. Kaltenbach K, Silverman N, Wapner RJ. Methadone maintenance during pregnancy. In: Parrino MW, ed. *State Methadone Treatment Guidelines.* Rockville, MD: U.S. Department of Health and Human Services, Center for Substance Abuse Treatment, 1992: 85–93. [Review III]

55. Oei J, Lui K. Management of the newborn affected by maternal opiates and other drugs of dependency. *J Paediatr Child Health* 2007; 43(1–2): 9–18. [Review; III]

56. Finnegan LP, Connaughton JF Jr., Kron RE et al. Neonatal abstinence syndrome: Assessment and management. *Addict Dis* 1975; 2(1–2): 141–58. [II-3]

57. Kraft WK, Gibson E, Dysart K et al. Sublingual buprenorphine for treatment of neonatal abstinence syndrome: A randomized trial. *Pediatrics* 2008; 122(3): e601–7. [RCT, *n* = 26; I]

58. Hunt RW, Tzioumi D, Collins E et al. Adverse neurodevelopmental outcome of infants exposed to opiates in-utero. *Early Hum Dev* 2008; 84(1): 29–35. [Review; III]

59. Holbrook BD, Rayburn WF. Teratogenic risks from exposure to illicit drugs. *Obstet Gynecol Clin North Am* 2014; 41(2): 229–39. [Review; III]

60. Mattick RP, Breen C, Kimber J et al. Buprenorphine maintenance versus placebo or methadone maintenance for opioid dependence. *Cochrane Database Syst Rev* 2008; 16(2): CD002207. [Systematic Review; I]

61. Dashe JS, Sheffield JS, Olscher DA et al. Relationship between maternal methadone dosage and neonatal withdrawal. *Obstet Gynecol* 2002; 100(6): 1244–9. [II-2]

62. Maas U, Kattner E, Weingart-Jesse B et al. Infrequent neonatal opiate withdrawal following maternal methadone detoxification during pregnancy. *J Perinat Med* 1990; 18(2): 111–8. [II-2]

63. Amato L, Davoli M, Minozzi S et al. Methadone at tapered doses for the management of opioid withdrawal. *Cochrane Database Syst Rev* 2005; 20(3): CD003409. [Systematic Review; I]

64. Maura S, Resemble A. Leaving methadone treatment: Lessons learned, lessons forgotten, lessons ignored. *Mt Sinai J Med* 2001; 68: 62–74. [Review; III]

65. Stewart RD, Nelson DB, Adhikari EH et al. The obstetrical and neonatal impact of maternal opioid detoxification in pregnancy. *Am J Obstet Gynecol* 2013; 209:e1–5 [II-1]

66. Rementeria JL, Nunag NN. Narcotic withdrawal in pregnancy: Stillbirth incidence with a case report. *Am J Obstet Gynecol* 1973; 116(8): 1152–5. [II-3]

67. Zuspan FP, Gumpel JA, Mejia-Zelaya A et al. Fetal stress from methadone withdrawal. *Am J Obstet Gynecol* 1975; 122(1): 43–6. [II-3]

68. Dashe JS, Jackson GL, Olscher DA et al. Opioid detoxification in pregnancy. Obstet Gynecol 1998; 92(5): 854–8. [II-3]

69. Blinick G, Wallach RC, Jerez E. Pregnancy in narcotics addicts treated by medical withdrawal. The methadone detoxification program. *Am J Obstet Gynecol* 1969; 105(7): 997–1003. [II]

70. Berghella V, Lim PJ, Hill MK et al. Maternal methadone dose and neonatal withdrawal. *Am J Obstet Gynecol* 2003; 189(2): 312–7. [II-2]

71. Seligman NS, Berghella V. Methadone maintenance therapy during pregnancy. In: *UpToDate*, Waltham MA. (Accessed on February 3, 2016). [Review; III]

72. Drozdick JD, Berghella V, Hill MK et al. Methadone trough levels in pregnancy. *Am J Obstet Gynecol* 2002; 187(5): 1184–8. [II-2]

73. Jones H, Kaltenbach K, Heil SH et al. Neonatal abstinence syndrome after methadone or buprenorphine exposure. *N Engl J Med* 2010; 363(24): 2320–31. [RCT, *n* = 131; I]

74. Strauss ME, Andresko M, Stryker JC et al. Relationship of neonatal withdrawal to maternal methadone dose. *Am J Drug Alcohol Abuse* 1976; 3(2): 339–45. [II-2]

75. Cleary BJ, Donnelly J, Strawbridge J et al. Methadone dose and neonatal abstinence syndrome-systematic review and meta-analysis. *Addiction* 2010; 105(12): 2071–84. [Meta-analysis]

76. Seligman NS, Almario CV, Hayes EJ et al. Relationship between maternal methadone dose at delivery and neonatal abstinence syndrome. *J Pediatr* 2010; 57(3): 428–33, 433.e1. [II-2]

77. Seligman NS, Salva N, Hayes EJ et al. Predicting length of treatment for neonatal abstinence syndrome in methadone-exposed neonates. *Am J Obstet Gynecol* 2008; 199(4): 396.e1–7. [II-2]

78. Hayes E, Seligman N, Horowitz K et al. 252: Dose-response relationship between maternal methadone dose and decreased neonatal head circumference. *Am J Obstet Gynecol* 2007; 197(6 Suppl.): s81. [II-2]

79. Hamilton R, McGlone L, MacKinnon JR et al. Ophthalmic, clinical, and visual electrophysiological findings in children born to mothers prescribed substitute methadone in pregnancy. *Br J Ophthalmol* 2010; 94(6): 696–700. [II-3]

80. Fischer G, Jagsch R, Eder H et al. Comparison of methadone and slow-release morphine maintenance in pregnant addicts. *Addiction* 1999; 94(2): 231–9. [RCT, *n* = 48; I]

81. Kashiwagi M, Arlettaz R, Lauper U et al. Methadone maintenance program in a Swiss perinatal center: (I): Management and outcome of 89 pregnancies. *Acta Obstet Gynecol Scand* 2005; 84(2): 140–4. [II-3]

82. Meyer M, Wagner K, Benvenuto A et al. Intrapartum and postpartum analgesia for women maintained on methadone during pregnancy. *Obstet Gynecol* 2007; 110(2, Pt. 1): 261–6. [II-2]

83. Pace CA, Kaminetzky LB, Winter M et al. Postpartum changes in methadone maintenance dose. *J Subst Abuse Treat* 2014; 47(3): 229–32. [II-3]

84. Lim S, Prasad MR, Samuels P et al. High-dose methadone in pregnant women and its effect on duration of neonatal abstinence syndrome. *Am J Obstet Gynecol* 2009; 200(1): 70.e1–5. [II-2]

85. Abdel-Latif ME, Pinner J, Clews S et al. Effects of breast milk on the severity and outcome of neonatal abstinence syndrome among infants of drug-dependent mothers. *Pediatrics* 2006; 117(6): e1163–9. [II-2]

86. Jansson LM, Choo R, Velez ML et al. Methadone maintenance and breastfeeding in the neonatal period. *Pediatrics* 2008; 121(1): 106–14. [II-2]

87. Ballard JL. Treatment of neonatal abstinence syndrome with breast milk containing methadone. *J Perinat Neonatal Nurs* 2002; 15(4): 76–85. [III]

88. Liu AJ, Nanan R. Letter to the editor: Methadone maintenance and breastfeeding in the neonatal period. *Pediatrics* 2008; 121(4): 869. [III]

89. Cain MA, Bornick P, Whiteman V. The maternal, fetal, and neonatal effects of cocaine exposure in pregnancy. *Clin Obstet Gynecol* 2013; 56(1): 124–32. [III]

90. DrugsFacts: *Cocaine*. Available at: https://www.drugabuse.gov /publications/drugfacts/cocaine. Last accessed February 3, 2016. [III]

91. Hernandez M, Birnbach DJ, Van Zundert AJ. Anesthetic management of the illicit-substance-using patient. *Curr Opin Anaesthesiol* 2005; 18(3): 3115–24. [Review; III]

92. Woods JR Jr. Pregnancy increases cardiovascular toxicity to cocaine. *Am J Obstet Gynecol* 1990; 162(2): 529–33. [II-2]

93. Plessinger MA, Woods JR Jr. Maternal, placental, and fetal pathophysiology of cocaine exposure during pregnancy. *Clin Obstet Gynecol* 1993; 36(2): 267–78. [Review; III]

94. Gaither K. Cocaine abuse in pregnancy: An evolution from panacea to pandemonium. *South Med J* 2008; 101(8): 783–4. [Editorial]

95. Plessinger MA, Woods JR Jr. Cocaine in pregnancy: Recent data on maternal and fetal risks. *Obstet Gynecol Clin North Am* 1998; 25(1): 99–118. [Review; III]

96. Richardson GA, Day NL, McGauhey PJ. Impact of prenatal marijuana and cocaine use on the infant and child. *Clin Obstet Gynecol* 1993; 36(2): 302–18. [Review; III]

97. Bauer CR, Langer JC, Shankaran S et al. Acute neonatal effects of cocaine exposure during pregnancy. *Arch Pediatr Adolesc Med* 2005; 159(9): 824–34. [II-2]

98. Bhuvaneswar CG, Chnag G, Epstein LA et al. Cocaine and opioid use during pregnancy: Prevalence and management. *Prim Care Companion J Clin Psychiatry* 2008; 10(1): 59–65. [Review III]

99. Hull L, May J, Farrell-Moore D et al. Treatment of cocaine abuse during pregnancy: Translating research to clinical practice. *Curr Psychiatry Rep* 2010; 12(5): 454–61. [Review III]

100. Monga M, Weisbrodt NW, Andres RL et al. The acute effect of cocaine exposure on pregnant human myometrial contractile activity. *Am J Obstet Gynecol* 1993; 169(4): 782–5. [II-3]

101. Oyelese Y, Ananth CV. Placental abruption. *Obstet Gynecol* 2006; 108(4): 1005–16. [Review III]

102. Day NL, Cottreau CM, Richardson GA. The epidemiology of alcohol, marijuana, and cocaine use among women of childbearing age and pregnant women. *Clin Obstet Gynecol* 1993; 36(2): 232–45. [Review III]

103. Cressman AM, Natekar A, Kim E et al. MOTHERISK ROUNDS: Cocaine Abuse During Pregnancy. *J Obstet Gynecol Canada* 2014; 36(7): 628–31. [Review; III]

104. Addis A, Moretti ME, Syed FA et al. Fetal effects of cocaine: An updated meta-analysis. *Reprod Toxicol* 2001; 15: 341–69. [Meta-analysis]

105. Meyer KD, Zhang L. Short- and long-term adverse effects of cocaine abuse during pregnancy on the heart development. *Ther Adv Cardiovasc Dis* 2009; 3(1): 7–16. [Review III]

106. Martinez A, Larrabee K, Monga M. Cocaine is associated with intrauterine fetal death in women with suspected preterm labor. *Am J Perinatol* 1996; 13: 163–6. [II-2]

107. Gouin K, Murphy K, Shah PS, and the Knowledge Synthesis Group on Determinants of Low Birth Weight and Preterm Births. Effects of cocaine use during pregnancy on low birth-weight and preterm birth: Systematic review and meta-analyses. *Am J Obstet Gynecol* 2011; 204: 304.e1–12. [Meta-analysis]

108. Bingol N, Fuchs M, Diaz V et al. Teratogenicity of cocaine in humans. *J Pediatr* 1987; 110(1): 93–6. [II-2]

109. Chasnoff IJ, Burns KA, Burns WJ. Cocaine use in pregnancy: Perinatal morbidity and mortality. *Neurotoxicol Teratol* 1987; 9: 291–3. [II-2]

110. DeLaney DB, Larrabee KD, Monga M. Preterm premature rupture of the membranes associated with recent cocaine use. *Am J Perinatol* 1997; 14(5): 285–8. [II-2]

111. Dinsmoor MJ, Iron SJ, Christmas JT. Preterm premature rupture of the membranes associated with recent cocaine use. *Am J Obstet Gynecol* 1994; 171(2): 305–8. [II-2]

112. Cordero DR, Medina C, Helfgott A. Cocaine body packing in pregnancy. *Ann Emerg Med* 2006; 48(3): 323–5. [II-3]

113. Bulterys M, Landesman S, Burns DN. Sexual behavior and injection drug use during pregnancy and vertical transmission of HIV-1. *J Acquir Immune Defic Syn Hum Retrovirol* 1997; 15: 76–82. [II-3]

114. Bada HS, Das A, Bauer CR et al. Gestational cocaine exposure and intrauterine growth: Maternal lifestyle study. *Obstet Gynecol* 2002; 100: 916–24. [II-2]

115. Shankaran S, Banh CM, Bauer CR et al. Prenatal cocaine exposure and BMI and blood pressure at 9 years of age. *J Hypertens* 2010; 28(6): 1166–75. [II-2]

116. Grewen K, Burchinal M, Vachet C et al. Prenatal cocaine effects on brain structure in early infancy. *Neuroimage* 2014; 101: 114–23. [II-2]

117. Elk R, Mangus L, Rhoades H et al. Cessation of cocaine use during pregnancy: Effects of contingency management interventions on maintaining abstinence and complying with prenatal care. *Addict Behav* 1998; 23(1): 57–64. [RCT, *n* = 12; I]

118. Svikis DS, Golden AS, Huggins GR et al. Cost-effectiveness of treatment for drug-abusing pregnant women. *Drug Alcohol Depend* 1997; 45(1–2): 105–13. [III]

119. Yonkers KA, Forray A, Nich C et al. Progesterone reduces cocaine use in postpartum women with a cocaine use disorder: A randomized, double-blinded study. *Lancet Psychiatry* 2014; 1(5): 360–7. [RCT, *n* = 50;I]

120. Izquierdo LA, Yonke N. Fetal surveillance in late pregnancy and during labor. *Obstet Gynecol Clin North Am* 2014; 41(2): 307–15. [Review III]

121. Kuczkowski KM. The cocaine abusing parturient: A review of anesthetic considerations. *Can J Anesth* 2004; 51(2): 145–54. [Review; III]

122. Berman S, O'Neill J, Fears S et al. Abuse of amphetamines and structural abnormalities in brain. *Ann N Y Acad Sci* 2008; 1141: 195–220. [Review; III]

123. Anglin MD, Burke C, Perrochet B et al. History of the methamphetamine problem. *J Psychoactive Drugs* 2000; 32(2): 137–41. [Review; III]

124. Skelton MR, Williams MT, Vorhees CV. Developmental effects of 3,4-methylenedioxymethamphetamine: A review. *Behav Pharmacol* 2008; 19(2): 91–111. [Review; III]

125. DrugsFacts: *Synthetic Cathinones*. Available at: https://www.drugabuse.gov/publications/drugfacts/synthetic-cathinones-bath-salts. Last accessed February 3, 2016. [III]

126. Plessinger MA. Prenatal exposure to amphetamines. Risks and adverse outcomes in pregnancy. *Obstet Gynecol Clin North Am* 1998; 25(1): 119–38. [Review III]

127. ACOG. Methamphetamine abuse in women of reproductive age. ACOG Committee Opinion No. 479. *Obstet Gynecol* 2011; 117(3): 751–5. [III]

128. Terplan M, Smith EJ, Kozloski MJ et al. Methamphetamine use among pregnant women. *Obstet Gynecol* 2009; 113(6): 1285–91. [II-3]

129. Green AR, Mechan AO, Elliott JM et al. The pharmacology and clinical pharmacology of 3,4-methylenedioxymethamphetamine (MDMA, "ecstasy"). *Pharmacol Rev* 2003; 55(3): 463–508. [Review; III]

130. Johnston LD, O'Malley PM, Bachman JG et al. *Monitoring the future national survey results on drug use, 1975–2006. Volume I: Secondary school students* (NIH Publication No. 07-6202). Bethesda, MD: National Institute on Drug Abuse, 2007. [II-3]

131. Gorman MC, Orme KS, Nguyen NT et al. Outcomes in pregnancies complicated by methamphetamine use. *Am J Obstet Gynecol* 2014; 211(4): 429-e1. [II-2]

132. Good MM, Solt I, Acuna JG et al. Methamphetamine use during pregnancy: Maternal and neonatal implications. *Obstet Gynecol* 2010; 116(2 Pt. 1): 330–4. [II-2, *n* = 276]

133. Cox S, Posner SF, Kourtis AP, Jamieson DJ. Hospitalizations with amphetamine abuse among pregnant women. *Obstet Gynecol* 2008; 111(2, Pt. 1): 341–7. [III]

134. Della Grotta S, LaGrasse LL, Arria AM et al. Patterns of methamphetamine use during pregnancy: Results from the Infant Development, Environment, and Lifestyle (IDEAL) study. *Matern Child Health J* 2010; 14(4): 519–27. [II-2]

135. Arria AM, Derauf C, Lagasse LL et al. Methamphetamine and other substance use during pregnancy: Preliminary estimates from the Infant Development, Environment, and Lifestyle (IDEAL) study. *Matern Child Health J* 2006; 10(3): 293–302. [II-3]

136. Nguyen D, Smith LM, LaGrasse LL et al. Intrauterine growth of infants exposed to prenatal methamphetamine: Results from the infant development, environment, and lifestyle study. *J Pediatr* 2010; 157(2): 337–9. [II-2]

137. Derauf C, LaGrasse LL, Smith LM et al. Demographic and psychosocial characteristics of mothers using methamphetamine during pregnancy: Preliminary results of the Infant Development, Environment, and Lifestyle Study (IDEAL). *Am J Drug Alcohol Abuse* 2007; 33(2): 281–9. [II-2]

138. Ho E, Karimi-Tabesh L, Gideon K. Characteristics of pregnant women who use Ecstasy (3, 4-methylenedioxymethamphetamine. *Neurotoxicol Teratol* 2001; 23(6): 561–7. [II-2]

139. Smith LM, LaGrasse LL, Derauf C et al. The Infant Development, Environment, and Lifestyle Study (IDEAL): Effects of prenatal methamphetamine exposure, polydrug exposure, and poverty on intrauterine growth. *Pediatrics* 2006; 118(3): 1149–56. [II-2]

140. Oei JL, Kingsbury A, Dhawan A et al. Amphetamines, the pregnant woman and her children: A review. *J Perinatol* 2012; 32(10): 737–47. [Review; III]

141. McElhatton PR, Bateman DN, Evans C et al. Congenital anomalies after prenatal ecstasy exposure. *Lancet* 1999; 354: 1441–2. [II-3]

142. Ladhani NN, Shah PS, Murphy KE, for the Knowledge Synthesis Group on Determinants of Preterm/LBW Births. Prenatal amphetamine exposure and birth outcomes: A systematic review and metaanalysis. *Am J Obstet Gynecol* 2011; 205: 219.e1–7. [Meta-analysis; III]

143. Oro AS, Dixon SD. Perinatal cocaine and methamphetamine exposure: Maternal and neonatal correlates. *J Pediatr* 1987; 111(4): 571–8. [II-2]

144. Shah R, Diaz SD, Arria A et al. Prenatal methamphetamine exposure and short-term maternal and infant medical outcomes. *Am J Perinatol* 2012; 29(5): 391–400. [II-2]

145. Cernerud L, Eriksson M, Jonsson B et al. Amphetamine addiction during pregnancy: 14-year follow-up of growth and school performance. *Acta Paediatr* 1996; 85(2): 204–8. [II-2]

146. Diaz SD, Smith LM, LaGasse LL et al. Effects of prenatal methamphetamine exposure on behavioral and cognitive findings at 7.5 years of age. *J Pediatr* 2014; 164(6): 1333–8. [II-2]

147. Chang L, Smith LM, LoPresti C et al. Smaller subcortical volumes and cognitive deficits in children with prenatal methamphetamine exposure. *Psychiatry Res* 2004; 132(2): 95–106. [II-2]

148. Singer LT, Moore DG, Fulton S et al. Neurobehavioral outcomes of infants exposed to MDMA (ecstasy) and other recreational drugs during pregnancy. *Neurotoxicol Teratol* 2012; 34(3): 303–10. [II-2]

149. Bolea-Alamanac BM, Green A, Verma G et al. Methylphenidate use in pregnancy and lactation: A systematic review of evidence. *Br J Clin Pharmacol* 2014; 77(1): 96–101. [Review; III]

150. McElhatton PR. The effects of benzodiazepine use during pregnancy and lactation. *Reprod Toxicol* 1994; 8(6): 461–75. [Review; III]

151. Wikner BN, Stiller CO, Källén B et al. Use of benzodiazepines and benzodiazepine receptor agonists during pregnancy: Maternal characteristics. *Pharmacoepidemiol Drug Saf* 2007; 16(9): 988–94. [II-2]

152. ACOG. Use of psychiatric medication during pregnancy and lactation. ACOG Practice Bulletin No. 92. *Obstet Gynecol* 2008; 111(4): 1001–20. [III]

153. Benzodiazepines and pregnancy [Internet]. Organization of Teratology Information Specialists; 2016. [Last accessed February 3, 2016]. Available from: http://mothertobaby.org/fact-sheets/benzodiazepines-pregnancy/. [III]

154. Enato E, Moretti M, Koren G. The fetal safety of benzodiazepines: An updated meta-analysis. *J Obstet Gynecol Can* 2011; 33(1): 46–8. [Meta-analysis; I]

155. Altshuler LL, Cohen L, Szuba MP et al. Pharmacologic management of psychiatric illness during pregnancy: Dilemmas and guidelines. *Am J Psychiatry* 1996; 153(5): 592–606. [III]

156. Bellantuono C, Tofani S, Sciascio GD, Santone G. Benzodiazepine exposure in pregnancy and risk of major malformations: A critical overview. *Gen Hosp Psychiatry* 2013; 35(1): 3–8. [Review; III]

157. Wikner BN, Stiller CO, Bergman U et al. Use of benzodiazepines and benzodiazepine receptor agonists during pregnancy: Neonatal outcome and congenital malformations. *Pharmacoepidemiol Drug Saf* 2007; 16(11): 1203–10. [II-2]

158. Sutton LR, Hinderliter SA. Diazepam abuse in pregnant women on methadone maintenance. Implications for the neonate. *Clin Pediatr* 1990; 29(2): 108–11. [II-3]

159. Lagreid L, Hagberg G, Lundberg A. Neurodevelopment in late infancy after prenatal exposure to benzodiazepines—A prospective study. *Neuropediatrics* 1992; 23(2): 60–7. [II-2]

160. Hartz SC, Heinonen OP, Shapiro S et al. Antenatal exposure to meprobamate and chlordiazepoxide in relation to malformations, mental development, and childhood mortality. *N Engl J Med* 1975; 292(14): 726–8. [II-2]

161. Kelly LE, Poon S, Madadi P, Koren G. Neonatal benzodiazepines exposure during breastfeeding. *J Pediatr* 2012; 16(3): 448–51. [II-3]

162. Baldridge EB, Bessen HA. Phencycldine. *Emerg Med Clin North Am* 1990; 8(3): 541–50. [Review III]

163. McCarron MM, Schulze BW, Thompson GA et al. Acute phencyclidine intoxication: Incidence of clinical findings in 1000 cases. *Ann Emerg Med* 1981; 10: 237. [II-3]

164. Golden NL, Kuhnert BR, Sokol RJ et al. Neonatal manifestation of maternal phencyclidine exposure. *J Perinat Med* 1987; 15(2): 185–91. [II-2]

165. Golden NL, Kuhnert BR, Sokol RJ et al. Phencyclidine use during pregnancy. *Am J Obstet Gynecol* 1984; 148(3): 254–9. [II-2]

166. Petrucha RA, Kaufman K, Pitts FN. Phencyclidine in pregnancy: A case report. *J Reprod Med* 1982; 27(5): 301–3. [II-3]

167. Golden NL, Sokol RJ, Rubin IL. Angel dust: Possible effects on the fetus. *Pediatrics* 1980; 65(1): 18–20. [II-3]

168. Deutsch SI, Mastropaolo, Rosse RB. Neurodevelopmental consequences of early exposure to phencyclidine and related drugs. *Clin Neuropharmacol* 1998; 21(6): 320–32. [Review; III]

169. Nicholas JM, Lipshitz J, Schreiber EC. Phencyclidine: Its transfer across the placenta as well as into breast milk. *Am J Obstet Gynecol* 1982; 18: 143–6. [II-3]

170. Kaufman KR, Petrucha RA, Pitts FN et al. PCP in amniotic fluid and breast milk: Case report. *J Clin Psychiatry* 1983; 44(7): 269–70. [II-3]

171. Kaufman KR, Petrucha RA, Pitts FN Jr. et al. Phencyclidine in umbilical cord blood: Preliminary data. *Am J Psychiatry* 1983; 140(4): 450–2. [II-3]

172. Strauss AA, Mondanlou HD, Bosu SK. Neonatal manifestations of maternal phencyclidine (PCP) abuse. *Pediatrics* 1981; 68(4): 550–2. [II-3]

173. Tabor BL, Smith Wallace T, Yonekura ML. Perinatal outcome associated with PCP versus cocaine use. *Am J Drug Alcohol Abuse* 1990; 16(3–4): 337–48. [II-2]

174. Mvula MM, Miller JM, Ragan FA. Relationship of phencyclidine and pregnancy outcome. *J Reprod Med* 1999; 44(12): 1021–4. [II-2]

175. Chasnoff IJ, Burns WJ, Hatcher RP et al. Phencyclidine: Effects on the fetus and neonate. *Dev Pharmacol Ther* 1983; 6(6): 404–8. [II-2]

176. Wachsman L, Schuetz S, Chan LS et al. What happens to babies exposed to phencyclidine (PCP) in utero? *Am J Drug Alcohol Abuse* 1989; 15(1): 31–9. [II-3]

177. Fico TA, VanderWende C. Phencyclidine during pregnancy: Behavioral and neurochemical effects in the offspring. *Ann NY Acad Sci* 1989; 562: 319–26. [II-3]

178. Howard J, Kropenske V, Tyler R. The long-term effects on neurodevelopment in infants exposed prenatally to PCP. *NIDA Res Monogr* 1986; 64: 237–51. [II-3]

179. McCarron MM. Phencyclidine intoxication. *NIDA Res Monogr* 1986; 64: 209–17. [II-3]

180. Madgula RM, Groshkova T, Mayet S. Illicit drug use in pregnancy: Effects and management. *Expert Rev Obstet Gynecol* 2011; 6(2): 179–92. [Review III]

181. Illinois Teratogen Information Service. *ITIS Newsletters: The effects of hallucinogen use during pregnancy.* 2000; 8(2). Available at: http://fetal-exposure.org/the-effects-of-hallucinogen-use-during-pregnancy/. Last accessed February 3, 2016. [II-3]

182. Long SY. Does LSD induce chromosomal damage and malformations? A review of the literature. *Teratology* 1972; 6(1): 75–90. [Review; III]

183. Jacobson CB, Berlin CM. Possible reproductive detriment of LSD users. *JAMA* 1972; 222(11): 1367–73. [II-2]

24

Respiratory diseases: asthma, pneumonia, influenza, and tuberculosis

Lauren A. Plante and Ryan K. Brannon

ASTHMA
Key Points
- Asthma is characterized by airway obstruction, inflammation, and increased responsiveness to stimuli. To be certain of diagnosis, once abnormal forced expiratory volume in one second (FEV_1) is found in a patient with historic and physical exam findings consistent with asthma, other differential diagnoses must be excluded.
- Asthma is classified as **mild intermittent, mild persistent, moderate persistent, and severe persistent** by symptoms and peak expiratory flow rate (PEFR) or spirometry.
- Asthma has historically been associated with small increased risks of preterm birth, low birth weight, perinatal mortality, and preeclampsia, but these risks are probably associated just with undertreatment of asthma; **if asthma is adequately treated, it is not associated with a significant increase in adverse perinatal outcomes**.
- Pregnancy has a variable effect on asthma severity with about two thirds getting better and one third worse.
- The **management** of asthma in pregnant women should follow the **same guidelines as for other nonpregnant patients**.
- Management is based on objective measurements of pulmonary function (PEFR) (Table 24.1). The management plan should include use of environmental control measures; adequate pharmacotherapy; and patient education regarding symptoms, management, and compliance.
- **Inhalation therapy is preferred to systemic treatments** with **inhaled corticosteroids, NOT inhaled β-agonist, the mainstay of therapy**.
- Prostaglandin F2α should be avoided. Ergonovine and indomethacin, sometimes used in obstetric care, may worsen bronchospasm.

Diagnosis
Asthma is characterized by reversible episodic symptoms of airway obstruction, in which alternative explanations have been excluded. For example, typical symptoms and a large reversibility (usually with betamimetic nebulizer treatment) of airflow obstruction on spirometry (increase in FEV_1 >15%) generally confirm the diagnosis of asthma. Airway inflammation with edema and remodeling rather than simply bronchospasm is the key. Increased airway responsiveness to stimuli is characteristic. Indicators that suggest a diagnosis of asthma include wheezing; history of recurrent cough; chest tightness or difficulty in breathing; worsening of symptoms with exercise; viral infection; exposure to animal fur or feathers, mold, pollen, house dust mites, tobacco or wood smoke;

changes in weather; airborne chemicals or dusts; or worsening of symptoms at night. Physical examination is not always reliable and may include thoracic hyperexpansion or chest deformity, hunching of shoulders or use of accessory muscles, audible wheezing or a prolonged expiratory phase, increased nasal discharge or nasal polyps, or any manifestation of an allergic skin condition. The more indicators present, the more likely the diagnosis; however, the absence of wheezing does not equal the absence of asthma. A clinical diagnosis of asthma can be confirmed with the use of spirometry, which can be used to determine whether airflow obstruction is present and, if so, whether it is reversible. Additionally, forced vital capacity (FVC), FEV_1, and FEV_1/FVC ratio are measured before and after administration of a short-acting bronchodilator. Reduced FEV_1 or FEV_1/FVC shows airflow limitation, and a 12% or greater improvement in FEV_1 after the administration of inhaled albuterol confirms reversibility [1].

To be certain of an asthma diagnosis, **once an abnormal FEV_1 is found in a patient with history and physical exam findings consistent with asthma, other differential diagnoses must be excluded**, such as chronic obstructive pulmonary disease, congestive heart failure, pulmonary embolus, laryngeal or vocal cord dysfunction, and mechanical airway obstruction.

Symptoms
Wheezing, shortness of breath, coughing, chest tightness, difficulty in breathing, dyspnea.

Incidence
Asthma affects approximately 8% of pregnant women [2]. Among U.S. women aged 18 to 44, 5% reported an asthma attack within the preceding 12 months. However, 12% to 14% had received a diagnosis of asthma at some point during their lifetimes [2]. Thus, this is a common disease among women of reproductive age.

Etiology and Basic Pathophysiology
Airway obstruction and inflammation, usually because of excessive response to stimuli, as described above.

Classification
Asthma severity, that is, the intrinsic intensity of the disease, is classified into four stages (Table 24.1) [1]. Severity is most easily measured in a patient who is not receiving long-term control therapy. Severity can also be measured, once asthma control is achieved, by the amount of medication required to maintain control (Tables 24.2 through 24.4).

Table 24.1   Classification of Asthma Severity

	Mild Intermittent	Mild Persistent	Moderate Persistent	Severe Persistent
Symptoms	≤2 times a week	>2 times a week but <1 time a day	Daily	Continuous
	Asymptomatic between exacerbations		Exacerbations occur ≥2 times a week	Frequent exacerbations
Pulmonary function	Normal PEFR between exacerbations		FEV$_1$ or PEFR 60% to 80% of predicted	FEV$_1$ or PEFR <60% of predicted
FEV$_1$ or PEFR in relation to predicted	≥80%	>80%		
PEFR variability	PEFR variability <20%	PEFR variability 20% to 30%	PEFR variability >30%	PEFR variability >30%
Nocturnal awakening	≤2 times a month	>2 times a month	>1 time a week	Nightly awakenings
Interference with daily activities	None	Mild	Some interference with normal activities but rare severe exacerbation	Limitations of physical activity
Treatment	Step 1	Step 2	Step 3 or Step 4	Step 5 or Step 6

Source: Adapted from National Asthma Education and Prevention Program. *Expert Panel Report 3: Guidelines for the diagnosis and management of asthma: Full report 2007.* http://www.nhlbi.nih. gov/guidelines/asthma/asthgdln.pdf.
Abbreviations: FEV$_1$, forced expiratory volume in one second; NAEPP, National Asthma Education and Prevention Program; PEFR, peak expiratory flow rate.

Table 24.2   Usual Drugs and Dosages for Long-Term Control Medication during Pregnancy

Medication	Dosage		
	Low Dose	Medium Dose	High Dose
Inhaled corticosteroid			
Beclomethasone CFC 42 or 84 µg/puff	168–504 µg TDD	504–840 µg TDD	>840 µg TDD
Beclomethasone HFA 40 or 80 µg/puff	80–240 µg TDD	240–480 µg TDD	>480 µg TDD
Budesonide dry powder 200 µg/puff	200–600 µg TDD	600–1200 µg TDD	>1200 mg TDD
Flunisolide 250 µg/puff	500–1000 µg TDD	1000–2000 µg TDD	>2000 µg TDD
Fluticasone Metered dose inhaler: 44, 88, 220 µg/puff	MDI: 88–264 µg TDD	MDI: 264–660 µg TDD	MDI: >660 µg TDD
Dry powder inhaler: 50, 100, 250 mg/ inhalation	DPI: 100–300 µg TDD	DPI: 300–750 µg TDD	DPI: >750 µg TDD
Triamcinolone acetonide 100 µg/puff	400–1000 µg TDD	1000–2000 µg TDD	>2000 µg TDD
Systemic corticosteroid	**How supplied**	**Daily dose** (all three drugs are dosed the same)	**Short burst to achieve control** (all dosed the same)
Methylprednisolone	Tablets: 2, 4, 8, 16, 32 mg	7.5–60 mg daily	40–60 mg/day
Prednisolone	Tablets: 5 mg Syrup: 5 mg/5 mL, 15 mg/5 mL	As a single dose in a.m.	As a single dose or as two divided doses
Prednisone	Tablets: 1, 2.5, 5, 10, 20, 50 mg oral solution: 5 mg/mL	Every other day as needed for control	For 3–10 days
Long-acting β-agonist (LAB A): Not for symptom relief, and not used alone; use with inhaled corticosteroids			
Salmeterol	MDI: 21 µg/puff DPI: 50 µg/blister	MDI: 2 puffs q12h DPI: 1 blister q12h	
Formoterol	DPI: 12 µg per single-use capsule	1 capsule q12h	
Combination: LABA plus inhaled corticosteroid			
Fluticasone/salmeterol	DPI: fluticasone dose varies 100, 250, or 500 µg/puff; Salmeterol always 50 µg/puff	One inhalation twice daily	Fluticasone dose depends on asthma severity
Cromolyn	MDI: 1 mg/puff Nebulizer 20 mg/amp	MDI: 2–4 puffs, 3–4 × daily or 1 ampule nebulized 3–4 × daily	
Leukotriene receptor antagonists			
Montelukast	10 mg tablet	10 mg qhs	
Zafirlukast	Tablet, 10 or 20 mg	40 mg daily	
Theophylline	Liquids; sustained-release tablets; capsules	Starting dose 10 mg/kg/day	Maximum dose 800 mg/day; serum drug monitoring, 5–12 µg/mL is therapeutic

Source: Adapted from National Asthma Education and Prevention Program. *Expert Panel Report 3: Guidelines for the diagnosis and management of asthma: Full report 2007.* http://www.nhlbi.nih. gov/guidelines/asthma/asthgdln.pdf.
Abbreviations: CFC, chlorofluorocarbons; DPI, dry powder inhaler; FEV$_1$, forced expiratory volume in one second; HFA, hydrofluoroalkane; MDI, metered-dose inhaler; NAEPP, National Asthma Education and Prevention Program; PEFR, peak expiratory flow rate; TDD, total daily dose.

Table 24.3 Quick-Relief Short-Acting β-Agonists

Medication	How Provided	Dose (All Same)
Albuterol CFC	90 µg/puff (200 puffs/canister)	Two puffs 5 min before anticipated exercise
Albuterol HFA	90 µg/puff (200 puffs/canister)	OR
Pirbuterol CFC	200 µg/puff (400 puffs/canister)	Two puffs q4–6h, as needed
Levalbuterol HFA	45 µg/puff (200 puffs/canister)	

Source: Adapted from National Asthma Education and Prevention Program. *Expert Panel Report 3: Guidelines for the diagnosis and management of asthma: Full report 2007.* http://www.nhlbi.nih.gov/guidelines/asthma/asthgdln.pdf.
Abbreviations: CFC, chlorofluorocarbons; HFA, hydrofluoroalkane.

Table 24.4 Medications for Treatment of Asthma Exacerbation

Medication	Dose	Comment
Short-acting inhaled β-agonist		
Albuterol nebulizer solutions 5 mg/mL, or 2.5 mg/3 mL, 1.25 mg/mL	Nebulizer: 2.5–5 mg q 20 min × 3 doses; follow with 2.5–10 mg q1–4h as needed or 10–15 mg/hr continuously	Dilute to minimum of 3 mL, use gas flow 6–8 L/min
MDI: 90 mg/puff	MDI: 4–8 puffs q20 min up to 4 hr; then q1–4h as needed	MDI is as effective as nebulizer if patient is able to coordinate
Levalbuterol nebulizer solutions 1.25 mg/3 mL, 0.63 mg/3 mL	1.25–2.5 mg q 20 min × 3 doses, then 1.25–5 mg q1–4h as needed, or 5–7.5 mg/hr continuously	
Bitolterol, pirbuterol		Has not been studied in severe exacerbations
Injected β-agonists		
Epinephrine 1:1000 (1 mg/mL)	0.3–0.5 mg sq q20 min × 3 doses	No proven advantage of injection over aerosol
Terbutaline 1 mg/mL	0.25 mg sq q20 min × 3 doses	No proven advantage of injection over aerosol
Anticholinergics		
Ipratroprium bromide Nebulizer solution 0.25 mg/mL	Nebulizer: 0.5 mg q30 min × 3 doses, then q2–4h as needed	Not as first-line monotherapy. May mix in nebulizer with albuterol
Ipratroprium plus albuterol nebulizer solution: each 3-mL vial contains 0.5 mg ipratroprium bromide þ 2.5 mg albuterol	Nebulizer: 3 mL q30 min × 3 doses, then q2–4h as needed	
MDI: each puff contains 18 µg ipratroprium bromide þ 90 µg albuterol	4–8 puffs as needed	
Systemic corticosteroids		
Prednisone	(dose all three the same) 120–180 mg/day, in three or four divided doses, × 48 hr	
Methylprednisolone	60–80 mg/day until	
Prednisolone	PEFR reaches 70% of predicted or 70% of personal best	

Source: Adapted from National Asthma Education and Prevention Program. *Expert Panel Report 3: Guidelines for the diagnosis and management of asthma. Section 5, Managing exacerbations of asthma. Full report, 2007.* http://www.nhlbi.nih.gov/files/docs/guidelines/11_sec5_exacerb.pdf.

National Heart, Lung, and Blood Institute (NHLBI) classification is as follows.

Mild Intermittent Asthma

- Fewer than two episodes per week AND fewer than two nocturnal episodes per month, plus
- PEFR better than 80% of personal best (or FEV$_1$ >80% of predicted), plus
- Less than 20% variation in PEFR in the course of a day.

Mild Persistent Asthma

- Symptoms more than twice a week (but not daily) or nocturnal symptoms more than twice per month, plus
- **Peak expiratory flow** (PEF) better than 80% of personal best (or FEV$_1$ >80% of predicted), plus
- No more than 20% to 30% variation in PEFR in the course of a day.

Moderate Persistent Asthma

- Daily symptoms or nocturnal symptoms more than once per week or
- PEF between 60% and 80% of personal best (FEV$_1$ 60%–80% of predicted) or
- PEF variation >30%.

Severe Persistent Asthma

- Continuous daytime symptoms or
- Frequent nocturnal symptoms or
- PEF <60% of personal best (FEV$_1$ <60% of predicted).
  - PEF variation is typically >30%.

Pregnancy Complications

Asthma has historically been associated with small increased risks of congenital malformations, preeclampsia, preterm birth, low birth weight, and perinatal mortality [3,4]. These risks are probably associated just with undertreatment of asthma: **If asthma is adequately controlled, it is not associated with a significant increase in adverse perinatal outcomes** [5,6]. A relationship has been reported between decreased FEV_1 during pregnancy and increased risk of low birth weight and prematurity [7]. In addition, women who required hospitalization for asthma during pregnancy or who reported their asthma control to be poor during pregnancy were at higher risk for preterm birth although not for growth restriction [6]. Large studies indicate that therapy tailored according to asthma severity can result in excellent infant and maternal outcomes [5,8]. There are no randomized prospective trials comparing pregnancy outcomes in treated and untreated asthmatics. Women who decrease their asthma medication during pregnancy deliver infants of lower birth weight and slightly shorter gestational age than those who either increase their medication or make no change [9].

Pregnancy Considerations

Pregnant women are less likely than others to receive appropriate asthma care [10]. Pregnant women are equally likely to be admitted for an asthma attack but are less likely to receive corticosteroids in the emergency department (ED), and those who are sent home are less likely to be prescribed outpatient steroids. Pregnant women are far more likely than nonpregnant counterparts to report ongoing symptoms two weeks after an ED visit, perhaps because of the difference in steroid use [10]. Adherence to treatment with inhaled corticosteroids has been reported to be poor in many studies. For example, women reported to decrease their use of inhaled corticosteroids during early pregnancy as compared with their use of these agents in the 20 weeks before their last menstrual period; this may be due to their reported concern regarding the safety of inhaled corticosteroids during pregnancy [3].

Pregnancy has a variable effect on asthma severity, which may improve, worsen, or remain unchanged. In general, **about two thirds get better, and one third get worse** [2]. **Most exacerbations occur between 24 and 36 weeks**, and the fewest symptoms occur at term. Of patients with mild disease, 2% were hospitalized during pregnancy, 13% were noted to have an exacerbation, and 13% had symptoms at time of delivery [7]. For patients with moderate asthma, 7% were hospitalized and 26% had an exacerbation during pregnancy with 21% symptomatic at delivery. Among severe asthmatics, 27% were hospitalized and 52% had an exacerbation during pregnancy, and 46% of severe asthmatics were symptomatic at delivery [7]. A number of factors have been proposed as predictors of disease worsening during pregnancy (smoking, carrying a female fetus, worsening of rhinitis), but studies are inconsistent [11–13].

Management

Principles

The management of asthma in pregnant women should follow the same guidelines as for other patients. The goal is to maintain asthma control during pregnancy. In 2004, the National Asthma Education and Prevention Program (NAEPP) stated, "It is safer for pregnant women with asthma to be treated with asthma medications than it is for them to have asthma symptoms and exacerbations" [14]. Recommendations for asthma management and control are available from the 2007

NAEPP Guidelines [1], the NAEPP update on managing asthma in pregnancy [14], and from the American College of Obstetricians and Gynecologists [15]. An expert panel of the NAEPP concluded in 2015 that an update to national asthma guidelines is warranted, but at the time of this writing no such update has yet been issued; the projected date for publication is 2018. [16] As is true for many guidelines, recommendations may be made on the basis of consensus or expert opinion rather than on level I evidence. A recent *Cochrane* review concluded that "no firm conclusions about optimal interventions for managing asthma in pregnancy can be made" [17].

Prevention

Eliminate or mitigate asthma triggers. Environmental control measures are shown in Table 24.5.

Preconception Care

Multidisciplinary care is recommended for preparation of pregnancy and during pregnancy. Education regarding prognosis, complications, and management of asthma therapy should be reviewed with emphasis on the fact that asthma therapy should not change in pregnancy compared to the nonpregnant state but should still aim for maximal relief of symptoms and best pulmonary function through attentive patient compliance with suggested management.

Prenatal Care

Achieving and maintaining asthma control requires four components of care:

1. Use of *objective* measures of lung function such as PEFR, to ascertain severity, assess asthma control, and to monitor therapy rather than relying on symptoms.
2. Control of environmental factors and comorbid conditions to eliminate or mitigate asthma triggers.
3. Pharmacotherapy designed to prevent or reverse airway inflammation typical of asthma, as well as drug treatment for exacerbations.
4. Patient education regarding symptoms, management, and compliance.

Table 24.5 Environmental Control Measures for Asthma Management

Reduce or eliminate allergens
   Cockroaches
   Pollen
   Mold
   Animal dander
   House dust mites
   Encase mattresses and pillows in allergen-impermeable
     covers
   Remove carpets from bedroom
   Reduce indoor humidity
Eliminate or reduce exposure to tobacco smoke
Reduce exposure to indoor and outdoor pollutants
   Wood-burning stoves, fireplaces
   Unvented stoves or heaters
   Irritants, such as perfumes and cleaning products

Source: Adapted from National Asthma Education and Prevention Program. *Expert Panel Report 3: Guidelines for the diagnosis and management of asthma*. Section 3, Control of environmental factors and comorbid conditions that affect asthma. http://www.nhlbi.nih.gov/files/docs/guidelines/06_sec3_comp3.pdf.

Workup of Asthma Control

Asthma control should be assessed on a regular basis (at least at each prenatal visit) by review of symptoms, medications used, and quality of life over the preceding weeks. The **PEF can be measured by peak flow meters**, which are portable, inexpensive, and disposable. Both FEV$_1$ and PEF remain unchanged in pregnancy in the normal state. **Predicted PEF values are based on age, gender, and height. For women, they range from 380 to 550 L/min. Each pregnant woman should establish her personal best during quiescent asthma. PEF >80% of personal best are normal; values between 50% and 80% are intermediate; values <50% are associated with severe asthma exacerbation.** Daily peak flow monitoring using an inexpensive home meter is advisable in cases of moderate or severe asthma in order to identify presymptomatic airflow obstruction, which may require escalation of therapy. Outcomes have not been proven to be different when symptom-based monitoring is used rather than PEF monitoring [1], but objective measures are particularly valuable for patients with a history of exacerbations, when evaluating a change in therapy, or for those patients whose perception of airflow is poor. **PEF results should be recorded in a log and brought to each prenatal visit.**

Therapy

General

Inhalation therapy is preferred to systemic treatments because of direct delivery to airway and fewer side effects. Spacer devices can increase delivery to the lungs and minimize oral absorption. For all except the mild intermittent type of asthma, **inhaled corticosteroids, NOT inhaled β-agonists, are the mainstay of therapy.**

Use of one or more canisters of β-agonist per month indicates inadequate asthma control. Gain control as quickly as possible; a short course of oral steroids may be helpful. Review symptoms monthly. Other indicators of a need for stepped-up

therapy are symptoms more than twice per week; three or more nighttime awakenings related to asthma symptoms; and limitation or interference with normal activity. Step-down therapy may be attempted only if symptoms are well controlled.

An individualized action plan should be generated for an asthmatic patient. This incorporates frequent self-assessment, a daily self-management plan, long-term self-management plan, and an asthma action plan based on symptoms, peak flow, and medications used. The action plan allows patients to step up therapy at home with exacerbations and provides criteria for contacting the physician or seeking care in an ED. Sample action plans can be found online at http://www.nhlbi.nih.gov/health/public/lung/asthma/asthma_actplan.pdf and http://www.nhlbi.nih.gov/health/public/lung/asthma/actionplan_text.htm.

If symptoms are not adequately controlled, review compliance, inhalation technique, and environmental control. If no room for improvement in these areas, step up to the next level of therapy. At step 3 or 4 (moderate or severe persistent disease) or if patient required >2 bursts of oral systemic corticosteroids in one year or has an exacerbation requiring hospitalization, refer to a specialist in asthma (if one is not already involved).

Goals

- No limitations at school or work
- Normal or near-normal pulmonary function assessed by PEF (or FEV$_1$)
- Prevent hypoxemia
- Minimal-to-no exacerbations, chronic symptoms, use of short-term β-agonists, or medication side effects

Suggested Medications

A stepwise approach to manage asthma is recommended to gain and maintain control (Figure 24.1). Usual drug doses are

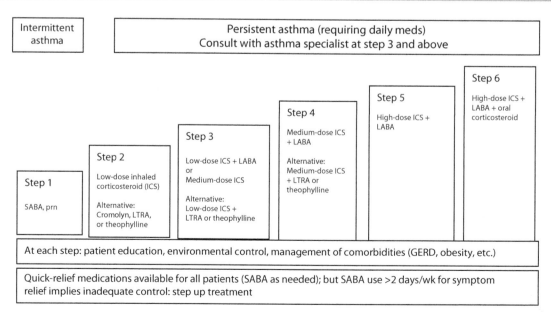

Figure 24.1 Stepwise approach to managing asthma medications. *Abbreviations*: SABA, short-acting β-agonist; LTRA, leukotriene receptor antagonist; LABA, long-acting β-agonist; GERD, gastroesophageal reflux disease. (Adapted from National Asthma Education and Prevention Program. *Expert Panel Report 3: Guidelines for the diagnosis and management of asthma: Full report 2007.* http://www.nhlbi.nih.gov/guidelines/asthma/asthgdln.pdf.)

shown in Table 24.2. Medications for exacerbation are shown in Tables 24.3 and 24.4 (all tables are adapted from the NAEPP) [1]. Algorithms for home and hospital management of exacerbation can be found in the NAEPP guidelines (Figures 24.2 and 24.3) [1]. Number and frequency of medications increase with increasing asthma severity. On the basis of clinical trials, medications are considered to be "preferred" or "alternative" at each step of therapy. For patients who are not already taking long-term control medications, assess asthma severity and initiate therapy according to level of severity. For patients who are already taking long-term control medications, assess asthma control and step-up therapy if the patient's asthma is not well controlled on current therapy. In general, **using short-acting β-agonists (SABA) >2 days a week indicates the need for starting or increasing long-term control medications**.

Mild intermittent asthma. These patients require **no daily medication** (step 1). Quick relief can be provided in the form of two to four puffs of a SABA bronchodilator as needed.

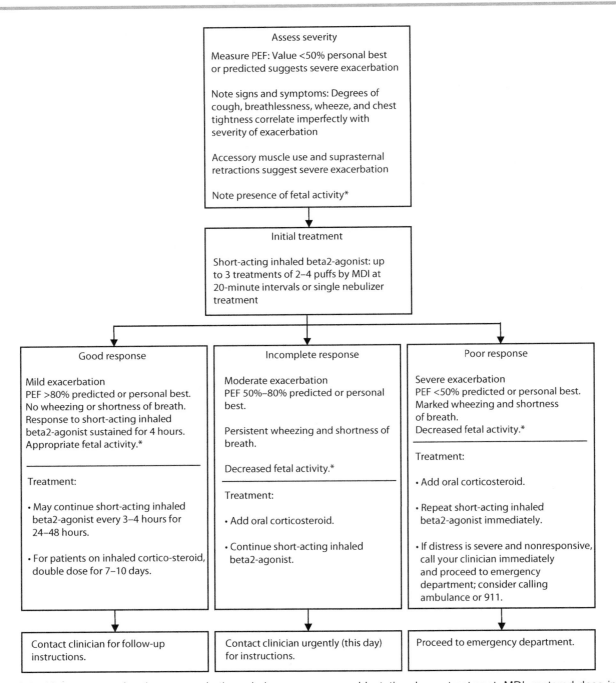

Figure 24.2 Management of asthma exacerbations during pregnancy and lactation: home treatment. MDI, metered-dose inhaler: PEF, peak expiratory flow. *Fetal activity is monitored by observing whether fetal kick counts decrease over time. (From National Asthma Education and Prevention Program. *NAEPP Working Group Report on managing asthma during pregnancy: recommendations for pharmacologic treatment—update 2004.* NIH Publication 05–3279. Available at: http://www.nhlbi.nih.gov/health/prof/lung /asthma/astpreg/astpreg_full.pdf, with permission from National Heart, Lung, and Blood Institute; National Institutes of Health; U.S. Department of Health and Human Services.)

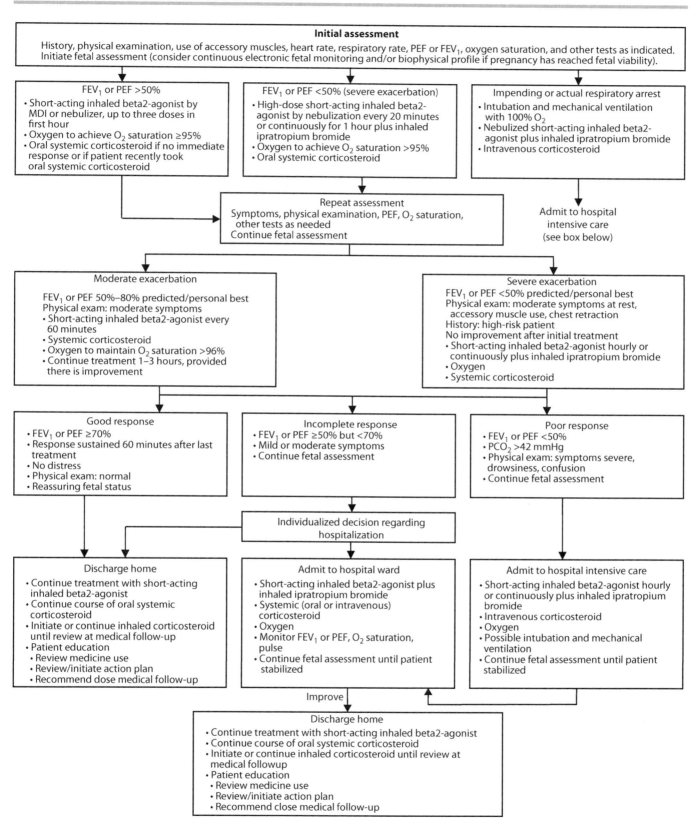

Figure 24.3 Management of asthma exacerbations during pregnancy and lactation: emergency department and hospital-based care. FEV_1, forced expiratory volume in 1 second: MDI, metered-dose inhaler: PCO_2, carbon dioxide partial pressure; PEF, peak expiratory flow. (From National Asthma Education and Prevention Program. *NAEPP Working Group Report on managing asthma during pregnancy: recommendations for pharmacologic treatment—update 2004.* NIH Publication 05–3279. Available at: http://www.nhlbi .nih.gov/health/prof/lung/asthma/astpreg/astpreg_full.pdf, with permission from National Heart, Lung, and Blood Institute; National Institutes of Health; U.S. Department of Health and Human Services.)

In the event of exacerbation, PEFR 50% to 80% of predicted should be treated with an inhaled short-acting β-mimetic immediately. Values <50% require the same therapy plus immediate visit to emergency room. However, the need to use rescue twice a week or more means a step up in therapy and a reclassification of severity. These patients can have severe exacerbations interrupting long periods of normal lung function, in which case systemic steroids should be offered.

Mild persistent asthma. Treat with a **daily inhaled corticosteroid** (low dose). Alternative therapies include inhaled cromolyn, leukotriene receptor antagonist (LTRA), or sustained-release theophylline adjusted to serum level of 5 to 12 μg/mL (step 2).

Moderate persistent asthma. Treat with either a **medium-dose inhaled corticosteroid or a low-dose inhaled corticosteroid plus a long-acting inhaled β-agonist** (step 3). If necessary, give the long-acting β-agonist (LABA) with a medium-dose corticosteroid (step 4).

Alternative therapies include low-dose or medium-dose inhaled corticosteroid in combination with either theophylline or a LTRA.

Severe persistent asthma. These patients require **both a high-dose inhaled corticosteroid and a long-acting inhaled β-agonist** (step 5) and may also require oral corticosteroids (step 6); when feasible, the oral corticosteroids should be discontinued and control maintained with inhaled agents.

An alternative therapy would be high-dose inhaled corticosteroid plus sustained-release theophylline titrated to therapeutic serum levels as above.

Inhaled Steroids

Anti-inflammatory agents decrease edema and secretions in the bronchioles. Indications are shown in Figure 24.1. They are used not for acute relief but for long-term management (four weeks for maximal benefit). **Inhaled corticosteroids are the most consistently effective long-term control medication at all steps of care for persistent asthma. If β-agonist (e.g., albuterol) is used two times a week, inhaled steroid therapy should be started.** Most of the data on inhaled steroids in human pregnancy come from budesonide (Pulmacort) [12]. Inhaled beclomethasone is associated with improved FEV_1 and fewer side effects compared to oral theophylline in the only trial comparing them in pregnancy [16]. In a large, double-blind, randomized trial, treatment with low-dose budesonide had no adverse effects on the outcome of pregnancy [17]. There is no evidence of increased rates of congenital malformations with the use of inhaled corticosteroids in pregnancy [4,14]. Nor is there an effect on fetal growth, preterm birth, rates of gestational hypertension, preeclampsia, and perinatal mortality [6,7,18–20] A meta-analysis concludes that they are safe in pregnancy [21].

β-Agonists

β-Agonists relax bronchiolar smooth muscle. There is no consistent evidence of increased rates of congenital malformations with the use of β-agonists in pregnancy [14] despite a recent case-control study suggesting an increased risk of gastroschisis when bronchodilators were used during the periconception period [22]. Without having adjusted for severity of maternal asthma, it would be premature to conclude that β-agonists correlate with gastroschisis. Use of inhaled β-agonists does not appear to increase perinatal risks in pregnant asthmatic patients (including gestational hypertension, preterm birth, low birth weight, fetal growth, and small for gestational age) [6,7].

Short-acting β-agonists. These are the treatment of choice for relief of acute symptoms. Regularly scheduled, daily, chronic use of SABA is **not** recommended. The onset of action is <5 minutes with a duration of only four to six hours.

Long-acting β-agonists. Produce bronchodilation for at least 12 hours after a single dose. They are not to be used as monotherapy for long-term control of asthma. Instead, they are used in combination with inhaled corticosteroids for long-term control and prevention of symptoms in moderate or severe persistent asthma. Long-acting β-agonists have been shown to be more effective than LTRA or theophylline as add-on therapy to inhaled corticosteroids [1].

Combination of Inhaled Corticosteroids and Long-Acting β-Agonists (Fixed-Drug Combination)

Fluticasone and salmeterol (Advair) combination is more effective than either drug alone in nonpregnant trials.

Cromolyn

Cromolyn sodium is a nonsteroidal anti-inflammatory agent used for chronic management of asthma, not acute exacerbations (four weeks for maximal benefit). There is **no evidence of increased rates of congenital malformations** with the use of cromolyn in pregnancy [14]; this is a safe drug in pregnancy as is nedocromil.

Theophylline

Theophylline has a long record of use in pregnancy and no teratogenic effects are known; however, the narrow therapeutic window and potential for maternal and fetal toxicity mandates close monitoring of serum levels. Low-dose theophylline is an alternative to a LABA when inhaled corticosteroids do not suffice to control symptoms, but this is not a preferred therapy [1]. Recommendations for target serum theophylline levels have been changed to 5 to 12 μg/mL.

Leukotriene Receptor Antagonists

Limited human data are available on the use of LTRA during pregnancy. Several small studies have not shown an increase in the rate of major malformations in offspring of women who took LTRA during pregnancy [23,24]. Mean birth weight was lower and risk of low birth weight and fetal distress was higher in the montelukast-exposed group, a difference that may have been related to asthma severity rather than drug effect. In nonpregnant individuals, these drugs are less effective than inhaled corticosteroids and do not add much benefit to women already on inhaled steroids. They do not reduce the risk of exacerbation requiring systemic steroids and are associated with modest improvement in PEF with very modest decrease in use of rescue short-acting b-2 agonists [25]. These drugs may be considered during pregnancy for women who had a good response to them prior to pregnancy, but they are not a preferred option when initiating therapy. Montelukast and zafirlukast are safe in pregnancy [26,27]. Zileuton, a 5-lipoxygenase inhibitor, has been advised against in pregnancy based on animal data: human data are lacking [14].

Anticholinergics

Anticholinergics inhibit muscarinic cholinergic receptors and reduce intrinsic vagal tone of the airway. Ipratropium bromide provides additive benefit to SABA in moderate or severe exacerbations in the emergency care setting, not the hospital setting.

Oral Corticosteroids

Oral corticosteroids are **indicated when combinations of inhaled steroids, β-agonists, and cromolyn do not control asthma.** Oral steroid use in the first trimester is associated with a possible increased risk of cleft lip (with or without cleft palate) from the background rate of 0.1% to 0.3%, a small excess risk. The use of oral corticosteroids during pregnancy is associated with an increase in incidence of gestational diabetes, preeclampsia, preterm delivery, and low birth weight. These outcomes may be attributed to either the drug or the severity of the disease process. Available data do not allow for the distinction [7].

Intravenous corticosteroids may be indicated in severe asthma exacerbation.

Status Asthmaticus

Recommendations for management are either anecdotal or extrapolated from management of status asthmaticus outside of pregnancy [28,29].

Acute Treatment of Asthma

The treatment of an acute asthma exacerbation should be the same, in general, as in nonpregnant adults. Oxygen, aerosolized albuterol, and ipratropium as well as systemic steroids should be initiated as described above [30].

Antepartum Testing

No specific indication.

Delivery

Asthma medications should be continued in labor. Although asthma is typically quiescent during labor and delivery, PEF should be measured upon admission and again every 12 hours in labor.

The idea of giving stress doses of steroids in labor or perioperatively is poorly supported by research (see Chapter 25). Individuals receiving long-term corticosteroids have not, in randomized studies, proven incapable of endogenous steroid production perioperatively. A recent systematic review concludes that there is no need to add stress-dose steroids in the perioperative period as long as patients continue to get their usual daily dose of steroids; this would not, however, be true for patients with primary adrenal failure or other primary dysfunction of the hypothalamic–pituitary axis, who would still require additional glucocorticoid coverage. Thus, extrapolating from work done on surgical patients, one would not expect adrenal crisis, and it would seem satisfactory to **continue their regular daily steroid dosing during labor for women who are on prednisone without adding additional "stress doses."** Blood pressure should, of course, be carefully monitored [31].

Prostaglandin E1 and E2 are safe. **Prostaglandin F2a should be avoided** as it can cause bronchospasm. Ergonovine, methylergonovine, and nonsteroidal anti-inflammatory agents (such as indomethacin, sometimes given for preterm labor) may precipitate bronchospasm.

Anesthesia

No specific changes; as a rule, regional anesthetics are preferred to general.

Postpartum/Breast-Feeding

The NAEPP found that the use of prednisone, theophylline, antihistamines, inhaled corticosteroids, β2-agonists, and cromolyn is not contraindicated for breast-feeding [14]. Breast-feeding does not protect against asthma in offspring [32]. Although nonsteroidal anti-inflammatory agents (NSAIDs) may precipitate bronchospasm in some asthmatics, the risk in the general asthmatic population is less than 1%. Thus, it is reasonable to treat patients during the postpartum period with NSAIDs especially if they have not previously exhibited an adverse reaction.

PNEUMONIA
Key Points

- The presence of an **infiltrate on chest X-ray** confirms the diagnosis of pneumonia.
- Complications of community-acquired pneumonia (CAP) include mechanical ventilation, maternal mortality, low birth weight infant, and perinatal mortality.
- **Prompt administration of** antibiotics without delay and **appropriate antibiotic therapy** are the most important principles for effective management.
- Hospitalization is indicated when a pregnant woman with CAP has coexisting medical conditions, such as malignancy, renal failure, immunosuppression, cerebrovascular disease, diabetes, or valvular heart disease, RR ≥30, diastolic BP ≤60, systolic BP ≤90, HR ≥125, altered mental status, $PaCO_2$ <60 on room air, presence of a pleural effusion, hematocrit <30, arterial pH <7.35, or multilobe involvement.
- **Most cases of low-risk CAP in pregnancy can be treated with a macrolide, and the more high-risk ones can be treated with a macrolide and a β-lactam.**
- Antibiotic therapy should not be changed within the first 72 hours unless clinical deterioration is overt or organism sensitivities become available.

Diagnosis

Pneumonia is an infectious process of the lower respiratory tract, which should be suspected if a patient presents with new respiratory symptoms of cough, dyspnea, or sputum production, particularly if fever and abnormal breath sounds are also present. The presence of an infiltrate on chest X-ray confirms the diagnosis.

Etiology/Basic Pathophysiology

Etiology is usually bacterial, viral, or fungal infection of the lungs. *Streptococcus pneumoniae* (5%–30%) and *Mycoplasma pneumoniae* (5%–30%) are the most common pathogens, but dozens of different organisms can cause pneumonia (Table 24.6) [33,34]. In CAP, the causative agent is identified in only 40% to 60% of the cases [35].

Classification

The distinction between CAP and hospital-acquired pneumonia is made in practice. In the majority of cases, clinical signs

Table 24.6 Pathogens Isolated in Patients with Community-Acquired Pneumonia

Bacterial
- *Common: Streptococcus pneumoniae, Mycoplasma pneumoniae, Haemophilus influenza, Staphylococcus aureus, Chlamydophila pneumoniae, and psittaci*
- *Less common: Pseudomonas aeruginosa, Legionella spp., Klebsiella spp., Moraxella catarrhalis, Bordetella pertussis, Escherichia coli, Enterobacter spp., Serratia spp.*

Viral
- Common: influenza A and B and varicella-zoster virus
- Less common: adenovirus species, enteroviruses (echovirus, coxsackievirus, poliovirus), Epstein-Barr virus, cytomegalovirus, respiratory syncytial virus (common in children), parainfluenza virus, human metapneumovirus, herpes simplex virus, coronaviruses, measles virus, hantavirus

Fungal
- *Uncommon: Histoplasma capsulatum, Coccidioides immitis, Cryptococcus neoformans, Blastomyces hominis, Aspergillus spp., Candida spp., Mucormycotic fungi*

Other Causes
- *Uncommon: Mycobacterium tuberculosis, Pneumocystis jirovecii, Toxoplasma gondii, Ascaris lumbricoides, Strongyloides stercoralis, Coxiella burnetii, Rickettsia rickettsii*

Source: Adapted from Sheffield JS, Cunningham FG. *Obstet Gynecol,* 114, 4, 915–22, 2009.

and symptoms do not distinguish one pathogen from another. **The vast majority of cases of pneumonia in pregnant women in clinical practice and in the literature are cases of CAP.**

The Infectious Diseases Society of America (IDSA) and The American Thoracic Society (ATS) use the Pneumonia Severity Index (PSI) to stratify CAP by comorbidity and mortality rates [36]. Most pregnant patients with CAP will fall into subset I; this is a group that, if nonpregnant, would be appropriately treated as outpatients. There are, however, **no reliable data as to inpatient versus outpatient therapy in pregnancy.**

Symptoms
Respiratory symptoms: cough, dyspnea, or sputum production; usually fever.

Epidemiology
The attack rate for CAP is no different among pregnant women than among women of reproductive age who are not pregnant, approximately 1.5 per 1000 [37]. Pregnant women hospitalized with CAP have lower severity scores than their nonpregnant counterparts; this may reflect either a tendency for the disease process to be less severe or a lower threshold for hospitalization during pregnancy. Pneumonia incidence is evenly distributed throughout pregnancy; that is, there is no specific period of vulnerability.

Risk Factors
Smoking; asthma.

Complications
Approximately **2% of pregnant women with pneumonia require intubation and mechanical ventilation** [38].

The risk of **maternal mortality with CAP was 2.9%** from reports in the 1990s [39]. Among women hospitalized for pneumonia during pregnancy, the risk of delivering a small-for-gestational-age infant is increased relative to controls although this may be confounded by different health behaviors in the two groups. Rates of preterm birth and perinatal mortality are increased after pregnancy complicated by pneumonia although not to statistical significance. Term and preterm premature rupture of membranes have been shown to be increased in women with viral and bacterial pneumonia [40].

Pregnancy Considerations
Women hospitalized for CAP during pregnancy appear to be less ill than their nonpregnant counterparts, measured by either severity score or length of stay, but this probably reflects a tendency to hospitalize for less severe disease because of the pregnancy. The rate of preterm delivery is higher among women with a diagnosis of pneumonia than among those with upper-tract respiratory infection or with no respiratory infection [41]. In addition, the risk of placental abruption is twice as high among pregnant women hospitalized for pneumonia compared to a control group without respiratory disease [42] although in this large data set obtained from the National Hospital Discharge Survey, the highest risk of abruption followed not pneumonia but chronic bronchitis.

Management
Principles
Prompt administration of antibiotics without delay and appropriate antibiotic therapy are the most important principles for effective management.

Prevention
Pneumococcal vaccine prevents 71% of cases of CAP and 32% of related mortality in nonpregnant adults [33]. **For details on recommended pneumococcal and influenza vaccines, see Chapter 38.**

Workup
Assess severity of illness by physical findings (blood pressure, respiratory rate, mental status, state of hydration) and by radiographic findings (e.g., multilobar involvement and pleural effusion). Laboratory testing for a specific cause is controversial and frequently nonrevealing. The IDSA and the ATS have recommended that diagnostic testing be initiated to determine the cause of CAP if the results would change treatment decisions, for example, antimicrobial regimens. This would be most useful in areas of high antibiotic resistance or if unusual pathogens are suspected. A list of clinical indications for more extensive diagnostic testing can be found in the IDSA/ATS Consensus Guidelines [36]. Routine diagnostic tests to identify an etiologic diagnosis are optional for the mildly ill, but **patients with severe CAP should have the following diagnostic tests: blood cultures, urinary antigen assays for *Legionella* spp. and *S. pneumoniae*, and expectorated sputum samples/endotracheal aspirates.**

Blood culture is positive in 5% to 11% of cases; positive blood cultures are more common in those with severe CAP [43]. Blood cultures should be obtained before antibiotic administration.

Treatment

Hospitalization

The initial management decision after diagnosis is to determine the site of care, that is, outpatient, hospital ward, or ICU. There are no trials addressing benefits of outpatient versus inpatient care for the pregnant woman with pneumonia. Keeping this in mind, physicians may still begin treatment decisions by using a prediction tool for increased mortality, such as the PSI, combined with clinical judgment [36]. The PSI was developed to assist physicians in identifying patients at a higher risk of complications and who are more likely to benefit from hospitalization, that is, those with comorbidities, hypoxemia, alteration in vital signs, etc. It has not been validated in pregnancy. Direct admission to ICU is required for patients with septic shock requiring vasopressors or with acute respiratory failure requiring intubation and mechanical ventilation.

The majority of obstetrical patients will fail to qualify as high risk by these criteria. Retrospectively applying ATS guidelines in place at the time of the study (similar to above), only 25% of pregnant patients with a diagnosis of CAP could have been assigned to outpatient care [38]. A 23-hour observation period might be useful in deciding whether inpatient treatment is warranted in the pregnant patient.

Antibiotics

There are no trials to determine which antibiotic regimen is most beneficial for the pregnant woman with pneumonia. No published treatment guidelines alter therapy for pneumonia because of pregnancy. Antibiotic selection should take into account the common causes of CAP, local antibiotic resistance patterns, clinical presentation, comorbid conditions, and recent antibiotic use. The fluoroquinolones are generally avoided in pregnancy because of concerns about interference with cartilage formation in the fetus, and the tetracyclines because of concerns about dentition. However, depending on drug allergies and microbiologic sensitivities, it may be necessary to alter these preferences. Initial choice of antimicrobial treatment is empirical. The ATS and IDSA recommend antibiotic regimens for adults with CAP [43]; they are adapted here to exclude, where possible, quinolones and tetracyclines. A joint ATS-IDSA updated guideline for antimicrobial therapies in CAP is expected late in 2016.

- Previously healthy patient, no recent antibiotic therapy, no risk factors for drug-resistant *S. pneumoniae*:
  - Erythromycin, azithromycin, or clarithromycin: only 1% of pregnant women with CAP remained febrile with erythromycin 500 mg every six hours [38].
- Previously healthy, but antibiotics within the past three months for any reason; or comorbidities (chronic heart/lung/liver/kidney disease, diabetes, or asplenia); or immunocompromise, including immunosuppressant drugs:
  - **β-lactam plus macrolide**; high-dose amoxicillin (1 g po tid) or high-dose amoxicillin clavulanate (2 g po bid) are preferred; alternatives include ceftriaxone, cefpodoxime, or cefuroxime (500 mg po bid).
- Inpatient, not in ICU:
  - β-lactam (cefotaxime, ceftriaxone, or ampicillin) **plus** a macrolide.
- Inpatient, ICU:
  - β-lactam **plus** azithromycin.

- *For Pseudomonas:*
  - Piperacillin-tazobactam, cefepime, imipenem, or meropenem **plus** ciprofloxacin or levofloxacin or
  - Piperacillin-tazobactam, cefepime, imipenem, or meropenem **plus** aminoglycoside **plus** azithromycin.
- For community-acquired methicillin-resistant *Staphylococcus aureus*:
  - Add vancomycin or linezolid

In summary, **most cases of low-risk CAP in pregnancy can be treated with a macrolide, and the more high-risk ones can be treated with a macrolide and a β-lactam**. Uncommon pathogens do exist and should be considered if response to therapy is inadequate or incomplete.

Typical responses to therapy include defervescence in two to four days with resolution of leukocytosis in the same time period. The chest X-ray may take longer to clear as may the auscultatory findings. **Antibiotic therapy should not be changed within the first 72 hours unless clinical deterioration is overt or organism sensitivities become available**. There is no evidence in nonpregnant adults that intravenous and oral therapy differ in efficacy. Patients should be switched from intravenous to oral therapy when hemodynamically stable and improving clinically, able to ingest medications and have a normally functioning GI tract. If the pathogen and sensitivities are known, the narrowest spectrum agent should be chosen for oral therapy, but in most cases, this will not be possible, and oral agents should duplicate the spectrum of the parenteral agents used. The American Thoracic Society and the Infectious Diseases Society of America recommend **discharge to home the same day that clinical stability is achieved (afebrile, no tachypnea nor tachycardia, normotensive, normoxemic, normal mental status, and able to tolerate oral intake) and the switch to oral agents is made**. Inpatient observation while receiving oral therapy is not necessary. A follow-up inpatient chest X-ray is not indicated.

There are inadequate data to determine the best duration of antimicrobial treatment for CAP. With older agents, a **duration of 10 to 14 days is commonly prescribed**, but newer agents have longer half-lives and therefore may be curative over shorter courses of therapy, for example, five to seven days; trials are under way. Regardless of the total duration, it is recommended that patients with CAP be treated for a minimum of five days, should be afebrile for 48 to 72 hours, and should be clinically stable before discontinuation of therapy [43].

Oxygen support should be provided as needed.

Antepartum Testing

No specific indication.

Delivery

No specific changes.

Anesthesia

No specific changes.

Postpartum/Breast-Feeding

No specific changes.

INFLUENZA
Key Points

- Trivalent inactivated influenza vaccine is recommended for all pregnant and postpartum women.
- **In addition to the protective effect of vaccination on women themselves, infants born to vaccinated mothers have fewer episodes of influenza, fever, and respiratory illness in their first six months of life.**
- Influenza antiviral medications should be started **as soon as possible after** symptom onset, ideally within 48 hours of symptom onset. **Treatment should not wait for laboratory confirmation of influenza.**
- Risk of severe illness and mortality because of influenza appear to be higher among pregnant women.

Epidemiology/Incidence

Annual epidemics of influenza typically occur during the late fall through early spring: in the northern hemisphere, flu season starts in September or October and may continue as late as May. In addition to seasonal flu, epidemics or pandemics arise unpredictably. The pattern of emergence is usually in the southern hemisphere first, during the austral winter, where influenza peaks in August.

Etiology/Basic Pathophysiology

Influenza illnesses are caused by infection with one of the three types of circulating RNA viruses: A, B, or C [44]. Although B and C are almost exclusive to humans, A is avian in origin, although capable of infecting a range of warm-blooded animals. Both A and B types cause epidemic human disease. Influenza A viruses are subtyped by their surface antigens hemagglutinin (H) and neuraminidase (N).

High mutation rates and the potential for cross-species genetic reassortment are characteristic of influenza A [44]. New influenza A subtypes have the potential to cause a pandemic as demonstrated most recently in the 2009 H1N1 pandemic. The 2009 pandemic influenza A (H1N) virus contained a combination of gene segments that had not been reported previously in animals or humans.

Influenza is spread by aerosolized droplets. The incubation period for influenza is one to four days; patients are likely infectious one day before symptom onset.

Symptoms

Infection with influenza virus can range from asymptomatic infection to uncomplicated upper respiratory tract disease to serious complicated illness, such as secondary bacterial pneumonia, sepsis, and organ failure. Symptoms include fever, cough, sore throat, nasal congestion or rhinorrhea, headache, myalgia, and malaise.

Diagnosis

A variety of laboratory tests are available (Table 24.7). Testing should occur if the result would influence clinical management. For screening during influenza season, antigen-based rapid testing is appropriate, but positive predictive value is poor when influenza prevalence is low.

Complications

Complications are largely maternal. In influenza pandemics, the maternal mortality case–fatality ratio is higher than that of the general population. In the most recent pandemic (2009), pregnant women, who represented approximately 1% of the U.S. population, accounted for 5% of deaths from 2009 influenza A (H1N1) [45,46]. In a case series from the 2009 H1N1 pandemic, 7% of deaths occurred in the first trimester, 27% in the second, and 64% in the third trimester [46]. This study is consistent with previous pandemics and seasonal influenza studies, which usually suggest that **the risk of influenza complications is higher in the second and third trimester** of pregnancy than in the first trimester [47,48].

Transplacental passage of influenza virus appears to be rare [49]. Infants born to women with laboratory-confirmed seasonal influenza during pregnancy do not have higher rates of low birth weight or lower Apgar scores [49,50]. The effect of influenza on perinatal outcomes is inconsistent. In most studies, there are no significant differences in mode of delivery, duration of delivery admission, episodes

Table 24.7 Influenza Testing Methods

Test	Method	Time	Comment
PCR	Gel-based reverse transcriptase PCR	≥2 hr	High sensitivity Very high specificity
Immunofluorescence	Direct or indirect fluorescent antibody stain	2–4 hr	Moderate-to-high sensitivity High specificity
Rapid tests	Antigen detection; enzyme immunoassay	10–30 min	Low-to-moderate sensitivity High specificity Limitations: may not distinguish influenza A and B Positive predictive value poor outside of influenza season
Viral culture	Shell vial culture or cell culture	2–10 days	Moderate-to-high sensitivity, highest specificity; useful for public health surveillance, not for clinician
Serology	Acute paired & convalescent samples: ELISA, complement fixation, hemagglutination, or neutralization	Weeks to months	Reference laboratories only; useful for public health surveillance, no help in clinical management

Source: Adapted from Harper SA, Bradley JS, Englund JA et al. *Clin Infect Dis*, 48, 1003–32, 2009.

of preterm labor, and adverse perinatal outcomes between the influenza and noninfluenza groups [51,52], although a large U.S. study of 2009 pandemic H1N1 influenza demonstrated a 30% risk of preterm birth among affected women [46], and another Norwegian study of 2009 pandemic H1N1 influenza reported a significant increase in fetal deaths [53]. Severe maternal illness, of course, such as overt respiratory failure, is associated with significantly worse perinatal outcome than in most seasonal or even pandemic influenza [54–56].

Pregnancy Considerations

Changes in the immune, respiratory, and cardiovascular systems result in pregnant women being more severely affected. Pregnant women are at higher risk for severe complications and death from influenza, both H1N1 influenza and seasonal influenza.

During periods of seasonal flu, pregnant women account for excess health care visits related to respiratory complaints and excess hospitalizations (above what would be expected outside of pregnancy); this is true for both healthy women and those with chronic conditions. The rate of hospitalization for seasonal (not pandemic) influenza among healthy nonpregnant women in Canada has been reported as 17/100,000, but 156/100,000 among healthy women who were pregnant. The tenfold difference in influenza hospitalization persisted among women with comorbidities, but as expected, the absolute rates are higher [57]. Pregnant women are at increased risk for hospitalization during influenza season, and those hospitalized for respiratory illness stay longer [46,57,58]. During the 2009 H1N1 influenza pandemic, pregnant and postpartum women with H1N1 influenza had a seven times higher risk of admission to ICU than nonpregnant women in the same age group, and after 20 weeks of pregnancy, the relative risk of ICU admission was 13 times higher [56]. The severity of disease is demonstrated by utilization of extracorporeal membrane oxygenation (ECMO): in 2009 in Australia and New Zealand, 16% of all ECMO interventions for respiratory failure in H1N1 were performed on pregnant or postpartum patients [59]; these are patients whom conventional mechanical ventilation could not adequately oxygenate.

Management

Prevention

Annual influenza vaccination is the most effective method for preventing influenza infection and its complications [60]. The vaccine is reformulated yearly to cover the strains predicted to be in circulation. The trivalent inactivated vaccine (TIV) for individuals is recommended for women who are pregnant, postpartum, or breast-feeding during the influenza season. TIV contains noninfectious killed viruses and cannot cause influenza. It can be given in any trimester of pregnancy. Safety is not a concern: there is no suggestion of fetal harm after TIV administration to pregnant women [61] and no difference in rate of preterm birth and cesarean delivery [62]. In fact, influenza vaccination in the first trimester is not associated with an increase in major malformation rates and is associated with a decrease in stillbirth rates [63]. The live attenuated influenza vaccine (given intranasally), like other live-virus vaccines, should not be given during pregnancy (see also Chapter 38).

In addition to the protective effect of vaccination on women themselves, infants born to vaccinated mothers have fewer episodes of influenza, fever, and respiratory illness in their first six months of life [64], which may represent antibody transfer [65]. Each season, influenza vaccines are reformulated. Vaccination providers may check updated information at the Centers for Disease Control and Prevention (http://www.cdc.gov/flu), Food and Drug Administration (http://www.fda.gov/BiologicsBloodVaccines/SafetyAvailability/vaccinesafety/default.htm), or World Health Organization (WHO) (http://ww.who.int/csr/disease/influenza/vaccine recommendations/en/index.html). However, national health authorities approve the specific composition and formulation of yearly vaccines for individual countries.

Prophylaxis after Suspected Exposure

Chemoprophylaxis after exposure to influenza is recommended for individuals at high risk of complications from influenza, which would include pregnant and postpartum women [66]. For household exposures, this means a 10-day course of either oseltamivir 75 mg once daily, or zanamivir as two 5-mg inhalations once daily. There are no RCTs of postexposure influenza prophylaxis among pregnant women. The efficacy of oseltamivir prophylaxis has, however, been called into question after a reanalysis of data obtained directly from the manufacturer [67]: See below.

Therapy

The neuraminidase inhibitors, oseltamivir and zanamivir, are modestly effective against both influenza A (including H1N1) and influenza B. Although the manufacturer has conducted no studies to assess safety of these medications for pregnant women, available risk–benefit data suggest that **pregnant women with suspected or confirmed influenza should receive prompt antiviral therapy. Information about peramivir in pregnancy is limited to a handful of cases treated under the FDA's Emergency Use Authorization, and no recommendation can be made about this drug**.

The standard dose for oseltamivir is 75 mg po bid for five days [68]. The standard dose for zanamivir is two inhalations twice daily for five days; this drug should be avoided in case of chronic respiratory disease, including asthma. If oseltamivir resistance is suspected, use zanamivir.

Treatment should be started as soon as possible, preferably within the first 48 hours. Delayed treatment of antiviral therapy has been associated with more severe illness and death in both seasonal influenza and 2009 influenza A (H1N1) whereas early initiation of treatment has been associated with reduced duration of illness, severity, mortality, and incidence of complications [46,54,69–71]. **Laboratory confirmation of influenza virus infection is not necessary for the initiation of treatment**. For uncomplicated influenza infection, a five-day course of antiviral medication is prescribed [68].

Several systematic reviews of neuraminidase inhibitors in nonpregnant adults [71–73] appeared to show an advantage for oseltamivir compared to placebo in reduction of symptoms (HR = 1.20; 95% CI, 1.06, 1.35) with a reduction in duration of illness of about one day. These reviews, however, have been called into question because of concerns of reporting bias. In order to perform the most recent systematic review, authors waged a four-year battle to obtain clinical trial results directly from the sponsoring pharmaceutical company and concluded that **oseltamivir, compared to placebo, shortened the time to** alleviation of symptoms by 16 hours (that is, from 7.0 days of symptoms to 6.3 days), **had no effect on hospital admission, and did not affect the risk of developing objectively verified pneumonia or any other complication deemed significant.** [70] When given as postexposure prophylaxis, oseltamivir reduced the probability of developing symptomatic influenza by 55% while increasing gastrointestinal disturbances, headache, psychiatric events, and renal compromise [70].

Epidemiologic data from the 2009–2010 pandemic showed that among pregnant women, later initiation of antiviral treatment (≥4 days after symptoms began) was associated with higher rates of hospital admission, ICU admission, and mechanical ventilation, compared to those who began treatment earlier. Women who received no antiviral drug had no increased risk of hospital admission but were more likely to be admitted to ICU and to receive mechanical ventilation, compared to those who began antiviral therapy at less than four days after symptom onset. "Late" or no treatment was also associated with higher risk of death although mortality was, surprisingly, higher with late treatment than with no treatment, perhaps reflecting small numbers [46].

There is limited evidence regarding the safety of oseltamivir use in pregnancy. A single cotyledon perfused placental model showed that oseltamivir is extensively metabolized by the placenta [74] with minimal accumulation of the metabolite on the fetal side. In a population of 90 Japanese women who received oseltamivir during pregnancy, the incidence of malformation (1.1%) was similar to the incidence of major malformations in the general population [75]. A retrospective cohort study of 239 pregnant women in Texas demonstrated no association of antepartum exposure to amantadine, rimantadine, or oseltamivir with adverse fetal outcomes [76]. As of 2015, **CDC continues to recommend oral oseltamivir for treatment of pregnant and postpartum women suspected of having influenza** and states that the decision to start antiviral treatment should not wait for laboratory confirmation, since "laboratory testing can delay treatment and because a negative rapid influenza diagnostic test does not rule out influenza" [77].

Antepartum Testing
No evidence for recommendations.

Delivery
No evidence for recommendations.

Postpartum/Breast-Feeding
Whether influenza viruses are passed into human milk is not known; however, respiratory droplets are believed to be the main mode of viral transmission. Because of the anti-infective benefits of human milk for infants, **continuation of breast-feeding is recommended while the mother is receiving treatment for influenza infection.** The concentration of oseltamivir found in breast milk equates to much lower doses than the therapeutic dose given to infants [78].

TUBERCULOSIS
Key Points
- Definite diagnosis of **active infection** is based on culture (of suspected site: sputum for pulmonary TB) for *Mycobacterium tuberculosis*. Sputum culture is also important for drug sensitivity testing.
- Diagnosis of **latent tuberculosis infection** is based on a positive tuberculin test (called tuberculin skin testing, TST, or purified protein derivative, PPD), or interferon gamma-release assay (IGRA), and the absence of signs, symptoms, or proof of active disease. The choice of diagnostic test is based on available resources and specific populations as noted below.
- Pregnancy does not influence the progression from latent to active disease.
- The treatment for latent tuberculosis infection in pregnancy is isoniazid 300 mg daily for six to nine months.
- Treatment of active tuberculosis consists of an initial two-month phase of therapy, including isoniazid, rifampin, pyrazinamide, and ethambutol. Directly observed therapy is usually recommended. For the following four months, continue isoniazid and rifampin. **Treatment for active tuberculosis is not altered by pregnancy.**

Epidemiology/Incidence
TB is rare in the developed world with, for example, approximately 9000 new cases in the United States in 2014. This is consistent with a rate of 3.0 cases per 100,000 persons. In comparison, there were more than nine million new TB cases in 2014 worldwide and 1.5 million deaths; TB is one of the top three causes of death for women of reproductive age [79]. HIV coinfection (about 12% worldwide) accounts for a significant portion of the tuberculosis burden. Even resource-rich countries have seen a resurgence of TB over the past few years as a result of an increase in immigrant populations. The national incidence of TB in pregnancy in the UK in 2008 was estimated at four per 100,000 maternities [80]. All but one of the TB patients in this study were non-Western immigrants and half had extrapulmonary disease. Few had undergone tuberculin skin testing despite recommendations to the contrary.

Symptoms (of Active Disease)
Cough, lethargy, dyspnea, malaise, fever, sweating, weight loss. Hemoptysis is a late finding.

Etiology/Basic Pathophysiology
The pathogenesis of tuberculosis infection and disease in pregnant women is similar to that in nonpregnant women. Spread (by airborne droplets) is facilitated by the ability of these small particles to remain airborne for hours after being emitted from an infected respiratory tract. Once the *Mycobacterium* is taken up by alveolar macrophages, the infection may either be contained by granuloma formation or may progress to active disease [81]. Most patients develop cell-mediated immunity, which is demonstrated by conversion of the tuberculin skin test and which constitutes latent tuberculosis infection. In some patients, the replication of *M. tuberculosis* cannot be contained, and active disease occurs. Latent tuberculosis infection can develop into active tuberculosis, especially in individuals with risk factors. Pulmonary disease is the most common but not the only form of active tuberculosis, which can manifest in 20% of cases (extrapulmonary tuberculosis) as meningitis, osteitis, genitourinary involvement, or disseminated disease.

Risk Factors/Associations

HIV is the most important risk factor. Poorly controlled diabetes, renal failure, malignancy, steroids, malnutrition, and vitamin A or D deficiency are other risk factors for acquiring active *M. tuberculosis* infection [81].

Diagnosis

Definitive diagnosis of **active** infection is still made by **culture** (of suspected site, e.g., sputum) for *M. tuberculosis*. Smear demonstrating acid-fast bacilli is a technique for rapid diagnosis [76]. Diagnosis of **latent tuberculosis** requires a positive **tuberculin skin test** (TST, also called purified protein derivative, PPD), in the absence of disease (thus no symptoms, X-ray findings, bacilli on smear, or positive culture). The **interferon gamma release assay (IGRA)** is an alternative method for diagnosing TB and can be used in all incidences in which the TST would be recommended. It is specifically preferred in populations who have previously received the BCG vaccination and those who historically have poor rates of return for TST reading.

The most widely used method to detect respiratory TB in most disease-endemic countries is the sputum smear microscopy test developed in the 19th century, drawbacks of which include low sensitivity (especially in children and in HIV-positive individuals), inability to determine drug susceptibility, and variable performance depending on operator training and skill. In December 2010, the WHO endorsed a novel rapid test for tuberculosis, a fully automated molecular test for TB case detection plus rifampicin resistance testing. Other than adding sputum and reagent to the cartridge, there is little for the technician to do [82]. In a multinational study of about 1500 nonpregnant adults, this assay identified 98% of patients with smear-positive and culture-positive tuberculosis (including more than 70% of patients with smear-negative and culture-positive disease) and correctly identified 98% of bacteria that were resistant to rifampin [82]. The effect of pregnancy on this test has not been extensively studied, but it is counterintuitive to assume pregnancy would affect test performance.

Pregnancy Considerations

Tuberculosis attack rates appear to be comparable in the pregnant and nonpregnant states. Presentation is similar among both pregnant and nonpregnant patients, but diagnosis may be delayed in pregnancy because of the ubiquity of constitutional complaints during early pregnancy. **Pregnancy is not known to influence the progression from latent to active disease**, nor has it been shown to affect the response to treatment. Pregnancy is not associated with higher (or lower) prevalence of anergy compared to other HIV-negative adults.

There are conflicting data on the effect of TB on maternal and neonatal outcomes. In a population-based study in Taiwan, women known to have TB during pregnancy—all of whom were treated—demonstrated an absolute increase of 2%–3% in the rate of low-birth-weight babies with no difference in preterm births compared to controls [83]. An earlier case-control study from India suggested higher rates of both preterm birth and small for gestational age newborns among women undergoing treatment for pulmonary TB, compared to matched controls [84], but a later Indian case-control study found no difference in perinatal outcome [85].

Congenital TB, which is very rare, is associated with maternal HIV infection, tuberculous endometritis, and miliary tuberculosis [86]. It can occur hematogenously via the placenta and umbilical vein or by fetal aspiration or ingestion of infected amniotic fluid. Neonatal TB develops following exposure of an infant to the mother's aerosolized respiratory sections. This is more common than congenital TB, and diagnosis of neonatal TB can lead to diagnosis of previously unrecognized TB in the mother [87].

Pregnancy Management

Principles

Management of *M. tuberculosis* infection in pregnancy should be multidisciplinary with involvement of obstetrician, maternal-fetal medicine, and infectious diseases specialists.

Screening

Tuberculin Skin Testing

Tuberculin skin testing (TST) is the method historically used to detect both latent and active disease. TST can be performed safely in pregnant women, and pregnancy does not alter the response to the TST [88]. Using standardized **purified protein derivative (PPD)**, 0.1 mL (5 tuberculin units) is administered intradermally in the volar surface of the forearm. The reaction is read 48 to 72 hours after the injection although reading is accurate up to a week after challenge. Targeted (not universal) tuberculin testing is recommended so as to identify individuals who are at increased risk for developing *M. tuberculosis* infection and who would benefit by treatment of latent tuberculosis infection. **Testing is discouraged among persons without risk factors** (Table 24.8). Persons at increased risk for development of active disease are those who were recently infected (i.e., converted from a positive to a negative skin test within the preceding two years) as well as those who have latent infection plus an increased risk of progression to overt disease. Table 24.8 shows some of the **indications for testing in pregnancy**: it is not an exhaustive list but is limited to those conditions that may be found in pregnancy. **Interpretation of PPD results** is shown in Table 24.9 [89].

A decision to test is a decision to treat. Therefore, do not test unless prepared to treat. With a positive skin test,

Table 24.8 Indications for Tuberculin Skin Testing in Pregnancy (Factors that Predispose to Progression from Latent to Active Disease)

Recent conversion
Household contacts of persons with infectious pulmonary TB
Recent immigration from parts of the world with high rates of TB
Homelessness
HIV infection
Living or working in institutional setting in which TB is common (hospital, jail, homeless shelter)
Injection drug use
Renal failure on hemodialysis
Diabetes
Solid organ transplantation
Certain cancers; certain surgeries, such as gastrectomy or jejunal bypass
High-dose corticosteroids for prolonged periods (lower limit not known)
Significantly underweight/poor nutrition

Table 24.9   Interpretation of Tuberculin Skin Testing

Size of Reaction	Persons in Whom Reaction Is Considered Positive
≥5 mm	HIV-infected persons Close contacts of persons with infectious tuberculosis Persons with an abnormal chest radiograph consistent with previous tuberculosis Immunosuppressed patients receiving the quivalent of ≥15 mg of prednisone per day for ≥1 month
≥10 mm	Foreign-born persons recently arrived (<5 years earlier) from country with high prevalence of tuberculosis Persons with a medical condition that increases the risk of tuberculosis[a] Injection-drug users Members of medically underserved, low-income populations (e.g., homeless persons) Residents and staff members of long-term care facilities (e.g., nursing homes, correctional institutions, and homeless shelters) Health care workers Children <4 years of age Persons with conversion on a tuberculin skin test (increase in duration of >10 mm within a 2-year period)
≥15 mm	All others

Source: Adapted from American Thoracic Society, CDC, and Infectious Diseases Society of America. Treatment of tuberculosis. *MMWR Recomm Rep*, 52, RR-11, 1–77, 2003.
[a]Medical conditions that increase the risk of tuberculosis: silicosis, end-stage renal disease, malnutrition, diabetes mellitus, carcinoma of the head and neck or lung, immunosuppressive therapy, lymphoma, leukemia, loss of >10% of ideal body weight, gastrectomy, and jejuno-ileal bypass.

chest X-ray (and perhaps additional testing) is indicated to differentiate latent from active infection as the therapy is different. The screening algorithm is shown in Figure 24.4.

Selective immunological testing (IGRA) for tuberculosis antigens, performed on whole blood, is available. IGRA appears to correlate better with recent TB exposure, is less likely to be affected by prior BCG vaccination, is more specific, at least as sensitive, is less likely to produce a false positive result, and may be a better predictor of progression, compared to TST [90,91]. Data in pregnancy are encouraging. A trial in Kenya of cryopreserved specimens obtained from HIV-positive pregnant women suggested that positive IGRA testing correlated strongly with the development of active TB postpartum [92]; a cross-sectional study in India showed that more pregnant women tested positive with IGRA than with TST, which may reflect higher sensitivity for latent tuberculosis infection. [93] IGRA may, in future, replace TST as the standard screen for TB exposure, latent infection, or disease. At this time **IGRA may be used to screen adults in any situation in which TST would be considered**, including women with prior BCG vaccine [94]. At this time, there are no studies that strongly support the use of one test versus the other. Although both tests are acceptable options for the diagnosis of TB, the ability to make a diagnosis in one visit with the IGRA does provide some logistical advantages.

Workup

Women with a cough lasting for >2 weeks or with symptoms as described above, especially with risk factors or from high-prevalence areas, should be worked up for tuberculosis. **Radiographic** findings suggesting tuberculosis include upper lobe infiltrate, cavitary lesions, and hilar adenopathy. Sputum smear can be negative even in active disease (15%–20% of cases). Sputum culture is required both for definite diagnosis

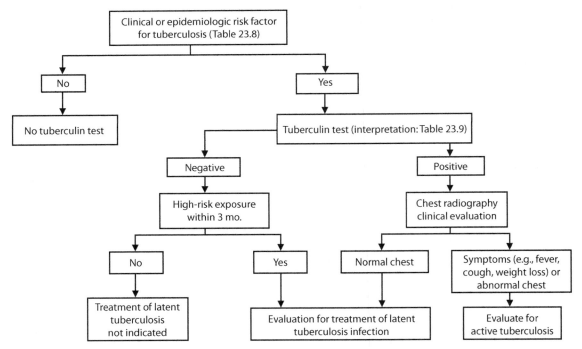

Figure 24.4   Tuberculosis screening algorithm. (Adapted from American Thoracic Society, CDC, and Infectious Diseases Society of America. Treatment of tuberculosis. *MMWR Recomm Rep*, 52, RR-11, 1–77, 2003.)

and for drug sensitivity testing [80] although both false positive and false negative results have been reported. Growth generally occurs in 7 to 21 days but may take 6 weeks or longer.

Management

Prevention

BCG (bacille Calmette-Guerin) vaccine has >70% efficacy in preventing *M. tuberculosis* **infection in children but not great efficacy in adults.** TST cannot distinguish between induration induced by BCG or *M. tuberculosis* infection. A history of BCG vaccination is ignored when administering and interpreting a tuberculin skin test. BCG should not be administered during pregnancy for the prevention of tuberculosis because it is a live vaccine. IGRA testing is useful in evaluating for TB in women with prior BCG vaccine.

Therapy

Latent Tuberculosis Infection

The treatment for latent tuberculosis infection in pregnancy is **isoniazid 300 mg daily for six to nine months** [87]. Alternative rifampin-based regimens have not been evaluated in pregnancy. Because isoniazid can interfere with pyridoxine metabolism and thereby precipitate peripheral neuropathy, **coadministration of pyridoxine 25 mg/day is advisable**. Isoniazid is 60% to 90% effective in reducing the risk of progression from tuberculosis latent infection to active disease. The most important but rare (1/1000) side effect of isoniazid is

Table 24.10 Recommended Daily Doses of First-Line Anti-Tuberculosis Drugs (Adults)

Isoniazid	4–6 mg/kg	Maximum 300 mg
Rifampicin	8–12 mg/kg	Maximum 600 mg
Pyrazinamide	20–30 mg/kg	
Ethambutol	12–18 mg/kg	

Source: Adapted from World Health Organization. *Treatment of Tuberculosis: Guidelines for National Programmes*. 4th ed, 2010. Available at: http://www.who.int/tb/publications/tb_treatmentguidelines /en/index.html.
Note: Daily dosing is optimal. Dosing three times a week instead of daily is an alternative for HIV-negative patients, assuming that therapy is directly observed. In the case of three times weekly treatment, doses of isoniazid, pyrazinamide, and ethambutol are higher than listed here.

hepatitis; the concern that this may be more common among pregnant women (which prompted a consideration of routinely deferring treatment to the puerperium) is based on a single investigation in which five cases of isoniazid hepatitis were identified among nearly 4000 pregnant women [95]: statistical significance was absent. Age >35 years is no longer considered a contraindication to isoniazid use [88]. **Pregnant and postpartum women should have pretreatment liver transaminases and bilirubin function tests,** and if these are normal, isoniazid can be started. Liver function tests should be obtained monthly. Isoniazid should be discontinued in a symptomatic or jaundiced patient if alanine aminotransferase (ALT) is more than three times the upper limit of normal and in an asymptomatic patient if ALT is more than five times the upper limit of normal [96].

Advantages of beginning treatment during pregnancy include better compliance and less loss to follow-up. A decision analysis suggests that antepartum treatment of latent tuberculosis infection is more efficient at preventing additional cases of TB within the population [97]. Recent infection with tuberculosis (i.e., a recent conversion of TST) or HIV coinfection increases the risk for transplacental spread of tubercle bacilli and thus for congenital tuberculosis, which implies that treatment for latent infection in these cases should be especially expeditious and compliant.

Active Tuberculosis Infection

Single-drug therapy is not acceptable for active TB. Multiple drugs for six months or more can cure >95% of patients (Tables 24.10 and 24.11) [90]. The treatment regimen is two-part, with an initial period of intensive therapy to kill actively growing bacilli, shortening the time the individual is infectious to others, followed by a second phase in which microbiologic cure is the goal. **The usual treatment for new patients with TB is an initial two-month phase of isoniazid, rifampin, pyrazinamide, and ethambutol.** Drugs may be given as fixed-dose combinations. Strict adherence to the regimen is important in minimizing drug resistance; for this reason, directly observed therapy is usually recommended. **For the following four months, isoniazid and rifampin are continued.** In settings in which isoniazid resistance is high and the patient's strain of TB has not been tested for isoniazid resistance, the four-month continuation phase should also include ethambutol.

Table 24.11 WHO-Recommended Treatment Regimens

Treatment Category	Patients	Tuberculosis Treatment[a]	
		Initial Phase	Continuation
I	New cases of smear-positive pulmonary TB, severe extrapulmonary TB, severe smear-negative pulmonary TB, or severe concomitant HIV disease	2 months $H_3R_3Z_3E_3$ or 2 months $H_3R_3Z_3S_3$	4 months H_3R_3
II	Previously treated smear-positive pulmonary TB, relapse, treatment failure, treatment after default	2 months HRZE or 2 months HRZS	4 months HR
		2 months $H_3R_3Z_3E_3S_3$/1 month $H_3R_3Z_3E_3$	5 months $H_3R_3E_3$
III	New cases of smear-negative pulmonary TB or with less severe forms of extrapulmonary TB	2 months HRZES/1 month HRZE	5 months HRE
		2 months $H_3R_3Z_3E_3$	4 months H_3R_3 4 months HR

Source: Adapted from World Health Organization. *Treatment of Tuberculosis: Guidelines for National Programmes*. 4th ed, 2010. Available at: http://www.who.int/tb/publications/tb_treatmentguidelines/en/index.html.
[a]Subscript refers to the number of doses per week; for daily dosing, no subscript. H, isoniazid; R, rifampicin; Z, pyrazinamide; S, streptomycin; E, ethambutol.

Treatment regimens and alternatives are available from the Centers for Disease Control and Prevention, the American Thoracic Society, the National Institute for Clinical Excellence, and the WHO. Those interested in these topics may bookmark the CDC's *Find TB Resources* website at http://www.fmdtbresources.org/scripts/index.cfm, which contains links to these sites.

In the case of multidrug-resistant (MDR) or extensively drug-resistant (XDR) tuberculosis, treatment becomes considerably more complex. Retreatment is beyond the scope of this chapter.

Tuberculosis treatment is not altered by pregnancy. Isoniazid, rifampin, pyrazinamide, and ethambutol are not teratogenic, and the WHO recommends their use in pregnant women [98]. Streptomycin exposure in utero has been associated with infant hearing loss, and so it is contraindicated in pregnancy. There are no adequate well-controlled reliable studies in human pregnancy. Although there has been some discussion in the literature about deferring treatment of latent tuberculosis infection to the postpartum period (see above), **there is no defensible argument for deferring treatment of active disease during pregnancy.** Pregnant women who are untreated pose an infection risk to the population at large as well as to their own infants.

Drug Resistance
MDR-TB—resistant to isoniazid and rifampin—accounts for about 1% of isolates in the United States [99]. Worldwide, MDR-TB accounts for about 4% of cases [100] although in some areas of the Russian Federation this rate is as high as 25%. Approximately 5% to 10% of MDR-TB strains are believed to be XDR, that is, also resistant to second-line anti-TB drugs. Pregnant women with MDR tuberculosis should be treated despite the limited safety data because of the grave public health implications. Tuberculosis strains that are known to be resistant to one or more of the first-line drugs are treated with alternative agents, for example, capreomycin, cycloserine, flu-oroquinolones, para-aminosalicylate, thiacetazone, amoxicillin-clavulanic acid, clofazimine, or clarithromycin. Kanamycin, streptomycin, and amikacin, which are ototoxic, have been associated with hearing loss in newborns whose mothers were treated during pregnancy. Ethionamide not only worsens nausea associated with pregnancy but has also been associated with congenital anomalies in animal studies: the WHO recommends against its use in pregnancy, if possible [101]. For all the second-line drugs, well-designed controlled studies in pregnant women are unavailable. The literature on treatment of drug-resistant TB during pregnancy is limited to case reports or case series [102–105]. Therapy of MDR tuberculosis during pregnancy should be driven by microbiologic susceptibility patterns (obtained by direct culture or known to be prevalent in the area), modified where possible by fetal concerns. For example, the WHO suggests that therapy of drug-resistant TB may be delayed until the second trimester after a discussion with the patient of the risks and benefits [99]. The individual practitioner is unlikely to make solo decisions about the treatment of MDR-TB as this is a role commonly filled by the health authority. The WHO maintains a tuberculosis gateway that provides links to epidemiology and to treatment of tuberculosis: http://www.who.int/tb/en/.

Coinfection with TB and HIV during Pregnancy
This is a large and growing public health problem, directly affecting global maternal mortality [106], which is nevertheless beyond the scope of this chapter. The interested reader is referred to a review of the topic [107] and to online resources at CDC (http://www.cdc.gov/tb/default.htm) and WHO (http://www.who.int/tb/publications/tb_women_factsheet_251013.pdf).

Infection Control Issues
Women with active pulmonary tuberculosis are infectious, but if the organism is sensitive, two weeks of multidrug therapy renders them noninfectious, so special precautions are not necessary thereafter. If the duration of therapy is shorter, or if MDR tuberculosis is present or suspected, the mother must be isolated in a negative pressure room for labor, and personal protective equipment should be worn by staff. Measures for the infant may include prophylactic isoniazid, BCG vaccination, or—in cases of MDR or XDR tuberculosis—separation from the mother.

Antepartum Testing
No specific indications.

Delivery
Cord blood and placenta should be tested for acid-fast bacilli.

Postpartum/Breast-Feeding
Maternal tuberculosis treatment is not altered by breast-feeding. Pyridoxine should be administered to the breast-feeding infant even if the infant is not receiving isoniazid therapy [85,87]. Neonate should undergo TST, chest X-ray, lumbar puncture, and *M. tuberculosis* smear and culture if mother had TB during pregnancy. If tuberculosis is suspected in the child, the child should be adequately treated.

REFERENCES
1. National Asthma Education and Prevention Program. *Expert Panel Report 3: Guidelines for the diagnosis and management of asthma: Full report 2007.* Available at: http://www.nhlbi.nih.gov/guidelines/asthma/asthgdln.pdf. [Guideline]
2. Kwon HL, Triche EW, Belanger K et al. The epidemiology of asthma during pregnancy: Prevalence, diagnosis, and symptoms. *Immunol Allergy Clin North Am* 2006; 26: 29–62. [III]
3. Enriquez R, Wu P, Griffin MR et al. Cessation of asthma medication in early pregnancy. *Am J Obstet Gynecol* 2006; 195: 149–53. [II-2]
4. Murphy VE, Wang G, Namazy JA et al. The risk of congenital malformations, perinatal mortality and neonatal hospitalization among pregnant women with asthma: A systematic review and meta-analysis. *BJOG* 2013; 120: 812–22. [II-1]
5. Dombrowski MP, Schatz M, Wise R et al., for the National Institute of Child Health and Human Development Maternal-Fetal Medicine Units Network and the National Heart, Lung and Blood Institute. Asthma during pregnancy. *Obstet Gynecol* 2004; 103: 5–12. [II-2]
6. Bakhireva LN, Schatz M, Jones KL et al. Asthma control during pregnancy and the risk of preterm delivery or impaired fetal growth. *Ann Allergy Asthma Immunol* 2008; 101: 137–43. [II-3]
7. Schatz M, Dombrowski MP, Wise R et al. Spirometry is related to perinatal outcomes in pregnant women with asthma. *Am J Obstet Gynecol* 2006; 194: 120–6. [II-3]

8. Bracken MB, Triche EW, Belanger K et al. Asthma symptoms, severity, and drug therapy; a prospective study of effects on 2205 pregnancies. *Obstet Gynecol* 2003; 102: 739–52. [II-2]

9. Olesen C, Thrane N, Nielsen GL et al. A population-based prescription study of asthma drugs during pregnancy: Changing the intensity of asthma therapy and perinatal outcomes. *Respiration* 2001; 68: 256–61. [II-2]

10. Cydulka RK, Emerman CL, Schreiber D et al. Acute asthma among pregnant women presenting to the emergency department. *Am J Respir Crit Care Med* 1999; 160: 887–92. [II-3]

11. Kircher S, Schatz M, Long B. Variables affecting asthma course during pregnancy. *Ann Allergy Asthma Immunol* 2002; 89: 463–6. [II-3]

12. Gluck JC, Gluck PA. The effect of pregnancy on the course of asthma. *Immunol Allergy Clin North Am* 2000; 20: 729–43. [II-3]

13. Beecroft N, Cochrane GM, Milburn HF. Effect of sex of fetus on asthma during pregnancy: Blind prospective study. *BMJ* 1998; 317(7162): 856–7. [II-3]

14. National Asthma Education and Prevention Program. *NAEPP Working Group Report on managing asthma during pregnancy: Recommendations for pharmacologic treatment—Update 2004.* NIH Publication 05–3279. Available at: http://www.nhlbi.nih.gov/health/prof/lung/asthma/astpreg/astpreg_full.pdf. Accessed November 15, 2010. [Guideline]

15. ACOG Committee on Practice Bulletins-Obstetrics. Asthma in pregnancy. ACOG Practice Bulletin No. 90. *Obstet Gynecol* 2008; 111(2 Pt. 1): 457–64. [III]

16. National Heart, Lung and Blood Advisory Council Asthma Expert Working Group. *Draft needs assessment report for potential update of the Expert Panel Report-3 (2007): Guidelines for the diagnosis and management of asthma, January 2015.* Available at: http://www.nhlbi.nih.gov/sites/www.nhlbi.nih.gov/files/NHLBAC_Asthma-WG-Report-2015%5B1%5D.pdf. Accessed September 21, 2015. [Guideline]

17. Bain E, Pierides KL, Clifton VL, Hodyl NA, Stark MJ, Crowther CA, Middleton P. Interventions for managing asthma in pregnancy. *Cochrane Database System Rev* 2014, 10: CD010660. doi:10.1002/14651858.CD010660.pub2. [Meta-analysis]

18. Dombrowski MP, Schatz M, Wise R et al. Randomized trial of inhaled beclomethasone dipropionate versus theophylline for moderate asthma during pregnancy. *Am J Obstet Gynecol* 2004; 190: 737–44. [I, n = 385]

19. Silverman M, Sheffer A, Diaz, P et al. Outcome of pregnancy in a randomized controlled study of patients with asthma exposed to budesonide. *Ann Allergy Asthma Immunol* 2005; 95: 566–70. [I, n = 313]

20. Namazy J, Schatz M, Long L et al. Use of inhaled steroids by pregnant asthmatic women does not reduce intrauterine growth. *J Allergy Clin Immunol* 2004; 113: 427–32. [II-2]

21. Martel M-J, Rey E, Beauchesne M-F et al. Use of inhaled corticosteroids during pregnancy and risk of pregnancy-induced hypertension: Nested case-control study. *BMJ* 2005; 330: 230–6. [II-2]

22. Breton MC, Beauchesne MF, Lemiere C et al. Risk of perinatal mortality associated with inhaled corticosteroid use for the treatment of asthma during pregnancy. *J Allergy Clin Immunol* 2010; 126: 772–7. [II-2]

23. Rahimi R, Nikfar S, Abdollahi M. Meta-analysis finds use of inhaled corticosteroids during pregnancy safe: A systematic meta-analysis review. *Hum Exp Toxicol* 2006; 25(8): 447–52. [I]

24. Lin S, Munsie JPW, Herdt-Losavio ML et al. Maternal asthma medication use and the risk of gastroschisis. *Am J Epidemiol* 2008; 168: 73–9. [II-2]

25. Bakhireva LN, Jones KL, Schatz M et al. Safety of leukotriene receptor antagonists in pregnancy. *J Allergy Clin Immunol* 2007; 119: 618–25. [II-2]

26. Sarkar M, Koren G, Kalra S et al. Montelukast use during pregnancy: A multicentre, prospective, comparative study of infant outcomes. *Eur J Pharmacol* 2009; 65: 1259–64. [II-2]

27. Ducharme FM. Addition of anti-leukotriene agents to inhaled corticosteroids for chronic asthma. *Cochrane Database System Rev* 2004; 1: CD003133. doi:10/1002/14651858.CD003133.pub2. [Meta-analysis]

28. Siddiqi AK, Gouda H, Multz AS et al. Ventilator strategy for status asthmaticus in pregnancy: A case-based review. *J Asthma* 2005; 42: 159–62. [II-3]

29. Elsavegh D, Shapiro JM. Management of the obstetric patient with status asthmaticus. *J Intensive Care Med* 2008; 23: 396–402. [II-3]

30. Lazarus SC. Emergency treatment of asthma. *NEJM* 2010; 363: 755–64. [III]

31. Marik PE, Varon J. Requirement of perioperative stress doses of corticosteroids: A systematic review of the literature. *Arch Surg* 2008; 143: 1222–26. [Review]

32. Rust GS, Thompson CJ, Minor P et al. Does breastfeeding protect children from asthma? Analysis of NHANES III survey data. *J Natl Med Assoc* 2001; 93: 139–48. [II-3]

33. File TM. Community-acquired pneumonia. *Lancet* 2003; 362: 1991–2001. [review]

34. Sheffield JS, Cunningham FG. Community-acquired pneumonia in pregnancy. *Obstet Gynecol* 2009; 114(4): 915–22. [Review]

35. Goodnight WH, Soper DE. Pneumonia in pregnancy. *Crit Care Med* 2005; 33(Suppl.): S390–7. [Review]

36. Fine MJ, Auble TE, Yealy DM et al. A prediction rule to identify low-risk patients with community-acquired pneumonia. *N Engl J Med* 1997; 336: 243–50. [II-3]

37. Jin Y, Carriere KC, Marrie TJ et al. The effects of community-acquired pneumonia during pregnancy ending with a live birth. *Am J Obstet Gynecol* 2003; 18: 800–6. [II-3]

38. Yost NP, Bloom SL, Richey SD et al. An appraisal of treatment guidelines for community-acquired pneumonia. *Am J Obstet Gynecol* 2000; 183: 131–5. [II-3]

39. Bloom SL, Ramin S, Cunningham FG. A prediction rule for community-acquired pneumonia. *N Engl J Med* 1997; 336: 1913–4. [Meta-analysis in letter to the editor]

40. Getahun D, Ananth CV, Oyelese Y et al. Acute and chronic respiratory diseases in pregnancy: Associations with spontaneous premature rupture of membranes. *J Matern Fetal Neonatal Med* 2007; 20: 669–75. [II-2]

41. Banhidy F, Acs N, Puho EH et al. Maternal acute respiratory infectious diseases during pregnancy and birth outcomes. *Eur J Epidemiol* 2008; 23: 29–35. [II-2]

42. Getahun D, Ananth CV, Peltier MR et al. Acute and chronic respiratory diseases in pregnancy: Associations with placental abruption. *Am J Obstet Gynecol* 2006; 195: 1180–4. [II-2]

43. Mandell LA, Wunderink RG, Anzueto A et al. Infectious Diseases Society of America/American Thoracic Society Consensus Guidelines on the management of community-acquired pneumonia in adults. *Clin Infect Dis* 2007; 44(Suppl.): S27–72. [Guideline]

44. Taubenberger JK, Morens DM. Influenza: The once and future pandemic. *Public Health Rep* 2010; 125(Suppl. 3): 16–26. [Review]

45. Jamieson DJ, Honein MA, Rasmussen SA et al. H1N1 2009 influenza virus infection during pregnancy in the USA. *Lancet* 2009; 374: 451–8. [II-3]

46. Siston AM, Rasmussen SA, Honein MA et al. Pandemic 2009 influenza A (H1N1) virus illness among pregnant women in the United States. *JAMA* 2010; 303: 1517–25. [II-3]

47. Dodds L, McNeil SA, Fell DB et al. Impact of influenza exposure on rates of hospital admissions and physician visits because of respiratory illness among pregnant women. *CMAJ* 2007; 176: 463–8. [II-2]

48. Tamma PD Steinhoff MC, Omer SB. Influenza infection and vaccination in pregnant women. *Expert Rev Respir Med* 2010; 4: 321–8. [Review]

49. Irving WL, James DK, Stephenson T et al. Influenza virus infection in the second and third trimesters of pregnancy: A clinical and seroepidemiological study. *BJOG* 2000; 107: 1282–9. [II-2]

50. Griffiths PD, Ronalds CJ, Heath RB. A prospective study of influenza infections during pregnancy. *J Epidemiol Community Health* 1980; 34: 124–8. [II-2]

51. Hartert TV, Neuzil KM, Shintani AK et al. Maternal morbidity and perinatal outcomes among pregnant women with respiratory hospitalizations during influenza season. *Am J Obstet Gynecol* 2003; 189: 1705–12. [II-2]

52. Acs N, Banhidy F, Puho E et al. Pregnancy complications and delivery outcomes of pregnant women with influenza. *J Matern Fetal Neonat Med* 2006; 19: 135–40. [II-2]

53. Haberg SE, Trogstad L, Gunnes N et al. Risk of fetal death after pandemic virus infection or vaccination. *NEJM* 2013; 368: 333–40. [II-1]

54. Louie KJ, Acosta M, Jamieson DJ et al. for the California Pandemic Working Group. Severe H1N1 influenza in pregnant and postpartum women in California. *N Engl J Med* 2010; 362: 27–35. [II-3]

55. ANZIC Influenza Investigators and Australasian Maternity Outcomes Surveillance System. Critical illness due to 2009 A/H1N1 influenza in pregnant and postpartum women: Population based cohort study. *BMJ* 2010; 340: c1279. [II-2]

56. Oluyomi-Obi T, Avery L, Schneider C et al. Perinatal and maternal outcomes in critically ill obstetrics patients with pandemic H1N1 influenza A. *J Obstet Gynaecol Can* 2010; 32: 443–7. [II-3]

57. Schanzer DL, Langley JM, Tam TWS. Influenza-attributed hospitalization rates among pregnant women in Canada 1994–2000. *J Obstet Gynecol Can* 2007; 29: 622–9. [II-2]

58. Cox S, Posner SF, McPheeters M et al. Hospitalizations with respiratory illness among pregnant women during influenza season. *Obstet Gynecol* 2006; 107: 1315–22. [III]

59. Davies AR, Jones D, Bailey M et al., for the Australia and New Zealand Extracorporeal Membrane Oxygenation (ANZ ECMO) Influenza Investigators. Extracorporeal membrane oxygenation for 2009 influenza A(H1N1) acute respiratory distress syndrome. *JAMA* 2009; 302(17): 1888–95. [II-3]

60. Cox NJ, Subbarao K. Influenza. *Lancet* 1999; 354: 1277–82. [III]

61. Mak TK, Mangtani P, Leese J et al. Influenza vaccination in pregnancy: Current evidence and selected national policies. *Lancet Infect Dis* 2008; 8: 44–52. [III]

62. Munoz FM, Greisinger AJ, Wehmanen OA et al. Safety of influenza vaccination during pregnancy. *Am J Obstet Gynecol* 2005; 192: 1098–106. [II-2]

63. Sheffield JS, Greer LG, Rogers VL et al. Effect of influenza vaccination in the first trimester of pregnancy. *Obstet Gynecol* 2012; 120: 532–7. [II-1])

64. Zaman K, Roy E, Arifeen SE et al. Effectiveness of maternal influenza immunization in mothers and infants. *N Engl J Med* 2008; 359: 1555–64. [RCT, *n* = 340]

65. Steinhoff MC, Omer SB, Roy E et al. Influenza immunization in pregnancy—Antibody responses in mothers and infants. *N Engl J Med* 2010; 362: 1644–6. [III]

66. Harper SA, Bradley JS, Englund JA et al. Seasonal influenza in adults and children: Diagnosis, treatment, chemoprophylaxis, and institutional outbreak management: Clinical practice guidelines of the Infectious Diseases Society of America. *Clin Infect Dis* 2009; 48: 1003–32. [Guideline]

67. Jefferson T, Jones M, Doshi P, Spencer EA, Onakpoya I, Heneghan CJ. Oseltamivir for influenza in adults and children: Systematic review of clinical study reports and summary of regulatory comments. *BMJ* 2014; 348: g2545. doi:10.1136/bmj.g2545. [II-2]

68. World Health Organization. *WHO guidelines for pharmacological management of pandemic (H1N1) 2009 influenza and other influenza viruses.* Available at: http://www.who.int/csr/resources/publications/swineflu/h1n1_use_antivirals_20090820/en/index.html. Accessed December 20, 2010. [Guideline]

69. Aoki FY, Macleod MD, Paggiaro P et al. IMPACT Study Group. Early administration of oral oseltamivir increases the benefits of influenza treatment. *J Antimicrob Chemother* 2003; 51: 123–9. [II-2]

70. Kaiser L, Wat C, Mills T et al. Impact of oseltamivir treatment on influenza-related lower respiratory tract complications and hospitalizations. *Arch Intern Med* 2003; 163(14): 1667–72. [I]

71. Nicholson KG, Aoki FY, Osterhaus AD et al. Efficacy and safety of oseltamivir in treatment of acute influenza: A randomised controlled trial. Neuraminidase Inhibitor Flu Treatment Investigator Group. *Lancet* 2000; 355(9218): 1845–50. [I]

72. Treanor JJ, Hayden FG, Vrooman PS et al. Efficacy and safety of the oral neuraminidase inhibitor oseltamivir in treating acute influenza: A randomized controlled trial. U.S. Oral Neuraminidase Study Group. *JAMA* 2000; 283: 1016–24. [I]

73. Jefferson T, Jones M, Doshi P et al. Neuraminidase inhibitors for preventing and treating influenza in healthy adults: Systematic review and meta-analysis. *BMJ* 2009; 339: b5106. [Review]

74. Worley KC, Roberts SW, Bawdon RE. The metabolism and transplacental transfer of oseltamivir in the ex vivo human model. *Infect Dis Obstet Gynecol* 2008; 2008: 927574. [II-3]

75. Tanaka T, Nakajima K, Murashima A et al. Safety of neuraminidase inhibitors against novel influenza A (H1N1) in pregnant and breastfeeding women. *CMAJ* 2009; 181(1–2): 55–8. [Review]

76. Greer, LG, Sheffield JS, Rogers VL et al. Maternal and neonatal outcomes after anterpartum treatment of influenza with antiviral medications. *Obstet Gynecol* 2010; 115: 711–6. [II-2]

77. Centers for Disease Control and Prevention. *Recommendations for obstetric health care providers related to use of antiviral medications in the treatment and prevention of influenza.* Available at: http://www.cdc.gov/flu/professionals/antivirals/avrec_ob.htm. Accessed September 22, 2015. [Guideline]

78. Wentges-van Holthe N, van Eijkeren M, van der Laan JW. Oseltamivir and breastfeeding. *Int J Infect Dis* 2008; 12: 451. [III]

79. World Health Organization. *Global tuberculosis control 2010.* Available at: http://whqlibdoc.who.int/publications/2010/9789241564069_eng.pdf. Accessed December 31, 2010. [III]

80. Knight M, Kurinczuk J, Nelson-Piercy C et al., on behalf of the United Kingdom Obstetric Surveillance System (UKOSS). Tuberculosis in pregnancy in the UK. *BJOG* 2009; 116: 584–8. [III]

81. Frieden TR, Sterling TR, Munsiff SS et al. Tuberculosis. *Lancet* 2003; 362: 887–92. [Review]

82. Boehme CC, Nabeta P, Hillemann D et al. Rapid molecular detection of tuberculosis and rifampin resistance. *N Engl J Med* 2010; 363: 1005–15. [II-2]

83. Lin HC, Lin HC, Chen SF. Increased risk of low birth weight and small for gestational age infants among women with tuberculosis. *BJOG* 2010; 117: 585–90. [II-2]

84. Jana N, Vasishta K, Jindal SK et al. Perinatal outcome in pregnancies complicated by pulmonary tuberculosis. *Int J Gynecol Obstet* 1994; 44: 119–24. [II-2]

85. Tripathy S. Tuberculosis and pregnancy. *Int J Gynaecol Obstet* 2003; 80: 247–53. [II-1]

86. American Thoracic Society, CDC, and Infectious Diseases Society of America. Treatment of tuberculosis. *MMWR Recomm Rep* 2003; 52(RR-11): 1–77. [Review]

87. Laibl V, Sheffield J. Tuberculosis in pregnancy. *Clin Perinatol* 2005; 32: 739. [Review]

88. American Thoracic Society. Targeted tuberculin testing and treatment of latent tuberculosis infection. *Am J Respir Crit Care Med* 2000; 161: S221–47. [Review]

89. Jasmer RM, Nahid P, Hopewell PC. Latent tuberculosis infection. *N Engl J Med* 2002; 347: 1860–6. [Review]

90. Royal College of Physicians, for the National Collaborating Centre for Chronic Conditions. *Tuberculosis: Clinical diagnosis and management of tuberculosis, and measures for its prevention and control.* National Institute for Clinical Excellence 2006. Available at: http://www.nice.org.uk/nicemedia/live/10980/30020/30020.pdf. Accessed December 28, 2010. [Guideline]

91. Lighter-Fisher J, Surette A-M. Performance of an interferon-gamma release assay to diagnose latent tuberculosis infection during pregnancy. *Obstet Gynecol* 2012; 119: 1088–95. [II-2]

92. Jonnalagadda S, Payne BL, Brown E et al. Latent tuberculosis detection by interferon g release assay during pregnancy predicts active tuberculosis and mortality in human immunodeficiency virus type 1-infected women and their children. *J Infect Dis* 2010; 202: 1826–35. [III]

93. Mathad JS, Bhosale R, Sangar V, Mave V et al. Pregnancy differentially impacts performance of latent tuberculosis diagnostics in a high-burden setting. *PLoS One* 2014; 9(3): e92308. doi:10.171/journal.pone.0092308. [II-2]

94. Mazurek GH, Jereb J, Vernon A et al. IGRA Expert Committee, Centers for Disease Control and Prevention (CDC). Updated guidelines for using Interferon Gamma Release Assays to detect *Mycobacterium tuberculosis* infection—United States, 2010. *MMWR Recomm Rep* 2010; 59(RR–5): 1–25. [Guideline]

95. Franks AL, Binkin NJ, Snider DE et al. Isoniazid hepatitis among pregnant and postpartum Hispanic patients. *Public Health Rep* 1989; 104: 151–5. [II-3]

96. Saukkonen J, Cohn D, Jasmer R et al. An official ATS statement: Hepatotoxicity of antituberculosis therapy. *Am J Respir Crit Care Med* 2006; 174: 935–52. [III]

97. Boggess KA, Myers ER, Hamilton CD. Antepartum or postpartum isoniazid treatment of latent tuberculosis infection. *Obstet Gynecol* 2000; 96: 757–62. [II-2]

98. World Health Organization. *Treatment of Tuberculosis: Guidelines for National Programmes.* 4th ed, 2010. Available at: http://www.who.int/tb/publications/tb_treatmentguidelines/en/index.html. Accessed December 26, 2010. [Guideline]

99. Centers for Disease Control and Prevention. *Reported Tuberculosis in the United States, 2009. Atlanta, GA: U.S. Department of Health and Human Services,* CDC, 2010. Available at: http://www.cdc.gov/tb/statistics/reports/2009/pdf/report2009.pdf. Accessed December 31, 2010. [Review]

100. World Health Organization. *Multidrug and extensively drug resistant TB (M/XDR-TB). 2010 Global Report on Surveillance and Response.* Available at: http://whqlibdoc.who.int/publications/2010/9789241599191_eng.pdf. Accessed December 31, 2010. [Review]

101. World Health Organization. *Guidelines for the programmatic management of drug-resistant tuberculosis. Emergency update 2008.* Available at: http://whqlibdoc.who.int/publications/2008/9789241547581_eng.pdf. Accessed December 30, 2010. [Guideline]

102. Lessnau K, Qarah S. Multidrug-resistant tuberculosis in pregnancy: Case report and review of the literature. *Chest* 2003; 123: 953–6. [III]

103. Shin S, Guerra D, Rich M et al. Treatment of multidrug-resistant tuberculosis during pregnancy: A report of 7 cases. *Clin Infect Dis* 2003; 36: 996–1003. [II-3]

104. Drobac P, delCastillo H, Sweetland A et al. Treatment of multidrug-resistant tuberculosis during pregnancy: Long-term followup of 6 children with intrauterine exposure to second-line agents. *Clin Infect Dis* 2005; 40: 1689–92. [II-3]

105. Palacios E, Dallman R, Munoz M et al. Drug-resistant tuberculosis and pregnancy: Treatment outcomes of 38 cases in Lima, Peru. *Clin Infect Dis* 2009; 48: 1413–9. [II-2]

106. Grange J, Adhikari M, Ahmed Y et al. Tuberculosis in association with HIV/AIDS emerges as a major nonobstetric cause of maternal mortality in Sub-Saharan Africa. *Int J Gynaecol Obstet* 2010; 108(3): 181–3. [III]

107. Adhikari M. Tuberculosis and tuberculosis/HIV co-infection in pregnancy. *Semin Fetal Neonatal Med* 2009; 234–240. [Review]

25

Systemic lupus erythematosus

Maria A. Giraldo-Isaza

KEY POINTS

- **Diagnosis**: ≥4/11 American College of Rheumatology (ACR) criteria **OR** 4/17 Systemic Lupus International Collaborating Clinics (SLICC) criteria with at least one clinical criteria and one immunologic criteria **OR** lupus nephritis by renal biopsy in the presence of ANA or anti ds-DNA antibodies.
- **Preconception counseling**: Feto-neonatal and maternal **complications** are primarily seen in systemic lupus erythematosus (SLE) patients **with active disease periconception or patients with hypertension, renal, heart, lungs, or brain disease or antiphospholipid or SSA/SSB antibodies**. Therefore, it is recommended to screen for all above and to start pregnancy with SLE in remission. Optimize medical therapy preconception.
- **Laboratories**: CBC with platelets, transaminases, creatinine, BUN, anti-Ro (SSA) and anti-La (SSB), anticardiolipin antibodies (ACA), lupus anticoagulant (LA) or dilute Russell's viper venom time (DRVVT), anti beta-2 glycoprotein-I, anti–ds DNA, C3, C4, CH50, urine sediment, 24-hour urine for total protein and creatinine clearance or spot urine protein-to-creatinine ratio.
- **Azathioprine and hydroxychloroquine (Plaquenil) are safe and effective in pregnancy. Currently hydroxychloroquine is the safest and most effective therapy for SLE pregnant women who need therapy. If stable with no recent flares on azathioprine and/or hydroxychloroquine (Plaquenil), it is recommended to continue them in pregnancy and postpartum.** Alternatively, they can also be started in pregnancy as needed.
- Low-dose aspirin (50–150 mg daily), if indicated, should be ideally initiated prior to 16 weeks for prevention of preeclampsia and fetal growth restriction (FGR).
- **For women with antiphospholipid syndrome (APS), see Chapter 26.**
- Women with **SSA/SSB antibodies** have about a **2% risk of congenital heart block (CHB)**. Preventive screening and therapy for CHB are not evidence based. Women with fetuses with CHB should be managed and delivered at a tertiary care center with the availability of immediate neonatal pacing.

DIAGNOSIS

SLE is a chronic multisystemic immunologic disease supported by the presence of autoantibodies in patients with clinical manifestations. The diagnosis can be challenging. Diagnostic criteria (ACR and SLICC) have been published. ACR criteria were developed in 1982 and revised in 1997: need ≥4/11 criteria to make diagnosis of SLE—either serially or simultaneously (Table 25.1) [1]. The ACR criteria were revised and validated to reflect new knowledge and attempt to reflect better clinical and immunologic aspects of the disease. The 2012 validated SLICC diagnosis needs 4/17 criteria with at least one clinical criteria and one immunologic criteria OR lupus nephritis by renal biopsy in the presence of ANA or anti ds-DNA antibodies (Table 25.2) [2]. The SLICC criteria were found to have better sensitivity (97% vs. 83%), less specificity (84% vs. 96%), and less misclassified cases (*n* = 62 vs. *n* = 74) when compared to the ACR criteria. Currently, either diagnostic criteria are used and acceptable.

SYMPTOMS

See diagnostic criteria in Tables 25.1 and 25.2. Also general (fatigue, fever, malaise, weight loss); GI (anorexia, ascites, vasculitis); thrombosis, Raynaud's phenomenon, among others.

EPIDEMIOLOGY/INCIDENCE

1:700 to 2000 general population (1:200 in African Americans), 90% in women, 1/500 in childbearing age. Table 25.3 has a list of incidence of abnormal laboratory tests and its associations with SLE; 25% of SLE patients meet criteria for antiphospholipid syndrome (APS) (see Chapter 26).

ETIOLOGY/BASIC PATHOPHYSIOLOGY

Autoantibody (Ab) to fixed tissue antigen (Ag) in vessel wall, nucleus, cytoplasmic membranes, etc.; Ag–Ab complexes in serum.

COMPLICATIONS
Maternal

Hypertension (4%–20%), preeclampsia (8%–20%), eclampsia (0.5%–1%), preterm birth (20%–50%) (spontaneous—preterm premature rupture of membranes [PPROM] and preterm labor [PTL]—and indicated), cesarean section (30%–40%), lupus flare (20%–30%), nephritis (10%–20%); hematologic complications including thrombocytopenia (4%), anemia (13%), antepartum bleeding (2%), blood transfusion (3%) [3–5]. There is also increased risk (1%–2%) for infections, thrombosis, and maternal death when compared with non-SLE pregnant women [5]. Increased risk of diabetes is associated with treatment with steroids during pregnancy.

Fetal/Neonatal

Increased incidence of first-trimester spontaneous pregnancy loss (10%–20%), fetal death (1%–5%), FGR (5%–20%), CHB (see below), neonatal lupus (see below) [3–5]. Independent risk factors for pregnancy loss in SLE women are proteinuria (≥500 mg in 24 hours), APS, thrombocytopenia (≤150,000/mm³), and hypertension (≥140/90 mmHg) [6].

Table 25.1 ACR Diagnostic Criteria[a]

1. Malar rash
2. Discoid rash
3. Photosensitivity
4. Oral ulcers: painless
5. Arthritis: nonerosive, involving two or more peripheral joints
6. Serositis: pleuritis or pericarditis
7. Renal disorder: persistent proteinuria >0.5 g/day or cellular casts
8. Neurologic disorder: seizure or psychosis
9. Immunologic disorder: positive lupus erythematosus cell preparation or anti-double-stranded (ds) DNA or anti-Smith (SM) antibody or false positive serologic test for syphilis
10. Hematologic disorder: hemolytic anemia with reticulocytosis or leukopenia <4000/mm³ or lymphopenia <1500/mm³ or thrombocytopenia <100,000/mm³
11. Antinuclear antibodies (ANA) in abnormal titers

[a]For diagnosis, need ≥4/11 criteria either serially or simultaneously.

Table 25.2 SLICC Diagnostic Criteria[a]

Clinical Criteria	Immunological Criteria
Acute cutaneous lupus: malar lupus rash, bullous lupus, toxic epidermal necrolysis, maculopapular lupus rash, photosensitivity	ANA (above laboratory reference)
Subacute cutaneous lupus	
Chronic cutaneous lupus: classic, hypertrophic, panniculitis, mucosal, lupus erythematosus tumidus, chilblains, discoid/lichen planus	Anti-ds DNA (above laboratory reference or ELISA twice above laboratory reference)
Oral ulcers: not explained by other causes	Anti-Smith
Nonscarring alopecia: not explained by other causes	Antiphospholipid antibody: Lupus anticoagulant OR false positive RPR OR medium/high titer of IgG, IgM, or IgA anticardiolipin; IgG, IgM, or IgA b2 glycoprotein
Synovitis: swelling/effusion = or >2 joints OR tenderness = or >2 joints with = or > 30 min morning stiffness	Low complement: C3, C4, or CH50
Serositis: Pleurisy, pleural effusions, or pleural rub >1 day OR pericardial pain, pericardial effusions, pericardial rub, or pericarditis by EKG >1 day	Direct coombs without hemolytic anemia
Renal: >500 mg protein/24 hr by urine protein/creatinine or 24 hr urine protein OR RBC casts	
Neurologic: seizures, psychosis, mononeuritis multiple, myelitis, peripheral or cranial neuropathy, acute confusional state not explained by other causes	
Hemolytic anemia	
Leukopenia (<4000/mm³) OR lymphopenia (<1000/mm³) not explained by other causes	
Thrombocytopenia (<100,000/mm³) not explained by other causes	

Abbreviations: ANA, antinuclear antibodies; RBC, red blood cell.
[a]For diagnosis, need 4/17 criteria, with at least one of the clinical criteria and one of the immunological criteria OR lupus nephritis by renal biopsy in the presence of ANA or anti ds-DNA antibodies.

These adverse outcomes are primarily seen in SLE patients with active disease periconceptionally or in patients with hypertension, renal, cardiac, pulmonary, or neurologic disease or antiphospholipid antibodies. APS is associated with most fetal deaths in SLE. Renal disease is present in 50% of SLE patients. Lupus nephritis and APS are associated with higher incidence of PTL and hypertensive disorders. Above complications may also be seen more frequently in multiple pregnancies with SLE.

PREGNANCY CONSIDERATIONS
Effect of Pregnancy on SLE

Pregnancy usually does not affect long-term prognosis of SLE. Incidence of flares varies widely, depending on the definition of flare, patient selection, and clinical status at conception. About 50% of patients will have measurable lupus activity during pregnancy. The overall rate of lupus flare is about 26.5% [3]. Flares can occur in any trimester, but are most common in late pregnancy and postpartum. Most flares in pregnancy are mild to moderate, musculoskeletal, cutaneous, and hematologic. Prednisone ≥20 mg only is usually required for severe flares.

Effect of SLE on Pregnancy

Increased incidence of complications (see above). If renal SLE, 50% have hypertension, 10% to 30% worsening but usually reversible renal disease. If creatinine ≥1.3 mg/dL and/or creatinine clearance <50 mL/min and/or proteinuria >3 g in 24 hours preconceptionally, there is a small risk of irreversible renal deterioration. Patients with SLE who undergo kidney transplant have a pregnancy outcome similar to those patients that have kidney transplants for other indications [7] (see Chapters 13 and 17).

Overall rate of renal flare is about 16% [8]. Proteinuria (>500 mg–1 g/day) and GFR <60 mL/min increase the risk of renal flares [9]. Pregnancy can worsen renal function. Mild renal insufficiency (creatinine <1.4 mg/dL): successful pregnancy outcome, no irreversible effect renal function. Moderate-to-severe renal insufficiency (creatinine >1.4 mg/dL): increased risk of OB complications, 43% worsening renal function, 10% irreversible renal deterioration [10]. Renal biopsy might

be indicated in selected women. Pregnancy by itself does not contraindicate renal biopsy.

MANAGEMENT
Principles

More than 90% of women without end-organ disease or antiphospholipid antibodies (APAs) do well and take home babies. Goal: pregnancy with SLE in remission. **Start pregnancy with SLE in remission.** To achieve this, usually **need**

Table 25.3 Selected Laboratory Tests for SLE

Test	Prevalence in SLE Patients	Associations/Comments
ANA	95%	Not specific or pathognomonic
Anti-double-stranded (ds) DNA	70%	Clinical activity and flares; renal
Anti-Ro (SSA)	30%	Congenital heart block (CHB), neonatal lupus, Sjogren's syndrome
Anti-La (SSB)	15%	CHB, neonatal lupus, Sjogren's syndrome
Anticardiolipin antibodies (ACA)	50%	APS (see Chapter 26), thrombosis
Lupus anticoagulant (LA)	26%	FGR, fetal death, preeclampsia
Anti-SM	20%	Specific for SLE
Anti-RNP	40%	Neonatal lupus, mixed connective tissue (CT) disorder
Anticentromere		90% in CREST variant of scleroderma

Abbreviations: ANA, antinuclear antibodies; SLE, systemic lupus erythematosus.

to optimize medical therapy preconceptionally. Most drugs are safe (see below) and should be continued throughout pregnancy.

Workup

Baseline prenatal laboratory tests in a woman with known SLE should include the following (Table 25.4): **CBC with platelets, transaminases, creatinine, blood urea nitrogen (BUN), anti-Ro (SSA), anti-La (SSB), ACA, LA, anti-beta 2-glycoprotein-I, anti–ds DNA, C3, C4, CH 50, urine sediment, 24-hour urine for total protein and creatinine clearance or** spot urine protein-to-creatinine ratio.

Differential diagnosis to distinguish SLE flare from preeclampsia includes the following: C3, C4 (↓ in SLE), and anti–ds DNA (↑ in SLE), urine sediment (red and white cells and cellular casts seen in SLE). Gestational age (GA) at onset of symptoms is also helpful with preeclampsia usually only after 20 weeks.

Preconception Counseling

Preconception, antepartum, intrapartum, and postpartum care are summarized in Table 25.4. Evaluate by history, physical exam, and laboratory tests. Obtain records. Discuss current medications. To ensure pregnancy is conceived with SLE quiescent, encourage patient to wait at least six months without flares/active disease before attempting conception. Review diagnosis, risks and complications, and management with patient and family. Discuss contraception. **If stable with no recent flares on azathioprine and/or hydroxychloroquine, it is recommended to continue them in pregnancy and postpartum**. Keep steroids, if needed, at lowest possible efficacious dose. Substitute teratogenic medications (e.g., mycophenolate mofetil) with safe medications prior to conception. Consider multidisciplinary management with rheumatologist/nephrologist if lupus nephritis. Based on baseline renal function, counsel regarding risks of progression of renal disease and irreversible renal damage (see Chapter 17, Renal disease). **Women with creatinine >2.5 mg/dL should be counseled regarding trying not to get pregnant and the alternatives of renal transplant, surrogacy, and/or adoption.**

Prenatal Care

For women with positive antiphospholipid antibody, see Chapter 26. Treatment decisions are based on the past obstetric history and any history of prior thromboembolic events. Identify and manage risk factors for early pregnancy loss.

Table 25.4 Proposed Management of SLE

Preconception
- Start pregnancy in remission (at least >6 months)
- Evaluate end-organ damage/prior laboratory
- Assess concurrent comorbidities (HTN, APS)
- Optimize medications, counsel regarding side effects
- Discontinue teratogenic medications
- Counseling maternal and fetal complications
- Baseline laboratory evaluation: CBC with platelets, transaminases, creatinine, blood urea nitrogen, anti-Ro (SSA), anti-La (SSB), ACA, LA, anti-beta 2-glycoprotein-I, anti–ds DNA, C3, C4, CH 50, urine sediment, 24-hour urine for total protein and creatinine clearance or spot urine protein-to-creatinine ratio
- Screen for diabetes if risk factors (long-term steroids)

Antepartum
- Multidisciplinary management (OB, MFM, rheumatology, nephrology, etc.)
- Continue hydroxychloroquine
- Consider starting hydroxychloroquine if prior child with CHB
- Initiate aspirin prior to 16 weeks gestation
- Baseline laboratory evaluation (same as preconception)
- Screen for diabetes if risk factors (e.g., on steroids)
- First trimester ultrasound for dating
- Ultrasound at 18–20 weeks for fetal anatomic survey
- Fetal echocardiogram at 20–22 weeks
- Serial growth ultrasounds every 3–4 weeks
- Ultrasounds weekly at 16–26 weeks and every 2 weeks at 26–34 weeks for PR interval measurement in SSA/SSB positive
- Antenatal testing weekly starting at 32 weeks, earlier as clinically indicated
- Surveillance for preeclampsia, worsening kidney disease
- Evaluation by pediatric cardiology if CHB
- For APS, see Chapter 26

Intrapartum
- Delivery at 39 0/7–39 6/7 weeks if no earlier indications
- Stress dose of steroids, if indicated
- Vaginal delivery ideal, cesarean section for OB indications/unable to monitor CHB
- Delivery at Level 3 NICU, pediatric cardiology/pacemaker availability if CHB
- Notify pediatric of SLE, especially if maternal SSA/SSB antibodies

Postpartum
- Contraception counseling
- Breast-feeding counseling
- Long-term follow-up

Abbreviations: ACA, anticardiolipin antibody; APS, anti-phospholipid syndrome; CHB, congenital heart block; HTN, hypertension; LA, lupus anticoagulant; MFM, maternal fetal medicine; NICU, neonatal intensive care unit; OB, obstetrician; SLE, systemic lupus erythematous.

The use of medications to treat or suppress SLE flares will need to be evaluated on an individual basis. If patients have been maintained on medication(s) throughout the pregnancy, these should be continued through the postpartum period. Counsel women regarding avoiding excessive sun exposure or fatigue.

Therapy (Table 25.5)

NSAIDs (Nonsteroidal Anti-Inflammatory Drugs)
Safe up to 28 to 30 weeks. Side effects: fetal ductal closure and oligohydramnios, especially after 30 weeks. **Low-dose aspirin (50–150 mg daily) should ideally be initiated prior to 16 weeks for prevention of preeclampsia and FGR** [11].

Hydroxychloroquine Sulfate (Plaquenil)
Antimalarian drug: 400 to 600 mg orally daily, then ↓ 200 to 400 mg daily. **Safe in pregnancy** [12]. No increased risk of miscarriage, stillbirth, pregnancy loss, and congenital anomalies in exposed pregnancies when compared to nonexposed group [13]. If stopped, 2.5 times risk of flare compared to placebo [14]. This is currently **the safest and most effective therapy for SLE pregnant women who need therapy. Important not to stop drug periconception** [13,15]. In fact, **if stable with no recent flares on hydroxychloroquine, it is recommended to continue it in pregnancy and postpartum**. No long-term effects. Safe in breast-feeding. Evolving data suggest hydroxychloroquine during pregnancy (200 mg/d initiated prior to 10 weeks gestation) decreases the recurrence of congenital heart block. Insufficient data for recommendation; current ongoing trial [16–18]. See below CHB Prevention.

Azathioprine (Azasan, Imuran)
Daily 50 to 100 mg orally or divided bid. Increase after six to eight weeks. Safe in pregnancy. FGR association is probably due to SLE not azathioprine. It induces chromosomal breaks, which disappear as the infant grows.

Corticosteroids
Mechanism of action: ↓ antibody levels. Prednisone: 5 to 80 mg usual daily dose. Try to keep maintenance doses ≤20 mg/day. For treatment of flares, usually need ≥60 mg/day for three weeks. Safe in pregnancy (metabolized by placenta, does not cross it). Animal studies report facial clefts. Safe for breast-feeding. High doses: risk of diabetes (perform early glucola), PPROM, hypertension, and FGR. Taper if used more than seven days. Side effects: increased bone loss, especially together with heparin (give calcium). Fluorinated corticosteroids (dexamethasone and betamethasone) cross the placenta and should not be used to treat lupus activity.

In general, there is no need for stress steroids peripartum. The usual oral daily dose should be given peripartum. **Stress dose of steroids are indicated only if prednisone ≥20 mg daily or equivalent dose of a different steroid given for >3 weeks** [19–21]. This is to prevent Addisonian collapse, manifested as general malaise, nausea/vomiting, and skin changes, which is extremely rare. If used, stress dose of steroids can be given as hydrocortisone 100 mg IV when patient is in active labor or prior to induction of anesthesia if cesarean delivery, followed by hydrocortisone 50 mg IV q8h for 24 hours. Usual oral dose should be restarted postpartum. If unexplained refractory hypotension, consider secondary hypotension and treat as needed.

Immunoglobulin
Used as 0.5 g/kg initiated after positive pregnancy test until 33 weeks of gestation. It has been associated in a nonrandomized study with decrease in the rate of miscarriage in patients with history of recurrent pregnancy loss (25% pregnancy loss in nontreated group vs. 0% in treated group) with or without

Table 25.5 Medications

Type of Medication	Drug	Pregnancy Category	Recommendation
NSAIDS		B (first to second trimester) D (third trimester)	Safe up to 28–30 weeks Aspirin (50–150 mg) <16 weeks for prevention of preeclampsia, FGR, and PTB
Corticosteroids	Prednisone Fluorinated corticosteroids (dexamethasone and bethametasone	C	Continue in pregnancy if efficacious Keep ≤20 mg/d as possible Fluorinated corticosteroids: Not for treatment of lupus activity Consider if CHB
Immunosuppressive agents	Hydroxychloroquine	C	Low risk Increased risk of flares if stopped
Immunosuppressive agents	Azathioprine	D	Continue in pregnancy if efficacious
Immunosuppressive agents: Calcineurin inhibitors	Cyclosporine Tacrolimus	C C	Limited data in the literature. Use only if benefits outweigh the risks Likely safe based on limited data
Immunosuppressive agents: TNF inhibitors	Infliximab Etanercept Rituximab	B B C	Likely safe based on limited data; long-term effects unknown Avoid as possible
Immunosuppressive agents	Methotrexate	X	Contraindicated, teratogenic
Immunosuppressive agents	Cyclophosphamide	D	Avoid, not safe in pregnancy
Immunosuppressive agents	Mycophenolate mofetil	D	Avoid, not safe in pregnancy
Immunosuppressive agents	Leflunomide	X	Contraindicated, teratogenic
Immunoglobulin		C	Limited data in the literature; use only if benefits outweigh the risks

Abbreviations: CHB, congenital heart block; FGR, fetal growth restriction; PTB, preterm birth.

associated APS, decrease in doses of concomitant medications including prednisolone, decrease in lupus activity, and improvement in laboratory values (anti-ds DNA, anti-Ro, and anti-LA antibodies) [22]. Insufficient data for recommendation; further studies are needed.

Cyclosporine
Calcineurin inhibitor (CNI). Limited data in the literature. Use only if benefits outweigh the risks in patients not responding to other therapy. No increased risk of congenital anomalies. Association with low birth weight, maternal diabetes, hypertension, and kidney graft rejection likely related to disease and not cyclosporine [23–25].

Tacrolimus
Calcineurin inhibitor (CNI). Limited data in the literature suggest reasonable use in pregnancy. Used for acute flare or maintenance of lupus nephritis. Data is mostly accumulating from case series and retrospective observational studies in women undergoing pregnancy after solid organ transplantation. Reported anomalies in observational studies include meningocele, urogenital anomalies (MCDK, unilateral polycystic renal disease, hypospadias) tracheoesophageal fistula, heart defects, ear defects, and cleft palate, however, not enough data to attribute to the use of Tacrolimus. Transient neonatal elevation of the potassium and creatinine level has been frequently observed after in utero exposure to Tacrolimus. Association with preterm delivery and low birth weight [26–31].

Tumor Necrosis Factors Inhibitors (TNF Inhibitors)
Etanercept, Infliximab: Limited data in the literature. Used only if benefits outweigh the risks. Data derived from patients with rheumatoid arthritis and inflammatory bowel disease. Even earlier data suggested possible association with VACTERL (vertebral, anorectal, cardiac, tracheoesophageal fistula, renal, limb defects) anomaly [32]; this has not been replicated by follow-up analyses [33–35].

Less data available with **Rituximab**, so avoid as possible. Reported decreased white blood cell counts in newborns exposed in utero. Ongoing trial by the Organization of Teratology Information Specialists-OTIS Project [35].

Other Agents
Acethaminophen or paracetamol: safe throughout pregnancy. Usually not as effective as other therapies.

Cyclophosphamide, methotrexate, penicillamine, Leflunomide and mycophenolate mofetil: avoid; not safe in pregnancy.

Leflunomide (antimetabolite, blocks pyrimidine synthesis by inhibiting the dihydroorotate dehydrogenase). **Avoid** as no data available and long half-life of its metabolite, Teriflunomide, is of concern. Wait two years after discontinuation of therapy to attempt conception. Cholestyramine can be used to accelerate clearance. Ongoing trial by The Organization of Teratology Information Specialists-OTIS Project [35].

Plasmapheresis: last resort, consult rheumatology.

ANTEPARTUM TESTING
Accurate gestational age assessment is important; therefore, a **first-trimester ultrasound** examination is indicated. Perform **fetal anatomic survey** between 18 and 20 weeks and **fetal echocardiogram** around 20–22 weeks. For women with SSA/

SSB, perform **serial PR interval measurements weekly from 16 to 26 weeks and every other week from 26 to 34 weeks**; see section titled "Congenital Heart Block." **Fetal growth** can be evaluated throughout the pregnancy with q 4 weeks ultrasound examinations. Patients in whom disease activity is quiescent and there is no evidence of hypertension, renal disease, FGR, or preeclampsia can **begin weekly fetal testing at 32 weeks**. Patients with active disease, antiphospholipid antibodies, renal disease, hypertension, or FGR can begin antepartum testing earlier.

DELIVERY
Delivery is recommended at 39 0/7–39 6/7 weeks, if no earlier indications. Vaginal delivery is ideal, and cesarean section should be reserved for obstetrical indications. Cesarean section might also be needed when unable to monitor fetuses with congenital heart block. Stress-dose steroids are indicated only if prednisone ≥20 mg daily or equivalent dose of a different steroid is given for >3 weeks. See section titled "Corticosteroids."

POSTPARTUM/BREAST-FEEDING
Flares are more common. Continue and consider increasing SLE therapies. Breast-feeding is usually safe depending on medications.

NEONATAL LUPUS
Neonatal lupus occurs in 1%–2% of babies born to mothers with SLE. It is caused by passage of maternal IgG (anti Ro/SSA and anti La/SSB) antibodies through the placenta. It is limited to fetuses of mothers who are positive for anti SSA/anti SSB antibodies (regardless of maternal diagnosis of lupus or other autoimmune disease). The female:male ratio is 14:1. It is transient, lasting up to 14 to 16 weeks. Neonatal death rate is 1% to 2%. The manifestations include cutaneous (photosensitive annular erythematous rash), hematologic (anemia, thrombocytopenia, pancytopenia), hepatic (elevated liver enzymes, cholestasis, fulminant liver disease), and cardiac (congenital heart block, dilated cardiomyopathy, endocardial fibroelastosis) abnormalities. Usually transient except cardiac manifestations.

CARDIAC NEONATAL LUPUS/CONGENITAL HEART BLOCK
Etiology
SSA/SSB antibodies bind to surface cardiomyocytes triggering inflammation, remodeling and fibrosis. Maternal SSA/SSB antibodies are necessary to cause CHB, but evidence suggests that there are other factors involved in the development of CHB. Cross reactivity of L-type calcium channels with SSA/SB antibodies has also been proposed as a mechanism altering calcium homeostasis [36].

Counseling
The risk of a fetus developing CHB and cardiac neonatal lupus (cardiac-NL) is about 2% in mothers with positive SSA/SSB and no prior affected pregnancy. It increases to 10%–15% if the mother has a prior child with cutaneous lupus and 19% if prior child with cardiac—NL. CHB is **most likely to occur between 18 and 24 weeks gestation**. It may be associated with

congestive heart failure (hydrops). CHB is usually permanent with a pacemaker needed in 60%–70% of surviving affected children. Cardiac-NL is associated with 18% neonatal mortality with 6% of these being in utero demises. The 10-year survival rate if born alive is 86%. Poor prognostic factors include diagnosis at <20 weeks gestation, hydrops, ventricular rate <50 bpm, left ventricular failure. Cardiac transplant is rare (1%) [37–39].

Management

Prenatal Care Evaluation

Evaluate for structural cardiac anomalies with **fetal echocardiogram**. CHB can be seen in CHD, but structural defects can also be seen in cardiac NL without CHB. Structural anomalies include persistent patent ductus arteriosus, ASD, VSD, and pulmonic and tricuspid valve abnormalities [40]. Of CHB cases, 10% to 20% have CHD and not SSA/SSB, but **95% of CHB without CHD have SSA/SSB**. For fetuses with hydrops, see also Chapter 54. If positive for SSA/SSB, consider following with **weekly fetal pulse Doppler echocardiography or fetal kinetocardiogram/tissue Doppler echocardiography (FKCG) from 16 to 26 weeks and every other week from 26 to 34 weeks to look for prolonged PR (AV) interval and any dysrrhythmia, especially looking for incomplete (first or second) degree block**. This screening may not be cost-effective given CHB is uncommon in prospective series even with positive SSA/SSB and is not evidence based [41]. The fetal mechanical PR interval is measured from simultaneous mitral and aortic Doppler waveforms. Fixed cutoff of PR interval measurement >150 ms have been used to diagnose first-degree heart block. For example, the PRIDE study [42,43] used a fixed cut of 150 ms. However, nomograms have been proposed adjusting by gestational age and fetal heart rate with normal PR interval ranging from 138 to 155 ms [44]. FKCG, a tissue velocity-based measurement of AV conduction, appears to be superior to the pulse Doppler echocardiography [45]. Data from prospective series revealed that the FKCG can detect first-degree AV block in ~8.5% of these high-risk fetuses and that Doppler can detect PR prolongation in only ~3% of these fetuses and did not precede the occurrence of third-degree block [42,46]. Even as it remains unclear if cardiac injury is progressive and could be prevented if diagnosed and treated early, prolongation of the PR interval >150 ms, moderate or severe tricuspide regurgitation, and/or atrial echodensity appear to be potential early biomarkers of reversible cardiac injury.

Prevention

A nonrandomized study suggests **hydroxychloroquine >200 mg/d initiated prior to 10 weeks** and continued through pregnancy decreases CHB recurrence in women with prior affected offspring (decreased risk by 64% in SSA/SSB positive mothers) [16]. Further research is needed for definitive conclusions. There is an ongoing prospective study [18]. Data is insufficient to recommend the use of hydroxychlroquine to decrease the risk of CHB in women with SSA/SSB antibodies without affected offspring. A cohort study showed decreased risk by 28% but statistical significance was no longer seen after multivariable analyses [17]. Maternal treatment with fluorinated steroids does not appear to impact fetal and neonatal mortality [39]. Data from an observational study suggested an increased mortality rate; however, this could have been influenced by severity of maternal disease itself [38]. IVIG is also ineffective for recurrence prevention [47,48].

Therapy

Treatment with fluorinated steroids (Betamethasone, Dexamethasone) upon detection has been reported as possibly associated with normalization of AV conduction. Studies (nonrandomized) suggest **dexamethasone 4 mg/day is likely beneficial in treating fetuses with first- and second-degree AV block and not beneficial and possibly harmful for third-degree block**. Risks–benefits of prolonged steroid treatment should be discussed with the patient. Once complete (third degree) CHB occurs, this is considered to be irreversible. No randomized trials have demonstrated the effectiveness of steroid, beta-mimetic, digoxin, IVIG, and other therapies to normalize conduction or improve outcome [38,39,42,43,46,49–53]. There is a potential benefit of IVIG (1 gram/kg, one to three doses) to improve survival rates and decrease the need of cardiac transplant in fetuses/neonates with cardiomyopathy and/or endocardial fibroelastosis [54]; however, further studies are needed before it can be recommended. Refer to Pediatric Cardiology if evidence of cardiac-NL.

Delivery

Women with fetuses with CHB should be managed and delivered at a tertiary care center with the availability of immediate neonatal pacing. Although trial of labor (TOL) by repeated scalp sampling to assure fetal well-being can be attempted, TOL is often difficult to manage clinically.

CONTRACEPTION

Combination oral contraceptives are safe for women with mild lupus who do not have antiphospholipid antibodies. Progestin only or copper IUDs are safe options for women with SLE with vascular disease, nephritis, or antiphospholipid antibodies [55–57].

REFERENCES

1. Tan EM, Cohan AS, Aries JF et al. The 1982 revised criteria for the classification of systemic lupus erythematosus. *Arthritis Rheum* 1982; 25: 1271. [III]
2. Petri M, Orbai AM, Alarcón GS et al. Derivation and validation of the Systemic Lupus International Collaborating Clinics classification criteria for systemic lupus erythematosus. *Arthritis Rheum* 2012; 64(8): 2677. [II-2]
3. Smyth A, Oliveira GH, Lahr BD et al. A systematic review and meta-analysis of pregnancy outcomes in patients with systemic lupus erythematosus and lupus nephritis. *Clin J Am Soc Nephrol* 2010; 5(11): 2060–8. [II-2]
4. Chakravarty EF, Nelson L, Krishnan E. Obstetric hospitalizations in the United States for women with systemic lupus erythematosus and rheumatoid arthritis. *Arthritis Rheum* 2006; 54(3): 899–907. [II-2]
5. Clowse ME, Jamison M, Myers E et al. A national study of the complications of lupus in pregnancy. *Am J Obstet Gynecol* 2008; 199(2): 127.e1–6. [II-2]
6. Clowse ME, Magder LS, Witter F et al. Early risk factors for pregnancy loss in lupus. *Obstet Gynecol* 2006; 107(2 Pt. 1): 293–9. [II-2]
7. McGrory CH, McCloskey LJ, DeHoratius RJ et al. Pregnancy outcomes in female renal recipients: A comparison of systemic lupus erythematosus with other diagnoses. *Am J Transplant* 2003; 3(1): 35–42. [II-2]

8. Huong DL, Wechsler B, Vauthier-Brouzes D et al. Pregnancy in past or present lupus nephritis: A study of 32 pregnancies from a single centre. *Ann Rheum Dis* 2001; 60(6): 599–604. [II-2]

9. Imbasciati E, Tincani A, Gregorini G et al. Pregnancy in women with pre-existing lupus nephritis: Predictors of fetal and maternal outcome. *Nephrol Dial Transplant* 2009; 24(2): 519–25. [II-2]

10. Jones DC, Hayslett JP. Outcome of pregnancy in women with moderate or severe renal insufficiency. *N Engl J Med* 1996; 335(4): 226–32. Correction published in *N Engl J Med* 1997; 336: 7. [II-2]

11. Bujold E, Roberge S, Lacasse Y et al. Prevention of preeclampsia and intrauterine growth restriction with aspirin started in early pregnancy: A meta-analysis. *Obstet Gynecol* 2010; 116(2 Pt. 1): 402–14. [I]

12. Costedoat-Chalumeau N, Amoura Z, Duhaut P et al. Safety of hydroxychloroquine in pregnant patients with connective tissue diseases: A study of one-hundred thirty-three cases compared to a control group. *Arthritis Rheum* 2003; 48: 3207–11. [II-1]

13. Clowse ME, Magder L, Witter F et al. Hydroxychloroquine in lupus pregnancy. *Arthritis Rheum* 2006; 54(11): 3640–7. [II-2]

14. The Canadian Hydroxychloroquine Study Group. A randomized study of the effect of withdrawing hydroxychloroquine sulfate in systemic lupus erythematosus. *N Engl J Med* 1991; 324: 150–4. [RCT]

15. Levy RA, Vilela VS, Cataldo MJ et al. Hydroxychloroquine in lupus pregnancy: Double-blind and placebo-controlled study. *Lupus* 2001; 10: 401–4. [RCT, *n* = 20]

16. Izmirly PM, Costedoat-Chalumeau N, Pisoni CN et al. Maternal use of hydroxychloroquine is associated with a reduced risk of recurrent anti-SSA/Ro-antibody-associated cardiac manifestations of neonatal lupus. *Circulation* 2012; 126(1): 76–82. [II-2]

17. Izmirly PM, Kim MY, Llanos C et al. Evaluation of the risk of anti-SSA/Ro-SSB/La antibody-associated cardiac manifestations of neonatal lupus in fetuses of mothers with systemic lupus erythematosus exposed to hydroxychloroquine. *Ann Rheum Dis* 2010; 69(10): 1827–30. [II-2]

18. Preventive Approach to Congenital Heart Block With Hydroxychloroquine (PATCH). http://www.clinicaltrials.org. [Review]

19. Marik PE, Varon J. Requirement of perioperative stress doses of corticosteroids: A systematic review of the literature. *Arch Surg* 2008; 143(12): 1222–6. [II-2]

20. The American College of Obstetricians and Gynecologists. Steroid use in pregnancy. *PROLOG Obstetrics, 6th ed.*, 46–47. [III]

21. Kelly KN, Domajnko B. Perioperative stress-dose steroids. *Clin Colon Rectal Surg* 2013; 26(3): 163–7. [Review; III]

22. Perricone R, De Carolis C, Kröegler B et al. Intravenous immunoglobulin therapy in pregnant patients affected with systemic lupus erythematosus and recurrent spontaneous abortion. *Rheumatology (Oxford)* 2008; 47(5): 646–51. [II-2]

23. Bar Oz B, Hackman R, Einarson T et al. Pregnancy outcome after cyclosporine therapy during pregnancy: A meta-analysis. *Transplantation* 2001; 71(8): 1051. [II-2]

24. Paziana K, Del Monaco M, Cardonick E et al. Cyclosporine use during pregnancy. *Drug Saf* 2013; 36(5): 279–94. [Review; III]

25. Armenti VT, Ahlswede KM, Ahlswede BA et al. National Transplantation Pregnancy Registry—Outcomes of 154 pregnancies in cyclosporine-treated female kidney transplant recipients. *Transplantation* 1994; 57(4): 502. [II-2]

26. Kainz A, Harabacz I, Cowlrick IS et al. Review of the course and outcome of 100 pregnancies in 84 women treated with tacrolimus. *Transplantation* 2000; 70(12): 1718–21. [II-3]

27. Kainz A, Harabacz I, Cowlrick IS et al. Analysis of 100 pregnancy outcomes in women treated systemically with tacrolimus. *Transpl Int* 2000; 13(Suppl. 1): S299–300. [II-3]

28. Jain A, Venkataramanan R, Fung JJ et al. Pregnancy after liver transplantation under tacrolimus. *Transplantation* 1997; 64(4): 559–65. [II-2]

29. Jain AB, Reyes J, Marcos A et al. Pregnancy after liver transplantation with tacrolimus immunosuppression: A single center's experience update at 13 years. *Transplantation* 2003; 76(5): 827–32. [II-2]

30. Webster P, Wardle A, Bramham K et al. Tacrolimus is an effective treatment for lupus nephritis in pregnancy. *Lupus* 2014; 23(11): 1192–6. [II-3]

31. Westbrook RH, Yeoman AD, Agarwal K et al. Outcomes of pregnancy following liver transplantation: The King's College Hospital experience. *Liver Transpl* 2015; 21(9): 1153–9. [II-2]

32. Carter JD, Ladhani A, Ricca LR et al. A safety assessment of tumor necrosis factor antagonists during pregnancy: A review of the Food and Drug Administration database. *J Rheumatol* 2009; 36(3): 635. [Review; III]

33. Crijns HJ, Jentink J, Garne E et al. EUROCAT Working Group. The distribution of congenital anomalies within the VACTERL association among tumor necrosis factor antagonist-exposed pregnancies is similar to the general population. *J Rheumatol* 2011; 38(9): 1871. [II-2]

34. Chambers C, Koren G, Tutuncu ZN et al. Are new agents used to treat rheumatoid arthritis safe to take during pregnancy? Organization of Teratology Information Specialists (OTIS) study. *Can Fam Physician* 2007; 53(3): 409–12. [Review; III]

35. Organization of Teratology Information Services (OTIS) Autoimmune Diseases in Pregnancy Project. http://www.clinicaltrials.org. [Online software; mostly II-3]

36. Izmirly PM, Buyon JP, Saxena A. Neonatal lupus: Advances in understanding pathogenesis and identifying treatments of cardiac disease. *Curr Opin Rheumatol* 2012; 24(5): 466–72. [Review; III]

37. Izmirly PM, Llanos C, Lee LA et al. Cutaneous manifestations of neonatal lupus and risk of subsequent congenital heart block. *Arthritis Rheum* 2010; 62(4): 1153. [II-2]

38. Izmirly PM, Saxena A, Kim MY et al. Maternal and fetal factors associated with mortality and morbidity in a multi-racial/ethnic registry of anti-SSA/Ro associated cardiac neonatal lupus. *Circulation* 2011; 124(18): 1927–35. [II-2]

39. Eliasson H, Sonesson SE, Sharland G et al. Fetal Working Group of the European Association of Pediatric Cardiology. Isolated atrioventricular block in the fetus: A retrospective, multinational, multicenter study of 175 patients. *Circulation* 2011; 124: 1919–26. [II-2]

40. Buyon JP, Hiebert R, Copel J et al. Autoimmune-associated congenital heart block: Demographics, mortality, morbidity and recurrence rates obtained from a national neonatal lupus registry. *J Am Coll Cardiol* 1998; 31: 1658. [II-2]

41. Van Bergen AH, Cuneo BF, Davis N. Prospective echocardiographic evaluation of atrioventricular conduction in fetuses with maternal Sjogren's antibodies. *Am J Obstet Gynecol* 2004; 191: 1014–8. [II-3]

42. Friedman DM, Kim MY, Copel JA et al. PRIDE Investigators Utility of cardiac monitoring in fetuses at risk for congenital heart block: The PR Interval and Dexamethasone Evaluation (PRIDE) prospective study. *Circulation* 2008; 117(4): 485–93. [II-1]

43. Friedman DM, Kim MY, Copel JA et al. Prospective evaluation of fetuses with autoimmune-associated congenital heart block followed in the PR Interval and Dexamethasone Evaluation (PRIDE) Study. *Am J Cardiol* 2009; 103(8): 1102–6. [II-1]

44. Wojakowski A, Izbizky G, Carcano ME et al. Fetal Doppler mechanical PR interval: Correlation with fetal heart rate, gestational age and fetal sex. *Ultrasound Obstet Gynecol* 2009; 34(5): 538–42. [II-2]

45. Nii M, Hamilton RM, Fenwick L et al. Assessment of fetal atrioventricular time intervals by tissue Doppler and pulse Doppler echocardiography: Normal values and correlation with fetal electrocardiography. *Heart* 2006; 92(12): 1831–7. [II-2]

46. Rein AJ, Mevorach D, Perles Z et al. Early diagnosis and treatment of atrioventricular block in the fetus exposed to maternal anti-SSA/Ro-SSB/La antibodies: A prospective, observational, fetal kinetocardiogram-based study. *Circulation* 2009; 119(14): 1867–72. [II-1]

47. Friedman DM, Llanos C, Izmirly PM et al. Evaluation of fetuses in a study of intravenous immunoglobulin as preventive therapy for congenital heart block: Results of a multicenter,

prospective, open-label clinical trial. (PITCH Study-Preventive IVIG Therapy for Congenital Heart Block). *Arthritis Rheum* 2010; 62(4): 1138–46. [II-1]

48. Pisoni CN, Brucato A, Ruffatti A et al. Failure of intravenous immunoglobulin to prevent congenital heart block: Findings of a multicenter, prospective, observational study. *Arthritis Rheum* 2010; 62(4): 1147–52. [II-2]

49. Saleeb S, Copel J, Friedman D et al. Comparison of treatment with fluorinated glucocorticoids to the natural history of auto-antibody-associated congenital heart block. *Arthritis Rheum* 1999; 42: 2335–45. [II-3]

50. Jaeggi ET, Fouron JC, Silverman ED et al. Transplacental fetal treatment improves the outcome of prenatally diagnosed complete atrioventricular block without structural heart disease. *Circulation* 2004; 110(12): 1542–8. [II-2]

51. Shinohara K, Miyagawa S, Fujita T et al. Neonatal lupus erythematosus: Results of maternal corticosteroid therapy. *Obstet Gynecol* 1999; 93: 952–7. [II-3]

52. Novi JM, Mulvihill BHK. Use of subcutaneous B-sympathomimetic pump for the treatment of fetal congenital complete heart block. *J Repro Med* 2003; 48: 893–5. [II-3]

53. Eronen M, Heikkila P, Teramo K. Congenital complete heart block in the fetus: Hemodynamic features, antenatal treatment, and outcome in six cases. *Pediatr Cardiol* 2001; 5: 385–92. [II-3]

54. Trucco SM, Jaeggi E, Cuneo B et al. Use of intravenous gamma globulin and corticosteroids in the treatment of maternal autoantibody-mediated cardiomyopathy. *J Am Coll Cardiol* 2011; 57: 715–23. [II-2]

55. Petri M, Kim MY, Kalunian KC et al. OC-SELENA Trial. Combined oral contraceptives in women with systemic lupus erythematosus. *N Engl J Med* 2005; 353(24): 2550–8. [RCT; I, *n* = 183]

56. Sánchez-Guerrero J, Uribe AG, Jiménez-Santana L, Mestanza-Peralta M et al. A trial of contraceptive methods in women with systemic lupus erythematosus. *N Engl J Med* 2005; 353(24): 2539–49. [RCT; I, *n* = 162]

57. ACOG Practice Bulletin Number 73. *Use of Hormonal Contraception in Women With Coexisting Medical Conditions.* [III]

26

Antiphospholipid syndrome

Tracy A. Manuck

KEY POINTS

- The **diagnosis** of antiphospholipid syndrome (APS) requires the presence of at least **one clinical and one laboratory** criteria (Tables 26.1 and 26.2).
- **APS is associated with venous thromboembolism (VTE), early onset preeclampsia, early pregnancy loss, fetal growth restriction (FGR), fetal death, preterm birth, and other complications.**
- Therapy should be as follows:
    - For APS with **≥3 unexplained consecutive pregnancy losses at <10 weeks or ≥1 fetal loss >10 weeks: low-dose ASA** and **prophylactic heparin** (either unfractionated or low molecular weight).
    - For APS with **VTE during the current pregnancy: therapeutic anticoagulation with heparin.**
    - For APS with **VTE prior to pregnancy: prophylactic anticoagulation with heparin.**
    - There are no trials to assess therapy for APS with a history of preeclampsia and/or FGR prior to 34 weeks gestation.
- If on low-molecular-weight heparin, regional anesthesia may need to be delayed until ≥24 hours after the last dose.

HISTORIC NOTES

Lupus anticoagulant (LA) was first described in the early 1950s as prolonging certain clotting assays. A few years later, LA was found to be associated with the false positive test for syphilis and, paradoxically, thrombosis.

DIAGNOSIS

The diagnosis of APS requires the presence of **at least one clinical** (Table 26.1) **and one laboratory** (Table 26.2) criteria [1,2]. Abnormal laboratory tests must occur on **more than two occasions, ≥12 weeks apart.** The two tests must occur within a five-year time frame. There are no time limits on the interval between the clinical and laboratory events. Once the diagnosis is established by the criteria above, subsequent negative results decrease but do not eliminate the risks of complications.

ANTIPHOSPHOLIPID ANTIBODY TESTING

Antiphospholipid antibodies (APAs) are directed against phospholipids and include anticardiolipin antibodies (ACAs), LA, and anti-beta-2 glycoprotein-I (B2GP-I) (Table 26.2). LA is a double misnomer. LA is seen in many patients without systemic lupus erythematosus (SLE) and is associated with thrombosis not anticoagulation (see Chapter 25). ACAs strongly correlate with LA and thrombosis. ACAs require the presence of plasma phospholipid-binding protein

B2 glycoprotein I to bind to cardiolipin. In contrast, ACAs from patients with syphilis or other infections are B2 glycoprotein I independent. Approximately 80% of patients with LA have ACAs, and 20% of patients with ACAs are found positive for LA [2]. Substantial **interlaboratory variation** when testing the same sera remains a **serious problem**.

SYMPTOMS

Clinical manifestations of APS may include any organ system, including vascular (arterial or venous), cardiac, cutaneous, endocrine/reproductive, gastrointestinal, hematologic, neurologic, obstetrical, ophthalmologic, pulmonary, renal, and others.

EPIDEMIOLOGY/INCIDENCE

Up to 11% of healthy controls with uncomplicated pregnancies have APAs with a median prevalence of about 2%. APAs have a very poor positive predictive value for adverse obstetric outcomes and a causal relationship between APAs and a single clinical event can be difficult to prove, given that many of the studied adverse obstetric outcomes are very common. Of SLE patients, 25% to 35% have APS (see Chapter 25). ACAs are present in 15% of women with recurrent miscarriage; LA is found in 8% of patients with recurrent miscarriage. In women with midtrimester fetal loss, LA is seen in up to 30%. Of definite APS patients, 70% have both ACAs and LA.

ETIOLOGY/BASIC PATHOPHYSIOLOGY

APAs may cause pregnancy loss by thrombosis of placental vessels, interference with coagulation factors (reduce levels of annexin V), inhibition of proliferation of trophoblasts, complement activation, or other yet unknown mechanisms. However, given that asymptomatic healthy women with APAs who do not meet criteria for APS have little to no increased risk, the mere presence of APAs is insufficient to cause these adverse pregnancy outcomes [3].

CLASSIFICATION

Primary APS refers to patients with APS but no other autoimmune disorders. *Secondary* APS refers to patients with other autoimmune disorders (e.g., SLE) [2].

COMPLICATIONS
Maternal

- **Venous and arterial thromboembolism:** Risk is 5% to 12% in pregnancy; there are no adequate cohort or case-control studies to validate these estimates of VTE with APS pregnant women [4], and 0.5% to 2% of

Table 26.1 Clinical Criteria for Diagnosis of Antiphospholipid Syndrome

1. *Vascular thrombosis*
   One or more clinical episodes of arterial, venous, or small vessel thrombosis, in any tissue or organ. Thrombosis must be confirmed by objective criteria (e.g., imaging or Doppler studies or histopathology)
   And/or

2. *Pregnancy morbidity*
   (A) **One or more unexplained deaths** of a morphologically normal fetus **at or beyond the 10th week** of gestation with normal fetal morphology documented by ultrasound or by direct examination of the fetus
   And/or
   (B) **One or more premature births** of a morphologically normal neonate **before the 34th week** of gestation **because of eclampsia or severe preeclampsia or features consistent with placental insufficiency** (e.g., abnormal Doppler flow, abnormal fetal testing, SGA <10%, oligohydramnios)
   And/or
   (C) **Three or more unexplained consecutive spontaneous abortions before the 10th week** of pregnancy with maternal anatomic or hormonal abnormalities and paternal and maternal chromosomal causes excluded

Sources: Modified from Miyakis S, Lockshin MD, Atsumi T et al. *J Thromb Haemost*, 4, 295–306, 2006; American College of Obstetricians and Gynecologists. Antiphospholipid syndrome. ACOG Practice Bulletin No. 132. *Obstet Gynecol*, 120, 6, 1514–21, 2012.
Abbreviations: AFI, amniotic fluid index; SGA, small for gestational age.

Table 26.2 Laboratory Criteria for the Diagnosis of Antiphospholipid Syndrome

1. **Lupus anticoagulant** present in plasma on two or more occasions **at least 12 weeks apart**. Examples are lupus anticoagulant, DRVVT, or aPTT test. Testing is ideally performed before the patient is treated with anticoagulants
   And/or

2. **Anticardiolipin antibody** of IgG and/or IgM isotype in serum or plasma, present as **>40 GPL or MPL** or >99th percentile on two or more occasions **at least 12 weeks apart**
   And/or

3. **Anti-B2 glycoprotein-I** of IgG and/or IgM isotype in serum or plasma (in titer **>99th percentile** for a normal population as defined by the laboratory performing the test), present on two or more occasions **at least 12 weeks apart**

Sources: Modified from Miyakis S, Lockshin MD, Atsumi T et al. *J Thromb Haemost*, 4, 295–306, 2006; American College of Obstetricians and Gynecologists. Antiphospholipid syndrome. ACOG Practice Bulletin No. 132. *Obstet Gynecol*, 120, 6, 1514–21, 2012.
Abbreviations: aPTT, activated partial thromboplastin time; DRVVT, dilute Russell's viper venom time.

asymptomatic nonpregnant people incidentally found to have APAs have thromboses each year. Most thrombotic events are venous (65%–70%). Arterial thromboses can occur in atypical sites, such as the retina, the subclavian artery, or the middle cerebral artery (the most common vessel involved when a stroke occurs in these patients).

- **Preeclampsia:** Incidence of preeclampsia is increased and ranges from 18% to 48% among women with APS. There is a statistically significant association especially between preeclampsia and ACA [4].

- **Autoimmune thrombocytopenia:** Risk is 40% to 50%. Thormbocytopenia secondary to APAs is difficult to distinguish from ITP and is treated in a similar fashion. Heparin-induced thrombocytopenia [less with low-molecular-weight heparin (LMWH)] can also occur as well as lupus flare in patients with coexisting SLE.

- **Other medical complications:** APS is also associated with autoimmune hemolytic anemia, livedo reticularis, cutaneous ulcers, chorea gravidarum, multi-infarct dementia, and transverse myelitis. These complications, although associated with APS, are insufficient for clinical diagnosis of APS.

- Rarely, catastrophic APS, resulting in progressive thromboses, multiorgan failure, and death may occur.

Fetal

- **Pregnancy loss and fetal death:** These complications can occur in any trimester and be recurrent. About 5% to 20% of women with recurrent pregnancy losses have APAs [2]. Although all APAs are associated with pregnancy loss and fetal death, early pregnancy loss has been associated in a review with both ACA and LA; recurrent first trimester with ACA; second trimester with LA; third trimester with ACA [4]. ACA IgM, ACA IgG, and anti-beta2-microglobulin-I are present in about 6%, 5%, and 2% of stillbirths, respectively, compared to 3%, 1%, and 0.6% of live births, respectively (three- to fivefold increased risk for stillbirth) [5].

- **FGR** (in particular with ACA) [4].

- **Preterm birth** (33%, secondary to gestational hypertension or placental insufficiency, either spontaneous or iatrogenic).

- **Placental abruption** (not associated with ACA or LA in a review) [4].

PREGNANCY CONSIDERATIONS

The likelihood of complications is lower if pregnancy starts when APS is "quiescent" without symptoms and with undetectable or lower levels of APAs. Complications are more frequent and severe if APS is active with high levels of APAs. As with other autoimmune disorders, APS can exacerbate postpartum: fever, pulmonary infiltrates, pleural effusion, occasionally renal, pulmonary complications, VTE; rarely DIC and mortality.

MANAGEMENT
Principles

Multidisciplinary management with rheumatologist or internal medicine specialist is recommended.

Who to Screen

Women with clinical criteria for APS (Table 26.1) should be screened for ACA, LA, and B2GP-I.

Other conditions associated with APS include autoimmune thrombocytopenia, amaurosis fugax, livdeo reticularis, systemic lupus erythematosus, and a false positive rapid plasma regain result (RPR). These conditions are not considered clinical criteria for APS; therefore, testing individuals for the presence of APA with these isolated conditions is not recommended. Testing women without clinical features of APS may lead to management dilemmas; this problem can be avoided by testing only individuals who meet clinical criteria for APS [2].

How to Screen

Laboratory tests include **ACA (IgG and IgM), LA, and B2GP-I (IgG and IgM) tests (Table 26.2)**. Initial positive results should be confirmed after a minimum of 12 weeks. Testing for APAs other than LA, ACA, and B2GP-I is not clinically useful in the diagnosis of APS and should not be performed.

Prevention

There is no preventive strategy available.

Therapy

Evidence

- Aspirin alone: Compared to placebo or usual care, low-dose aspirin *alone* is not associated with any difference in outcome in pregnant women with APS [6–8]. The summary relative risk for recurrent pregnancy loss is 1.05, 95% CI 0.66, 1.68 [9].
- **Combination of unfractionated heparin (UFH) and low-dose aspirin** in APS patients **with recurrent first-trimester losses** is associated with significant **reduction in early pregnancy loss** (OR 0.26, 95% CI 0.14–0.48; number needed to treat 4) [9–12] compared to low-dose aspirin alone. **Low molecular weight heparin** (LMWH) did not show a benefit when combined with aspirin (OR 0.70, 95% CI 0.34–1.45) [13,14]. This could be attributed to the lower efficacy of LMWH or to several other parameters, such as the paucity of studies on LMWH and small study samples, low cutoff threshold for APAs positivity, coexistence of other thrombophilic disorders within the same study, late entry into the studies that may preclude many early losses, nonacceptance of randomization, and the crossover from assigned treatments [13,14]. These five studies have been reviewed and published as a systematic review [15].
- Two small RCTs have directly compared LMWH to UFH, and despite the small number of patients recruited, **effectiveness of LMWH appears comparable with that of UFH** [16,17]. One additional small open-label RCT randomized women with APS and recurrent abortion to receive LMWH plus low dose aspirin or UFH plus low dose aspirin and found similar live rates (80% vs. 66.7%, *p* = 0.243) [18].
- A meta-analysis of five studies demonstrated **improved overall live-birth rates among women treated with UFH and low-dose aspirin** (74.3%) compared to low-dose aspirin alone (55.8%; RR 1.30, 95% CI 1.04–1.63, NNT 5.6) [19].
- The addition of glucocorticoids does not improve outcomes and is associated with an increased risk of preterm birth. Compared to low-dose aspirin alone or placebo, prednisone and low-dose aspirin are not associated with a significant difference in pregnancy loss (RR 0.85, 95% CI 0.53, 1.36) [20,21]. However, there were significant higher rates of preterm birth in the prednisone

groups in both trials and higher NICU admissions in one study [21]. There were also lower birth weights in the prednisone group in one of the studies [20]. In another study, when compared to heparin and low-dose aspirin, prednisone and low-dose aspirin were associated with no difference in pregnancy loss rates, but again the prednisone group had a significantly higher rate of preterm birth [22].

- Severe and/or resistant APS and alternative therapy:
  - IVIG: In women already on heparin and aspirin, the addition of IVIG does not affect pregnancy loss rates in a very small trial, but is associated with a significantly higher preterm birth rate [23]. This therapy is very expensive, and is the only treatment shown to lower anticardiolipin levels.
  - Hydroxychloroquine: theoretical benefits, as it reverses platelet activation induced by APA, but no human data are available.
  - Plasma exchange: limited case reports and a small case series have investigated the role of therapeutic plasma exchange in improving pregnancy outcomes among women who have failed first-line therapy. The largest report included 18 women who received prednisone (10 mg/day) and plasma exchange (3x/week) and reported a 100% live birth rate, but the majority had at least one major complication such as PTB (22%), oligohydramnios (16%), fetal growth restriction (11%), and/or preeclampsia (5%) [24]. Additional studies are needed before this strategy can be routinely recommended.

Actual Therapy (Table 26.3)

- **APS with early (usually <10 weeks) recurrent pregnancy loss: low-dose aspirin (ASA)** and **prophylactic heparin (either** UFH or LMWH although most data in UFH) [9,25,26].

  Therapy is usually begun once fetal viability is established, but **there is insufficient evidence regarding best time of initiation of therapy**. Low-dose aspirin dose is usually about 75 to 100 mg daily (and some experts recommend starting it even preconception in severe cases) [25]. Dose for prophylactic UFH is usually 5000 to 7500 U first trimester, 7500 to 10,000 U second trimester, 10,000 U third trimester SQ q12h. Dose for prophylactic LMWH is usually enoxaparin (Lovenox) 30 to 40 mg SQ q12h or dalteparin (Fragmin) 5000 U SQ q12h. One may adjust prophylaxis in high-risk cases to a heparin (anti-Xa) level range of 0.2 to 0.4. Anti-Xa level is usually drawn four hours after injection. Anti-Xa levels have not been adequately evaluated prospectively to show a reduction in the incidence of complications.

- **APS with VTE during the current pregnancy: therapeutic anticoagulation** [25,26].

  Therapeutic intravenous UFH doses need to be adjusted to keep activated partial thromboplastin time (aPTT) two to three times normal. Therapeutic LMWH is usually enoxaparin 1 mg/kg q12h SQ or dalteparin 200 U/kg q12h SQ. Therapeutic LMWH must be adjusted to heparin (anti-Xa) level 0.5 to 1.2. After initial therapy, subcutaneous therapeutic LMWH or UFH should be continued for a minimum total duration of

Table 26.3 Suggested Prophylaxis for APS during Pregnancy and Postpartum Based on Selected Clinical Scenarios

	Antepartum	Postpartum
APS characterized by laboratory criteria and fetal loss (≥3 recurrent consecutive first trimester miscarriages or ≥1 unexplained fetal loss >10 weeks) but no history of arterial or venous thrombosis	Low-dose aspirin with either: • UFH 5000–7500 U first trimester; 7500–10,000 U second trimester; 10,000 U third trimester SQ q12h or • LMWH, e.g., enoxaparin (Lovenox) 30–40 mg SQ q12h or dalteparin (Fragmin) 5000 U SQ q12h	LMWH and low-dose aspirin
APS characterized by laboratory criteria and obstetric morbidity of ≥1 preterm deliveries of a morphologically normal infant <34 weeks due to placental insufficiency (IUGR or severe preeclampsia) but no history of arterial or venous thrombosis	• Clinical surveillance and low dose aspirin or • Low-dose aspirin and UFH or LMWH in cases of recurrent placental insufficiency or evidence of extensive decidual inflammation, vasculopathy, and/or thrombosis on placental pathology[a]	• Clinical surveillance or • Low-dose aspirin and UFH or LMWH[a]
Laboratory criteria for APS but no clinical criteria for APS	Clinical surveillance	• Clinical surveillance, or • Postpartum anticoagulation only if family history of thrombosis
APS with previous arterial or venous thrombosis	Low-dose aspirin with either • UFH 5000–7500 U first trimester; 7500–10,000 U second trimester; 10,000 U third trimester SQ q12h or • LMWH, e.g., enoxaparin (Lovenox) 30–40 mg SQ q12h or dalteparin (Fragmin) 5000 U SQ q12h	Warfarin (lifelong)

Abbreviations: APS, antiphospholipid syndrome; LMWH, low-molecular-weight heparin; SQ, subcutaneous; UFH, unfractionated heparin.
[a]There is no level 1 evidence for this management, but it may be considered in select cases and in consultation with maternal fetal medicine.

six months. Anticoagulation should also be used for six weeks postpartum. Postpartum anticoagulation could be at therapeutic doses if the VTE occurred late in pregnancy, or it could be at prophylactic doses if the VTE occurred early in pregnancy.

- **APS with VTE in a prior pregnancy: prophylactic heparin (either UFH or LMWH) both in the antepartum and postpartum period (six weeks)** [25,26].

    Therapy is usually begun once fetal viability is established, but there is insufficient evidence regarding the best time of initiation of therapy. Low-dose aspirin dose is usually about 75 to 100 mg daily. Prophylactic UFH dose is usually 5000 to 7500 U first trimester, 7500 to 10,000 U second trimester, 10,000 U third trimester SQ q12h. Prophylactic LMWH dose are usually enoxaparin (Lovenox) 30 to 40 mg SQ q12h, or dalteparin (Fragmin) 5000 U SQ q12h. One may adjust prophylaxis in high-risk cases to a heparin (anti-Xa) level range of 0.2 to 0.4. Anti-Xa level is usually drawn four hours after injection. Anti-Xa levels have not been adequately evaluated prospectively to show a reduction in the incidence of complications.

- **APS with late fetal death:** Treatment trials have not shown a significant benefit at this time. The two trials that addressed this issue had some weaknesses, and thus no recommendations can be made at this time [13,14].

- **APS with a medically indicated preterm birth secondary to early onset intrauterine growth restriction (IUGR) or severe preeclampsia:** There are no treatment trials to assess any therapy, and recommendations are based primarily on expert opinion. Some experts have suggested prophylaxis similar to that shown in Table 26.3 [26]. Clinical surveillance alone is a reasonable strategy given the lack of evidence in this group of women [2].

Other Issues with Therapy

Heparin is associated with a 5% decrease in bone mass density and, therefore, osteoporosis. Supplemental **calcium (calcium gluconate/carbonate 1500 mg daily) and vitamin D, as well as resistance exercise**, should be encouraged. Idiosyncratic thrombocytopenia known as **heparin-induced thrombocytopenia (HIT)** occurs in <5% of women on heparin therapy, is usually mild, and starts usually three to 15 days after initiation of therapy. HIT is less common with LMWH. If on heparin (either type), consider checking an anti-Xa level at least once in three weeks after initiating heparin. **Check platelet counts initially and then weekly in the first three weeks to assure that there is no evidence of HIT.** There is no evidence to assess warfarin therapy for women with extreme thrombotic histories, including recurrent thromboses or cerebral thrombosis (see also Chapter 28).

ANTEPARTUM TESTING

- Early ultrasound is essential for accurate dating.
- Detailed fetal anatomic survey ultrasound at 18 to 20 weeks and follow-up ultrasounds approximately every four to six weeks for growth, fluid volume, and (if necessary) Doppler evaluation of the fetus.

- Fetal surveillance testing (e.g., NSTs and/or BPPs) starting at 32 weeks. The optimal regimen for fetal testing is unclear, and the entire clinical scenario must be considered when determining the optimal testing regimen for an individual patient.

PREPARATIONS FOR DELIVERY

- If on LMWH, switch to UFH at 36 weeks to allow regional anesthesia.
- Delivery should be considered at 39 0/7–39 6/7 weeks gestation to control timing of anticoagulation discontinuation.
- Anticoagulation should be discontinued 24 hours prior to planned induction of labor or cesarean section.

DELIVERY

Consider sending the placenta to pathology to check for decreased placental weight, ischemic-hypoxic changes— infarctions, decidual and fetal thrombi, chronic villitis.

ANESTHESIA

If on UFH, regional anesthesia can be administered usually six to eight hours after the dose, or at least when the aPTT is within normal limits. **If on LMWH, regional anesthesia should be delayed until ≥24 hours after the last dose because** there is a risk of spinal hematoma if regional anesthesia is performed within 24 hours. That is why a woman on LMWH might be switched off LMWH on to UFH weeks before any chance of labor or delivery (usually around 36 weeks if no other risk of preterm birth).

POSTPARTUM/BREAST-FEEDING

- In women with APS based on recurrent embryonic loss <10 weeks, the use of anticoagulation in the postpartum period has never been shown to be helpful.
- In women with APS based on fetal loss ≥10 weeks and no thrombotic events, anticoagulation for six weeks is usually recommended in the United States [2] (only three to five days in the United Kingdom).
- Women with APS based on prior thrombotic events should remain on lifelong anticoagulation therapy, and postpartum should be switched to warfarin therapy. Warfarin therapy is safe in breast-feeding women. An INR of 3.0 is desirable.

Estrogen-containing contraceptives are contraindicated as they further increase the VTE risk.

It is imperative that women with APS be followed closely by a medical or hematological specialist after pregnancy. Women with APS based on obstetric history and no history of thrombosis have an **increased postpartum risk of deep venous thrombosis** (adjusted hazard ratio [aHR] 1.85, 95% CI 1.50–2.28, annualized rate 1.46%) and **stroke** (aHR 2.10, 95% CI 1.08–4.08, annualized rate 0.17%) [27]. Additionally, about 10% with APS will later develop SLE [2].

REFERENCES

1. Miyakis S, Lockshin MD, Atsumi T et al. International consensus statement on an update of the classification criteria for definite antiphospholipid syndrome (APS). *J Thromb Haemost* 2006; 4: 295–306. [Review]
2. American College of Obstetricians and Gynecologists. Antiphospholipid syndrome. ACOG Practice Bulletin No. 132. *Obstet Gynecol* 2012; 120(6): 1514–21. [Review]
3. Infante-Rivard C, David M, Gauthier G, Rivard GE. Lupus anticoagulants, anticardiolipin antibodies, and fetal loss: A case-control study. *N Engl J Med* 1991; 325(15): 1063–6. [Case control, n = 55]
4. Robertson L, Wu O, Langhorne S et al. Thrombophilia in pregnancy: A systematic review. *Br J Haematol* 2006; 132: 171–96. [Review]
5. Silver RM, Parker CB, Reddy UM et al. Antiphospholipid antibodies in stillbirth. *Obstet Gynecol* 2013; 122: 641–57. [II-1]
6. Pattison NS, Chamley LW, Birdsall M et al. Does aspirin have a role in improving pregnancy outcome for women with the antiphospholipid syndrome? A randomized controlled trial. *Am J Obstet Gynecol* 2000; 183: 1008–12. [RCT, n = 50]
7. Cowchock S, Reece EA. Do low-risk pregnant women with antiphospholipid antibodies need to be treated? *Am J Obstet Gynecol* 1997; 176: 1099–100. [RCT, n = 19]
8. Tulppala M, Marttunen M, Soderstrom-Anttila V et al. Low-dose aspirin prevention of miscarriage in women with unexplained or autoimmune related recurrent miscarriage: Effect on prostacyclin and thromboxane A2 production. *Hum Reprod* 1997; 12: 1567–72. [RCT, n = 66]
9. Empson M, Lassere M, Craig JC et al. Recurrent pregnancy loss with antiphospholipid antibody: A systematic review of therapeutic trials. *Obstet Gynecol* 2002; 99: 135–44. [Meta-analysis; 10 RCTs; includes Refs. 2, 3, 4, 6, 8, 9, 10, 11, 12; n = 627]
10. Rai R, Cohen H, Dave M et al. Randomised controlled trial of aspirin and aspirin plus heparin in pregnant women with recurrent miscarriage associated with phospholipids antibodies. *BMJ* 1997; 314: 253–7. [RCT, n = 90]
11. Kutteh WH. Antiphospholipid antibody-associated recurrent pregnancy loss: Treatment with heparin and low dose aspirin is superior to low-dose aspirin alone. *Am J Obstet Gynecol* 1996; 174: 1584–9. [RCT, n = 50]
12. Goel N, Tuli A, Choudhry R. The role of aspirin versus aspirin and heparin in cases of recurrent abortions with raised anticardiolipin antibodies. *Med Sci Monit* 2006; 12: CR132–6. [RCT, n = 72]
13. Farquharson RG, Quenby S, Greaves M. Antiphospholipid syndrome in pregnancy: A randomized controlled trial of treatment. *Lupus* 2002; 100: 408–13. [RCT, n = 98]
14. Laskin CA, Spitzer KA, Clark CA et al. Low molecular weight heparin and aspirin for recurrent pregnancy loss: Results from the randomized, controlled HepASA trial. *J Rheumatol* 2009; 36: 279–87. [RCT, n = 88]
15. Ziakas P, Pavlou M, Voulgarelis M. Heparin treatment in antiphospholipid syndrome with recurrent pregnancy loss. *Obstet Gynecol* 2010; 115: 1256–62. [Review]
16. Noble LS, Kutteh WH, Lashey N et al. Antiphospholipid antibodies associated with recurrent pregnancy loss: Prospective, multicenter, controlled pilot study comparing treatment with low-molecular-weight heparin versus unfractionated heparin. *Fertil Steril* 2005; 83: 684–90. [RCT, n = 50]
17. Stephenson MD, Ballem PJ, Tsang P et al. Treatment of antiphospholipid antibody syndrome (APS) in pregnancy: A randomized pilot trial comparing low molecular weight heparin to unfractionated heparin. *J Obstet Gynaecol Can* 2004; 26: 729–34. [RCT, n = 26]

18. Fouda UM, Sayed AM, Abdou AM, Ramadan DI, Fouda IM, Zaki MM. Enoxaparin versus unfractionated heparin in the management of recurrent abortion secondary to antiphospholipid syndrome. *Int J Gynaecol Obstet* 2011; 112(3): 211–5. BMID 21251653. [RCT, *n* = 60]

19. Mak A, Cheung MW, Cheak AA, Ho RC. Combination of heparin and aspirin is superior to aspirin alone in enhancing live births in patients with recurrent pregnancy loss and positive antiphospholipid antibodies: A meta-analysis of randomized controlled trials and meta-regression. *Rheumatology* 2010; 49(2): 281–8. [Meta-analysis, 334 women in 5 studies – references 5, 8, 9, 11, 12]

20. Silver RK, MacGregor SN, Sholl JS et al. Comparative trial of prednisone plus aspirin vs. aspirin alone in the treatment of anticardiolipin antibody positive obstetric patients. *Am J Obstet Gynecol* 1993; 169: 1411–7. [RCT, *n* = 39]

21. Laskin CA, Bombardier C, Hannah ME et al. Prednisone and aspirin in women with autoantibodies and unexplained recurrent fetal loss. *N Engl J Med* 1997; 337: 148–53. [RCT, *n* = 202]

22. Cowchock FS, Reece EA, Balaban D et al. Repeated fetal losses associated with antiphospholipid antibodies: A collaborative randomized trial comparing prednisone with low-dose heparin treatment. *Am J Obstet Gynecol* 1992; 166: 1318–23. [RCT, *n* = 45]

23. Branch DW, Peaceman AM, Druzin M et al. A multicenter placebo-controlled pilot study of intravenous immune globulin treatment of antiphospholipid syndrome during pregnancy. The Pregnancy Loss Study Group. *Am J Obstet Gynecol* 2000; 182: 122–7. [RCT, *n* = 16]

24. El-Haieg AU, Zanati MF, El-Foual FM. Plasmapheresis and pregnancy outcome in patients with antiphospholipid syndrome. *Int J Gynaecol Obstet* 2007; 99(3): 236. [Case series, *n* = 18]

25. Bates S, Greer I, Pabinger I et al. Venous thromboembolism, thrombophilia antithrombotic therapy and pregnancy. *Chest* 2008; 133: 844–86. [Review]

26. Ruiz-Irastorza G, Crowther M, Branch W et al. Antiphospholipid syndrome. *Lancet* 2010; 376: 1498–509. [Review; III]

27. Gris JC, Bouvier S, Molinari N, Galanaud JP, Cochery-Nouvellon E, Mercier E, Fabbro-Peray P, Balducchi JP, Marès P, Quéré I, Dauzat M. Comparative incidence of a first thrombotic event in purely obstetric antiphospholipid syndrome with pregnancy loss: The NOH-APS observational study. *Blood* 2012; 119(11): 2624–32. [Case control, *n* = 1592]

27

Inherited thrombophilia

Robert M. Silver and James A. Airoldi

KEY POINTS

- **Inherited thrombophilias** are genetic conditions that increase the risk of thromboembolism.
- **The risk of thrombotic events is affected by numerous factors**, including thrombophilia, personal history of deep vein thrombosis (DVT), family history of DVT, surgery, age over 35 years, high parity, high body mass index, smoking, trauma, and immobilization.
- The **prevalence** and **thrombogenic potential** of the **inherited thrombophilias** are shown in **Tables 27.1 and 27.2**.
- **Venous thromboembolism (VTE)** is associated with **factor V Leiden (FVL), prothrombin 20210A gene mutation (PGM), antithrombin III (ATIII) deficiency, decreased protein C (PC) and protein S (PS)** in retrospective cohort studies.
- **The presence of inherited thrombophilias has been weakly associated with adverse pregnancy outcomes** such as stillbirth, preeclampsia, and fetal growth restriction **in retrospective studies**. However, there has been **NO or minimal association in several large prospective studies**.
- Fetal carriage of inherited thrombophilia mutations also have been weakly associated with adverse pregnancy outcomes, but quality data are lacking.
- **Screening** for inherited thrombophilias:
  - Universal screening for inherited thrombophilias is not recommended.
  - It is recommended to screen any pregnant woman with a **prior personal history of VTE** as this could affect anticoagulation recommendations, especially if the event was "unprovoked." Screening should include **FVL, PGM, ATIII, PS, and PC although ATIII, PC, and PS deficiencies are rare in the absence of a family history of VTE**.
  - In a woman with **VTE in the current pregnancy**, screening can be performed for **FVL, PGM, and ATIII. PC and PS assessment is less reliable in pregnancy**.
  - In an otherwise **healthy pregnant woman** with no personal history of VTE or adverse pregnancy outcomes but whose **first-degree relative has a genetic thrombophilia or VTE**, there is **insufficient evidence** to recommend for or against any type of screening. Given a lack of proven benefit, screening such women is not advised. In an otherwise **healthy pregnant woman** with a **prior adverse pregnancy outcome** but no major risk factors for VTE, there is **insufficient evidence** to support thrombophilia screening.
- **Treatment** for inherited thrombophilias and related conditions:
  - If **PC, PS, heterozygous FVL, or PGM** are detected in a woman with **prior VTE, prophylactic anticoagulation is reasonable**.
- If **homozygous FVL or PGM or an ATIII deficiency or a compound heterozygote** is detected in a woman with a **prior VTE, full therapeutic anticoagulation** is reasonable although prophylactic anticoagulation may be adequate.
- In a woman with a **prior personal history of a VTE** and a **recurring etiology (e.g., estrogen containing oral contraceptives or pregnancy), prophylactic anticoagulation** is recommended.
- Among **women with a nonrecurring cause for the prior VTE (e.g., orthopedic surgery) and no thrombophilia,** the risk of recurrent antepartum VTE is low; therefore, **routine antepartum prophylaxis with heparin may not be warranted.** Anticoagulation could still be given postpartum.
- Thromboprophylaxis is not advised for women with thrombophilia in hopes of improving obstetric outcomes.

See also Chapters 25, 26, and 28.

HISTORIC NOTES

Antithrombin deficiency and dysfibrinogenemia, the first inherited thrombophilias to be described (1965), were discovered in studies of families in which several members were affected by venous thrombosis [1,2]. Later, heterozygous deficiencies of protein C (PC) [3] and protein S (PS) [4] were identified as causes of inherited thrombophilia. In 1993, resistance to activated PC, the most common cause of inherited thrombophilia, was discovered [5,6]. In most cases, it results from a mutation of the factor V gene (G1691A), resulting in an abnormal factor V protein, termed factor V Leiden (FVL) [7]. In 1996, the G20210A mutation of the prothrombin gene was found to be another cause of thrombophilia [8].

DEFINITION

Inherited thrombophilias are genetic conditions that increase the risk of VTE [9].

EPIDEMIOLOGY/INCIDENCE

VTE is one of the leading causes of pregnancy-related maternal morbidity and mortality in the developed world [10]. Estimates for the incidence of thrombotic events occurring during pregnancy and the puerperium vary from 0.2 to 2 per 1000 births [10,11]. During pregnancy, women have a fivefold increased risk of VTE compared with nonpregnant women [11], and cesarean delivery carries a fivefold higher risk of thrombosis relative to vaginal delivery [12,13]. The incidence of thrombotic events is equal in the antepartum and postpartum periods. However, the rate of VTE per day is relatively higher postpartum. Also, the increased risk may persist for

Table 27.1 Prevalence of Different Thrombophilias in the General and At-Risk Populations

	Prevalence in General Population (%)	Prevalence in Patients with History of Thrombosis (%)
Factor V Leiden (heterozygous)	1–15	10–50
Prothrombin gene (heterozygous)	2–5	6–18
ATIII deficiency	0.02	1–3
Protein S deficiency	0.1–1.3	1–5
Protein C deficiency	0.2–0.4	3–5
Hyperhomocysteinemia	5	10
MTHFR (C677T heterozygous)	5–14	–

Source: Derived from Grandone E, Margaglione M, Colaizzo D et al. *Am J Obstet Gynecol*, 179, 1324–8, 1998; Franco RF, Reitsma PH. *Hum Genet*, 109, 369–84, 2001.

up to 12 weeks after delivery [14]. Antepartum risk is equally divided for each trimester [11]. Pulmonary embolism is more common postpartum [11].

Up to 50% of women who have thrombotic events during pregnancy possess an underlying **congenital or acquired thrombophilia** [15]. The frequency of major inherited thrombophilias varies substantially within healthy populations and among patients with previous venous thrombosis (Table 27.1) [16,17]. The most common inherited thrombophilias are heterozygosity for the FVL gene mutation, the prothrombin G20210A gene mutation (PGM), and the thermolabile variant of methylenetetrahydrofolate reductase (C677T MTHFR), the most common cause of hyperhomocysteinemia. However, this latter thrombophilia is only weakly associated with VTE [18]. Less common thrombophilias include autosomal-dominant deficiencies of antithrombin, PC, and PS. Factor V Leiden and the G20210A mutation in the prothrombin gene are common among Caucasians but are less common among Asians and Africans [18,19]. For example, a recent prospective cohort study of the factor V Leiden noted a carrier rate of 6.1% in Caucasians, 0.8% in African-Americans, 1.7% in Hispanics, and 1.9% in others [20] (Table 27.1).

ETIOLOGY/BASIC PATHOPHYSIOLOGY

Changes in the coagulation system, an increase in venous stasis, and vascular injury at delivery (Virchow's triad) substantially increase the risk of developing VTE in pregnancy compared with the nonpregnant state [10]. Changes in the coagulation system during pregnancy include increases in fibrinogen and factors II, VII, VIII, IX, X, and XII; an increase in the activity of the fibrinolytic inhibitors as evidenced by increases in plasminogen-activator inhibitor 1 (PAI-1) and 2 (PAI-2); a decrease in PS activity (because of estrogen-induced decreases in total PS and increases in the complement 4b binding protein, which binds PS); and an increase in resistance to activated PC in the second and third trimesters [21,22] (see Chapter 3 of *Obstetric Evidence Based Guidelines*). In approximately 50% of patients with a hereditary thrombophilia, the initial thrombotic event occurs in the presence of an additional risk factor, such as pregnancy, personal or family history, high body mass index, smoking, oral contraceptive use, orthopedic trauma, immobilization, or surgery [23,24]. Histologic examination of uteroplacental vessels and intervillous architecture from pathologic pregnancies typically display increased fibrin deposition, thrombosis, and hypoxia-associated endothelial and trophoblast changes [25]. However, these findings are not consistent in placentas of women with thrombophilias [26].

GENETICS/CLASSIFICATION OF EACH INHERITED THROMBOPHILIA (TABLES 27.1 AND 27.2)
Factor V Leiden

The FVL mutation arises from a (G to A) mutation in nucleotide 1691 of the factor V gene's 10th exon, resulting in a substitution of a glutamine for an arginine at position 506 in the factor V polypeptide (factor V Q506). The resultant amino acid substitution impairs the inactivation of factor Va by the complex activated PC and PS. This defect is termed the FVL mutation and is primarily inherited in an **autosomal-dominant** fashion. It is the most common cause of activated PC resistance. Its prevalence is about 5% to 10% in Europeans, 3% in Afro-Americans, and rare in Asian and African populations (Table 27.1). Homozygosity for the mutation, although rare, confers a far higher risk of thromboembolism. Compound

Table 27.2 Risk of VTE with Different Thrombophilias

	VTE Potential (RR of VTE)	VTE Risk per Pregnancy		% of All VTE
		No History (%)	*Prior VTE* (%)	
Factor V Leiden heterozygote	5–7	0.25	10	40
Factor V Leiden homozygote	25	1.5	17	2
Prothrombin gene heterozygote	3–9	0.5	>10	17
Prothrombin gene homozygote	25	2–3	>17	0.5
FVL/prothrombin compound heterozygote	84	4.5–5	>20	1–3
Antithrombin III activity <60%	50–100	0.4–7	40	1
Protein C activity <50%	10–13	0.1–0.8	4–17	14
Protein S free antigen <55%	2–10	0.1	0–22	3
Hyperhomocysteinemia (>16 mM)	3–6	0.2	NA	<5%

Sources: Derived from Grandone E, Margaglione M, Colaizzo D et al. *Am J Obstet Gynecol*, 179, 1324–8, 1998; Franco RF, Reitsma PH. *Hum Genet*, 109, 369–84, 2001; Gerhardt A, Scharf RE, Beckmann MW et al. *N Engl J Med*, 342, 374–80, 2000.
Abbreviations: RR, risk ratio; VTE, venous thromboembolism.

heterozygotes (FVL heterozygotes and prothrombin gene heterozygotes; see below) should be treated similar to homozygous women [18,19].

Prothrombin G20210A

Heterozygosity for a mutation in the promoter of the prothrombin gene (G20210A) leads to increased (150%–200%) circulating levels of prothrombin and an increased risk of thromboembolism. Homozygosity for the prothrombin mutation confers a risk of thrombosis equivalent to that of FVL homozygosity. It is inherited in an **autosomal-dominant** fashion [19].

Antithrombin III

Antithrombin III (ATIII) deficiency is the **most thrombogenic** of the inherited thrombophilias with a 70% to 90% lifetime risk of thromboembolism. Deficiencies in AT result from numerous point mutations, deletions, and insertions, and are usually inherited in an **autosomal-dominant** fashion. Because the prevalence of AT deficiency is low, 1/1000 to 1/5000, it is only present in 1% of patients with thromboembolism [19]. The appropriate **threshold for abnormally low activity is <60%**.

Protein C

PC is a vitamin K-dependent polypeptide synthesized primarily in the liver. Activated PC combines with free PS to inhibit factors V and VIII (see Figure 28.1). PC levels can be decreased by warfarin. PC deficiency can result from numerous mutations, which have highly variable procoagulant sequelae, making it extremely difficult to predict which patients with PC or PS deficiencies will develop thromboembolism [19]. The inheritance is **autosomal dominant**. PC deficiency is best diagnosed by a **functional assay activity cutoff of <50%**, found in only 0.3% of the population.

Protein S

PS is a vitamin K-dependent polypeptide synthesized primarily in the liver. PS is present in plasma in its free (40%) and bound (60%) forms, but it is the free form that is functional. PS functions as a cofactor with PC (see Figure 28.1). PS deficiency has three distinct phenotypes: 1) type I, marked by reduced total and free immunoreactive forms; 2) type II, characterized by normal free immunoreactive levels but reduced activated protein C (APC) cofactor activity; and 3) type III, in which there is normal total immunoreactive but reduced free immunoreactive levels. The inheritance is **autosomal dominant. Protein S decreases normally** by about 40% **during pregnancy**, and thus screening during pregnancy is not recommended. The decrease in pregnancy is due to estrogen-induced decreases in total PS and increases in the complement 4b binding protein, which binds PS. A **free PS antigen <55%** in nonpregnant women should be detected at least twice to document PS deficiency, and best correlates with PS mutations. If screening in pregnancy is performed, cutoff values in the second and third trimesters of <30% and <24%, respectively, may be valid [27].

MTHFR/Homocysteinemia

The most common form of genetic hyperhomocysteinemia results from the production of a thermolabile variant of **methylenetetrahydrofolate reductase (MTHFR)** with reduced enzymatic activity (T mutation) [28]. The gene encoding for this variant contains an alanine-to-valine substitution at amino acid 677 (C677T) [29]. The responsible mutation is common, with a population frequency for homozygosity estimated between 5% and 14% [30,31]. A MTHFR polymorphism at A1298C is less common. Homozygosity for the thermolabile variant of MTHFR (TT genotype) is a relatively common cause of mildly elevated plasma homocysteine levels in the general population, often occurring in association with low serum folate levels [32,33]. Increased blood levels of homocysteine may reflect deficiency of folate, vitamin B_6, and/or vitamin B_{12} [34–37]. Plasma folate and B_{12} levels, in particular, are strong determinants of the homocysteine concentration. Homocysteine levels are inversely related to folate consumption, reaching a stable baseline level when folate intake exceeds 400 mg/day [38,39]. Vitamin B_6 is a weaker determinant [39]. **Isolated MTHFR mutations (in the setting of normal homocysteine levels) are not associated with increased risk of VTE, and therefore should not be categorized as thrombophilias [11,40,41].**

RISK FACTORS/ASSOCIATIONS

The risk of thrombotic events is affected by numerous factors including **thrombophilia, personal history of DVT, family history of DVT, surgery, age over 35 years, high parity, high body mass index, smoking, edema, proteinuria, tissue trauma, and immobilization** [42,43].

COMPLICATIONS
VTE

The thrombogenic potential of inherited thrombophilias and the estimated probability of thrombosis per pregnancy in affected individuals are shown in Table 27.2 [16,17,44,45]. If a woman is a heterozygote for both FVL and PGM, the probability of thrombosis per pregnancy is estimated at 4.6% [44]. Data from older case-control studies show significant associations between thrombophilias and VTE in women with no personal history [14] as well as in those with prior VTE [45]. In a prospective study [29], the frequency of FVL in women with a history of thrombosis was higher than expected, (15% vs. 2%), but not for MTHFR (about 505 in cases and controls). In another prospective study [46], pregnant women with a single previous episode of VTE without antepartum anticoagulation had a 2.4% antepartum recurrence of VTE. There were **no recurrences in the 44 women who had no evidence of thrombophilia and who also had a previous episode of thrombosis that was associated with a nonrecurring risk factor.** However, the small numbers of women meeting these criteria do not allow a definitive conclusion that there is no increased risk of recurrent thrombosis. Among the 51 women with abnormal laboratory results or a previous episode of idiopathic thrombosis, or both, 5.9% had an antepartum recurrence of VTE [46]. **Although there was no association between thrombophilias and VTE in several prospective studies in asymptomatic women, they included too few individuals to make conclusions regarding the risk of VTE [20,47].**

Adverse Pregnancy Outcome (Table 27.3)

To assess the true association between thrombophilias and pregnancy complications, prospective cohort studies are preferred over retrospective cohort and case-control studies.

Table 27.3 Associations between Inherited Thrombophilias and Adverse Pregnancy Outcomes

	Factor V	PT 20210	MTHFR (C677T)
First trimester loss	No [18,58,60,63] Yes [59]	No [56,63]	No [59]
Second or third trimester loss	No [18,58,60,63] Yes [57]	No [56,57,63]	No [57] Yes [61]
IUGR	No [18,57–60,63]	No [56,57,63]	No [57,59]
Preeclampsia	No [18,55,57–60,63]	No [56,57,63]	No [55,57,59] Yes [61]
Placental abruption	No [18]	No [55–57,63]	No [56] Yes [57]	No [57]

Sources: Derived from Inherited thrombophilias in pregnancy. American College of Obstetricians and Gynecologists Practice Bulletin Number 138, September 2013. *Obstet Gynecol*, 122, 706–17, 2013; Facco F, You W, Grobman W. *Obstet Gyneco*, 113, 1206–16, 2009; Kist W, Janssen N, Kalk, J et al. *Thromb Haemost*, 99, 77–85, 2008; Kahn S, Platt R, McNamara H et al. *Am J Obstet Gynecol*, 200, 151–9, 2009; Said JM, Higgins J, Moses E et al. *Obstet Gynecol*, 115, 5–13, 2010; Clark P, Walker I, Govan L et al. *Br J Haematol*, 140, 236–40, 2008; Murphy RP, Donoghue R, Nallen R. *Arterioscler Thromb Vasc Biol*, 20, 266–70, 2000; Lindqvist PG, Svensson PJ, Marsal K et al. *Thromb Haemost*, 81, 532–7, 1999; Rodger MA, Walker MC, Smith GC et al. *J Thromb Haemost*, 12, 469–78, 2014.
Note: Based on prospective cohort studies and large case-control studies.
Abbreviations: MTHFR (C677T), methylenetetrahydrofolate reductase, PT, prothrombin.

Meta-analyses of retrospective cohort and case-control studies show associations between various thrombophilias and adverse pregnancy outcomes [48–55]. Confounders were assessed and included ethnicity, genetic testing only, and severity of illness [56]. Thrombophilias tended to be more strongly associated with later pregnancy loss (e.g., after 10 or 20 weeks) gestation than early pregnancy loss [48,49]. However, there was no association found between thrombophilias and adverse pregnancy outcomes in several prospective cohort studies. In a large multicenter study in the United States conducted through the MFMU, neither the FVL or prothrombin gene mutations were related to pregnancy loss (any trimester), placental abruption, preeclampsia, or fetal growth restriction [20,47]. In another large case-control study, there was no significant association between preeclampsia and four different thrombophilias (FVL, prothrombin gene mutation, MTHFR C677T mutation, or homocysteine) [57].

Seven prospective cohort studies are noted in the most current literature. **All were performed in low-risk women, which should be distinguished from women with thromboembolism and/or obstetric complications.**

In the first study, there was no association between the factor V Leiden mutation or the prothrombin G20210A mutation and pregnancy loss, preeclampsia, abruption, or SGA neonates in a low-risk, prospective cohort [20,47].

In the second study, some associations between thrombophilias and adverse outcomes were noted [58]:

- Women who carried the prothrombin gene mutation had an odds ratio (OR) of 3.58 (95% confidence interval [CI] 1.20–10.61, $p = 0.02$) for the development of the composite primary outcome (abruption, stillbirth, or neonatal death).
- Homozygous carriers of the MTHFR 1298 polymorphism had an odds ratio of 0.26 (95% CI 0.08–0.86, $p = 0.03$) for the composite outcome, denoting a protective effect.
- None of the other polymorphisms studied showed a significant association with the composite outcome.
- Placental abruption was significantly associated with prothrombin gene mutation (OR 12.15, 95% CI 2.45–60.39, $p = 0.002$).
- FVL conferred an increased risk of stillbirth (OR 8.85, 95% CI 1.60–48.92, $p = 0.01$).

In the third study, there was no association between FVL and preeclampsia, intrauterine growth restriction, or pregnancy loss. FVL was associated with birth weights >90th percentile (OR 1.81; 95% CI 1.04–3.31) and neonatal death (OR 14.79; 95% CI 2.71–80.74) [59].

In the fourth study, the frequency of FVL and MTHFR was no higher in those who subsequently developed preeclampsia or intrauterine growth retardation, and none of the screened population developed thrombosis [60].

In the fifth study, the APC-resistant subgroup did not differ from the non-APC-resistant subgroup in terms of pregnancy complications but was characterized by an eightfold higher risk of VTE (3/270 vs. 3/2210), a lower rate of profuse intrapartum hemorrhage (3.7% vs. 7.9%) ($p = 0.02$) and less intrapartum blood loss (340 mL vs. 361 mL) ($p = 0.04$) [61].

In the sixth study, women with hyperhomocysteinemia had severe preeclampsia (2/35 vs. 5/714, $p < 0.01$) and stillbirth (2/35 vs. 10/714, $p < 0.05$) more frequently than normohomocysteinemia [62].

The seventh study was performed in three tertiary care centers in Canada. Women were assessed for thrombophilias in the early second trimester of pregnancy. Placenta-mediated pregnancy complications occurred in 11.64% of women testing positive for thrombophilias compared to 11.23% in those testing negative (RR 1.04 [95% CI, 0.81–1.33]) [63].

In summary, there are no consistent results from these prospective cohort studies **with most showing no or little association between thrombophilias and adverse pregnancy outcomes. Importantly, the vast majority of women with thrombophilias and no prior adverse pregnancy outcomes have uncomplicated normal pregnancies.** *Accordingly, such women should not be screened for thrombophilias and should be reassured regarding pregnancy.*

Other than the potential for selection bias in case-control studies, it is unclear why results differ in retrospective and prospective studies. At worst, thrombophilias should be considered a minor "risk factor" rather than a "cause" of obstetric complications. It also seems that women with thrombophilias and prior adverse pregnancy outcomes comprise a different population than those with no prior complications. Indeed, the obstetric history is more predictive of subsequent obstetric risk than the thrombophilia.

FETAL THROMBOPHILIAS

Fetal carriage of thrombophilic mutations may also have adverse clinical consequences. A case-control study evaluated abortuses for the presence of FVL [64]. The mutation was present more frequently among abortuses than in unselected pregnancies. If the placenta showed >10% infarction, the fetus was 10 times more likely to have the mutation than when the placenta was normal. Carriers of multiple or homozygous thrombophilic defects were at increased risk of having a birth weight in the lowest quartile or lowest decile in a retrospective study [65]. In a prospective study [20], there was no statistical significance between fetal thrombophilia and any adverse pregnancy outcome. However, fetal FVL mutation carriage was associated with more frequent preeclampsia among African-American women and Hispanic women compared to Caucasian women.

DOSE DEPENDENCY OF THROMBOPHILIA

A case-control study nested in the European Prospective Cohort on Thrombophilia (EPCOT) compared 571 women with thrombophilia with 395 control patients and reported an increased risk of fetal loss (miscarriage and stillbirth) among the former patients (29.4% vs. 23.5%; $p = 0.04$) [66]. The risk of loss was greater after 28 weeks than at or before 28 weeks (OR 3.6; 95% CI 1.4–9.4 vs. OR 1.27; 95% CI 0.94–1.71). **The highest risk for stillbirth was observed in women with combined thrombophilic defects and antithrombin and PC deficiencies.** This suggests that often single genetic defects, such as FVL, may not lead to thrombosis, but rather it is the presence of multiple defects that causes a problem.

In another study [67], the FVL homozygous genotype increased the risk of late fetal loss. However, the overall likelihood of a positive outcome was high in women who were homozygous for factor V.

MANAGEMENT
Screening (Table 27.4)
The decision to perform screening should be influenced by the following:

- Prevalence of the risk factor in the studied population (e.g., personal and family history of thrombosis or thrombophilia).
- If the information gathered will impact clinical management in the short and long term.

There is **insufficient evidence to support universal screening** given the overall low prevalence of thrombophilias in the general population and the low prevalence of VTE and adverse pregnancy outcomes even in women with thrombophilias.

It is reasonable to screen any pregnant women with a **current or prior personal history of VTE**, especially when the VTE was not associated with a clear precipitating event such as immobilization after surgery. In a small prospective

study [66], pregnant women with a single previous episode of VTE without antepartum anticoagulation had a 2.4% antepartum recurrence of VTE. There were **no recurrences in the 44 women who had no evidence of thrombophilia and who also had a previous episode of thrombosis that was associated with a nonrecurring risk factor.** However, there have been numerous subsequent exceptions with recurrent VTE in this population. Nonetheless, they are at lower risk than women with VTE and thrombophilias. Among the 51 women with abnormal laboratory results or a previous episode of idiopathic thrombosis, or both, 5.9% had an antepartum recurrence of VTE.

In an otherwise **healthy pregnant woman** with no personal history of VTE, but whose **first-degree relative has a genetic thrombophilia or prior VTE**, there is **insufficient evidence** to recommend for or against screening. Thrombophilia screening in this population is advised by some authorities [18]. However, given a lack of proven benefit, we do not advise screening such women.

In an otherwise **healthy pregnant woman** with a **prior adverse pregnancy outcome** but no major risk factors for VTE, there is **insufficient evidence** to support screening either antepartum or postpartum.

Screening for MTHFR mutations is not recommended.

Diagnosis
It is important to be cognizant of potential inaccuracy when testing for thrombophilias. In general, DNA or antibody-based tests are reliable in most circumstances. However, some clotting assays may be affected by anticoagulant therapy, pregnancy, and other conditions. Table 27.5 describes testing of thrombophilias. The following are some potential causes of false positive results when testing for thrombophilias [68]:

- *Hyperhomocysteinemia*: deficiencies of folic acid, vitamin B_{12}, or vitamin B_6; older age, renal failure, smoking
- *Protein C activity*: pregnancy, liver disease, childhood, use of oral anticoagulants, vitamin K deficiency, disseminated intravascular coagulation (DIC), the presence of antibodies against PC
- *Protein S total and free antigen*: pregnancy, liver disease, childhood, use of oral anticoagulants, vitamin K deficiency, DIC, use of oral contraceptives, nephrotic syndrome, the presence of antibodies to PS
- *Antithrombin III activity*: liver disease, use of heparin therapy, nephrotic syndrome, DIC

Treatment
The primary goal of clinical management is to **reduce the risk of VTE.** As with many pregnancy-related conditions, there are few data from properly designed clinical trials to guide evidence based management. **Accordingly, recommendations are based on observational studies and extrapolation of data derived from nonpregnant populations.** Expert based recommendations from the most recent ACOG bulletin are shown in Table 27.6. Treatment can be divided into "prevention of VTE" and "prevention of obstetrical complications."

Prevention of VTE
Among **women with a nonrecurring cause for the prior VTE and no thrombophilia**, the risk of recurrent antepartum

Table 27.4 Who to Consider Screening (or Not Screening) for Inherited Thrombophilias

	Screen For
Prior VTE with nonrecurrent etiology	Factor V, PT 20210, ATIII, PC, PS
Prior VTE with recurrent etiology	Factor V, PT 20210, ATIII, PC, PS
VTE in current pregnancy	Factor V, PT 20210, ATIII, PC
General population	No screening
Relative with inherited thrombophilia but no personal history of VTE	No screening
Prior adverse pregnancy outcome	No screening

Abbreviations: ATIII, antithrombin III; PC, protein C; PS, protein S; PT, prothrombin; VTE, venous thromboembolism.

Table 27.5 Testing Characteristics for Different Thrombophilias

	Testing Method	Can Patients Be Tested during Pregnancy?	Is the Test Reliable during Acute Thrombosis?	Is the Test Reliable while on Anticoagulation?
Factor V Leiden	APC resistance assay	No	Yes	Yes
	DNA analysis	Yes	Yes	Yes
Prothrombin gene mutation G20210A	DNA analysis	Yes	Yes	Yes
Protein C deficiency	Protein C activity (<50%)	Yes	No	No
Protein S deficiency	Free protein S antigen (<55%)	No[a]	No	No
ATIII deficiency	ATIII activity (<60%)	Yes	No	No
Hyperhomocysteinemia	Fasting plasma homocysteine	Yes	Unclear	Yes

Source: Adapted from Inherited thrombophilias in pregnancy. American College of Obstetricians and Gynecologists Practice Bulletin Number 138, September 2013. *Obstet Gynecol,* 122, 706–17, 2013.
Abbreviation: ATIII, antithrombin III.
[a]Protein S cutoffs in pregnancy may be reliable if lower thresholds are used (testing should be repeated more than six weeks postpartum): [69].

Table 27.6 Recommended Thromboprophylaxis for Pregnancies Complicated by Inherited Thrombophilias[a]

Clinical Scenario	Antepartum Management	Postpartum Management
Low-risk thrombophilia[b] without previous VTE	Surveillance without anticoagulation therapy	Surveillance without anticoagulation therapy or postpartum anticoagulation therapy if the patient has additional risk factors[c]
Low-risk thrombophilia with a family history (first-degree relative) of VTE	Surveillance without anticoagulation therapy	Postpartum anticoagulation therapy or intermediate-dose LMWH/UFH
Low-risk thrombophilia[b] with a single previous episode of VTE—not receiving long-term anticoagulation therapy	Prophylactic or intermediate-dose LMWH/UFH or surveillance without anticoagulation therapy	Postpartum anticoagulation therapy or intermediate-dose LMWH/UFH
High-risk thrombophilia[d] without previous VTE	Surveillance without anticoagulation therapy or prophylactic LMWH or UFH	Postpartum anticoagulation therapy
High-risk thrombophilia[d] with a single previous episode of VTE or an affected first-degree relative—not receiving long-term anticoagulation therapy	Prophylactic, intermediate-dose or adjusted-dose LMWH/UFH regimen	Postpartum anticoagulation therapy or intermediate or adjusted-dose LMWH/UFH for 6 weeks (therapy level should be at least as high as antepartum treatment)
No thrombophilia with previous single episode of VTE associated with transient risk factor that is no longer present—excludes pregnancy- or estrogen-related risk factor	Surveillance without anticoagulation therapy	Postpartum anticoagulation therapy[i]
No thrombophilia with previous single episode of VTE associated with transient risk factor that was pregnancy- or estrogen-related	Prophylactic-dose LMWH or UFH[e]	Postpartum anticoagulation therapy
No thrombophilia with previous single episode of VTE without an associated risk factor (idiopathic)—not receiving long-term anticoagulation therapy	Prophylactic-dose LMWH or UFH[e]	Postpartum anticoagulation therapy
Thrombophilia or no thrombophilia with two or more episodes of VTE—not receiving long-term anticoagulation therapy	Prophylactic or therapeutic-dose LMWH or Prophylactic or therapeutic-dose UFH	Postpartum anticoagulation therapy or Therapeutic-dose LMWH/UFH for 6 weeks
Thrombophilia or no thrombophilia with two or more episodes of VTE—receiving long-term anticoagulation therapy	Therapeutic-dose LMWH or UFH	Resumption of long-term anticoagulation therapy

Source: Reprinted with permission from Inherited thrombophilias in pregnancy. American College of Obstetricians and Gynecologists Practice Bulletin Number 138, September 2013. *Obstet Gynecol,* 122, 706–17, 2013.
Abbreviations: LMWH, low molecular weight heparin; UFH, unfractionated heparin; VTE, venous thromboembolism.
[a]Postpartum treatment levels should be greater or equal to antepartum treatment. Treatment of acute VTE and management of antiphospholipid syndrome are addressed in other Practice Bulletins.
[b]Low-risk thrombophilia: factor V Leiden heterozygous; prothrombin *G20210A* heterozygous; protein C or protein S deficiency.
[c]First-degree relative with a history of a thrombotic episode before age 50 years or other major thrombotic risk factors (e.g., obesity or prolonged immobility).
[d]High-risk thrombophilia: antithrombin deficiency; double heterozygous for prothrombin *G20210A* mutation and factor V Leiden; factor V Leiden homozygous or prothrombin *G20210A* mutation homozygous.
[e]Surveillance without anticoagulation therapy is supported as an alternative approach by some experts.

VTE is low; therefore, **routine antepartum prophylaxis with heparin may not be warranted**. Prophylactic anticoagulation should still be given postpartum, especially if there is a cesarean delivery. **If moderate risk thrombophilias such as PC, PS, heterozygous FVL, or PGM are detected in this group of women, prophylactic anticoagulation is advised. If high-risk thrombophilias, such as homozygous FVL or PGM; a compound heterozygote; or ATIII deficiency is detected, full therapeutic anticoagulation is recommended.** An elevated homocysteine and a low folate, B_6, or B_{12} level should prompt replacement.

In a woman with a **prior personal history of a VTE** and no prior sporadic precipitating event (e.g., unprovoked, oral contraceptives, or pregnancy), **prophylactic anticoagulation** antepartum and postpartum is usually recommended. Full anticoagulation is advised in women with high-risk thrombophilias. An elevated homocysteine and a low folate, B_6, or B_{12} level should prompt replacement.

In a woman with a **VTE in the current pregnancy, full anticoagulation is typically advised for three to six months. At that time, women with low-risk thrombophilias are then given prophylactic doses of anticoagulation through six weeks postpartum. Those with high-risk thrombophilias** (homozygous FVL, homozygous PGM, compound heterozygote, ATIII deficiency) **or recurrent VTE are treated with full anticoagulant doses through six weeks postpartum and often for life.**

Prevention of Obstetrical Complications (See Table 28.5)

On balance, anticoagulant therapy in women with thrombophilias does not appear to be efficacious for improving obstetric outcomes. However, there are scant high-quality data, and definitive conclusions cannot be made. A prospective randomized, nonblinded non-placebo-controlled randomized trial evaluated the effect of thromboprophylaxis in women with **one unexplained pregnancy loss** at ≥10th week of amenorrhea and either heterozygous **FVL mutation, prothrombin G20210A** mutation, or **PS deficiency** (free antigen <55%) [70]. Women were given 5 mg folic acid daily before conception to be continued during pregnancy, and either **low-dose aspirin** 100 mg daily **or LMWH** enoxaparin 40 mg starting at eight weeks. LMWH was associated with a higher (86% vs. 29%) incidence of a **healthy live birth** and lower incidence of low birth weight (10% vs. 30%). No significant side effects of the treatments could be evidenced in patients or newborns. This trial led to enthusiasm about the potential benefits of thromboprophylaxis. However, this was not a blinded trial, and outcomes in untreated women were considerably worse than expected. Thus, results should be interpreted with caution.

Since that time, results have not been as encouraging. A retrospective, nonrandomized study noted no improvement in pregnancy outcomes in women with trhombophilias who were and were not treated with thromboprophylaxis [71]. A cohort study showed that in women with a **thrombophilia** (heterozygous factor V, activated PC resistance, MTHFR 677 TT genotype, PS deficiency, heterozygous prothrombin 20210, antithrombin II deficiency, hyperhomocysteinemia, and/or PC deficiency) and a **history of ≥3 first trimester losses, ≥2 second trimester losses, or a fetal death in the third trimester,** enoxaparin 40 mg/day was associated with an approximate 80% rate of live births, similar to enoxaparin 80 mg/day [72]. Recent meta-analyses and reviews also found

no increase in live birth rates in women with thrombophilias and pregnancy loss treated with anticoagulant therapy [73,74]. The FRUIT trial compared low-dose aspirin with and without dalteparin in 139 women with thrombophilia and prior adverse pregnancy outcome. Dalteparin decreased the risk of recurrent hypertensive disease prior to 34 weeks gestation (risk reduction 8.7% (95% CI 1.9–15.5%) but had no effect on fetal growth [75,76].

Finally, a recent, large, multicenter, multinational study, the TIPPS trial, compared antepartum prophylactic dalteparin versus no dalteparin for the prevention of pregnancy complications in 289 women with thrombophilia [77]. There was no difference in adverse obstetric outcomes between groups. There also was a similar rate of major bleeding although minor bleeding was more common in the dalteparin group [78]. Taken together, these data do NOT support the use of thromboprophylaxis in women with thrombophilias in order to improve pregnancy outcomes.

Hyperhomocysteinemia

There are no trials to assess interventions for the pregnant woman with hyperhomocysteinemia. It might be reasonable to suggest safe therapy aimed to normalize the homocysteine level, with folic acid 4 mg once a day, in addition to vitamin B_6 25 mg three to four times a day and vitamin B_{12} 100 mg once a day, but counseling should emphasize that this therapy has not been tested in trials in pregnant women. This therapy has been tested in the nonpregnant population. The Vitamins and Thrombosis (VITRO) study investigated the effect of homocysteine lowering by daily supplementation of B vitamins on the risk reduction of DVT and pulmonary embolism (PE) [78]. The results did not show that homocysteine lowering by vitamin B supplementation prevents recurrent venous thrombosis even though homocysteine levels were lowered back to the normal range with therapy.

For **antepartum testing, delivery, anesthesia,** and **postpartum/breast-feeding,** see Chapter 28.

REFERENCES

1. Egeberg O. Inherited antithrombin III deficiency causing thrombophilia. *Thromb Diath Haemorrh* 1965; 13: 516–30. [II-3]
2. Beck EA, Charache P, Jackson DP. A new inherited coagulation disorder caused by an abnormal fibrinogen ("fibrinogen Baltimore"). *Nature* 1965; 208: 143–5. [II-3]
3. Griffin JH, Evatt B, Zimmerman TS et al. Deficiency of protein C in congenital thrombotic disease. *J Clin Invest* 1981; 68: 1370–3. [II-3]
4. Comp PC, Esmon CT. Recurrent venous thromboembolism in patients with a partial deficiency of protein S. *N Engl J Med* 1984; 311: 1525–8. [II-2]
5. Koeleman BP, Reitsma PH, Bertina RM. Familial thrombophilia: A complex genetic disorder. *Semin Hematol* 1997; 34: 256–64. [II-2]
6. Dahlback B, Carlsson M, Svensson PJ. Familial thrombophilia due to a previously unrecognized mechanism characterized by poor anticoagulant response to activated protein C: Prediction of a cofactor to activated protein C. *Proc Natl Acad Sci U S A* 1993; 90: 1004–8. [II-3]
7. Bertina RM, Koeleman BP, Koster T et al. Mutation in blood coagulation factor V associated with resistance to activated protein C. *Nature* 1994; 369: 64–7. [II-2]
8. Poort SR, Rosendaal FR, Reitsma PH et al. A common genetic variation in the 3'-untranslated region of the prothrombin gene is associated with elevated plasma prothrombin levels and an increase in venous thrombosis. *Blood* 1996; 88: 3698–703. [II-2]
9. Lockwood CJ. Inherited thrombophilias in pregnant patients. *Prenat Neonat Med* 2001; 6: 3–14. [Review]

10. Greer IA. Thrombosis in pregnancy: Maternal and fetal issues. *Lancet* 1999; 353: 1258–65. [Review]

11. Inherited thrombophilias in pregnancy. Practice bulletin No. 113. American College of Obstetricians and Gynecologists. *Obstet Gynecol* 2010; 116: 212–22. [Review]

12. Lindqvist P, Dahlback B, Marsal K. Thrombotic risk during pregnancy: A population study. *Obstet Gynecol* 1999; 94: 595–9. [II-2]

13. Macklon NS, Greer IA. Venous thromboembolic disease in obstetrics and gynaecology: The Scottish experience. *Scott Med J* 1996; 41: 83–6. [II-2]

14. Kamel H, Navi BB, Sriram N et al. Risk of a thrombotic event after the 6 week postpartum period. *N Engl J Med* 2014; 370: 1307–15. [II-2]

15. Grandone E, Margaglione M, Colaizzo D et al. Genetic susceptibility to pregnancy-related venous thromboembolism: Roles of factor V Leiden, prothrombin G20210A, and methylenetetrahydrofolate reductase C677T mutations. *Am J Obstet Gynecol* 1998; 179: 1324–8. [II-2]

16. Franco RF, Reitsma PH. Genetic risk factors of venous thrombosis. *Hum Genet* 2001; 109: 369–84. [II-2]

17. Haverkate F, Samama M. Familial dysfibrinogenaemia and thrombophilia. Report on a study of the SSC Subcommittee on fibrinogen. *Thromb Haemost* 1995; 73: 151–61. [II-2]

18. Inherited thrombophilias in pregnancy. American College of Obstetricians and Gynecologists Practice Bulletin Number 138, September 2013. *Obstet Gynecol* 2013; 122: 706–17. [Review]

19. Lockwood C. Inherited thrombophilias in pregnant patients: Detection and treatment paradigm. *Obstet Gynecol* 2002; 99: 333–41. [Review]

20. Dizon-Townsend D, Miller C, Sibai B et al. The relationship of the factor V Leiden mutation and pregnancy outcomes for mother and fetus. *Obstet Gynecol* 2005; 106: 517–24. [II-2]

21. Lockwood CJ. Heritable coagulopathies in pregnancy. *Obstet Gynecol Surv* 1999; 54: 754. [Review]

22. Walker MC, Garner PR, Keely EJ et al. Changes in activated protein C resistance during normal pregnancy. *Am J Obstet Gynecol* 1997; 77: 162. [II-3]

23. De Stefano V, Leone G, Mastrangelo S et al. Clinical manifestations and management of inherited thrombophilia: Retrospective analysis and follow-up after diagnosis of 238 patients with congenital deficiency of antithrombin III, protein C, protein S. *Thromb Haemost* 1994; 72: 352–8. [II-3]

24. Middledorp S, Henkens CM, Koopman MM et al. The incidence of venous thromboembolism in family members of patients with factor V Leiden mutation and venous thrombosis. *Ann Intern Med* 1998; 128: 15–20. [II-2]

25. Kingdom JC, Kaufmann P. Oxygen and placental villous development: Origins of fetal hypoxia. *Placenta* 1997; 18: 613–21. [II-3]

26. Many A, Schreiber L, Rosner S et al. Pathologic features of the placenta in women with severe pregnancy complications and thrombophilia. *Obstet Gynecol* 2001; 98(6): 1041–4. [II-3]

27. Paidas MJ, Ku DH, Lee MJ et al. Protein Z, protein S levels are lower in patients with thrombophilia and subsequent pregnancy complications. *J Thromb Haemost* 2005; 3:497–501. [II-2]

28. Kang SS, Wong PWK, Susmano A et al. Thermolabile methylenetetrahydrofolate reductase: An inherited risk factor for coronary artery disease. *Am J Hum Genet* 1991; 48:536. [II-3]

29. Frosst P, Blom HJ, Milos R et al. A candidate genetic risk factor for vascular disease: A common mutation in methylenetetrahydrofolate reductase. *Nat Genet* 1995; 10: 111. [II-3]

30. Gallagher PM, Meleady R, Shields DC et al. Homocysteine and risk of premature coronary heart disease: Evidence for a common gene mutation. *Circulation* 1996; 94: 2154. [II-3]

31. Guttormsen AB, Ueland PM, Nesthus I et al. Determinants and vitamin responsiveness of intermediate hyperhomocysteinemia (40 mmol/L). *J Clin Invest* 1996; 98: 2174. [II-3]

32. Harmon DL, Woodside JV, Yarnell JW et al. The common "thermolabile" variant of methylenetetrahydrofolate reductase is a major determinant of mild hyperhomocysteinemia. *QJM* 1996; 89: 571. [II-3]

33. Kluijtmans LA, Young IS, Boreham CA et al. Genetic and nutritional factors contributing to hyperhomocysteinemia in young adults. *Blood* 2003; 101: 2483. [II-3]

34. Robinson K, Arheart K, Refsum H et al., for the European COMCAC Group. Low circulating folate and vitamin B6 concentrations. Risk factors for stroke, peripheral vascular disease, and coronary artery disease. *Circulation* 1998; 97: 437. [II-2]

35. Rimm EB, Willett WC, Hu FB et al. Folate and vitamin B6 from diet and supplements in relation to risk of coronary heart disease among women. *JAMA* 1998; 279: 359. [II-2]

36. Voutilainen S, Rissanen TH, Virtanen J et al. Low dietary folate intake is associated with an excess incidence of acute coronary events: The Kuopio Ischemic Heart Disease Risk Factor Study. *Circulation* 2001; 103: 2674. [II-1]

37. Vermeulen EG, Stehouwer CD, Twisk JW et al. Effect of homocysteine-lowering treatment with folic acid plus vitamin B6 on progression of subclinical atherosclerosis: A randomised, placebo-controlled trial. *Lancet* 2000; 355: 517. [RCT, n = 158, I]

38. Selhub J, Jacques PF, Wilson PW et al. Vitamin status and intake as primary determinants of homocysteinemia in an elderly population. *JAMA* 1993; 270: 2693. [II-1]

39. Ubbink JR, Vermaak WJ, van der Merwe A et al. Vitamin B-12, vitamin B-6, and folate nutritional status in men with hyperhomocysteinemia. *Am J Clin Nutr* 1993; 57: 47. [II-2]

40. McColl MD, Ellison J, Reid F et al. Prothrombin 20210, MTHFR C677T mutations in women with venous thromboembolism associated with pregnancy. *BJOG* 2000; 107: 565–9. [III]

41. Ziakas PD, Poulou LS, Pavlou M, Zintzaras E. Thrombophilia and venous thromboembolism in pregnancy: A meta-analysis of genetic risk. *Eur J Obstet Gynecol and Reprod Biol* 2015; 191: 106–11. [II-2]

42. Zotz RB, Gerhardt A, Scharf RE. Inherited thrombophilia and gestational venous thromboembolism. *Best Pract Res Clin Haematol* 2003; 16: 243. [Review]

43. British Society of Hematology. Investigation and management of heritable thrombophilia. *Br J Haematol* 2001; 114: 512. [Review]

44. Gerhardt A, Scharf RE, Beckmann MW et al. Prothrombin and factor V mutations in women with a history of thrombosis during pregnancy and the puerperium. *N Engl J Med* 2000; 342: 374–80. [II-2]

45. Simioni P, Tormene D, Prandoni P et al. Pregnancy related recurrent events in thrombophilic women with previous venous thromboembolism. *Thromb Haemost* 2001; 86: 929. [II-2]

46. Brill-Edwards P, Ginsberg JS, Gent M et al. Safety of withholding heparin in pregnant women with a history of venous thromboembolism. *N Engl J Med* 2000; 343: 1439–44. [II-1, n = 125]

47. Silver R, Zhao Y, Spong Y et al. Prothrombin gene G20210A mutation and obstetric complications. *Obstet Gynecol* 2010; 115: 14–20. [II-2]

48. Robertson L, Wu O, Langhorne S et al. Thrombophilia in pregnancy: A systematic review. *Br J Haematol* 2006; 132: 171–96. [Review]

49. Rey E, Kahn SR, David M et al. Thrombophilic disorders and fetal loss: A meta-analysis. *Lancet* 2003; 361: 901. [II-2]

50. Howley HE, Walker M, Rodger MA. A systematic review of the association between factor V Leiden or prothrombin gene variant and intrauterine growth restriction. *Am J Obstet Gynecol* 2005; 192: 694. [II-2]

51. Lin J, August P. Genetic thrombophilias and preeclampsia: A meta-analysis. *Obstet Gynecol* 2005; 105: 182–92. [II-2]

52. Roque H, Paidas MJ, Funai EF et al. Maternal thrombophilias are not associated with early pregnancy loss. *Thromb Haemost* 2004; 91: 290. [II-2]

53. Infante-Rivard C, Rivard GE, Yotov WV et al. Absence of association of thrombophilia polymorphisms with intrauterine growth restriction. *N Engl J Med* 2002; 347: 1. [II-2]

54. Prochazka M, Happach C, Marsal K et al. Factor V Leiden in pregnancies complicated by placental abruption. *BJOG* 2003; 110: 462–6. [II-2]

55. Facco F, You W, Grobman W. Genetic thrombophilias and intrauterine growth restriction. A meta-analysis. *Obstet Gynecol* 2009; 113: 1206–16. [Review]

56. Kist W, Janssen, N, Kalk, J et al. Thrombophilias and adverse pregnancy outcome—A confounded problem. *Thromb Haemost* 2008; 99: 77–85. [II-3]

57. Kahn S, Platt R, McNamara H et al. Inherited thrombophilia and preeclampsia within a multicenter cohort: The Montreal Preeclampsia study. *Am J Obstet Gynecol* 2009; 200: 151–9. [II-3]

58. Said JM, Higgins J, Moses E et al. Inherited thrombophilia polymorphisms and pregnancy outcomes in nulliparous women. *Obstet Gynecol* 2010; 115: 5–13. [II-2]

59. Clark P, Walker I, Govan L et al. The GOAL study: A prospective examination of the impact of factor V Leiden and ABO(H) blood groups on haemorrhagic and thrombotic pregnancy outcomes. *Br J Haematol* 2008; 140: 236–40. [II-2]

60. Murphy RP, Donoghue R, Nallen R. Prospective evaluation of the risk conferred by factor V Leiden and thermolabile methylenetetrahydrofolate reductase polymorphisms in pregnancy. *Arterioscler Thromb Vasc Biol* 2000; 20: 266–70. [II-2]

61. Lindqvist PG, Svensson PJ, Marsal K et al. Activated protein C resistance (FVQ506) and pregnancy. *Thromb Haemost* 1999; 81: 532–7. [II-2]

62. Murakamis S, Matsubara N, Miyakaw S et al. The relation between homocysteine concentration and methylenetetrahydrofolate reductase genetic polymorphism in pregnant women. *J Obstet Gynaecol Res* 2001; 27: 349–52. [II-2]

63. Rodger MA, Walker MC, Smith GC et al. Is thrombophilia associated with placenta-mediated pregnancy complications? A prospective cohort study. *J Thromb Haemost* 2014; 12: 469–78. [II-2]

64. Dizon-Townson DS, Meline L, Nelson LM et al. Fetal carriers of the factor V Leiden mutation are prone to miscarriage and placental infarction. *Am J Obstet Gynecol* 1997; 177: 402. [II-2]

65. von Kries R, Junker R, Oberle D et al. Foetal growth restriction in children with prothrombotic risk factors. *Thromb Haemost* 2001; 86: 1012. [II-2]

66. Preston FE, Rosendaal FR, Walker ID et al. Increased fetal loss in women with heritable thrombophilia. *Lancet* 1996; 348: 913–6. [II-2]

67. Biron-Andréani C, Bauters A, Le Cam-Duchez V et al. Factor V Leiden homozygous genotype and pregnancy outcomes. *Obstet Gynecol* 2009; 114: 1249–53. [II-2]

68. Seligsohn U, Lubetsky A. Medical progress: Genetic susceptibility to venous thrombosis. *N Engl J Med* 2001; 344: 1222–31. [Review]

69. Said JM, Igniatovic V, Monagle PT et al. Altered reference ranges for protein C and protein S during early pregnancy: Implications for the diagnosis of protein C and protein S deficiency during pregnancy. *Thromb Haemost* 2010; 103: 984–8. [II-3]

70. Gris JC, Mercier E, Quere I et al. Low molecular weight heparin verses low-dose aspirin in women with one fetal loss and a constitutional thrombophilic disorder. *Blood* 2004; 103: 3695. [RCT, n = 160, I]

71. Warren JE, Simonsen SE, Branch DW, Porter TF, Silver RM. Thromboprophylaxis and pregnancy outcome in asymptomatic women with inherited thrombophilias. *Am J Obstet Gynecol* 2009; 200.e1–5. [II-2]

72. Brenner B, Hoffman R, Carp H et al. Efficacy and safety of two doses of enoxaparin in women with thrombophilia and recurrent pregnancy loss: The LIVE-ENOX study. *J Thromb Haemost* 2005; 3: 227–9. [II-2]

73. de Jong PG, Kaandorp S, Di Nisio M, Goddijin M, Middledorp S. Aspirin and/or heparin for women with unexplained recurrent miscarriage with or without inherited thrombophilia (Review). *The Cochrane Library* 2014; 7: 1–73. [Review]

74. Areia AL, Fonseca E, Areia M, Moura P. Low-molecular weight heparin plus aspirin versus aspirin alone in pregnant women with hereditary thrombophilia to improve live birth date; meta-analysis of randomized controlled trials. *Arch Gynecol Obstet* 2015; doi:10.1007/s00404-015-3782-2. [Review; I]

75. de Vries JI, van Pampus MG, Hague WM, Bezemer PD, Joosten JH. Low-molecular weight heparin added to aspirin in the prevention of recurrent early-onset preeclampsia in women with inheritable thrombophilia in the FRUIT-RCT. *J Thromb Haemost* 2012; 10: 64–72. [I]

76. Abheiden CNH, Van Hoorn ME, Hague WM et al. Does low molecular weight heparin influence fetal growth or uterine and umbilical arterial Doppler in women with a history of early-onset uteroplacental insufficiency and an inheritable thrombophilia? Secondary randomized controlled trial results. *BJOG* 2015; doi:10.1111/1471-0528.13421. [I]

77. Rodger MA, Hague WM, Kingdom J et al. Antepartum dalteparin versus no antepartum dalteparin for the prevention of pregnancy complications in pregnant women with thrombophilias (TIPPS): A multinational open-label randomized trial. *Lancet* 2014; 384: 1673–83. [I]

78. den Heijer M, Willems H, Blom H et al. Homocysteine lowering by B vitamins and the secondary prevention of deep vein thrombosis and pulmonary embolism: A randomized, placebo-controlled, double-blind. *Blood* 2007; 109: 139–44. [RCT, n = 325, I]

28

Venous thromboembolism and anticoagulation

Melissa Chu Lam and James A. Airoldi

KEY POINTS

- Venous thromboembolism is one of the **leading causes of pregnancy-related maternal morbidity and mortality in high-income countries.**
- Risk factors are listed in Table 28.2 and include pregnancy, **increased parity, prior thromboembolism, age of 35 years or more, increased maternal weight, instrumented-assisted deliveries or cesarean section, prolonged immobilization, smoking, and the presence of an acquired or inherited thrombophilia.**
- **Compressive ultrasonography** is the **primary modality for the diagnosis of deep vein thrombosis (DVT)** in pregnancy.
- The **ventilation/perfusion (V/Q) scan** or a **computed tomography pulmonary angiography (CTPA)** are fairly equivalent first-line imaging tests **for the diagnosis of pulmonary embolism (PE)** in pregnant patients although some experts favor V/Q scans.
- The three anticoagulants typically used are **unfractionated heparin (UFH), low-molecular weight heparin (LMWH),** and **warfarin.**
- **Platelet counts** should be **checked** five days **after the initiation of UFH** and periodically for the first three weeks of heparin therapy.
- **LMWH is at least as effective and safe as UFH** for the treatment of patients with acute DVT and for the prevention of DVT. **LMWH and UFH do not cross the placenta** and are safe for the fetus. The incidences of bleeding, osteopenia, and heparin-induced thrombocytopenia with LMWH are probably decreased compared to UFH in pregnant patients. Pregnant women may require higher doses, and the risks could be dose related. **The dosing of LMWH in pregnancy remains controversial.**
- **Warfarin** derivatives **cross the placenta** and have the potential to cause both **bleeding in the fetus and teratogenicity.** Warfarin use is believed to be safe in the first 6 weeks of gestation but has been **associated with warfarin embryopathy in 4%–5% of fetuses when maternal exposure occurs between six and nine weeks gestation.**
- In the pregnant patient with **acute VTE, either therapeutic LMWH throughout pregnancy or intravenous UFH** for at least five days, followed by therapeutic UFH or LMWH for a **minimum of 6 months,** is the recommended approach. Anticoagulants should be administered for at least six weeks postpartum.
- There are three general approaches to the antepartum management of pregnant patients with **previous VTE: UFH, LMWH, or close surveillance** (Table 28.4).
- Among women with a nonrecurring cause for the prior VTE and no thrombophilia, the risk of recurrent antepartum VTE is low, and therefore routine antepartum prophylaxis with heparin is not warranted. However, postpartum low-dose prophylaxis is still recommended.
- If there is a **potential recurring cause, prophylactic anticoagulation is recommended.**
- In pregnant women with a **prior VTE with history of a low-risk thrombophilia (heterozygous Factor V or prothrombin gene, protein C or S), prophylactic anticoagulation** is recommended.
- **Therapeutic anticoagulation is recommended for prior VTE and high-risk thrombophilia (ATIII deficiency, homozygous factor V or prothrombin gene, or compound heterozygote).**
- **Therapeutic anticoagulation** should be used in pregnant women if the woman has **recurrent VTE episodes, life-threatening thrombosis, or thrombosis while receiving chronic anticoagulation.** Filters of the inferior vena cava should be considered in these situations as well.
- It is recommended that pregnant patients with **recurrent early pregnancy losses and antiphospholipid syndrome (APS)** who do not have a history of VTE receive **prophylactic regimen of heparin and low-dose aspirin** and that those with previous VTE and APS receive a similar prophylactic dose of heparin.
- In pregnant women with **mechanical heart valves,** it appears reasonable to use one of these four regimens: 1) therapeutic LMWH or UFH between 6 and 12 weeks and close to term only and vitamin K antagonists (VKAs) at other times, 2) careful therapeutic UFH throughout pregnancy, 3) careful therapeutic LMWH throughout pregnancy, or 4) VKAs throughout pregnancy.

DEFINITION

Venous thromboembolism (VTE) refers to a condition in which blood clots inappropriately and includes deep vein thrombosis (DVT, when a clot forms in the deep veins of the body) and pulmonary embolism (PE, when a clot in the deep veins breaks free and is carried to the arteries of the lung), which are the most common, and others, such as cerebrovascular events (CVA or stroke) [1].

SYMPTOMS

The two most common initial symptoms (80% of pregnant patients with DVT) are **unilateral pain and edema** of an extremity [2]. Other symptoms include discoloration and color of the leg. Pain with foot dorsiflexion (Homans' sign) is neither sensitive nor specific in nonpregnant patients, but data are lacking in patients who are pregnant. Compared with the nonpregnant patient, in whom distal vein thrombosis is more common, **most events in pregnancy are ileofemoral,** and patients may manifest with unusual symptoms, such as isolated buttock, groin, flank, or abdominal pain [3]. PE is not detected clinically in 70%–80% of patients in whom it is detected postmortem. Most patients who die of PE do so within 30 minutes of the event, reinforcing the need for rapid and accurate diagnosis [4]. Clinical presentation of PE can range from low-grade pyrexia, dyspnea, tachypnea, chest pain, or hemoptysis to cardiovascular collapse. Due to common nonspecific symptoms during pregnancy, diagnosis of VTE can be challenging. Clinical suspicion of DVT is confirmed in 10% of pregnant patients compared with 25% of nonpregnant patients, and PE is confirmed in only 4% of pregnant patients [5].

EPIDEMIOLOGY AND INCIDENCE

VTE is **one of the leading causes of pregnancy-related maternal morbidity and mortality in high-income countries** [6]. Fatal PE accounts for **9.8% of all pregnancy related deaths in the United States** [7]. Due to physiological and anatomical changes normally associated with pregnancy, the risk of VTE in women during pregnancy and immediately postpartum is higher than women who are the same age and not pregnant. **The risk of VTE is increased fivefold during pregnancy and 60-fold during the first three months after birth** [8]. A systematic review to evaluate the risk of VTE during the postpartum period demonstrated a substantially higher risk during the first six weeks postpartum with a gradual decline with every week after delivery; however, it is not entirely clear from these data exactly when a woman's risk of VTE returns to baseline levels [9]. This **risk might persist until at least 12 weeks postpartum** [10]. Although the relative risk of VTE is greatly increased, the **absolute risk is estimated at around one to two in 1000 pregnancies** [11]. Although much of the evidence suggests an incidence is equally distributed throughout all trimesters, a recent study suggested an exponential increase in the risk across the duration of pregnancy [12]. The **highest risk is in the puerperium** likely because of the addition of trauma to the pelvic vessels during delivery. Unlike nonpregnant women, in which distal DVT is more common, the anatomic distribution of DVT in pregnant women differs from that for nonpregnant patients. In addition to what was previously known—that **left-sided DVT is more common** in pregnancy—this study also found that proximal DVT restricted to the **femoral or iliac veins** is also more common (>60% of cases) [13]. **PE occurs in 15% of untreated DVTs with a mortality rate of 1% and in 4.5% of treated DVTs with a mortality rate of 1%** [14]. Death from PE occurs in about every 1.1–1.5 per 100,000 pregnancies [15].

GENETICS

Thrombophilic disorders can be inherited or acquired. About 50% of patients with thrombosis have an identifiable underlying genetic disorder [16]. Approximately 50%–60% of patients with a hereditary basis for thrombosis or a thrombophilia do not experience a thrombotic event until one other risk factor is present [17]. Tables 27.1 through 27.4 summarize the prevalence, risk of VTE, testing characteristics, and management for the different inherited thrombophilias [18] (see Chapter 27).

Antiphospholipid syndrome (APS) is the most important acquired thrombophilia of pregnancy and is defined by specific levels of circulating antiphospholipid antibodies and one of the clinical criteria, which include vascular thrombosis or recurrent miscarriages, unexplained death of a fetus after 10 weeks of gestation, or premature birth before 34 weeks due to eclampsia or preeclampsia [18] (see Chapter 26). Current evidence does not support inherited thrombophilia or APS

screening [19]. However, expert opinion suggest screening may be considered in cases of personal history of VTE that was associated with a noncurrent risk factor (e.g., fractures, surgery, and prolonged immobilization) or a first-degree relative with a high-risk thrombophilia [20].

ETIOLOGY/BASIC PATHOPHYSIOLOGY

The coagulation cascade is briefly and schematically shown in Figure 28.1. Pregnancy is associated with marked alterations in the proteins of the coagulation and fibrinolytic systems [20–22] (see Chapter 3 in *Obstetric Evidence Based Guidelines*) (Table 28.1). A tendency for excessive clotting seems to be an adaptive mechanism to prevent excessive bleeding at delivery. At delivery, about 120 spiral arteries are denuded while carrying about 12% of the woman's cardiac output every minute. Much of the prevention in bleeding is due to myometrial contraction, but there are also marked increased clotting capacity, impaired fibrinolysis, and decreased natural anticoagulant activity in pregnancy. Pregnancy and postpartum are characterized by the presence of the three components of Virchow's triad, which contribute to the increased risk of VTE:

1) **Hypercoagulable blood**: Increased clotting potential, decreased anticoagulant activity, and decreased fibrinolysis occurs during pregnancy to prepare for the hemostatic challenges of delivery. Mechanisms driving this state include the following:
   - Increase in the levels of Fibrinogen (factor II) and factor V, VII, VIII, IX, X, and XII levels [23]. The generation of fibrin also increases markedly.
   - The anticoagulant activity of protein S is decreased by about 40% although the levels of protein C remain normal [24].
   - Thrombus dissolution (fibrinolysis) is decreased from increased plasminogen activator inhibitor type 1 and 2 activity and decreased tissue plasminogen activator activity [23].
2) **Venous stasis**: Caused by progesterone-induced venodilatation, venous compression by the gravid uterus, compression of the left iliac vein by the right iliac artery, and immobilization.
3) **Vascular damage**: Due to venous distention, vaginal, assisted vaginal, and cesarean deliveries [25].

RISK FACTORS/ASSOCIATIONS

Risk factors are shown in Table 28.2, with the most common in pregnancy including a **personal history of thrombosis** [4] (15%–25% of all cases of VTE are recurrent events) [26], **age 35 years or more, multiparity, obesity, multiple pregnancy, assisted vaginal or cesarean delivery, immobilization, smoking, and the presence of inherited or acquired thrombophilia** (see Chapters 26 and 27) [27]. About 50% of cases of VTE in pregnancy are associated with an inherited or acquired thrombophilia [15].

COMPLICATIONS

DVT: Risk of PE, post-thrombotic syndrome from venous hypertension due to thrombotic obstruction, which presents with signs and symptoms of chronic venous insufficiency [28].

PE: Risk of death, pulmonary hypertension, and right ventricular failure [29].

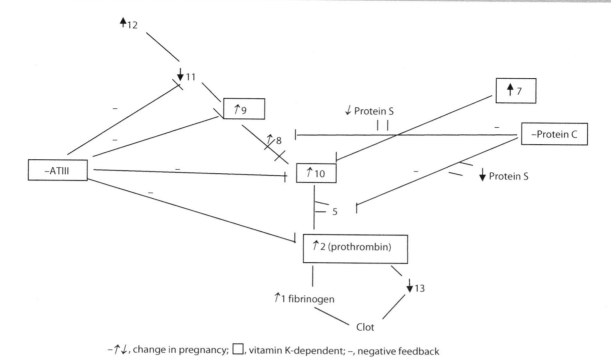

−↑↓, change in pregnancy; □, vitamin K-dependent; −, negative feedback

Figure 28.1 Coagulations cascade and some pregnancy changes.

Table 28.1 Changes in the Normal Functioning of the Coagulation System during Pregnancy

Coagulant Factors	Change in Pregnancy
Procoagulants	
Fibrinogen	Increased
Factor VII	Increased
Factor VIII	Increased
Factor X	Increased
von Willebrand factor	Increased
Plasminogen activator inhibitor-1	Increased
Plasminogen activator inhibitor-2	Increased
Factor II	No change
Factor V	No change
Factor IX	No change
Anticoagulants	
Free protein S	Decreased
Protein C	No change
Antithrombin III	No change

MANAGEMENT
Principles

Given the paucity of data regarding diagnosis and treatment in pregnancy, most data are derived from the nonpregnant general population.

Diagnosis

A full history and physical examination should be the initial steps in the diagnoses of DVT or PE, but objective testing is essential because **clinical assessment alone is unreliable** and the consequences of misdiagnosis are serious. To diagnose VTE, clinical suspicion must remain high. Only about 25% of

patients who present with symptoms of DVT have a definitive diagnosis of DVT on objective testing [30]. However, in symptomatic pregnant women, DVT and PE appear less prevalent due to the fact that symptoms such as lower extremity edema, chest pain, and dyspnea can be common in pregnancy. The **prevalence of DVT is about 8% in pregnant women with suspected DVT, and the prevalence of PE is about 5% in pregnant women with suspected PE** [31]. A concern with diagnostic tests has been the potential side effects of fetal radiation exposure. Epidemiologic studies have shown that exposure to radiation of less than a cumulative dose of 5 rads has not been associated with significant risk for fetal injury [32]. The diagnostic tests shown in Table 28.3 are all below the safe limit. Some case-controlled studies, however, have shown a slight increase of childhood cancers [33]. No increase in pregnancy loss, growth retardation, or mental retardation has been found [34].

Deep Vein Thrombosis

During pregnancy, thrombosis most frequently begins in the veins of the calf or in the iliofemoral segment of the deep venous system and has a striking predilection for the left leg [35–37] (85%–90%), possibly because of the compressive effects on the left iliac vein by the right iliac artery where they cross [38]. Although clinical assessment using clinical decision rules has been demonstrated to be very successful in assigning pretest probability outside of pregnancy, the studies deriving and validating this model did not include pregnant patients [39].

In nonpregnant women, D dimer can also be used in combination with clinical probability score to diagnose DVT [40]. However, **D Dimer values increase progressively throughout pregnancy, limiting its utility** [41]. Although **a low D dimer may be helpful in ruling out DVT**, a positive (high) D Dimer result will be common in pregnancy and

Table 28.2   Conditions Associated with Increased Risks for VTE (Pregnant and Nonpregnant Women)

Previous VTE
Thrombophilia
Advancing age
Obesity
Surgery
Trauma
Active cancer
Acute medical illnesses, e.g., acute myocardial infarction, heart
  failure, respiratory failure, infection
Inflammatory bowel disease
Antiphospholipid syndrome
Dyslipoproteinemia
Nephrotic syndrome
Paroxysmal nocturnal hemoglobinuria
Myeloproliferative diseases
Behcets syndrome
Varicose veins
Superficial vein thrombosis
Congenital venous malformation
Long-distance travel
Prolonged bed rest
Immobilization
Limb paresis
Chronic care facility stay
Pregnancy/puerperium
Oral contraceptives
Hormone replacement therapy
Heparin-induced thrombocytopenia
Other drugs
  -Chemotherapy
  -Tamoxifen
  -Thalidomide
  -Antipsychotics
Central venous catheter
Vena cava filter
Intravenous drug abuse

Source: Modified from American College of Obstetrics and Gynecology. Thromboembolism in pregnancy. *ACOG* 2011; 123, Reaffirmed 2014.

Table 28.3   Radiation Exposures of Diagnostic Tests for VTE

Test	Radiation Exposure (Rads)
Chest X-ray	0.001
Perfusion scan	0.018
Ventilation scan	0.019
Helical CT	0.005
Limited venography	0.050
Pulmonary angiography	0.221
Compression u/s	none
MRI	none

always require confirmatory testing [42]. **Compressive ultrasonography is now the primary modality for the diagnosis of DVT in pregnancy** (Figure 28.2). This method is noninvasive, and there is no radiation exposure to the fetus. It has a sensitivity of 97% and a specificity of 94% for the diagnosis of proximal DVT in nonpregnant patients [43,44]. The sensitivity and specificity is lower for distal DVT (i.e., DVT isolated to the paired calf veins, peroneal, anterior tibial, and posterior tibial veins) and for iliac vein thrombosis [45]. When iliac vein thrombosis is suspected, the available options include 1) venography, 2) magnetic resonance imaging, or 3) pulse

Doppler and/or direct visualization of the iliac vein [44]. In cases of confirmed DVT with compression ultrasonography, treatment should be initiated. In cases of negative results and no suspicion of iliac vein process, surveillance is recommended. When tests are negative or equivocal and there is **suspicion of thrombosis, patients can either have additional imaging studies, such as venography or serial noninvasive testing,** or have presumptive anticoagulation therapy started [45].

Pulmonary Embolism

The accurate diagnosis of PE in pregnancy is imperative. If undiagnosed, it can be fatal whereas treating patients with anticoagulation can expose them to unnecessary risks of such therapy. **The approach to diagnosing PE in pregnancy is similar to that of the nonpregnant patient** (Figure 28.3).

If the clinical features are compatible with PE, **V/Q scan is one of the tests of choice** [46]. If the test is normal, PE is excluded. If a segmental defect in perfusion with normal ventilation (high probability lung scan) is seen, the diagnosis of PE is confirmed [31]. About 40%–60% of V/Q scans are diagnostic (either high probability or normal). **Patients with nondiagnostic lung scans can undergo compression ultrasound or CT pulmonary angiography (CTPA)**. A limitation of V/Q scan in the nonpregnant population is that most scans are nondiagnostic, in which the incidence of PE varies widely from 10% to 30%. In pregnant patients, however, fewer patients will have nondiagnostic scans, likely due to less concomitant respiratory disease and hyperdynamic pulmonary circulation [47].

CTPA is also an additional first line-imaging test available. It is usually preferred in nonpregnant patients for several reasons: 1) the specificity is higher than V/Q (>90% vs. 10%), 2) CTPA may identify alternative diagnosis as cause of the symptoms, and 3) CTPA is more widely accessible [48]. Despite its advantages, the sensitivity and specificity of CTPA can be affected by the location of the embolus. CTPA is more sensitive for the detection of central arteries and can miss subsegmental emboli [49]. CTPA has also been associated with increased risk of breast cancer [50]. Regardless of the method chosen for diagnosing PE, both are not associated with high-dose radiation exposure to the fetus. Doppler US of the lower extremities can also be initially performed because the diagnosis of DVT may confirm PTE indirectly and the therapy is the same for both conditions [51].

Pulmonary angiography remains the gold standard for ruling out PE. This test requires expertise for performance and interpretation and is invasive. Thus, it is held in reserve for patients in whom the diagnosis cannot be made or excluded on the basis of less invasive testing.

MANAGEMENT: CLINICAL SCENARIOS AND ANTICOAGULATION

Despite an increased risk of DVT/PE associated with pregnancy and the postpartum period, routine anticoagulation therapy is not currently recommended due to possible complications that can arise with this therapy [52,53]. Anticoagulation is recommended in those patients with an acute thromboembolism or with risk factors including a prior history of DVT/PE or a diagnosed thrombophilia. **Table 28.4 shows proposed management of patients based on risk factors for VTE in pregnancy.**

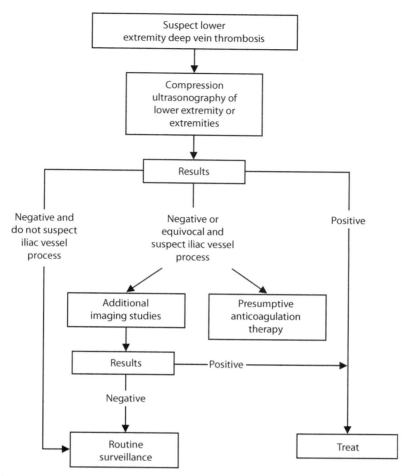

Figure 28.2   Diagnosis of DVT during pregnancy. (Courtesy of Leo R. Brancazio; American College of Obstetrics and Gynecology. Thromboembolism in pregnancy. *ACOG* 2011; 123, Reaffirmed 2014.)

The anticoagulants that have been evaluated for the prevention and treatment of VTE in pregnancy include heparin and heparin-like compounds (UFH, LMWH, heparinoids, and pentasaccharide) and coumadin derivatives (warfarin). There is limited evidence for safety and efficacy on new oral anticoagulants, such as rivaroxaban, apixaban, or edoxaban [54]. UFH and LMWH are the anticoagulants most often used given their safety and efficacy during pregnancy.

Unfractionated Heparin (UFH)

The word heparin derives from the Greek "hepar," liver, the organ in which it was first isolated from. UFH exerts its anticoagulation action by two mechanisms of action: 1) stimulation of anti-thrombin III (ATIII) activity, which inhibits factor 2, 9, 10, and 11 and 2) direct factor 10 inhibition [55]. It does not cross the placenta and is safe for the fetus; however, it has been associated with adverse effects in the mother, including bleeding, skin reactions, heparin-induced thrombocytopenia (HIT) and osteoporosis [56].

Bleeding
The rate of major maternal bleeding in pregnant patients treated with UFH therapy is about 2%, which is consistent with the reported rates of bleeding associated with heparin therapy in nonpregnant patients [57] and with warfarin [58].

UFH half-life is about 1.5 hours. This short half-life makes it the preferred anticoagulation around the time of delivery or surgery. The anticoagulant effect lasts for about 8–12 hours and its effect can be reversed with protamine sulfate if necessary. PTT can be obtained to verify clearance. Recent UFH administration is not a contraindication to regional anesthesia as long as the PTT is not prolonged.

Heparin Induced Thrombocytopenia (HIT)
Approximately 3% of nonpregnant patients receiving UFH acquire HIT [59]. HIT is very rare in pregnancy and is an adverse reaction to heparin in which antibodies to platelets form. These antibodies can activate platelets and lead to life-threatening arterial and venous thrombosis. It should be suspected with a fall in platelet count >50% from baseline or <100,000/microL, antibodies to heparin, skin lesions at the injection site, and systemic reaction after IV injection **5–15 days after commencing heparin** [59]. It should be differentiated from a transient thrombocytopenia that can occur with initiation of UFH due to platelet clumping. **Platelet counts should be checked about five days after initiation of UFH and periodically for the first two weeks.** Definitive laboratory data using HIT antibody testing (e.g., immunoassay and sometimes functional assay) may not be available for several days, and it may be necessary to make a presumptive diagnosis of HIT while awaiting these data. In

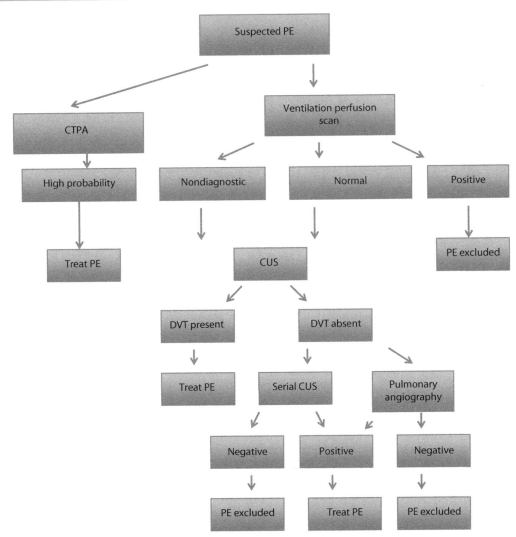

Figure 28.3　Workup for suspected pulmonary embolus. (From American College of Obstetrics and Gynecology. Thromboembolism in pregnancy. *ACOG* 2011; 123, Reaffirmed 2014.)

pregnant women who are diagnosed with HIT and require anticoagulation, **alternative options** include use of the heparinoid, danaparoid sodium (does not cross the placenta but unavailable in the United States [60], or **fondaparinux**, a synthetic pentasaccharide and selective factor Xa inhibitor. A retrospective study comparing fondaparinux with enoxaparin found no effects of fondaparinux on mother or infant; however, some anticoagulant activity has been detected in umbilical cord blood of exposed infants [61–63]. Fondaparinux has been recommended by the Pregnancy and Thrombosis Working Group as an alternative for patients with HIT [64].

Heparin-Induced Osteoporosis
Symptomatic vertebral fractures have been reported to occur in about 2% to 3% of heparin-treated patients and significant reductions in bone mineral density in up to 30% of patients receiving **long-term** UFH [65]. The mean bone loss is about 5% with unclear reversibility. **LMWH has a lower risk of osteopenia than UFH.**

Low Molecular Weight Heparin (LMWH)

LMWH has become **the anticoagulant of choice during pregnancy.** LMWH exerts its anticoagulation action by stimulation of antithrombin III activity, inhibiting in particular factor 10 (not factor 2). Multiple studies have found LMWH to be more effective, associated with lower risk of hemorrhagic complications and with lower mortality than UFH in the treatment of DVT in nonpregnant women [66,67]. In a *Cochrane* review of 22 studies with more than 8000 patients with DVT and PE, **LMWH was associated with lower rates of VTE recurrence or extension, lower mortality, and less bleeding during the initial treatment period** [68]. Also, **the risk of HIT is substantially lower with LMWH as well as the risk of heparin-induced osteoporosis** [69], and there are **fewer allergic skin reactions**. The other advantage is a longer plasma life and a more predictable response than UFH [70]. LMWH does not cross the placenta, and studies have supported its safety on maternal and fetal outcomes [71].

The dosing of LMWH remains controversial. The anticoagulant effect of LMWH lasts for 18–24 hours. Pregnant

Table 28.4 Recommended Thromboprophylaxis for Pregnancies Complicated by Inherited Thrombophilias and/or History of VTE

Clinical Scenario	Antepartum Management	Postpartum Management[a]
Low-risk thrombophilia[b] without previous VTE	Surveillance without anticoagulation therapy or prophylactic LMWH or UFH	Surveillance without anticoagulation therapy or postpartum anticoagulation therapy if the patient has additional risks factors[c]
Low-risk thrombophilia[b] with a single previous episode of VTE—not receiving long-term anticoagulation therapy	Prophylactic or intermediate-dose LMWH/UFH or surveillance without anticoagulation therapy	Postpartum anticoagulation therapy or intermediate-dose LMWH/UFH
High-risk thrombophilia[d] without previous VTE	Prophylactic LMWH or UFH	Postpartum anticoagulation therapy
High-risk thrombophilia[d] with a single previous episode of VTE—not receiving long-term anticoagulation therapy	Prophylactic, intermediate-dose, or adjusted-dose LMWH/UFH regimen	Postpartum anticoagulation therapy or intermediate or adjusted-dose LMWH/UFH for 6 weeks (therapy level should be at least as high as antepartum treatment)
Previous single episode of VTE associated with transient risk factor that is no longer present—excludes pregnancy- or estrogen-related risk factor but no thrombophilia	Surveillance without anticoagulation therapy	Postpartum anticoagulation therapy[e]
Previous single episode of VTE associated with transient risk factor that was pregnancy- or estrogen-related, but no thrombophilia	Prophylactic-dose LMWH or UFH[e]	Postpartum anticoagulation therapy
Previous single episode of VTE without an associated risk factor (idiopathic)—Not receiving long-term anticoagulation therapy but no thrombophilia	Prophylactic-dose LMWH or UFH[e]	Postpartum anticoagulation therapy
Two or more episodes of VTE—not receiving long-term anticoagulation therapy with or without thrombophilia	Prophylactic or therapeutic-dose LMWH or Prophylactic or therapeutic-dose UFH	Postpartum anticoagulation therapy or Therapeutic-dose LMWH/UFH for 6 weeks
Two or more episodes of VTE—Receiving long-term anticoagulation therapy, with or without thrombophilia	Therapeutic-dose LMWH or UFH	Resumption of long-term anticoagulation therapy

Source: Modified from American College of Obstetrics and Gynecology. Thromboembolism in pregnancy. *ACOG* 2011; 123, Reaffirmed 2014.

Abbreviations: LMWH, low molecular weight heparin; UFH, unfractionated heparin; VTE, venous thromboembolism.

[a]Postpartum treatment levels should be greater or equal to antepartum treatment. Treatment of acute VTE and management of antiphospholipid syndrome are addressed in other Practice Bulletins.

[b]Low-risk thrombophilia: factor V Leiden heterozygous; prothrombin *G20210A* heterozygous; protein C or protein S deficiency.

[c]First-degree relative with a history of a thrombotic episode before age 50 years or other major thrombotic risk factors (e.g., obesity, prolonged immobility).

[d]High-risk thrombophilia: antithrombin deficiency; double heterozygous for prothrombin *G20210A* mutation and factor V Leiden; factor V Leiden homozygous or prothrombin *G20210A* mutation homozygous.

[e]Surveillance without anticoagulation is supported as an alternative approach by some experts.

women may require increases in dalteparin dose of 10%–20% compared with doses of nonpregnant women to reach the target anti-Xa levels [72–74]. Anticoagulation with LMWH may need to be monitored in pregnant women and the dose adjusted to reach the target Xa level, which decreases the logistical and financial benefits of LMWH. The therapeutic anti-Xa level for adjusted-dose therapy is 0.5–1.2 U/mL. The target anti-Xa level for prophylactic dose therapy is 0.2–0.4 U/mL. To achieve these levels, often dosing every 12 hours is necessary even for prophylaxis in pregnancy. Twice-daily dosing of enoxaparin may be necessary to maintain anti-Xa activity above 0.1 IU/mL throughout a 24-hour period in pregnant women [6,65,67]. Enoxaparin 40 mg every 12 hours (instead of once daily) has been suggested for prophylactic anticoagulation in women at or above 90 kg [6]. It is not known whether a specific minimum level of anti-Xa activity is necessary throughout the day to prevent thrombosis in pregnancy or whether maintaining a specific minimum level of anti-Xa activity for only a portion of the day is sufficient. Anti-Xa levels may be used especially for obese and for renal disease patients [6].

Warfarin (Coumadin)

Vitamin K derives its name from the German word *koagulation*. Warfarin derivatives are vitamin K antagonists (VKAs) and inhibit vitamin K-dependent factors (2, 7, 9, 10, and proteins C and S). VKA **crosses the placenta** and **can cause bleeding and teratogenicity in the fetus** [75]. Warfarin is believed to be safe in the first six weeks of gestation, but has been associated with **warfarin embryopathy in 4%–5% of fetuses when maternal exposure is between six and nine weeks**. Warfarin embryopathy is characterized by **skeletal (stippled epiphyses), nasal, and limb (hypoplasia) involvement. Bleeding in the fetus can occur in all trimesters**. There are cases in which warfarin is the preferred anticoagulation despite its risks. These include women with mechanical heart valves, those who have a recurrence while receiving heparin, and those with contraindications to heparin therapy. In a systematic review of observational studies between 1966 and 1997 that reported outcome with various anticoagulant regimens in pregnant women with **mechanical prosthetic heart valves**, VKAs were associated with the lowest risk of valve thrombosis and systemic embolism (3.9%)

[76]. In general, four possible regimens can be considered in patients with mechanical heart valves: 1) VKAs throughout pregnancy, 2) either therapeutic LMWH or UFH between six and 12 weeks and close to term only and VKAs at other times, 3) careful therapeutic UFH throughout pregnancy, or 4) careful therapeutic LMWH throughout pregnancy. Patient should understand the risks and benefits and options before making a decision. Warfarin does not induce an anticoagulant effect in the breast-fed infant when the drug is given to a nursing mother [77,78]. Therefore, the use of warfarin in breast-feeding women who require postpartum anticoagulant therapy is safe.

Aspirin

Low dose aspirin (60–150 mg) can be administered safely during the second and third trimesters in women at risk for hypertensive complications and/or fetal growth restriction (FGR) [79,80]. The safety of higher doses of aspirin and/or aspirin ingestion during the first trimester remains uncertain with potential reported complications during the first trimester including birth defects (e.g., gastroschisis) and bleeding.

TREATMENT OF NEW ONSET DVT AND PE IN PREGNANCY

There are no RCTs for treatment of DVT specific to pregnant women. **Therapeutic doses** are recommended in patients with an acute VTE [81]. As previously mentioned, **LMWH is the preferred option. Weight-adjusted doses** are used for the treatment of acute VTE, and requirements may alter as pregnancy progresses because the volume of distribution of LMWH changes and glomerular filtration rate increased in the second trimester [81]. **Bid or daily regimens (1.5 mg/kg) can be used** without a risk of recurrence with the once daily dosing vs. the bid regimen [82]. Table 28.5 shows recommended heparin doses. **It is not clear whether adjustment of dosing is necessary**; however, based on conclusions of some small studies, dose can be increased to maintain a **therapeutic anti-Xa LMWH level in the range of 0.6–1.0 units/ml**, and slightly higher doses may be needed for a once daily regimen. **Measurement of anti-Xa levels can be done every one to three months, four to six hours after injection.** Patients are usually **converted to a subcutaneous therapeutic dose of UFH in the last month of pregnancy.** In this case, aPTT should be obtained six hours after injection and dose modified to achieve an aPTT of 1.2–2.5 [25]. Platelets should be checked for HIT in cases of UFH, but data is less clear regarding LMWH [83,84]. Intravenous UFH may be preferred in cases in which delivery, surgery, or thrombolysis (indicated for severe PE with hemodynamic compromise) [85] is necessary. Other options for treatment of life-threatening PE include catheter-assisted thrombus removal and surgical embolectomy. Embolectomy has been associated with a 20%–40% incidence of fetal loss, so this treatment should be restricted to cases in which the woman's life is endangered [86].

Duration of therapeutic anticoagulation treatment after an acute episode of VTE in pregnancy and postpartum should be a minimum of three months with many experts recommending six months [81]. Controversy exists on whether the dose of LMWH or UFH can be reduced after the initial therapeutic anticoagulation. Some suggest continuation of therapeutic doses during pregnancy and postpartum, and others have proposed lowering the dose to an intermediate dose regimen [87] or 75% of a full-treatment

Table 28.5 Anticoagulation Regimens

Management Type	Dosage
Prophylactic LMWH[a]	Enoxaparin, 40 mg SC once[b] daily
	Dalteparin, 5000 units SC once daily
	Tinzaparin, 4500 units SC once daily
Therapeutic LMWH[c] (also referred to as weight-adjusted, full-treatment dose)	Enoxaparin, 1 mg/kg every 12 hours
	Dalteparin, 200 units/kg once daily
	Tinzaparin, 175 units/kg once daily
	Dalteparin, 100 units/kg every 12 hours
Minidose prophylactic UFH	UFH, 5000 units SC every 12 hours
Prophylactic UFH	UFH, 5000–10,000 units SC every 12 hours
	UFH, 5000–7500 units SC every 12 hours in first trimester
	UFH, 7500–10,000 units SC every 12 hours in the second trimester
	UFH, 10,000 units SC every 12 hours in the third trimester, unless the aPTT is elevated
Therapeutic UFH (also referred to as weight-adjusted, full-treatment dose)	UFH, 10,000 units or more SC every 12 hours in doses adjusted to target aPTT in the therapeutic range (1.5–2.5, 6 hours after injection)
Postpartum anticoagulation	Prophylactic LMWH/UFH for 4–6 weeks
	or
	Vitamin K antagonists for 4–6 weeks with a target INR of 2.0–3.0, with initial UFH or LMWH therapy overlap until the INR is 2.0 or more for 2 days
Surveillance[d]	

Source: Modified from American College of Obstetrics and Gynecology. Thromboembolism in pregnancy. *ACOG* 2011; 123, Reaffirmed 2014.
Abbreviations: aPTT, activated partial thromboplastin time; INR, international normalized ratio; LMWH, low molecular weight heparin; SC, subcutaneously; UFH, unfractionated heparin.
[a]Although at extremes of body weight, modification of dose may be required.
[b]Some advocate twice a day.
[c]May target an anti-Xa level in the therapeutic range of 0.6–1.0 units/mL for twice daily regimen; slightly higher doses may be needed for a once-daily regimen.
[d]Clinical vigilance and appropriate objective investigation of women with symptoms suspicious of deep vein thrombosis or pulmonary embolism may be needed.

dose [88], which has been successfully used in patients at high risk, such as cancer patients.

Women with antithrombin deficiency, antiphospholipid antibodies, homozygous or combined thrombophilias, or previous VTE may benefit from indefinite anticoagulation, but this should be decided by an internist after pregnancy [89]. Long-term, low-intensity warfarin therapy is associated with an about 50% prevention of recurrent VTE, major hemorrhage, or death in patients with a prior idiopathic VTE [90].

Inferior vena cava (IVC) filters should be restricted to women with proven VTE and either recurrent PE despite adequate anticoagulation or contraindications to anticoagulation [51]. Suprarenal placement is recommended. Careful evaluation should be undertaken because filter placement is associated with complications, such as migration, filter fracture, and IVC perforation [51].

In the initial management of DVT, the leg should be elevated and a gradual elastic compression stocking applied to reduce edema. Traditionally, it was thought that mobilization could dislodge an unstable thrombus and cause PE. Randomized controlled trials have shown the opposite. **Early ambulation with leg compression does not increase PE or thrombus propagation, and leg pain and edema improve faster** [89].

The **use of thrombolytic agents** during pregnancy has been limited to life-threatening situations because of the risk of substantial maternal bleeding, especially at the time of delivery and immediately postpartum [91]. The risk of placental abruption and fetal death due to these drugs is currently unknown.

Embolectomy, another treatment option when conservative treatment fails, is indicated to prevent death in patients who are hemodynamically unstable despite anticoagulation and treatment with vasopressors [92]. Embolectomy has been associated with a 20%–40% incidence of fetal loss [93], so this treatment must be restricted to cases in which the woman's life is endangered.

PREVENTION OF VTE

Avoidance of risk factors (Table 28.2) is the key to the prevention of VTE and its complications. **Preconception counseling** should review preventative measures as well as review in detail any prior history of VTE or known thrombophilia. In general, for a pregnant patient with a prior VTE, prophylactic anticoagulation is recommended, but this can be modified based on the cause of the VTE and the presence of a thrombophilia. See Table 28.4 for further recommendations.

Women with a history of VTE (with or without thrombophilia) are believed to have a higher **risk of recurrence** in subsequent pregnancies. Estimates of the rate of recurrent venous thrombosis during pregnancy in women with a history of VTE have varied **between 1% and 10%** [94–97]. The higher of these estimates has prompted recommendation for anticoagulant prophylaxis during pregnancy and the postpartum period in women with a history of VTE. However, the risk is likely to be lower than has been suggested by some of these studies because they were retrospective with the possibility of significant bias. The risk is dramatically influenced by risk factors, in particular the presence of thrombophilias (Table 28.2 and Chapter 27).

There are very few randomized controlled trials (RCTs) for the prevention of VTE in pregnancy (both antepartum and postpartum). The sample sizes of all trials are small and often cannot be combined.

For antenatal prophylaxis, none of the RCTs included in the latest *Cochrane Review* reported on maternal mortality, and no differences were detected for the other primary outcomes of symptomatic thromboembolic events, symptomatic PE, and symptomatic DVT when LMWH or UFH was compared with no treatment/placebo or when LMWH was compared with UFH [98]. The RR for symptomatic VTE was antenatal LMWH/UFH versus no heparin, RR 0.33; 95% confidence interval (CI) 0.04 to 2.99 (two trials, 56 women); and antenatal LMWH versus UFH, RR 0.47; 95% CI 0.09 to 2.49 (four trials, 404 women). No differences were shown when antenatal LMWH or UFH was compared with no treatment/placebo for any secondary outcomes. Antenatal LMWH was associated with fewer adverse effects sufficient to stop treatment (RR 0.07; 95% CI 0.01 to 0.54; two trials, 226 women), and fewer fetal losses (RR 0.47; 95% CI 0.23 to 0.95; three trials, 343 women) when compared with UFH. In two trials, antenatal LMWH compared with UFH was associated with fewer bleeding episodes (defined in one trial of 121 women as bruises >1 inch, RR 0.18, 95% CI 0.09 to 0.36, and in one trial of 105 women as injection site hematomas of ≥2 cm, bleeding during delivery, or other bleeding, RR 0.28; 95% CI 0.15 to 0.53). The results for these secondary outcomes should be interpreted with caution, being derived from small trials that were not of high methodological quality [98].

In general, in pregnant women with a **prior VTE**, **prophylactic anticoagulation** can be used. This may be modified based on the cause of the first VTE and the presence of a thrombophilia. **If the prior VTE was related to a nonrecurrent cause** (i.e., broken bone and immobilization) **and the thrombophilia workup is negative**, the risk of recurrence is very low, and **prophylaxis may be avoided**, especially in women without other risk factors except pregnancy. In fact, the risk of recurrence was 0% in 44 such women followed without antepartum anticoagulation [99].

Approximately 50%–80% of gestational VTEs are associated with **heritable thrombophilia** (Chapter 27). Given that the background rate of VTE during pregnancy is approximately 1:1000, the absolute risk of VTE remains modest for the majority of these thrombophilias except antithrombin deficiency, homozygosity for the factor V Leiden mutation and for the prothrombin mutation, and combined defects. The absolute risk of pregnancy-associated VTE has been reported to range from 9% to 16% in homozygotes for the factor V Leiden mutation [100–103]. Double heterozygosity for the factor V Leiden and prothrombin gene mutations has been reported to have an absolute risk of pregnancy-associated VTE of 4.0% (95% CI, 1.4 to 16.9%) [104]. These data suggest that women with antithrombin deficiency, homozygosity for the factor V Leiden mutation, or the prothrombin mutation as well as double heterozygotes, should be managed more aggressively than those with other low-risk inherited thrombophilias, and thus **adjusted-dose therapeutic anticoagulation is recommended for prior DVT and a high risk thrombophila** (ATIII deficiency, homozygous factor V or prothrombin gene mutation, or double heterozygote). Therapeutic anticoagulation may also be used in pregnant women if the woman has had recurrent VTE episodes, life-threatening thrombosis, or thrombosis while receiving chronic anticoagulation. Filters in the inferior vena cava should be considered in this situation as well. In pregnant women with a **history of a prior VTE with history of a low risk thrombophilia** (heterozygous factor V or prothrombin gene, protein C or S), **prophylactic anticoagulation is recommended**. Persistent antiphospholipid antibodies are associated with an increased risk of VTE during pregnancy and the puerperium. It has been suggested that pregnant patients with the antiphospholipid syndrome who do not have a history of venous thrombosis receive a low-dose prophylactic regimen of heparin as well as those with previous thrombosis [65] (Chapter 26). The antepartum management of pregnant women with known thrombophilia and no prior VTE remains controversial because of our limited knowledge of the natural histories of various thrombophilias and a lack of trials of VTE prophylaxis. Prospective data is lacking regarding the issue of the incidence of VTE in a large group of pregnant women with known thrombophilia and no prior VTE. Currently, there is no evidence to suggest prophylactic low-dose anticoagulation in this group. If there is a very strong family history of VTE (especially at young ages), consideration can be made for low-dose prophylactic anticoagulation. Individualized risk assessment should be performed in this situation.

PROPHYLAXIS IN WOMEN WITH MECHANICAL HEART VALVES

Women who anticipate ultimately needing valve replacement surgery should be encouraged to complete childbearing before valve replacement. The highest risk for VTE is with first-generation mechanical valves (Starr-Edwards, Bjork-Shiley) in the mitral position, followed by second-generation valves (St Jude) in the aortic position. (Chapter 2). These women need to be **therapeutically anticoagulated throughout pregnancy and postpartum with blood levels frequently (usually weekly) checked to ensure therapeutic levels of anticoagulation**. Pregnant women with prosthetic heart valves pose a problem because of the **lack of trials** regarding the efficacy and safety of antithrombotic therapy during pregnancy. There is insufficient data to make definitive recommendations about optimal anticoagulation in pregnant patients with mechanical heart valves.

There are, in general, **four regimens** that can be considered: 1) VKAs throughout pregnancy, 2) either therapeutic LMWH or UFH between six weeks and 12 weeks and close to term only and to use VKAs at other times, 3) careful therapeutic UFH throughout pregnancy, and 4) careful therapeutic LMWH throughout pregnancy. Before any of these approaches is used, it is crucial to explain the risks/benefits carefully to the patient.

In a review, **VKAs throughout pregnancy** was the **regimen associated with the lowest risk of valve thrombosis/ systemic embolism** (3.9%); using UFH only between six and 12 weeks gestation was associated with an increased risk of valve thrombosis (9.2%) [105]. This analysis suggests that VKAs are more efficacious than UFH for thromboembolic prophylaxis of women with mechanical heart valves in pregnancy; however, coumarins increase the risk of **embryopathy**. In the first trimester coumarin is associated with a 10%–15% teratogenic risk (nasal hypoplasia, optic atrophy, digital anomalies, mental impairment). European experts have recommended warfarin therapy throughout pregnancy in view of the reports of poor maternal outcomes with heparin and their impression that the risk of embryopathy with coumarin derivatives has been overstated [106]. If coumarin is used, the dose should be adjusted to attain a target INR of 3.0 (range, 2.5 to 3.5).

A common option utilizes unfractionated **heparin during the first trimester to minimize teratogenesis, warfarin** for the majority of pregnancy (12–36 weeks), and unfractionated heparin again in the last month to prepare for delivery and allow for epidural anesthesia. Although this may be efficacious, fetal risk is not completely eliminated. **Substituting VKAs with heparin between six and 12 weeks** reduces the risk of fetopathic effects but possibly subjects the woman to an increased risk of thromboembolic complications. The reported high rates of thromboembolism with **UFH** might be explained by inadequate dosing and/or the use of an inappropriate target therapeutic range.

The use of **weight-adjusted therapeutic UFH** warrants careful monitoring and appropriate dose adjustment. A target aPTT ratio of at least twice the control should be attained [107]. If used, SC UFH should be initiated in high doses, usually every eight hours, and adjusted to prolong a six-hour postinjection aPTT into the therapeutic range (usually 60–80 seconds); strong efforts should be made to ensure an adequate anticoagulant effect. **LMWH** use in pregnant women with prosthetic heart valves has been associated with treatment failures [108–111], and the use of LMWH for this indication has recently become controversial due to a warning from a LMWH manufacturer regarding their safety in this situation [112]. If used, LMWH should be administered twice daily and dosed to achieve anti-Xa levels of 1.0 to 1.2 U/mL four to six hours (peak) after SC injection, with trough 0.6–0.7.

Extrapolating from data in nonpregnant patients with mechanical valves receiving warfarin therapy [113], for some high-risk women, **the addition of low-dose aspirin**, 75 to 162 mg/d, can be considered in an attempt to reduce the risk of thrombosis, recognizing that it increases the risk of bleeding.

ANTEPARTUM TESTING

No specific recommendations.

DELIVERY AND ANESTHESIA

For women on anticoagulation, a planned delivery, either through induction of labor or by cesarean delivery, may optimize timing of events and prevent the risks of an unplanned delivery. Patients can be recommended to withhold anticoagulation 12–24 hours (depending on the type of heparin used) prior to induction or scheduled cesarean delivery. Women are **usually converted to UFH near term** (e.g., 36 weeks) with the purpose of preventing the rare possibility of an epidural or spinal hematoma with regional anesthesia [114]. If regional anesthesia is planned and/or desired, UFH is usually stopped about 12 hours before the start of induction or cesarean delivery. The American Society of Regional Anesthesia and Pain Medicine Guidelines **support the use of neuraxial anesthesia in patients receiving 5000 Units of UFH bid**, but safety is unknown in higher doses, and individualized evaluation is recommended on a case-by-case basis. If spontaneous labor occurs after adjusted UFH doses occur, aPTT should be obtained and, if prolonged, reversal can be performed with protamine sulfate [31]. For LMWH, the American Society of Regional Anesthesia and Pain Medicine guidelines recommend **withholding neuraxial anesthesia for 10–12 hours after a prophylactic dose of LMWH or 24 hours after the last therapeutic dose of LMWH** [114].

For women not receiving regional anesthesia, if vaginal or cesarean delivery occurs more than four hours after a prophylactic dose of UFH, the patient is not at significant risk of hemorrhagic complications.

Pneumatic compression devices are recommended in patients in whom anticoagulation therapy has been temporarily withheld during delivery [4].

In cases in which VTE was diagnosed within two to four weeks prior to delivery, intravenous UFH can be used just prior to delivery and reversed with protamine. Removable filters can be placed to provide protection from PE during the time anticoagulation is stopped [31].

In women with mechanical heart valves, therapeutic anticoagulation can be continued IV (half-life: 1.5 hours) until active labor and then stopped during active labor and for delivery with therapeutic heparin restarted about 6–12 hours after delivery and warfarin restarted in an overlapping fashion (to avoid paradoxical thrombosis) 24–36 hours after delivery (the night after delivery). Extensive counseling on all these options and risks is required.

PROPHYLAXIS AFTER CESAREAN DELIVERY

Available data suggests that the risk of VTE is higher after **cesarean section** (especially emergent surgery) than after vaginal delivery [115]. The presence of additional risk factors for pregnancy-associated VTE (for example, prior VTE, thrombophilia, age >35 years, obesity, prolonged bed rest, and concomitant acute medical illness) may exacerbate this risk. Clinical judgment should be used to decide on anticoagulation after cesarean section, taking into account all of the patient's risk factors.

For postcaesarean/postnatal prophylaxis, only one RCT comparing five-day versus 10-day LMWH after caesarean section reported on maternal mortality, observing no deaths. No differences were seen across any of the comparisons for the other primary outcomes (symptomatic thromboembolic events, symptomatic PE, and symptomatic DVT). The RRs for symptomatic thromboembolic events were postcesarean LMWH/UFH versus no heparin, RR 1.30; 95% CI 0.39 to 4.27 (four trials, 840 women); postcesarean LMWH versus UFH, RR 0.33; 95% CI 0.01 to 7.99 (three trials, 217 women); postcesarean five-day versus 10-day LMWH, RR 0.36; 95% CI 0.01 to 8.78 (one trial, 646 women); postnatal UFH versus no heparin, RR 0.16; 95% CI 0.02 to 1.36 (one trial, 210 women). For prophylaxis after cesarean section, in one trial (of 580 women), women receiving UFH and physiotherapy were more likely to have bleeding complications than women receiving physiotherapy alone (RR 5.03; 95% CI 2.49 to 10.18) [98].

Use of a **pneumatic compression device** after cesarean delivery has been shown to provide a VTE risk reduction similar to universal prophylaxis with heparin while reducing the risks associated with anticoagulation [116]. Routine anticoagulation is not recommended in the universal population in the United States, but it is currently in the United Kingdom and other countries. For patients with additional risk factors from VTE, individual risk assessment may require prophylaxis with LMWH or UFH [82]. In women undergoing cesarean delivery with BMI >50 kg/m^2, previous VTE, or two or more additional risk factors for VTE (such as smoking, multiple gestation, BMI >30 kg/m^2, prolonged immobility, and infection), adding to mechanical prophylaxis pharmacological VTE prophylaxis, with either enoxaparin 40 mg daily or UH 5000 every 12 hours, should be considered. This pharmacological prophylaxis can start postoperatively, at 6 to 12 hours, after concerns for hemorrhage have decreased and can continue until full ambulation [117]. In certain cases, for example, women with anti-thrombin deficiency,

anti-thrombin concentrates can be used [4] (see Chapter 13 in *Obstetric Evidence Based Guidelines*).

POSTPARTUM MANAGEMENT OF ANTICOAGULATION

To minimize bleeding complications, anticoagulation with UFH or LMWH should be **restarted 4–6 hours after a vaginal delivery or 6–12 hours after cesarean delivery** and no sooner than **2 hours after epidural removal** [114]. Pneumatic compression devices should be left in place until patient is ambulating and anticoagulation is restarted. It has been proposed that anticoagulant therapy should be continued for at least 6 weeks postpartum and to allow a total duration of treatment of at least 3 months after a VTE [82].

Women who require more than 6 weeks of therapeutic anticoagulation postpartum can be bridged to warfarin, which is safe during breast-feeding [118]. Warfarin can be started with a 5-mg dose. If desired, warfarin can be started in an overlapping fashion (to avoid paradoxical thrombosis) 24–36 hours after delivery (the night after delivery). Daily testing of the international normalized ratio (INR) is recommended starting on day 2 of warfarin therapy and subsequent doses titrated to maintain the INR between 2.0 and 3.0. Heparin should be continued for the first five to seven days and can be discontinued once the INR is greater than 2.0 for at least 24 h [119]. In general, postpartum anticoagulation should be at levels at or higher those antepartum (Table 28.5).

Breast-feeding is safe while on anticoagulation (with either UFH, LMWH, or warfarin).

Thrombophilia testing should be considered once anticoagulation has been discontinued and only if this will influence the patient's future management [120].

CONTRACEPTION

Combined estrogen–progestin oral contraceptives have been associated with higher efficacy than progestin-only pills but have the disadvantage of an increased risk of VTE. This risk has been attributed to the estrogen component. In women taking estrogen-containing oral contraceptives, the risk of VTE increases 39-fold to 99-fold among those heterozygous for factor V Leiden and prothrombin G20210A mutations [121]. A meta-analysis of eight observational studies assessing the risk of VTE in women prescribed progestin oral contraception showed no increased risk compared with nonusers of hormonal contraception [122]. In a subanalysis of women prescribed injectable progestins, there was a twofold increase in thrombotic risk. Also, the type of progestin might influence this risk with newer progestins, such as desogestrel, gestodene, and norgestimate associated with a greater risk than older ones, such as levonorgestrel, lynestrenol, and noresthisterone [123–125]. Better contraceptive options for women at risk for VTE include the **intrauterine device (including those with estrogen) and progestin implants**. Barrier methods of contraception are also safe but less effective [126].

REFERENCES

1. Kesieme E, Chinenye K, Jebbin N, Irekpita E, Dongo A. Deep vein thrombosis: A clinical review. *J Blood Medicine* 2011; 2: 59–69. [Review]
2. James A. Venous thromboembolism in pregnancy. *Asterioscler Thromb Vasc Biol* 2009; 29: 326–31. [Review]

3. Rodger M. Evidence based for the management of venous thromboembolism in pregnancy. *Hematology* 2010. [Review]

4. American College of Obstetrics and Gynecology. Thromboembolism in pregnancy. *ACOG* 2011; 123, Reaffirmed 2014. [Review]

5. Dresang L, Fontaine P, Leeman L, King V. Venous thromboembolism during pregnancy. *Am Fam Physician* 2008; 77(12): 1709–16. [Review]

6. Geer IA. Thrombosis in pregnancy: Maternal and fetal issues. *Lancet* 1999; 353: 1258–65. [Review]

7. Pregnancy Mortality Surveillance System. CDC. [Review]

8. Pomp ER, Lenselink AM, Rosendaal FR, Doggen CJ, Dogge CJM. Pregnancy, the postpartum period and prothrombotic defects: Risks of venous thrombosis in the MEGA study. *J Thrombosis Haemostasis* 2008; 6940: 632–7. [II-2]

9. Jackson E, Curtis K, Gaffield M. Risk of venous thromboembolism during the postpartum period. A systematic review. *Obstet and Gynecol* 2011; 117: 691–703. [Review]

10. Kamel H, Navi BB, Siriam N, Hovsepian DA, Devereux RB, Elkind MS. Risk of thrombotic event after the 6-week postpartum period. *N Engl J Med* 2014: 370(14): 1307. [II-3]

11. Lussana F, Coppens M, Cattaneo M, Middeldorp S. Pregnancy-related venous thromboembolism: Risk and the effect of Thromboprophylaxis. *Thrombosis Res* 2012: 129: 673–80. [Review]

12. Virkus, RA, Lokkegaard EC, Bergholt T, Mogensen U, Langhoff-Ross J, Lidegaard O. Venous thromboembolism in pregnant and puerperal women in Denmark 1995–2005. A national cohort study. *Thromb Haemost* 2011; 106(2): 204–309. [II-2]

13. Chan WS, Spencer F, Ginsberg J. Anatomic distribution of deep vein thrombosis in pregnancy. *CMAJ* 2010; 182(7): 657–60. [Review]

14. Gherman RB, Goodwin TM, Leung B et al. Incidence, clinical characteristics and timing of objectively diagnosed venous thromboembolism during pregnancy. *Obstet Gynecol* 1999; 94: 730–4. [II-2]

15. Marik P, Plante L. Venous thromboembolic disease and pregnancy. *N Engl J Med* 2008; 359: 2025–33. [III]

16. Grandone E, Margaglione M, Colaizzo D et al. Genetic susceptibility to pregnancy-related thromboembolism: Roles of Factor V Leiden, Prothrombin G20210A, and methylenetetrahydrofolate reductase C677T mutations. *Am J Obstet Gynecol* 1998; 179:1324–8. [II-2]

17. National Institutes of Health Consensus Development Conference. Prevention of venous thrombosis and pulmonary embolism. *JAMA* 1986; 256: 744–9. [Review]

18. Antiphosphlipidsyndrome. Practice Bulletin, December 2012. The American College of Obstetrics and Gynecology. [Review]

19. Robertson L, Wu O, Langhorne P, Twaddle S, Clark P, Lowe GD, Walker ID, Greaves M, Brenkel I, Regan L, Greer IA. Thrombophilia in pregnancy: A systematic review. *Br J Haematol* 2006: 132: 171–96. [Review]

20. Inherited thrombophilias in pregnancy. Practice Bulletin September 2013. The American College of Obstetrics and Gynecology. [Review]

21. Lockwood CJ. Heritable coagulopathies in pregnancy. *Obstet Gynecol Surv* 1999; 54: 754. [Review]

22. Walker MC, Garner PR, Keely EJ et al. Changes in activated protein C resistance during normal pregnancy. *Am J Obstet Gynecol* 1997; 77: 162. [II-3]

23. Rosenkranz A, Hiden M, Leschnik B et al. Calibrated automated thrombin generation in normal uncomplicated pregnancy. *Thromb Haemost* 2008; 99: 331–7. [II-3]

24. Clark P, Brennand J, Conkie JA et al. Activated protein C sensitivity, protein C, protein S and coagulation in normal pregnancy. *Thromb Haemost* 1998; 79: 1166–70. [II-3]

25. Thromboembolism in pregnancy. Practice Bulletin August 2011. The American College of Obstetrics and Gynecology. [Review]

26. Pabinger I, Grafenhofer H, Quehenberger KP, Mannhalter C, Lechner K et al. Temporary increase in the risk of recurrence during pregnancy in women with a history of venous thromboembolism. *Blood* 2002; 100: 1060–2. [II-3]

27. Investigation and management of heritable thrombophilia. *Br J Haematol* 2001; 114–512. [Review]

28. Henke PK, Camerota AJ. An update on etiology, prevention and therapy of post thrombotic syndrome. *J Vasc Surg* 2011; 53(2): 500–9. [II-3]

29. Benotti JR, Ockene IS, Alpert JS, Dalen JE. The clinical profile of unresolved pulmonary embolism. *Chest* 1983; 84(6): 669. [II-3]

30. Hirsh J, Lee A. How we diagnose and treat deep vein thrombosis. *Blood* 2002; 99: 3102–10. [II-2]

31. Bates, S, Ginsberg J. How we manage venous thromboembolism during pregnancy. *Blood* 2002; 3470–8. [II-2]

32. Pabinger I, Grafnhofer H. Thrombosis during pregnancy: Risk factors, diagnosis and treatment. *Pathophysiol Haemost Thromb* 2002; 32: 322–4. [II-3]

33. Doll R, Wakefield R. Risk of childhood cancer from fetal radiation. *Br J Radiol* 1997; 70: 130–9. [II-2]

34. Ginsberg JS, Hirsh J, Ranbow AJ, Coates G. Risks to the fetus of radiologic procedures used in the diagnosis of maternal venous thromboembolic disease. *Thromb Haemost* 1989; 61: 189–96. [II-3]

35. Bergqvist D, Hedner U. Pregnancy and venous thromboembolism. *Acta Obstet Gynecol Scand* 1983; 62: 449–53. [Review]

36. Bergqvist A, Bergqvist D, Hallbook T. Deep vein thrombosis during pregnancy: A prospective study. *Acta Obstet Gynecol Scand* 1983; 62: 443–8. [II-1]

37. Hull RD, Raskob GE, Carter CJ. Serial impedance plethysmography in pregnant patients with clinically suspected deep-vein thrombosis: Clinical validity of negative findings. *Ann Intern Med* 1990; 112: 663–7. [II-2]

38. Cockett FB, Thomas ML, Negus D. Iliac vein compression: Its relation to iliofemoral thrombosis and the post-thrombotic syndrome. *BMJ* 1967; 2: 14–6. [II-2]

39. Wells PS, Owen C, Doucette S, Fergusson D, Tran H. Does this patient have deep vein thrombosis? *JAMA* 2006; 295: 199–207. [III]

40. Bates S, Jaeschke R, Stevens S, Goodacre S, Wells P, Stevenson M, Kearon C, Schunemann H, Crowther M, Pauker S, Makdissi R, Guyatt G. Antithrombotic therapy and prevention of thrombosis, 9th ed: American College of Chest Physicians evidence-based clinical practice guidelines. *Chest* 2012; e351S-e418S. [Review]

41. Kjellberg U, Anderson NE, Rosen S, Tenghorn L, Hellgren M. APC resistance and other haemostatic variables during pregnancy and puerperium. *Thromb Haemost* 1999; 81: 527–31. [II-3]

42. Michiels JJ, Freyburger G, van der Graaf F, Janssen M, Oortwijn W, Van Beek E. Strategies for the safe and effective exclusion and diagnosis of deep vein thrombosis by sequential use of clinical score, D-dimer testing, and compression ultrasonography. *Semin Thromb Hemost* 2000; 26(6): 657–67. [II-3]

43. Kearon C, Julian JA, Newman TE et al. Noninvasive diagnosis of deep vein thrombosis: McMaster diagnostic imaging practice guidelines initiative. *Ann Intern Med* 1998; 128: 663–77. [Review]

44. Chan WS, Ginsberg JS. Diagnosis of deep vein thrombosis and pulmonary embolism in pregnancy. *Thromb Res* 2002; 107: 85–91. [II-2]

45. Heijboer C, Beuler HR, Lensing AQ et al. A comparison of real time diagnosis of deep vein thrombosis in symptomatic outpatients. *N Engl J Med* 1993; 329: 1365–9. [II-2]

46. Bourjely G, Paidas M, Khalil H et al. Pulmonary embolism in pregnancy *Lancet* 2010; 375: 500–12. [Review]

47. Chan WS, Ray JG, Murray S et al. Suspected pulmonary embolism in pregnancy: Clinical presentation, results of lung scanning and subsequent maternal and pediatric outcomes. *Arch Intern Med* 2002; 162: 1170–5. [II-2]

48. Roy PM, Meyer G, Vielle B et al. Appropriateness of diagnostic management and outcomes of suspected pulmonary embolism. *Ann Intern Med* 2006; 144: 157–64. [Review]

49. Goodman LR, Curtin JJ, Mewissen MW et al. Detection of pulmonary embolism in patients with unresolved clinical and scintigraphic diagnosis: Helical CT vs angiography. *Am J Roentgenol* 1995; 164: 1369–74. [II-2]

50. Remy-Jardin M, Remy. Spiral CT angiography of the pulmonary circulation. *Radiology* 1999; 212: 615–36. [Review]

51. Greer IA. Thrombosis in pregnancy: Updates in diagnosis and management. *Hematology* 2012; 203–7. [Review]

52. Tooher R, Gates S, Dowswell T, Davis LJ. Prophylaxis for venous thromboembolic disease in pregnancy and the early postnatal period. *Cochrane Database System Rev* 2010; 5. [Review]

53. Che Yaakob CA, Dzarr AA, Ismail AA, Zuky Nik Lah NA, HoJJ. Anticoagulant therapy for deep vein thrombosis (DVT) in pregnancy. *Cochrane Database System Rev* 2010; 6. [Review]

54. Wells S, Forgie M, Rodger M. Treatment of venous thromboembolism. *JAMA* 2014; 311(7): 717–28. [Review]

55. Hirsh J, Anand S, Halperin J, Fuster V. Mechanism of action and pharmacology of unfractionated heparin. *Arterioscler Thromb Vascular Biol* 2001; 21: 1094–6. [II-3]

56. Nelson-Piercy C. Hazards of heparin: Allergy, heparin-induced thrombocytopenia and osteoporosis. *Bailliere's Clinical Obstet Gynaecol* 1997; 11: 489–509. [II-2]

57. Hull RD, Delmore TJ, Carter CJ et al. Adjusted subcutaneous heparin vs warfarin sodium in the long-term treatment of venous thrombosis. *N Engl J Med* 1982; 306: 189–94. [II-1]

58. Hull RD, Hirsh J, Jay R et al. Different intensities of oral anticoagulant therapy in the treatment of proximal-vein thrombosis. *N Engl J Med* 1982; 307: 1676–81. [II-3]

59. Warkentin TE, Levine MN, Hirsh J et al. Heparin-induced thrombocytopenia in patients treated with low molecular weight heparin or unfractionated heparin. *N Engl J Med* 1995; 332: 1330–5. [II-2]

60. Greinacher A, Eckhart T, Mussmann J, Mueller-Eckhardt C. Pregnancy complicated by heparin associated thrombocytopenia: Management by a prospectively in vitro selected heparinoid (Org 10172). *Thromb Res* 1993; 71: 123–6. [II-3]

61. Widmer M, Blum J, Hofmeyr GJ, Carroli G, Abdel-Aleem H, Lumbiganon P et al. Misoprostol as an adjunct to standard uterotonics for treatment of postpartum haemorrhage: A multicenter, double-blinded randomised trial. *Lancet* 2010; 375: 1808–13. [I]

62. Knol HM, Schultinge L, Erwich JJHM, Meijer K. Fondaparinux as an alternative anticoagulant therapy during pregnancy. *J Thromb Haemost* 2010; 8: 1876–9. [Review]

63. Dempfle CE. Minor transplacental passage of fondaparinux in vivo. *N Engl J Med* 2004; 350: 1914–5. [II-3]

64. Duhl AJ, Paidas MJ, Ural SH, Branch W, Casele H, Cox-Gill J et al. Pregnancy and Thrombosis working group. Antithrombotic therapy and pregnancy: Concensus report and recommendations for prevention and treatment of venous thromboembolism and adverse pregnancy outcomes. *Am J Obstet Gynecol* 2007; 197: 457 e1–21. [Review]

65. Ginsberg JS, Greer I, Hirsh J. Use of antithrombotic agents during pregnancy. *Chest* 2001; 119: 122–31. [Review]

66. Dolovich I, Ginsberg JS. Low molecular weight heparin in the treatment of venous thromboembolism: An updated meta-analysis. *Vessels* 1997; 3: 4–11. [Review]

67. Gold MK, Dembitzer AD, Doyle RI, Hastie TJ, Garber AM. Low molecular weight heparins compared with unfractionated heparin for treatment of acute deep vebous thrombosis. A meta-analysis of randomized controlled trials. *Ann Intern Med* 1999; 130: 800–9. [Meta-Analysis]

68. Van Dongen CJ, van den Belt AG, Prins MH, Lensing AW. Fixed dose subcutaneous low molecular weight heparins versus adjusted dose unfractionated heparin for venous thromboembolism. *Cochrane Database Syst Rev* 2004; 4. [Review]

69. Greer IA, Nelson-Piercy C. Low-molecular-weight heparins for thromboprophylaxis and treatment of venous thromboembolism in pregnancy: A systematic review of safety and efficacy. *Blood* 2005; 106: 401–7. [Review]

70. Weitz J. Low-molecular-weight heparins. *N Engl J Med* 1997; 337: 688–98. [Review]

71. Nelson-Piercey C, Letsky EA, de Michaeal Swiet. Low-molecular-weight heparin for obstetric thromboprophylaxis: Experience of sixty-nine pregnancies in sixty-one women at high risk. *Am J Obstet Gynecol* 1997; 176(5): 1062–8. [II-2]

72. Barbour LA, Oja JL, Schultz LK. A prospective trial that demonstrates that dalteparin requirements increase in pregnancy to maintain therapeutic levels of anticoagulation. *Am J Obstet Gynecol* 2004; 191: 1024–9. [II-1]

73. Casele HL, Laifer SA, Wolkers DA et al. Changes in the pharmacokinetics of the low-molecular-weight heparin enoxaparin sodium during pregnancy. *Am J Obstet Gynecol* 1999; 181: 1113–7. [II-2]

74. Sephton V, Farquharson RG, Topping J et al. A longitudinal study of maternal dose response to low molecular weight heparin in pregnancy. *Obstet Gynecol* 2003; 101: 1307–11. [II-2]

75. Hall JAG, Paul RM, Wilson KM. Maternal and fetal sequelae of anticoagulation during pregnancy. *Am J Med* 1980; 68: 122–40. [II-3]

76. Han WS, Anand S, Ginsberg JS. Anticoagulation of pregnant women with mechanical heart valves: A systematic review of the literature. *Arch Intern Med* 2000; 160(2): 191–6. [Review]

77. Orme L'E, Lewis M, de Swiet M et al. May mothers given warfarin breast-feed their infants? *BMJ* 1977; 1: 1564–5. [II-3]

78. McKenna R, Cole ER, Vasan V. Is warfarin sodium contraindicated in the lactating mother? *J Pediatr* 1983; 103: 325–7. [II-3]

79. Imperiale TF, Petrulis AS. A metanalysis of low dose aspirin for prevention of pregnancy induced hypertensive disease. *JAMA* 1991; 266: 260–4. [Review]

80. CLASP Collaborative Group. CLASP: A randomized trial of low dose aspirin for the prevention of preeclampsia among 9,364 pregnant women. *Lancet* 1994; 343: 619–29. [I]

81. Bates SM, Greer IA, Pabinger I, Sofaer S, Hirsh J. Venous thromboembolism, thrombophilia, antithrombotic therapy, and pregnancy: American College of Chest Physicians Evidence-Based Clinical Practice Guidelines. 8th ed. American College of Chest Physicians. *Chest* 2008; 133: 844S–86S. [Review]

82. Knight M; UKOSS. Antenatal pulmonary embolism: Risk factors, management and outcomes. *BJOG* 2008; 115(4): 453–61. [Review]

83. Warketin TE, Greinacher A, Koster A, Lincoff AM. Treatment and prevention of heparin-induced thrombocytopenia: American College of Chest Physicians Evidence-Based Clinical Guidelines, 8th ed. American College of Chest Physicians. *Chest* 2008; 133: 340S–80S. [Review]

84. Walenga JM, Prechel M, Jeske WP, Bakhos M. Unfractionated heparin compared with low molecular weight heparin as related to heparin-induced thrombocytopenia. *Curr Opin Pulm Med* 2005; 11: 385–91. [Review]

85. Jaff MR, McMurtry MS, Archer SI, Cushman M, Goldenberg N, Goldhaber SZ et al. American Heart Association Council on Cardiopulmonary, Critical Care. Management of massive and submassive pulmonary embolism, iliofemoral deep vein thrombosis, and chronic thromboembolic pulmonary hypertension: A scientific statement from the American Heart Association. *Circulation* 2011; 123: 1788–830. [Review]

86. Ahearn GS, Hadjiliadis D, Govert JA et al. Massive pulmonary embolism during pregnancy successfully treated with recombinant tissue plasminogen activator: A case report and review of treatment options. *Arch Intern Med* 2002; 162: 1221–7. [Review]

87. Monreal M, Lafoz E, Olive A, del Rio IVC. Comparison of subcutaneous unfractionated heparin with low-molecular-weight heparin (Fragmin) in patients with venous thromboembolism and contraindications to coumarin. *Thromb Haemost* 1994; 7(1): 7–11. [II-1]

88. Lee AYY, Levine MN, Baker RI et al. Randomized comparison of low-molecular-weight heparin versus oral anticoagulant therapy for the prevention of recurrent venous thromboembolism in patients with cancer. *N Engl J Med* 2003; 349(2): 146–53. [I]

89. Aschwanden M, Labs KH, Engel H, Schob A, Jeannerret C, Mueller-Brand J et al. Acute deep vein thrombosis: Early mobilization does not increase the frequency of pulmonary embolism. *Thromb Haemost* 2001; 85: 42–6. [II-3]

90. Greenfield LJ, Cho KJ, Proctor MC et al. Late results of suprarenal Greenfield vena cava filter placement. *Arch Surg* 1992; 127: 969–73. [II-2]

91. Riedel M. Acute pulmonary embolism 2: Treatment. *Heart* 2001; 85: 351–60. [Review]

92. Ahearn GS, Hadjiliadis D, Govert JA et al. Massive pulmonary embolism during pregnancy successfully treated with recombinant tissue plasminogen activator: A case report and review of treatment options. *Arch Intern Med* 2002; 162: 1221–7. [II-3]

93. De Swiet M, Floyd E, Letsky E. Low risk of recurrent thromboembolism in pregnancy. *Br J Hosp Med* 1987; 38: 264. [Review]

94. Howell R, Fidler J, Letsky E et al. The risk of antenatal subcutaneous heparin prophylaxis: A controlled trial. *BJOG* 1983; 90: 1124–8. [II-1]

95. Badaracco MA, Vessey M. Recurrent venous thromboembolic disease and use of oral contraceptives. *BMJ* 1974; 1: 215–7. [II-2]

96. Tengborn L. Recurrent thromboembolism in pregnancy and puerperium: Is there a need for thromboprophylaxis? *Am J Obstet Gynecol* 1989; 160: 90–4. [II-2]

97. Pettila V, Kaaja R, Leinonen P et al. Thromboprophylaxis with low molecular weight heparin (dalteparin) in pregnancy. *Thromb Res* 1999; 96: 275–82. [II-2]

98. Bain E, Wilson A, Tooher R, Gates S, Davis LJ, Middleton P. Prophylaxis for venous thromboembolic disease in pregnancy and the early postnatal period. *Cochrane Database System Rev* 2014; 2. [Meta-analysis; 19 RCTs, *n* = >2600, Review]

99. Middledorp S, Van der Meer J, Hamulyak K et al. Counseling women with factor V Leiden homozygosity: Use absolute instead of relative risks. *Thromb Haemost* 2001; 87: 360–1. [Review]

100. Middledorp S, Libourel EJ, Hamulyak K et al. The risk of pregnancy-related venous thromboembolism in women who are homozygous for factor V Leiden. *Br J Haematol* 2001; 113: 553–5. [II-2]

101. Martinelli I, Legnani C, Bucciarelli P et al. Risk of pregnancy-related venous thrombosis in carriers of severe inherited thrombophilia. *Thromb Haemost* 2001; 86: 800–3. [II-2]

102. Pabinger I, Nemes L, Rintelen C et al. Pregnancy-associated risk for venous thromboembolism and pregnancy outcome in women homozygous for factor V Leiden. *Hematol J* 2000; 1: 37–41. [II-2]

103. Hill NCW, Hill JG, Sargent JM et al. Effect of low dose heparin on blood loss at caesarean section. *BMJ* 1988; 296: 505–6. [II-3]

104. Brill-Edwards. Safety of withholding heparin in pregnant women with a history of venous thromboembolism. *N Engl J Med* 2000; 343: 1439–44. [II-2]

105. Sbarouni E, Oakley CM. Outcome of pregnancy in women with valve prostheses. *Br Heart J* 1994; 71: 196–201. [II-2]

106. Brill-Edwards P, Ginsberg JS, Johnston M et al. Establishing a therapeutic range for heparin. *Ann Intern Med* 1993; 119: 104–9. [II-2]

107. Arnaout MS, Kazma H, Khalil A et al. Is there a safe anticoagulation protocol for pregnant women with prosthetic valves? *Clin Exp Obstet Gynecol* 1998; 25: 101–4. [II-2]

108. Leyh RG, Fischer S, Ruhparwar A et al. Anticoagulation for prosthetic heart valves during pregnancy: Is low-molecular-weight heparin an alternative? *Eur J Cardiothorac Surg* 2002; 21: 577–9. [II-2]

109. Mahesh B, Evans S, Bryan AJ. Failure of low molecular-weight heparin in the prevention of prosthetic mitral valve thrombosis during pregnancy: Case report and review of options for anticoagulation. *J Heart Valve Dis* 2002; 11: 745–50. [II-3]

110. Lev-Ran O, Kramer A, Gurevitch J et al. Low-molecular-weight heparin for prosthetic heart valves: Treatment failure. *Ann Thorac Surg* 2000; 69: 264–5. [II-3]

111. Lovenox Injection. Bridgewater, NJ: Aventis Pharmaceuticals, 2004. [Review]

112. Turpie AGG, Gent M, Laupacis A et al. A comparison of aspirin with placebo in patients treated with warfarin after heart-valve replacement. *N Engl J Med* 1993; 329: 524–9. [I]

113. Anderson DR, Ginsberg JS, Burrows R et al. Subcutaneous heparin therapy during pregnancy: A need for concern at the time of delivery. *Thromb Haemost* 1991; 63: 248–50. [II-2]

114. Horlocker TT. Low molecular weight heparin and neuraxial anesthesia. *Thromb Res* 2001; 101: 141–54. [II-3]

115. Lindqvist P, Dahlback B, Marsal K. Thrombotic risk during pregnancy: A population study. *Obstet Gynecol* 1999; 94: 595–9. [II-2]

116. Quinones J, James D, Stamilio D, Lawrence Cleary K, Macones G. Thromboprophylaxis after cesarean delivery. A decision analysis. *Obstet Gynecol* 2005; 106(4): 733–40. [Review]

117. Society for Maternal Fetal Medicine (SMFM), Varner MW. Thromboprophylaxis for cesarean delivery. *Cont Obstet Gynecol* 2011; 6: 30–3. [Review]

118. Orme ML, Lewis PJ, de Swiet M, Serlin MJ, Sibeon R, Baty JD et al. May mothers given warfarin breastfeed their infants? *Br Med J* 1977; 1: 1564–5. [II-3]

119. Keeling D, Baglin T, Tait C, Watson H, Perry D, Baglin C et al. British Committee for Standards in Haeatology Guidelines on oral anticoagulation with warfarin-fourth edition. *Br J Haematol* 2011; 154: 311–24. [Review]

120. Thromboembolic Disease in Pregnancy and the Puerperium: Acute Management. Green-top Guideline No. 37b, April 2015. [Review]

121. Gomes MP, Deitcher SR. Risk of venous thromboembolic disease associated with hormonal contraceptives and hormone replacement therapy: A clinical review. *Arch Intern Med* 2004; 164: 1965–76. [Review]

122. Mantha S, Karp R, Raghavan V, Terrin N, Bauer KA, Zwicker JI. Assesing the risk of venous thromboembolic events in women taking progestin-only contraception: A meta-analysis. *BMJ* 2012; 345: e4944. [Review]

123. Lidegaard O, Lokkegaard E, Svendsen AL, Agger C. Hormonal Contraception and risk of venous thromboembolism: A national follow-up study. *BMJ* 2009; 339: b2921. [II-3]

124. Van Hylckama Vlieg A, Helmerhorst FM, Vandenbroucke JP, Doggen CJ, Rosendaal FR. The venous thrombotic risk of oral contraceptives, effects of estrogen dose and progestogen type, results of the MEGA case-control study. *BMJ* 2009; 339. [II-2]

125. Kemmeren JM, Algra A, Gorbee DE. Third generation oral contraceptives and risk of venous thrombosis: Meta-analysis *BMJ* 2001; 323: 131–4. [Review]

126. US medical eligibility criteria for contraceptive use, 2010. Centers for Disease Control and Prevention (CDC). *MMWR Recomm Rep* 2010; 59(RR-4): 1–86. [Review]

29

Hepatitis A

Neil Silverman and Steven K. Herrine

KEY POINTS

- **The vast majority of hepatitis A virus (HAV) infections** are **self-limited.**
- There is **no perinatal transmission of HAV.**
- The inactivated HAV **vaccine** can be **safely used for prevention**, can be safely used and should be given during prevention during pregnancy if a patient is at risk for HAV exposure.
- **Exposed pregnant women** can receive immune globulin **injections**, which are >85% effective in preventing HAV infection if given within 2 weeks of exposure.
- Therapy of acute HAV infection in pregnancy is supportive.

DIAGNOSIS

Anti-HAV IgM is the diagnostic criterion for acute hepatitis A virus (HAV) infection.

SYMPTOMS

Fever, malaise, decreased appetite, nausea, abdominal discomfort, dark urine, jaundice.

EPIDEMIOLOGY/INCIDENCE

Hepatitis A infection is seen in <1/1000 pregnancies [1]. Worldwide, geographic areas can be characterized by high, intermediate, or low levels of endemicity (Figure 29.1). Levels of endemicity are related to hygienic and sanitary conditions in the geographic areas. HAV infection is common (high or intermediate endemicity) throughout the developing world, where infections most frequently are acquired during early childhood and usually are asymptomatic or mild. In areas of high endemicity, adults are usually immune and epidemics of hepatitis A are uncommon.

There were about 17,000 cases in the United States in 1999 (down almost 50% from 1995) although rates have been shown to decline nationally even more lately as a result of implementation of vaccine protocols, particularly among children [2]. In fact, acute hepatitis A national incidence (new cases) has recently declined 92%, from 12.0 cases per 100,000 persons in 1995 to 1.0 per 100,000 persons in 2007—the lowest rate ever recorded [3]. About 40% of the population is HAV IgG+ (usually immune from an old infection).

GENETICS

RNA within the genus hepatovirus of the piconavirus family.

ETIOLOGY/BASIC PATHOPHYSIOLOGY

Fecal/oral contact with infected person or contaminated food/water; rarely from blood transmission. Most U.S. cases are from person to person or sexual contact transmission during outbreaks. Average incubation period is 28 (15–49) days, then abrupt onset. HAV infection can be symptomatic (adults) but also asymptomatic (mostly children <6 years old). Symptoms last usually less than 2 months (up to 6 months in 10%–15% patients). **The vast majority of cases are self-limited.**

RISK FACTORS/ASSOCIATIONS

Increased risk of acquiring HAV infection in travelers to developing/high-prevalence countries; men who have sex with men; intravenous drug users; people who work with nonhuman primates; people with chronic liver disease.

COMPLICATIONS

Mortality is <0.3%. Chronic carrier state does not exist.

PREGNANCY CONSIDERATIONS

No perinatal transmission.

PREGNANCY MANAGEMENT
Workup

HAV IgM and IgG. HAV IgM is detectable 5–10 days before the onset of symptoms and usually decreases to undectable concentrations within 6 months after recovery [4]. Consider rest of hepatitis workup (see Hepatitis B and C guidelines). Check AST/ALT, bilirubin. HAV IgG is associated with immunity.

Prevention/Preconception Counseling

Avoid fecal-oral contamination by washing all foods and keeping hands clean. Be aware of frequent source (40%) being contact with children. Havrix (Smith Kline Beecham) and Vaqta (Merck) are **inactive live virus vaccines**. Two doses IM (Havrix 1 ml [50 u] or Vaqta 1 g [1440 u]), given 6–12 months apart, are needed to confer immunity. They can be **safely used during pregnancy if a patient is at risk for HAV exposure**. HA vaccine is also available in combination with HB vaccine. Immunity after vaccination lasts >10 years.

Prenatal Care
Therapy

Acute infection. No anti-HAV drug is available at present. Supportive therapies can be offered as outpatient. Consider hospitalization only in rare cases of severe dehydration, encephalopathy, or coagulopathy.

Exposed pregnant women can receive immune globulin injections (0.02 mg/kg IM), which are >85% effective in preventing HAV infection if given within 2 weeks of exposure (close

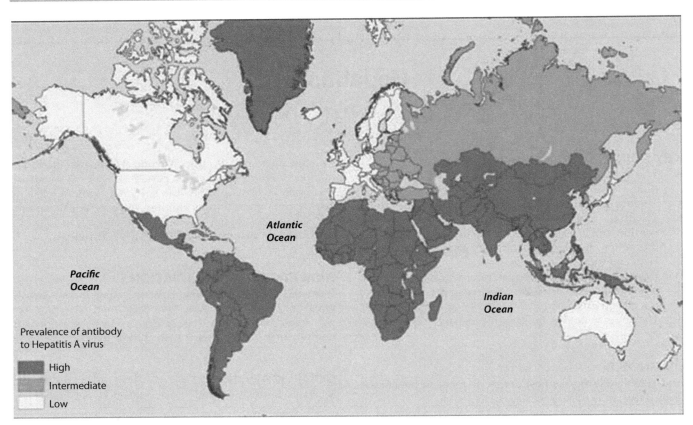

Figure 29.1   Endemicity of hepatitis A in the world. (From www.CDC.gov.)

personal or sexual contact). The HAV vaccine series should also be initiated [1]. In June 2007, U.S. guidelines were revised to allow for Hepatitis A vaccine to be used after exposure to prevent infection in healthy persons aged 1–40 years.

ANTEPARTUM TESTING
Not indicated.

DELIVERY
Follow obstetrical indications.

ANESTHESIA
No particular precautions necessary.

POSTPARTUM/BREAST-FEEDING
Breast-feeding is not contraindicated.

REFERENCES
1. Viral hepatitis in pregnancy. *ACOG Educational Bulletin* 86, October 2007. [Review; III]
2. APGO Educational Series on Women's Health. *Hepatitis B and C: The Ob/Gyn's role.* APGO, Maryland, 2002. [Review; III]
3. Daniels D, Grytdal S, Wasley A. Surveillance for acute viral hepatitis—United States, 2007. *MMWR Surveillance Summary* 2009; 58(SS03): 1–27. [Guideline]
4. Centers for Disease Control and Prevention. Prevention of hepatitis A through active or passive immunization: Recommendations of the Advisory Committee on Immunization Practices (ACIP). *MMWR Recomm Rep* 2006; 55(RR-07); 1–23. [Guideline; III]

30

Hepatitis B

Neil Silverman and Steven K. Herrine

KEY POINTS

- **Universal precautions, proper hygiene, avoidance of high-risk behavior** with contact with potentially infectious body fluids (blood, semen, and saliva) must be employed by the mother (or potential mother) to avoid acquiring the infection.
- **Hepatitis B virus (HBV) vaccine should be administered preconception or early in pregnancy to every reproductive age woman** who is susceptible.
- **All women** should be **screened for HBV infection during pregnancy: HBsAg is the appropriate screening test.**
- Vertical transmission of HBV occurs in 90% to 95% of women with HBeAg+ and 90% of women with acute hepatitis in the third trimester in the absence of neonatal immunoprophylaxis.
- Vertical transmission can occur in about 20% to 30% of women who are HBsAg+ but HBeAg– in the absence of neonatal immunoprophylaxis.
- **In pregnant women with HBV infection, HBV viral load testing should be considered in the third trimester.**
- **In pregnant women with HBV infection and viral load >6–8 log 10 ($10^{6–8}$) copies/mL, HBV-targeted maternal antiviral therapy should be considered for the purpose of decreasing the risk of intrauterine fetal infection.**
- 90% of newborns infected with HBV develop chronic HB without intervention with 25% of chronic HB carriers eventually dying of complications (cirrhosis, hepatocellular cancer) of HBV infection.
- Hepatitis B vaccine and HBIG should be given within 12 hours of birth to all newborns of HBsAg positive mothers or those with unknown or undocumented HBsAg status regardless of whether maternal antiviral therapy has been given during the pregnancy.
- **Breast-feeding is not contraindicated as long as the newborn receives appropriate immunoprophylaxis.**

DIAGNOSIS/DEFINITION
Adults (Table 30.1)

Acute: HBsAg+, HBcAb+, HBcIgM+, HBsAb–.
Chronic: HBsAg+ >6 months, HBsAb– [1,2].

The virus can be found by PCR in blood, urine, feces, seminal fluid, saliva, and the GI tract. Serum, semen, and saliva are infectious. The initial differential diagnosis of hepatitis includes hepatitis A, B, or C viruses (HAV, HBV, HCV), cytomegalovirus (CMV), Epstein-Barr virus (EBV), varicella zoster virus (VZV), coxsackie B virus, herpes simplex virus (HSV), rubella, autoimmune hepatitis, and drug- or herbal-induced hepatotoxicity.

Infants

The diagnosis is made by detection of persistent (e.g., >9 months of age) HBsAg. Only HBsAb is attributable to newborn vaccination: HBcAb arises only as the result of actual HBV infection.

SYMPTOMS

Only 30% to 50% of acutely infected adult patients have symptoms, such as loss of appetite, malaise, nausea, and vomiting. About 10% have jaundice. The onset is usually insidious.

EPIDEMIOLOGY/INCIDENCE

More than 400 million worldwide have chronic HBV infection. Most acquire the infection at birth or in the first one to two years of life. More than 300,000 liver cancers per year are due to HBV (>50% of 530,000 cases—118,000 cases due to HCV—so hepatitis is responsible for 82% of all liver cancer). One third of the world's population (two billion people) have been infected with HBV [3]: 90% have complete resolution, and about 10% overall develop **chronic HBV infection**. But this incidence is age-specific: **90% in children who are infected at <1 year of age** and only 2% in persons >5 years old. **About 25% of HBV chronic infection patients die** of liver disease (4000/yr in the United States, >1 million/yr worldwide—0.5% mortality) [4].

    The vaccine is about 95% effective against HBV. More than 90 countries implement universal vaccination: the worldwide eradication of HBV is a distinct possibility but far away at present. More than 75% of chronic HBV infection patients are Chinese, second is sub-Saharan Africa (10%–20% incidence in these countries). Incidence is 0.2% to 0.5% in North America, Europe, and Australia. The absolute annual incidence of acute HBV infection has decreased in the United States from 8000 to 3500 cases over the 2000–2013 interval with a stabilized rate of 0.9–1.1 cases/100,000 population in the United States from 2009 to 2013. In endemic areas where universal childhood HBV vaccination has been instituted, decreases in HBsAg carrier rates were associated with subsequent reductions, up to 70%, in the incidence of hepatocellular carcinoma in children and adolescents [5,6].

GENETICS

Small partially double-stranded DNA virus.

Table 30.1   Interpretation of the Hepatitis B Panel

Test	Results	Interpretation	Vertical transmission[a]
HbsAg Anti-HBc Anti-HBs	Negative Negative Negative	Susceptible	0%
HbsAg Anti-HBc Anti-HBs	Negative Positive Positive	Immune because of natural infection	0%
HbsAg Anti-HBc Anti-HBs	Negative Negative Positive	Immune because of hepatitis B vaccination	0%
HbsAg Anti-HBc Anti-HBc IgM Anti-HBs	Positive Positive Negative Negative	Acutely infected	First trimester: 10% Third trimester: 80%–90% HBeAg–: 10%–20% HBeAg+:90%
HbsAg Anti-HBc Anti-HBc IgM Anti-HBs	Positive Positive Negative Negative	Chronically infected	HBeAg–: 2%–10% HBeAg+: 80%–90%

HbsAg
Anti-HBc
Anti-HBs
	Negative
	Positive
	Negative
		Four interpretations possible:
		  1. May be recovering from acute HBV infection
		  2. May be distantly immune and test is not sensitive enough to detect very low level of anti-HBs in serum
		  3. May be susceptible with false positive anti-HBc
		  4. May be an undetectable level of HBsAg present in the serum and the person is actually a carrier
			0%

Source: Adapted from APGO Educational Series on Women's Health. Hepatitis B and C. In: *Sexually Transmitted Infections: The Ob/Gyn's Role.* Maryland: APGO, 2003.
[a]Assuming HIV negative and no HB vaccine and immunoprophylaxis of neonate.

ETIOLOGY/BASIC PATHOPHYSIOLOGY

HB virus exposure, then incubation of about 60 to 90 days (depends on the amount of viral exposure), then laboratory changes (Table 30.1; Figure 30.1).

- Antigens
  - "s" surface—infected. If present >6 months, chronic
  - HBV infection
  - "c"—core
  - "e"—envelope—connotes higher infectivity
- Antibodies
  - "s"—immune
  - "c"—core—positive in "window" period and usually precedes HBsAb conversion

The presence of HBsAb is diagnostic for immunity whether it results from vaccination or from natural (but cleared or resolved) infection. HBcAb arises only as a result of natural infection and coexists with HBsAb in individuals who have cleared their acute infection. In contrast, HBsAb and HBsAg do not coexist in standard clinical testing because HBsAg is the clearance, or neutralizing antibody, for the antigen.

About 5% of HBV infections in adults become chronic. This can lead to cirrhosis, hepatocellular carcinoma, and death. (http://www.cdc.gov/vaccines/pubs/pinkbook/hepb.html)

CLASSIFICATION
See Table 30.1.

RISK FACTORS/ASSOCIATIONS
Transmission is parenteral (blood borne) and sexual (mucosal). The greatest source of chronic HBV infection worldwide

is perinatal transmission from HBV-infected mothers. Twenty-five percent of sexual contacts become positive. Intravenous drug use (IVDU), sexually transmitted diseases (STDs), multiple sex partners, household contacts, time in a mental institution/prison, and acupuncture are other risk factors as is the rare HBV-infected blood transfusion. The risk of transfusion-attributable HBV infections is about 1 per 137,000 transfused units of screened blood [1]. HBV-infected patients are more likely to be infected with HIV and HCV.

COMPLICATIONS
Ninety percent of adult patients resolve the infection (clear both HBsAg and HBeAg) and develop HBsAb; 10% develop chronic hepatitis B infection (maintain HBsAg). Of these, most are asymptomatic with normal liver function tests (LFTs), with no HBV detectable by PCR. The other 15% to 30% of chronic HB has persistent viral replication: These patients can develop cirrhosis and hepatocellular cancer. Mortality is 0.5% to 1%. About 5% to 10% of all HBV transmission is transplacental hematogenous.

The outcome of acute HBV infection is age-dependent. About **95% of neonates**, 20%–30% of children age 1–5 years old, and <5% of adults **develop chronic infection. Up to 40% of men and 15% of women with perinatally acquired HBV infection will die of liver cirrhosis or hepatocellular carcinoma** [7].

PREGNANCY CONSIDERATIONS
Vertical transmission occurs in about **20% to 30% of children born to HbsAg+/HBeAg– mothers** if no neonatal immunoprophylaxis is given. **If the woman is also HBeAg+, the risk for vertical transmission is about 90% to 95% with 90% of**

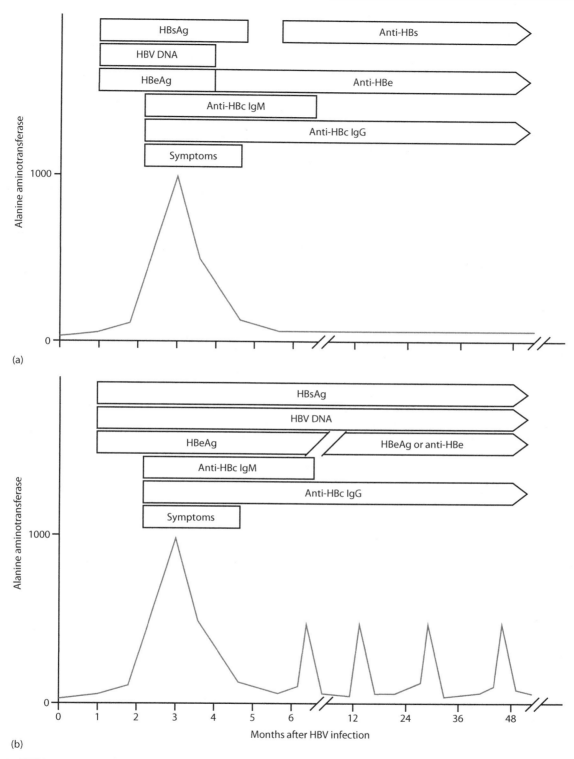

Figure 30.1 HBV markers during natural course resolved acute HBV infection (a) and transition of acute to chronic HBV infection (b). A subset of chronic patients might seroconvert from HBeAg to anti-HBe despite persistence of HBV DNA. HBV = hepatitis B virus. (From Trepo C, Chan HLY, Lok A. *Lancet* 384, 2053–63, 2014. With permission.)

infected neonates becoming chronic carriers as a result if no neonatal immunoprophylaxis is given. Vertical transmission is lowest (<10%) if HBeAb negative. **Vertical transmission is also trimester-dependent: first trimester 10%, third trimester 80% to 90%**, of which 90% occurs because of intrapartum exposure to blood and secretions. Although the use of HBIG and HBV vaccine neonatally has shown a dramatic impact in lowering rates of perinatal HBV transmission, concern persists regarding the **5%–15% of newborns who are infected despite receiving appropriate neonatal immunoprophylaxis**. This subgroup has been thought to represent a cohort of newborns infected in utero but, until recently, no measures had been shown to have an impact on HBV viremia in infected individuals. Maternal HBV-DNA level has been demonstrated to be the strongest predictor of neonatal immunoprophylaxis failure, representing intrauterine infection, with a lower **prophylaxis effective rate (PER)** directly related to a higher maternal viral load. Earlier studies showed a PER **close to 100% if prelabor HBV-DNA levels were <5.5 log 10 (or <316,000) copies/mL** (equivalent to 56,000 or 4.8 log 10, IU/mL) [8,9] with more recent prospective studies showing a stepwise decrease in PER as HBV-DNA levels rose above 6–8 log 10 (1 million–100 million) copies/mL [10,11].

Risk of vertical transmission of HBV appears not to be higher in HBV-infected women who undergo amniocentesis versus HBV-infected women who do not [1] although most data are obtained from studies conducted before the routine use of HBV viral load testing as a disease marker; therefore, it may not apply to women with very high viral load. In fact, a recent series did demonstrate an **increase in risk for in utero infection after amniocentesis in women with viral titers >7 log 10 copies/mL** compared to those women with titers below that cutoff (50% vs. 4%, OR 21.3, $p = 0.006$) [12]. There are insufficient data to assess the risk of in utero infection related to chorionic villus sampling in HBV-infected women [13]. Such emerging data may have an impact on counseling surrounding invasive prenatal testing as data accumulate from more series using maternal HBV viral load as a predictor of procedural risk. Pregnancy course is otherwise not altered by HBV (same incidences of pregnancy loss, congenital anomalies, etc.), except for higher preterm birth rates for acute third-trimester HBV infection.

MANAGEMENT
Principles
Main goal is prevention of vertical transmission.

Workup
HBsAg, HBsAb, HBcAb, HBcIgM, HBeAg, HBeAb. See Table 30.1 for interpretation of diagnosis, disease stage. **HBV DNA by quantitative PCR is recommended in the early third trimester** for women diagnosed as chronic carriers. This test is used to counsel women regarding the risk of intrauterine infection/neonatal immunization failure and to discuss options related to maternal antiviral therapy during pregnancy to decrease the risk of fetal infection [14,15]. Liver biopsy can be considered for initial assessment of severity of disease for chronic HBV.

Prevention/Preconception Counseling [1,4]
Universal precautions, proper hygiene, and avoidance of high-risk behavior with contact with potentially infected fluids (e.g., serum, semen, and saliva) must be employed by the mother (or potential mother) to avoid acquiring the infection.

HBV vaccine should be administered preconception or early in pregnancy to every reproductive age woman who is susceptible.

Universal maternal screening with HBsAg is recommended at first visit or preconception.

If HBsAg+, test for HBsAb, eAg, eAb, cAb. Also test **quantitative HBV-DNA level in early third trimester**. Consideration should be given to offering maternal antiviral therapy for very high maternal viral loads, which is discussed below. All HBsAg+ women should also have their neonate receive HBIg and HB vaccine within 12 hours of birth regardless of whether maternal antiviral therapy was used during pregnancy. This combination prevents >90% of vertical transmission.

If HBsAg–, consider vaccine in pregnancy for all and especially high-risk groups such as STDs, HIV+, HepC+, and IVDU.

Women who are known to be or found to be chronically HBV infected (HBsAg+) should also be screened for prior hepatitis A virus infection (test: HAV-IgG) and vaccinated if nonimmune because coinfection with other hepatitis viruses has additive morbidity.

Prenatal Care
Universal maternal screening with HBsAg at first visit or preconception. If HBsAg+, send workup as above. If HBsAg–, no further workup. **Consider repeating in early third trimester in high-risk groups**, such as sex with acutely or chronically HBV-infected person, sex workers, multiple/new partners, multiple STDs, HIV, IVDU, occupational contact with blood, receivers of unscreened blood, hemodialysis patients, household contacts of infected patients, persons in prisons or institutions, or countries with high rates of HBV infection.

Therapy
Main intervention therapies [1,2,4,16,17]:

Hepatitis B Vaccine
Series of three IM injections in deltoid muscle over six months of recombinant DNA; 95% seroconversion (HBsAb+ and immune) rate. It is safe in pregnancy and for neonate. Two vaccines available:

1. Recombivax HB (Merck and Co, Inc., New Jersey, U.S.): adults >20 years old = 10 mg (1 mL); 11–19 years old = 5 (0.5); <11 years old = 2.5 (0.25); within 12 hours of delivery and maternal HBeAg+ = 5; within 12 hours of delivery and maternal HBeAg– = 2.5.
2. Engerix-B (Smith Kline Beecham Biologicals, Belgium): adults >20 years old = 20 mg (1 mL); 11 to 19 years old = 20 (1); <11 years old = 10 (0.5); within 12 hours of delivery and maternal HBeAg+ = 10; within 12 hours of delivery and maternal HBeAg– = 10.

There is also one combination (HA and HB) vaccine available (Twinrix) [1].

HBIg
Immunoglobulins specific for HB (0.5 mL/kg IM for adult; 0.13 mL/kg for neonate). It is safe in pregnancy and for neonate.

Nucleoside/Nucleotide Analogs (Table 30.2)
Safety: generally safe. A recent analysis of antiretroviral registry data looking specifically at the fetal safety profiles of

Table 30.2 FDA Pregnancy Category of Hepatitis B Drugs

Drug	Class	Pregnancy Category
Interferon alpha-2b	interferon	C
Peginterferon alpha	interferon	C
Lamivudine	nucleoside analog	C
Adefovir dipivoxil	nucleotide analog	C
Entecavir	nucleoside analog	C
Telbivudine	nucleoside analog	B
Tenofovir	nucleotide analog	B

the subgroup of anti-HIV agents also effective against HBV demonstrated **no increase in exposure risk.** For tenofovir, for example, the registry had compiled data on a sufficient number of first trimester exposures to detect at least a twofold increase risk in birth defects with none demonstrated [18].

HBV viral load has been shown to be directly related to the risk of disease progression in infected adults. Randomized controlled trials have shown that use of antivirals in HBV-infected adults can lower viremia and, in turn, lower long-term disease risks. Some of the single-agent antivirals studied are those used to treat HIV infection, specifically lamivudine and tenofovir. One of the earlier nonpregnant adult trials using lamivudine demonstrated significantly less progression of hepatic fibrosis and cirrhosis over 32 months compared to placebo but also that drug resistance developed in a high proportion of patients [19]. A meta-analysis compiling data on the use of lamivudine during pregnancy for this purpose included 10 trials although only three were placebo-controlled; compared to placebo, treatment with lamivudine starting at 24–32 weeks of gestation through 4 weeks postpartum resulted in a (significant) 80% decrease in intrauterine fetal HBV infection (OR 0.2 [0.10–0.39]; $p < 0.001$) [20].

Subsequent trials using tenofovir and entecavir, another reverse transcriptase inhibitor, showed sustained viral suppression below detectable levels and reversal of hepatic histopathology without similar levels of resistance in nonpregnant adults [21].

More recent reports have demonstrated that in chronically infected nonpregnant adults, tenofovir monotherapy has maintained HBV-DNA suppression when used for up to 6 years of continuous treatment with no evidence of tenofovir resistance even in patients whose virus became resistant to lamivudine [22,23]. The most recent treatment guidelines issued by the American Association for the Study of Liver Diseases (AASLD) in 2009 for the treatment of chronic HBV infection moved **tenofovir and entecavir** to **first-line therapies** with lamivudine not a first-line agent due to resistance concerns [24].

Regarding pregnancy data, in a recent multicenter prospective observational study, HBV antiviral therapy was given to pregnant women with elevated HBV DNA levels (>7 log10 IU/mL) after 32 weeks of gestation. All newborns received recommended active and passive immunization. Lamivudine and tenofovir were both associated with a reduction in vertical transmission risk (0% and 2%, respectively) compared to no antiviral therapy (20% transmission) [25].

Based on these studies and others, **the use of HBV-specific antivirals after 28–32 weeks of gestation for HBV infected women with high viral load (>10^6–10^8 copies/ mL) has been suggested** in addition to administration of both HBV vaccine and HBIG within 12–24 hours of birth to

minimize in utero infection and to maximize neonatal HBV prevention. In Europe, both the European Association for the Study of the Liver (EASL) and the UK's National Institute for Health and Care Excellence have published such guidelines in 2012 and 2013, respectively [14,26]. Both agencies currently advocate discussion of antiviral therapy with HBV infected pregnant women with viral loads >6–7 log 10 IU/mL (6.7–7.7 log 10 copies/mL) with treatment to be offered in the third trimester. As more data are published in larger trials, this will inevitably lead to development of perinatal treatment protocols in the United States [15,27].

Conditions

- *Acute Hepatitis B in pregnancy*: diagnosis: document conversion from HBsAg– to HBsAg+. Check all labs as above. Outpatient supportive therapy. Consider hospitalization for severe anemia, diabetes mellitus, severe dehydration, coagulopathy, bilirubin >15. Consider nucleoside/ nucleotide and/or HBIg therapy. Vitamin K 10 mg IM (or po) q8h × 3 can be given to pregnant women with coagulopathy. Mortality is about 1% [1]. Sexual, needle, and household contacts should be informed by the patient.
- *Exposure to HB in pregnancy*: Check all labs as above. If HBsAg– and sAb–, give HBIg and begin the HB vaccine series (preferably within 24 hours of exposure): this combination will prevent 75% of transmission. Must give HBIg within 14 days of sexual contact. Repeat HBIg within one month if blood or mucous membrane exposure.
- *Vertical transmission prevention*: **In pregnant women with HBV infection and viral load >6–8 log 10 (10^{6-8}) copies/mL, HBV-targeted maternal antiviral therapy should be considered for the purpose of decreasing the risk of intrauterine fetal infection. All newborns born to women with HBsAg+ should receive HBIg and HB vaccine** within 12 hours of birth given simultaneously at different sites IM [1,2] **regardless of whether maternal antiviral therapy was also used during pregnancy**.

ANTEPARTUM TESTING

Not indicated.

DELIVERY

Per obstetrical indications.

ANESTHESIA

No particular precautions necessary.

POSTPARTUM/BREAST-FEEDING

Breast-feeding is not contraindicated as long as the neonate receives HBIg and HB vaccine as above [1,28].

RARE/RELATED

Hepatitis D virus: incomplete RNA virus, which can superinfect 20% to 25% of chronic HBV-infected patients. HDV infection worsens chronic HBV infection so that 25% may die from disease. If HBV is prevented, HDV infection is prevented too. HDV has no effect on pregnancy or fetus/neonate.

REFERENCES

1. American College of Obstetricians and Gynecologists. Viral hepatitis in pregnancy. ACOG Practice Bulletin No. 86. *Obstet Gynecol* 2007; 110(4): 941–56. [Review]

2. APGO Educational Series on Women's Health. Hepatitis B and C. In: *Sexually Transmitted Infections: The Ob/Gyn's Role.* Maryland: APGO, 2003. [Good pregnancy review]

3. WHO 2014; Trepo C, Chan HLY, Lok A. Hepatitis B virus infection. *Lancet* 2014; 384: 2053–63. [Review]

4. Mast EE, Weinbaum CM, Fiore AE et al. A comprehensive immunization strategy to eliminate transmission of hepatitis B virus infection in the United States: Recommendations of the advisory committee on immunization practices (ACIP) part II: Immunization in adults. *MMWR Recomm Rep* 2006; 55(RR–16): 1–33; quiz CE1. [Review]

5. Ni YH, Chang MH, Wu JF, Hsu HY, Chen HL, Chen DS. Minimization of hepatitis B infection by a 25-year universal vaccination program. *J Hepatol* 2012; 57: 730–5. [II-2]

6. Chang MH, You SL, Chen CJ et al. Taiwan Hepatoma Study Group. Decreased incidence of hepatocellular carcinoma in hepatitis B vaccines: A 20-year follow-up study. *J Natl Cancer Inst* 2009; 101: 1348–55. [II-2]

7. Trepo C, Chan HLY, Lok A. Hepatatis B virus infection. *Lancet* 2014; 384: 2053–63. [Review]

8. Burk RD, Hwang LY, Ho GY, Shafritz DA, Beasley RP. Outcome of perinatal hepatitis B virus exposure is dependent on maternal virus load. *J Infect Dis* 1994; 170: 1418–23. [II-2]

9. del Canho R, Grosheide PM, Mazel JA et al. Ten-year neonatal hepatitis B vaccination program, The Netherlands, 1982–1992: Protective efficacy and long-term immunogenicity. *Vaccine* 1997; 15: 1624–30. [II-2]

10. Xu WM, Cui YT, Wang L, Yang H, Liang ZQ, Li XM et al. Lamivudine in late pregnancy to prevent perinatal transmission of hepatitis B virus infection: A multicentre, randomized, double-blind, placebo-controlled study. *J Viral Hepat* 2009; 16: 94–103. [II-2]

11. Wiseman E, Fraser MA, Holden S et al. Perinatal transmission of hepatitis B virus: An Australian experience. *Med J Aust* 2009; 190: 489–92. [II-2]

12. Yi W, Pan CQ, Hao J et al. Risk of vertical transmission of hepatitis B after amniocentesis in HBs antigen-positive mothers. *J Hepatol* 2014; 60: 523–9. [II-2]

13. Towers CV, Asrat T, Rumney P. The presence of hepatitis B surface antigen and deoxyribonucleic acid in amniotic fluid and cord blood. *Am J Obstet Gynecol* 2001; 184: 1514–20. [II-3]

14. Hepatitis B (chronic): Diagnosis and management of chronic hepatitis B in children, young people and adults. NICE guidelines [CG165] Published date: June 2013. https://www.nice.org.uk/guidance/cg165/resources/guidance-hepatitis-b-chronic-pdf (retrieved Sept. 25, 2015). [II-3]

15. Sarkar M, Terrault NA. Ending vertical transmission of hepatitis B: The third trimester intervention. *Hepatology* 2014; 60: 448–51. [Review, II-3]

16. Lai CL, Ratziu V, Yuen MF et al. Viral hepatitis B. *Lancet* 2003; 362: 2089–94. [General review, nonpregnant]

17. Lai C-L, Yuen M-F. Chronic hepatitis B—New goals, new treatments. *N Engl J Med* 2008; 359: 2488–91. [Review, nonpregnant, III]

18. Brown RS Jr, Verna EC, Pereira MR et al. Hepatitis B virus and human immunodeficiency virus drugs in pregnancy: Findings from the Antiretroviral Pregnancy Registry. *J Hepatol* 2012; 57: 953–9. [II-2]

19. Liaw YF, Sung JJ, Chow WC et al. Cirrhosis Asian Lamivudine Multicentre Study Group. Lamivudine for patients with chronic hepatitis B and advanced liver disease. *N Engl J Med* 2004; 351: 1521–31. [RCT]

20. Shi Z, Yang Y, Ma L, Li X, Schreiber A. Lamivudine in late pregnancy to interrupt in utero transmission of hepatitis B virus: A systematic review and meta-analysis. *Obstet Gynecol* 2010; 116: 147–59. [Meta-analysis; 10 RCTs, n = 951]

21. Chang TT, Liaw YF, Wu SS, Schiff E, Han KH, Lai CL et al. Long-term entecavir therapy results in the reversal of fibrosis/cirrhosis and continued histological improvement in patients with chronic hepatitis B. *Hepatology* 2010; 52: 886–93. [RCT]

22. Kitrinos KM, Corsa A, Liu Y et al. No detectable resistance to tenofovir disoproxil fumarate after 6 years of therapy in patients with chronic hepatitis B. *Hepatology* 2014; 59: 434–42. [RCT]

23. Corsa AC, Liu Y, Flaherty JF et al. No resistance to tenofovir disoproxil fumarate through 96 weeks of treatment in patients with lamivudine-resistant chronic hepatitis B. *Clin Gastroenterol Hepatol* 2014; 12: 2106–12. [RCT]

24. Lok AS, McMahon BJ. Chronic hepatitis B: Update 2009. *Hepatology* 2009; 50: 661–2. [Guideline]

25. Greenup AJ, Tan PK, Nguyen V et al. Efficacy and safety of tenofovir disoproxil fumarate in pregnancy to prevent perinatal transmission of hepatitis B virus. *J Hepatol* 2014; 61: 502–7. [II-1]

26. European Association for the Study of the Liver. EASL clinical practice guidelines: Management of chronic hepatitis B virus infection. *J Hepatol* 2012; 57: 167–85. [Review]

27. Society for Maternal-Fetal Medicine (SMFM); Dionne-Odom J, Tita AT, Silverman NS. Hepatitis B in pregnancy: Screening, treatment, and prevention of vertical transmission. *Am J Obstet Gynecol* 2016; 214: 6–14. [Guideline]

28. Hill JB, Sheffield JS, Kim MJ et al. Risk of hepatitis B transmission in breast-fed infants of chronic hepatitis B carriers. *Obstet Gynecol* 2002; 99: 1049–52. [II-1]

31

Hepatitis C

Neil Silverman, Raja Dhanekula, and Jonathan M. Fenkel

KEY POINTS

- Chronic hepatitis C virus (HCV) infection is defined as a **reactive HCV antibody with detectable HCV RNA for >6 months duration**.
- Chronic hepatitis C virus (HCV) infection is one of the most common chronic liver diseases and accounts for 5 deaths per 100,000 population in the United States in the most recent data survey from 2014 [1]. The majority of liver transplants performed in the United States are for chronic HCV-related liver disease or hepatocellular carcinoma (liver cancer).
- Complications of chronic HCV infection include **cirrhosis, liver failure, and hepatocellular carcinoma**.
- HCV is **primarily acquired** via **infected blood-to-blood contact, but mother-to-infant (vertical transmission) can occur about 5% of the time an HCV-infected mother delivers a newborn.**
- Transmission occurs from mothers who are HCV-RNA positive (as opposed to those who are anti-HCV positive but HCV-RNA negative). The risk of transmission is, as with HIV, in part related to the level of viremia at the time of birth.
- **Mother-to-infant transmission** is most commonly diagnosed by **the presence of HCV-antibody and/or HCV RNA in the infant after 18 months of age but can also be diagnosed by detectable HCV RNA on two occasions 3–4 months apart after the infant is 2 months old. Coinfection with HIV and high maternal viral load** are associated with higher risk of transmission.
- **Risk factors** (Table 31.1) for HCV should be avoided to prevent HCV infection and be **used for screening**.
- HCV-positive pregnant women should be **screened for** coinfection with HIV (**HIV antibody**) and hepatitis B (**hepatitis B surface antigen**) as well as other sexually transmitted infections. Blood tests to measure liver function (**AST, ALT**, total bilirubin, albumin, platelet count, prothrombin time/INR) are also recommended. Strong consideration should be given for **hepatology referral** and **measurement of HCV quantitative RNA ("viral load") and/or HCV genotype** for counseling regarding risk of mother-to-infant transmission, risk reduction behaviors, and eventual treatment consideration.
- Patients with chronic HCV infection are at high risk of liver failure if they become infected with other forms of viral hepatitis. Screening for immunity to hepatitis A (**hepatitis A total ab/IgG**) and hepatitis B (**hepatitis B surface antibody**) **and vaccinating if not immune** is also recommended.
- **Treatment** for chronic HCV infection has changed dramatically since 2011. HCV can be cured >90% of the time with combination **direct-acting antiviral agents (DAAs)**, such as ledipasvir/sofosbuvir, paritaprevir/ritonavir/dasabuvir/ombitasvir, or sofosbuvir+daclatasvir, with few side effects and all oral administration. Safety and efficacy of treatment in pregnant patients has not been established or studied and is not recommended at this time. Older treatments including pegylated interferon are no longer recommended, and ribavirin is contraindicated in pregnancy due to teratogenicity concerns.
- **In women of reproductive age with chronic HCV, treatment before conception should be strongly considered with as short as an 8–12 weeks regimen of DAAs**, particularly if they have advanced liver fibrosis, compensated cirrhosis, severe extrahepatic complications of HCV, or prior children infected with HCV via mother-to-infant transmission. Pregnancy is not recommended in patients with decompensated cirrhosis.
- **In HCV-positive but HIV-negative women, cesarean delivery should be reserved for obstetric indications** as it does not decrease the risk of vertical transmission of HCV infection.
- **Breast-feeding** is generally not considered to be a risk factor for vertical transmission of HCV in non-HIV infected women. Breast-feeding is instead contraindicated in women coinfected with both HCV and HIV infections.
- **Treatment of HCV should be considered postpartum in all infected patients.**

DIAGNOSES/DEFINITIONS/CLASSIFICATION
Adults

Chronic hepatitis C virus (HCV) infection is defined as a **reactive HCV antibody with detectable HCV RNA for more than 6 months duration**. Patients often have elevated liver enzyme tests although this is not required to make the diagnosis and does not occur in all patients with chronic HCV infection.

HCV can cause both acute and chronic hepatitis. The acute process is self-limited with flu-like symptoms, rarely causes hepatic failure, and usually leads to chronic infection. Chronic HCV infection often follows a progressive course over many years and can ultimately result in cirrhosis, liver failure, hepatocellular carcinoma, and the need for liver transplantation.

Acute HCV hepatitis is not common in pregnancy, but would be most likely to occur in women who use intravenous drugs while pregnant. The incubation time is usually 30 to 60 days. Diagnosis is made by **detectable HCV RNA in the blood. HCV antibody is usually nonreactive** in acute hepatitis C, at least for the first 2–3 months of infection. Treatment is supportive and up to 20% may clear infection spontaneously. Patients who develop symptoms, and in particular jaundice, from acute HCV are more likely to clear infection spontaneously than those without symptoms. **Once the infection has been present for >6 months, it is considered chronic** and will not clear without antiviral therapy.

Table 31.1   Risk Factors for HCV Infection

Risk Factor	Odds Ratio[a]
Intravenous drug use	49.6
Blood transfusion	10.9
Sex with an intravenous drug user	6.3
Having been in jail more than three days	2.9
Religious scarification	2.8
Having been struck or cut with a bloody object	2.1
Pierced ears or body parts	2.0
Immunoglobulin injection	1.6
History of multiple sexually transmitted diseases	
HIV infection	
Hepatitis B infection	
Sexual partner who abuses intravenous drugs or has HIV, HBV, or HCV infection	
Recipient of organ transplants before 1992	
Unexplained elevated transaminases	
History of hemodialysis	
Participant in in vitro fertilization programs from anonymous donors	

[a]Odd ratios from Murphy EL et al. NHLBI Retrovirus Epidemiology Donor Study (REDS) *Hepatology*, 31, 3, 756, 2000.

HCV can be found by PCR in blood, urine, feces, seminal fluid, saliva, and GI tract [2,3].

The initial **differential diagnosis of acute hepatitis** includes hepatitis A, B, or C virus (HAV, HBV, or HCV), cytomegalovirus (CMV), Epstein-Barr, varicella (VZV), coxsackie B, herpes (HSV), rubella, autoimmune, etc.

Infants

Mother-to-infant transmission is most commonly diagnosed by **the presence of HCV-antibody and/or HCV RNA in the infant after 18 months of age but can also be diagnosed by detectable HCV RNA on two occasions 3–4 months apart after the infant is 2 months old**.

SYMPTOMS

Most (about 75%) patients with chronic infection are asymptomatic or have only mild nonspecific symptoms.

Among those who have symptoms, the most frequent complaint is fatigue; other less common manifestations include nausea, anorexia, myalgia, arthralgia, weakness, and weight loss [4].

Extrahepatic manifestations: A number of extrahepatic diseases have been associated with chronic HCV infection. Most cases appear to be directly related to the viral infection [5]. These include the following:

- Hematologic diseases, such as essential mixed cryoglobulinemia and lymphoma
- Renal disease, particularly membranoproliferative glomerulonephritis
- Autoimmune disorders, such as thyroiditis and the presence of autoantibodies
- Dermatologic conditions, such as porphyria cutanea tarda and lichen planus
- Diabetes mellitus

NATURAL HISTORY

The majority of patients who acquire HCV do not spontaneously clear the virus and thus **develop chronic HCV infection**. Chronic infection results in chronic inflammation of the liver, which heals with scar tissue formation or fibrosis and **ultimately cirrhosis** in a subset of patients although the **rate of disease progression is variable**. Patients who develop cirrhosis are at further risk for decompensating events (such as variceal hemorrhage, ascites, and encephalopathy) and hepatocellular carcinoma although many patients with compensated cirrhosis remain stable for years (Figure 31.1) [6].

The risk of chronic infection after HCV acquisition is high. In most studies, **50% to 85%** of patients chronically remain HCV RNA positive following infection and seroconversion, depending on the population and the source of infection. Of those who are able to spontaneously clear HCV, most do so within 12 weeks of seroconversion although spontaneous clearance after a longer period of follow-up has been described.

The mechanism responsible for the high prevalence of viral persistence, and thus chronic infection, is unclear, but both viral and host factors are likely to contribute.

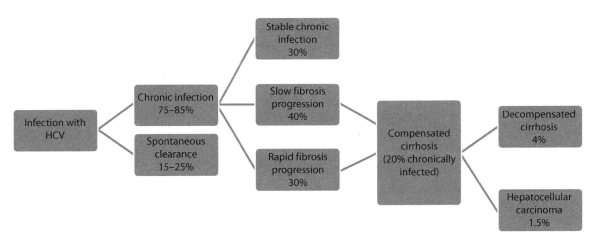

Figure 31.1   Natural history of Hepatitis C. (Derived from Merican I, Sherlock S et al. *Q J Med*, 86, 2, 119, 1993; Grebely J, Page K, Sacks-Davis R et al. *Hepatology*, 59, 1, 109–20, 2014; Montes-Cano MA, García-Lozano JR, Abad-Molina C et al. *Hepatology*, 52, 1, 33, 2010.)

EPIDEMIOLOGY/INCIDENCE

In the United States, **0.6% to 4.5% of pregnant women have HCV antibodies** with considerable worldwide geographic variation. HCV is the most common chronic blood-borne infection in the United States (although HBV is worldwide). Globally, it was estimated that in 2005, more than 185 million people had HCV antibodies, a prevalence of 2.8 percent [6,7]. Of noninstitutionalized U.S. citizens, 1.3% (3.6 million) carry HCV antibodies; 74% of these (2.7 million) have detectable viral RNA in their serum (chronic disease) [8]. The prevalence of antibodies to hepatitis C virus (anti-HCV) in the United States is approximately 1.6% (equating to about 4.1 million anti-HCV positive persons), and the prevalence of positive HCV RNA is approximately 1.3% (or about 3.2 million persons who are HCV RNA-positive). The peak prevalence is observed among persons born between 1945 and 1964 (baby boomers) and the Centers for Disease Control (CDC) recently recommended one-time screening for HCV in all Americans born between 1945 and 1965 [9,10]. The prevalence is projected to decrease from the current about 1.6% to about 1% by the year 2030. On the contrary, the prevalence of liver disease caused by HCV is on the rise. This is because of the significant lag time, often 20 years or longer, between the onset of infection and clinical manifestations of liver disease.

Chronic HCV is one of the most common chronic liver diseases and accounts for **8–13,000 deaths in the United States each year**. The majority of liver transplants performed in the United States are for chronic HCV-related liver disease or hepatocellular carcinoma (liver cancer). Chronic HCV infection is usually slowly progressive and may not result in clinically apparent liver disease in many patients. Approximately 20%–50% of chronically infected individuals develop cirrhosis over a 20- to 30-year period of time.

GENETICS

Single-stranded RNA virus; striking genetic heterogeneity, including six major genotypes with rapid accumulation of mutations. At least **six different genotypes of HCV** have been identified with multiple subtypes among the genotypes. Current treatments are targeted to specific genotypes and subtypes.

ETIOLOGY/BASIC PATHOPHYSIOLOGY

HCV is **primarily acquired** via **infected blood-to-blood contact, but mother-to-infant (vertical transmission) can occur about 5% of the time an HCV-infected mother delivers a newborn** [11]. Sexual contact is a very weak risk factor. Table 31.1 delineates **risk factors** associated with HCV acquisition. Sexual contact is a very uncommon source of HCV infection. The risk of infecting a noninfected partner in monogamous couples in which one partner is HCV infected is thought to be <1% with regular sexual contact. Personal care items such as razors, toothbrushes, and nail clippers can also present household risk for HCV infection through infected blood. See Figure 31.1 for the natural history of HCV infection and likelihood of developing chronic hepatitis.

RISK FACTORS/ASSOCIATIONS

In the United States, the primary risk factor for HCV infection is parenteral (injected or inhaled) drug abuse (Table 31.1) [12]. The risk of HCV infection via blood transfusion is now <1/million transfused units in the United States [2]. Up to 40% of HCV-infected women may have no risk factors. HCV can be found in semen [3] and acquired through artificial insemination [13]. As with HIV, IVF with ICSI (after sperm washing and separation) can avoid the risk of an HCV-infected male partner from infecting his female partner via unprotected intercourse [14].

COMPLICATIONS

The most common maternal long-term complications of chronic infection include **cirrhosis** (20%–50%) and **hepatocellular carcinoma** (1%–5%). Chronic HCV is associated with increased all-cause mortality not only related to liver disease. Renal disease, malignancy, and cardiovascular diseases are also more common in chronic HCV infected patients [15]. Extra-hepatic complications of chronic HCV are detailed above under "Symptoms." Perinatal complications of maternal HCV infection include perinatal transmission (see below).

PREGNANCY CONSIDERATIONS
Mother-to-Infant (Perinatal) Transmission

HCV perinatal (also called vertical) transmission rates have been reported between **2% and 10%**. HCV chronically infects an estimated 25,000–50,000 U.S. children with 750 new cases a year acquired through vertical transmission [16–18]. Table 31.2 summarizes transmission rates compiled from 77 studies and 383 cases of mother-to-infant transmission cases [2,11]. **Coinfection with HIV greatly increases** vertical transmission [11]. The risk of infection is approximately **at least twofold higher or more** in infants born to women coinfected **with** HCV and **HIV**. Highly active antiretroviral HIV therapy has been shown to decrease HCV transmission in HCV–HIV coinfected women [19]. Mothers must be viremic to transmit the virus to the infant. Although maternal HCV antibody can be passively transmitted to the infant, viremia is required for transmission of the virus. Vertical transmission correlates with **high maternal HCV viral load** [20], but a specific cutoff that predicts transmission has not been identified. **The higher the maternal HCV viral titer, the higher the risk of perinatal transmission.**

Other maternal risk factors reported to be possibly associated with an increased rate of vertical HCV transmission include prolonged membrane rupture during labor (6 hours or longer) and use of internal fetal monitoring during labor [16,17]. Nonetheless, it is controversial whether prolonged rupture of the membranes (i.e., for >6 hours) increases risk. **The use of scalp electrodes is discouraged.** There is no association between gestational age and risk of transmission. Amniocentesis does not appear to significantly increase the risk [21], but very few studies have addressed this. If

Table 31.2 Rate of Vertical Transmission of Hepatitis C

	Weighted Rate (%)[a]
Anti-HCV only (RNA negative)	1–2
Viremic (HCV RNA positive)	4–6
HIV positive	19–40
HIV negative	3–5
Anti-HCV and injection drug use	9

[a]Weighted rate adjusts for sample size of study and variance. (See Poynard T, Yuen M-F, Ratziu V et al. *Lancet*, 362, 2095–100, 2003; Hoofnagle JH. *N Engl J Med*, 360, 1899–901, 2009.)

amniocentesis is requested, transplacental needle insertion should be avoided. There are no data regarding CVS and in utero transmission: appropriate counseling should be undertaken if an HCV-infected woman requests CVS, and the availability of amniocentesis should be discussed as a potentially less invasive and vasodisruptive procedure.

Vertical transmission **does not correlate with mode of delivery** in non-HIV-infected pregnant women. Therefore, in these women, cesarean delivery has not been shown to independently decrease the risk of perinatal transmission and should be considered only for obstetrical reasons. HIV coinfected women delivered by cesarean section were 60% less likely to have a HCV-infected child than those delivered vaginally [22].

Diagnostic confirmation of vertical transmission is obtained with **positive serum HCV RNA on two occasions 3 to 4 months apart after the infant is 2 months old or anti-HCV detected after the child is 18 months old.**

MANAGEMENT
Prevention
There is no HCV vaccine available. **Risk factors** for HCV (Table 31.1) should be **avoided, and risk reduction counseling should be performed for HCV-infected patients.** Prevention of complications of liver disease includes avoidance of alcohol and hepatotoxic medicines (including alternative and herbal remedies) and certain foods, such as raw shellfish.

Principles
Effect of Pregnancy on Hepatitis C
Pregnancy does not affect the clinical course of acute or chronic hepatitis C. There is an improvement in biochemical markers of liver damage in HCV-positive women during pregnancy [23]. There is a linear increase in HCV viremia throughout pregnancy [3], 50% above baseline [23].

Effect of Hepatitis C on Pregnancy
Chronic active hepatitis in the pregnant woman is associated with an increased incidence of preterm delivery, intrauterine growth restriction, small for gestational age, and NICU admission [24–26]. HCV vertical transmission and its consequences can affect the neonate. Long-term complications of HCV infection for either the mother or the baby can lead to cirrhosis, cancer, and death.

Screening
It is neither cost-effective nor appropriate to screen universally for HCV among low-risk pregnant women. **Screening is recommended in women with risk factors for HCV infection** (Table 31.1). Screening is performed with anti-HCV (HCV IgG) antibody. Universal screening may become recommended when therapy for HCV in pregnancy is deemed safe and effective.

Workup
Any woman who tests positive for anti-HCV antibody should have **HCV RNA quantitative viral load** (via polymerase chain reaction, PCR) to confirm the diagnosis of chronic hepatitis C. She should be screened for coinfection with HIV (**HIV antibody**) and hepatitis B (**hepatitis B surface antigen**) as well as other **sexually transmitted infections.**

Blood tests to measure liver function (**AST, ALT**, total bilirubin, albumin, platelet count, prothrombin time/INR) are also recommended. Strong consideration should be given for **hepatology referral** for counseling regarding risk of vertical transmission, risk reduction behaviors, and eventual treatment consideration. An HCV genotype is also recommended if treatment is being considered as treatment is tailored to the genotype/subtype. Additionally, patients with chronic HCV infection are at high risk of liver failure if they become infected with other forms of viral hepatitis. Screening for immunity to hepatitis A (**hepatitis A total Ab/IgG**) and hepatitis B (**hepatitis B surface antibody**) and **vaccinating if not immune** is also recommended.

Preconception/Pregnancy Counseling
Effect of pregnancy on HCV infection and vice versa should be reviewed. Counseling of the pregnant woman with HCV infection should include **review of risk factors known to increase mother-to-infant transmission** (HIV coinfection, HCV viremia especially with high viral loads, vaginal delivery in HIV coinfected women, scalp electrode, and breastfeeding in HIV coinfected women), and reassurance for factors known not to increase transmission (vaginal delivery in HIV-negative women, gestational age at time of infection, chorioamnionitis, and breast-feeding in HIV-negative women). Amniocentesis, especially nontransplacental, is associated with minimal risk of HCV vertical transmission. Counseling should also include other possible complications, management, and postpartum follow-up.

Other disease-specific counseling tips include avoid sharing personal care items, such as toothbrushes and dental or shaving equipment, and be cautioned to cover any bleeding wound in order to keep their blood away from others. Patients should be counseled to stop using illicit drugs and alcohol. Those who continue to inject drugs should be counseled to avoid reusing or sharing syringes, needles, water, and cotton or other paraphernalia; to clean the injection site with a new alcohol swab; and to dispose safely of syringes and needles after one use.

HCV-infected patients should be counseled that the risk of sexual transmission is low and that the infection itself is not a reason to change sexual practices (i.e., those in long-term relationships need not start using barrier precautions and others should always practice "safer" sex). Still, some sexual behaviors including sex during menses, sex with toys, and anal intercourse are associated with an increased risk of sexual transmission compared to vaginal intercourse.

In women of reproductive age with chronic HCV, **treatment before conception should be strongly considered with a short (8–12 weeks) regimen of direct-acting antiviral agents (DAAs)**, particularly if they have advanced liver fibrosis, compensated cirrhosis, severe extrahepatic complications of HCV, or prior children infected with HCV via mother-to-infant transmission. Pregnancy is not recommended in patients with decompensated cirrhosis. Liver transplant may be considered in some of these cases.

Therapy
Treatment for all nonpregnant adults with HCV chronic HCV infection has changed dramatically since 2011 after the introduction of the first **HCV-specific direct DAAs**, telaprevir and boceprevir. Since then, many other DAAs have been FDA

approved, and more are expected to market in the next few years. **Three general classes of HCV antiviral activity are now available, including HCV protease inhibitors, HCV polymerase inhibitors, and NS5A inhibitors. By using DAAs from at least two of the three categories, HCV can be cured >90% of the time** with as little as one pill/day for 8–24 weeks in most patients regardless of prior treatment experience. Some of the available combinations for genotype 1 include ledipasvir/sofosbuvir, simeprevir + sofosbuvir, paritaprevir/ritonavir/ombitasvir + dasabuvir, and sofosbuvir + daclatasvir. Using a + instead of a/distinguishes combination of two agents rather than a combination pill. In addition, recent trials have demonstrated the efficacy of a regimen combining the polymerase inhibitor sofosbuvir with a newer NS5A inhibitor, veltpatasvir, across all HCV genotypes when used for 12 weeks as a once-daily, fixed-dose therapy [27,28]. These combinations have very few and generally mild side effects, including headache, nausea, fatigue, and insomnia and are given all by oral administration. In nonpregnant adults, indications for treatment include patients with cirrhosis as well as all HCV-positive patients for the prevention of developing advanced fibrosis and cirrhosis.

The main goal of treatment for chronic HCV is now cure. This is typically defined as a sustained virologic response (SVR): an undetectable viral load (less than the lower limit of quantification) at 12–24 weeks after completing therapy, which is associated with reduction of both all-cause and liver-related mortality from HCV [29,30].

Safety and efficacy of this treatment in pregnant patients has not been established and is not recommended at this time. Older treatments, including pegylated interferon, are no longer recommended, and ribavirin is contraindicated in pregnancy due to teratogenicity concerns. Both the apparent safety profile and the potential ribavirin- and interferon-free nature of these regimens make them particularly **attractive for potential use in pregnancy**. The short duration (12 weeks or less for most patients) is also an attractive duration for use during the third trimester. **Sofosbuvir and ledipasvir are both category B drugs** given there was no evidence of fetal harm in animal studies. NS5A inhibitors' profile in pregnancy is promising, but further animal and patient studies are warranted before use in pregnant patients commences. As research evolves, interferon-free combination DAA regimens will most likely become first-line treatment options in pregnancy with better efficacy and lower rates of side effects for both treatment-naïve patients as well as previous interferon nonresponders [31]. Pregnancy is a unique opportunity to not only cure the mother of her HCV, but also to prevent her child from becoming infected.

ANTEPARTUM TESTING
Not indicated for HCV infection alone.

DELIVERY
In HCV-positive women not coinfected with HIV, mode of delivery does not affect vertical transmission, so **cesarean delivery should be reserved for obstetric indications**. In HCV- and HIV-coinfected women, mode of delivery should be cesarean delivery if the HIV viral load is ≥1000 [23].

ANESTHESIA
No particular precautions necessary.

POSTPARTUM
Patients with hepatitis C should be immunized against hepatitis A and B during pregnancy if not already immune as these vaccines are safe. If immunization has not occurred antenatally, hepatitis A and B vaccines (or their combination) should be given postpartum even if breast-feeding [32].

BREAST-FEEDING
Breast-feeding is generally not considered to be a risk factor for vertical transmission of HCV in non-HIV infected women [2]. The safety of breast-feeding operates on the assumption that traumatized, cracked, or bleeding nipples are not present. However, with HIV coinfection, those who breast-fed were four times more likely to infect their children than those who bottle-fed [23]. **Breast-feeding is therefore contraindicated in women with HCV/HIV coinfection** [33,34].

REFERENCES
1. CDC. Surveillance for Viral Hepatitis—United States, 2014. Accessed on CDC.gov, August 1, 2016.
2. Viral hepatitis in pregnancy. ACOG Educational Bulletin No. 86. American College of Obstetricians and Gynecologists. *Obstet Gynecol* 2007; 110: 941–55. [Review]
3. Leurez-Ville M, Kunstmann JM, De Almeida M et al. Detection of hepatitis C virus in the semen of infected men. *Lancet* 2000; 356: 42–3. [II-2]
4. Conry-Cantilena C. Routes of infection, viremia, and liver disease in blood donors found to have hepatitis C virus infection. *N Engl J Med* 1996; 334(26): 1691. [II-2]
5. Cacoub P. Extrahepatic manifestations associated with hepatitis C virus infection. A prospective multicenter study of 321 patients. The GERMIVIC. Grouped'Etude et de Recherche en Medecine Interne et Maladies Infectieuses sur le Virus de l'Hepatite C. *Medicine (Baltimore)* 2000; 79(1): 47–56. [II-1]
6. Merican I, Sherlock S et al. Clinical, biochemical and histological features in 102 patients with chronic hepatitis C virus infection. *Q J Med* 1993; 86(2): 119. [II-3]
7. Mohd Hanafiah K. Global epidemiology of hepatitis C virus infection: New estimates of age-specific antibody to HCV seroprevalence. *Hepatology* 2013; 57(4): 1333. [II-2]
8. Denniston MM. Chronic hepatitis C virus infection in the United States, National Health and Nutrition Examination Survey 2003 to 2010. [II-3]
9. Smith BD. Recommendations for the identification of chronic hepatitis C virus infection among persons born during 1945–1965. Centers for Disease Control and Prevention. *MMWR Recomm Rep* 2012; 61(RR-4): 1. [II-2]
10. Moyer VA, U.S. Preventive Services Task Force. Screening for hepatitis C virus infection in adults: U.S. Preventive Services Task Force recommendation statement. *Ann Intern Med* 2013; 159(5): 349. [II-2]
11. Yeung LT. Mother-to-infant transmission of hepatitis C virus. *Hepatology* 2001; 34(2): 223–9. [II-2]
12. Murphy EL et al. Risk factors for hepatitis C virus infection in United States blood donors. NHLBI Retrovirus Epidemiology Donor Study (REDS). *Hepatology* 2000; 31(3): 756. [II-2]
13. Lesourd F, Izopet J, Mervan C et al. Transmission of hepatitis C during the ancillary procedures for assisted conception: Case report. *Hum Reprod* 2000; 15: 1083–5. [II-3]
14. American Society for Reproductive Medicine, Practice Committee. Recommendations for reducing the risk of viral transmission during fertility treatment with the use of autologous gametes: A committee opinion. *Fertil Steril* 2013; 99: 340. [III]
15. Lee MH, Yang HI, Lu SN et al. Chronic hepatitis C virus infection increases mortality from hepatic and extrahepatic diseases: A community-based long-term prospective study. *J Infect Diseases* 2012; 2(3): 99–107. doi:10.1093/infdis/jis385. [II-2]

16. American College of Obstetricians and Gynecologists. AOCG Practice Bulletin No. 86. Viral hepatitis in pregnancy. *Obstet Gynecol* 2007; 110: 941–56. [III]

17. Dunkelburg JC. Hepatitis B and C in pregnancy: A review and recommendations for care. *J Perinatol* 2014; 34: 882–91. [II-3]

18. Jhaveri R. Diagnosis and management of hepatitis C virus-infected children. *Pediatr Infect Dis J* 2011; 30: 983–5. [Review]

19. Zanetti AR, Tanzi E, Paccagnini S et al. Mother-to-infant transmission of hepatitis C virus. Lombard Study Group on vertical HCV transmission. *Lancet* 1995; 345: 289–91. [II-2]

20. Ohto H, Terazawa S, Sasaki N et al. Transmission of hepatitis C virus from mothers to infants. *N Engl J Med* 1994; 330: 744–50. [II-2]

21. Delamare C, Carbonne B, Heim N et al. Detection of hepatitis C virus RNA (HCV RNA) in amniotic fluid: A prospective study. *J Hepatol* 1999; 31: 416–20. [II-2]

22. European Paediatric Hepatitis C Virus Network. Effects of mode of delivery and infant feeding on the risk of mother-to-child transmission of hepatitis C virus. *Br J Obstet Gynecol* 2001; 108: 371–7. [II-2]

23. Conte D, Fraquelli M, Prati D et al. Prevalence and clinical course of chronic hepatitis C virus (HCV) infection and the rate of vertical transmission in a cohort of 15,250 women. *Hepatology* 2000; 31: 751–5. [II-2]

24. Simms J, Duff P. Viral hepatitis in pregnancy. *Semin Perinatol* 1993; 17: 384–93. [Review]

25. Zanetti AR, Tanzi E, Newell ML. Mother-to-infant transmission of hepatitis C virus. *J Hepatol* 1999; 3(Suppl. 1): S96–S100. [II-2]

26. Pergam S, Wang C, Gardella CM et al. Pregnancy complications associated with Hepatitis C: Data from 2003–2005 Washington state birth cohort. *Am J Obstet Gynecol* 2008; 199: 38.e1–9. [II-3]

27. Feld JJ, Jacobson IM, Hezode C et al. Sofosbuvir and velpatasvir for HCV genotype 1, 2, 4, 5, and 6 infection. *N Engl J Med* 2015; 373: 2599–607. doi:10.1056/NEJMoa1512610. [I]

28. Foster GB, Afdhal N, Roberts SK et al. Sofosbuvir and velpatasvir for HCV genotype 2 and 3 infection. *N Engl J Med* 2015; 373: 2608–17. doi:10.1056/NEJMoa1512612. [I]

29. Van der Meer AJ, Veldt BJ, Feld JJ et al. Association between sustained virological response and all-cause mortality among patients with chronic hepatitis C and advanced hepatic fibrosis. *JAMA* 2012; 308: 2584–93. [II-2]

30. Bruno S, Stroffolini T, Colombo M et al., and the Italian Association of the Study of Liver Disease (AISF). Sustained virological response to interferon-alpha is associated with improved outcome in HCV-related cirrhosis: A retrospective study. *Hepatology* 2007; 45: 579–87. [II-3]

31. Webster DP, Klenerman P, Dusheiko. Hepatitis C. *Lancet* 2015; 385(9973): 1124–35. doi:10.1016/S0140-6736(14)62401-6. Epub Feb 14, 2015. [Review]

32. Pelham J, Berghella V. Alpha interferon use in pregnancy. *Obstet Gynecol* 2004; 103: 77s. [II-3]

33. Poynard T, Yuen M-F, Ratziu V et al. Viral hepatitis C. *Lancet* 2003; 362: 2095–100. [Review]

34. Airoldi J, Berghella V. Hepatitis C and pregnancy. *Obstet Gynecol Surv* 2006; 61: 10. [Review]

HIV

William R. Short

KEY POINTS

- **Identification** of HIV infection in pregnancy is **essential for the prevention of perinatal transmission. Therefore, universal screening is recommended in the first trimester or at entry into prenatal care.** An **opt-out approach** has been shown to increase acceptance rates for HIV testing in pregnant women and is the recommended approach to universal prenatal screening.
- Screening should be **repeated preferably before 36 weeks in cases of high-risk behavior, high prevalence area, or previously declined testing.**
- **Rapid testing** is recommended for previously untested women presenting in labor or those expected to be delivered for maternal or fetal indications before results of conventional testing can be obtained. If a rapid HIV test result is positive, antiretroviral prophylaxis should be offered without waiting for the results of the confirmatory conventional tests.
- **Goal** of HIV treatment in pregnancy is to **prevent vertical transmission** primarily by reducing maternal **viral load to <1000 copies/mL or preferably below the limit of detection of the assay.**
- **Rate of perinatal transmission** is directly **correlated to maternal viral load, but other factors also appear to play a role. Perinatal transmission can occur at any HIV RNA level, including in women with an undetectable viral load.**
- All HIV positive women should be recommended **a combination antiretroviral therapy (ART)** regardless of clinical or immunological diagnosis to maximally suppress viral replication, reduce the risk of perinatal transmission, and minimize the risk of development of resistant virus.
- Plasma **HIV-1 RNA levels** should be **monitored serially, at least initially, and in each trimester to both assess effectiveness of ART and assess options for best mode of delivery.**
- Women with a **viral load >1000 copies/mL at ≥34–36 weeks gestation** should be counseled regarding the **benefit of planned cesarean delivery at 38 weeks** to reduce the risk of transmission. In addition, intrapartum intravenous Zidovudine should be administered.
- With effective antiretroviral therapy leading to undetectable viral load, planned cesarean delivery for viral load ≥1000, and formula feeding, the risk of perinatal transmission is reduced to <2%.

HISTORIC NOTES

The first report in the Centers for Disease Control and Prevention's (CDC) *Morbidity and Mortality Weekly Report* (*MMWR*), dated June 5, 1981, discussed five young men, all active homosexuals who were treated for biopsy confirmed *Pneumocystis carinii* pneumonia (PCP) at three different hospitals in Los Angeles. The authors speculated that there was some aspect of a homosexual's lifestyle or some disease that was acquired through sexual contact that had a role in these unusual cases [1]. This disease was eventually called the acquired immune deficiency syndrome (AIDS), and human immunodeficiency virus (HIV) was identified as the etiologic agent. In 1983, cases of women who were steady sexual partners of men with AIDS were identified [2].

In 1994, the landmark study conducted by the Pediatric AIDS Clinical Trial group (PACTG-076) concluded that a regimen of antepartum and intrapartum Zidovudine (AZT) administered to the mother and then to the newborn for six weeks resulted in a reduction of maternal–infant transmission of HIV-1 from 25.5% to 8% [2]. This was followed by a dramatic change in the landscape of preventing mother-to-child transmission of HIV. Subsequent studies demonstrated that the use of combination antiretroviral therapy resulted in transmission rates of 1%–2% [3].

DIAGNOSIS

Diagnosis is made when a screening **ELISA is positive** and is followed by a **confirmatory positive Western blot**. Regarding **rapid testing**, the sensitivity and specificity of each of the available rapid testing assays ranges from 95% to 100%, and the positive predictive value depends on the prevalence of disease in the population. In a population with low prevalence of disease, the positive predictive value is low and the false positive rate is high. For example, with a prevalence of disease of ~1% in the population, the positive predictive value of the test may be as low as 60%.

The fourth-generation HIV test begins with testing for antibodies to HIV-1 and HIV-2 as well as for the p24 viral antigen. Samples that are found to be reactive to this initial step are then tested to determine if HIV-1 and HIV-2 antibodies are present. This qualitative immunoassay for HIV antibodies is known as the HIV Multispot. If the Multispot testing for HIV-1 and HIV-2 is negative or indeterminate, a viral nucleic acid amplification test is next performed. If the patient is Multispot negative but viral RNA positive, the patient is considered to have an acute HIV infection. Using the new fourth-generation testing algorithm, HIV can be diagnosed at approximately day 15 of acute infection or 5 days prior to the earliest diagnosis with third-generation antibody testing [4]. The time course for production of HIV RNA, HIV-1 p24 antigen, and HIV antibodies are visually represented in Figure 32.1 [5]. Testing using this algorithm has shown a specificity rate of 99.85% and has shown a reduction of false positives when compared to the previous generation modality [6]. The fourth-generation algorithm provides a more accurate way of screening for acute infection and also makes the clear distinction between infection with HIV-1 and HIV-2.

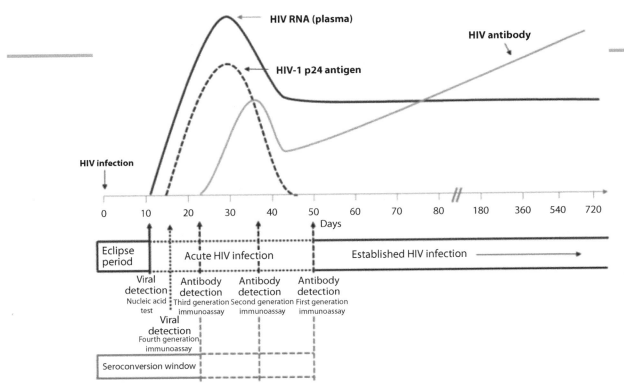

Figure 32.1 A comparison of generations 1–4 in detecting HIV in human serum. (Graph reprinted from Branson BM, Owen SM, Wesolowski L et al. Centers for Disease Control and Prevention. Laboratory Testing for the Diagnosis of HIV Infection: Updated Recommendations. Available at http://stacks.cdc.gov/view/cdc/23447. 2014.)

EPIDEMIOLOGY

Unlike the early years of the epidemic, the management of HIV in the United States today is not just about preventing death and treating opportunistic infections, but also about selecting and implementing long-term treatment strategies that will enable patients to live long, healthy, and productive lives as well as about ways to prevent the occurrence of new HIV infections.

In the United States, HIV was first reported in women in 1983 and was found among those who had been steady sexual partners of males with acquired AIDS [2]. Although men still represent the majority of people living with HIV, the number of women increased rapidly, and at the end of 2011, an estimated one in four individuals living with HIV in the United States was female. Minority women bear a disproportionate burden of the disease. At the end of 2010, **women** accounted for an estimated 9500 or **20%** of the approximate 45,000 new infections occurring in the United States. Of these new infections among women, 64% were among **black/African Americans** compared to 18% white and 15% Hispanic/Latinas compared to their makeup in the entire U.S. population of 12%, 68%, and 14%, respectively, showing how black women are disproportionally affected by the HIV epidemic. Regardless of race or ethnicity, **unprotected heterosexual contact** is the most common mode of transmission [7].

In the early years, an HIV diagnosis was essentially a death sentence. In an analysis from the North American AIDS Cohort Collaboration on Research and Design (NA-ACCORD), Hogg and colleagues estimated the change in life expectancy from 2000 to 2007 among individuals who were prescribed ART in the United States and Canada. In their analysis, **life expectancy increased from 36.1 to 51.4 years** from 2000–2002 to 2006–2007 with the greatest increases seen in those who started with a baseline CD4 count above 350 cells/mm³; in this situation, a 20-year-old HIV-positive person with a CD4 count >350 cells/mm³ can **expect to live into their early 70s** [8]. These benefits may not be achieved by all individuals for numerous reasons. In 2009, despite all the major advances in diagnosis and treatment, HIV was the fourth leading cause of death among African American women aged 25 to 44 years, causing about 800 deaths, or 9% of all deaths in this group [9].

The Women's Interagency HIV Study (WIHS), a representative cohort, studied deaths over a 10-year period among its participants. From 1995 through 2004, deaths from non-AIDs causes increased and accounted for a majority of the deaths by 2001–2004. The most common non-AIDs causes of death were trauma or overdose, liver disease, cardiovascular disease, and malignancy. Independent predictors of mortality besides HIV-associated variables were depressive symptoms and active Hepatitis B or C [10].

The **reduction in perinatal transmission of HIV** is one of the most important achievements in HIV medicine; however, perinatal transmissions continue to occur. In a landmark study, AIDS Clinical Trial Group 076 demonstrated that zidovudine monotherapy administered during pregnancy, labor, and delivery and to the newborn reduced the risk of HIV transmission to the infant by 67%, from 25% to 8% [9]. Additional studies have demonstrated the effectiveness of combination therapy, further decreasing the risk of HIV transmission to 1%–2% [10]. The Department of Health and Human Services (DHHS) perinatal guidelines **recommend that all HIV-positive women who are pregnant receive** an effective combination ART regardless of CD4 count to minimize the risk of mother-to-child transmission [10]. In 2010, an estimated 217 children younger than the age of 13 years were diagnosed with HIV in the 46 states with long-term, confidential name-based HIV infection reporting since at least 2007; **162 (75%)** of those **children were perinatally infected**. Missed opportunities included primary prevention strategies for women and girls, lack of prenatal testing, failure to prescribe antiretroviral medication during pregnancy, lack of cesarean section for women with viral loads above 1000 copies/mL, and breast-feeding [11]. In summary, treating women with HIV provides unique opportunities and challenges for providers. Understanding the epidemiologic trends in HIV-infected women in the United States is crucial because these trends are not only complex, but also dynamic.

PATHOPHYSIOLOGY

HIV primarily infects T lymphocytes that express the CD4 antigen, resulting in a progressive loss of these cells over time and impairment of cellular immunity as well as humoral immunity. When CD4 lymphocytes are sufficiently depleted, there is the progression to AIDS, characterized by the development of opportunistic infections and malignancies.

CLASSIFICATION

The CDC classification is based on clinical and laboratory evaluations (Table 32.1). There are three clinical categories: asymptomatic (A), symptomatic (B), or an AIDS-defining condition (C); and three ranges of CD4 count: >500 [1], 200–499 [2], <200 cells/mm^3. Regardless of symptoms, a CD4 <200 cells/mm^3 or the presence of an AIDS-defining illness in an HIV-positive person is an AIDS diagnosis [12].

RISK FACTORS

Risk of perinatal transmission is closely related to viral load (VL) at the time of delivery [13,14]. Other risk factors include low CD4+ T lymphocyte count, lack of antiretroviral (ARV) therapy, biologic phenotype of the virus, substance abuse, prolonged duration of membrane rupture, HCV coinfection, sexually transmitted infections (STIs), preterm birth, and chorioamnionitis [15,16]. Risk factors for maternal infection include unprotected sexual contact with an infected person, sharing drug needles or syringes, sexual contact with someone whose HIV status is unknown, and transfusions of contaminated blood or blood components. The presence of ulcerating or nonulcerating STIs, including syphilis, genital herpes, chlamydial infection, gonorrhea, or bacterial vaginosis, increases susceptibility to HIV infection during sex with infected partners. There is no evidence that HIV is spread through sweat, tears, urine, feces, or by insect bites, such as mosquito bites.

COMPLICATIONS
Maternal

Increased risks of chorioamnionitis, postpartum endometritis, and wound infection have been reported. The risk of peripartum infection is inversely proportional to the CD4+ count at the time of delivery.

Fetal

Possible increased risk of preterm delivery if on a protease inhibitor (PI)-containing regimen, but no increased risk of FGR, stillbirth, or low Apgar scores [17–19].

PREGNANCY CONSIDERATIONS

Effect of pregnancy on disease: Pregnancy has no clear effect on HIV progression. A transient but clinically insignificant decrease in the CD4+ T lymphocyte count has been described.

Effect of disease on pregnancy: Perinatal transmission can occur antepartum (25%–40%), intrapartum (60%–75%), or postpartum with breast-feeding (14%). **Perinatal transmission appears closely related to viral load.** There is a strong correlation between high maternal VL at delivery and risk of transmission, but transmission has occurred at all levels of VL [20]. Transmission rates are about 1.2% on HAART, 10.4% on AZT monotherapy, and 25% on no ARV [11].

PREGNANCY MANAGEMENT
Screening

Regulations and policies about HIV screening in pregnancy vary from state to state. Given the effectiveness of intervention, **standard serologic testing with counseling is recommended for all pregnant women at the initiation of prenatal care** with a screening ELISA, which, if positive, is followed by a confirmatory Western blot or the new approach using a fourth-generation assay. An **opt-out approach** in which the patient is informed that she will be tested for HIV along with other standard prenatal labs unless she declines has been shown in several studies to significantly increase testing rates from less than 40% to 85%–98% [21–24]. Screening should be **repeated at 28 to 32 weeks in the case of high-risk behavior, high-prevalence area, or previously declined testing** [24]. **Rapid testing** is recommended for previously untested women presenting in labor or those expected to be delivered for maternal or fetal indications before results of conventional testing can be obtained [25,26]. If a rapid HIV test result is positive, ARV prophylaxis should be offered without waiting for the results of the confirmatory conventional tests.

Table 32.1 Classification for HIV Infection

	Clinical Categories		
CD4 Count	A Asymptomatic, Acute (Primary) HIV, or PGL	B Symptomatic, Not A or C Conditions	C AIDS-Indicator Conditions
1. ≥500/μL	A1	B1	C1
2. 200–499/μL	A2	B2	C2
3. <200/μL AIDS-indicator T cell count	A3	B3	C3

Source: Data from Centers for Disease Control and Prevention. *MMWR Morb Mortal Wkly Rep*, 41, 1–19, 1992.

Principles

The goal of HIV therapy is to achieve a HIV-1 RNA level <1000 copies/mL or below the limit of detection of the assay. The **risk of perinatal transmission can be <2%** with effective ART therapy, planned cesarean delivery (CD) as appropriate, and avoidance of breast-feeding. ART therapy is recommended in pregnancy predominantly to decrease maternal VL and thereby decrease the risk of perinatal transmission and to improve maternal health. **Combination ART therapy is indicated in pregnancy regardless of clinical or immunological status.** When combination ART therapy is not available or the patient chooses not to undertake this therapy, several short-course peripartum drug regimens have been shown to significantly decrease the risk of vertical transmission to ~10%.

Preconception Counseling

Many HIV-positive women enter pregnancy aware of their diagnosis, and more than half of these women enter the first trimester on ART therapy. Preconception counseling should include the following:

- Initiate or modify ART therapy, avoiding potentially teratogenic agents
- Opportunistic infection prophylaxis as indicated by CD4 count
- Appropriate immunizations
- Optimize maternal nutritional status, initiating folic acid supplementation
- Screen for and treat STIs
- Screen for psychological and substance abuse disorders
- Prevent unwanted/unintended pregnancies

Prenatal Care

Care in pregnancy should be **multidisciplinary** with close collaboration between the obstetrician, maternal-fetal medicine team, and infectious disease specialists. A specialist with experience in the treatment of pregnant women with HIV-1 infection should be involved in the prenatal care.

Initial prenatal visit history

- Complete medical and obstetric/gynecologic history.
- Document history of prior or current ART use, including resistance to regimens.
- Assess the need for prophylaxis against opportunistic infections, such as pneumocystis pneumonia (PCP), toxoplasmosis, or mycobacterium avium complex (MAC).

Physical examination

Complete physical exam at initial visit. During subsequent visits, screen for HIV disease progression. With CD4 <200 cells/mm³, specifically evaluate for thrush, HSV, lymphadenopathy, or a rash.

Laboratory tests

Baseline (and follow-up) laboratory investigations should include the following:

- Hepatitis B surface antigen and antibody, hepatitis B core antibody, hepatitis C antibody.
- CBC with differential, liver, and renal profile.

- VDRL/RPR, gonorrhea, and chlamydia testing. PPD.
- Early diabetes screening of patients with a history of prolonged protease inhibitor (PI) exposure.
- Pap smear (all abnormal Pap smears require colposcopy). **CD4 cell count** (should be monitored at the initial visit and at least every trimester in pregnancy).
- Plasma **HIV RNA levels** (should be monitored at the initial visit, 2 to 4 weeks after initiating or changing therapy, monthly until HIV RNA levels are undetectable, and then at about 34 to 36 weeks gestation to make a decision regarding mode of delivery. The VL should decrease by 1 to 2 logs within 4 weeks of starting therapy).
- Resistance testing should be performed prior to starting ART in women who enter pregnancy with a HIV RNA level above the threshold for resistance testing on therapy; in women with suboptimal viral suppression after initiation of therapy; and in women with a persistently detectable plasma VL on therapy, which previously suppressed the virus to below the assay level of detection. Genotyping is preferable to phenotyping because it is less expensive and it has a faster turnaround time and a greater sensitivity for detecting mixtures of wild-type and resistant virus.
- HLA B-5701 testing if abacavir use is anticipated.

Counseling

- Discuss risk of transmission and factors that modify those risks.
- Discuss risk and benefits of ART for both the patient and the fetus.
- Educate on safe sex practices with condoms.

PROPHYLAXIS FOR OPPORTUNISTIC INFECTIONS (TABLE 32.2)
Antiretroviral Therapy

A landmark study, AIDS Clinical Trial Group 076, demonstrated that zidovudine monotherapy administered during pregnancy, labor, and delivery and to the newborn reduced the risk of HIV transmission to the infant by 67%, from 25% to 8% [3]. Additional studies have demonstrated the effectiveness of combination therapy, further decreasing the risk of HIV transmission to 1%–2% [20]. The Department of Health and Human Services (DHHS) perinatal guidelines recommend that all HIV-positive women who are pregnant receive effective combination ART regardless of CD4 count to minimize the risk of mother-to-child transmission [27].

The goals of HIV treatment during pregnancy are to maintain the woman's health, restore her immune system, suppress viral replication, and decrease the risk of perinatal transmission. The choice of preferred ART for the pregnant female differs from the nonpregnant female and is based on evolving experience and information about safety, efficacy, and tolerability in pregnancy (Table 32.3). Women who present for prenatal care on a suppressive regimen should continue that regimen as long as it is tolerated because there is a risk of loss of virologic control when switching regimens, and this may increase risk of perinatal transmission [27].

There are physiologic changes that occur during pregnancy that may alter drug disposition and that could potentially lead to decreased drug exposure. Some of the changes include total body water increase, decreased protein binding, induction of hepatic metabolic pathways, and increased clearance

Table 32.2 Prophylaxis for Opportunistic Infections

Infection	Indication	First-Line Tx	Alternate Tx

Pneumocystis jiroveci pneumonia[a]	• CD4 count <200
	  • CD4% <14
	• History of AIDS-defining illness
	  • History of oropharyngeal candidiasis
	• History of Pneumocystis jiroveci pneumonia (secondary prophylaxis)
		Trimethoprim-sulfamethoxazole (TMP-SMZ) one DS tablet daily
		or
		Trimethoprim-sulfamethoxazole (TMP-SMZ) one SS tablet daily
			TMP-SMZ one DS tablet 3×/wk
			or
			Dapsone 50 mg bid or 100 mg daily
			Dapsone 50 mg po daily + (Pyrimethamine 50 mg + Leucovorin 25 mg) po weekly
			or
			Dapsone 200 mg + Pyrimethamine 75 mg + Leucovorin 25 mg po weekly
			Atovaquone 750 mg bid or 1500 mg daily
			Aerosolized pentamadine 300 mg monthly

Toxoplasmic encephalitis[b]	CD4 <100 cells/µl and Seropositive for T. gondii IgG	Trimethoprim-sulfamethoxazole (TMP-SMZ) one DS tablet daily	TMP-SMZ one SS tablet daily TMP-SMZ one DS 3×/week Dapsone 50 mg po daily + (Pyrimethamine 50 mg + Leucovorin 25 mg) po weekly Dapsone 200 mg po + leucovorin 25 mg po weekly and pyrimethamne 75 mg weekly Atovaquone 1500 mg po daily Atovaquone 1500 mg + Pyrimethamine 25 mg + Leucovorin 10 mg po daily
Disseminated *Mycobacterium avium* complex[c] *Mycobacterium tuberculosis*	CD4 count <50 cells/µl PPD ≥5 mm or Prior positive PPD without adequate treatment or Contact with person with active TB regardless of PPD status	Azithromycin 1200 mg po/week Clarithromycin 500 mg bid or Azithromycin 600 mg twice weekly INH sensitive: INH 300 mg po + pyridoxine 50 mg po daily for 9 months or INH 900 mg po twice weekly by DOT + pyridoxine 25 mg po daily for 9 months INH resistant: Rifampin 600 mg po daily or rifabutin 300 mg po daily for 4 months	Rifabutin 300 mg po daily or Rifabutin 300 mg po daily + Azithromycin 1200 mg po weekly Rifampin 600 mg po daily or rifabutin (dose dependent on drug interactions with ART) po daily for 4 months
Varicella zoster virus	Varicella nonimmune and exposed to chicken pox or shingles	Varicella zoster immune globulin— 5 vials (1.25 mL each) within 48–96 hours of exposure	

[a]Primary prophylaxis should be discontinued after sustained response to ART with a CD4 count >200 cells/µl for >3 months. Secondary prophylaxis should be discontinued if CD4 count increases from <200 cells/µl to >200 cells/µl for >3 months in response to ART.
[b]Discontinue primary prophylaxis after sustained response to ART with CD4 count >200 cells/µl for >3 months. Discontinue secondary prophylaxis when initial therapy completed and asymptomatic with sustained CD4 count >200 cells/µl for >6 months in response to ART.
[c]Discontinue primary prophylaxis after sustained response to ART with CD4 count >100 cells/µl for >3 months.

of drugs that are renally eliminated [28]. These changes may be associated with incomplete virologic suppression, virologic failure, and/or development of drug resistance, so altered doses of some ART should be considered or careful monitoring with viral load, particularly in the second and third trimesters.

IMMUNIZATIONS [29]

Although HIV infection is primarily a disease of cell-mediated immunity, humoral immunity is also impaired in HIV-positive individuals. Serologic response to vaccination may be suboptimal, especially in those with advanced disease. Live virus vaccines have historically been withheld from HIV-positive individuals because of the risk of contracting the disease from the vaccine. Vaccines should be administered early in the course of HIV infection if possible to increase the likelihood of adequate responses and to minimize the risk of

disseminated infection from live vaccines in immunocompromised patients.

All patients should receive Prevnar-13, **Pneumovax, Hepatitis B** vaccine series, and inactivated **Influenza** vaccine. Patients who are HCV positive should also be offered the **Hepatitis A** vaccine series.

Tetanus and diphtheria (Td) immunization should be updated. Substitute Tdap once for Td, then Td booster every 10 years.

Inactivated polio vaccine as a primary series or booster should be administered to those at risk of exposure.

If risk of exposure to yellow fever is high and CD4 count is >200, yellow fever vaccine may be administered; however, serologic response may be as low as 35% [27].

Patients who are Rubella nonimmune and have a CD4 count >200 should be offered vaccination in the postpartum period [30].

Table 32.3   Initial Combination Regimens for Antiretroviral-Naïve Pregnant Women

Drug	Comments
Preferred regimens	
Regimens with clinical trial data in adults demonstrating optimal efficacy and durability with acceptable toxicity and ease of use, PK data available in pregnancy, and no evidence to date of teratogenic effects or established adverse outcomes for mother/fetus. To minimize the risk of resistance, a PI regimen is preferred for women who may stop ART during the postpartum period.	
Preferred two-NRTI backbone	
ABC/3TC	Available as FDC. Can be administered once daily. ABC **should not be used** in patients who test positive for HLA-B*5701 because of the risk of hypersensitivity reaction. ABC/3TC with ATV/r or with EFV is not recommended if pretreatment HIV RNA >100,000 copies/mL.
TDF/FTC or 3TC	TDF/FTC available as FDC. Either TDF/FTC or TDF and 3TC can be administered once daily. TDF has potential renal toxicity, thus TDF-based dual NRTI combinations should be used with caution in patients with renal insufficiency.
ZDV/3TC	Available as FDC. NRTI combination with most experience for use in pregnancy but has disadvantages of requirement for twice-daily administration and increased potential for hematologic toxicities.
Preferred PI regimens	
ATV/r plus a preferred two-NRTI backbone	Once daily administration. Extensive experience in pregnancy. Maternal hyperbilirubinemia.
DRV/r plus a preferred two-NRTI backbone	Better tolerated than LPV/r. PK data available. Increasing experience with use in pregnancy. Must be used twice daily during pregnancy.
Preferred NNRTI regimen	
EFV plus a preferred two-NRTI backbone Note: May be initiated **after the first 8 weeks of pregnancy.**	Concern because of birth effects seen in primate study; risk in humans is unclear. Postpartum contraception must be ensured. Preferred regimen in women who require coadministration of drugs with significant interactions with PIs or the convenience of coformulated, single tablet, once-daily regimen.
Preferred integrase inhibitor regimen	
RAL plus a preferred two-NRTI backbone	PK data available and increasing experience in pregnancy. Rapid viral load reduction. Useful when drug interactions with PI-based regimens are a concern. Twice-daily dosing required.

Source: Panel on Treatment of HIV-Infected Pregnant Women and Prevention of Perinatal Transmission. *Recommendations for Use of Antiretroviral Drugs in Pregnant HIV-1-Infected Women for Maternal Health and Interventions to Reduce Perinatal HIV Transmission in the United States. March 28, 2014.* Available at: http://aidsinfo.nih.gov/contentfiles/PerinatalGL.pdf. Accessed December 29, 2015. [Guideline]
Abbreviations: 3TC, lamivudine; ABC, abacavir; ART, antiretroviral therapy; ARV, antiretroviral; ATV/r, atazanavir/ritonavir; CD4, CD4 T lymphocyte cell; DRV/r, darunavir/ritonavir; EFV, efavirenz; FDC, fixed-dose combination; FTC, emtricitabine; NNRTI, non-nucleoside reverse transcriptase inhibitor; NRTI, nucleoside reverse transcriptase inhibitor; PI, protease inhibitor; PK, pharmacokinetic; RAL, raltegravir; RTV, ritonavir; TDF, tenofovir disoproxil fumarate; ZDV, zidovudine.

Varicella vaccine is indicated in HIV-positive adults with a CD4 cell count >200 cells/ul in the postpartum period for varicella nonimmune women.

BCG vaccine should **not** be administered to HIV-infected women or their newborns—even if the risk of acquiring TB is high. Disseminated BCG has been reported after immunization [31,32].

ANEUPLOIDY SCREENING
There is limited evidence on the effect of HIV infection on prenatal aneuploidy screening. Currently, serum screening appears **not affected** sufficiently **by HIV infection** to alter its accuracy. Routine counseling should occur regarding noninvasive prenatal aneuploidy screening [33] (see Chapter 5 in *Obstetric Evidence Based Guidelines*).

ANTEPARTUM TESTING
Ultrasound evaluation should be performed for the usual obstetric indications including confirmation of gestational age and to assess fetal anatomy [34]. Invasive procedures, such as amniocentesis, chorionic villus sampling, and cordocentesis indicated for diagnostic or therapeutic purposes, may place the

fetus at increased risk of transmission of the HIV virus, and appropriate counseling with review of indication for these interventions is recommended [35]. Among women on HAART, no perinatal transmissions have been reported after **amniocentesis**, but a small risk of transmission cannot be ruled out [35]. If an amniocentesis is planned, it **should be performed after initiation of an effective combination ART regimen and when the VL is nondetectable, avoiding traversing the placenta.**

PRETERM PREMATURE RUPTURE OF MEMBRANES
The risks of prematurity-related morbidity/mortality must be balanced against the risk of vertical transmission with prolonged rupture of membranes. If PPROM occurs prior to 32 weeks, expectant management with administration of corticosteroids for fetal maturity and antibiotics for latency are recommended. At a gestational age ≥32 weeks, delivery without the benefit of corticosteroids should be considered if appropriate support is immediately available to care for the premature infant. Consultation with a neonatologist should be sought if considering delivery prior to 32 weeks without the benefit of steroids as prognosis is dependent on resources available for care of the preterm infant [16].

DELIVERY AND INTRAPARTUM CARE

Use the most recent VL level to counsel regarding **mode of delivery**. Risk of perinatal transmission with persistently undetectable VL on antiretroviral therapy is <2% regardless of mode of delivery. Honor the woman's decision regarding mode of delivery. Women who have a viral load greater than 1000 copies/mL at the time of delivery should undergo a cesarean delivery scheduled at 38 weeks gestation with the addition of preoperative intravenous zidovudine to maximize prevention of perinatal transmission. It remains unclear how soon after the onset of labor or rupture of membranes that the benefit of cesarean delivery is lost; the delivery plan in these situations should be individualized. For women who have viral loads below the threshold of 1000 copies/mL, there is no proven added benefit to a cesarean section, and in this situation, cesarean should be performed only for standard obstetrical indications. ART should be continued during labor [27]. The benefits of intrapartum AZT in this situation are not clear, and the recommendation is not to administer it.

Maintain universal body fluid precautions for all deliveries. Inform pediatrician of mother's status. Bulb suction for the baby at delivery and washing off maternal secretions as soon as possible after birth are suggested.

Induction of labor should be reserved for obstetric indications. Admit in early labor and augment labor to expedite delivery. **Continue the oral ART regimen in labor; administer intravenous AZT in labor with loading and maintenance dosing continuously until the umbilical cord is clamped if the viral load is >1000 copies/mL at or near delivery.** Continue ART therapy as usual and initiate **AZT infusion for 3 hours prior to CD** and continue until cord clamped. Delay amniotomy; however, it is not contraindicated and may be used to augment labor later in the active phase. Avoid invasive fetal monitoring, intrauterine pressure catheter (IUPC), fetal scalp electrode (FSE), fetal scalp blood sampling (FSBS), episiotomy, forceps, or vacuum delivery [27].

BREAST-FEEDING

Women with HIV infection who have access to an adequate supply of infant formula or other suitable source of nutrition **should not breast-feed** [36]. If access to an alternate nutrition source is not sufficient to completely replace breast-feeding, then exclusive breast-feeding is preferable to alternating breast-feeding/formula-feeding regimens. Any woman considering breast-feeding should be aware of her HIV status. A decision not to breast-feed may raise issues regarding confidentiality of a mothers' HIV diagnosis and requires sensitivity and supportive interventions [37,38].

MATERNAL POSTPARTUM CARE

Maternal postpartum care is essential to establish ongoing primary care for HIV disease. Long-term planning is essential to ensure that the woman does not fall out of the health care system. Following delivery, considerations regarding **continuation of the ART regimen for maternal therapeutic indications are the same as for nonpregnant individuals.** The pros and cons of continuing versus discontinuing therapy postpartum should be discussed with the woman so that she can make an educated decision prior to delivery regarding postpartum ART use. In general, once ART is commenced, it is continued for lifetime.

Family planning is critical to the prevention of perinatal transmission. **Condom use should be strongly encouraged.** Monitor for gynecological manifestations associated with disease progression.

Rubella vaccines should be administered postpartum to those women with CD4 count >200 [30].

FOLLOW-UP OF INFANTS

The baby should be bathed soon after delivery to remove potentially infectious maternal secretions. **All HIV-exposed infants should receive postpartum ART drugs to reduce perinatal transmission of HIV.** Infant prophylaxis should be **initiated as soon as possible postdelivery.** HIV diagnostic testing to establish or rule out HIV infection as early as possible is suggested. Initiate PCP prophylaxis at six weeks (until there are two consecutive negative HIV results). Long-term follow-up of HIV- and ARV-exposed infants is important [27].

DIAGNOSIS OF HIV INFECTION IN THE INFANT

Early diagnosis of HIV infection is crucial in infants; however, establishing the diagnosis is complicated by the presence of transplacentally acquired maternal antibodies, which make serological testing unreliable. The mean time to clear maternal antibodies is 10.3 months, but it can take up to 18 months [39]. For this reason, early pediatric diagnosis relies on identification of the virus usually via HIV-1 DNA or RNA PCR (polymerase chain reaction) techniques. The former measures integrated virus in the host genome, and the latter measures circulating plasma virus. HIV-1 coculture is not routinely performed because of cost and time although it is also a reliable diagnostic method. HIV viral load testing should be performed at a minimum age of 14 to 21 days, 1 to 2 months, and 4 to 6 months after birth. Some experts also test at birth, especially if there is poor control in pregnancy. **HIV may be presumptively excluded with two or more negative PCR tests with one at ≥14 days and another at ≥1 month of age.** Many experts confirm HIV-negative status with an HIV antibody test at 12 to 18 months [40].

ACUTE HIV INFECTION

Primary or acute HIV infection in pregnancy is associated with an increased risk of perinatal transmission. When acute retroviral syndrome is suspected in pregnancy or during breast-feeding, a plasma HIV RNA test should be performed, which is usually >10,000,000 copies/mL with a negative HIV antibody test [41]. All pregnant women with acute or recent HIV infection should start ART as soon as possible to prevent perinatal transmission aiming to suppress the VL to undetectable. Resistance testing should be performed but initiation should not be delayed pending the results. Because clinically significant resistance to protease inhibitors (PI) is less common than resistance to non-nucleoside reverse transcriptase inhibitor (NNRTI) in naïve patients, a Ritonavir-boosted PI-based regimen should be used if initiated prior to resistance testing results becoming available.

REFERENCES

1. CDC. Pneumocystis pneumonia—Los Angeles. *MMWR Morb Mortal Wkly Rep* 1981; 30: 250–2. [Epidemiologic data]
2. CDC. *Immunodeficiency among female sex partners of males with Acquired Immune Deficiency Syndrome (AIDS).* 1983; 31: 697–8. [II-2]

3. Connor EM, Sperling RS, Gelber R et al. Reduction of maternal-infant transmission of human immunodeficiency virus type 1 with zidovudine treatment. Pediatric AIDS Clinical Trials Group Protocol 076 Study Group. *N Engl J Med* 1994; 331(18): 1173–80. [II-2]

4. Hutchinson AB, Ethridge SF, Wesolowski LG et al. Costs and outcomes of laboratory diagnostic algorithms for the detection of HIV. *J Clin Virology* 2013; 58 (Suppl. 1): e2–7. [II-2]

5. Branson BM, Owen SM, Wesolowski L et al. Centers for Disease Control and Prevention. Laboratory Testing for the Diagnosis of HIV Infection: Updated Recommendations. Available at http://stacks.cdc.gov/view/cdc/23447. Published June 27, 2014. [Guideline]

6. Lee K, Park HD, Kang ES. Reduction of HIV seroconversion window period and false positive rate by using ADVIA Centaur HIV antigen/antibody combo assay. *Ann Laboratory Med* 2013; 33960: 420–5. [II-2]

7. CDC. Estimated HIV incidence among adult and adolescents in the United States, 2007–2010. *HIV Surveillance Supplemental Report* 2012; 17(4). [Epidemiologic data]

8. Samji H, Cescon A, Hogg RS et al. Closing the gap: Increases in life expectancy among treated HIV-positive individuals in the United States and Canada. *PLoS ONE* 8(12): e81355. doi:10.1371/journal.pone.0081355. [II-2]

9. CDC. HIV Mortality (through 2009). Accessed at http://www.cdc.gov/hiv/library/slideserts/index/html. [Epidemiologic data]

10. French A, Gawel SH, Hershow R et al. Trends in mortality and causes of death among women with HIV in the US: A ten-year study. *JAIDS* 2009; 51(4): 399–406. [II-2]

11. Cooper ER, Charurat M, Mofenson L et al. Combination antiretroviral strategies for the treatment of pregnant HIV-1-infected women and prevention of perinatal HIV-1 transmission. *J Acquir Immune Defic Syndr* 2002; 29(5): 484–94. [II-2]

12. Castro KG, Ward JW, Slutsker L et al. 1993 revised classification system for HIV infection and expanded surveillance case definition for AIDS among adolescents and adults. *MMWR Recomm Rep* 1992; 41(RR-17): 1–19. [Guideline]

13. Garcia PM, Kalish LA, Pitt J et al. Maternal levels of plasma human immunodeficiency virus type 1 RNA and the risk of perinatal transmission. Women and infants transmission study group. *N Engl J Med* 1999; 341(6): 394–402. [II-2]

14. Mofenson LM, Lambert JS, Stiehm ER et al. Risk factors for perinatal transmission of human immunodeficiency virus type 1 in women treated with zidovudine. Pediatric AIDS Clinical Trials Group Study 185 Team. *N Engl J Med* 1999; 341(6): 385–93. [II-2]

15. Landesman SH, Kalish LA, Burns DN et al. Obstetrical factors and the transmission of human immunodeficiency virus type 1 from mother to child. The women and infants transmission study. *N Engl J Med* 1996; 334(25): 1617–23. [II-2]

16. International Perinatal HIV Group. Duration of ruptured membranes and vertical transmission of HIV-1: A meta-analysis from 15 prospective cohort studies. *AIDS* 2001; 15(3): 357–68. [Meta-analysis of II-2 data]

17. European Collaborative Study, Swiss Mother and Child HIV Cohort Study. Combination Antiretroviral Therapy and duration of pregnancy. *AIDS* 2000; 14(18): 2913–20. [II-2]

18. Cotter A, Gonzales Garcia A, Dutheley L et al. Is antiretroviral therapy associated with an increased risk of preterm delivery, low birthweight or stillbirth? *J Infect Dis* 2006; 193: 1195–201. [II-2]

19. Tuomala RE, Shapiro DE, Mofenson L et al. Antiretroviral therapy during pregnancy and the risk of an adverse outcome. *N Engl J Med* 2002; 346(24): 1863–70. [II-2]

20. Ioannidis JP, Abrams EJ, Ammann A et al. Perinatal transmission of human immunodeficiency virus type 1 by pregnant women with RNA virus loads <1000 copies/ml. *J Infect Dis* 2001; 183(4): 539–45. [II-2]

21. Stanley B, Fraser J, Cox NH. Uptake of HIV screening in genitourinary medicine after change to "opt-out" consent. *Br Med J* 2003; 326(7400): 1174. [II-2]

22. Mossman CL, Ratnam S. Opt-out prenatal HIV testing in Newfoundland and Labrador. *Can Med Assoc J* 2002; 167(6): 630; author reply 630–1. [II-2]

23. Jayaraman GC, Preiksaitis JK, Larke B. Mandatory reporting of HIV infection and opt-out prenatal screening for HIV infection: Effect on testing rates. *Can Med Assoc J* 2003; 168(6): 679–82. [II-2]

24. Center for Disease Control and Prevention. HIV testing among pregnant women United States and Canada, 1998–2001. *MMWR* 2002. [Epidemiologic data]

25. Prenatal and perinatal human immunodeficiency virus testing: Expanded recommendations. American College of Obstetricians and Gynecologists committee opinion number 418. *Obstet Gynecol* 2008; 112: 739–42. [Guideline]

26. Bulterys M, Jamieson DJ, O'Sullivan MJ et al. Rapid HIV-1 testing during labor: A multicenter study. *J Am Med Assoc* 2004; 292(2): 219–23. [II-2]

27. Panel on Treatment of HIV-Infected Pregnant Women and Prevention of Perinatal Transmission. *Recommendations for Use of Antiretroviral Drugs in Pregnant HIV-1-Infected Women for Maternal Health and Interventions to Reduce Perinatal HIV Transmission in the United States*. March 28, 2014. Available at: http://aidsinfo.nih.gov/contentfiles/PerinatalGL.pdf. Accessed December 29, 2015. [Guideline]

28. Mirochnick M, Capparelli E. Pharmacokinetic antiretrovirals in pregnant women. *Clin Pharmacokinetics* 2004; 43(15): 1071–87. [II-2]

29. Aberg JA, Gallant JE, Ghanem KG et al. Primary care guidelines for the management of persons infected with HIV: 2013 update by the HIV Medical Association of the Infectious Diseases Society of America. *CID* 2013. [Guideline]

30. Kim DK, Bridges CB, Harriman KH. Advisory Committee on Immunization practices recommended immunization schedule for adults 19 years or older: United States, 2016. *Ann Internal Med* 2016; 164(3): 184–94. [Guideline]

31. CDC. Division of Tuberculosis Elimination. *Fact Sheet BCG vaccine*. 2005. [Guideline]

32. Hussey G, Hawkridge T, Eley B et al. Adverse effects of bacilli calmette-Guerin vaccination in HIV-positive infants. *CID* 2004; 38(9): 1333–4. [II-2]

33. LaVigne KA, Seligman NS, Berghella V. Offering aneuploidy screening to HIV infected women: Routine counseling. *Br J Obstet Gynecol* 2011; 118(7): 775–8. [II-2]

34. ACOG Committee on Practice Bulletin 2004. ACOG Practice Bulletin No. 58. Ultrasonography in pregnancy. *Obstet Gynecol* 2004; 104(6): 1449–58. [Guideline]

35. Mandelbrot L, Jasseron C, Ekoukou D et al. Amniocentesis and mother to child HIV transmission in the Agence Nationale de Recherches sur le SIDA et les Hepatites Virales French Perinatal Cohort. *Am J Obstet Gynecol* 2009; 200(2): 160.e1–9. [II-2]

36. Coutsoudis A. Breastfeeding and the HIV positive mother: The debate continues. *Early Hum Dev* 2005; 81(1): 87–93. [Review]

37. Dunn DT, Newell ML, Ades AE et al. Risk of human immunodeficiency virus type 1 transmission through breastfeeding. *Lancet* 1992; 340(8819): 585–8. [II-2]

38. Tess BH, Rodrigues LC, Newell ML et al. Infant feeding and risk of mother-to-child transmission of HIV-1 in Sao Paulo State, Brazil. Sao Paulo collaborative study for vertical transmission of HIV-1. *J Acquir Immune Defic Syndr Hum Retrovirol* 1998; 19(2): 189–94. [II-2]

39. Louisirirotchanakul S, Kanoksinsombat C, Likanonsakul S et al. Patterns of anti-HIV IgG3, IgA and p24Ag in perinatally HIV-1 infected infants. *Asian Pac J Allergy Immunol* 2002; 20(2): 99–104. [II-2]

40. Centers for Disease Control and Prevention. Revised surveillance case definitions for HIV infection among adults, adolescents and children aged <18 months and for HIV infection and AIDS among children aged 18 months to <13 years, United States, 2008. *MMWR* 2008; 57(RR-10): 1–12. [Epidemiologic data]

41. Hecht FM, Busch MP, Rawal B et al. Use of laboratory tests and clinical symptoms for identification of primary HIV infection. *AIDS* 2002; 16(8): 1119–29. [II-2]

33

Gonorrhea

A. Marie O'Neill

KEY POINTS

- Gonorrhea has been associated with an increased risk of spontaneous abortion, preterm birth, early rupture of fetal membranes, chorioamnionitis, and perinatal mortality as well as neonatal conjunctivitis leading to blindness, increased HIV transmission, and postpartum infection.
- Prevention strategies shown to be effective include use of **condoms, screening high-risk populations, early diagnosis and treatment,** and **partner notification and treatment without clinical assessment.**
- There is insufficient evidence to recommend screening of low-risk pregnant women.
- Pregnant women at **high risk** for gonorrhea are those of **age <25 years, with prior sexually transmitted infection (STI), having multiple sexual partners, having a partner with a past history of any sexually transmitted infections (STI), sex work, drug use, or inconsistent condom use.** These women should be **screened** in pregnancy **for gonorrhea.**
- Definitive **diagnosis** requires isolation by **culture or positive nucleic acid amplification test.**
- Because of the potential for concomitant infection, **testing for *Chlamydia trachomatis*, syphilis, HIV, and hepatitis B is recommended.**
- First-line treatment for gonorrhea in pregnancy in the United States and most of Western Europe is **ceftriaxone 250 mg IM plus a single dose of azithromycin 1 g orally.** Due to increasing drug resistance, single agent therapy is no longer considered adequate.
- Patients presenting with preterm premature rupture of membranes and having active gonorrheal infection can be managed expectantly as long as prompt treatment for gonorrhea is instituted.
- The emergence of **multidrug-resistant organisms** is causing a worldwide crisis in the treatment of gonorrhea and of all STIs. The prevalence of multidrug-resistant gonorrhea is greatest in low- and middle-income countries but is increasing in all countries. Overuse and inappropriate use of antibiotics in health care and farming is a major and preventable contributor to the emergence of drug-resistant organisms. Responsible use of antibiotics must become a priority for all health care professionals.

EPIDEMIOLOGY/INCIDENCE

Worldwide, it is estimated that 106.1 million new cases of gonorrhea occur annually [1]. The highest incidences of gonorrhea and its complications occur in developing countries. As a result of a national gonorrhea control program implemented in the United States in the 1970s, the national rate of gonorrheal infection has decreased >75% over the last three decades. The number of cases reported in the United States reached a low of **301,174 cases, or 99.1/100,000**; however, the rate has increased slightly each year since. In 2013, there were 333,004 cases of gonorrhea reported to the Centers for Disease Control (CDC) with approximately 44,000 of these infections occurring in pregnant women. The CDC estimated that fewer than half of all infections are reported, and the true rate is estimated to be 820,000 cases annually [2]. The incidence is substantially lower in all countries of Western Europe than in the United States, but high and rising rates have been documented in Eastern Europe. Gonorrhea disproportionately affects African-Americans with the reported rate of infection in this population being 12.4 times greater than that in whites; however, as a result of both declining rates of infection in blacks and increasing rates in whites, this disparity is declining [2,3]. The median prevalence of gonorrhea in unselected populations of pregnant women has been estimated to be 10% in Africa, 5% in Latin America, and 4% in Asia [4].

ETIOLOGY

Neisseria gonorrhoeae is a gram-negative diplococcus that primarily infects the nonciliated, columnar, or cuboidal epithelium of the endocervix, urethra, rectum, or pharynx. Gonococci are obligate human pathogens and can survive only briefly outside of the human reservoir.

PATHOPHYSIOLOGY/TRANSMISSION

N. gonorrhoeae is easily transmitted during oral, vaginal, or anal sex. The transmission rate from male to female during vaginal intercourse is approximately 50% per contact, rising to 90% after three exposures [5,6]. The incubation period for *N. gonorrhoeae* is on average 2 to 7 days but may vary between 1 and 14 days. **Vertical transmission to the infant occurs in 30% to 47% cases if cervical infection is present at the time of delivery.** The eye is the most common site of neonatal infection, but disseminated gonococcal infection or gonococcal arthritis may also occur in the newborn [7,8]. The vast majority of vertical transmission occurs **during vaginal delivery**; however, transmission has been reported after cesarean delivery in patients with ruptured membranes.

SYMPTOMS

The clinical manifestations of gonorrhea are unchanged in pregnant women except that pelvic inflammatory disease (PID) and perihepatitis are uncommon after the first trimester. Cervical infection is **asymptomatic in up to 80% of women** [9]. When symptoms are present, they include a purulent or mucopurulent cervical exudate, edema, and easily induced cervical or endocervical bleeding. Urethral infection is present in 70% to 90% of women who have gonococcal cervicitis—most will present with dysuria [9,10]. *N. gonorrhoeae* does not cause vaginitis; however, coinfection with bacterial vaginosis, trichomonas, or *C. trachomatis* is common and often causes abnormal vaginal discharge. Pharyngeal infection is typically asymptomatic but may cause exudative pharyngitis and cervical lymphadenopathy. This occurs in 10% to 20% of women with cervical gonorrhea [11,12]. Rectal infection is typically asymptomatic but may cause anal pruritus; mucopurulent discharge; and sometimes pain, tenesmus, and bleeding. This occurs in about 40% of women with cervical gonorrhea [9]. Disseminated gonococcal infection occurs in 0.5% to 3% of infected individuals and usually causes septic arthritis accompanied by a rash of hemorrhagic papules and pustules [13]. There are conflicting reports as to whether pregnancy is a risk factor for disseminated infection; however, a recent publication reports an incidence of 0.04% to 0.09% in pregnancy [14].

COMPLICATIONS

- Gonorrhea has been associated with an increased risk of **spontaneous abortion, preterm birth, early rupture of fetal membranes, chorioamnionitis, and perinatal mortality**. It is not clear if these complications are a direct result of gonococcal infection or if infection is a marker for other high-risk factors [15–18].
- Vertical transmission to the infant can cause conjunctivitis, which if left untreated may result in **blindness**. Prior to routine prophylaxis of all infants at the time of birth, approximately 25% of congenital blindness in the United States was caused by gonorrheal conjunctivitis, and it remains a major cause of congenital blindness in underdeveloped countries [7,8].
- Epidemiologic and biologic studies provide strong evidence that gonococcal infections **facilitate the transmission of HIV infection**, which has major implications for the pregnancy [18,19].
- Women with active cervical infection at the time of delivery are at increased risk for **postpartum infection** [15,17].

MANAGEMENT
Prevention

Condoms, when used correctly and consistently, provide a high degree of protection from gonorrheal infection as well as from other STIs [20,21]. Other important practices for prevention of gonorrhea are **screening to identify asymptomatic cases in high-risk populations, early diagnosis and treatment, and partner notification and treatment.** Several recent randomized trials reported a **reduction in the rate of reinfection with an expedited approach to partner therapy (EPT)** whereby **partners are treated without a clinical assessment.** In this approach, the patient delivers either medication or prescriptions to their partner [22–25]. The legal status of such an approach varies in the United States with some states prohibiting EPT. Legal status should be verified prior to providing EPT. Another complicating factor in providing EPT is the most recent recommendation of combination intramuscular and oral medications as first-line treatment for uncomplicated gonorrhea in the United States. **Evaluation of all sex partners from the previous 60 days and treatment with the recommended regimen (ceftriaxone 250 mg IM plus a**

single dose of azithromycin 1 g orally) is the best course of action.** However, if this is not possible, EPT with oral cefixime 400 mg and azithromycin 1 g should be considered as not treating partners is significantly more harmful than is the use of oral EPT for gonorrhea [24,25].

Screening (Table 33.1) [26–31]

There is no evidence that screening low-risk pregnant women is beneficial. Screening pregnant **women at high risk** for gonorrhea may prevent other complications associated with gonococcal infection during pregnancy. **Risk factors include age <25, prior STI, multiple sexual partners, having a partner with a past history of any STI, sex work, drug use, or inconsistent condom use.** Because *N. gonorrhoeae* can cause infection at a variety of body sites, the decision of which sites to test should be guided by sexual history and physical exam findings.

Diagnosis (Table 33.1) [26–31]

Isolation of *N. gonorrhoeae* by culture is the historic mainstay of gonorrhea diagnosis; however, this method is somewhat limited by the difficulty of maintaining viability of organisms during transport and storage from a variety of settings in which screening programs are established and the time delay from specimen collection to result reporting [5,26]. In most laboratories, culture has been replaced by **nucleic acid amplification tests** (**NAATs**), including ligase (LCR), polymerase chain reaction (PCR), transcription-mediated amplification (TMA), and strand-displacement amplification (SDA). The sensitivity, specificity, and ease of specimen collection and transport with NAAT technology is better than that of any other test available, and these tests have been shown to be cost-effective in preventing sequelae due to *N. gonorrhea* infection [26]. A significant limitation of these tests is the risk of specimen contamination—the presence of a single viable or nonviable organism will lead to a positive test result; therefore, workflow and lab cleaning procedures are of extreme importance [31]. Non-NAAT testing utilizing DNA probes is available but is NOT recommended due to significantly lower sensitivity [30]. For NAAT testing, **a self-collected or clinician-collected vaginal swab is the preferred specimen type; however, a first catch voided urine or endocervical swab is acceptable** for most available assays—confirm specimen requirements for each assay used [30]. NAAT tests are not FDA approved for use on rectal, pharyngeal, or conjunctival specimens; however, most labs have developed performance specifications for using NAATs on these specimens, and they are currently the recommended testing method for rectal and oropharyngeal specimens with the caveat that the testing lab must be in compliance with the Clinical Laboratory Improvement Amendments (CLIA) for test modifications [28–30]. Conjunctival specimens should be cultured. Some assays can detect *C. trachomatis* or *N. gonorrhoeae* in a single specimen. Several of these combined assays do not differentiate between the two organisms, so a positive result should be followed by tests for each organism to obtain an organism-specific result [31]. Clinicians who perform STI screening tests should be aware of the prevalence of STIs in the population being screened and have a conceptual understanding of positive predictive value and the impact of screening low-risk individuals with a test that has limited specificity. The positive predictive value of nucleic acid-based tests is <60% when

Table 33.1 Screening and Diagnostic Tests for Gonorrhea

	Sensitivity	Specificity	Advantages	Disadvantages
NAAT	96.7% compared to culture	98%	• High sensitivity • Is the current gold standard for screening and diagnosis • Approved for testing on voided urine • Approved for testing on liquid-based pap medium • Rapid results • Specimen less affected by handling and transport • Currently the preferred testing method for rectal and oropharyngeal specimens if lab is CLIA compliant	• Most expensive option • No isolate preserved for forensics or sensitivity testing • Highest false-positive rate when persons at low risk are tested • Limited to cervical or urine specimens • Nonviable organisms or contaminants will give false-positive result
Culture	80%–90%	100%	• Can obtain specimen from any potentially infected site • Preserve and isolate for antimicrobial sensitivity testing and forensics	• Organism is especially fastidious—can be difficult to grow in culture • Overgrowth of contaminating microorganisms can give a false negative result • Organism can be rendered nonviable during transport if incorrect media used or delay in transport • 48–72 hr to complete
Gram stain	40%–60% compared to culture	70%–90%	• Rapid results • Negative predictive value is 99%–100% • In setting of limited resources can be used for screening with follow-up testing of screen positives	• Least sensitive/specific • Higher false negative rate results in more failure to treat
Non-NAAT	92.1% compared to culture	99%	• Inexpensive • Rapid results • Specimen less affected by handling and transport	• Nonviable organisms or contaminants will give false-positive result • Limited to cervical specimens • NOT RECOMMENDED

Sources: Crotchfelt KA, Welsh LE, DeBonville D et al. *J Clin Microbiol*, 35, 6, 1536–40, 1997; Koumans EH, Black CM, Markowitz LE et al. *J Clin Microbiol*, 41, 4, 1507–11, 2003; Martin DH, Cammarata C, Van Der Pol B et al. *J Clin Microbiol*, 38, 10, 3544–9, 2000; Bachmann LH, Johnson RE, Cheng H, Markowitz LE, Papp JR, Hook EW III. *J Clin Microbiol*, 47, 902–7, 2009; Bachmann LH, Johnson RE, Cheng H et al. *J Clin Microbiol*, 48, 1827–32, 2010; Papp JR, Schachter J, Gaydos C, Van Der Pol B. Recommendations for the laboratory-based detection of *Chlamydia trachomatis* and *Neisseria gonorrhea*, 2014.

Abbreviation: NAAT, nucleic acid amplification test.

the prevalence of infection in the population is <1%. **Routine test of cure is not recommended except in cases in which an alternate treatment is used to treat pharyngeal infections; then a test of cure by either culture or NAAT is recommended in 14 days** [31,32]. Because of the continued increase in antibiotic-resistant strains, **suspected treatment failures must be evaluated with culture rather than a NAAT so that antibiotic sensitivity can be evaluated** [31,32].

Treatment

Due to increasing multidrug resistance, awareness of local antimicrobial resistance data is of utmost importance in the treatment of gonorrhea. The Gonococcal Isolate Surveillance Project (GISP) of the CDC and the European Gonococcal Antimicrobial Surveillance Programme (Euro-GASP) have reported resistance to penicillins, tetracyclines, and fluoroquinolones. From 2006 to 2011, the minimum concentrations of cefixime needed to inhibit in vitro growth of the *N. gonorrhoeae* strains circulating in the United States and many other countries increased, suggesting that the susceptibility may be decreasing. In addition, treatment failures with cefixime or other oral cephalosporins have been reported in Asia, Europe, South Africa, and Canada [32–37].

Current CDC recommendations for treatment are presented in Table 33.2 [32,33]. Currently, only one regimen consisting of **dual treatment with ceftriaxone and azithromycin is recommended** for treatment of gonorrhea in the United States, but as resistance patterns change, so too will treatment recommendations. There are no published trials evaluating

Table 33.2 Current CDC Recommendations for Treatment of Gonorrhea Infection

Site of Infection	Recommended	Alternate
Cervix/urethra/rectum	Ceftriaxone 250 mg IM single dose (99.1% efficacy) **PLUS** Azithromycin 1 g po single dose	Spectinomycin 2 g IM single dose if allergic to cephalosporins (98.2% efficacy)[a]
Pharynx	Ceftriaxone 250 mg IM single dose (99% efficacy) **PLUS** Azithromycin 1 g orally in a single dose	Spectinomycin 2 g IM single dose (only 50% efficacy)[a]
Conjunctiva	Ceftriaxone 1 g IM in a single dose **PLUS** Azithromycin 1 g orally in a single dose	
Expedited partner therapy (EPT)	Ceftriaxone 250 mg IM single dose **PLUS** Azithromycin 1 g po single dose	Cefixime 400 mg po single dose **PLUS** Azithromycin 1 g po single dose[b]

Sources: From Papp JR, Schachter J, Gaydos C, Van Der Pol B. Recommendations for the laboratory-based detection of *Chlamydia trachomatis* and *Neisseria gonorrhea*. 2014; Centers for Disease Control & Prevention (CDC). Update to CDC's sexually transmitted, diseases treatment Guidelines, 2010: Oral cephalosporins no longer no longer a recommended treatment for gonococcal infections. *MMWR*, 61, 590–4, 2012.
[a]Consultation with an infectious disease specialist is recommended prior to treatment with an alternate regimen.
[b]Oral regimen for expedited partner treatment is considered appropriate ONLY when partner cannot be present for first-line IM/PO regimen.

this regimen in a pregnant population; however, efficacy of cephalosporins in a pregnant population has previously been demonstrated [38–40]. Dual therapy using two antimicrobials with different mechanisms of action (e.g., a cephalosporin plus azithromycin) is expected to improve treatment efficacy and potentially slow the emergence and spread of resistance to cephalosporins. Persons infected with *N. gonorrhoeae* are frequently coinfected with *C. trachomatis*. **Of women who have endocervical gonorrhea, 35% to 50% are coinfected with *C. trachomatis*,** so there is a longstanding recommendation that persons treated for gonococcal infection also be treated with a regimen that is effective against uncomplicated genital *C. trachomatis* infection, further supporting the use of dual therapy that includes azithromycin [32,33]. Patients should be advised to **abstain from sexual activity for 7 days after treatment and until all partners are adequately treated** and complete 7 days of abstinence to prevent transmission and reinfection.

Allergic reactions to first-generation cephalosporins occur in only <2.5% of persons with a history of penicillin allergy and are uncommon with third-generation cephalosporins (e.g., ceftriaxone and cefixime). Use of ceftriaxone or cefixime is contraindicated in persons with a history of an IgE-mediated penicillin allergy (e.g., anaphylaxis, Stevens-Johnson syndrome, and toxic epidermal necrolysis). Data are limited regarding alternative regimens for treating gonorrhea among persons who have either a cephalosporin or IgE-mediated penicillin allergy. Spectinomycin can be considered for treatment of urogenital and anorectal gonorrhea; however, it is not widely available. An infectious disease specialist should be consulted for advisement in treating persons with cephalosporin or IgE-mediated penicillin allergy [41,42]. Updates can be found at http://www.cdc.gov/STD/treatment/ [33].

For uncomplicated gonococcal infection treated with the recommended regimen, a test of cure is *not* necessary. However, if alternate treatment regimens are used, consider performing a test of cure with either a NAAT or culture two weeks after completing the treatment.

If a patient fails the recommended treatment regimen, a culture should be obtained for antimicrobial susceptibility testing. Treatment is considered to have failed if the patient

reports compliance with medication regimen, simultaneous treatment of her partner, and no sexual activity without barrier protection after completing treatment. It is difficult to exclude reinfection as the cause of a positive result on repeat testing. In the United States, clinicians should contact their local or state health department or the CDC for guidance and assistance in follow-up of these patients as part of the ongoing GISP. In European countries, the European Centre for Disease Prevention and Control (ECDC) should be made aware of apparent treatment failures [34,35].

Patients presenting with preterm premature rupture of membranes who are found to have active gonorrheal infection can be managed expectantly as long as treatment for gonorrhea is initiated promptly [38].

Because of the potential for concomitant infection, testing for *C. trachomatis*, syphylis, HIV, and hepatitis B is recommended.

REFERENCES

1. *Prevalence and incidence of selected sexually transmitted infections, Chlamydia trachomatis, Neisseria gonorrhoeae, syphilis and Trichomonas vaginalis. Methods and results used by WHO to generate 2005 estimates.* Geneva, World Health Organization, 2011. [Epidemiologic data]
2. Centers for Disease Control and Prevention. *Sexually transmitted disease surveillance 2014.* Atlanta: U.S. Department of Health and Human Services; 2015. [Epidemologic data]
3. Satterwhite CL, Torrone E, Meites E et al. Sexually transmitted infections among US women and men: Prevalence and incidence estimates, 2008. *Sexually Transmitted Dis* 2013; 40(3): 187–93. [Epidemologic data]
4. *Prevalence and incidence of selected sexually transmitted infections, Chlamydia trachomatis, Neisseria gonorrhoeae, syphilis and Trichomonas vaginalis. Methods and results used by WHO to generate 2005 estimates.* Geneva, World Health Organization, 2011. [Epidemiologic data]
5. Handsfield HH, Sparling FP. *Neisseria gonorrhoeae*. In: Mandell GL, Bennett JE, Dolin R, eds. *Principles and Practices of Infectious Diseases. 6th ed.* Philadelphia, PA: Churchill and Livingstone, Inc., 2005: 2514–27. [Review]
6. Lin JS, Donegan SP, Heeren TC et al. Transmission of *Chlamydia trachomatis* and *Neisseria gonorrhoeae* among men with urethritis and their female sex partners. *J Infect Dis* 1998; 178(6): 1707–12. [II-2]

7. Fransen L, Nsanze H, Klauss V et al. Ophthalmia neonatorum in Nairobi, Kenya: The roles of *Neisseria gonorrhoeae* and *Chlamydia trachomatis*. *J Infect Dis* 1986; 153(5): 862–9. [II-3]

8. Galega FP, Heymann DL, Nasah BT. Gonococcal ophthalmia neonatorum: The case for prophylaxis in tropical Africa. *Bull World Health Organ* 1984; 62(1): 95–8. [Review]

9. McCormack WM, Stumacher RJ, Johnson K et al. Clinical spectrum of gonococcal infection in women. *Lancet* 1977; 1(8023): 1182–5. [Review]

10. Brunham RC, Paavonen J, Stevens CE et al. Mucopurulent cervicitis—The ignored counterpart in women of urethritis in men. *N Engl J Med* 1984; 311(1): 1–6. [II-2]

11. Wiesner PJ. Gonococcal pharyngeal infection. *Clin Obstet Gynecol* 1975; 18(1): 121–9. [II-2]

12. Wiesner PJ, Tronca E, Bonin P et al. Clinical spectrum of pharyngeal gonococcal infection. *N Engl J Med* 1973; 288(4): 181–5. [II-3]

13. Holmes KK, Counts GW, Beaty HN. Disseminated gonococcal infection. *Ann Intern Med* 1971; 74(6): 979–93. [II-3]

14. Phupong V, Sittisomwong T, Wisawasukmongchol W. Disseminated gonococcal infection during pregnancy. *Arch Gynecol Obstet* 2005; 273(3): 185–6. [II-3]

15. Edwards LE, Barrada MI, Hamann AA et al. Gonorrhea in pregnancy. *Am J Obstet Gynecol* 1978; 132(6): 637–41. [II-3]

16. Schulz KF, Cates W Jr, O'Mara PR. Pregnancy loss, infant death, and suffering: Legacy of syphilis and gonorrhoea in Africa. *Genitourin Med* 1987; 63(5): 320–5. [II-3]

17. McGregor JA, French JI, Richter R et al. Antenatal microbiologic and maternal risk factors associated with prematurity. *Am J Obstet Gynecol* 1990; 163(5 Pt. 1): 1465–73. [II-2]

18. Alger LS, Lovchik JC, Hebel JR et al. The association of *Chlamydia trachomatis*, *Neisseria gonorrhoeae*, and group B streptococci with preterm rupture of the membranes and pregnancy outcome. *Am J Obstet Gynecol* 1988; 159(2): 397–404. [II-2]

19. Fox KK, Whittington WL, Levine WC et al. Gonorrhea in the United States, 1981–1996. Demographic and geographic trends. *Sex Transm Dis* 1998; 25(7): 386–93. [Epidemiologic data]

20. Cohen MS, Hoffman IF, Royce RA et al. Reduction of concentration of HIV-1 in semen after treatment of urethritis: Implications for prevention of sexual transmission of HIV-1. AIDSCAP Malawi Research Group. *Lancet* 1997; 349(9069): 1868–73. [II-2]

21. Paz-Bailey G, Koumans EH, Sternberg M et al. The effect of correct and consistent condom use on chlamydial and gonococcal infection among urban adolescents. *Arch Pediatr Adolesc Med* 2005; 159(6): 536–42. [II-2]

22. Golden MR, Whittington WL, Handsfield HH et al. Effect of expedited treatment of sex partners on recurrent or persistent gonorrhea or chlamydial infection. *N Engl J Med* 2005; 352(7): 676–85. [II-2]

23. Kissinger P, Mohammed H, Richardson-Alston G et al. Patient-delivered partner treatment for male urethritis: A randomized, controlled trial. *Clin Infect Dis* 2005; 41(5): 623–9. [RCT]

24. Expedited partner therapy in the management of gonorrhea and chlamydial infection. Committee Opinion No. 632. American College of Obstetricians and Gynecologists. *Obstet Gynecol* 2015; 125: 1526–8. [III]

25. *Guidance on the Use of Expedited Partner Therapy in the Treatment of Gonorrhea. Division of STD Prevention, National Center for HIV/AIDS, Viral Hepatitis, STD, and TB Prevention,* Centers for Disease Control and Prevention, 2015. [Review]

26. Crotchfelt KA, Welsh LE, DeBonville D et al. Detection of *Neisseria gonorrhoeae* and *Chlamydia trachomatis* in genitourinary specimens from men and women by a coamplification PCR assay. *J Clin Microbiol* 1997; 35(6): 1536–40. [II-2]

27. Koumans EH, Black CM, Markowitz LE et al. Comparison of methods for detection of *Chlamydia trachomatis* and *Neisseria gonorrhoeae* using commercially available nucleic acid amplification tests and a liquid pap smear medium. *J Clin Microbiol* 2003; 41(4): 1507–11. [II-2]

28. Martin DH, Cammarata C, Van Der Pol B et al. Multicenter evaluation of AMPLICOR and automated COBAS AMPLICOR CT/NG tests for *Neisseria gonorrhoeae*. *J Clin Microbiol* 2000; 38(10): 3544–9. [II-2]

29. Bachmann LH, Johnson RE, Cheng H, Markowitz LE, Papp JR, Hook EW III. Nucleic acid amplification tests for diagnosis of *Neisseria gonorrhea* oropharyngeal infections. *J Clin Microbiol* 2009; 47: 902–7. [II-2]

30. Bachmann LH, Johnson RE, Cheng H et al. Nucleic acid amplification tests for diagnosis of *Neisseria gonorrhea* and *Chlamydia trachomatis* rectal infections. *J Clin Microbiol* 2010; 48: 1827–32. [II-2]

31. Papp JR, Schachter J, Gaydos C, Van Der Pol B. Recommendations for the laboratory-based detection of *Chlamydia trachomatis* and *Neisseria gonorrhea*. 2014. [Review]

32. Centers for Disease Control & Prevention (CDC). Update to CDC's sexually transmitted Diseases treatment Guidelines, 2010: Oral cephalosporins no longer no longer a Recommended treatment for gonococcal infections. *MMWR* 2012; 61: 590–4. [III]

33. Centers for Disease Control and Prevention. *Sexually Transmitted Disease Surveillance 2013: Gonococcal Isolate Surveillance Project (GISP) Supplement and Profiles.* Atlanta: U.S. Department of Health and Human Services; 2015. [Review]

34. Unemo M, Golparian D, Syversen G et al. Two cases of verified clinical failures using internationally recommended first-line cefixime for gonorrhea treatment, Norway, 2010. *Euro Surveillance* 2010; 15: 19721. [III]

35. Ison CA, Hussey J, Sankar KN et al. Gonorrhea treatment failures to cefixime and Azithromycin in England, 2010. *Euro Surveillance* 2011; 16: 19833. [III]

36. Ohnishi M, Saika T, Hoshina S et al. Ceftriaxone-resistant *Neisseria gonorrhoeae*, Japan. *Emerg Infect Dis* 2011; 17: 148–9. [III]

37. Allen VG, Mitterni L, Seah C et al. *Neisseria gonorrhoeae* treatment failure and susceptibility to cefixime in Toronto, Canada. *JAMA* 2013; 309: 163–70. [III]

38. Maxwell GL, Watson WJ. Preterm premature rupture of membranes: Results of expectant management in patients with cervical cultures positive for group B streptococcus or *Neisseria gonorrhoeae*. *Am J Obstet Gynecol* 1992; 166(3): 945–9. [II-3]

39. Ramus RM, Sheffield JS, Mayfield JA et al. A randomized trial that compared oral cefixime and intramuscular ceftriaxone for the treatment of gonorrhea in pregnancy. *Am J Obstet Gynecol* 2001; 185(3): 629–32. [RCT]

40. Brocklehurst P. Antibiotics for gonorrhea in pregnancy. *Cochrane Database Syst Rev* 2002; (2): CD000098. [Meta analysis; 2 RCTs, *n* = 346]

41. Novalbos A, Sastre J, Cuesta J et al. Lack of allergic cross-reactivity to cephalosporins among patients allergic to penicillins. *Clin Exp Allergy* 2001; 31: 438–43. [II-2]

42. Romano A, Gaeta F, Valluzzi RL et al. IgE-mediated hypersensitivity to cephalosporins: Cross-reactivity and tolerability of penicillins, monobactams, and carbapenems. *J Allergy Clin Immunol* 2010; 126: 994–9. [II-2]

34

Chlamydia

Rebecca J. Mercier

KEY POINTS

- Untreated maternal genital *Chlamydia trachomatis* has been associated with increased **preterm premature rupture of membranes, preterm birth, low birth weight, and decreased perinatal survival**.
- **Neonatal infection** is associated with neonatal **conjunctivitis** and **pneumonitis**.
- **Prevention strategies shown to be effective include condoms, screening to identify asymptomatic cases in high-risk populations, early diagnosis and treatment, and partner notification and treatment without a clinical assessment.**
- Screening and treatment of women at risk for chlamydial infection improves pregnancy outcome.
- **Pregnant women with risk factors should undergo screening: age <25 years** (strongest risk factor), **multiple sex partners, new partner within last 3 months, single marital status, inconsistent use of barrier contraception, previous or concurrent sexually transmitted infection (STI), vaginal discharge, mucopurulent cervicitis, friable cervix, or signs of cervicitis on physical examination.**
- There is insufficient evidence to recommend for or against routine screening of asymptomatic, low-risk pregnant women aged 26 years and older for chlamydial infection although several national organizations, including the American College of Obstetricians and Gynecologists (ACOG) and the Centers for Disease Control (CDC), do recommend **universal screening in pregnancy**.
- **A nucleic acid amplification (NAAT) (e.g., LCR or PCR) screening test, confirmed by another NAAT test**, achieves highest predictive accuracy for the diagnosis of maternal genital *chlamydial* infection and is therefore the gold standard.
- **Azythromycin 1 g orally as a single dose**, amoxicillin, and erythromycin (in order of preference) are all accepted treatments of maternal genital *chlamydial* infection. **Partner notification and treatment without a clinical assessment** increases the rates of partner treatment and decreases the rates of maternal reinfection for various STIs and is therefore supported.
- A **test of cure** approximately three weeks after completion of therapy with a recommended regimen and **repeat testing in the third trimester** as well as **testing for** *N. gonorrhea*, **syphilis, HIV, and hepatitis B** are recommended for those women with positive testing earlier in pregnancy.

BACKGROUND

The major sexually transmitted diseases caused by *C. trachomatis* are cervicitis, urethritis, proctitis, and lymphogranuloma venerum (LGV). *C. trachomatis* is also a significant pathogen causing conjunctivitis in both the newborn and in sexually active adolescents and adults.

EPIDEMIOLOGY/INCIDENCE

Worldwide it is estimated that more than 105.7 million chlamydial infections occur annually with approximately half of those in women; at any given time, 100.4 million adults are infected [1]. The incidence of chlamydial infections in the United States and worldwide continues to rise annually. In 2013, a total of 1,401,906 chlamydial infections were reported to the Centers for Disease Control (CDC) in the United States; more than 900,000 of these cases were among females, and approximately 200,000 of these occur in pregnant women [2]. Higher rates among women compared to men likely reflects more frequent screening, and the increase in the number of cases reported annually is thought to be due in part to expansion of screening programs for at-risk women.

The age-specific rate for chlamydial infection is highest in the 15- to 24-year-old age category. The rate of chlamydia in African-American females in the United States is 6.4 times higher than the rate among white females. Estimates of the prevalence of chlamydia in pregnancy in the United States vary widely, ranging from 2.8% to 19% with the highest prevalence tending to be found in urban populations [3,4]. The prevalence of chlamydia varies significantly across the world. The rates of genital *C. trachomatis* infection in pregnant women are shown in Table 34.1 [5].

Ocular trachoma, a chronic keratoconjunctivitis caused by *C. trachomatis*, is rare in the developed world, but worldwide it is estimated that 7 to 9 million people are blind as a result of this condition [6].

LGV occurs sporadically in developed countries but is endemic in Africa, India, Southeast Asia, South America, and the Caribbean. The WHO and several partner organizations have initiated a program for global elimination of ocular trachoma as a disease of public health importance by the year 2020. Infection with *C. trachomatis* confers little protection against reinfection, and the limited protection that is conferred is short lived.

SYMPTOMS

C. trachomatis infections can be divided into **four clinical categories:**

- **Classic ocular trachoma**
- **Other ocular and genital diseases in adults**
- **LGV**
- **Perinatal infection—primarily conjunctivitis and pneumonia**

In pregnant women, genital infection including LGV and conjunctivitis are the most clinically significant.

Table 34.1 The Rates of Chlamydial Infection in Pregnant Women

United States	5%	India	17%
Italy	2.7%	Papua New Guinea	26%
Iceland	8%	Tanzania	6%
Brazil	2.1%	Cape Verde	13%
Thailand	5.7%		

Source: World Health Organization. *Global Prevalence and Incidence of Selected Curable Sexually Transmitted Infections.* Geneva: World Health Organization, 2001.

Maternal Genital Infection

The clinical manifestations of *C. trachomatis* are unchanged in pregnant women except that pelvic inflammatory disease and perihepatitis are uncommon after the first trimester. **About 70% to 90% of women with cervical or urethral *C. trachomatis* infection are asymptomatic.**

Cervicitis/Urethritis
Mucopurulent cervicitis that may be perceived as vaginal discharge, cervical edema and friability, dysuria if urethritis present, and low abdominal pain if upper genital tract infection present.

Proctitis/Proctocolitis
Results from anal intercourse or secondary spread of secretions from the cervix.

- Serovars D through K—anal pruritus and a mucous rectal discharge that may become mucopurulent. The infection remains superficial, is limited to the rectum, and closely resembles gonococcal proctitis. Infection is often asymptomatic.
- LGV strains—rectal pain, tenesmus, rectal bleeding, and fever. The disease extends into the colon. The rectal and colonic mucosa become ulcerated, and a granulomatous inflammatory process occurs in the bowel wall with both noncaseating granulomas and crypt abscesses. Sinus tract formation can lead to rectovaginal fistulas in women.

Chlamydial Conjunctivitis
Chlamydia is the most common cause of chronic follicular conjunctivitis. Common manifestations are a unilateral or bilateral asymmetric conjunctivitis associated with moderate hyperemia and mucopurulent discharge.

LGV
Often a difficult diagnosis to make because it is not thought of in the differential.

- The first stage is the formation of a primary lesion—a small papule or herpetiform ulcer—usually on genital mucosa or adjacent skin and causes little or no symptoms.
- The secondary stage occurs days to weeks later and is characterized by painful inguinal lymphadenopathy and systemic symptoms.
- The third stage manifests as hypertrophic chronic granulomatous enlargement with ulceration of the external genitalia. Lymphatic obstruction may also lead to elephantiasis of the genitalia.

PATHOPHYSIOLOGY/ETIOLOGY

C. trachomatis is an **obligate intracellular** pathogen that exhibits morphologic and structural similarities to gram-negative bacteria. The organism has a unique life cycle that includes an extracellular infectious form and an intracellular replicative form. The target cells of *C. trachomatis* are the squamocolumnar epithelial cells of the endocervix and upper genital tract, the conjunctiva, urethra, and rectum.

Target cells of the trachoma biovar of *C. trachomatis* are the squamocolumnar epithelial cells of the endocervix and upper genital tract, conjunctiva, urethra, and rectum. LGV biovar of *C. trachomatis* penetrates breaks in the skin or infects epithelial cells of the mucous membranes of the genital tract or rectum. It is then carried by lymphatic drainage to the regional lymph nodes, where it multiplies inside mononuclear phagocytes. *C. trachomatis* serovars D through K cause conjunctivitis in neonates as well as in adults. The incubation for *C. trachomatis* is variable depending on the type of infection but in general is 7 to 21 days.

TRANSMISSION

- *C. trachomatis* is readily transmitted during vaginal, oral, or anal sex, and mother-to-infant transmission commonly occurs at delivery.
- The risk of acquisition of *C. trachomatis* with a single episode of sexual intercourse with an infected partner is not known. However, it appears to be substantially less than that for *Neisseria gonorrhoeae* [7].
- Between 22% and 44% of infants born to infected women develop neonatal conjunctivitis [8].
- Between 11% and 20% of infants born to infected mothers develop pneumonia caused by *C. trachomatis* [9].

COMPLICATIONS/RISKS

Untreated maternal genital *C. trachomatis* has been associated to be an independent risk factor for the statistically significant increase in **preterm premature rupture of membranes, preterm birth, low birth weight, and decreased perinatal survival** when compared to either treated women or controls without the infection [10]. Successful treatment is therefore associated with prevention of premature rupture of membranes and small-for-gestational-age infants [11]. Treatment early in pregnancy with sustained eradication is associated with better outcomes compared to diagnosis and treatment later in pregnancy [12]. **Neonatal infection** acquired from an infected maternal genital tract at the time of delivery is associated with neonatal **conjunctivitis** and **pneumonitis**.

MANAGEMENT
Prevention

Condoms, when used correctly and consistently, provide a high degree of protection from chlamydia and other STIs [13]. Other important practices for prevention of chlamydia are **screening to identify asymptomatic cases in high-risk populations, early diagnosis and treatment**, and **partner notification and treatment**. Expedited partner treatment (EPT) is an approach to therapy with which the patient delivers either medication or prescriptions to their partner without requiring the partner to present for clinical assessment. EPT is known to increase the rates of partner treatment and to decrease the rates of maternal reinfection for various STIs [14,15]; the impact on specifically chlamydial reinfection is uncertain [16–18]. ACOG supports the provision of EPT for all STIs [19]. In the United States, EPT is explicitly permissible in 38 states, is potentially allowable in eight states, and is illegal in four states (Florida, Kentucky, Ohio, and West Virginia) [20].

Screening

There is no trial to assess the efficacy of universal or risk-based screening for *chlamydial* genital infection in pregnancy. The Canadian Task Force, the CDC, the American College of Obstetricians and Gynecologists (ACOG), and the American Academy of Pediatrics (AAP) recommend that all pregnant women be screened for chlamydial infection at the first prenatal visit with repeat testing in the third trimester for women age <25 or with risk factors for infection [21–23]. The U.S. Preventative Services Task Force recommends screening only pregnant women aged 24 and younger and those over age 24 who have risk factors for infection [24]. **Risk factors for acquiring chlamydial infection (extrapolated mainly from nonpregnant studies) are age <25 years (strongest risk factor), multiple sex partners, new partner within last 3 months, single marital status, inconsistent use of barrier contraception, previous or concurrent STI, vaginal discharge, mucopurulent cervicitis, friable cervix, and cervical ectopy.**

Diagnosis

A nucleic acid amplification (NAAT) (e.g., ligase chain reaction [LCR] or polymerase chain reaction [PCR]) screening test, confirmed by another NAAT test, achieves highest predictive accuracy for the **diagnosis of maternal genital** *chlamydial* **infection [25,26]. Therefore, NAAT testing is the gold standard for the diagnosis of maternal genital** *chlamydial* **infection.**

- *Anti-Chlamydia* IgM is uncommon in adults with genital tract infection. The prevalence of *anti-Chlamydia* IgG is high in sexually active adults (30%–60%) even in those who do not have an active infection and is probably due to past infection. The sensitivity, specificity, and predictive values of serologies are not high enough to make them clinically useful in the diagnosis of active disease. Thus, **chlamydial serologies are not recommended for diagnosis** of active disease except in suspected cases of LGV.
- When endocervical culture is compared with endocervical DFA, EIA, and PCR, **nonculture tests have a higher sensitivity** even in a population with a prevalence rate as low as 4.3% [27,28].
- Clinicians who perform STD screening tests should be aware of the prevalence of STDs in the population being screened and have a conceptual understanding of positive predictive value and the implications of screening low-risk individuals with a test that has limited specificity. In low-prevalence populations (<5% infected), a significant proportion of positive test results are false positives. For example, with a prevalence of 3%, out of 1000 patients, 30 are infected. A test with a sensitivity of 80% and a specificity of 99% detects 24 of the infected people but falsely identifies 10 uninfected as infected. The positive predictive value in this example is 70%.

- The Centers for Disease Control and Prevention recommended confirming positive screening tests for *C. trachomatis* when positive predictive values are <90%.
- **A positive result on a nonculture test should be considered presumptive evidence of infection in a low-prevalence population. Consideration should be given to performing an additional test after a positive screening test and requiring that both the screening test and additional test be positive to make a diagnosis of** *C. trachomatis* **infection.**
- Except for using culture to obtain an isolate, a non-NAAT should not be used as an additional test after a NAAT because of the lower sensitivity of the non-NAAT.
- The majority of commercial NAATs have been cleared by the Food and Drug Administration (FDA) to detect *C. trachomatis* in endocervical swabs and urine from women.
- Two prospective studies compared LCR NAAT performed on voided urine to endocervical culture in pregnant women, and found the LCR NAAT to be more sensitive [29,30]; voided urine NAAT has been shown to be equivalent to endocervical NAAT in pregnant women [31].
- Commercial NAAT performed with vaginal swabs are equivalent to cervical swabs in detecting chlamydia [28], and one trial has found them to be equivalent in pregnant women [32].
- Patient-collected vaginal swabs have been found to have sensitivity equal to endocervical swabs collected by a health care provider in nonpregnant patients [28]; only one small trial has assessed their performance in pregnant patients [33].

TREATMENT

- **Azithromycin, amoxicillin,** and **erythromycin** (in order of preference) are all accepted treatments of maternal genital *chlamydial* infection (Table 34.2). Azithromycin has the highest efficacy, highest compliance, and fewest reported side effects in pregnant women [34–38].
- Amoxicillin is associated with similar efficacy to erythromycin in achieving a negative test of cure and is better tolerated in pregnant women than erythromycin [39–42].
- Although in vitro studies suggest that *C. trachomatis* may have resistance to amoxicillin, two randomized trials have demonstrated that it is efficacious in pregnant patients [43,44]. Amoxicillin is less expensive than azithromycin. However, because azithromycin is a single dose and amoxicillin requires a thrice-daily dosing for a seven day course, compliance with amoxicillin is often lower than with azithromycin [43].
- Clindamycin may be considered if azithromycin, erythromycin, and amoxicillin are contraindicated or not tolerated [45].
- Doxycycline is one treatment of choice in nonpregnant women, but is not recommended in pregnancy because it may cause permanent discoloration in developing fetal teeth.
- Treatment for LGV and conjunctivitis caused by *C. trachomatis* has not been studied in pregnancy. Recommendations are based on treatment recommendations in nonpregnant populations.

Table 34.2 Treatment of Chlamydial Infection in Pregnancy

	Recommended	Alternate
Cervicitis/urethritis/proctitis	**Azithromycin** 1 g orally single dose **OR** **Amoxicillin** 500 mg orally three times a day for 7 days	**Erythromycin base** 500 mg orally four times a day for 7 days **OR** **Erythromycin base** 250 mg orally four times a day for 14 days **OR** **Erythromycin ethylsuccinate** 800 mg orally four times a day for 7 days **OR** **Erythromycin ethylsuccinate** 400 mg orally four times a day for 14 days
Conjunctivitis	**Azithromycin** 1 g orally single dose	**Erythromycin base** 250 mg orally four times a day for 21 days
Lymphogranuloma venerum	**Erythromycin base** 500 mg orally four times a day for 21 days	

Source: Centers for Disease Control and Prevention. Sexually Transmitted Diseases Treatment Guidelines 2015. *MMWR*, 64, 3, 10–11, 2015.

- Concurrent treatment for gonorrhea is not indicated unless a positive test for this organism is obtained. **Because of the potential for concomitant infection, testing for *N. gonorrhea*, syphilis, HIV, and hepatitis B is recommended.**

Treatment of sexual partners may decrease reinfection rates [16–18]. Common partner-management options include partner notification (partners are notified and instructed to seek evaluation and treatment) and patient-delivered partner therapy (partner is provided with either medication or prescriptions directly via the index patient). Expedited partner treatment (EPT) is the approach to therapy with which the patient delivers either medication or prescriptions to their partner without requiring the partner to present for clinical assessment. EPT is known to increase the rates of partner treatment and to decrease the rates of maternal reinfection for various STIs [14,15]; the impact on specifically chlamydial reinfection is uncertain [16–18]. ACOG supports the provision of EPT for all STIs [19]. No single partner management strategy has been shown to be more effective than any other in reducing reinfection rates. In the United States, EPT is currently explicitly permissible in 38 states, is potentially allowable in eight states, and is illegal in four states (Florida, Kentucky, Ohio, and West Virginia) [20].

A follow-up test of cure is recommended in pregnant women treated for *chlamydia*. If a nucleic acid-based test is used, follow-up testing should be performed at least three weeks post-treatment because nonviable organisms may remain present for some days after successful treatment and can give a false positive test result. **Repeat testing in the third trimester of pregnancy is recommended for women who test positive earlier in pregnancy** to reduce transmission to the neonate at birth [24].

One prospective study of cervical chlamydial infection in women presenting with preterm premature rupture of membranes who were conservatively managed and not treated for *Chlamydia* showed no effect on duration of latency and no increase in the incidence of chorioamnionitis or early endometritis [46].

REFERENCES

1. World Health Organization. *Global Prevalence and Incidence of Selected Curable Sexually Transmitted Infections*. Geneva: World Health Organization, 2008. [Epidemiologic Data]
2. *CDC Sexually Transmitted Disease Surveillance, 2013*. Atlanta, GA. U.S. Department of Health and Human Services. Dec 2014. [Epidemiologic Data]
3. *CDC Sexually Transmitted Disease Surveillance, 2011*. Atlanta, GA. U.S. Department of Health and Human Services. Dec 2012. [Epidemiologic Data]
4. Berggren EK, Patchen L. Prevalence of Chlamydia trachomatis and Neisseria gonorrhoeae and repeat infection among pregnant urban adolescents. *Sex Transm Dis* 2011; 38(3): 172–4. [II-2]
5. World Health Organization. *Global Prevalence and Incidence of Selected Curable Sexually Transmitted Infections*. Geneva: World Health Organization, 2001. [Epidemiologic data]
6. Chidambaram JD, Melese M, Alemayehu W et al. Mass antibiotic treatment and community protection in trachoma control programs. *Clin Infect Dis* 2004; 39(9): e95–7. [II-2]
7. Lycke E, Lowhagen GB, Hallhagen G et al. The risk of transmission of genital *Chlamydia trachomatis* infection is less than that of genital *Neisseria gonorrhoeae* infection. *Sex Transm Dis* 1980; 7(1): 6–10. [II-2]
8. Hammerschlag MR, Roblin PM, Gelling M et al. Use of polymerase chain reaction for the detection of *Chlamydia trachomatis* in ocular and nasopharyngeal specimen from infants with conjunctivitis. *Pediatr Infect Dis J* 1997; 16(3): 293–7. [II-2]
9. Schachter J, Grossman M, Sweet RL et al. Prospective study of perinatal transmission of *Chlamydia trachomatis*. *J Am Med Assoc* 1986; 255(24): 3374–7. [II-2]
10. Ryan GM Jr, Abdella TN, McNeeley SG et al. *Chlamydia trachomatis* infection in pregnancy and effect of treatment on outcome. *Am J Obstet Gynecol* 1990; 162(1): 34–9. [II-2]
11. Cohen I, Veille JC, Calkins BM. Improved pregnancy outcome following successful treatment of chlamydial infection. *J Am Med Assoc* 1990; 263(23): 3160–3. [II-2]
12. Folger AT. Maternal Chlamydia trachomatis infections and preterm birth: The impact of early detection and eradication during pregnancy. *Matern Child Health J* 2014; 18(8): 1795–802. [II-3]
13. Paz-Bailey G, Koumans EH, Sternberg M et al. The effect of correct and consistent condom use on chlamydial and gonococcal infection among urban adolescents. *Arch Pediatr Adolesc Med* 2005; 159(6): 536–42. [II-2]
14. Schillinger JA, Kissinger P, Calvet H, Whittington WL et al. Patient-delivered partner treatment with azithromycin to prevent repeated Chlamydia trachomatis infection among women: A randomized, controlled trial. *Sex Transm Dis* 2003; 30(1): 49–56. [RCT, *n* = 1787; I]
15. Golden MR, Kerani RP, Stenger M, Hughes JP et al. Uptake and population-level impact of expedited partner therapy (EPT) on Chlamydia trachomatis and Neisseria gonorrhoeae: The Washington State community-level randomized trial of EPT. *PLoS Med* 2015; 12(1). [RCT, *n* = 24 health jurisdictions; I]

16. Golden MR, Whittington WL, Handsfield HH et al. Effect of expedited treatment of sex partners on recurrent or persistent gonorrhea or chlamydial infection. *N Engl J Med* 2005; 352(7): 676–85. [II-2]

17. Ferreira A, Young T, Mathews C, Zunza M, Low N. Strategies for partner notification for sexually transmitted infections, including HIV. *Cochrane Database System Rev* 2013; 10. [Meta-analysis, 26 RCT, n > 17000; I]

18. Trelle S, Shang A, Nartey L, Cassell JA, Low N. Improved effectiveness of partner notification for patients with sexually transmitted infections: Systematic review. *BMJ* 2007; 334(7589): 354. [Meta-analysis, 14 RCT, n > 12000; I]

19. American College of Obstetricians and Gynecologists Expedited partner therapy in the management of gonorrhea and chlamydia infection. Committee Opinion Number 632. 2015. [Review; III]

20. Centers for Disease Control and Prevention. *Legal status of expedited partner therapy.* Accessed on July 27, 2015 at http://www.cdc.gov/std/ept/legal/default.htm. [Review; III]

21. Public Health Agency of Canada. *Canadian Guidelines on Sexually Transmitted Infections—Management and Treatment of Specific Infections, Chlamydia.* Accessed on August 4, 2015 at http://www.phac-aspc.gc.ca/std-mts/sti-its/cgsti-ldcits/section-5-2-eng.php. [Review; III]

22. American Academy of Pediatrics and American College of Obstetricians and Gynecologists. *Guidelines for Perinatal Care. 7th ed.* Washington, DC: American College of Obstetricians and Gynecologists, 2012. [Guideline]

23. Centers for Disease Control and Prevention. Sexually Transmitted Diseases Treatment Guidelines 2015. *MMWR* 2015; 64(3): 10–11. [Guideline]

24. U.S. Preventative Services Tasks Force. Screening for chlamydial infection: U.S. Preventative Services Tasks Force Recommendation Statement. *Ann Intern Med* 2014; 162: 902–11. [Guideline]

25. Dille BJ, Butzen CC, Birkenmeyer LG. Amplification of *Chlamydia trachomatis* DNA by ligase chain reaction. *J Clin Microbiol* 1993; 31(3): 729–31. [II-3]

26. Ossewaarde JM, Rieffe M, Rozenberg-Arska M et al. Development and clinical evaluation of a polymerase chain reaction test for detection of *Chlamydia trachomatis. J Clin Microbiol* 1992; 30(8): 2122–8. [II-3]

27. Thejls H, Gnarpe J, Gnarpe H et al. Expanded gold standard in the diagnosis of *Chlamydia trachomatis* in a low prevalence population: Diagnostic efficacy of tissue culture, direct immunofluorescence, enzyme immunoassay, PCR and serology. *Genitourin Med* 1994; 70(5): 300–3. [II-2]

28. Papp JR, Schachter J, Gaydos CA, Van Der Pol B. Centers for Disease Control and Prevention Recommendations for the laboratory-based detection of Chlamydia trachomatis and Nisseria gonorrhoeae 2014. *MMWR* 2014; 63(2). [Review III]

29. Andrews WW, Lee HH, Roden WJ et al. Detection of genitourinary tract *Chlamydia trachomatis* infection in pregnant women by ligase chain reaction assay. *Obstet Gynecol* 1997; 89(4): 556–60. [II-3]

30. Gaydos CA, Howell MR, Quinn TC et al. Use of ligase chain reaction with urine versus cervical culture for detection of *Chlamydia trachomatis* in an asymptomatic military population of pregnant and nonpregnant females attending papanicolaou smear clinics. *J Clin Microbiol* 1998; 36(5): 1300–4. [II-2]

31. Roberts SW, Sheffield JS, McIntire DD, Alexander JM. Urine screening for Chlamydia trachomatis during pregnancy. *Obstet Gynecol* 2011; 117(4): 883–5. [II-2]

32. Witkin SS, Inglis SR, Polaneczky M. Detection of Chlamydia trachomatis and Trichomonas vaginalis by polymerase chain reaction in introital specimens from pregnant women. *Am J Obstet Gynecol* 1996; 175(1): 165–7. [II-2]

33. Oakeshott P, Hay P, Hay S, Steinke F, Rink E, Thomas B, Oakeley P, Kerry S. Detection of *Chlamydia trachomatis* infection in early pregnancy using self-administered vaginal swabs and first pass urines: A cross-sectional community-based survey. *Br J Gen Pract* 2002; 52(483): 830–2. [II-3]

34. Adair CD, Gunter M, Stovall TG et al. *Chlamydia* in pregnancy: A randomized trial of azithromycin and erythromycin. *Obstet Gynecol* 1998; 91(2): 165–8. [RCT, n = 106]

35. Bush MR, Rosa C. Azithromycin and erythromycin in the treatment of cervical chlamydial infection during pregnancy. *Obstet Gynecol* 1994; 84(1): 61–3. [II-2]

36. Edwards MS, Newman RB, Carter SG et al. Randomized clinical trial of azithromycin vs erythromycin for the treatment of *Chlamydia* cervicitis in pregnancy. *Infect Dis Obstet Gynecol* 1996; 4: 333–7. [RCT, n = 140]

37. Rosenn MF, Macones GA, Silverman NS. Randomized trial of erythromycin and azithromycin for treatment of chlamydial infection in pregnancy. *Infect Dis Obstet Gynecol* 1995; 3: 241–4. [RCT, n = 48]

38. Pitsouni E, Iavazzo C, Athanasiou S, Falagas ME. Single-dose azithromycin versus erythromycin or amoxicillin for Chlamydia trachomatis infection during pregnancy: A meta-analysis of randomised controlled trials. *Int J Antimicrob Agents* 2007; 30(3): 213–21. [Meta-analysis, 8 RCT, n > 500]

39. Alary M, Joly JR, Moutquin JM et al. Randomised comparison of amoxycillin and erythromycin in treatment of genital chlamydial infection in pregnancy. *Lancet* 1994; 344(8935): 1461–5. [RCT, n = 210]

40. Silverman NS, Sullivan M, Hochman M et al. A randomized, prospective trial comparing amoxicillin and erythromycin for the treatment of *Chlamydia trachomatis* in pregnancy. *Am J Obstet Gynecol* 1994; 170(3): 829–32. [RCT, n = 74]

41. Magat AH, Alger LS, Nagey DA et al. Double-blind randomized study comparing amoxicillin and erythromycin for the treatment of *Chlamydia trachomatis* in pregnancy. *Obstet Gynecol* 1993; 81(5 Pt. 1): 745–9. [RCT, n = 143]

42. Turrentine MA, Troyer L, Gonik B. Randomized prospective study comparing erythromycin, amoxicillin, and clindamycin for the treatment of *Chlamydia trachomatis* in pregnancy. *Infect Dis Obstet Gynecol* 1995; 2: 205–9. [RCT, n = 174]

43. Kacmar J, Cheh E, Montagno A, Peipert JF. A randomized trial of azithromycin versus amoxicillin for the treatment of Chlamydia trachomatis in pregnancy. *Infect Dis Obstet Gynecol* 2001; 9(4): 197–202. [RCT, n = 39]

44. Jacobson GF, Autry AM, Kirby RS, Liverman EM et al. A randomized controlled trial comparing amoxicillin and azithromycin for the treatment of Chlamydia trachomatis in pregnancy. *Am J Obstet Gynecol* 2001; 184(7): 1352–4; discussion 1354–6. [RCT, n = 129]

45. Brocklehurst P, Rooney G. Interventions for treating genital *Chlamydia trachomatis* infection in pregnancy. *Cochrane Database of Syst Rev* 2009; 4. [Meta-analysis, 11 RCT, n > 300]

46. Ismail MA, Pridjian G, Hibbard JU et al. Significance of positive cervical cultures for *Chlamydia trachomatis* in patients with preterm premature rupture of membranes. *Am J Perinatol* 1992; 9(5–6): 368–370. [II-3]

35

Syphilis

A. Marie O'Neill

KEY POINTS

- **Prenatal screening** and treatment of pregnant women for syphilis is **cost-effective even in areas of low prevalence of the disease** (<0.1%).
- **All pregnant women should be screened with a serologic test for syphilis at the first prenatal visit. Women who are at high risk, live in areas of high syphilis morbidity, or are previously untested should be screened at 28 weeks and again at delivery.**
- **Penicillin** (parenteral penicillin G, 2.4 million units IM, either once or repeated weekly for three weeks depending on stage) remains the only recommended **treatment** for syphilis in pregnancy.
- Pregnant women with a **penicillin allergy** should be **desensitized** and then treated with penicillin.
- Staging of disease and penicillin dosing are not altered by pregnancy.
- Current treatment regimens are based on more than 50 years of clinical experience with penicillin, expert opinion, and observational clinical studies rather than on randomized clinical trials.

DEFINITION

Treponema pallidum is the causative agent of syphilis.

INCIDENCE/EPIDEMIOLOGY

- Worldwide, it is estimated that **more than 5.6 million new cases of syphilis occur annually** [1].
- In 2007 the World Health Organization (WHO) estimated there are **more than 2 million active syphilis infections in pregnant women annually worldwide**. More than 90% of new cases occur in developing countries with the greatest burden of disease seen in sub-Saharan Africa and Southeast Asia. Approximately 80% of infected women have had at least one antenatal visit; however, >66% were not screened or treated [2]. Since 1989, the newly independent states of the former Soviet Union have experienced a 43-fold increase in reported cases with rises proportionally larger among reproductive-aged women [3].
- **Each year at least half a million infants are born with congenital syphilis worldwide, and another half million stillbirths and spontaneous abortions occur as a result of maternal infection.**
- The rate of primary and secondary syphilis in the United States declined by 89.7% between 1990 and 2000 but then increased almost every year from 2001 to 2014. In 2014, there were 19,999 cases of primary and secondary syphilis reported to the Centers for Disease Control (CDC). Approximately 22% of these infections occur in reproductive-aged women [4]. The number of cases of **congenital syphilis in the United States** decreased from 446 cases (10.5/100,000 live births) in 2008 to 334 cases (8.4/100,000) in 2012 but then began to increase annually with **458 cases** (11.6/100,000) **in 2014** [4]. Syphilis disproportionately affects African-Americans with the reported rate of infection in this population being 5.4 times greater than that in whites and 57% of infants with congenital syphilis being born to black women [4,5]. The Syphilis Elimination Effort (SEE) is a national initiative launched by the Centers for Disease Control and Prevention in 1999 to reduce or eliminate syphilis in the United States. Updates on the progress of this project can be found at http://www.cdc.gov/stopsyphilis/.
- In 2007 the WHO launched the Initiative for Global Elimination of Congenital Syphilis with a goal of achieving a prenatal screen rate of ≥90% and providing adequate treatment to ≥90% of seropositive women and their partners [2].

PATHOPHYSIOLOGY AND TRANSMISSION

T. pallidum is a gram-negative spirochete unable to survive outside the human host and therefore has never been grown in culture. Unlike most other infectious diseases, it is rarely if ever diagnosed by isolation and characterization of the causative organism. *T. pallidum* can survive in the human host for several decades.

T. pallidum is easily transmitted by sexual contact, and an overwhelming majority of cases are transmitted by **sexual intercourse**. Endemic syphilis is transmitted nonvenerally by close contact with an active lesion and occurs in communities living under poor hygiene conditions. Syphilis is rarely transmitted during transfusion of blood or blood products or through needle sharing by intravenous drug abusers. The organism generally enters the body through small breaches in epithelial surfaces of genital, anorectal, oropharyngeal, or other cutaneous sites; however, penetration of intact mucous membranes can occur. Once inside the body, it rapidly disseminates. The **incubation period** for *T. pallidum* averages 3 weeks but can range from 10 to 90 days. During the incubation period, infected patients have, by definition, neither clinical nor serologic evidence of disease but are potentially infectious. The period of greatest infectivity is early in the disease when a chancre, mucous patch, or condyloma latum is present. Infectivity decreases over time, and after four years, it is very unlikely that an untreated individual will spread syphilis even by sexual contact. The risk of infection during a single sexual encounter with an infected individual is up to 60% depending on the stage of disease and approaches 100% after five sexual encounters [6].

Fetal syphilis occurs as a result of transplacental passage of the spirochete that enters fetal circulation causing infection. **Neonates** may acquire syphilis at the time of delivery by contact with infectious maternal secretions, blood, or genital lesions. Perinatal transmission may occur during any stage of maternal disease; however, it is most common in cases of maternal primary, secondary, or early latent syphilis with up to 83% of fetuses and newborns being affected [7].

SYMPTOMS AND CLASSIFICATION

Syphilis has been called "the great pretender" because of the **myriad of clinical manifestations** it can produce. It is a chronic, systemic infection characterized by several stages. The immune response to *T. pallidum* plays a significant role in the manifestations of all stages of syphilis. Much of the pathology observed in the disease is attributable to **vascular abnormalities caused by proliferative endarteritis** that occurs in all stages of syphilis. The pathophysiology of the endarteritis is not known although the scarcity of treponemes and the intense inflammatory infiltrate suggest that the immune response plays a role in the development of these lesions. **Manifestations of syphilis are not altered by pregnancy.**

Incubation Period

- Asymptomatic with no serologic evidence of disease. Transmission can occur during this period.

Primary Syphilis [6,8–10]

- Symptoms develop at the site of initial treponemal invasion as a result of local replication of the organism.
- Treponemes also spread throughout the body by hematologic and lymphatic dissemination even before the appearance of the chancre.
- Regional **adenopathy** often develops within the first week and usually consists of several discrete nontender, rubbery nodes. Inguinal adenopathy is often bilateral.
- Primary lesions are popular, but rapidly ulcerate to form a chancre.
- The classic **chancre** is a solitary, painless lesion with raised, firm, everted edges, central ulceration, and a granular base. However, up to 40% of individuals have multiple chancres.
- The most common site is the labia or cervix in females, but primary lesions may also occur on the lips, breasts, mouth, and anus.
- Without treatment, the local lesion **spontaneously resolves within three to six weeks**.
- Approximately 25% of individuals will have an adequate immune response and the infection will be spontaneously cleared.

Secondary Syphilis [6,8–10]

- If the primary infection is untreated, **secondary syphilis develops two to eight weeks later in approximately 75% of untreated individuals**.
- Secondary infection demonstrates a wide diversity in physical features involving virtually any organ and is often not thought of early in the diagnostic process.

- It generally begins with a **nonspecific constitutional illness** that commonly includes a sore throat, low-grade fever, myalgias, and generalized lymphadenopathy.
- **Skin rashes** are the classic and most commonly recognized lesions, but the appearance is highly variable, and differential diagnosis is often challenging.
- Rash is often initially macular and nonpruritic and becomes papular by three months.
- Rash frequently involves the **palms of the hands** and **soles of the feet**, and may be accompanied by mucous patches in the mouth, pharynx, or cervix and condyloma lata in the anogenital region or axilla. **Condyloma lata** are hypertrophic lesions resembling flat warts that occur in moist areas.
- Individuals are highly contagious during this stage, especially upon contact with mucous patches or condyloma lata.
- Secondary disease **lasts for an average of 3.6 months** and spontaneously resolves. Approximately 25% of individuals experience a relapse of secondary disease during the first year of infection.

Latent Syphilis [6,8–10]

- In latent syphilis, by definition, there are **no clinical stigmata of active disease** although disease remains detectable by **positive specific treponemal serologic tests** [FTA-ABS (fluorescent treponemal antibody absorption) or MHA-TP (microhemagglutination assay for *T. pallidum*)]. Latent syphilis is further subdivided into stages based on the duration of infection: early latent, late latent, and latent of unknown duration.

Early Latent Syphilis

- Early latency is defined as the time period within one year of initial infection.
- 90% of relapse occurs during this time period; mucocutaneous lesions are most common. Patient *is* infectious when lesions are present.
- Patients are believed to be potentially infectious in the absence of lesions.
- Vertical transmission of infection may occur.

Late Latent Syphilis

- Initial infection has occurred greater than one year previously.
- Associated with host resistance to reinfection.
- Sexual transmission is unlikely.
- Transplacental infection of the fetus can occur but is less likely than with earlier stages of disease.
- Infection via blood transfusion is possible.

Latent Syphilis of Unknown Duration

- Date of initial infection cannot be established as having occurred within the previous year *and* patient is aged 13 to 35 years *and* has a nontreponemal titer ≥1:32.

Late Benign Syphilis (Tertiary Syphilis) [6,8–10]

- Without treatment at earlier stages of disease, tertiary syphilis eventually develops in 30% to 40% of infected patients.

- Usually becomes clinically manifest **after a period of 15 to 30 years** of untreated infection.
- Characteristic manifestations of tertiary disease include cardiovascular and gummatous lesions.
- **Cardiovascular** syphilis typically presents as inflammatory lesions of the cardiovascular system—especially aortitis.
- **Gummas** are granulomatous, nodular lesions that can occur in a variety of organs, most commonly skin and bone.
- In patients with untreated syphilis, about 10% develop cardiovascular syphilis, 16% develop gummatous syphilis, and 6.5% develop symptomatic neurosyphilis [9].
- The diagnosis of late syphilis is confounded by the lack of sensitivity of the nontreponemal tests in these conditions.
- If a patient suspected of having late syphilis has a nonreactive nontreponemal test, a confirmatory treponemal test should be performed.
- Approximately one third of patients will remain seroreactive for decades but will *not* develop clinical manifestations of tertiary syphilis.
- Treatment of tertiary syphilis achieves a microbiologic cure, but many of the clinical manifestations will be irreversible.

Neurosyphilis [6,8–10]

- The diagnosis of neurosyphilis is made at **any** stage of disease when *both* clinical and laboratory criteria are met.
- *T. pallidum* disseminates widely after initial infection. Examination of **cerebrospinal fluid** will reveal evidence of infection [elevated lymphocytes and protein, **positive VDRL (venereal disease research laboratory)**] in approximately 15% of patients with primary syphilis and as many as 40% of patients with secondary syphilis.
- Many patients with CSF evidence of infection will be asymptomatic in the early stages of disease.
- Persistence of CSF abnormalities for more than five years in the untreated patient is highly predictive of the development of clinical neurosyphilis.
- Clinical evidence of central nervous system infection with *T. pallidum* includes the following:
  - Acute syphilitic meningitis
  - Meningovascular syphilis/seizures/stroke syndrome
  - General paresis/dementia/depression/memory loss/change in personality
  - Argyle Robertson pupils—small fixed pupils that do not react to light but do react to convergence accommodation
  - Tabes dorsalis—paresthesias, abnormal gait, shooting pains in the extremities or trunk, diminished peripheral reflexes, loss of position and vibration senses
- Laboratory evidence of neurosyphilis includes a reactive serologic test for syphilis and a reactive VDRL in the CSF.
- The CSF-VDRL is a highly specific test but has a **sensitivity of only about 30%**.
- Treponemal-specific **testing of CSF is helpful only when negative**—this rules out neurosyphilis. IgG

antibodies cross the blood–brain barrier and can give a positive result in the absence of neurosyphilis, so **a positive treponemal-specific test is not helpful in making the diagnosis**.
- CSF examination is essential in patients with signs or symptoms of neurologic involvement at any stage of *T. pallidum* infection and is also recommended in **all patients with untreated syphilis of unknown duration or of duration greater than one year**.
- CSF evaluation should include a cell count, protein level, and VDRL. Elevated lymphocytes and protein and positive VDRL are typical findings.
- Treatment of neurosyphilis achieves a microbiologic cure, but many of the neurologic manifestations will be irreversible.

RISK FACTORS

Risk factors for maternal infection include multiple sexual partners, unprotected sex, sex in exchange for money or drugs, presence of other sexually transmitted infections, African-American race, and spending time in a correctional facility.

The **single most significant risk factor for congenital syphilis infection is the maternal stage of disease**. With early-stage disease (primary, secondary, and early latent), up to 83% of fetuses and newborns are affected [7].

COMPLICATIONS

- Untreated syphilis can profoundly affect pregnancy outcome resulting in **spontaneous abortion, stillbirth, nonimmune hydrops fetalis, preterm birth, or perinatal morbidity and mortality. Fetal syphilis** has similar complications and manifestations to those seen in neonatal syphilis: hepatomegaly, ascites, elevated transaminases, anemia, and thrombocytopenia are common [7].
- The longer the interval between infection and pregnancy, the more benign the outcome for the infant [11].
- In general, infection during early gestation ends in spontaneous abortion or stillbirth; infection in late gestation results in full-term delivery of an infant with congenital syphilis, and infection in the distant past often results in an unaffected infant [11].
- The greatest risk of stillbirth caused by congenital syphilis occurs at 24 to 32 weeks gestation [12].
- Rates of **vertical transmission** in untreated women based on stage of disease [13]:
  - 70% to 100% in primary syphilis
  - 40% in early latent syphilis
  - 10% in late latent disease

MANAGEMENT
Prevention

Important practices for prevention of syphilis are early diagnosis and treatment, partner notification and treatment, and screening to identify asymptomatic cases in high-risk populations.

Screening (Table 35.1) [12,14]

- Most pregnant women with syphilis are asymptomatic and can only be identified through serological screening.

Table 35.1 Screening Tests for Syphilis

	Sensitivity (%)	Specificity (%)	Advantages	Disadvantages
Serology	85.5	97.1	• Relatively inexpensive • Rapid	• Not useful in primary disease • RPR and VDRL detect antigens NOT specific to treponemes
Dark-field microscopy	80	99–100	• Technically simple • Useful in evaluating lesions of primary disease	• Not widely available—requires special equipment and an experienced operator
ICS	84.1–95.3	92	• Immediate diagnosis if positive findings • Point-of-care testing	• Slightly lower sensitivity than other methods
PCR	95.8	95.7	• Inexpensive • Can be used in the most resource-poor settings • In trials PCR does differentiate syphilis from other treponematoses	• Expensive
Point of care	98.2	97.3	• Considered a valid test for primary and secondary infection • Inexpensive, rapid result reduces risk of patient lost to follow-up	• Investigational–not yet available for clinical use • Positive result should be confirmed with diagnostic testing

Sources: Derived from Montoya PJ, Lukehart SA, Brentlinger PE et al. *Bull World Health Organ*, 84, 2, 97–104, 2006; Young H. *Dermatol Clin*, 16, 4, 691–8, 1998.
Abbreviations: ICS, immunochromatographic strip; PCR, polymerase chain reaction; RPR, rapid plasma reagin; VDRL, venereal disease research laboratory.

- Prenatal screening and treatment programs are limited or nonexistent in many developing countries where the incidence and burden of disease is greatest.
- **Screening all pregnant women for syphilis and appropriately treating those found to be reactive effectively reduces complications associated with infection during pregnancy** [15].
- In the United States, serologic screening during pregnancy has been legislated since the 1930s; however, only 90% of states currently have statutes requiring antepartum syphilis screening [16]. Of those states with mandatory screening, 76% require one prenatal test early in pregnancy, and 24% require repeat screening in the third trimester. The most cost-effective approach is to screen all pregnant women at their initial prenatal visit, and to repeat screening in the third trimester in those women with significant risk factors [15].
- **The CDC and** American College of Obstetricians and Gynecologists **(ACOG) recommend screening all pregnant women with a serologic test at the first prenatal visit. Women who are at high risk, live in areas of high syphilis morbidity, or are previously untested should be screened at 28 weeks and again at delivery** [5,17].
- The genus *Treponema* includes *T. carateum*, the causative agent of *pinta*, and T. *pallidum*. The latter species is subdivided into three subspecies: *T. pallidum* subspecies *pallidum*, which causes *syphilis*; *T. pallidum* subspecies *pertenue*, which causes *yaws*; and *T. pallidum* subspecies *endemicum*, which causes *bejel*. The subspecies causing pinta, yaws, and bejel are morphologically and serologically indistinguishable from *T. pallidum pallidum* (syphilis), so there is no test in current clinical use that can differentiate one of these treponemal infections from another. The transmission of yaws, pinta, or bejal is

not via sexual contact and the clinical course of each disease is significantly different, which differentiates them from syphilis.

- **Serologic testing** remains the mainstay for screening and laboratory diagnosis of secondary, latent, and tertiary syphilis. These tests include nontreponemal and treponemal antibody detection.
- Nontreponemal tests are useful for screening. These include the rapid plasma reagin **(RPR)** card test and the **VDRL**.
- Nontreponemal tests are also useful for monitoring treatment as titers drop over time and often revert to negative; however, with repeated infection, complete seroreversion may not occur.
- Point of care testing is now being used, primarily in resource-poor settings. Syphilis Health Check is the only point of care test currently FDA approved. It was approved in 2011 and received waiver from the Clinical Laboratory Improvement Amendment (CLIA) to allow the test to be used by untrained personnel and outside of conventional lab settings in 2015. It is a rapid immunochromatographic test that qualitatively screens for antibodies to *T. pallidum* in serum, plasma, or whole blood. It can be performed on a finger stick whole blood specimen and yields result in 12 minutes. It is a *screening* test, so positive results should be followed up with confirmatory diagnostic testing. If confirmatory testing is not possible, immediate treatment of screen positive women and their partners has the potential to reduce transmission to the fetus and to sexual contacts. A number of logistical and technical problems have been reported with this approach, and so far no clear reduction in perinatal death has been observed. More trials are needed to adequately assess the risks and benefits of this strategy [18].

Diagnosis

- Treponemal tests are used to confirm the diagnosis. These include the serum **FTA-ABS** and the **MHA-TP** tests.
- Treponemal tests remain reactive for many years in more than 85% of persons adequately treated, and they give a false positive result in about 1% of the general population and should therefore not be used for screening [19].
- Serologic tests are generally not reactive until several weeks after the appearance of the primary lesion and therefore are not useful in diagnosing primary syphilis.
- Dark-field microscopy and direct fluorescent-antibody testing for *T. pallidum* (DFA-TP) are diagnostic options for primary syphilis.
- **Dark-field microscopy** is the most specific technique for diagnosing syphilis when an active chancre or condyloma latum is present. Its sensitivity is limited by the experience of the operator performing the test, the number of live treponemes in the lesion, and the presence of nonpathologic treponemes in oral or anal lesions. Given the inherent difficulties of dark-field microscopy, negative examinations on three different days are necessary before a lesion may be considered negative for *T. pallidum* [20].
- A new screening test that consists of an immunochromatographic strip (ICS) impregnated with treponemal antigen, which tests blood obtained by finger prick and offers immediate results, is available [14]. It has been found to be cost-effective and has the potential to have a significant impact on the epidemiology of this disease in undeveloped, resource-poor countries.
- The complete genome of *T. pallidum* has been sequenced, and specific PCR primers have been developed; however, PCR is not yet available for routine clinical use [21,22].

Workup

- **Lumbar puncture** is indicated with the following:
  - Neurologic/ophthalmologic signs
  - Aortitis/gummas
  - Treatment failure/treatment with agent other than penicillin
  - HIV infection
  - Titer >1:32
- Cerebral spinal fluid with a positive VDRL is diagnostic for neurosyphilis

Treatment (Table 35.2) [23]

- The efficacy of penicillin for the treatment of syphilis was well established through clinical experience before the value of randomized controlled clinical trials was recognized. Therefore, almost all the recommendations for the treatment of syphilis are based on the opinions of persons having knowledge about STDs and are reinforced by case series, clinical trials, and more than 50 years of clinical experience.
- Although erythromycin, azithromycin, and ceftriaxone are routinely used to treat syphilis in nonpregnant patients, they have not been shown to reliably cure maternal infection or prevent congenital syphilis [24].
- **Parenteral penicillin G** is the only therapy with documented efficacy for syphilis during pregnancy. The success of therapy is >98% [25].

Table 35.2 Treatment of Syphilis

Primary syphilis	**Benzathine penicillin G** 2.4 million units IM in a single dose
Secondary syphilis	**Benzathine penicillin G** 2.4 million units IM in a single dose
Early latent syphilis	**Benzathine penicillin G** 2.4 million units IM in a single dose
Late latent syphilis[a]	**Benzathine penicillin G** 2.4 million units IM each at 1-wk intervals × 3 wk 7.2 million units total
Tertiary syphilis	**Benzathine penicillin G** 2.4 million units IM each at 1-wk intervals × 3 wk 7.2 million units total
Neurosyphilis	**Aqueous crystalline penicillin G** 18–24 million units per day, administered as 3–4 million units IV every 4 hr or continuous infusion, for 10–14 days OR **Procaine penicillin** 2.4 million units IM once daily PLUS **Probenecid** 500 mg orally four times a day, both for 10–14 days

Source: Centers for Disease Control and Prevention. Sexually Transmitted Diseases Treatment Guidelines 2015. *Morb Mort Week Re*, 64, 36–7, 2015.
[a]Or syphilis of unknown duration.

- The highest risk of fetal treatment failure exists with maternal secondary syphilis [24].
- High VDRL titers at treatment and delivery, earlier maternal stage of syphilis, the interval from treatment to delivery, and delivery of an infant at ≤36 weeks gestation are associated with the delivery of a congenitally infected neonate after adequate treatment for maternal syphilis [25].
- Pregnant women with syphilis in any stage who report **penicillin allergy** should be evaluated to determine the need for **desensitization and treated with penicillin** (Table 35.3) [26].

Table 35.3 Oral Desensitization Protocol for Patients with a Positive Skin Test

Penicillin V Suspension Dose No.	Units	Cumulative Dose (Units)
1	100	100
2	200	300
3	400	700
4	800	1500
5	1600	3100
6	3200	6300
7	6400	12,700
8	12,000	24,700
9	24,000	48,700
10	48,000	96,700
11	80,000	176,700
12	160,000	336,700
13	320,000	656,700
14	640,000	1,296,700

Source: Adapted from Wendel GD Jr, Stark BJ, Jamison RB et al. *N Engl J Med*, 312, 19, 1229–32, 1985.
Note: Observation period: 30 minutes before parenteral administration of penicillin. Interval between doses, 15 minutes; elapsed time, 3 hours and 45 minutes; cumulative dose, 1.3 million units.

- Women with a penicillin reaction other than anaphylaxis should undergo skin testing. Those with a history of anaphylaxis or a positive skin test to one of the penicillin determinants should be desensitized and treated with penicillin.
- Desensitization is a straightforward, relatively safe procedure that can be done orally or intravenously. Oral desensitization is regarded as safer and is easier to perform. Patients should be desensitized in a hospital setting because serious IgE-mediated allergic reaction can rarely occur. Desensitization is typically completed in approximately four hours, after which the first treatment dose of penicillin is administered. After desensitization, patients must be maintained on a penicillin regimen for the duration of therapy if multiple weekly doses are indicated by stage of disease.
- The **Jarisch–Herxheimer** reaction is an acute febrile reaction frequently accompanied by headache, myalgias, and other symptoms that usually occurs within the first 24 hours after any therapy for syphilis. It occurs most often in early disease—especially primary—and is thought to represent massive lysis of treponemes. The reaction begins within one to two hours of treatment, peaks at eight hours, and typically resolves within 24 to 48 hours. It **occurs in up to 45%** of pregnant women treated for syphilis. The Jarisch–Herxheimer reaction may induce labor or cause fetal distress in pregnant women; however, these concerns should **not** prevent or delay therapy.
- Ultrasonography provides a noninvasive means to evaluate the fetus for signs of syphilis. Abnormal findings indicate a risk for obstetric complications and fetal treatment failure [27].
- **Sexual contacts must be elicited, tracked, and treated** (by law in the United States).

Follow-Up after Treatment

- Nontreponemal antibody serologic titers should be checked at 1, 3, 6, 12, and 24 months following treatment [11].
- Among patients with primary and secondary syphilis, **a fourfold decline** (two dilutions) **by 6 months and an eightfold decline** (four dilutions) **by 12 months are expected**.
- Among patients with early latent syphilis a fourfold decline by 12 months is expected.
- Titers that show a fourfold rise or do not decrease appropriately suggest either treatment failure or reinfection. The treatment regimen should be repeated in these cases.
- It is important that the same testing method (RPR or VDRL) be used for all follow-up examinations because titers may vary by one to two dilutions if different tests are used.
- Patients with neurosyphilis should have repeat CSF evaluation every six months for the first two years, or until the CSF shows no evidence of disease [11].
- Treponemal tests usually stay positive for life.

NEONATAL

Neonatal congenital syphilis is characterized by macopapular rash, hepatosplenomegaly, osteochondritis/periostosis (do X ray of long bones: 95% of these infants will have osteochondritis),

jaundice, ascites/hydrops, petechiae/purpura, lymphadenopathy, chorioretinitis, anemia, thrombocytopenia, hyperbilirubinemia, elevated liver enzymes, and reactive syphilis serologic tests in blood/cerebral spinal fluid. Babies can be asymptomatic. Out of the congenitally affected babies, 50% are born to mothers without prenatal care. **Infants of mothers with** untreated syphilis, relapse/reinfection, treated with erythromycin, treated <1 month before delivery, without good history of treatment, without fourfold decrease in titers, or without enough serologic follow-up **should be treated.** **Lumbar puncture** should be done on any infant suspected to have congenital syphilis.

REFERENCES

1. World Health Organization Department of HIV/AIDS. *Global Incidence and Prevalence of four curable sexually transmitted infections (STIs): New estimates from WHO.* Geneva: World Health Organization, 2009. [Epidemiologic data]
2. World Health Organization Department of Reproductive Health and Research. *The global elimination of syphilis: Rationale and strategy for action.* Geneva: World Health Organization, 2007. [Epidemiologic data]
3. Borisenko KK, Tichonova LI, Renton AM. Syphilis and other sexually transmitted infections in the Russian federation. *Int J STD AIDS* 1999; 10(10): 665–8. [Epidemiologic data]
4. Centers for Disease Control and Prevention. *Sexually Transmitted Disease Surveillance, 2014.* Atlanta, GA: U.S. Department of Health and Human Services, 2015. [Review]
5. Centers for Disease Control and Prevention. *STDs and Pregnancy Fact Sheet.* Atlanta, GA: Department of Health and Human Services, 2015. [Review]
6. Garnett GP, Aral SO, Hoyle DV et al. The natural history of syphilis. Implications for the transmission dynamics and control of infection. *Sex Transm Dis* 1997; 24(4): 185–200. [Review]
7. Hollier LM, Harstad TW, Sanchez PJ et al. Fetal syphilis: Clinical and laboratory characteristics. *Obstet Gynecol* 2001; 97(6): 947–53. [II-2]
8. Clark EG, Danbolt N. The Oslo study of the natural history of untreated syphilis; An epidemiologic investigation based on a restudy of the Boeck-Bruusgaard material; A review and appraisal. *J Chronic Dis* 1955; 2(3): 311–44. [II-2]
9. Danbolt N, Clark EG, Gjestland T. The Oslo study of untreated syphilis; A re-study of the Boeck-Bruusgaard material concerning the fate of syphilitics who receive no specific treatment; A preliminary report. *Acta Derm Venereol* 1954; 34(1–2): 34–8. [II-2]
10. Rockwell DH, Yobs AR, Moore MB Jr. The Tuskegee study of untreated syphilis; The 30th year of observation. *Arch Intern Med* 1964; 114: 792–8. [II-2]
11. Singh AE, Romanowski B. Syphilis: Review with emphasis on clinical, epidemiologic, and some biologic features. *Clin Microbiol Rev* 1999; 12(2): 187–209. [Review]
12. Montoya PJ, Lukehart SA, Brentlinger PE et al. Comparison of the diagnostic accuracy of a rapid immunochromatographic test and the rapid plasma reagin test for antenatal syphilis screening in Mozambique. *Bull World Health Organ* 2006; 84(2): 97–104. [II-3]
13. Fiumara NJ. Review of congenital syphilis. *Sex Transm Dis* 1984; 11(1): 49–50. [Review]
14. Young H. Syphilis serology. *Dermatol Clin* 1998; 16(4): 691–8. [II-3]
15. United States Preventive Services Task Force. *Screening for syphilis infection: Recommendation statement.* Rockville, MD: Agency for Healthcare Research and Quality, 2004. [Guideline]
16. Hollier LM, Hill J, Sheffield JS et al. State laws regarding prenatal syphilis screening in the United States. *Am J Obstet Gynecol* 2003; 189(4): 1178–83. [Review]

17. American College of Obstetricians and Gynecologists and American Academy of Pediatrics. *Guidelines for Perinatal Care. 7th ed.* Elk Grove Village, IL: AAP; Washington, DC: ACOG, 2012. [III]

18. Tucker JD, Bu J, Brown LB et al. Accelerating worldwide syphilis screening through rapid testing: A systematic review. *Lancet Infect Dis* 10(6): 381–6. [Review]

19. Larsen SA, Steiner BM, Rudolph AH. Laboratory diagnosis and interpretation of tests for syphilis. *Clin Microbiol Rev* 1995; 8(1): 1–21. [II-3]

20. Cummings MC, Lukehart SA, Marra C et al. Comparison of methods for the detection of *Treponema pallidum* in lesions of early syphilis. *Sex Transm Dis* 1996; 23(5): 366–9. [II-1]

21. Liu H, Rodes B, Chen CY et al. New tests for syphilis: Rational design of a PCR method for detection of *Treponema pallidum* in clinical specimens using unique regions of the DNA polymerase I gene. *J Clin Microbiol* 2001; 39(5): 1941–6. [II-2]

22. Serwin AB, Kohl PK, Chodynicka B. The centenary of Wassermann reaction—The future of serological diagnosis of syphilis, up-to-date studies. *Przegl Epidemiol* 2005; 59(3): 633–40. [Review]

23. Centers for Disease Control and Prevention. Sexually Transmitted Diseases Treatment Guidelines 2015. *Morb Mort Week Rep* 2015; 64(RR): 36–7. [Guidelines]

24. Alexander JM, Sheffield JS, Sanchez PJ et al. Efficacy of treatment for syphilis in pregnancy. *Obstet Gynecol* 1999; 93(1): 5–8. [II-2]

25. Sheffield JS, Sanchez PJ, Morris G et al. Congenital syphilis after maternal treatment for syphilis during pregnancy. *Am J Obstet Gynecol* 2002; 186(3): 569–73. [II-2]

26. Wendel GD Jr, Stark BJ, Jamison RB et al. Penicillin allergy and desensitization in serious infections during pregnancy. *N Engl J Med* 1985; 312(19): 1229–32. [II-2]

27. Wendel GD Jr, Sheffield JS, Hollier LM et al. Treatment of syphilis in pregnancy and prevention of congenital syphilis. *Clin Infect Dis* 2002; 35(Suppl. 2): S200–9. [II-2]

36

Trichomoniasis

Tino Tran

KEY POINTS

- Pregnant women colonized with *Trichomonas vaginalis* in the second trimester have a **higher risk of delivering an infant with low birth weight** or **delivering before term,** but unfortunately **metronidazole treatment** has been **associated with an increased risk of preterm birth.**
- *T. vaginalis* infection is a **risk factor for sexual transmission of HIV-1 with a twofold increase reported.**
- **Condoms,** when used correctly and consistently, provide a high degree of **protection from many STIs, including** *T. vaginalis.*
- There is no evidence that identifying asymptomatic *T. vaginalis* is beneficial in reducing the associated risk of preterm delivery or delivery of a low-birth-weight infant. Therefore, **there is insufficient evidence to recommend screening of asymptomatic pregnant women** and some evidence that **treatment of these patients may in fact be harmful.**
- **Metronidazole as a single 2-g oral dose or 500 mg twice a day for seven days at any gestational age** is the treatment of choice for **symptomatic** *T. vaginalis* infection.
- **Concurrent treatment of sexual partners** is recommended to prevent reinfection.
- Currently, trichomoniasis diagnosis by PCR and NAAT is the gold standard in diagnosis.

EPIDEMIOLOGY/INCIDENCE

Worldwide, it is estimated that the incidence of trichomoniasis is 240 million new cases annually between men and women. The prevalence worldwide was estimated to be around 152 million [1]. Developing countries account for a disproportionate number of cases. Trichomoniasis affects approximately 3.7 million and 80,000 nonpregnant and pregnant women in the United States annually [2]. The frequency of infection in European women is similar. The WHO estimates 78 million new infections annually in Africa [3]. In contrast to bacterial sexually transmitted infections (STIs), such as *Neisseria gonorrhoeae* and *Chlamydia trachomatis, T. vaginalis* infection rates are as high or higher in middle-aged women when compared to adolescents. Incidence is highest among women with multiple sexual partners and in populations with high rates of other sexually transmitted infections.

SYMPTOMS/SIGNS

The clinical manifestations of trichomoniasis are unchanged in pregnant women. Infection is **asymptomatic in up to 50% of women.** The most common symptoms include vulvovaginal pruritis (23%–82%), vaginal discharge (50%–75%), dysuria (30%–50%), and dyspareunia (10%–50%). The most common signs are copious vaginal discharge (50%–75%) (yellow/green in 5%–20%, frothy in 10%–50%), inflammation of vaginal mucosa (40%–75%), vulvar erythema (10%–20%), and abdominal pain (1%–5%).

PATHOPHYSIOLOGY/ETIOLOGY

Trichomoniasis is caused by the protozoan *T. vaginalis,* which had been previously thought to be a harmless commensal. *T. vaginalis* can infect the vagina and the Skene's glands of the urethra along with the urethra itself. Less common sites of infection include the cervix, bladder, and bartholins gland. The incubation period for *T. vaginalis* is 4 to 7 days on average but ranges from 2 to 28 days. The mechanism on how trichomoniasis infection causes preterm labor is unknown. Some studies have linked infection to a maternal inflammatory response. This was demonstrated by findings of elevated cervical interleukin-9 and vaginal defensing in pregnant asymptomatic patients, which causes a neutrophilic response to release mixed metalloproteinases [4].

TRANSMISSION

T. vaginalis is easily transmitted during **vaginal intercourse.** The organism will survive for several hours in a moist environment outside the host and is rarely transmitted nonvenerally. The transmission rate from male to female during vaginal intercourse has been reported to be 66% to 100% [5]. Vertical transmission to a female infant occurs in 2% to 17% if vaginal infection is present at the time of delivery [6].

COMPLICATIONS/RISKS

Pregnant women colonized with *T. vaginalis* in the second trimester had a 30%–40% **higher risk of delivering an infant with low birth weight** or **delivering before term** and a 40% higher risk of giving birth to an infant who was both preterm *and* of low birth weight [7]. In a meta-analysis, infection with trichomoniasis yielded an increased relative risk of 1.42 for preterm birth, 1.41 for preterm premature rupture of membranes, and 1.51 for small for gestational age [4]. In pregnant women with *T. vaginalis,* unfortunately **metronidazole treatment,** as given in the trial (two 2-g doses given 48 hours apart at 16–23 weeks, which is twice the usual dose for treatment) has been **associated with an 80% increase of preterm birth** compared to no treatment with the majority of the increase in preterm delivery attributed to spontaneous preterm labor [8–10]. The proposed mechanism for treatment with metronidazole causing preterm labor is that lysis of dying trichomonads elicits an inflammatory response that triggers labor [8–10] (see also chapter 17 of *Obstetric Evidence Based Guidelines*). Other nonrandomized studies have not shown this association. A retrospective study found no association between metronidazole use and increase risk of preterm birth, low birth weight, or congenital abnormalities [11]. Another retrospective cohort of 4274 women diagnosed with trichomoniasis found treatment was not associated with an increased risk of preterm birth and may even be protective (HR 0.69, CI 0.52–0.92, $p = 0.010$) [12].

$T.$ $vaginalis$ infection is a **risk factor for sexual transmission of HIV-1** in women. Studies from Africa have suggested that $T.$ $vaginalis$ infection approximately doubles the rate of HIV transmission [13]. The proposed mechanism for this increased risk is twofold: local infiltration of large number of leukocytes including CD4+ lymphocytes—the primary target of HIV infection—and disruption in the integrity of the vaginal mucosa allowing access to viral particles. HIV-positive women who become infected with $T.$ $vaginalis$ have been shown to shed more HIV virus in their vaginal secretions and therefore pose a higher risk for transmission.

Epidemiologic studies of $T.$ $vaginalis$ infection in the neonate have reported vertical transmission rates ranging from 2% to 17% [6], causing vaginal, urinary, and respiratory infection in these neonates.

MANAGEMENT
Prevention
Condoms, when used correctly and consistently, provide a high degree of protection from many STIs [14].

Most cases of reinfection result from sexual contact with an untreated partner. Adequate treatment of sexual partners has been shown to decrease reinfection [15].

Screening
There is no evidence that identifying asymptomatic $T.$ $vaginalis$ in the general population is beneficial in reducing the associated risk of preterm delivery or delivery of a low-birth-weight infant. However, there is mounting evidence that all **women with HIV should be screened for trichomoniasis** as there is a high rate of coinfection (up to 53%). Treatment of trichomoniasis in women with concomitant HIV has been shown to decrease genital tract viral shedding and load [16].

Diagnosis
Wet mount preparation of vaginal secretions suspended in normal saline with microscopic observation of motile trichomonads is the most **commonly utilized** method of diagnosing trichomoniasis in women. Cost is minimal with wet preparation; however, the **sensitivity** of this method is **low**. Providers using wet mount to diagnose trichomoniasis should also attempt to interpret slides immediately as decreases in sensitivity have been found with slides interpreted >1 hr after retrieval [16].

Isolation of $T.$ $vaginalis$ by **culture was the prior gold standard**, but the greater cost and longer time to diagnosis make this an underutilized diagnostic option. Commonly used culture media [17,18] include the following:

- Modified Diamond's broth media (sensitivity 95%)
- InPouch™ transport and test system (sensitivity 87%)
- Modified Columbia agar (sensitivity 98%)

To increase the detection rate in a high-risk population without substantially increasing cost, culture could be performed on those symptomatic patients with a negative wet mount.

Conventional Pap smear is not considered accurate for the identification of $T.$ $vaginalis$. Confirmatory testing is necessary for those cases reported by Pap: sensitivity = 60% to 70%, specificity = 88%. Liquid-based Pap smear is accurate for the identification of $T.$ $vaginalis$ and warrants treatment without further testing; however, the sensitivity is low (61.4%) [19]. Clinicians who perform STI screening tests should be aware of the prevalence of STIs in the population being screened and have a conceptual understanding of positive predictive value and the impact screening low-risk individuals has with a test that has limited specificity (Table 36.1) [20–22].

Nucleic acid-based tests are currently considered the gold standard for detection of trichomonads. PCR and nucleic acid amplification tests that can be performed as rapid point of care testing are commercially available in the United States. Recently, multiple assays such as the APTIMA T. Vaginalis assay (Hologic Gen-Probe, San Diego CA) and the BD Probe tec TV Qx have been FDA cleared for detection of trichomonas vaginalis from vaginal, cervical, or urine specimens for women. The sensitivity and specificity of NAAT testing has been found to be as high as 95.3%–99% and 95.2%–99% respectively [23]. Rapid Swabs for trichomoniasis are also readily available and can be read in as quickly as 10 minutes.

Table 36.1   Screening/Diagnostic Tests for $T.$ $vaginalis$

	Sensitivity (%)	Specificity (%)	Advantages	Disadvantages
Wet mount	62–80	>99	• Rapid results • Inexpensive	• Low sensitivity compared to culture • Sensitivity and specificity are strongly dependent on the skills and experience of the microscopist and also on the quality of the sample
Culture	95	100	• High specificity • High sensitivity and specificity	• Organism can be rendered nonviable if incorrect media used or delay in transport • 3–7 days to complete • Not available in most clinical labs
PCR/NAAT	95	98	• Results available more quickly than with culture	• Most expensive option

Sources: From Radonjic IV, Dzamic AM, Mitrovic SM et al. *Eur J Obstet Gynecol Reprod Biol*, 126, 116–20, 2006; Aslan DL, Gulbahce HE, Stelow EB et al. *Diagn Cytopathol*, 32, 6, 341–4, 2005; Patel SR, Wiese W, Patel SC et al. *Infect Dis Obstet Gynecol*, 8, 5–6, 248–57, 2000.
Abbreviations: NAAT, nucleic acid amplification test; PCR, polymerase chain reaction.

Treatment

The nitroimidazoles are the only class of drugs useful for the oral or parenteral treatment of trichomoniasis. In randomized clinical trials, oral nitroimidazoles have resulted in parasitologic cure rates of 90% to 95%. Metronidazole and tinidazole are most commonly used. **Metronidazole can be given as a single 2-g oral dose or 500 mg twice a day for seven days** and can be given to symptomatic women **at any gestational age** [9]. In patients with coinfection with HIV, studies have shown the twice-a-day dosing to be more effective and thus should be the treatment of choice. All patients, regardless of HIV status, should also be rescreened for a test of cure approximately three months out from initial infection [16,24]; this can be done as soon as two weeks with PCR amplification. Multiple studies and meta-analyses have not demonstrated a definitive association between metronidazole use during pregnancy and teratogenic or mutagenic effects in infants [25,26]. Tinidazole is given as a single 2-g oral dose. Its use is contraindicated in the first trimester of pregnancy. Metronidazole resistance is increasingly common. The CDC estimated that **5% of clinical isolates of *T. vaginalis* exhibit** some degree of **metronidazole resistance**. An escalated dosing regimen of metronidazole 2 g daily for three to five days has been successful in some cases of resistant infection, but in general, **not more than a single 2-g dose should be given to prevent possible increase in preterm birth** [9]. Tinidazole is effective in treating up to 60% of metronidazole-resistant *T. vaginalis* infections. **Concurrent treatment of sexual partners** is recommended to prevent reinfection. In those rare cases with a confirmed metronidazole allergy, patients should go through desensitization of their allergy before being treated with metronidazole.

REFERENCES

1. World Health Organization. *Prevalence and incidence of selected sexually transmitted infections.* 2005. [Epidemiologic data]
2. Satterwhite CL, Torrone E, Meites E et al. Sexually transmitted infections among US women and men: Prevalence and incidence estimates, 2008. *Sex Transm Dis* 2013; 40: 187–93. [Epidemiologic data]
3. Gerbase AC, Mertens TE. Sexually transmitted diseases in Africa: Time for action. *Afr Health* 1998; 20(3): 10–2. [Review]
4. Silver BJ, Guy RJ, Kaldor JM et al. Trichomonas vaginalis as a cause of perinatal morbidity: A systematic review and meta-analysis. *Sex Transm Dis* 2014; 41(6): 369–76. [Meta-analysis; 11 studies]
5. Krieger JN. Trichomoniasis in men: Old issues and new data. *Sex Transm Dis* 1995; 22(2): 83–96. [II-3]
6. Danesh IS, Stephen JM, Gorbach J. Neonatal *Trichomonas vaginalis* infection. *J Emerg Med* 1995; 13(1): 51–4. [II-3]
7. Cotch MF, Pastorek JG II, Nugent RP et al. *Trichomonas vaginalis* associated with low birth weight and preterm delivery. The Vaginal Infections and Prematurity Study Group. *Sex Transm Dis* 1997; 24(6): 353–60. [II-2]
8. Klebanoff MA, Carey JC, Hauth JC et al. Failure of metronidazole to prevent preterm delivery among pregnant women with asymptomatic *Trichomonas vaginalis* infection. *N Engl J Med* 2001; 345(7): 487–93. [RCT; *n* = 617. 2 g metronidazole q48h × 2 doses]
9. Gulmezoglu AM. Interventions for trichomoniasis in pregnancy. *Cochrane Database Syst Rev* 2011; 1. [Meta-analysis; two RCTs; *n* = 842]
10. Ross SM, Van Middelkoop A. Trichomonas infection in pregnancy: Does it affect outcome? *S Afr Med J* 1983; 63: 566–7. [RCT; *n* = 225; 2 g metronidazole × 1 dose to women and their partners]
11. Koss C, Baras D, Lane S et al. Investigation of metronidazole use during pregnancy and adverse birth outcomes. *Antimicrob Agents Chemother* 2012; 56: 4800–5. [II-11, 2, 3, …]
12. Mann JR, McDermott SD, Zhou L et al. Treatment of trichomoniasis in pregnancy and preterm birth: An observational study. *J Women's Health* 2009; 18(4): 493–7. [II-2]
13. Laga M, Manoka A, Kivuvu M et al. Non-ulcerative sexually transmitted diseases as risk factors for HIV-1 transmission in women: Results from a cohort study. *AIDS* 1993; 7(1): 95–102. [II-2]
14. Paz-Bailey G, Koumans EH, Sternberg M et al. The effect of correct and consistent condom use on chlamydial and gonococcal infection among urban adolescents. *Arch Pediatr Adolesc Med* 2005; 159(6): 536–42. [II-3]
15. Schwebke JR, Desomnd RA. A randomized controlled trial of partner notification methods for prevention of *Trichomonas* in women. *Sex Transm Dis* 2010; 37: 392–6. [RCT, *n* = 484]
16. Workowski K, Bolan G et al. Sexually Transmitted Diseases Treatment Guidelines 2015. Center for Disease Control and Prevention. *MMWR* 2015. [Guideline]
17. Borchardt KA, Zhang MZ, Shing H et al. A comparison of the sensitivity of the InPouch TV, diamond's and trichosel media for detection of Trichomonas vaginalis. *Genitourin Med* 1997; 73(4): 297–8. [II-2]
18. Stary A, Kuchinka-Koch A, Teodorowicz L. Detection of *Trichomonas vaginalis* on modified Columbia agar in the routine laboratory. *J Clin Microbiol* 2002; 40(9): 3277–80. [II-2]
19. Lara-Torre E, Pinkerton JS. Accuracy of detection of *Trichomonas vaginalis* organisms on a liquid-based Papanicolaou smear. *Am J Obstet Gynecol* 2003; 188(2): 354–6. [II-2]
20. Radonjic IV, Dzamic AM, Mitrovic SM et al. Diagnosis of *Trichomonas vaginalis* infection: The sensitivities and specificities of microscopy, culture and PCR assay. *Eur J Obstet Gynecol Reprod Biol* 2006; 126: 116–20. [II-2]
21. Aslan DL, Gulbahce HE, Stelow EB et al. The diagnosis of *Trichomonas vaginalis* in liquid-based pap tests: Correlation with PCR. *Diagn Cytopathol* 2005; 32(6): 341–4. [II-3]
22. Patel SR, Wiese W, Patel SC et al. Systematic review of diagnostic tests for vaginal trichomoniasis. *Infect Dis Obstet Gynecol* 2000; 8(5–6): 248–57. [Review]
23. Hollman D, Coupey SM, Fox AS et al. Screening for Trichomonas Vaginalis in high-risk adolescent females with a new transcription- mediated nucleic acid amplification test (NAAT): Associations with ethnicity, symptoms, and prior and current STIs. *J Pediatr Adolesc Gynecol* 2010; 23: 312–6. [II-2]
24. Kissinger P, Mena L, Levison J et al. A randomized treatment trial: Single versus 7-day dose of metronidazole for the treatment of *Trichomonas vaginalis* among HIV-infected women. *J Acquir Immune Defic Syndr* 2010; 55: 565–71. [RCT, *n* = 270]
25. Burtin P, Taddio A, Ariburnu O et al. Safety of metronidazole in pregnancy: A meta-analysis. *Am J Obstet Gynecol* 1995; 172(2 Pt. 1): 525–9. [Meta-analysis]
26. Sorensen HT, Larsen H, Jensen ES et al. Safety of metronidazole during pregnancy: A cohort study of risk of congenital abnormalities, preterm delivery and low birth weight in 124 women. *J Antimicrob Chemother* 1999; 44(6): 854–6. [II-2]

37

Group B *Streptococcus*

Laura Carlson and M. Kathryn Menard

KEY POINTS

- Asymptomatic group B streptococcus (GBS) colonization in the mother is associated with an incidence of neonatal GBS disease of ~1% to 2% without intervention. **Neonatal disease** is divided into **early onset** or **late onset** with possible complications being **sepsis, pneumonia, meningitis**, and less frequently **focal infections** and death.
- Major **risk factors** for neonatal GBS sepsis are **prolonged rupture of membranes (≥18 h), preterm delivery**, and **temperature ≥100.4°F (≥38°C).**
- **Universal prenatal maternal screening and intrapartum antibiotic treatment** is the most efficacious of the current strategies for prevention of early-onset disease and >50% more effective than a risk factor-based strategy. There is no known effective preventive strategy for late-onset GBS sepsis.
- **Women with GBS bacteriuria (>10,000 colony-forming units [CFU])** in the current pregnancy or who had a **prior infant with GBS sepsis** are candidates for **intrapartum antibiotics prophylaxis** and should be the only two groups **not screened** in the third trimester.
- **Screening** involves collecting an **anovaginal specimen at 35 to 37 weeks** (labeled penicillin-allergic if appropriate).
- Women who are GBS positive are treated with **penicillin in labor.** Ampicillin is a reasonable alternative. If the patient is penicillin-allergic but not at high risk for anaphylaxis, cefazolin is the agent of choice. **For the woman at high risk for anaphylaxis to penicillin and a cultured isolate sensitive to both clindamycin and erythromycin, treatment with clindamycin is indicated. If the culture is resistant to either clindamycin or erythromycin or the results are unknown, then treatment with vancomycin is recommended.**
- **Intrapartum treatment for chorioamnionitis is recommended regardless of GBS maternal status.**

DIAGNOSIS/DEFINITION

GBS is a bacterium also known as *Streptococcus agalactiae*. Infection with GBS is a cause of morbidity and mortality in pregnant or postpartum women as well as fetuses and newborns.

SYMPTOMS

In the **mother**, GBS colonization is usually **asymptomatic.** It can cause urinary tract infection, chorioamnionitis, endometritis, and bacteremia. In the fetus, it can be associated with stillbirth. Two forms of infection occur in **newborns: early onset** and **late onset**. Early-onset neonatal GBS disease usually causes illness within the first 24 hours of life. However, illness can occur up to six days after birth. Late-onset neonatal disease usually occurs at three to four weeks of age; it

can occur any time from seven days to three months of age. Symptoms of neonatal GBS include breathing problems, not eating well, irritability, extreme drowsiness, unstable temperature (low or high), weakness, or listlessness (in late onset).

EPIDEMIOLOGY/INCIDENCE (FIGURE 37.1)

GBS is a major cause of infectious morbidity among infants. In the United States, it is the most common cause of serious neonatal bacterial sepsis, including neonatal meningitis. The prevalence of asymptomatic GBS anovaginal colonization in pregnant women is **about 20%** with a range of 10% to 30% [1]. GBS colonization during pregnancy can be transient or persistent. A substantial portion of women who are colonized during one pregnancy will not have GBS colonization during a subsequent pregnancy. Usually 40% to 75% of neonates born to colonized mothers are colonized themselves [2]. As a result of prevention efforts employing screening and antibiotic prophylaxis, the incidence of **early-onset GBS sepsis** fell in the United States from 1.7 cases per 1000 live births in 1990 to **0.25 per 1000 live births in 2013** [3].

ETIOLOGY/BASIC PATHOPHYSIOLOGY

GBS is an encapsulated gram-positive coccus that colonizes the vaginal and gastrointestinal tract (reservoir) in 10% to 30% of healthy pregnant women [2,4–6]. GBS may cause maternal urinary tract infection, amnionitis, endomyometritis, and maternal sepsis. Neonates acquire the organism as a result of **vertical transmission from the maternal genital tract** to the infant in utero or **usually at delivery**.

CLASSIFICATION

Disease in the neonate is divided into early and late disease (Table 37.1). **Early neonatal sepsis** with GBS often is observed within 24 hours of delivery. Early-onset disease presents within the first six days of life with breathing difficulty, shock, pneumonia, and occasionally meningitis [1]. Nothing specific regarding the clinical presentation in early disease differentiates GBS as the etiology from other pathogens. Pneumonia with bacteremia is common and meningitis less likely. **Late-onset GBS disease** is defined as infection after one week and before three months after birth. Late-onset disease is commonly characterized by bacteremia and meningitis. Infections in the infant can be localized or systemic.

RISK FACTORS/ASSOCIATIONS

For early-onset GBS disease, risk factors include **prolonged rupture of membranes (ROM) (≥18 hours), preterm delivery (but >80% GBS neonates are term), temperature ≥100.4°F (≥38°C),** maternal GBS colonization between 35 and 37 weeks,

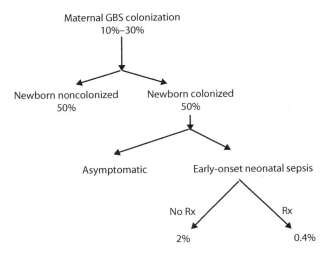

Figure 37.1 GBS infection: maternal to infant transmission. Rx, treatment.

birth of a previous infant with invasive GBS disease, maternal chorioamnionitis, young maternal age, African-American race, Hispanic ethnicity, and GBS bacteriuria during pregnancy. Diabetes or maternal GBS colonization in a previous pregnancy are not risk factors for early-onset GBS disease although GBS colonization in a previous pregnancy is a risk factor for recurrent maternal GBS colonization [7].

COMPLICATIONS (TABLE 37.1)

In newborns, GBS can cause **sepsis, pneumonia, meningitis,** and less frequently **focal infections,** such as osteomyelitis, septic arthritis, or cellulitis. Early-onset GBS sepsis is defined as occurring within the first week of life, usually around 48 hours and within 72 hours. Neonatal death occurs in 4% to 6% of cases of early-onset disease. Mortality is higher among preterm infants, 20% to 30% if <33 weeks gestation, compared with 2% to 3% among full-term infants [1].

MANAGEMENT
Principles/Prevention

Several approaches to the prevention of **early-onset** GBS neonatal infection have been studied or devised [8]. There

are **no trials** to assess the effectiveness of any of these approaches, probably because they would have to include about >100,000 screened pregnancies to show a difference in early-onset GBS sepsis given the current incidence of the disease (<0.5%). Potential strategies are outlined in the following sections.

Maternal Vaccination

Vaccination against GBS is potentially the most effective method of preventing the morbidity and mortality caused by infection. GBS vaccines have been investigated as a tool to reduce maternal colonization and prevent transmission to the neonate; however, a licensed vaccine is not yet available with few trials ongoing [1]. GBS capsular polysaccharide (CPS)-based protein conjugate vaccines have been produced and tested in animals [9]. The first capsular polysaccharide vaccine was poorly immunogenic, so a trial of protein conjugate vaccines followed, using tetanus toxoid as the conjugate. They were shown to be safe and well tolerated, and the antibody response was persistent for over a year in the mother, and the passive protection in the neonate protected him/her against late onset disease [10]. There is need for a phase III randomized trial recording neonatal disease events [1,11]. Vaccination is the only strategy that would have the potential to protect against late-onset disease, which current strategies do not cover.

Universal Maternal Treatment

There is insufficient data to evaluate universal treatment of all women during birth.

Prenatal Maternal Screening and Prelabor Maternal Treatment

Antibiotics should not be used before the intrapartum period to treat asymptomatic maternal GBS colonization except if GBS is present in the urine (2%–4% of pregnancies). Asymptomatic women with GBS in the urine culture at 27 to 31 weeks gestation have decreased preterm birth (PTB) <37 weeks when treated with penicillin 1 million IU three times per day for six days compared to placebo [12]. GBS bacteriuria during pregnancy should be treated at the time of diagnosis. In fact, every urine specimen sent in pregnancy should be labeled "pregnant," so to alert the laboratory to report any isolation of GBS. GBS identified in urine is a marker for heavy maternal colonization and is associated with a higher risk for early-onset GBS sepsis and is also an indication for intrapartum antibiotic prophylaxis [1]. Antibiotic therapy (with erythromycin) does not prevent PTB or affect stillbirths in women with GBS colonization [13].

Table 37.1 Early- vs. Late-Onset GBS Characteristics

	Early Onset	Late Onset
Definition	Occurs <1 wk	≥1 wk
Usual timing of manifestation after birth	24–48 hr	≥1 wk
Incidence (of all neonatal GBS sepsis)	80% (natural); 50% (screen and treat)	20% (natural); 50% (screen and treat)
Most common/predominant clinical signs/ symptoms	Sepsis, pneumonia (meningitis 10%–30%)	Meningitis, localized infections (ears, eyes, breasts, bone, joints, skin, etc.)
Serotype		III (95%)
Case-fatality ratio	Overall = 5%	<2%
	Full-term = 2%–3%	
	<33 wk = 30%	
Long-term morbidity		If meningitis—15%–50% can have neurologic sequelae

No Prenatal Maternal Screening and Intrapartum Treatment Based on Risk Factors

Risk factors used for this strategy are delivering <37 weeks, intrapartum temperature ≥100.4°F (≥38°C), or ROM ≥18 hours [1]. More than 20% of neonates with early-onset GBS sepsis are born to women without risk factors. As shown below, although this was a popular strategy in the past, it is less effective than a screening-based strategy [10,12]. A risk factor-based strategy is still recommended in the United Kingdom [14,15]. Intrapartum treatment for chorioamnionitis is recommended regardless of maternal GBS status.

Universal Prenatal Maternal Screening and Intrapartum Treatment (Figure 37.2)

A screening-based strategy is >50% more effective than a risk factor-based strategy [16]. This is the protocol with the most evidence for efficacy [1,17]. After the Centers for Disease Control (CDC) recommended this screening strategy compared to either the risk factor-based strategy in 2002, the incidence of early-onset GBS sepsis declined from 0.47/1000 live births (1999–2001) to 0.25/1000 live births [3]. A screening-based strategy involves an incidence of intrapartum antibiotic prophylaxis similar (24%) to that of the risk-factor approach [18]; thus, the treatment risks should be similar. This approach of screening for GBS colonization and intrapartum treatment **does not affect incidence of late-onset GBS sepsis**. A screening-based strategy is recommended in the United States [1,19] (see section titled "Screening" below for more details).

Neonatal (Screening and) Treatment Only

Screening and/or treatment of just the neonate without some form of in utero prophylaxis is a much inferior approach than the maternal screening approaches just described (screening or risk factor–based). Neonatal treatment only is "too little, too late" as 40% of neonates with GBS are already bacteremic at birth. Evaluation of neonates born to GBS-positive mothers who were not treated or to mothers with risk factors is imperative [20].

Screening/Diagnosis (Figure 37.2)

Detection

Detecting vaginal GBS colonization of pregnant women is a way of detecting women at high risk for early-onset GBS infection. Because colonization can be intermittent, a swab done earlier in pregnancy is less predictive of intrapartum status and early-onset GBS disease than a culture performed near term. The recommended time frame for performing the culture is 35 to 37 weeks gestation [1]. The negative predictive values of GBS cultures performed at 35 to 37 weeks (prevalence about 20%) are 95% to 98% [1]. **Women with GBS bacteriuria** in the current pregnancy or who had a **prior infant with GBS sepsis** are candidates for **intrapartum antibiotics prophylaxis**, and **should not be screened** [1]. Notably, cultures obtained after prophylactic antibiotic administration may not accurately reflect GBS status [21].

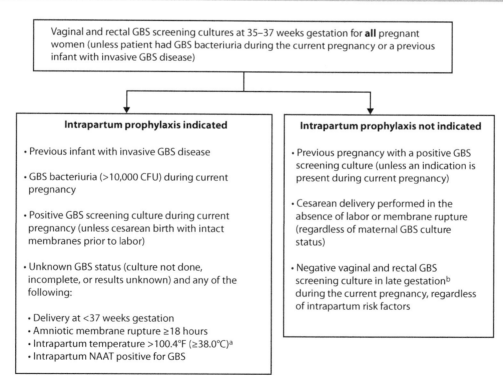

Figure 37.2 Indications for intrapartum antibiotic prophylaxis to prevent perinatal GBS disease under a universal prenatal screening strategy based on combined vaginal and rectal cultures collected at 35 to 37 weeks gestation from all pregnant women. If nucleic acid amplification test (NAAT) is negative and any of the above risk factors are present, then intrapartum prophylaxis is indicated. [a]If amnionitis is suspected, broad-spectrum antibiotic therapy that includes an agent known to be active against GBS should replace GBS prophylaxis. [b]Optimal timing 35–37 weeks gestation. (From Verani JR, McGee L, Schrag SJ. Prevention of perinatal group B streptococcal disease—Revised guidelines from CDC, 2010. Division of Bacterial Diseases, National Center for Immunization and Respiratory Diseases, Centers for Disease Control and Prevention (CDC). *MMWR Recomm Rep*, 59, RR–10, 1–3, 2010.)

Collection of Screening Specimen

A vaginal-rectal swab, collected at 35 to 37 weeks gestation. **Sampling the lower vagina, followed by the anorectal area gives highest yield for GBS** [1]. Vaginal-rectal swabs, during which >70% of women report at least mild pain, do not increase GBS detection rates compared to vaginal-perianal swabs [22]. The swab is transported in special medium (e.g., Amies or Stuart's without charcoal), which maintains GBS viability for up to one to four days. It is labeled "penicillin allergy" when applicable. The swab is cultured using a selective enrichment broth media (e.g., Todd-Hewitt with antibiotics) over 18 to 24 hours. For penicillin-allergic patients, clindamycin and erythromycin disk susceptibility is done [1].

The availability of a sensitive rapid screening test to accurately detect women in labor who are colonized with GBS would make prevention strategies more efficient, but the available **rapid tests still lack acceptable performance characteristics to be applied in all circumstances.** However, for women who present at term with unknown GBS status and without risk factors for GBS sepsis, application of real-time PCR has adequate specificity (92%–99%) to appropriately identify women in whom antibiotics are indicated [23–26].

Intrapartum Prophylaxis (Table 37.2)

The incidence of early-onset GBS infection is reduced with use of intrapartum antibiotic prophylaxis in women colonized with GBS. Treatment is associated with a 90% decreased incidence of infant colonization and 83% decreased incidence of early-onset neonatal infection with GBS [27]. The rate of

Table 37.2 Recommended Regimens for Intrapartum Antimicrobial Prophylaxis for Perinatal GBS Disease Prevention[a]

Recommended	Penicillin G, 5 million units IV initial dose, then 2.5–3 million units IV every 4 hr until delivery
Alternative	Ampicillin, 2 g IV initial dose, then 1 g IV every 4 hr until delivery
If penicillin allergic[b]	
Patients not at high risk for anaphylaxis	Cefazolin, 2 g IV initial dose, then 1 g IV every 8 hr until delivery
Patients at high risk for anaphylaxis[c]	
GBS susceptible to clindamycin and erythromycin[d]	Clindamycin, 900 mg IV every 8 hr until delivery
GBS resistant to clindamycin or erythromycin or susceptibility unknown	Vancomycin, 1 g IV every 12 hr until delivery

Source: From Verani JR, McGee L, Schrag SJ. Prevention of perinatal group B streptococcal disease—Revised guidelines from CDC, 2010. Division of Bacterial Diseases, National Center for Immunization and Respiratory Diseases, Centers for Disease Control and Prevention (CDC). *MMWR Recomm Rep*, 59, RR–10, 1–3, 2010.
[a]Broader-spectrum agents, including an agent against GBS, may be necessary for treatment of chorioamnionitis.
[b]History of penicillin allergy should be assessed to determine whether a high risk for anaphylaxis, angioedema, respiratory distress, or urticaria is present.
[c]If laboratory facilities are adequate, clindamycin and erythromycin susceptibility testing should be performed on prenatal GBS isolates from penicillin-allergic women at high risk for anaphylaxis.
[d]Resistance to erythromycin is often, but not always, associated with clindamycin resistance. If a strain is resistant to erythromycin but appears susceptible to clindamycin, it may still have inducible resistance to clindamycin. Treatment with erythromycin is not recommended.

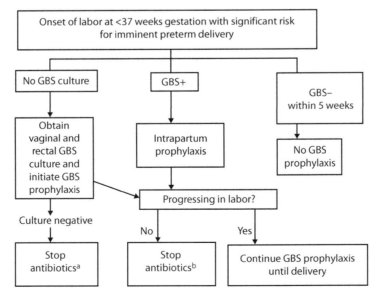

Figure 37.3 Algorithm for GBS prophylaxis for women with threatened preterm delivery. This algorithm is not an exclusive course of management. Variations that incorporate individual circumstances or institutional preferences may be appropriate. [a]If delivery has not occurred within 4 weeks, a vaginal and rectal GBS screening culture should be repeated and the patient should be managed as described, based on the result of the repeat culture. [b]GBS prophylaxis at onset of true labor. (From National Institute for Health and Clinical Excellence: *Antibiotics for early-onset neonatal infection. CG149.* London: National Institute for Health and Clinical Excellence, 2012.)

infant GBS sepsis in the control groups of the studies where this outcome was reported ranged from 2% to 9%. This is higher than the overall infection rates of 1% to 3% that are reported in babies whose mothers are colonized with GBS, raising questions as to how representative the populations studied were.

Penicillin is the first-line agent for intrapartum GBS prophylaxis (Table 37.2). When antibiotics are given ≥2 hours before delivery, neonatal GBS colonization is minimized [1]. A retrospective study further evaluated timing of antibiotic prophylaxis and found a further reduction in early onset sepsis if antibiotics were administered at least 4 hours prior to delivery [28]. **For women with penicillin allergy not at high risk for anaphylaxis, cefazolin is recommended. For**

the woman at high risk for anaphylaxis to penicillin and a cultured isolate sensitive to both clindamycin and erythromycin, treatment with clindamycin is indicated. If the culture is resistant to either clindamycin or erythromycin or the results are unknown, then treatment with vancomycin is recommended [1]. If intrauterine infection is diagnosed, broad-spectrum antibiotic therapy (e.g., ampicillin and gentamicin) is recommended. Women with preterm premature rupture of membranes at or after 34 weeks who are colonized with GBS should be counseled to proceed with delivery [29].

Adverse consequences of prophylaxis are anaphylaxis to penicillin (4–40/100,000), drug resistance, and neonatal infection from agents different than GBS. Penicillin is the preferred antibiotic to decrease emerging resistance. Early-onset

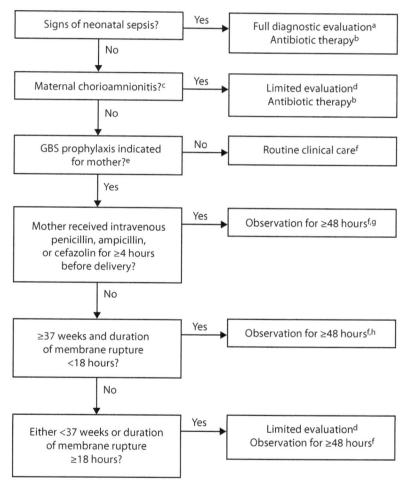

Figure 37.4 Algorithm for secondary prevention of early-onset GBS disease in the newborn. [a]Blood culture, a complete blood count (CBC) with white blood cell differential and platelet counts, chest radiograph (if respiratory abnormalities are present), and lumbar puncture (if patient is stable enough to tolerate procedure and sepsis is suspected). [b]Directed toward the most common causes of neonatal sepsis, including intravenous ampicillin for GBS and coverage for other organisms (including *Escherichia coli* and other gram-negative pathogens) and should take into account local antibiotic-resistance patterns. [c]Consultation with obstetric providers is important to determine the level of clinical suspicion for chorioamnionitis. [d]Blood culture (at birth) and CBC with differential and platelets (at birth and/or at 6–12 hours of life). [e]See Table 37.2 for indications for intrapartum GBS prophylaxis. [f]If signs of sepsis develop, a full diagnostic evaluation should be conducted and antibiotic therapy initiated. [g]If ≥37 weeks gestation, observation may occur at home after 24 hours if other discharge criteria have been met, access to medical care is readily available, and a person who is able to comply fully with instructions for home observation will be present. If any of these conditions is not met, the infant should be observed in the hospital for at least 48 hours and until discharge criteria are achieved. [h]Some experts recommend a CBC with differential and platelets at age 6–12 hours. (From Verani JR, McGee L, Schrag SJ. Prevention of perinatal group B streptococcal disease—Revised guidelines from CDC, 2010. Division of Bacterial Diseases, National Center for Immunization and Respiratory Diseases, Centers for Disease Control and Prevention (CDC). *MMWR Recomm Rep*, 59, RR–10, 1–3, 2010.)

sepsis from pathogens other than GBS requires continuous surveillance.

Newborns of women undergoing **cesarean delivery** before labor or ROM have an extremely low risk for early-onset GBS disease. Antibiotic prophylaxis is not recommended in this circumstance. However, women planning to be delivered by cesarean should still undergo screening for GBS at 35 to 37 weeks in case they present in labor or with ROM.

For women with **threatened preterm delivery**, see Figure 37.3.

Vaginal chlorhexidine has not been shown to be associated with reductions in neonatal early-onset GBS infection, pneumonia, sepsis, or mortality [30]. The lack of efficacy may be due to insufficient data (type II error).

Antepartum Testing

No specific indication for GBS carriers.

Delivery

Intrapartum antibiotic prophylaxis is described in Figure 37.2 and Table 37.2. There is insufficient evidence to assess whether digital vaginal examinations or intrauterine fetal monitoring affect incidence of GBS sepsis [1]. There seems to be no increase in GBS sepsis in pregnancies undergoing stripping of membranes [31], but none of the studies reported screening or results for GBS.

NEONATAL MANAGEMENT

See Figure 37.4 [1].

REFERENCES

1. Verani JR, McGee L, Schrag SJ. Prevention of perinatal group B streptococcal disease—Revised guidelines from CDC, 2010. Division of Bacterial Diseases, National Center for Immunization and Respiratory Diseases, Centers for Disease Control and Prevention (CDC). *MMWR Recomm Rep* 2010; 59(RR–10): 1–3. [Review/guideline; Accessible at: http://www.cdc.gov/groupb strep]
2. Regan JA, Klebanoff MA, Nugent RP. The epidemiology of GBS colonization in pregnancy. Vaginal infections and prematurity study group. *Obstet Gynecol* 1991; 77(4): 604–10. [II-2]
3. Centers for Disease Control and Prevention. 2013. *Active Bacterial Core Surveillance Report, Emerging Infections Program Network, Group B Streptococcus*, 2013. [Epidemiologic data]
4. Anthony BF, Okada DM, Hobel CJ. Epidemiology of group B *Streptococcus*: Longitudinal observations during pregnancy. *J Infect Dis* 1978; 137: 524–30. [II-3]
5. Dillon HC Jr, Gray E, Pass MA et al. Anorectal and vaginal carriage of group B streptococci during pregnancy. *J Infect Dis* 1982; 145: 794–9. [II-3]
6. Boyer KM, Gadzala CA, Kelly PD et al. Selective intrapartum chemoprophylaxis of neonatal group B streptococcal early-onset disease. II. Predictive value of prenatal cultures. *J Infect Dis* 1983; 148: 802–9. [II-2]
7. Page-Ramsey SM, Johnstone SK, Kim D, Ramsey PS. Prevalence of group B *Streptococcus* colonization in subsequent pregnancies of group B *Streptococus*-colonized versus noncolonized women. *Am J Perinatol* 2013; 30: 383–8. [II-2]
8. Rouse DJ, Goldenberg RL, Oliver SP et al. Strategies for the prevention of early-onset neonatal group B streptococcal sepsis: A decision analysis. *Obstet Gynecol* 1994; 83: 483–94. [Decision analysis]
9. Paoletti LC, Mafoff LC. Vaccines to prevent neonatal GBS infection. *Semin Neonatal* 2002; 7(4): 315–23. [Review]
10. Lin FY, Philips III JB, Azimi PH. Level of maternal antibody required to protect neonates against early onset disease caused by group B *Streptococcus* type Ia: A multicenter, seroepidemiology study. *J Infect Dis* 2001; 184: 1022–8. [II-1]
11. Law MR, Palomaki G, Alfiveric Z et al. The prevention of neonatal group B streptococcal disease: A report by a working group of the medical screening society. *J Med Screen* 2005; 12: 60–8. [III]
12. Thomsen AC, Morup L, Hansen KB. Antibiotic elimination of group-B streptococci in urine in prevention of preterm labour. *Lancet* 1987; 591–3. [RCT; *n* = 69]
13. Klebanoff MA, Regan JA, Rao AV et al. Outcome of the vaginal infections and prematurity study: Results of a clinical trial of erythromycin among pregnant women colonized with group B streptococci. *Am J Obstet Gynecol* 1995; 172: 1540–5. [RCT; *n* = 938; vaginal–cervical GBS at 23–26 weeks: Erythromycin 333 mg tid or placebo for 10 weeks or up to 35 6/7 weeks, whichever came first]
14. National Institute for Health and Clinical Excellence: *Antibiotics for early-onset neonatal infection. CG149*. London: National Institute for Health and Clinical Excellence, 2012. [Review/guideline; available at: http://www.nice.org/uk/cg149]
15. National Institute for Health and Clinical Excellence: *Antenatal Care. CG62*. London: National Institute for Health and Clinical Excellence, 2008. [Review/guideline; available at: http://www.nice.org/uk/cg62]
16. Schrag SJ, Zell ER, Lyndfield R et al. A population-based comparison of strategies to prevent early-onset group B streptococcal disease in neonates. *N Engl J Med* 2002; 347: 233–9. [II-1]
17. Locksmith GJ, Clark P, Duff P. Maternal and neonatal infection rates with three different protocols for prevention of group B streptococcal disease. *Am J Obstet Gynecol* 1999; 180: 416–22. [II-1]
18. Gibbs RS, Schrag S, Schuchat A. Perinatal infections due to group B streptococci. *Obstet Gynecol* 2004; 104: 1062–76. [Review]
19. American College of Obstetrics and Gynecologists. Prevention of early-onset group B streptococcal disease in newborns. Committee Opinion No. 485. *Obstet Gynecol* 2011; 117. [III, guideline, reaffirmed in 2015]
20. Puopolo KM, Madoff LC, Eichenwald EC. Early-onset group B streptococcal disease in the era of maternal screening. *Pediatrics* 2005; 115(5): 1240–6. [II-2]
21. Mackay G, House MD, Bloch E, Wolfberg AJ. A GBS culture collected shortly after GBS prophylaxis may be inaccurate. *J Mat Fetal Neonatal Med* 2012; 25(6): 736–8. [II-2]
22. Jamie WE, Edwards RK, Duff P. Vaginal-perianal compared with vaginal-rectal cultures for identification of group B *Streptococcus*. *Obstet Gynecol* 2004; 104: 1058–61. [II-2]
23. Chan WSW, Chua SC, Gidding HF, Ramjan D, Wong MYW, Olma T, Thomas L, Gilberg GL. Rapid identification of group B streptococcus carriage by PCR to assist in the management of prelabour rupture of membranes in term pregnancy. *Aust N Z J Obstet Gynaecol* 2014; 54(2): 138–45. [II-2]
24. Poncelet-Jasserand E, Forges F, Varlet M-N, Chauleur C, Seffert P, Siani C, Pozzetto B, Ros A. Reduction of the use of antimicrobial drugs following the rapid detection of *Streptococcus agalactiae* in the vagina at delivery by real-time PCR assay. *BJOG*; 120: 1098–109. [II-2]
25. Young BC, Dodge LE, Gupta M, Rhee JS, Hacker MR. Evaluation of a rapid, real-time intrapartum group B *streptococcus* assay. *Am J Obstet Gynecol* 2011; 205: 37231–6. [II-2]
26. Abdelazim IA. Intrapartum polymerase chain reaction for detection of group B streptococcus colonization. *Aust N Z J Obstet Gynaecol* 2013; 53: 236–42. [II-2]
27. Ohlsson A, Shah VS. Intrapartum antibiotics for known maternal Group B streptococcal colonization. *Cochrane Database Syst Rev* 2014; 6: CD007467. [Three RCTs, *n* = 488 infants. Overall poor-quality RCTs]

28. Turrentine MA, Greisinger AJ, Brown KS, Wehmanen OA, Mouzoon ME. Duration of intrapartum antibiotics for group B streptococcus on the diagnosis of clinical neonatal sepsis. *Inf Dis Obstet Gynecol* 2013; 2013: 525878. doi:10.1155/2013/525878. [II-2]

29. Tajik P, van der Ham DP, Zafarmand MH et al. Using vaginal Group B *Streptococcus* colonization in women with preterm premature rupture of membranes to guide the decision for immediate delivery: A secondary analysis of the PPROMEXIL trials. *BJOG* 2014; 121: 1263–73. [I]

30. Ohlsson A, Shah VS, Stade BC. Vaginal chlorhexidine during labour to prevent early-onset neonatal group B streptococcal infection. *Cochrane Database Syst Rev* 2014; 12: CD003520. [Meta-analysis; five RCTs, *n* = 2190]

31. Boulvain M, Stan CM, Irion O. Membrane stripping for induction of labor. Jan *Cochrane Database Syst Rev* 2010. [Meta-analysis]

38

Vaccination

Amber S. Maratas, Edward M. Buchanan, and Joshua H. Barash

KEY POINTS

- Evaluation of a woman's immune status should occur in the preconception period. Optimally, immunization with indicated vaccines should occur prior to pregnancy.
- Immunity to **rubella, varicella, influenza, and hepatitis B** should be determined and administered as necessary in the **preconception period**.
- Nonetheless, in most cases, vaccines should be administered to pregnant women believed to be at high risk for acquiring a vaccine-preventable illness, as there is **no vaccine** that is **more dangerous to a pregnant woman or her fetus than the disease it is designed to prevent.**
- Recombinant, inactivated, and subunit vaccines as well as toxoids and immunoglobulins pose no threat to a developing fetus.
- **Inactivated influenza vaccine should be given (by injection as killed virus) to all pregnant women during the influenza season. The live attenuated form of the vaccine (intranasal spray) should not be given during pregnancy.**
- **Hepatitis B** vaccine can be safely given in pregnancy.
- **Tdap** vaccine should be administered **to all pregnant women in every pregnancy** regardless of previous vaccination history. Optimal timing of Tdap vaccination is **27–36 weeks gestation.**
- **Live, attenuated vaccines are contraindicated in pregnancy** because of the theoretical concern for fetal infection. However, if inadvertent vaccination occurs during pregnancy, no adverse fetal outcomes have been described with rubella, varicella, or BCG vaccination.
- **Rubella and varicella immunity should be determined in all women of childbearing age.** MMR (measles–mumps–rubella) and varicella vaccination should be avoided in pregnancy as they are live attenuated vaccines and **administered to all nonimmune women in the preconception or postpartum period.**
- **Breast-feeding** does not adversely affect immunization and **is not a contraindication for any vaccine with the exception of smallpox vaccine.**
- No vaccine is 100% safe and 100% effective in nonpregnant or pregnant adults.

HISTORICAL NOTES

Vaccination is **one of the most cost-effective and clinically successful medical interventions available.** The incidence of vaccine-preventable diseases drops precipitously upon initiating an effective vaccination program within a population [1]. Although traditionally targeted for children, adult vaccination programs are critically important to prevent disease in pregnant women and their offspring.

PREGNANCY AND VACCINE-PREVENTABLE DISEASES

Pregnancy is an important part of the life cycle when certain infections can play a particularly destructive role. Pregnancy creates a relative immune suppression, which places a woman at greater risk of complications from illnesses such as influenza and varicella. Likewise, maternal infections with such viruses as varicella and rubella can cause a spectrum of fetal effects including congenital anomalies, fetal morbidities, and even fetal death. Finally, neonates are highly susceptible to complications from vaccine-preventable diseases at a time when they do not receive full protection from vaccination themselves. By **immunizing close contacts of a newborn**, the risk of exposure is reduced, a strategy known as **"cocooning."** Maternal **vaccination also provides protection of the neonate through passive immunization**, in which maternal antibodies (IgG) are transmitted transplacentally, particularly in the last four to six weeks of gestation [2]. An additional benefit may occur with the passage of antibodies (IgA) via breast milk.

GENERAL GUIDELINES FOR VACCINATION AND PREGNANCY
Preconception

Evaluation of a woman's immune status should occur in the preconception period. Optimally, immunization with indicated vaccines should occur prior to pregnancy. For the reproductive age female, immunity to **rubella, varicella, influenza, tetanus, pertussis, hepatitis B, and HPV** are particularly beneficial for the health of the woman and her offspring (Tables 38.1 through 38.4). **If live, attenuated vaccines are administered, the patient should avoid pregnancy for four weeks** because of the theoretical concern for transplacental infection of the fetus [32].

In addition, **family members of a newborn should be immunized against influenza and pertussis.** Although vaccination does not have to occur preconception as is optimal for the mother, these vaccinations should be administered to family members before or during a woman's pregnancy to provide a protective barrier to disease from the moment of birth.

Pregnancy

If a woman is pregnant at the time of evaluation, careful selection of appropriate vaccinations should be made on the basis of the clinical situation to reduce morbidity from high-risk infections. Recombinant, **inactivated, and subunit vaccines as well as toxoids and immunoglobulins pose no threat to a developing fetus** [33–35]. These medications may be administered at any time in pregnancy although delaying until the second trimester will avoid false associations with adverse events in the first trimester.

Table 38.1   Recommended for All Women of Childbearing Age (Preconception, Postpartum, and Considered Safe in Pregnancy)

Vaccine	Vaccine Type	Dosing Regimen	Indications/Comments
Influenza [3,4] Trivalent inactivated vaccine (TIV)	Inactivated subunit (IM injection)	Annually	Vaccinate all adults and children >6 mo. Pregnant women should be immunized during the influenza season at any gestation. Do not administer live vaccine (LAIV, FluMist) during pregnancy.
Tetanus/diphtheria Td [5]	Toxoids	Booster every 10 yr after primary series completed	Uncertain history or incomplete primary series, administer three-dose primary series (Td): • Vaccines given at 0, 4 weeks, and 6–12 months. • Tdap should replace one dose of Td, preferably during the late second or third trimester of pregnancy [6].
Tdap [5]	Toxoids/acellular	Single dose of Tdap to replace one Td booster (see Indication/ Comments for details)	No history of prior Tdap vaccination: • Tdap should be administered as a one-time booster regardless of interval since the last tetanus- or diphtheriatoxoid containing vaccine. Tdap and pregnancy: • Women who have not received Tdap should receive it during pregnancy, preferably between 27 and 36 weeks gestation.
Hepatitis B [7]	Recombinant	*Pre-exposure prophylaxis:* • Three-dose series: 0, 1, and 4 mo[a] • Third dose at least 2 mo after second dose AND at least 4 mo after initial dose *Postexposure prophylaxis:* • Either vaccinate, give HBIG, or both (depends on exposure type, vaccine status, time from exposure)	Exposure to blood in workplace, dialysis/ESRD patients, current or history of injection drug use, more than one sexual partner in the past 6 months, other sexually transmitted infections, hepatitis C, household contact or sexual partner of person with chronic Hepatitis B, health care personnel, travel to area of high prevalence for >6 mo[b]
Human papilloma (HPV) [8,9]	Recombinant	Three-dose series • Second dose 1–2 mo after the first dose • Third dose 6 mo after the initial dose	Although HPV vaccine has not been causally associated with adverse outcomes during pregnancy (category B), it is not recommended during pregnancy. If a woman becomes pregnant after starting the series, the remainder of the series should be delayed until after delivery. No interventions are needed if a dose is inadvertently administered during pregnancy.

[a]Special dosing required for dialysis and immunocompromised patients.
[b]Diseases related to travel, available at http://wwwnc.cdc.gov/travel/content/diseases.aspx.

Live, attenuated vaccines are contraindicated in pregnancy because of the theoretical concern for fetal infection. However, if inadvertent vaccination occurs during pregnancy, no adverse fetal outcomes have been described with rubella, varicella, or BCG vaccination [29,36–40].

SPECIFIC VACCINES
Influenza
Inactivated influenza vaccine should be administered in any trimester during the flu season because of the risk that infection poses to a pregnant woman [41] (Table 38.1). Given incomplete immunity against influenza with vaccination, close contacts of the pregnant woman should also be immunized. Pregnant women and young infants are at significant increased risk for serious consequences of influenza. During pregnancy, women have a fourfold increased rate of serious illness and hospitalization [42]. The increased morbidity related to influenza during pregnancy is related to physiologic changes that include decreased pulmonary volume, increased cardiac output, and suppression of cell-mediated immunity [43]. Following the 2009 H1N1 pandemic, a retrospective cohort found an association with

influenza infection and increased rates of stillbirth and prematurity [44]. A randomized controlled trial of 314 mothers and infants demonstrated immunization benefits to both mother and child. Immunized pregnant women had 30% less respiratory febrile illnesses. Infants less than six months old born to immunized mothers had 63% fewer cases of influenza [45]. Influenza vaccine has been routinely administered during pregnancy since 1957. No study to date has shown an adverse consequence of inactivated influenza vaccine in pregnant women or their offspring [3,4,46] (see also Chapter 24).

Td/Tdap
Td (**tetanus** toxoid, reduced inactivated **diphtheria** toxoid) is a tetanus vaccine containing diphtheria toxoid as well (Table 38.1). Tetanus in newborn infants, once common, is prevented if the mother has been immunized because the immune mother passes antibodies to the fetus across the placenta. Maternal tetanus toxoid vaccination has been shown to be up to 98% effective in preventing neonatal tetanus [47].

Td effectiveness in preventing neonatal deaths was 62% [5]. The WHO estimates that 1.5 million cases of neonatal

Table 38.2   Recommended for Pregnant Women at Significant Risk for Exposure

Vaccine	Subtype	Dosing Regimen	Indications/Comments
Hepatitis A [10,11]	Inactivated	*Pre-exposure prophylaxis*: • Two-dose vaccine series, second dose 6–18 mo after the first dose *Postexposure prophylaxis*: • Either vaccinate, give IG, or both depending on exposure type, age, health status[a]	Chronic liver disease, clotting disorders requiring clotting factor precipitates, illicit drug users (both injection and noninjection), men who have sex with men, travel/live/work in endemic areas Unvaccinated persons in contact with an infected person (both sexual and household contacts), members of child care centers with an infected employee or child, to be considered for hospital workers in close contact with infected patients
Pneumococcal [12]	Polysaccharide	Single dose	Smoking (adults 19 yr and older), chronic pulmonary disease including smoking, asthma, chronic liver disease, chronic alcoholism, chronic cardiovascular disease, chronic renal failure or nephrotic syndrome, functional or anatomic asplenia (e.g., sickle cell disease or splenectomy), diabetes mellitus, immunosuppressive conditions (e.g., HIV)
		One time revaccination after 5 yr	Chronic renal failure or nephrotic syndrome, functional or anatomic asplenia (e.g., sickle cell disease or splenectomy), chronic high-dose steroids, immunosuppressive conditions
Rabies [13–15]	Inactivated	*Pre-exposure prophylaxis*: • Three doses: day 0, 7, 21, or 28 • Test Ab titer every 6 mo for continuous exposure or every 2 yr for intermittent exposure • Booster vaccination if titer < acceptable level *Postexposure prophylaxis*: • *Not previously vaccinated*: single dose of rabies immune globulin (RIG) + four doses of vaccine on days 0, 3, 7, and 14[c] • *If previously vaccinated*: one dose of vaccine immediately, and repeat 3 days later	Veterinary workers, persons having frequent contact with animal species at risk for rabies,[b] spelunkers, travelers to areas where dog rabies is enzootic and rapid access to medical care may not be available Indicated for any wound/scratch/bite caused by a possibly rabid animal[b] Multiple studies on the vaccine and RIG in pregnant women failed to show an elevated risk, vaccine felt to be overall safe in pregnancy [13,14].
Meningococcal [16–21]	Polysaccharide, conjugate, recombinant	Single dose, revaccination after 5 yr recommended if continued high risk for infection	Anatomic or functional asplenia, terminal complement component deficiency, military recruits, boarding school or college students, travel or reside in endemic or epidemic area Safety data with the quadrivalent polysaccharide vaccine in pregnancy is limited; however, more safety data is available for the polysaccharide than the conjugated version of the vaccine. Of note, conjugated vaccine has not been associated with any increase risk of adverse effects when given inadvertently in pregnancy. No pregnancy data exists for Serogroup B meningococcal vaccines.
Polio (IPV, *inactivated polio vaccine*) [22]	Inactivated	Three-dose primary series if not previously completed • Second dose 1–2 mo after first dose • Third dose 6–12 mo after second dose Booster—if risk of exposure and primary series completed more than 10 yr previously: • Single dose of IPV	Travel to or live in areas where polio is endemic or epidemic, lab worker who might handle poliovirus, health care workers who might care for polio infected persons, unvaccinated adults whose children will receive OPV • IPV is used exclusively for routine vaccination in the United States and other nations where polio is not endemic. OPV is still used for outbreaks [22]. • *Pregnancy*: Vaccination should be avoided on theoretical grounds, but if at increased risk for infection, IPV can be administered. No adverse effects have been found in pregnant women or their fetuses.

(Continued)

Table 38.2 (Continued) Recommended for Pregnant Women at Significant Risk for Exposure

Vaccine	Subtype	Dosing Regimen	Indications/Comments
Polio (OPV, *oral polio vaccine*)	Live	If less than 4 wk available to immunize, a single dose of OPV may be given [22] Three-dose primary series and booster recommendations are same as above	[d]OPV has a risk of causing *vaccine-related paralytic poliomylitis*. It is used in countries endemic for polio where the superior secretory immunity in the gastrointestinal tract induced by OPV is an advantage. OPV is the only product available in many developing nations and should be used in pregnancy as indicated. No adverse effects have been found to mother/fetus
Anthrax [23]	Inactivated, acellular vaccine	*Pre-exposure*: 5 IM doses (0 wk, 4 wk, 6 mo, 12 mo, and 18 mo [IM]) + annual booster to maintain immunity	*Pre-exposure*: Military personnel in high-risk areas, persons who perform high-risk laboratory work, handle animal product/hides and unable to adhere to standards of prevention (Although likely safe in pregnancy, CDC recommends deferment in vaccine administration in pregnant persons even if high risk of exposure)
		Postexposure: three doses SC (0, 2, 4 wk) with 60-day antimicrobial postexposure prophylaxis	*Postexposure*: Given to persons exposed including pregnant and breast-feeding women, children <18 yr decided case by case
Japanese encephalitis [24]	Inactivated	Three-dose series • 0, 7, and 30 days	Travelers with significant risk of exposure based on destination, duration of travel, season, and activities [24]
Typhoid OralTY21a Injectable Vi Whole-cell vaccine Yellow fever [25–27]	Live attenuated Polysaccharide Inactivated Live virus	Oral: three-dose series • One dose every 2 days Injection Vi: • Single dose Inactivated injection: • Two doses 4 wk apart Single dose • Booster every 10 yr for continued risk/exposure	Given to those at high risk: travel to or live in area where typhoid is endemic, close contact of typhoid carrier, lab exposure to *Salmonella typhi* bacteria. Information on safety in pregnancy is not available, on theoretical grounds avoid vaccination in pregnancy Given to those at high risk: live in or travel to area where yellow fever is endemic, or lab exposure to the virus. Not well studied in pregnancy, pregnant women who must travel to areas where risk of yellow fever infection is high should be vaccinated

Abbreviation: IG, immunoglobulin.
[a]Recommendations for hepatitis A postexposure prophylaxis: http://www.cdc.goV/mmwr/preview/mmwrhtml/mm5641a3.htm#box.
[b]Animals at high risk for carrying rabies: http://www.cdc.gov/mmwr/preview/mmwrhtml/rr57e517a1.htm.
[c]For persons with immunosuppression, rabies post-exposure prophylaxis should be administered using all five doses of vaccine on days 0, 3, 7, 14, and 28.
[d]Diseases related to travel: http://wwwnc.cdc.gov/travel/content/diseases.aspx.

tetanus have been prevented since a 1989 initiative to eliminate maternal and neonatal tetanus.

Tdap vaccine (tetanus toxoid, reduced inactivated **diphtheria** toxoid, and **acellular pertussis**) was first licensed in 2005 and now recommended for use in persons age ≥7 years old (Table 38.1). Pertussis protection was added to Td vaccine due to a resurgence of pertussis cases in the United States. Family members with pertussis are the source of infection in 75% of cases in early infancy when complications and fatalities are high [48]. Infants less than 12 months old account for most of the morbidity and mortality related to pertussis [47].

Tdap administration is recommended for all women in each pregnancy between 27 and 36 weeks gestation regardless of previous immunization timing. With peak maternal antibody titers occurring at least two weeks after vaccination, this timing allows for maximal transplacental antibody passage to the fetus during the third trimester [49]. Consequently, the newborn will benefit from passive immunity to pertussis until active immunization takes effect via the childhood immunization program schedule. This strategy, recommended by the CDC since 2013, has been shown more cost-effective and clinically superior to the previous strategy of postpartum and household contact Tdap vaccination by mathematical modeling [47,50].

Hepatitis B

Hepatitis B is a serious problem in pregnancy because of the possibility of vertical transmission to the neonate (see Chapter 30) (Table 38.1). Vertical transmission occurs in up to 90% of infected women depending on their viral status, and 90% of the children who become infected develop chronic infection [51,52]. Nonimmune women at high risk for HBV infection during pregnancy should be immunized. This includes women who have had more than one sexual partner in the past six months, illicit drug users (both injection and noninjection), those with an HBsAg-positive sex partner, and those being evaluated or treated for a sexually transmitted disease [7]. Women at risk should also be counseled on safe sexual practices to prevent HBV infection. HBV is also spread through oral secretions; therefore, it is also recommended to vaccinate women who have household members that are Hepatitis B sAg positive [7]. Although reports are limited, this vaccine has not been shown to have any adverse effects on the developing fetus [21,51,52].

Streptococcus pneumoniae

In Table 38.2, pneumococcal vaccine indications are presented, which includes maternal asthma and smoking. Studies are

Table 38.3 Not Recommended in Pregnancy

Vaccine	Type	Dosing Regimen	Comments
Varicella	Live attenuated	Two-dose series: • Second dose 4–8 wk after first Postexposure prophylaxis: • Varicella zoster immune globulin (VZIG) within 96 hr of exposure to varicella or herpes zoster If VZIG is not available: • IVIG can be used at a dose of 400 mg/kg given IV as a single dose OR • Closely monitor for development of disease and treat with acyclovir if disease develops	Not given to pregnant women or women planning to become pregnant within 4 wk **Initiate series in the immediate postpartum period to those women determined to be varicella nonimmune** on prenatal evaluation VZIG and IVIG are safe in pregnancy and breast-feeding Acyclovir in Pregnancy Registry was completed in 1999. Data on 124,748 exposures in pregnancy did not find an association with any adverse pregnancy outcome [28]
MMR (measles–mumps–rubella)	Live attenuated	Single dose	Not given to pregnant women or women planning to become pregnant within 4 wk **Administer this MMR vaccine in the immediate postpartum period to those women determined to be rubella nonimmune** on prenatal evaluation
BCG	Live attenuated	Single dose	Consider giving to health care workers in areas where drug resistant strains of TB persist. No harmful fetal effects have been associated with BCG, but its use is not recommended in pregnancy [29]
Smallpox [30,31]	Live attenuated	Single inoculation Immunity decreases 3–5 yr after vaccination *Postexposure prophylaxis:* Vaccination within 3 days of exposure will completely prevent or significantly modify smallpox in the vast majority of persons. Vaccination 4–7 days after exposure likely offers some protection from disease or decreases severity	Pregnant women, or women planning to become pregnant within 4 wk, should not be vaccinated in the absence of exposure to active disease Close contacts of pregnant women or women planning to become pregnant within 4 wk should not be vaccinated unless exposed to active disease—exposure to the resulting lesion can cause vaccinia viral infection in the pregnant woman and/or fetus

Note: CDC's Advisory Committee on Immunization Practices does not recommend preventive use of vaccinia immune globulin (VIG) for pregnant women. However, if a woman has a complication from smallpox vaccine that could be treated with VIG, she should receive it while pregnant [30,31].

Table 38.4 Vaccination Clinical Guide Summary

Preconception	Pregnancy	Postpartum[g]
Influenza[a]	Any trimester	Influenza[a]
MMR[b]	Influenza[a]	MMR[b]
Varicella[b]	Gestational age 27–36 weeks	Varicella[b]
Td/Tdap	Tdap[e]	Tdap[h]
HPV[c]	Maternal indications benefit > risk	HPV[c]
Hepatitis B[d]	Hepatitis B	Hepatitis B[d]
Pneumococcal[d]	Pneumococcal	Pneumococcal[d]
Meningococcal[d]	Meningococcal[f]	Meningococcal[d]
Hepatitis A[d]	Hepatitis A	Hepatitis A[d]

Note: See Table 38.2 for further details about travel vaccines or vaccines related to high risk conditions.
[a]Administer 1 dose of inactivated vaccine during influenza season.
[b]If demonstrated nonimmune, preconception advise to avoid pregnancy for 4 weeks.
[c]Age 13–26 years.
[d]When maternal indications are present.
[e]Administer every pregnancy regardless of vaccination history.
[f]Tetravalent polysaccharide preferred based on safety data [21].
[g]Postpartum vaccines listed are not contraindicated in breast feeding [32].
[h]If not already given intrapartum.

limited, but this vaccine has not shown any adverse effects on developing fetus [21]. In pregnancy, studies lack sufficient statistical power to prove effectiveness in newborn protection. However, pneumococcal vaccination during pregnancy appears to reduce the risk of neonatal infection (RR 0.51; 95% CI 0.18–1.41) and pneumococcal colonization in infants by 16 months of age (RR 0.33; 95% CI 0.11–0.98) [12]. At the present time, **pneumococcal vaccination is recommended for maternal indications only.**

CONTRAINDICATIONS TO VACCINATION

The only true contraindication applicable to all vaccines is a history of a *severe* allergic reaction after a prior dose of vaccine or to a vaccine component unless the recipient has been desensitized. An extensive listing of vaccine components, their use, and the vaccines that contain each component is available from CDC's National Immunization Program website at http://www.cdc.gov/vaccines.

REFERENCES

1. Roush SW, Murphy TV. Vaccine-Preventable Disease Table Working Group. Historical comparisons of morbidity and mortality for vaccine-preventable diseases in the United States. *JAMA* 2007; 298(18): 2155–63. [III, Review]
2. Insel RA. Maternal immunization to prevent neonatal infection. *N Engl J Med* 1988; 319(18): 1219–20. [III, Review]
3. Munoz FM, Greisinger AJ, Wehmanen OA et al. Safety of influenza vaccination during pregnancy. *Am J Obstet Gynecol* 2005; 192(4): 1098–106. [II-2]
4. Grohskoph LA, Sokolow LZ, Olsen SJ et al. Centers for Disease Control and Prevention (CDC). Prevention and control of influenza with vaccines: Recommendations of the Advisory Committee on Immunization Practices (ACIP), United States, 2015–16 Influenza Season. *MMWR Recomm Rep* 2015; 64(30): 818–25. [Guideline]
5. Demicheli V, Barale A, Rivetti A. Vaccines for women to prevent neonatal tetanus. *Cochrane Database Syst Rev* 2005; (4): CD002959. [Meta-analysis; two RCTs, *n* = 10,560]
6. Centers for Disease Control and Prevention: *ACIP Provisional Recommendations for Pregnant Women on Use of Tetanus Toxoid, Reduced Diphtheria Toxoid and Acellular Pertussis Vaccine (Tdap).* Posted August 2011. Available at: http://www.cdc.gov/vaccines/recs/provisional/default/htm. Accessed September 1, 2011. [Guideline]
7. Mast EE, Weinbaum CM, Fiore AE; CDC. A comprehensive immunization strategy to eliminate transmission of hepatitis B virus infection in the United States: Recommendations of the Advisory Committee on Immunization Practices (ACIP). *MMWR Recomm Rep* 2006; 55(RR16): 1–25. [Guideline]
8. Garland S, Ault K, Gall S et al. Pregnancy and infant outcomes in the clinical trials of a human papilloma virus type 6/11/16/18 vaccine: A combined analysis of five randomized controlled trials. *Obstet Gynecol* 2009; 114: 1179–88. [Meta-analysis: Five RCTs, *n* = 25,551]
9. Markowitz LE, Dunne EF, Saraiya M et al. Centers for Disease Control and Prevention. Human Papillomavirus Vaccination: Recommendations of the Advisory Committee on Immunization Practices (ACIP). *MMWR Recomm Rep* 2014; 63(RR05): 1–30. [Guideline]
10. Fiore AE, Wasley A, Bell BP, Advisory Committee on Immunization Practices (ACIP). Prevention of hepatitis A through active or passive immunization: Recommendations of the Advisory Committee on Immunization Practices (ACIP). *MMWR Recomm Rep* 2006; 55(RR-7): 1–23. [Guideline]
11. Duff B, Duff P. Hepatitis A vaccine: Ready for prime time. *Obstet Gynecol* 1998; 91(3): 468–71. [Review]
12. Chaithongwongwatthana S, Yamasmit W, Limpongsanurak S et al. Pneumococcal vaccination during pregnancy for preventing infant infection. *Cochrane Database Syst Rev* 2006; (1): CD004903. [Meta-analysis; three RCTs, *n* = 280]
13. Chabala S, Williams M, Amenta R et al. Confirmed rabies exposure during pregnancy: Treatment with human rabies immune globulin and human diploid cell vaccine. *Am J Med* 1991; 91(4): 423–4. [II-3]
14. Sudarshan MK, Madhusudana SN, Mahendra BJ. Post-exposure prophylaxis with purified vero cell rabies vaccine during pregnancy—Safety and immunogenicity. *J Commun Dis* 1999; 31(4): 229–36. [Review]
15. Manning SE, Rupprecht CE, Fishbein D et al. Advisory Committee on Immunization Practices Centers for Disease Control and Prevention (CDC). Human rabies prevention—United States, 2008: recommendations of the Advisory Committee on Immunization Practices (ACIP). *MMWR* 2008; 57(RR-3): 1–28. [Guideline]
16. Cohn AC, MacNeil JR, Clark TA. Centers for Disease Control and Prevention. Prevention and control of meningococcal disease: Recommendations of the Advisory Committee on Immunization Practices (ACIP). *MMWR Recomm Rep* 2013; 62(RR02): 1–22. [Guideline]
17. Adam I, Abdalla MA. Is meningococcal polysaccharide vaccine safe during pregnancy? *Ann Trop Med Parasitol* 2005; 99(6): 627–8. [Review]
18. Shahid NS, Steinhoff MC, Roy E et al. Placental and breast transfer of antibodies after maternal immunization with polysaccharide meningococcal vaccine: A randomized, controlled evaluation. *Vaccine* 2002; 20(17–18): 2404–9. [II-2, RCT; *n* = 157]
19. Leston GW, Little JR, Ottman J et al. Meningococcal vaccine in pregnancy: An assessment of infant risk. *Pediatr Infect Dis J* 1998; 17: 261–3. [II-3]
20. MacNeil JR, Rubin L, Folaranmi T et al. Centers for Disease Control and Prevention. Use of Serogroup B Meningococcal Vaccines in Adolescents and Young Adults: Recommendations of the Advisory Committee on Immunization Practices (ACIP), 2015. *MMWR Recomm Rep* 2015; 64(41): 1171–6. [Guideline]
21. Makris, MC, Polyzos KA, Mavros MN, Athanasiou S, Rafailidis PI, Falagas ME. Safety of Hepatitis B, pneumococcal polysaccharide and meningococcal polysaccharide vaccines in pregnancy: A systematic review. *Drug Saf* 2012; 35: 1–14. [Review]
22. Centers for Disease Control and Prevention. Poliomyelitis prevention in the United States: Updated recommendations of the Advisory Committee on Immunization Practices (ACIP). *MMWR Recomm Rep* 2000; 49(RR05): 1–22. [Guideline]
23. Wright JG, Quinn CP, Shadomy S et al. Center for Disease Control and Prevention. Use of anthrax vaccine in the United States: Recommendations of the Advisory Committee on Immunization Practices (ACIP), 2009. *MMWR Recomm Rep* 2010; 59(RR06): 1–30. [Guideline]
24. Fischer M, Lindsey N, Staples JE, Hills S. Centers for Disease Control and Prevention. Japanese encephalitis vaccines: Recommendations of the Advisory Committee on Immunization Practices (ACIP). *MMWR Recomm Rep* 2010; 59(RR-1): 1–27. [Guideline]
25. Tsai TF, Paul R, Lynberg MC et al. Congenital yellow fever virus infection after immunization in pregnancy. *J Infect Dis* 1993; 168(6): 1520–3. [II-3]
26. Nasidi A, Monath TP, Vandenberg J et al. Yellow fever vaccination and pregnancy: A four-year prospective study. *Trans R Soc Trop Med Hyg* 1993; 87(3): 337–9. [II-2]
27. Nishioka Sde A, Nunes-Araujo FR, Pires WP et al. Yellow fever vaccination during pregnancy and spontaneous abortion: A case-control study. *Trop Med Int Health* 1998; 3(1): 29–33. [II-2]
28. Stone KM, Reiff-Eldridge R, White AD et al. Pregnancy outcomes following systemic prenatal acyclovir exposure: Conclusions from the international acyclovir pregnancy. *MMWR Recomm Rep* 2003; 52(RR04): 1–28. [Guideline]

29. Centers for Disease Control and Prevention. The role of BCG vaccine in the prevention and control of tuberculosis in the United States. A joint statement by the Advisory Council for the Elimination of Tuberculosis and the Advisory Committee on Immunization Practices. *MMWR Recomm Rep* 1996; 45(RR-4): 1–18. [Guideline]

30. Centers for Disease Control and Prevention. Smallpox vaccination and adverse reactions. *MMWR Recomm Rep* 2003; 52(RR04): 1–28. [Guideline]

31. Centers for Disease and Control and Prevention. *Smallpox vaccination information for women who are pregnant or breastfeeding.* Available at: http://www.bt.cdc.gov/agent/smallpox/faq /pregnancy.asp, 2009. Accessed September 1, 2011. [Guideline]

32. Centers for Disease Control and Prevention. *Guidelines for vaccinating pregnant women.* Available at: http://www.cdc. gov/vaccines /pubs/preg-guide.htm. Accessed January 21, 2016. [Guideline]

33. Kroger AT, Sumaya CV, Pickering LK et al. General recommendations on immunization—Recommendations of the Advisory Committee on Immunization Practices (ACIP). *MMWR Recomm Rep* 2011; 60(2): 1–61. [Guideline]

34. Grabenstein JD. Pregnancy and lactation in relation to vaccines and antibodies. *Pharm Pract Manag Q* 2001; 20(3): 1–10. [III, review]

35. Koren G, Pastuszak A, Ito S. Drugs in pregnancy. *N Engl J Med* 1998; 338(16): 1128–37. [III, review]

36. Bar-Oz B, Levichek Z, Moretti ME et al. Pregnancy outcome following rubella vaccination: A prospective controlled study. *Am J Med Genet* 2004; 130A: 52–4. [II-1]

37. Bart SW, Stetler HC, Preblud SR et al. Fetal risk associated with rubella vaccine: An update. *Rev Infect Dis* 1985; 7(Suppl. 1): S95–102. [III, review]

38. Centers for Disease Control and Prevention. Rubella vaccination during pregnancy—United States, 1971–1988. *MMWR Morb Mortal Wkly Rep* 1989; 38(17): 289–93. [III, review]

39. Sheppard S, Smithells RW, Dickson A et al. Rubella vaccination and pregnancy: Preliminary report of a national survey. *Br Med J (Clin Res Ed)* 1986; 292(6522): 727. [Survey]

40. Wilson E, Goss MA, Marin M et al. Varicella vaccine exposure during Pregnancy: Data from 10 years of the pregnancy registry. *J Infect Dis* 2008; 197(Suppl. 2): S178–84. [II-2]

41. Mak TK. Influenza vaccination in pregnancy: Current evidence and selected national policies. *Lancet Infect Dis* 2008; 8(1): 44–52. [III, review]

42. MacDonald NE, Riley LE, Steinhoff MC. Influenza immunization in pregnancy. *Obstet Gynecol* 2009; 114(2 Pt. 1): 365–8. [III, review]

43. Tamma PD, Ault KA, del Rio C et al. Safety of influenza vaccination during pregnancy. *Am J Obstet Gynecol* 2009; 201(6): 547–52. [III, review]

44. Pierce M, Kurinczuk JJ, Spark P, Brocklehurst P, Knight M. UKOSS. Perinatal outcomes after maternal 2009/H1N1 infection national cohort study. *BMJ* 2011; 342: d3214. [II-2]

45. Zaman K, Roy E, Arifeen SE et al. Effectiveness of maternal influenza immunization in mothers and infants. *N Engl J Med* 2008; 359(15): 1555–64. [I, RCT, n = 340]

46. American College of Obstetricians and Gynecologists Committee on Obstetric Practice. Influenza vaccination during pregnancy. Committee Opinion No. 608. American College of Obstetricians and Gynecologists. Obstet Gynecol 2014; 124:648–51. [III, review]

47. Centers for Disease Control and Prevention. Updated recommendations for use of tetanus toxoid, reduced diphtheria toxoid, and acellular pertussis vaccine (Tdap) in pregnant women—Advisory Committee on Immunization Practices (ACIP), 2012. *MMWR Morb Mortal Wkly Rep* 2013; 62(7): 131–5. [Guideline]

48. Bisgard K, Pascual FB, Ehresmann KR et al. Infant pertussis: Who was the source? *Pediatr Infect Dis J* 2004; 23: 985–9. [II-3]

49. Munoz FM, Bond, NH, Maccato M et al. Safety and immunogenicity of tetanus diphtheria and acellular pertussis (Tdap) immunization during pregnancy in mothers and infants: A randomized clinical trial. *JAMA* 2014; 311(17): 1760–9. [I, RCT, n = 48]

50. Terranella A, Asay GRB, Messonnier ML et al. Pregnancy dose Tdap and postpartum cocooning to prevent infant pertussis: A decision analysis. *Pediatrics* 2013; 131(6). [III]

51. Gupta I, Ratho RK. Immunogenicity and safety of two schedules of hepatitis B vaccination during pregnancy. *J Obstet Gynaecol Res* 2003; 29(2): 84–6. [II-2]

52. Levy M, Koren G. Hepatitis B vaccine in pregnancy: Maternal and fetal safety. *Am J Perinatol* 1991; 8: 227–32. [Review]

39

Trauma

Lauren A. Plante

KEY POINTS

- Trauma during pregnancy is a common complication and accounts for a significant fraction of maternal deaths as well as perinatal mortality.
- Changes in physiology related to pregnancy must be borne in mind when managing trauma care.
- Care of the pregnant trauma patient:
  - **There is no level I evidence** to dictate the initial care of the traumatized pregnant patient, the type and duration of monitoring, the type of testing required, or the follow-up care of ongoing pregnancy after trauma.
  - **Initial maternal stabilization takes priority over fetal assessment**.
  - Transfer to a trauma center should be considered for severe cases. This decision is usually made at the scene.
  - Multidisciplinary approach is important as obstetrician, maternal-fetal specialist, trauma surgeon, intensivist, anesthesiologist, neonatologist, and others may need to be involved.
  - **Maternal stabilization: "ABCs"** (airway, breathing, circulation).
  - **Appropriate radiologic or other studies should not be withheld because of pregnancy**.
  - Ultrasound, fetal monitoring, tocodynamometer (contraction) monitoring, and Kleihauer–Betke (KB) test can be considered in the management of the pregnant woman with trauma.
- After hospital discharge following trauma, there remains an increased probability of worse perinatal outcome. Ongoing fetal assessment may be indicated although the exact type of surveillance has not been established.

DEFINITION

Trauma includes both intentional harm and accidents. Intentional harm encompasses assault, blunt force trauma, and penetrating trauma. Accidents include, predominantly, motor vehicle crashes and falls.

INCIDENCE

Incidence of trauma in pregnancy is unclear, and both the burden and the breakdown of cause vary by region and socioeconomic factors. A commonly quoted figure of 8% from the United States is of uncertain reliability [1,2]. Estimates vary widely from **8% (any physical trauma) to 0.2% to 2% (evaluation for trauma) to 0.4–2/10,000 (hospitalization for trauma)** [3–5]. A population-based study in Sweden, using both the national birth registry and the national traffic accident registry, calculated a ratio of 207 motor vehicle crashes per 100,000

pregnancies [6]. The probability of hospital admission after maternal trauma increases with increasing gestational age [7]. **Domestic violence** against pregnant women ranges from **4% to 9%** [8]. Published figures are probably affected by reporting bias and undercounting of the total number of injuries. Not all cases of maternal trauma are seen at a trauma center or even referred to a hospital. Available literature on trauma is generally biased toward more serious injury whenever data are collected from hospital visits or admissions rather than from traffic records. A recent analysis of the National Inpatient Sample (NIS) demonstrates that, among women admitted to hospital following MVA, pregnant women had a *lower* risk of fracture, open wounds, intracranial, internal and spinal cord injury, transfusion, operations (other than those coded as genitourinary, a grouping that includes cesarean), and death than a matched group of nonpregnant controls [9]. This may represent either a difference in the type or severity of MVA in which a pregnant woman is involved, a difference in seatbelt use, or a differential willingness on the part of physicians to admit a pregnant patient for observation even with minor or no discernable injury. The NIS data set also showed that 3.8% of MVA involved pregnant women although it could not show the overall incidence of MVA in pregnancy. Motor vehicle crashes involving pregnant women are, roughly, evenly distributed by trimester [10,11].

ETIOLOGY/BASIC PATHOPHYSIOLOGY

Causes of trauma in pregnancy in the United States:

- **73% motor vehicle accident**, including auto vs. pedestrian (MVA; 3%–4% of all MVA involve a pregnant woman) [9,12]
- 12% assault
- 9% fall
- 2% bicycle
- <1% suicide
- 3% other (unintentional)

These reflect American data and cannot be taken as universally representative. By way of comparison, assault accounted for more than half of admissions of pregnant patients to a metropolitan trauma service in South Africa [13].

PROGNOSTIC FACTORS

Factors that predispose injured women to a worse pregnancy outcome, defined as delivery, pregnancy loss, or hysterectomy, are as follows:

- Higher degree of severity, e.g., injury severity score (ISS) >9 (For an online calculator of injury severity score, see http://www.trauma.org/index.php/main/article/383/)
- Lactate >2 mmol/L

- Altered mental status at admission (Glasgow Coma Score <8)
- Lack of proper seatbelt use
- Severe head injury
- Injury to thorax, abdomen, lower extremities, or spine

Drug use and shock at admission are also correlated with worse outcome although to a lesser extent [3,14]. Individual risk factors associated with fetal demise include penetrating injury, severity of injury, maternal hypotension, and need for laparotomy [13,15].

In cases of minor trauma (ISS = 0), classically described risk factors, such as Kleihauer–Betke, fibrinogen <200, contraction pattern by tocodynamomoter, direct abdominal trauma, placenta location, and abdominal pain are not reliable predictors of adverse pregnancy outcomes [16]. Although the evaluation of each patient should be individualized, extensive evaluation measures that are routine in practice may be reconsidered in cases of minor trauma in pregnancy.

COMPLICATIONS

Complications are more common if there is severe injury (ISS ≥9) [4] or if the woman is delivered during the hospitalization for trauma [5]. Delayed complications may occur even when there is no injury diagnosed at the time of hospitalization and when the woman is discharged home undelivered.

Maternal Death

Maternal mortality associated with trauma is about 0.1% to 1.4% [3,5]: This is 10 to 100 times increased over the background U.S. maternal mortality ratio. Among pregnant women hospitalized after trauma, the case fatality rate is 2%–4% [9,17–21].

Trauma is a leading cause of maternal death as **about 27% of maternal deaths are injury related** [22]. Of these deaths, the largest fraction is attributed to MVAs (44%), followed by homicide (31%), unintentional injuries (13%), and suicide (10%). Data from the Pregnancy Mortality Surveillance System in the 1990s suggested that the majority of pregnancy-associated homicides occurred in the postpartum period [22], but figures drawn a decade later from the National Violent Death Reporting System showed that 77% of pregnancy-associated homicides occurred, in fact, during pregnancy [23]. Trauma and other forms of violence are the leading cause of death in nonpregnant women of reproductive age.

Hospitalization

Women in the third trimester are more likely to be admitted to the hospital than women in the first or second trimester [10]; 3% of all trauma admissions are pregnant [24].

Transfusion

0.6% to 4%.

Hysterectomy

0.5% to 2%. May be indicated in cases of penetrating injury to the uterus or in cases of uterine rupture, resulting from blunt force trauma when surgical repair is not reasonable [25], or in cases in which coagulopathy follows placental abruption.

Fetal/Neonatal Outcomes

Nonreassuring fetal testing: 5% to 20%; preterm birth (PTB) <37 weeks: 14% to 20% [4].

Abruptio Placentae

1% to 13%. Severity of maternal injury does not reliably correlate with abruption [26].

Fetal Injury

Very few cases have been reported of fetal injury from maternal gunshot or stab wounds and of fetal fractures, visceral ruptures, and intracranial hemorrhage after blunt trauma. Penetrating abdominal injury, which, in the second half of pregnancy, usually involves the uterus, is associated with fetal death in up to 73% of cases [27] and has been proposed as an indication to explore the abdomen or effect cesarean delivery.

Fetal Death

0.4% to 1.5%. The rate of fetal death among women *hospitalized* for trauma is about 11% [17–21]. About 5/1000 fetal deaths can be attributed to trauma or approximately four traumatic fetal deaths per 100,000 live births [28]. **The single most salient risk factor for fetal death is maternal death.** The majority (>80%) of these fetal deaths in the United States are associated with MVA, and 6% are related to firearms and another 3% to falls: This does not mean that MVA is uniquely lethal to fetuses, only that it is more common than other mechanisms of injury. Less than half of fetal deaths are designated as due to placental injury (42%), 20% as placental abruption. Fetal death is more likely in cases of maternal death, hemorrhagic shock, or no seatbelt use. Aside from maternal death, the most significant associations with fetal death after blunt trauma are maternal ejection from a vehicle, maternal tachycardia (HR >110), maternal ISS >9, and fetal bradycardia (FHR <120) [29]. However, even minor maternal injuries from MVA have been associated with fetal death. Swedish data showed the risk of fetal death to be 93% with fatal maternal injury, 5% with major maternal injury, and 1% with minor maternal injury, but because there are so many more minor injuries, these still contributed significantly to fetal outcome statistics [6]. The odds ratio for fetal demise was 3.55 among all women involved in a motor vehicle crash; excluding early pregnancy losses, the odds ratio for fetal death was 2.49 when only third-trimester crashes were taken into account.

Neonatal Death

0.4% to 1.5%; highly related to preterm birth.

SPECIAL CONSIDERATIONS FOR COMPLICATIONS FROM ASSAULT

The rate of hospitalization for assault during pregnancy is 0.04% to 0.1% [30,31]. In California, 46% of assaults were related to an unarmed fight, 12% to firearms or bomb, and 9% to stab injuries. Women assaulted during pregnancy had higher rates of preterm delivery, low birth weight, placental abruption, stillbirth, and uterine rupture compared to women who were never hospitalized for assault during pregnancy. Thirteen percent of women hospitalized after assault delivered during the hospitalization. These women had worse outcomes than either women who were not assaulted or women who were assaulted but discharged undelivered [30]. In New Zealand, assault during pregnancy and assault after pregnancy were both associated with long-term danger for women, including injury and death within a 5-year period [31].

Intimate-partner violence accounted for 20% of the assaults in women who were discharged undelivered and for 50% of the assaults in women who delivered during the hospitalization [30]. Sadly, over a 15-year period in Maryland, homicide was the leading cause of pregnancy-associated maternal death, most often perpetrated by a current or former intimate partner and most often by gunshot [32].

PREGNANCY CONSIDERATIONS

Causes of trauma in pregnancy differ from nonpregnant trauma in that more are attributed to motor vehicles and fewer to other causes. Pregnancy is generally protective in relation to suicide. Compared to women of the same age who are not pregnant, pregnant women who sustained trauma were younger, had lower ISS and lower mortality (1% vs. 4%), had shorter length of stay, and lower rates of alcohol and drug use; however, 12% had been drinking and 20% had been using drugs [10]. A crash rate of 13/1000 person-years was calculated for pregnant women aged 15 to 39, which is half the rate for nonpregnant women in this age group (26/1000) [10].

In 11% of pregnancy trauma cases [24], the **pregnancy status was unknown** at admission to the receiving trauma team, and in two thirds of those, the pregnancy was newly diagnosed by serum hCG screening—that is, the status had possibly not been known by the patient either. Of those pregnancies unknown to the trauma team at admission but presumably known to the patient (although she did not or could not communicate the status to the team), fetal mortality was >75%, including both spontaneous and elective abortion. Incidental pregnancies that were news to the trauma team although *not* to the patient carried a 25% probability of fetal mortality [24]. One third of the nonsurvivors in the newly diagnosed group were voluntary abortions, in which the women reported they were fearful of nonspecific damage because of either injury or radiation. It must be cautioned, however, that the stated rationale for elective abortion is not always true.

PREGNANCY MANAGEMENT
Prevention of Injury
Seatbelts

Rates of seatbelt use are now similar among pregnant and nonpregnant individuals involved in MVAs, based on the National Automotive Sampling System/Crashworthiness Data System: approximately two thirds used a lap and shoulder belt [11]. **Three-point seatbelts should always be worn with the shoulder belt over the shoulder, collar bone, and across the chest, between the breasts, and the lap belt as low as possible under the abdomen and the uterus.** Seat belts **save maternal lives** by preventing ejection. Correct seat belt use is also associated with **better fetal outcomes**: an in-depth physical and mechanical analysis of 57 MVAs involving pregnant women demonstrated adverse fetal outcomes (death or damage) in 29% of correctly seatbelted, 50% of improperly restrained, and 80% of unrestrained women [33]. However,

severity of the crash was an independent predictor of poor fetal outcome: 85% of severe crashes (≥30 mph) in this sample were followed by fetal death, direct fetal injury, uterine rupture, or preterm delivery. A large study that linked birth records with state crash records in North Carolina concluded that the risk of stillbirth was tripled when a crash involved an unbelted pregnant driver compared to a belted pregnant driver [34]. Seatbelt restraints also have a protective role in low-velocity collisions. Impact testing using a crash-test dummy modeled to represent a woman at 30 weeks of pregnancy demonstrated two to three times higher peak abdominal pressure when the dummy was unrestrained compared to properly belted [35].

Air Bags

A cohort study in Washington State cross-referenced state patrol crash data with birth certificate and fetal death certificate data and found no statistically significant differences in maternal or fetal outcomes among 198 women whose airbag deployed compared to 622 women whose airbag did not deploy [36]. The **rates of preterm labor and of fetal death were higher in the no-airbag group**, and the lack of statistical significance may be a function of small numbers. In the North Carolina study, the rate of placental abruption was 58% higher when the pregnant driver's vehicle was not equipped with airbags [34] although rates of preterm birth and stillbirth were not significantly different.

In a case series of 30 women past 20 weeks of pregnancy who were hospitalized after crashes in which their air bags deployed, 67% of whom were also restrained with a seat belt, 90% had obstetrical signs or symptoms at admission (contractions, abdominal pain, abnormal fetal heart rate, or vaginal bleeding), but there was only one fetal death. All with a live fetus were discharged home undelivered after a mean length of stay of 24 hours although unfortunately most were lost to follow-up [37]. **On the available evidence, no definitive statement can be made as to the utility or safety of air bags specifically in pregnancy, but because they save maternal lives, they would, on balance, be expected to save fetal lives.**

Intimate Partner Violence

Prevention is key. ACOG recommends screening for intimate partner violence at the initial prenatal visit, at least once per trimester, and again in the postpartum period. ACOG also encourages gun safety and firearm restrictions as a way of reducing pregnancy-associated homicide [38,39].

Care of the Pregnant Trauma Patient

There are no trials assessing effectiveness of initial care and interventions for the pregnant patient following trauma, including the type and duration of monitoring, the type of testing required, or the follow-up care of ongoing pregnancy after trauma. The Society of Obstetricians and Gynaecologists of Canada has recently released guidelines for care of the pregnant trauma patient [40]. Guidelines have also been published by the Eastern Association for the Surgery of Trauma [7], and the American College of Surgeons includes a section on trauma in pregnancy in the Advanced Trauma Life Support (ATLS) course and manual [41]. These recommendations are level II and level III, given lack of randomized trials in pregnancy.

Workup and Management

An algorithm for evaluation and management of trauma in pregnancy, specifically, is shown in Figure 39.1 [2]. Electronic resources are also available online at www.myatls.com and as the MyATLS app for smartphones: search iPhone's AppStore or GooglePlay for Android devices.

Stabilization

The American College of Surgeons [42], the American College of Obstetricians and Gynecologists [1], and the Society of Obstetricians and Gynaecologists of Canada [40] are unanimous in declaring that **maternal stabilization takes priority over fetal assessment**. The ATLS algorithm lays out, in order,

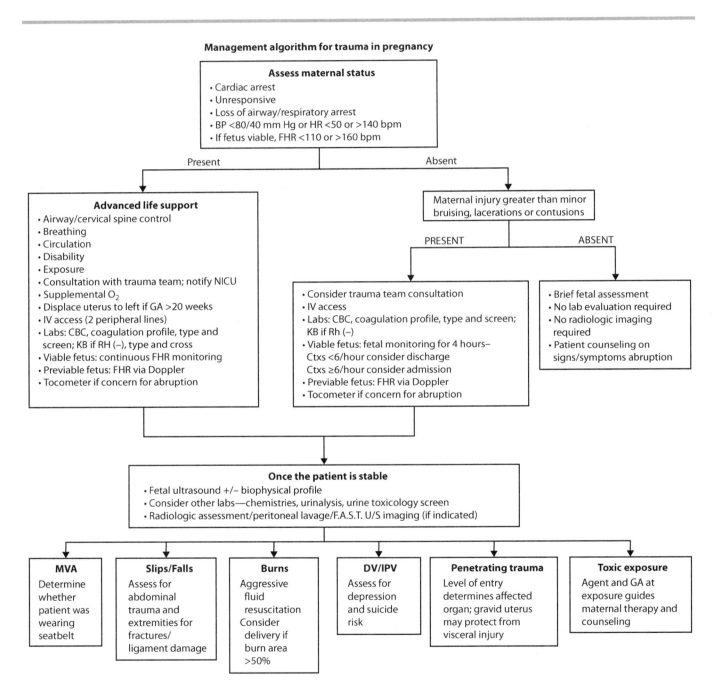

Proposed algorithm for evaluation and management of trauma in pregnancy.

Figure 39.1 Management algorithm for trauma in pregnancy. *Abbreviations*: *BP*, blood pressure; *CBC*, complete blood cell count; *Ctxs*, contractions; *DV*, domestic violence; *FAST*, focused assessment with sonography for trauma; *FHR*, fetal heart rate; *GA*, gestational age; *HR*, heart rate; *IPV*, intimate partner violence; *ISS*, injury severity score; *IV*, intravenous; *KB*, Kleihauer-Betke; *MVA*, motor vehicle accident; *NICU*, neonatal intensive care unit; *O₂*, oxygen; *U/S*, ultrasound. (Reprinted from Mendez-Figueroa H, Dahlke JD, Vrees RA, Rouse DJ. *Am J Obstet Gynecol*, 208, 4, 321.e1–9, 2013. With permission.)

Table 39.1 Maternal Stabilization after Trauma in Pregnancy

- **A**irway
- **B**reathing
- **C**irculation
- **D**isability (neurological evaluation)
- **E**xposure, environmental control (undress the patient, look everywhere for injuries, but keep them warm)
- (**F**etus)

Source: Modified from American College of Surgeons, ACS Committee on Trauma. *Advanced Trauma Life Support. ATLS Student Course Manual, 9th edition.* ACS, Chicago, IL. 2012.

assessment and stabilization as shown in Table 39.1. These are addressed briefly, in regard to pregnant patients especially, in the following subsections.

Airway. Airway edema is more common in pregnant women, so smaller endotracheal tube size is required. Airway reflexes are not changed in pregnancy, but longer gastric emptying times and diminished function of the lower esophageal sphincter leave pregnant women more prone to aspiration of gastric contents.

Breathing. In pregnancy, minute ventilation is increased and functional residual capacity is decreased, so periods of apnea or hypopnea lead more quickly to hypoxemia.

Circulation. Physiologic changes in pregnancy include increased cardiac output, expanded plasma volume, peripheral vasodilation, and a decrease in systolic and diastolic blood pressure. As a result, the signs of hypovolemia are seen later in pregnant women because of these compensatory mechanisms. Tachycardia and narrowed pulse pressure are late findings as pregnant women progress through the stages of hypovolemic shock. Fetal heart rate should be evaluated as an additional vital sign. A normal fetal heart rate suggests normal uterine perfusion, and an abnormal FHR may reflect compromised perfusion and function as an early warning sign of decreased circulatory volume. Maintenance of left uterine displacement is important in maintaining preload and cardiac output after midpregnancy because of the effect of the gravid uterus on compressing the inferior vena cava. If the patient is visibly pregnant to the prehospital provider, the supine position should be avoided.

After maternal stabilization, history (medical/surgical/pregnancy history, gestational age, trauma mechanism, etc.) should be obtained, a thorough physical examination should be performed (including vital signs, signs of trauma, uterine tenderness, speculum examination, and bimanual exam), and available records (e.g., ultrasounds, laboratory tests) should be reviewed. Problems with history or physical examination, however, must be borne in mind. In severe trauma, history may be unobtainable if the patient's neurologic status is compromised; information may be obtained from family members or emergency responders as an alternative. The absence of uterine tenderness cannot be construed as the absence of uterine or placental injury. Speculum/manual exam may be difficult or impossible if the patient is in c-spine immobilization or has pelvic fractures.

The **focused abdominal sonogram for trauma (FAST)** is commonly undertaken as part of an initial assessment in the emergency department. This is a quick four-quadrant ultrasound to look for free fluid in the abdomen and pelvis; sensitivity is reported to be 80% and specificity 100% in the pregnant patient following blunt-force abdominal trauma [34]. The FAST scan, although not originally designed for fetal assessment, presents an obvious opportunity to ascertain fetal cardiac activity and other relevant factors.

Evaluation and Diagnostic Studies

Appropriate studies should not be withheld because of pregnancy.

1. CT is recommended for evaluation of **hemodynamically stable** patients with associated neurological injury, multiple nonabdominal injury, or equivocal physical examination. Patients with a negative CT should nonetheless be admitted for observation [43] (radiation concerns, see below and Tables 39.2 and 39.3) [33].
2. **Blunt abdominal trauma**
   a. **FAST ultrasound:** The maternal abdomen can be evaluated for the presence of intraperitoneal blood with diagnostic peritoneal lavage (DPL) or with ultrasound; the FAST scan has supplanted DPL in most institutions [7,41]. FAST scan has 80% sensitivity and 100%

Table 39.2 Estimates of Fetal Radiation Dose for the Following Examinations

Examination	Mean Fetal Dose (mGy)	Maximum Fetal Dose (mGy)
Skull	<0.01	<0.01
Chest	<0.01	<0.01
Abdomen	1.4	4.2
Thoracic spine	<0.01	<0.01
Lumbar spine	1.7	10
Pelvis	1.1	4
IVP	1.7	10

Source: From Health Protection Agency, the Royal College of Radiologists and the College of Radiographers. Protection of pregnant patients during diagnostic medical exposures to ionizing radiation: Advice from the Health Protection Agency, the Royal College of Radiologists and the College of Radiographers. 2009.

Table 39.3 Estimates of Fetal Radiation Exposure with Computed Tomography (CT)

CT Examination	Mean Fetal Dose (mGy)	Maximum Fetal Dose (mGy)
Head	<0.005	<0.005
Chest	0.06	0.96
Abdomen	8.0	49
Lumbar spine	2.4	8.6
Pelvis	25	79
Pelvimetry	0.2	0.4

Source: From Health Protection Agency, the Royal College of Radiologists and the College of Radiographers. Protection of pregnant patients during diagnostic medical exposures to ionizing radiation: Advice from the Health Protection Agency, the Royal College of Radiologists and the College of Radiographers. 2009.

specificity for intra-abdominal injury in the pregnant patient following blunt abdominal trauma [41]. If DPL is elected, it is typically performed with an open technique in pregnancy. Both these techniques can be performed quickly and therefore are suitable for evaluation of an unstable patient and avoid transport and ionizing radiation altogether.

   b. Exploratory laparotomy is indicated for a positive DPL [43] and in most cases of a positive FAST scan. Suspicion of uterine rupture is also an indication for laparotomy [40].

3. In hemodynamically stable patients with positive FAST scan, follow-up CT scan may be considered so as to identify the source: Some solid viscus injuries may be managed nonoperatively [43].

4. **Penetrating abdominal wound: Single preoperative** dose of broad-spectrum **antibiotic** [43]. Laparotomy is indicated if hypotension is present with a penetrating abdominal wound; gunshot wound to abdomen; bleeding from GI or GU tract after penetrating trauma; peritonitis; evisceration; free air. The pregnant uterus tends to shield maternal viscera, so stab wounds to the abdomen are less likely to injure bowel unless the site is the upper abdomen. In contrast, the fetus is often injured. As is true outside of pregnancy, the trajectory of a bullet or other missile is unpredictable and therefore laparotomy is generally indicated.

5. **Open fractures**: Prophylactic **antibiotics** with gram-positive coverage, administered as soon as possible after injury [42].

6. **Traumatic brain injury**: Head CT is generally required. Broad-spectrum prophylactic antibiotics if penetrating brain injury [42].

7. **Spine trauma suspected: immobilization and imaging, generally CT** [42].

8. **Special pregnancy-specific evaluations/studies:**

   a. **Fetal ultrasound**: Although there is insufficient formal evidence to assess the effectiveness of performing a fetal ultrasound in the woman with trauma in pregnancy, it is near universal and is without risk as long as it does not delay definitive maternal care. Assessment of fetus, AFV, and placenta by ultrasound may be beneficial for management. Ultrasound is insufficiently sensitive to detect placental abruption unless it involves >50% of the placenta, so that negative ultrasound does not exclude abruption, especially because abruption may develop days after the initial trauma.

   b. **Fetal monitoring**: There is insufficient evidence to assess fetal monitoring and especially its duration in the woman with trauma in pregnancy. Assessment of fetal status may be beneficial as the fetoplacental unit is often one of the most sensitive "organs" to be affected by maternal circulatory compromise. If fetal monitoring is to be undertaken, continuous monitoring is probably preferable to intermittent. **More than one third of third-trimester women with trauma have ominous findings on monitoring** [19]. The fact that maternal and fetal outcomes are worse in women who do not have electronic monitoring in some reports [19] reflects the team priorities (more severely injured mothers require interventions that preclude fetal monitoring, or electronic monitoring is deemed of low priority).

   c. **Tocodynamometer or contraction monitoring**: An oft-cited study [26] found that at >20 weeks gestation, >90% of women with trauma presenting for evaluation demonstrate some uterine contractions in the first four hours with uterine activity decreasing over time. Within the first hour, 64% were contracting with a frequency of every five minutes or more, declining to 29% by hour 4. Patients without contractions or whose contractions never exceeded q10 minute frequency were discharged at the end of four hours, and none had abruption [26]. Those who had been contracting at more than q11 minute frequency were all kept for at least 24 hours. There was one placental abruption at six hours, resulting in emergent delivery for fetal distress, and among the patients hospitalized beyond 24 hours, there was a 40% delivery rate with one stillborn infant. Total abruption rate was 8% [26]. From these data comes the common recommendation for **monitoring at least four hours after maternal trauma** [40,44]. Others have recommended a minimum of six hours of monitoring, acknowledging that the best duration of monitoring is unknown [7]. **In nearly 5% of trauma in pregnancy cases, fetal compromise or placental abruption becomes evident only after prolonged monitoring (6–48 hours or more)** [45].

   d. The **Kleihauer–Betke (KB)** test assesses presence of fetal red blood cells in the maternal circulation. It has been proposed as an adjunct to predict preterm labor after trauma [46]. A study of 233 women found that 20% of pregnant trauma patients who had KB drawn had positive results although **the test proved neither sensitive nor specific for a poor outcome** [45]: 96% of women with a positive KB (defined as >0.01 mL of fetal blood in the maternal circulation) had preterm contractions, half of whom also had cervical change, and none of those with a negative test had any contractions during the period of surveillance, which encompassed a minimum of four hours. A smaller study evaluating 73 women with KB after trauma calculated the likelihood ratio of a positive KB for predicting preterm labor as greater than 20 [46]; none of the KB-negative women had contractions. The authors proposed that if the KB were negative, duration of monitoring could be limited to the time it took to get the test back, that is, 1–2 hrs. Although the test is inexpensive and simple to perform, it has been criticized for its **subjectivity and lack of reproducibility** [47]. Using known admixtures of fetal and maternal blood, KB testing overestimates the volume of fetomaternal hemorrhage and has been demonstrated to vary more than tenfold with repeat testing of a single sample [47]. Some have advocated **substitution of flow cytometry (using a fluorescence-activated cell sorter) or monoclonal antibodies to Hb F** as a test for fetomaternal hemorrhage; although these are both sensitive and more precise, they are expensive and not widely available.

   e. **Rh status** must be tested after maternal trauma. Rh negative women should receive Rh immune globulin after maternal trauma of any degree because even minor maternal trauma may be associated with maternofetal hemorrhage sufficient to cause sensitization. KB is particularly helpful with Rh-negative women to determine dose of Rh immune globulin needed to prevent rhesus isoimmunization.

   f. **Coagulation studies** (e.g., fibrinogen, D-dimer, PT, and PTT): There is no evidence of benefit of routine coagulation studies unless massive hemorrhage has occurred or is expected.

g. **Admission**: Admission to the hospital for **longer observation (≥24 hours)** should be considered for women with **uterine tenderness, continued abdominal pain, a high-risk mechanism of injury (such as auto vs. pedestrian or high-speed crash), persistent (>4/hour) contractions, rupture of membranes, positive KB, bleeding, abnormal fetal heart rate tracing** [40].

The indication for **tetanus prophylaxis** does not change during pregnancy (see Chapter 38). All traumatic wounds are at risk for development of tetanus, and passive immunization should be considered in all cases with human tetanus immune globulin 250 units given IM [42].

Radiation in the Pregnant Trauma Patient

Estimates of **fetal radiation dose** for the following examinations are shown in Table 39.2 [33]. Gray is the unit of measurement for absorbed dose of radiation; it is defined as 1 J of energy deposited in 1 kg of material. This has replaced the rad or roentgen-absorbed dose, which is the dose delivered to an object of 100 ergs of energy per gram of material. One Gray = 100 rads (or, 1 rad = 10 mGy). **Teratogenic effects are of no concern until after 5 to 10 mGy.** Plain radiographs of the spine and chest can be performed in pregnancy with minimal radiation exposure to the fetus with abdomen and pelvis shielding. The American College of Radiology considers that some radiological examinations expose a pregnant uterus to so low a dose that pregnancy does not affect the decision to proceed [48]: these include chest X-ray in the first and second trimester, X-ray or CT of the extremities, and any imaging of the head or neck. With CT scanning, the total radiation dose to the fetus depends on the site imaged, the machine and technique used, and on the distance between cuts.

Estimates of fetal radiation exposure with **computed tomography** (CT) are shown in Table 39.3 [49]. Because the actual fetal dose given in a procedure may be as much as tenfold higher than the published mean dose, depending on the patient's size and the technique used, **actual dose should be ascertained** wherever possible by contacting the institution's radiation physicists for dosimetry. The ACR suggests that unused personnel monitors for radiation dose could be placed above and below the patient's pelvis so as to document the uterine dose [48]. The proxy for fetal radiation dose is uterine dose.

Concerns about radiation effects on the embryo or fetus include death, malformation, growth restriction, abnormal development of the brain with cognitive sequelae, and cancer. No data are available for cellular effects per se, only for clinical effects. Threshold doses for the appearance of death or malformation are shown in Table 39.4 [49]. Data for cognitive impairment (mental retardation), based on survivors of the atomic bomb exposed in utero, suggest no effect with exposure before 10 weeks or after 27 weeks. These data do raise the possibility of a dose-response (rather than threshold) model between 10 and 17 weeks with a loss of 30 IQ points per Gy (1000 mGy). Diagnostic radiologic procedures are orders of magnitude below these limits. Even in the 10- to 17-week fetus in which a dose-response curve may be postulated for cognitive impairment, an 80-mGy study, such as CT of the pelvis, would have only minimal potential to compromise intellectual function, for example, 2 IQ points.

Table 39.4 Threshold Doses by Gestational Age for the Appearance of Embryo/Fetus Death or Congenital Malformation

Weeks from LMP	Embryo/Fetus Death	Congenital Malformation
No threshold at conception		
4 to 7	250–500 mGy	200 mGy
7 to 9	500 mGy	500 mGy
9 to 23	>500 mGy	Very few observed
23 to term	>1000 mGy	Very few observed

Source: From Health Protection Agency, the Royal College of Radiologists and the College of Radiographers. Protection of pregnant patients during diagnostic medical exposures to ionizing radiation: Advice from the Health Protection Agency, the Royal College of Radiologists and the College of Radiographers. 2009.

Concerns have also been raised about the possibility of **cancer** induction in children exposed to intrauterine radiation. Unlike death or malformation, the induction of cancers is believed to be a dose-response rather than threshold phenomenon. Because childhood cancers are rare events, even a doubling or quadrupling of the risk has little impact on cancer deaths. Excess risk of fatal childhood cancer attributed to fetal exposure with typical diagnostic procedures range from 1 in 30,000 to 1 in 1700. The derived risk is estimated at one excess case per 33,000 per mGy of exposure. The highest risks, which remain quite small on a population basis, are seen with the highest exposures, for example, CT of the pelvis [49]. This concern is not a reason to routinely offer termination of pregnancy [49,50]. Recent estimates of conceptus radiation dose with a single anteroposterior chest radiograph (assuming an average maternal size: dose increases with increasing maternal size) range from 0.0021 to 0.0028 mGy in the first trimester to 0.1 to 5.9 mGy in the second and 0.1 to 1.9 mGy in the third trimester [51]. This corresponds to an excess risk of childhood cancer of approximately 10 per million.

Ultrasound and magnetic resonance imaging (MRI) do not utilize radiation energy and are not associated with adverse effects on the embryo or fetus. MRI is used infrequently in the setting of trauma.

Iodinated contrast medium is not known to be harmful to fetuses: It is not teratogenic and does not suppress fetal thyroid function. The American College of Radiology states, "We do not recommend withholding the use of iodinated contrast agents in pregnant or potentially pregnant patients when it is needed for diagnostic purposes" [52].

Unfortunately, **pregnant women are less likely to undergo recommended imaging after trauma** [53], a situation one author group has called "**radiation fear**" and which **can only be decried**.

CARDIOPULMONARY RESUSCITATION

Indications for beginning cardiopulmonary resuscitation (CPR) are **no different in pregnant patients**. Algorithms for treatment, including drugs and defibrillation, are unchanged by the fact of pregnancy [54]. After midpregnancy, **left uterine displacement** should be effected so as to avoid caval compression: This may be done with a wedge under the right hip, manual displacement of the uterus from above, or with a human wedge in which the patient's right hip is lifted onto a rescuer's knees. The 2015 American Heart Association (AHA) guidelines advocate manual uterine displacement in preference to the other techniques because of easier access for defibrillation and airway management and the potential for more effective chest compressions when the patient is not tilted [54]. Survival among pregnant women undergoing CPR in the emergency department after traumatic injury has been reported as 17% in a national administrative data set, worse than age-matched nonpregnant controls [55].

PRENATAL CARE

If the pregnant patient who has had trauma can be discharged undelivered, she should be counseled that **abruption, PTB, and other complications can occur even days to weeks after discharge of a stable woman after trauma** [5,16]. Even if they have been discharged from the hospital, women who suffered trauma in pregnancy should be aware that a normal baby outcome cannot be guaranteed. The optimal strategy for ongoing pregnancy surveillance is not known, but heightened suspicion for pregnancy complications is reasonable.

ANTEPARTUM TESTING

There is no trial to assess effectiveness of testing in this population.

DELIVERY

There are no specific recommendations as to delivery of women who have had some trauma earlier in pregnancy, which is a more common situation than the one of catastrophic trauma.

If efforts to resuscitate the pregnant patient having had major trauma are unsuccessful and there is *no return of spontaneous circulation*, **perimortem cesarean delivery (PMCD)** should be performed for patients at later gestational ages. The gestational age at which this intervention should be undertaken is subject to dispute, probably reflecting confusion about the purpose of PMCD: The goal has sometimes been understood as fetal salvage and sometimes as an adjunct to maternal resuscitation. If aortocaval compression by the gravid uterus impedes venous return to the heart or renders chest compressions ineffective, and PMCD alleviates both by emptying the uterus, it may allow for return of spontaneous circulation. Intervention for the sake of the fetus does not make sense before viability—depending on local practice, much before 24 weeks—but intervention for maternal resuscitation may be considered even at earlier gestational ages. Some have advocated PMCD in such circumstances if the uterus extends to the fundus or above, corresponding to about 20 weeks in a singleton pregnancy because the potential for aortocaval compression is present. The 2015 AHA guidelines [54] are circumspect, stating, "**Not every pregnant woman in cardiac arrest is a candidate for PMCD; the decision depends on whether the gravid uterus is thought to interfere with maternal hemodynamics.**"

Although no trials exist, it has been reported that **the best fetal outcomes occur with delivery within 4–5 minutes after arrest** and **higher fetal mortality rates occurring at greater than 10 minutes of cardiopulmonary arrest** [56]. Data are quite limited, however. A review of literature published from 1980 to 2010 turned up a total of 94 cases of maternal cardiac arrest: In 87% of viable pregnancies, PMCD was undertaken with an average time from arrest to delivery of 16 minutes [57]. Very few were delivered in under 4 minutes; neonatal survival was noted to occur even when arrest-to-delivery times were appreciably longer. Return of spontaneous circulation in the mother was more common without PMCD (93%) than after PMCD (54%), but the odds of maternal survival were fivefold higher when PMCD occurred less than 10 min from arrest. The authors of this review stated that PMCD clearly contributed to maternal survival in 32% of cases, and in no case was it deleterious to maternal survival. **Overall neonatal survival after PMCD was 64% even when delivery occurred more than 10 minutes after maternal arrest.** A surveillance project in the UK has been collecting data on all cardiac arrests in pregnancy over a 3-year period, including information on PMCD, but results have not yet been published [58].

Time should not be wasted moving a patient to any other location for PMCS, nor should preparations be extensive. To quote the 2015 AHA guidelines [54]: "**The only equipment needed to start a PMCD is a scalpel.**"

ANESTHESIA

No specific recommendations regarding anesthesia for delivery in women who have sustained trauma earlier in pregnancy.

POSTPARTUM/BREAST-FEEDING

No specific recommendations.

REFERENCES

1. American College of Obstetricians (Webb) Gynecologists. *Obstetric aspects of trauma management.* ACOG Educational Bulletin No. 251, 1998, Washington DC: ACOG. [Level III evidence. Expert opinion. The American College of Obstetricians and Gynecologists quotes trauma rates of 1 in 12 pregnancies, but it is unclear how the figure was obtained.]
2. Mendez-Figueroa H, Dahlke JD, Vrees RA, Rouse DJ. Trauma in pregnancy: An updated systematic review. *Am J Obstet Gynecol* 2013; 208(4): 321.e1–9. [Systematic review]
3. Ikossi DG, Lazar AA, Morabito D et al. Profile of mothers at risk: An analysis of injury and pregnancy loss in 1195 trauma patients. *J Am Coll Surg* 2005; 200: 49–56. [Level II-2. Cohort. The American College of Surgeons maintains a National Trauma Data Bank (NTDB)—Data collected from 130 trauma centers in the United States, including level I, level II, and level III facilities. Review of the NTDB between 1994 and 2001 compared 1195 female admissions that were additionally coded as pregnant to a control group of 76,126 injured women in the same age group. Because during this time there were approximately 27 million live births in the United States (NCHS), that equates to four trauma center admissions per 100,000 live births.]
4. Schiff MA, Holt VL. Pregnancy outcomes following hospitalization for motor vehicle crashes in Washington State from 1989 to 2001. *Am J Epidemiol* 2005; 161: 503–10. [Level II-2. Cohort. State of Washington hospitalizations for MVA in pregnancy from 1989 to 2001, *n* = 625]
5. El Kady D, Gilbert WM, Anderson J et al. Trauma during pregnancy: An analysis of maternal and fetal outcomes in a large population. *Am J Obstet Gynecol* 2004; 190(6): 1661–8. [Level II-2. Cohort. California: 10,316 women who sustained trauma during a pregnancy of at least 20 weeks gestation identified via a statewide hospital discharge database from 1991 to 1999]

6. Kvarnstrand L, Milsone I, Lekander T, Druid H, Jacobsson B. Maternal fatalities, fetal and neonatal deaths related to motor vehicle crashes during pregnancy: A national population-based study. *Acta Obstet Gynecol Scand* 2008; 87: 946–52. [Level II-2. Cohort]

7. Barraco RD, Chiu WC, Clancy TV et al., EAST Practice Management Guidelines Work Group. Practice management guidelines for the diagnosis and management of injury in the pregnant patient: The EAST Practice Management Guidelines Workgroup. *J Trauma* 2010; 69(1): 211–4. [III, review]

8. Saltzman LE, Johnson CH, Gilbert BC et al. Physical abuse around the time of pregnancy: An examination of prevalence and risk factors in 16 states. *Matern Child Health J* 2003; 7(1): 31–43. [II-3]

9. Azar T, Longo C, Oddy L, Abenhaim HA. Motor vehicle collision-related accidents in pregnancy. *J Obstet Gynaecol Res* 2015; 41: 1370–76. [Level II-2. Cohort, retrospective; administrative data set]

10. Weiss HB, Strotmeyer S. Characteristics of pregnant women in motor vehicle crashes. *Inj Prev* 2002; 8: 207–10. [1995–1999 National Automotive Sampling System Crashworthiness Data System, drawn from police-reported traffic accidents]

11. Manoogian S. Comparison of pregnant and non-pregnant occupant crash and injury characteristics based on national crash data. *Accident Analysis and Prevention* 2015; 69–76. [Level II-2. Administrative data set]

12. Hyde LK, Cook LJ, Olson LM et al. Effect of motor vehicle crashes on adverse fetal outcome. *Obstet Gynecol* 2003; 102: 279–86. [II-3]

13. Wall SL, Figueirido F, Laing GL, Clarke DL. The spectrum and outcome of pregnant trauma patients in a metropolitan trauma service in South Africa. *Injury* 2014; 45: 1220–3. [Level III. Case series]

14. Aboutanos SZ, Aboutanos MB, Dompokowski D et al. Predictors of fetal outcome in pregnant trauma patients: A five-year institutional review. *Am Surg* 2007; 73(8): 824–7. [II-3]

15. Petrone P, Talving P, Browder T et al. Abdominal injuries in pregnancy: A 155-month study at two level 1 trauma centers. *Injury* 2011; 42(1): 47–9. [II-3]

16. Cahill AG, Bastek JA, Stamilio DM et al. Minor trauma in pregnancy—Is the evaluation warranted? *Am J Obstet Gynecol* 2008; 198: 208.e1–5. [II-2. Prospective cohort of 256 complete records of patients with minor trauma. Rate of positive KB at presentation 2.8%. Adverse pregnancy outcome in this cohort consisted of 19.2% with no statistically significant association of any single predictor variable or in combination.]

17. Corsi PR, Rasslan S, de Oliveira LB et al. Trauma in pregnant women: Analysis of maternal and fetal mortality. *Injury* 1999; 30: 239–43. [II-3. Fetal death: Corsi's 315; Shah's 14% if you don't count elective abortions; Rogers was 9%; Warner's—A fairly small study—was 6%; and Theodorou's 18%. Maternal death: Corsi 12%, Shah 9%, Rogers 4%, and Warner 3%]

18. Shah KH, Simons RK, Holbrook T et al. Trauma in pregnancy: Maternal and fetal outcomes. *J Trauma* 1998; 45: 83–6. [II-3]

19. Rogers FB, Rozycki GS, Osler TM et al. A multi-institutional study of factors associated with fetal death in injured pregnant patients. *Arch Surg* 1999; 134: 1274–7. [II-3]

20. Warner MW, Salfinger SG, Rao S et al. Management of trauma during pregnancy. *ANZ J Surg* 2004; 74: 125–8. [II-3]

21. Theodorou DA, Velmahos GC, Souter I et al. Fetal death after trauma in pregnancy. *Am Surg* 2000; 66: 809–12. [II-3]

22. Chang J, Berg CJ, Saltzmann LE et al. Homicide: A leading cause of injury deaths among pregnant and postpartum women in the United States, 1991–1999. *Am J Public Health* 2005; 95: 471–7. [Level II-3. Administrative data set. Pregnancy Mortality Surveillance System, established in 1989 by the Center for Disease Control, identified 7342 deaths among women who were pregnant or within one year postpartum]

23. Palladino CL, Singh V, Campbell J, Flynn H, Gold KJ. Homicide and suicide during the perinatal period. *Obstet Gynecol* 2011; 118: 1056–63. [Level II-3. Administrative data set]

24. Boccichio GV, Napolitano LM, Hann J et al. Incidental pregnancy in trauma patients. *J Am Coll Surg* 2001; 192: 566–9. [II-3]

25. Brown HL. Trauma in pregnancy. *Obstet Gynecol* 2009; 114(1): 147–60. [III, review]

26. Pearlman MD, Tintinalli JE, Lorenz RP. A prospective controlled study of outcome after trauma during pregnancy. *Am J Obstet Gynecol* 1990; 162: 1502–10. [II-2; n = 60. Recommendations for at least four hours of monitoring]

27. Petrone P, Talving P, Browder T, Teixeira PG, Fisher O, Lozornio A et al. Abdominal injuries in pregnancy: 1 155-month study at two level 1 trauma centers. *Injury* 2011; 42: 47–9. [Level III. Case series]

28. Weiss HB, Songer TJ, Fabio A. Fetal deaths related to maternal injury. *JAMA* 2001; 286: 1863–8. [Level III. Administrative data. Fetal death certificates in 16 U.S. States, 1995–1997]

29. Curet MJ, Schermer CR, Demarest GB et al. Predictors of outcome in trauma during pregnancy: Identification of patients who can safely be monitored for less than 6 hours. *J Trauma* 2000; 49: 18–24. [Level III. Case series. Eight years' experience at a large level I trauma center; 271 pregnant women who were admitted after blunt trauma; reviewed delivery outcomes in approximately half]

30. El Kady D, Gilbert WM, Xing G et al. Maternal and neonatal outcomes of assaults during pregnancy. *Obstet Gynecol* 2005; 105: 357–63. [II-3, n = 2070 pregnant women hospitalized following an assault]

31. Gulliver PJ, Dixon RS. Immediate and long-term outcomes of assault in pregnancy. *Austr NZ J Obstet Gynaecol* 2014; 54: 256–62. [Level II-2, Case-control]

32. Cheng D, Horon IL. Intimate-partner homicide among pregnant and postpartum women. *Obstet Gynecol* 2010; 115: 1181–6. [Level III, Case series]

33. Klinich KD, Flannagan CAC, Rupp JD et al. Fetal outcome in motor-vehicle crashes: Effects of crash characteristics and maternal restraint. *Am J Obstet Gynecol* 2008; 198: 450.e1–9. [II-3]

34. Vladutiu CJ, Marshall SW, Poole C, Casteel C, Menard MK, Weiss HB. Adverse pregnancy outcomes following motor vehicle crashes. *Am J Prev Med* 2013; 45: 629–36. [II-2. Cohort]

35. Motozawa Y, Hitosugi M, Abe T et al. Effects of seat belts worn by pregnant drivers during low-impact collisions. *Am J Obstet Gynecol* 2010; 203: 62.e1–8. [II-3]

36. Schiff MA, Mack CD, Kaufman RP et al. The effect of air bags on pregnancy outcomes in Washington State, 2002–2005. *Obstet Gynecol* 2010; 115: 85–92. [II-2]

37. Metz TD, Abbott JT. Uterine trauma in pregnancy after motor vehicle crashes with airbag deployment: A 30-case series. *J Trauma* 2006; 61: 658–61. [II-3]

38. American College of Obstetricians and Gynecologists. Committee on Health Care for Underserved Women. The Hidden Causes of Maternal Mortality, in press 2015. ACOG, Washington, DC. [III, Expert opinion]

39. American College of Obstetricians and Gynecologists Statement of Policy. *Gun Violence and Safety.* Feb 2014. Online at http://www.acog.org/-/media/Statements-of-Policy/Public/2014GunViolence AndSafety.pdf?dmc=1&ts=20150925T2306541535. (Accessed September 25, 2015). [Guideline]

40. Jain V, Chari R, Maslovitz S, Farine D et al. Guidelines for the management of a pregnant trauma patient. *J Obstet Gynaecol Can* 2015; 37: 553–74. [III, Guideline, expert opinion, evidence-based where possible]

41. Brown MA, Sirlin CB, Farahmand N et al. Screening sonography in pregnant patients with blunt abdominal trauma. *J Ultrasound Med* 2005; 24: 175–9. [II-3]

42. American College of Surgeons, ACS Committee on Trauma. *Advanced Trauma Life Support. ATLS Student Course Manual, 9th edition.* ACS, Chicago, IL. 2012. [III, Guideline]

43. Hoff WS, Holevar M, Nagy KK, Patterson L et al. Practice management guidelines for the evaluation of blunt abdominal trauma: The EAST Practice Management Guidelines Work Group. *J Trauma* 2002; 53: 602–15. [III, Guideline, expert opinion]

44. American College of Emergency Physicians. *Trauma in the obstetric patient: A bedside tool.* http://www.acep.org/Clinical—Practice-Management/Trauma-in-the-Obstetric-Patient—A-Bedside-Tool. Accessed September 20, 2015. [Guideline]

45. Dahmus MA, Sibai BM. Blunt abdominal trauma: Are there any predictive factors for abruptio placentae or maternal-fetal distress? *Am J Obstet Gynecol* 1993; 169: 1054–9. [II-2; 1988–1991; 233 patients >20 weeks gestation admitted after noncatastrophic abdominal trauma. Unusually, in this population assaults and falls each outnumbered motor vehicle accidents. Duration of monitoring ranged from 0 to 120 hours with a mean of 13 hours]

46. Muench MV, Baschat AA, Reddy UM et al. Kleihauer–Betke testing is important in all cases of maternal trauma. *J Trauma* 2004; 57: 1094–8. [II-2]

47. Ochsenbein-Imhof N, Ochsenbein AF, Seifert B et al. Quantification of fetomaternal hemorrhage by fluorescence microscopy is equivalent to flow cytometry. *Transfusion* 2002; 42: 947–53. [II-3]

48. American College of Radiology and Society for Pediatric Radiology. ACR-SPR Practice parameter for imaging pregnant or potentially pregnant adolescents and women with ionizing radiation. Amended 2014 (Resolution 39.) Online at http://www.acr.org/~/media/9E2ED55531FC4B4FA53EF3B6D3B25DF8.pdf. Accessed September 25, 2015. [Guideline]

49. Health Protection Agency, the Royal College of Radiologists and the College of Radiographers. Protection of pregnant patients during diagnostic medical exposures to ionizing radiation: Advice from the Health Protection Agency, the Royal College of Radiologists and the College of Radiographers. 2009. Available at: https://www.ipem.ac.uk/Portals/0/Images/Protection%20of%20pregnant%20patients.pdf. Accessed November 20, 2010. [III, review]

50. American College of Obstetricians and Gynecologists. Committee on Obstetric Practice. Guidelines for diagnostic imaging during pregnancy and lactation. In press 2015. Alternative citation: ACOG. Guidelines for diagnostic imaging during pregnancy. ACOG Committee Opinion No. 299. *Obstet Gynecol* 2004; 104: 647–51. [III]

51. Damilakis J, Perisinakis K, Prassopoulos P et al. Conceptus radiation dose and risk from chest screen-film radiography. *Eur Radiol* 2003; 13: 406–12. [II-2]

52. ACR Committee on Drugs and Contrast Media. ACR Manual on Contrast Media—Version10.1, 2015. http://www.acr.org/~/media/ACR/Documents/PDF/QualitySafety/Resources/Contrast%20Manual/2015_Contrast_Media.pdf. [Guideline]

53. Shakerian R, Thomson BN, Judson R, Skandarajah AR. Radiation fear: Impact on compliance with trauma imaging guidelines in the pregnant patient. *J Trauma Acute Care Surg* 2015; 78: 88–93. [39% got no imaging; in the high-risk mechanism group, compliance with imaging guidelines only 19%! Level II-3. Cross-sectional]

54. Jeejeebhoy FM, Zelop CM, Lipman S, Carvalho B, Joglar J, Mhyre JM et al., on behalf of the American Heart Association Emergency Cardiovascular Care Committee, Council on Cardiopulmonary Critical Care, Perioperative and Resuscitation, Council on Cardiovascular Diseases in the Young, and Council on Clinical Cardiology. Cardiac arrest in pregnancy: A scientific statement from the American Heart Association. *Circulation* 2015; 132. doi:10.1161/CIR.0000000000000300. [Guideline, evidence-based where possible]

55. Lavecchia M, Abenhaim HA. Cardiopulmonary resuscitation in the emergency department. *Resuscitation* 2015; 91: 104–7. [Level II-2, cohort, retrospective]

56. Katz VL, Dotters DJ, Droegemueller W. Perimortem cesarean delivery. *Obstet Gynecol* 1986; 68: 571–6. [III]

57. Einav S, Kaufman N, Sela HY. Maternal cardiac arrest and perimortem cesarean delivery: Evidence or expert-based? *Resuscitation* 2012; 83: 1191–200. [III]

58. National Perinatal Epidemiology Unit. UK Obstetric Surveillance Project. https://www.npeu.ox.ac.uk/ukoss/current-surveillance/cap?highlight=YTozOntpOjA7czo3OiJjYXJkaWFljtpOjE7czo2OiJhcnJlc3QiO2k6MjtzOjE0OiJjYXJkaWFjIGFycmVzdCI7fQ==. (Accessed September 24, 2015). [Level II-2, cohort]

40

Critical care

Lauren A. Plante

KEY POINTS

- In the developed world, <1% of maternity admissions require admission to intensive care but up to 5% require admission to intermediate care or a high-dependency unit.
- Most maternal admissions to ICU are postpartum.
- Antepartum admission to ICU is associated with high rates of preterm birth.
- Standard of care for acute respiratory distress syndrome is a low-tidal-volume strategy although this has not been formally tested in pregnancy.
- Delayed recognition and treatment of sepsis increases mortality.

BACKGROUND

The field of maternal critical care remains insufficiently researched. Although many recommendations in critical care are based on good evidence, little is specifically focused on pregnant or postpartum women. Much of this chapter, perforce, addresses general critical care, extrapolating to maternal critical care whenever possible.

INCIDENCE

In the developed world, between **1 and 8/1000 obstetric admissions are managed in an intensive care unit (ICU)** [1–11]. Among this population, the risk of death ranges from 2% to 11%, a figure that, although better than average ICU mortality in a general population, is orders of magnitude higher than the maternal mortality ratio in the developed world.

Figures on ICU admission do *not* include women with similarly life-threatening conditions who are treated within the confines of a labor and delivery unit or specialized obstetric care unit. Another 1% to 5% of all women admitted for delivery require this type of care [12–14].

Definitions of maternal mortality (and related terms) and severe maternal morbidity (also called, at times, near-miss mortality) are shown in Table 40.1. Audits of near-miss maternal mortality or severe acute maternal morbidity have been used to quantitate life-threatening conditions and therefore constitute a proxy for intensive care utilization. In Scotland, severe morbidity and near-miss events were recorded in 4/1000 deliveries although only one third of these ended up in the ICU [8]. Severe maternal morbidity also occurred in 4/1000 deliveries between 1991 and 2001 in Canada [15] but increased to 14/1000 between 2003 and 2007 [16]. This increase in Canadian figures may represent differential classification, different data sets, or a real increase in severe acute maternal morbidity over time. Analysis of year-by-year data shows a steady increase in rates of acute renal failure, assisted ventilation, and major obstetrical hemorrhage in Canada [17].

Admission to an ICU was reported in 2.4/1000 deliveries in the Netherlands, but only one third of women with serious maternal morbidity were cared for in the ICU [18]. Population-based estimates put rates of severe maternal morbidity during hospitalizations for delivery at 5.1/1000 in the United States between 1991 and 2003 [19]. Using the same methodology, the same researchers calculated rates of severe maternal morbidity in 2-year intervals from 1998 through 2009, this time analyzing both delivery and postpartum hospitalizations: Severe morbidity rates during delivery hospitalizations rose by 75% and during postpartum hospitalizations by 114% [20]. By 2009, **the frequency of severe maternal morbidity during hospitalization for delivery was 129.1 per 10,000 delivery hospitalizations and during postpartum hospitalizations was 29 per 10,000 or about a tripling of the 1991–2003 rate**. With 4 million births per year in the United States [21], these figures imply **more than 50,000 episodes of severe acute maternal morbidity** among pregnant and postpartum women in this country. **The need for maternal critical care appears to be increasing in the developed world**, influenced largely by an increase in both the rate of postpartum hemorrhage and the risk of adverse outcomes among women with postpartum hemorrhage [22,23]. One may predict that the need will continue to rise in parallel with a rising cesarean rate [24,25].

LEVELS OF CRITICAL CARE

The American College of Critical Care Medicine (ACCM) describes **three levels of adult ICUs** [26]:

Level I critical care: Typically found in university medical centers; provide comprehensive, sometimes specialized, critical care. They require continuous availability of sophisticated technologies (Table 40.2), highly trained nursing staff, and physicians with critical care training immediately available at the bedside. Comprehensive support services are in place.

Level II critical care: Although level II centers can provide comprehensive critical care, they lack resources for highly specialized subpopulations, such as cardiothoracic patients, and must have arrangements in place to transfer out patients who exceed their expertise.

Level III critical care: Level III ICUs provide only initial stabilization of critically ill patients, followed by transfer for comprehensive critical care to a level I or II facility.

An alternative to the ICU is the **intermediate care or high-dependency unit (HDU)** [27]. Patients who require frequent monitoring of vital signs or frequent nursing interventions but do not need specific ICU life support treatments may be admitted to such a unit. The intermediate care unit is staffed at lower nursing levels and includes less complex technology than the ICU, which makes it less expensive to run, frees up beds in the ICU, and has been associated with

Table 40.1 Definitions of Maternal Mortality (and Related Terms) and Severe Maternal Morbidity (or Near-Miss Maternal Mortality)

	Definition	Reference
Maternal mortality	Death of a woman while pregnant or within 42 days of termination of pregnancy, irrespective of the duration and the site of the pregnancy from any cause related to or aggravated by the pregnancy or its management but not from accidental or incidental causes	World Health Organization and CDC, both ICD-9 and ICD-10 (Source: Hoyert DL. Maternal mortality and related concepts. National Center for Health Statistics. *Vital Health Stat* 2007; 3(33). http://www.cdc.gov/nchs/data/series/sr_03/sr03_033.pdf. (Accessed 11/3/15).
Pregnancy-related deaths	Death while pregnant or within 42 days of termination of pregnancy regardless of cause of death	Same as above
Direct obstetric deaths	Death resulting from obstetric complications (pregnancy, labor, puerperium)	Same as above
Indirect obstetric deaths	Death resulting from previous existing disease or disease developed during pregnancy not due to direct obstetric causes but aggravated by physiology of pregnancy	Same as above
Late maternal deaths	Death from direct OR indirect obstetric causes >42 days but <1 year after termination of pregnancy	Same as above
Severe maternal morbidity	A woman who nearly died but survived a complication that occurred during pregnancy, childbirth, or within 42 days of termination of pregnancy	Pattinson R, Sale L, Souza JP, van den Broek N, Rooney C, on behalf of the WHO Working Group on Maternal Mortality and Morbidity Classifications. *Bull World Health Org* 2009; 87: 734.
Severe maternal morbidity	A woman receiving 4 or more units of red blood cells and/or ICU admission	Joint Commission (JCAHO) as: (http://www.acog.org/About-ACOG/News-Room/Statements/2015/Severe-Maternal-Morbidity-Clarification-of-the-New-Joint-Commission-Sentinel-Event-Policy; also http://www.jointcommission.org/assets/1/23/jconline_February_4_151.PDF. (Accessed 11/4/15).

Table 40.2 Equipment and Support That an ICU Should Be Prepared to Provide

- Continuous ECG monitoring (with high/low alarms), all patients
- Continuous arterial pressure monitoring (invasive and noninvasive)
- Central venous pressure monitoring
- Transcutaneous oxygen monitoring or pulse oximetry for all patients receiving supplemental oxygen
- Airway equipment, including laryngoscopes and endotracheal tubes
- Ventilatory equipment: Ambu bags, ventilators, oxygen, compressed air
- Emergency resuscitation equipment
- Equipment to support hemodynamically unstable patients: infusion pumps, blood/fluid warmers, pressure bags, blood filters
- Beds with removable headboard and adjustable position; various specialty beds
- Adequate lighting for bedside procedures
- Suction
- Cooling/warming blankets
- Scales
- Temporary pacemakers (transcutaneous and transvenous)
- Temperature monitoring devices
- Pulmonary artery pressure monitoring
- Cardiac output monitoring
- Continuous and intermittent dialysis and ultrafiltration
- Peritoneal dialysis
- Capnography
- Fiberoptic bronchoscopy
- Intracranial pressure monitoring
- Continuous EEG monitoring capability
- Positive and negative pressure isolation rooms
- Immediate access to information (medical books, journals, drug information, poison control, personnel phone and page numbers, patient lab and test data, medical record information)

Source: Adapted from Haupt MT, Bekes CE, Brilli RJ et al. *Crit Care Med*, 31: 2677–83, 2003.

greater family satisfaction. Intermediate care units include post-ICU step-down units, telemetry units for cardiac patients, etc.

Low-risk monitor patients are those predicted to be at low risk of requiring active life-saving treatment, such as mechanical ventilation or vasopressors. The most frequent monitoring services deployed in the care of such patients in the ICU are **ECG (>99%), intra-arterial BP monitoring (51%), and pulse oximetry (33%)**, and the most frequent labor-intensive nursing interventions were intake/output measurement, hourly vital signs, and hourly neurologic checks [28]. When planning obstetric critical care services, the intermediate care unit is a good approximation of the type and acuity of services generally needed. However, recent experience in 2009 with novel influenza should remind us that pregnant women are at higher risk of respiratory failure in some circumstances, and a contingency plan for epidemic flu (and other respiratory infections) must be made, including provision of mechanical ventilatory support [29–31].

An alternate schema for levels of critical care comes from the Intensive Care Society (ICS) in the United Kingdom [32]. Unfortunately, this numbering system runs in reverse from the ACCM levels: level 0 refers to normal ward care, level 1 to patients at risk of deterioration, level 2 to patients with single-organ failure, and level 3 to patients with more than a single organ failure or those requiring mechanical ventilation (Table 40.3) [32]. The Maternal Critical Care Working Group, convened in London in 2011, explicitly adapted the ICS guidelines to maternal care: see Table 40.4 [33].

ORGANIZATION OF OBSTETRIC CRITICAL CARE SERVICES

If the discipline of critical care is young, that of obstetric critical care is younger still. **There are no evidence based recommendations published specifically for critical care in**

Table 40.3   Levels of Adult ICU Care

Level 0	Patients whose needs can be met through normal ward care in acute hospital.
Level 1	Patients at risks of their condition deteriorating, or those recently relocated from higher levels of care, whose needs can be met on an acute ward with additional advice and support from the Critical Care Team.
Level 2	Patients requiring more detailed observation or intervention including support for a single failing organ system or postoperative care and those "stepping down" from higher levels of care.
Level 3	Patients requiring advanced respiratory support alone or basic respiratory support together with support of at least two organ systems. This level includes all complex patients requiring support for multiorgan failure.

Source: Intensive Care Society. Guidelines for the provision of intensive care services, 2015. http://www.ics.ac.uk/ics-homepage /guidelines-and-standards/, accessed October 10, 2015 (Guideline). With permission.

pregnancy. The interested practitioner must extrapolate from the general critical care literature instead [34,35] or rely on expert opinion.

Hemorrhage and hypertension are, consistently, the **most common causes of admission from obstetrical services to intensive care** [1–11,15,18,36–53]. The majority of these patients require monitoring and only simple interventions. The degree of nursing care involved, although higher-acuity than on most general wards, is well within the abilities of most labor and delivery nurses in a specialty or subspecialty care facility, that is, levels of maternal care II and III as described by the American College of Obstetricians and Gynecologists and Society for Maternal-Fetal Medicine [54]. The intermediate care unit or HDU is also designed to provide care of this type.

A smaller number of obstetrical patients have non-obstetric causes for ICU admission: these amount to 20% to 30% of the total [1,5,7,13]. **Most obstetric patients who are admitted to the ICU are sent there postpartum rather than undelivered** [5,6,39]. The preponderance of postpartum over antepartum admissions may stem from postpartum vulnerability (e.g., postpartum hemorrhage, postpartum decompensation of cardiac disease) or to ascertainment bias: Obstetricians may be reluctant to transfer or intensivists to accept a patient whose fetus must be considered in management. In the rare case of an "obstetrical ICU" existing within a labor/delivery unit, there is a higher percentage of both antepartum admissions and primary medical (nonobstetric) admissions [7,44]. This may reflect a lower threshold for admission to the obstetrical ICU (as no transfer or travel is involved), a need to justify the continuation of the service, or a preference to transfer out postpartum patients: Labor and delivery (L&D) beds are a scarce commodity, and a postpartum patient requiring intensive care ties up space and personnel when she could be adequately cared for outside of the obstetric unit.

Table 40.4   Levels of Care According to the Maternal Critical Care Working Group

Level of Care	Maternity Example
Level 0: Normal ward care	Care of low-risk mother
Level 1: Additional monitoring or intervention, or step down from higher level of care	» Risk of hemorrhage » Oxytocin infusion » Mild pre-eclampsia on oral antihypertensives/fluid restriction, etc. » Woman with medical condition such as congenital heart disease, diabetic on insulin infusion
Level 2: Single organ support	Basic respiratory support (BRS) » 50% or oxygen via face mask to maintain oxygen saturation » Continuous positive airway pressure (CPAP), bilevel positive airway pressure (BIPAP) Basic cardiovascular support (BCVS) » Intravenous antihypertensives, to control blood pressure in pre-eclampsia » Arterial line used for pressure monitoring or sampling » CVP line used for fluid management and CVP monitoring to guide therapy Advanced cardiovascular support (ACVS) » Simultaneous use of at least two intravenous, anti-arrhythmic/antihypertensive/vasoactive drugs, one of which must be a vasoactive drug » Need to measure and treat cardiac output Neurological support » Magnesium infusion to control seizures (not prophylaxis) » Intracranial pressure monitoring Hepatic support » Management of acute fulminant hepatic failure, e.g., from HELLP syndrome or acute fatty liver, such that transplantation is being considered
Level 3: Advanced respiratory support alone, or support of two or more organ systems above	Advanced respiratory support » Invasive mechanical ventilation Support of two or more organ systems » Renal support and BRS » BRS/BCVS and an additional organ supported[a]

Source: Maternal Critical Care Working Group. The Royal College of Obstetricians and Gynaecologists, the Royal College of Anaesthetists, the Royal College of Midwives, the Intensive Care Society, the British Maternal and Fetal Medicine Society, the Obstetric Anaesthetists' Association, and the Department of Health. Providing equity of critical and maternity care for the critically ill pregnant or recently pregnant woman. July 2011, https://www.rcog.org.uk/globalassets/documents/guidelines/prov_eq_matandcritcare.pdf, accessed September 25, 2015 (Guideline). With permission from The Royal College of Anaesthetists. Adapted from Wheatly S, *Int J Ob Anesth* 2010;19:353–355.
[a]A BRS and BCVS occurring simultaneously during the episode count as single organ support.

Most obstetrical services would be unable to implement a full-service obstetrical ICU. Both the technology and the personnel mandated by ICU guidelines are impracticable. The HDU or intermediate care unit, however, is a reasonable model for much of obstetric critical care. Published experience, albeit limited, is encouraging. A high-volume public hospital in Dallas admitted 1.7% of maternity cases to a five-bed obstetrics intermediate care unit, usually postpartum (80%), with a mean length of stay less than 24 hours [13]. Of these 500 women, 15% subsequently were transferred to a full-service medical or surgical ICU, most for mechanical ventilation. A referral maternity hospital in Dublin opened a "high-dependency" or intermediate care unit [12]. Prior to debut of the HDU, patients requiring intensive care services (0.1% of maternity admissions) were transferred out to another hospital with a medical/surgical ICU. After the obstetric HDU was established, the referral rate to the off-site ICU dropped by 50%, but the HDU was busier than one might have expected: 1% of maternity patients were admitted thereto, a tenfold increase in the percentage of patients who were managed as higher acuity. The question as to whether this represents underutilization of needed services before the advent of the obstetric intermediate care unit or overutilization after cannot be answered. In a large women's hospital in Birmingham without an on-site ICU, a three-bed HDU within the delivery suite accommodated between 1% and 5% of all obstetric patients: The percentage has steadily been increasing over time [14]. Among women admitted to this HDU, 3.5% were then transferred out to intensive care.

The American College of Obstetricians and Gynecologists, jointly with the Society for Maternal-Fetal Medicine, produced an obstetric care consensus on **levels of maternal care**, the stated goal being a reduction in maternal morbidity and mortality [54]. **Critical care services are specifically mentioned in level III and IV facilities.** Level III facilities are expected to have

> an on-site intensive care unit...and critical care providers on-site to actively collaborate with maternal-fetal specialists at all times. Equipment and personnel with expertise must be available on-site to ventilate and monitor women in the labor and delivery unit until they can be safely transferred to the ICU.

The concept of critical care in pregnancy is more explicitly spelled out in the description of level IV facilities, which are to be regional perinatal health care centers:

> A level IV facility is distinct from a level III facility in the approach to the care of pregnant women and women in the postpartum period with complex and critical illnesses. In addition to having ICU care on-site for obstetric patients, a level IV facility must have...a maternal-fetal medicine care team that has the expertise to assume responsibility for pregnant women and women in the postpartum period who are in critical condition or have complex medical conditions. The maternal-fetal medicine team collaborates actively in the comanagement of all obstetric patients who require critical care and ICU services. This includes comanagement of ICU-admitted obstetric patients...The team should be led by a board-certified maternal-fetal medicine subspecialist with expertise in critical care obstetrics...The maternal-fetal medicine team must have expertise in critical care at the physician level, nursing level, and ancillary services level...There should be institutional support for the routine involvement of a maternal-fetal medicine care team with the critical care units and specialists...The director of obstetric services is a board-certified maternal-fetal medicine subspecialist or a board-certified obstetrician–gynecologist with expertise in critical care obstetrics.

The American College of Critical Care Medicine states, "The Physician Director should meet guidelines for the definition of an intensivist and the practice of critical care medicine" [55]. **The definition of an intensivist is one few obstetricians or maternal-fetal medicine specialists would be able to meet because** it includes not only skills, interest, and availability but also completion of an approved training program in critical care medicine. Mabie has suggested several ways in which an obstetrician might obtain some critical care training [44]: a critical care fellowship, a residency in internal medicine, or a maternal-fetal medicine fellowship. A plea to put the "M" back into MFM [56] resulted in a new ABOG requirement for MFM fellows to complete 1 month of ICU training, which cannot be considered adequate in itself. Critical care medicine fellowships run 12 months under the aegis of anesthesiology or surgery (both of which are open to individuals who have completed residency in OBGYN) or 2 years after completion of an emergency medicine or internal medicine residency or 3 years after a pediatrics residency. Having acquired formal training would, of course, be insufficient if there is not enough clinical material to maintain skills and expertise: This is an even higher hurdle. Zeeman et al. [13] mention only that a maternal-fetal medicine faculty member was director of the OB intermediate care unit without specifying whether this individual had any critical care qualifications or training. Despite the patient volume, it appears that no mechanical ventilation, pulmonary artery catheterization, or vasopressor therapy was carried out in this unit: This is appropriate for an intermediate care unit but ensures that providers' skills decay. The Birmingham HDU, which also appears to exclude mechanical ventilation [14], is described only as "staffed by qualified midwives" with anesthetic and obstetric teams covering.

Recommendations for nursing care in an ICU [26,55] state that all nurses working in critical care should complete a clinical and didactic course in critical care before taking on patient responsibilities, participate in continuing education, and assume nurse-to-patient ratios either 1:2 *or* based on patient acuity. High nurse-to-patient ratios are already standard on labor/delivery units and would, therefore, be rather easy to implement. As above, acquiring and maintaining critical care skills would be considerably more difficult.

ACOG and SMFM have recommended that nursing services in maternal level III hospitals have "continuously available...RNs with special training and expertise in managing women with complex maternal illnesses" and that level IV facilities should also have "nursing leadership [with] expertise in maternal intensive and critical care" [54].

Competence in core procedural skills is expected of any physician practicing in critical care [57]:

1. Maintenance of airway (nonintubated patient)
2. Ventilation (bag and mask)
3. Endotracheal intubation
4. Management of pneumothorax
5. Arterial puncture; insertion of an arterial line
6. Central venous cannulation
7. Pulmonary artery catheterization (insertion, maintenance, interpretation)—little used now
8. ECG interpretation
9. Cardioversion, defibrillation

Some critical care techniques are used less frequently now than in the past. **Utilization of the pulmonary artery catheter dropped** by two thirds in the first decade of the 21st century [58], after demonstration that its use is not associated with improvement in outcomes. **Noninvasive methods of ventilation have replaced mechanical ventilation in some cases.** More recent competencies for critical care training and practice now also include ultrasound imaging (lung, abdominal, and heart as well as procedural guidance), advanced airway management (including supraglottic airway), bronchoscopy, and thoracentesis [59,60]. As some techniques are phased out, new ones appear; thus, the list here can only be taken as a snapshot of current critical care practice. Skill maintenance may not be feasible unless alternative means are sought, such as simulation-based or supervised experience.

CONSIDERATIONS IN TRANSFER (INTERHOSPITAL)

Preterm delivery may occur concurrently with critical illness because of underlying medical or obstetric conditions, spontaneous preterm labor, or iatrogenic interventions. One case-control study [6] puts at 36 weeks the mean gestational age achieved by antepartum patients admitted to ICU. For respiratory failure in pregnancy, median gestational age achieved is 31 to 32 weeks [61,62]. The Mayo series of 93 antepartum admissions to ICU reported that one third resulted in fetal losses and one half in preterm births [54]. Thus, **it would appear prudent that a pregnant woman requiring ICU services, after achieving a gestational age compatible with extrauterine viability, should be managed in a facility with both adult and neonatal ICU capability.** Because some hospitals maintain adult intensive care services but no maternity services and others, specifically women's hospitals, do not have adult intensive care, **arrangements should be in place for seamless transfer to a facility that maintains appropriate levels of care for mothers and neonates.** Guidelines for perinatal transfers have advocated antenatal over neonatal transfer when feasible. In the event that maternal transport is unsafe or impossible, alternative arrangements for neonatal transport must be made.

Transfer in cases of critical illness is more complex than the usual perinatal transfer. The transport process increases risk of morbidity and mortality for the critically ill [64] and therefore cannot be embarked upon lightly. Once the decision to transfer has been made and the patient (or her designated decision maker) has consented, she should be transferred as expeditiously as possible to the receiving facility that has agreed to accept her. If the patient is unstable, she should be stabilized and/or resuscitated to the best possible condition prior to transport albeit with the understanding that complete stabilization may not be possible outside of the receiving facility. Transport may be by ground or air, based on the urgency of the patient's condition, the distance between facilities, weather conditions, potential interventions during transport, and equipment or personnel available. **The minimum monitoring of a critically ill patient during transport includes continuous pulse oximetry and ECG as well as regular assessment of vital signs** [64]. Patients who already have arterial or central lines should have those monitored as well. Women who are mechanically ventilated must have the endotracheal tube position confirmed and secured before transport and must be assessed for adequacy of oxygenation and ventilation.

All critically ill patients must have secure venous access before transport.

Opinion, but no data, guides us as to additional monitoring during transport of the critically ill obstetrical patient. Patients at high risk of delivering en route should be held at the initial hospital until delivered because there is unlikely to be access to both the patient's head and her vagina in tight transport quarters, most transport teams lack expertise in delivery and neonatal resuscitation, and a dedicated neonatal transport team can be summoned for the newborn. There is little benefit in tocodynamometry during the transport process with information insufficient to make a recommendation. Fetal monitoring during transport may be feasible to perform but is of unproven utility. Because fetal monitoring equipment takes up space in tight quarters and there is little or nothing the transport team can do en route for an ominous tracing, it seems preferable to avoid fetal monitoring when transporting a critically ill obstetric patient. Simple measures, such as left uterine displacement and supplemental oxygen, should be routine during transport of the critically ill pregnant patient.

ADMISSION TO INTENSIVE CARE

The commonest reasons for transfer to ICU are, reliably, hemorrhage and hypertension, and most admissions are postpartum. Level II and level III maternity units [54] may be able to care for such patients on the labor and delivery unit, particularly if an intermediate care unit or HDU is located there. Level I facilities, however, should consider transfer either to a higher-level perinatal center or to the ICU at their own facility. In cases in which both obstetric and critical care services are at the most basic level, transfer of such patients to another facility may be the best approach. A small number of OB-GYN specialty hospitals exist in the United States [65]: These usually have limited critical care support or consultation available in-house and probably should also have a low threshold for transfer. Obstetrics services in such hospitals should have a set of **site-specific guidelines established at the hospital level.**

The American College of Obstetricians and Gynecologists has suggested using an objective parameters model [66,67] when deciding need for maternal critical care: see Table 40.5. This simplifies the process of triage in that any patient meeting those criteria becomes a candidate for admission or transfer to ICU. Alternate models are diagnosis-driven or priority-driven, which are less useful in this patient population.

In any center, a decision to transfer to ICU should be made on the basis of need for site-specific care. An obstetric service should adopt guidelines for transfer based on the level of care required, modified by the level of care that could be provided on the labor floor or within an existing obstetric intermediate care unit. **Necessary care must not be withheld while awaiting transfer.** The Maternal Critical Care Working Group has called for equity of care for pregnant and puerperal women with critical illness, meaning that the same standard of care applies for both their obstetrical and critical care needs regardless of where that care must be delivered [33].

LOGISTICS

The Maternal Critical Care Working Group provides useful guidance about service organization, competencies, and

Table 40.5 Objective Parameters Model: Criteria for Admission to ICU

Vital signs
Heart rate <40 or >150 bpm
Blood pressure <80 mmHg systolic (or 20 mmHg below the patient's usual BP)
Mean arterial pressure <60 mmHg
Blood pressure >120 mm diastolic
Respiratory rate >35/min

Laboratory values (new)
Serum sodium <110 or >170 mEq/L
Serum potassium <2.0 or >7.0 mEq/L
PaO_2 <50 mmHg
pH <7.1 or >7.7
Serum calcium >15 mg/dL
Serum glucose >800 mg/dL
Toxic drug level in a hemodynamically or neurologically compromised patient

Imaging (new)
Cerebrovascular hemorrhage, contusion, or subarachnoid hemorrhage with altered mental status or focal neurologic findings
Ruptured viscus or esophageal varices with hemodynamic instability
Dissecting aortic aneurysm

ECG
MI with complex arrhythmia, hemodynamic instability or congestive heart failure
Sustained ventricular tachycardia or ventricular fibrillation
Complete heart block with hemodynamic instability

Physical findings (new)
Airway obstruction
Anuria
Burns >10% of body surface area
Cardiac tamponade
Coma
Continuous seizures, cyanosis
Unequal pupils (unconscious patient)

Source: Adapted from American College of Obstetricians and Gynecologists. Critical care in pregnancy. ACOG Practice Bulletin No. 100, 2009. Washington DC: ACOG 2009 Compendium of Selected Publications.

workforce development [33]. This document is indispensable to anyone contemplating setting up maternal critical care services.

Zeeman proposed a "blueprint" for obstetric critical care [13,68], that is, an intermediate care unit in the obstetric setting. She lists as advantages the "concurrent availability of expert obstetric care and critical care management... the option of continuous fetal monitoring with on-hand expertise in its interpretation... the advantages of keeping mother and infant together combined with the improved continuity of antenatal and postnatal care" [68]. This seems indisputable for units that are big enough to keep up expertise. For lower-volume centers, however, it is not always feasible, and for even the largest services, there will be patients who are best treated in a full-service ICU.

Better outcomes are demonstrated in a general medical/surgical ICU population when specialized ICU physicians staff the unit. High-intensity ICU physician staffing (either a closed ICU model or mandatory intensivist consultation) is associated with lower ICU mortality, lower hospital mortality, and decreased length of stay in both ICU and hospital compared to models in which intensivist consultation is optional [69]. Although there are **limited data specifically addressing**

the critical care obstetric patient, it would be odd indeed if intensivist input did not improve outcomes in this population as well [70,71].

If a patient who is still pregnant requires critical care services, the first question to answer is: where is she best cared for? If the pregnancy is early or the duration of ICU services is anticipated to be lengthy, the labor floor is not likely the best location. If she is in active labor, the labor floor is probably the best choice. Most patients, however, will fall into neither of these categories; factors affecting the decision include degree of instability, interventions required, staffing and expertise available, anticipated duration of ICU stay, probability of delivery, access for family, etc.

The obstetrician transferring a patient to an ICU must be familiar with the types of units available within the facility, that is, general medical/surgical ICU or specialty unit (cardiothoracic, neurologic/neurosurgical, etc.), and understand whether the ICU is open, closed, or hybrid/transitional [72]. In an open unit, any physician can write orders or perform procedures; management or consultation by an intensivist is not mandatory. In a closed ICU, only the critical care staff writes orders and manages patients: The primary team gives over control. The hybrid or transitional model allows all physicians to write orders but requires an on-site critical care physician to consult, round on, or comanage all patients in the unit. As above, **involving the intensivist improves outcome**.

Despite the need for expertise, it is acknowledged that **critical care requires a multidisciplinary approach** [55] to achieve best outcomes. The usual ICU team comprises physicians, nurses, pharmacists, and respiratory therapists. In the case of maternal critical care, the ICU team must also include obstetricians, obstetric/perinatal nurses, and, sometimes, pediatricians. Commonly, the physician cohort would be subspecialty-trained, for example, maternal-fetal medicine and neonatology.

When an undelivered patient is transferred to ICU, efforts should be made to map out the anticipated course of her condition or disease, look ahead to possible complications, and set parameters for delivery (except in cases of too-early gestational age). Modifications of physical and laboratory assessment related to pregnancy must be known and taken into account; the obstetrician will be more familiar with these than the intensivist. The plan should be clear to the medical team and to the patient's family and to the patient herself if she is able to understand. The risk–benefit balance for a given intervention will change as pregnancy progresses, so it is important to revisit the care plan on a regular basis.

Fetal monitoring will often, but not always, be appropriate. If plans are made for fetal monitoring outside of the labor and delivery unit, the team should strategize about the type and frequency of monitoring as well as the expected interventions. It is not appropriate to commit to continuous fetal monitoring unless the strip can be interpreted in real time by someone qualified to read it and empowered to take corrective action. In some cases, this will entail an obstetric or perinatal nurse at the bedside in ICU. Alternatively, remote access monitoring can be used to transmit the tracing to a display on the obstetrical unit. Changes in the fetal monitor tracing often reflect alterations in maternal physiology rather than in the fetal status per se and thus may function as an early warning system for derangements in maternal end-organ status (acid–base balance, volume status, etc.). This means that the response that is a reflex on the labor floor—in which the nonreassuring fetal tracing is immediately evaluated for delivery—must be suppressed long enough to look for alternate explanations that would be better addressed by correcting maternal status.

The **plan for delivery** should be made long before delivery is imminent and address preferred location for delivery, mode of delivery, requirement for analgesia or anesthesia, and access for the neonatal team. It must also include alternatives in case matters do not go as anticipated.

The patient in an HDU or intermediate care unit on the labor floor can easily be delivered there. Many critically ill obstetric patients will, however, be elsewhere. Advantages of vaginal delivery in ICU include ready availability of critical care interventions and staff, plus avoidance of potentially destabilizing transport. Disadvantages include lack of space to conduct delivery, unfamiliarity of critical care personnel with obstetric management, space constraints for the pediatric team and equipment, and inadequate privacy. The alternative, transport to L&D, ensures familiarity with obstetric issues but unfamiliarity with critical care issues. The process of transport itself is risky for a critically ill patient [64].

When considering delivery in ICU, the increased likelihood of instrumental delivery must be kept in mind. Patients with translaryngeal intubation cannot close the glottis to push and therefore may have a prolonged second stage, often requiring delivery via vacuum or forceps. Patients with cardiac, respiratory or neuromuscular compromise are at risk of decompensation during labor, especially in second stage. Women with altered mental status may not tolerate pain or obstetric manipulation. Pain relief cannot be forgone in ICU even when a patient cannot verbalize discomfort, but patients may not qualify for regional analgesia techniques because of issues with positioning, hemodynamic instability, or coagulopathy. Intravenous analgesia is, of course, an alternative to epidural, but is not as effective in protecting a medically fragile patient from hemodynamic derangements associated with pain.

Cesarean delivery in ICU is fraught with hazards. The ICU does, on occasion, host surgical procedures performed under local anesthesia, such as tracheostomy, percutaneous gastrostomy, insertion of vena cava filters, or diagnostic laparoscopy [73–76]. Some cardiothoracic units allow emergency re-exploration in ICU for bleeding or tamponade rather than retransport back to the operating room [77], and resuscitative laparotomy has, rarely, been performed at the bedside when patients have been deemed too unstable for transport to OR although with very high mortality rates [78]. For the most part, however, surgical procedures are avoided in ICU when possible. Disadvantages of performing cesarean in the ICU include inadequate space for anesthetic and surgical equipment (to say nothing of required neonatal resuscitation gear), inadequate lighting, unfamiliarity of attendant personnel with the operation, the accumulation of a crowd of onlookers, and the risk of nosocomial infection with drug-resistant organisms: ICUs have the highest rates of health care-associated infections in a hospital [79,80]. In the special condition of perimortem cesarean, of course, these concerns would be ignored.

ROLE OF OB-GYN

In an intermediate care unit on a labor/delivery floor, **the lead physician** will typically be an obstetrician-gynecologist (Ob-Gyn) with or without subspecialty maternal-fetal medicine training; sometimes this function will be fulfilled instead by an obstetric anesthesiologist. The team leader would coordinate and manage the patient's care, in addition to providing hands-on care as necessary. It is essential that the lead physician be immediately available to the critically ill obstetrical patient and that coverage arrangements are adequate in order to avoid interference with prompt and timely delivery of care. When other specialty consultation is required, the lead physician must coordinate and integrate such consultation as appropriate. He/she must also be able to clearly decide when the patient's condition is no longer appropriate for intermediate care and then transfer up for intensive care or down for routine ward care.

When obstetric patients are transferred to the ICU, the obstetrician's role will depend on the ICU model (open or closed) and the patient's status (antepartum or postpartum). The Ob-Gyn's anxiety about a patient in the ICU is easily matched by the ICU team's anxiety about a fetus in the uterus, and even in a closed unit, the obstetrician's input is welcomed. Decisions about care for a pregnant patient in the ICU should be made in concert by the multidisciplinary team and should involve the patient and her family insofar as this is feasible. **No matter what the ICU model, the obstetrician should continue to see the patient and consult with the primary ICU team daily**, offering pregnancy-specific knowledge necessary to give the best care to these complex patients.

If a patient is transferred to the ICU postpartum, the obstetrician's role becomes simpler medically although the patient and family may have concerns regarding any obstetrical event that precipitated transfer. Anger, dissatisfaction, or legal action often follow a perceived bad outcome: In case of a postpartum complication or condition requiring critical care, the obstetrician may bear the brunt of questions. This is likely to be stressful even when there has been no evident error as the fear of litigation is prominent in such cases [81].

The medical issues with a postpartum admission to the ICU typically relate to uncertainty (on the part of the primary ICU team) about vaginal bleeding, evaluation of fever, therapies such as magnesium, and feasibility of breast-feeding, especially compatibility with various medications. There may be surgical issues, such as re-exploration or reclosure of incisions. Under some circumstances, the Ob-Gyn will be the advocate for bringing together the critically ill mother and her new baby.

Fetal surveillance is often employed when a pregnant patient is admitted to ICU. The obstetrician who is used to reviewing fetal heart rate tracings as an indicator of fetal status should consider that the fetal heart rate tracing reflects maternal end-organ (uteroplacental) perfusion and maternal acid–base status as well. If baseline variability disappears or decelerations are seen, a reason should be sought in maternal physiology, such as hypotension, acidemia, or compression of the inferior vena cava by the gravid uterus in supine position. Correction of these factors may result in improvement of the tracing.

The potential for preterm delivery is high in the ICU [6,61–63]. Attempts to suppress preterm contractions are ill advised in the case of critical illness in pregnancy: Aside from the equivocal efficacy of tocolytic drugs, preterm labor may represent an adaptive response. No drug is devoid of side effects, which must be carefully monitored in the setting of critical illness (tachycardia and decreased BP with β-agonists, effects on platelet function and renal perfusion with indomethacin, magnesium's effects on cardiac function, etc.). But because of the potential for preterm birth, the threshold for administration of a course of antenatal corticosteroids to promote fetal lung maturity should be low. Corticosteroids are often given in an ICU setting for reasons, such as sepsis and spinal cord injury: It may be feasible to substitute betamethasone or dexamethasone for the usual hydrocortisone in these circumstances in order to obtain additional fetal benefit.

Physicians who deal with the critically ill are familiar with the difficulties of informed consent and with the frequent need to identify a designated decision maker. This is not typically a problem with which obstetricians have much experience, but in critical care obstetrics, the designated decision maker must assume the role for both mother and fetus when the woman herself cannot. Even if a woman has previously made her wishes known with a living will or advance directive, state law varies: Advance directives may be specifically invalidated if a patient is pregnant [82]. The hospital ethics committee may be called upon for guidance as needed.

SPECIFIC CONDITIONS FOR WHICH CRITICAL CARE MAY BE REQUIRED

Reviews of severe acute maternal morbidity [1–11,15,18,36–53] suggest the following conditions are of most concern: **hemorrhage, eclampsia, cardiac arrest, pulmonary edema, respiratory failure, renal failure, sepsis, shock** (multiple types), **cerebrovascular event, coma, anesthetic complications** (e.g., aspiration, difficult/failed intubation), **and other cardiac conditions**. Most obstetricians will be familiar with hemorrhage, preeclampsia, and eclampsia—in fact, more familiar than most intensivists—and these conditions are frequently handled on a labor and delivery unit without transfer. The remainder of the chapter addresses a few critical care topics with which the obstetrician is likely to be less familiar. With the understanding that critical care medicine, like any other branch of medicine, is constantly evolving, current evidence based practice in critical care is described below.

Acute Respiratory Distress Syndrome and Mechanical Ventilation

The **acute respiratory distress syndrome (ARDS)** is a nonspecific response of the lung to a variety of inciting events. It is the extreme form of a spectrum of **acute lung injury (ALI)** and has been defined as "a syndrome of inflammation and increased permeability that is associated with a constellation of clinical, radiology, and physiologic abnormalities that cannot be explained by, but may coexist with, left atrial or pulmonary capillary hypertension" [83]. In other words, **ARDS is a type of noncardiogenic pulmonary edema**. Criteria for ARDS diagnosis were revised in 2012 [84] and are shown in Table 40.6. The lungs are poorly compliant and resist expansion. Positive-pressure ventilation, the mainstay of treatment, itself may cause further damage to the lung.

ARDS is an uncommon disorder in pregnancy with an incidence frequently quoted from case series as between 1/3000 and 1/6000 deliveries [61,85]. More recent population-level data, however, show that ARDS was coded in six delivery hospitalizations and three postpartum hospitalizations per 10,000 deliveries in 2008–2009 [86]. Not only is this much higher than the estimates from old case series, but the incidence appears to be rising with time as figures from the same data set in 1998–99 were 3.6 (delivery hospitalizations) and 1.1 (postpartum hospitalizations) per 10,000 deliveries. Data from

Table 40.6   Berlin Definition of ARDS

	Acute Respiratory Distress Syndrome
Timing	Within 1 week of a known clinical insult or new or worsening respiratory symptoms
Chest imaging[a]	Bilateral opacities—not fully explained by effusions, lobar/lung collapse, or nodules
Origin of edema	Respiratory failure not fully explained by cardiac failure or fluid overload Need objective assessment (e.g., echocardiography) to execute hydrostatic edema if no risk factor present
Oxygenation[b]	
Mild	200 mmHg < PaO_2/FIO_2 ≤ 300 mmHg with PEEP or CPAP ≥5 cm H_2O[c]
Moderate	100 mmHg < PaO_2/FIO_2 ≤ 200 mmHg with PEEP ≥5 cm H_2O
Severe	PaO_2/FIO_2 ≤ 100 mmHg with PEEP ≥5 cm H_2O

Source: The ARDS Definition Task Force, *JAMA* 2012; 307: 2526–33 (Consensus guideline). With permission.
Abbreviations: CPAP, continuous positive airway pressure; FIO_2, fraction of inspired oxygen; PaO_2, partial pressure of arterial oxygen; PEEP, positive end-expiratory pressure.
[a]Chest radiograph or computed tomography scan.
[b]If altitude is higher than 1000 m, the correction factor should be calculated as follows: [PaO2/FIO2×(barometric pressure/760)].
[c]This may be delivered noninvasively in the mild acute respiratory distress syndrome group.

Canada, however, showed a rate of ARDS of 0.6 per 10,000 among pregnancy hospitalizations from 2003–2007 [87]. It is possible that this represents not an epidemiologic difference in North America, but a difference in data capture: U.S. data relied on ICD-9 codes and Canadian on ICD-10. ARDS itself is not always captured in administrative data sets but may be approximated by the number of cases of mechanical ventilation. In the Netherlands, between 2004 and 2006, 291 women of the 358,874 delivered required mechanical ventilation for a rate of about 8 per 10,000 [18].

Among pregnant women with H1N1 influenza, the rate of ARDS was nearly twice as high as among nonpregnant women (9.7% vs. 5.4%) [88]; the difference in severity is demonstrated in a report from Australia and New Zealand in which extracorporeal membrane oxygenation was required in 45% of pregnant or postpartum women with severe H1N1 respiratory disease [89].

The mortality rate for ARDS among obstetrical patients was estimated to be 24% to 44% in older case series [61,85,90,91] and 33% in a more recent series [92], neither greatly different from the general population case fatality rate of 38% [93]. A review of Canadian hospital admissions between 1991 and 2002, however, found that the case fatality rate among obstetric patients with ARDS in the absence of any major preexisting condition was only 6% [15], and between 2003 and 2007, the case fatality rate was under 3% [87].

In managing ARDS in pregnancy, many authorities recommend **maintaining maternal SpO_2 >95% or PaO_2 >60 mmHg** in an effort to promote fetal well-being, but it is unclear what evidence supports this recommendation. The gradient between maternal and fetal oxygen content drives transfer. Because the oxygen content of fetal blood is quite low, the gradient is easily preserved: normal fetal umbilical venous pO_2 is only 31 to 42 mmHg [94]. Oxygen delivery to the fetus and to fetal organs, as to the adult, is the product of blood flow and oxygen content. Adaptive strategies in the fetus include higher affinity of fetal hemoglobin for oxygen and high cardiac output relative to size.

There is one experimental trial of deliberate hypoxia in human pregnancy [95]. Ten women with normal pregnancies near term were exposed to a hypoxic gas mixture with an FIO_2 approximately 0.1 (50% room air, 50% nitrogen) for 10 minutes during which time maternal oxygen saturation (SpO_2) decreased by 15%. Fetal heart rate baseline and variability, umbilical artery Doppler indices, and middle cerebral artery Doppler indices did not change during experimental maternal hypoxia. Direct sampling of fetal blood was not performed in this study.

In ARDS, the **use of lower tidal volumes in mechanical ventilation was associated with lower mortality and more ventilator-free days in nonpregnant adults** [96] in a randomized controlled trial in a general medical–surgical ICU population. This strategy allows hypercapnia and respiratory acidosis but minimizes inflation pressures and stretch-induced lung injury. There are no data on outcomes of a lung-protective or lower-tidal-volume-ventilation strategy for pregnant women with ARDS. In fact, **there are no randomized controlled trials of ventilator strategies in an obstetrical population**. Maternal acidemia does affect fetal acid–base status, which suggests that continuous fetal monitoring could be useful, specifically in determining the lower acceptable limits of maternal pH.

After the publication of the ARDSNet trial, which demonstrated better survival when low-tidal-volume ventilation was employed [96], strategies for mechanical ventilation swung away from normalizing arterial blood gases to limiting barotrauma, volutrauma, and other types of ventilator-induced lung injury. No trials have been performed on ARDS in pregnant patients, and few publications describe ventilator settings in the case of ARDS in pregnancy. In case series from the era preceding low-tidal-volume ventilation for ARDS, barotrauma rates were high in obstetric patients who were mechanically ventilated: 36% to 44% [61,85]. This compares unfavorably with the background rate of barotrauma of 11% among nonobstetric patients ventilated with "traditional" tidal volumes in ARDS [96]. There is, however, no head-to-head trial among pregnant patients with ARDS.

When contemplating a low-tidal-volume ventilation strategy for pregnant women with ARDS, the maternal $PaCO_2$ must also be considered. CO_2 transfer across the placenta also requires a gradient; in this case, the higher PCO_2 of fetal blood diffuses across placental interface to the lower PCO_2 of maternal blood. High maternal PCO_2, as in permissive hypercapnia, might be expected to impede transfer and allow fetal acidemia. In a small trial of CO_2 rebreathing in 35 healthy pregnant women, a rise in the maternal end-tidal CO_2 as high as 60 torr was associated with a loss of fetal heart rate variability in 57% of fetuses monitored, this being a proxy for fetal acidemia; 90% of fetuses thus affected normalized the tracing posttest [97]. A few case reports describe women with status asthmaticus during pregnancy in whom permissive hypercapnia was implemented so as to decrease the risk of barotrauma [98,99]. In most cases, there appeared to be no immediate or long-term ill effects on the fetuses, but one of six exhibited a nonreassuring fetal heart rate tracing after seven days' hypercapnia and was therefore delivered. There is also a small case series of airway pressure release ventilation (ARPV) in pregnancy, an alternative lung-protective strategy, in which the lungs were kept inflated to a high PEEP (28–33 cm H_2O) and interrupted for brief periods with low PEEP (8–10 cm H_2O). This was well tolerated by mothers and fetuses, and maternal oxygenation immediately improved [100].

The author suggests that a **pregnant woman ventilated with a low tidal volume strategy should have the fetal heart rate tracing continuously monitored once viability has been reached, and if the tracing is suspicious for fetal acidemia, consider increasing minute ventilation by increasing frequency or tidal volume (to increase maternal pH, decrease PCO_2) or switch to airway pressure release ventilation.** This is an example of using the fetal heart rate tracing as another maternal vital sign.

Delivery does not improve maternal survival in ARDS [61,62,101]. Fetal survival, however, is tightly linked to gestational age at delivery: This would imply a fetal benefit to continuing rather than interrupting pregnancy, assuming maternal and fetal condition permits.

Sepsis

Sepsis, a leading cause of maternal death in the era before the introduction of aseptic technique and antibiotics, is again resurgent. In the most recent triennial report of maternal deaths in the United Kingdom, 25% of maternal deaths were due to sepsis [102]. **There are no randomized trials on sepsis specific to the obstetric population.** In most trials, pregnant patients are explicitly barred from enrollment.

Table 40.7 lists older criteria for sepsis with which the reader may be familiar, **but the paradigm has recently been revised. The Sepsis-3 consensus panel has radically simplified both categorization and diagnosis (see Table 40.8).** Sepsis must be conceptualized neither as infection nor as bacteremia, but should be understood as "life-threatening organ dysfunction caused by a dysregulated host response to infection" [103].

In this context, organ failure is paramount: it may be circulatory failure, respiratory or renal failure, gastrointestinal or hepatic dysfunction, coagulopathy, etc. The old categories of systemic inflammatory response syndrome and severe sepsis have disappeared; because sepsis is now understood to incorporate organ failure, the previous concept of "severe sepsis" is redundant. Only the categories of sepsis and septic shock have been retained.

There is no gold-standard diagnostic test for sepsis, so the clinician must look for clinical criteria rather than biomarkers. The clinical measures that have been found to best correlate with sepsis [104,105] are any two of the following three findings:

1. Systolic BP ≤100 mmHg
2. Respiratory rate ≥22/min
3. Altered mental status

Fever is not included, as it is neither necessary nor sufficient to a sepsis diagnosis. This triad, a modification of the Sequential Organ Failure Assessment (SOFA) score, is known as the quick SOFA, or qSOFA, score, and can be easily applied to patients outside of the ICU. (For patients currently in ICU, a 2-point increase in the full SOFA score should be taken to represent sepsis.) Because a qSOFA score of 2 or 3 has been shown to predict mortality or prolonged ICU stay, one would then carefully look for signs of organ dysfunction, begin or escalate treatment, increase acuity of observations, or consider transfer to a higher level of care. These cutoffs have not been studied in pregnancy and the puerperium, and given

Table 40.7 Former Diagnostic Criteria for Sepsis (Now Supplanted by Sepsis-3: See Table 40.8)

Infection, documented or suspected, and some of the following:

General variables

Fever (>38.3°C)

Hypothermia (core temperature <36°C)

Heart rate >90/min or more than 2 standard deviations above the normal value for age

Tachypnea

Altered mental status

Significant edema or positive fluid balance (>20 mL/kg over 24 hr)

Hyperglycemia (plasma glucose >140 mg/dL) in the absence of diabetes

Inflammatory variables

Leukocytosis (WBC >12,000/μL)

Leukopenia (WBC <4000/μL)

WBC in the normal range with >10% bands

Plasma C-reactive protein more than 2 standard deviations above the normal value

Plasma procalcitonin more than 2 standard deviations above normal

Hemodynamic variables

Arterial hypotension (SBP <90 mmHg, MAP <70 mmHg, or SBP decrease >40 mmHg)

Organ dysfunction variables

Arterial hypoxemia (PaO_2/FIO_2 <300)

Acute oliguria (urine output <0.5 mL/kg/hr for at least 2 hrs despite adequate fluid resuscitation)

Creatinine increase >0.5 mg/dL

Coagulation abnormalities (INR >1.5 or aPTT >60 sec)

Ileus

Thrombocytopenia (platelet count <100,000/μL)

Hyperbilirubinemia (total bilirubin >4 mg/dL)

Tissue perfusion variables

Hyperlactatemia (>1 mmol/L)

Decreased capillary refill or mottling

Unclear how these criteria should be modified for the physiologic changes of pregnancy.

Source: Dellinger RP, Levy MM, Rhodes A, Annane D et al., for the Surviving Sepsis Campaign Guidelines Committee. *Crit Care Med*, 41, 580–637, 2013. With permission.

Table 40.8 Current Classification and Criteria for Sepsis (from Sepsis-3)

Categories:

Sepsis: life-threatening organ dysfunction caused by a dysregulated host response to infection. Organ dysfunction is identified as an acute change in SOFA score of >2 points, consequent to the infection.

Septic shock: a subset of sepsis in which underlying circulatory and cellular metabolism abnormalities are profound enough to substantially increase mortality.

Diagnosis:

Sepsis: quick SOFA (qSOFA) score

Any two of the following:

Respiratory rate > 22/min

Altered mentation

Systolic BP < 100 mmHg

For a patient already in ICU, use the full SOFA score.

Septic shock: persistent hypotension requiring vasopressors to maintain mean arterial pressure >65 mmHg and a serum lactate level > 2 mmol/L (18 mg/dL), despite adequate volume resuscitation.

Source: Umo-Etuk J et al. *Int J Obstet Anesth*, 5, 79–84, 1996.

the well-known changes in pregnancy physiology, the BP criterion may be too strict.

The only additional category in Sepsis-3 is that of septic shock, now defined as "a subset of sepsis in which underlying circulatory and cellular metabolism abnormalities are profound enough to substantially increase mortality" [103]. Mortality rates with septic shock are 35%–54% [104,105]. Circulatory failure is diagnosed by hypotension (mean arterial pressure ≤65 mmHg) requiring vasopressors, and cellular metabolic abnormalities as hyperlactatemia (>2 mmol/L), despite adequate volume resuscitation.

Several recent publications describe the epidemiology of maternal sepsis and suggest that **rates of the most severe forms of sepsis are increasing among pregnant and postpartum patients**. A case-control study performed by the UK Obstetric Surveillance System gave the incidence of severe sepsis as approximately 5 per 100,000 maternities in 2011–12 [106]. In the United States, although the total incidence of sepsis among women hospitalized for delivery remained at about 30 cases per 100,000 deliveries over the decade from 1998 to 2008, the incidence of severe sepsis, which accounted for about one third of cases, increased 10% per year, as did the rate of maternal death from sepsis [107,108]. That is, between 1998 and 2008, the rate of severe sepsis increased 112% and the rate of death from sepsis 129% among women hospitalized for delivery. Linking California vital statistics records to hospitalizations between 2005 and 2007, Acosta et al. reported the incidence of maternal sepsis as 10 per 10,000 live births with severe sepsis being about 5 per 10,000 [109]: This represents a doubling of the rate calculated by Callaghan between 1991 and 2003 [19]. The case fatality rate for maternal sepsis in the United States was calculated [105] as 4.4%. National ascertainment of all maternal deaths in the Netherlands from 2004 to 2006 gave an overall case fatality rate for maternal sepsis as 7.7% with nonobstetric etiologies being 12.2% [110]. Increasing maternal mortality from sepsis contrasts poorly with observations in a general adult population: A meta-analysis of sepsis mortality among adult (nonpregnant) patients in the control arms of randomized controlled trials—that is, getting standard care for sepsis—showed a 38% decline in mortality between 1991 and 2009 [111]. The case fatality rate for septic abortion is as high as 20% [112], but in the developed world, this condition is seen almost exclusively where abortion is illegal.

Sepsis may be obstetric or nonobstetric. Obstetric sepsis includes uterine infection, both chorioamnionitis and endomyometritis, septic abortion, and wound infection; in addition, sepsis may follow invasive procedures, such as amniocentesis, chorionic villus sampling, cervical cerclage, or percutaneous umbilical blood sampling. The UK Obstetric Surveillance System reported on all cases of severe maternal sepsis in 2011–12, determining that 20% of cases arose from the genital tract, 34% from the urinary tract, 9% were respiratory in origin, and in 30% the source remained unidentified [109]. In the Netherlands, among women with severe maternal morbidity from sepsis in 2004–06, 56% of causes were attributed to the genital tract, 14% from the urinary tract, and 8% pneumonia [110] although the study design did not allow for complete ascertainment. **Survival is better in obstetric than nonobstetric causes of sepsis [105,108], which may reflect either expedited awareness and treatment or the amenability of the uterus to source control.** During influenza pandemics, as in the H1N1 pandemic in 2009–10, respiratory causes of sepsis become more prominent among pregnant women as among the population generally. See Chapter 24 for a more detailed discussion of influenza in pregnancy.

The diagnosis of sepsis may be more challenging in obstetric patients, particularly when normal alterations in pregnancy physiology are taken into account. Blood pressure in normal pregnancy tends to be lower and heart rate higher, and leukocytosis is common both in the third trimester and in labor [113]. Thus, the specificity of usual criteria for sepsis has been called into question. The more salient problem, however, would be the possibility of under-recognition of sepsis in pregnancy and the puerperium. In a series of maternal deaths from sepsis in the state of Michigan between 1999 and 2006, **only 18% were febrile at presentation**, and 25% were never febrile during hospitalization [114].

Delay contributes to death in sepsis [115]. This may be blamed on delay in diagnosis, delay in starting appropriate antibiotics, or delay in escalation of care. A review of maternal deaths due to sepsis revealed a delay in antibiotics in 73% and a delay in escalation of care (e.g., consultation with infectious disease specialist or transfer to critical care) in 53% [114]. Similarly, the most recent triennial review of maternal deaths in the United Kingdom identified a delay in recognition or management in 70% of maternal deaths from sepsis [105]; sadly, two thirds of those delays occurred in the obstetric unit.

The Surviving Sepsis Campaign (SSC) [116] is a multiorganizational effort to improve mortality in sepsis and septic shock based on best available evidence. It proposes a number of therapeutic goals and recommends care bundles (see Table 40.9). **Adherence to SSC goals has been shown to improve mortality in septic shock** [117]. SSC guidelines, originally codified in 2003, were revised in 2008 and again in 2012; a revision is planned for 2017. The website is available at www.survivingsepsis.org. There are no guidelines geared specifically toward pregnancy, though it seems reasonable to apply these recommendations until pregnancy-specific guidance becomes available.

1. **Broad-spectrum antimicrobial therapy should be begun within one hour of diagnosis of sepsis or septic shock** (see below); cultures, including blood cultures, should be obtained as appropriate, providing this does not delay the start of antimicrobials. Mortality increases as time to appropriate antibiotics increases [118–120]. Initial therapy will be empiric, commonly requires more than one drug for broad coverage, and should be active against all likely inciting pathogens, bacterial, viral and/or fungal. Regimen should be reassessed daily for possible de-escalation based on clinical response and culture results; empiric therapy should be limited to 3–5 days. Specific regimens for identified pathogens are not provided here, being both beyond the scope of this chapter and subject to rapid change as organisms evolve resistance. Usual print and/or online resources may be accessed, or consultation may be sought from an expert in infectious disease. Total duration of therapy should usually be 7–10 days although may need to be longer if *S. aureus* bacteremia, slow clinical response, undrainable focus of infection, etc. Broad-spectrum coverage is appropriate in OB patients: In a large study of peripartum sepsis, more than 40 organisms were cultured, including aerobic gram-positive and gram-negative as well as anaerobic bacteria [121]. When narrowing coverage, consideration should be given to whether transplacental coverage is needed; some drugs do not cross placenta well and result in inadequate fetal treatment, such as azithromycin in the treatment of syphilis [122].

2. **Blood cultures before antibiotic therapy as long as antimicrobial therapy is not delayed more than 45 minutes.** At least two sets of blood cultures should be obtained. No reason this would not apply in obstetric patients. One study in Finland described this specific policy for obstetric patients: 2% (of more than 40,000) were cultured for fever and had broad-spectrum antibiotics instituted immediately. Bacteremia was confirmed in 5% of cases; only 1 of the 798 patients cultured developed septic shock, for an incidence of 0.1% [121].

3. **Source control.** SSC recommends "a specific anatomical diagnosis of infection requiring consideration for emergent source control be sought and diagnosed or excluded as rapidly as possible, and intervention be undertaken for source control within the first 12 hr after the diagnosis is made, if feasible." The intervention undertaken should be the one with the least potential for physiologic derangement, e.g., percutaneous rather than surgical drainage of an abscess. There is limited data specific to pregnancy. Up to half of cases of sepsis in pregnant/postpartum women localize to the uterus [106,109–112,123] and would therefore require the uterus be emptied. **There are no data on antibiotics without delivery for women diagnosed with clinical sepsis attributed to intra-amniotic infection.** Women with a diagnosis of *subclinical* intra-amniotic infection, treated with antibiotics alone in the hope of delaying delivery to a more favorable gestational age, have had pregnancy prolonged by days to weeks with the only maternal morbidity a 3% rate of postpartum endometritis [124] but with an infant death rate of 33% and major infant morbidity >75%. It should be emphasized that patients with subclinical chorioamnionitis, who typically present with preterm labor or membrane rupture, are unlikely to come to the ICU; if these nonseptic patients cannot be managed without delivery, there is no argument for managing clinical chorioamnionitis without it. There is no evidence for deferring source control in pregnancy.

Table 40.9 Core Bundles for Management of Sepsis (SSC)

To be completed within 3 hours of presentation with sepsis or septic shock:
1. Measure lactate level
2. Obtain blood cultures prior to administration of antibiotics
3. Administer broad spectrum antibiotics
4. Administer 30 mL/kg crystalloid for hypotension or lactate ≥4 mmol/L

To be completed within 6 hours of presentation
1. Begin vasopressors for hypotension that does not respond to initial fluid resuscitation; maintain MAP > 65 mm Hg.
2. In the event of persistent hypotension after initial fluid load, or if initial lactate was >4 mmol/L, reassess volume status and tissue perfusion.
3. Repeat lactate measurement if initial lactate was elevated.

Source: Surviving Sepsis Campaign, http://www.survivingsepsis.org /SiteCollectionDocuments/SSC_Bundle.pdf Accessed 8/16/16

After 2001, there sprang up a recommendation for a protocolized form of aggressive fluid resuscitation known as "early goal-directed therapy" (EGDT), first popularized after a small randomized trial in an adult non-pregnant population showed a benefit in mortality among severe forms of sepsis [125]. EGDT required invasive monitoring of central venous pressure and central venous oxygen saturation, which were targeted with extensive fluid resuscitation, transfusion, vasopressors, and inotropes. Despite the lack of pregnancy-specific data, EGDT had subsequently been recommended in pregnancy as well [126–128]. More recently, however, three much larger RCTs have demonstrated no mortality benefit at all to EGDT, and to the contrary, show more organ failure, more interventions, greater length of stay, and higher cost [129–131]. It has been removed from the SSC bundle. Again, we have no pregnancy-specific data, but since EDGT was never tested in pregnant patients in the first place and has now been disproven in a general adult population, it should not be implemented as standard sepsis care.

In addition to the recommendations for initial resuscitation and antimicrobial treatment, SSC weighs in on **hemodynamic support and adjunctive therapy** in severe sepsis and septic shock, as follows:

1. **Crystalloid as the fluid of choice**, rather than colloid: no survival benefit to colloid, additional cost, and a disadvantage in outcome specifically with hydroxyethyl starch (HES) [116]. No evidence to recommend crystalloid versus colloid in pregnancy. Decreased oncotic pressure in pregnancy and decreased gradient between colloid oncotic pressure and pulmonary artery occlusion pressure [132] may increase risk of pulmonary edema in pregnancy when crystalloid resuscitation is chosen. If colloid resuscitation is elected in pregnancy, use albumin rather than hydroxyethyl starch (HES), because of evidence of harm with HES.

2. **Initial fluid challenge with sepsis-induced tissue hypoperfusion: 30 mL/kg** [116]. No data specific to pregnancy; however, the gradient between colloid oncotic pressure and pulmonary artery occlusion pressure is lower in pregnancy [132], so there is more risk of inducing pulmonary edema. Not all patients are fluid responders anyway, so a quick test of fluid responsiveness using either passive leg raising or point-of-care ultrasound (diameter of the inferior vena cava, extravascular lung water) might be useful as a first step in determining how much of a fluid load to try [133–135]. These techniques are not specifically validated in pregnancy, however.

3. **Vasopressor to target initial mean arterial pressure >65 mmHg but individualized for the patient**. The goal is to maintain tissue perfusion even if hypovolemia has not yet been resolved. Supplemental clinical end points are also important: BP, mental status, urine output, blood lactate. **Norepinephrine is the vasopressor of choice** [116]. No data exist to make a recommendation about the lower limit of mean arterial pressure in pregnancy, but because mean arterial pressure is normally lower in pregnancy [136], a target MAP ≥65 may be too stringent. Although MAP is approximately 4 to 5 mmHg lower in pregnancy, one cannot extrapolate a target of 60 mmHg instead. The uteroplacental circulation does not autoregulate, and compromised placental perfusion is expected to affect the fetus. Use of clinical end points, as described above, is crucial in making a decision for an individual patient; if the patient is still pregnant, the electronic fetal heart rate tracing may help with individualization of target MAP. There is little data as to use of vasopressors in septic pregnancy in general. Norepinephrine has been studied, in a randomized trial, as an agent to maintain maternal BP during cesarean under spinal anesthesia [137]. Compared to the commonly used agent phenylephrine, norepinephrine maintained BP equally well with a more favorable chronotropic profile and a higher cardiac output. There was no difference in Apgar scores or cord gases; a significantly lower concentration of epinephrine in the cord blood of norepinephrine-exposed than phenylephrine-exposed infants suggested at least the possibility of decreased physiologic stress. Although the dose used in this study was constrained to a maximum of 5 mcg/min and the duration of fetal exposure generally less than 30 min, which are both less than would be required in septic shock, **this study nevertheless represents early evidence that norepinephrine does not seem to impair uteroplacental perfusion in and of itself**. This supports preclinical work that showed, in a dual-perfused single-cotyledon model of human placenta, no change in fetal arterial perfusion with administration of norepinephrine [138].

4. **Trial of dobutamine in either myocardial dysfunction (high filling pressures and low cardiac output) or ongoing hypoperfusion despite adequate intravascular volume and MAP** [116]. Normal cardiac output in pregnancy is increased and the systemic vascular resistance decreased [132]; thus, it is unclear what would constitute a "low" cardiac output in pregnancy. In addition, this is probably outdated, as current critical care practice seldom makes use of invasive monitoring of cardiac output or filling pressures; in the recent ProCESS trial, only 1% of septic shock patients in the control arm received dobutamine [129]. Dobutamine has little effect on resting uterine tone even at high doses but decreases uterine blood flow in gravid ewes [139]. Human data are lacking. It is unlikely that fetal concerns would be paramount in a situation in which the maternal condition was sufficiently dire to consider adding dobutamine to vasopressor therapy.

5. **Corticosteroids are sometimes used in septic shock when fluid resuscitation and vasopressors have been unsuccessful**. The SSC guidelines are now less than lukewarm in this recommendation [116]. There are no specific data in pregnancy. Many pregnant patients will have been given betamethasone or dexamethasone for fetal indications; these steroids have not been studied extensively in septic shock.

SSC also makes recommendations for **blood product administration** (defer RBC transfusion until hemoglobin concentration is less than 7.0 g/dL, prophylactic platelets when platelet count <10,000 or, if at high risk of bleeding, 20,000), **thromboprophylaxis**, and **stress ulcer prophylaxis. Oral or enteral feeding** is preferred over parenteral nutrition or fasting. A former recommendation for tight glucose control (≤110 mg/dL), using insulin infusion as necessary, has been updated to **maintain blood glucose ≤180 mg/dL** in adult patients with sepsis. Obstetricians are already accustomed to targeting glucose control in diabetic pregnancy, frequently use insulin infusions in labor, and should find glycemic control an easy recommendation to adopt. It must be cautioned, however, that the ideal range for glucose in critically ill pregnant patients has not been studied; obstetricians may be tempted to aim for the usual range recommended in diabetes of 80–120 mg/dL in an effort to minimize fetal hyperinsulinemia and neonatal hypoglycemia, but this may or may not be correct in the management of sepsis.

The final recommendations in the SSC guidelines are universally applicable and underappreciated. These state that **the prognosis and goals of care should be discussed with the patient and family** as soon as feasible and that **the goals of care should be incorporated into treatment, including end-of-life planning** [116]. Goals for a pregnant or postpartum patient in ICU may be challenging to set or may be painful for the patient, her family members, or the health care professionals involved, but they cannot be shunted aside. Some women may prioritize the outcome for the fetus/neonate above their own health; in other cases, the family may need to make unwelcome choices between the critically ill woman and the potential new baby. It may be helpful to bring in multiple perspectives, including, in some cases, a palliative care team or an ethicist.

What is missing from this discussion are the voices of women themselves who have survived a stay in the intensive care unit. A small qualitative survey of women's experiences in maternal critical care elucidated several themes: the distance between their expectations about childbirth and the reality they experienced, the pain of being separated from their newborn regardless of how sick they were, and the difficulty of being transferred out of ICU to a maternity ward [140]. Many women were shocked or frightened to wake up in the ICU, slow in understanding why, disturbed or powerless being in the ICU, and unsupported in their specific needs once out of ICU. **The long-term outcome of women who have survived maternal critical care remains unreported in the medical literature** although physical and psychiatric sequelae are common among ICU survivors in general.

REFERENCES

1. Panchal S, Arria AM, Labhsetwar SA. Maternal mortality during hospital admission for delivery: A retrospective analysis using a state-maintained database. *Anesth Anal* 2001; 93: 134–411. [II-2; case control; *n* = 135]
2. Keizer JL, Zwart JJ, Meerman RH et al. Obstetric intensive care admissions: A 12-year review in a tertiary care centre. *Eur J Obstet Gynecol Reprod Biol* 2006; 128: 152–6. [II-3; case series; *n* = 142]
3. Umo-Etuk J, Lumley J, Holdcroft A. Critically ill parturient women and admission to intensive care: A 5-year review. *Int J Obstet Anesth* 1996; 5: 79–84. [II-3; case series, *n* = 39]
4. Hazelgrove JF, Price C, Pappachan VJ et al. Multicenter study of obstetric admissions to 14 intensive care units in southern England. *Crit Care Med* 2001; 29: 770–5. [II-3; case series, *n* = 210]
5. Lapinsky SE, Kruczynski K, Seaward GR et al. Critical care management of the obstetric patient. *Can J Anaesth* 1997; 44: 325–9. [II-3; case series, *n* = 65]
6. Selo-Ojeme DO, Omosaiye M, Battacharjee P et al. Risk factors for obstetric admissions to the intensive care unit in a tertiary hospital: A case-control study. *Arch Gynecol Obstet* 2005; 272: 207–10. [II-2; case control, 33 cases]
7. Munnur U, Karnad DR, Bandi VD et al. Critically ill obstetric patients in an American and an Indian public hospital: Comparison of case-mix, organ dysfunction, intensive care requirements, and outcomes. *Intensive Care Med* 2005; 31(8): 1087–94. [II-3; case series, 174 in Houston, 754 in Mumbai]
8. Brace V, Penney G, Hall M. Quantifying severe maternal morbidity: A Scottish population study. *BJOG* 2004; 111: 481–4. [II-2; audit, *n* = 196]
9. Heinonen S, Tyrvainen E, Saarikoski S et al. Need for maternal critical care in obstetrics: A population-based analysis. *Int J Obstet Anesth* 2002; 11: 260–4. [II-3; case series, *n* = 22]
10. Baskett TF, O'Connell CM. Maternal critical care in obstetrics. *J Obstet Gynaecol Can* 2009; 31: 218–21. [II-3; case series, *n* = 117]
11. Pollock W, Rose L, Dennis CL. Pregnant and postpartum admissions to the intensive care unit: A systematic review. *Intensive Care Med* 2010; 36: 1465–74. [Review, 40 studies, *n* = 7887 patients]
12. Ryan M, Hamilton V, Bowen M et al. The role of a high-dependency unit in a regional obstetric hospital. *Anaesthesia* 2000; 55: 1155–8. [II-3; case series, *n* = 123]
13. Zeeman GG, Wendel GD, Cunningham FG. A blueprint for obstetric critical care. *Am J Obstet Gynecol* 2003; 188: 532–6. [II-3; case series, *n* = 483]
14. Saravanakumar K, Davies L, Lewis M et al. High dependency care in an obstetric setting in the UK. *Anaesthesia* 2008; 63: 1081–6. [II-3; case series, 3551]
15. Wen SW, Liston R, Heaman M et al., for the Maternal Health Study Group, Canadian Perinatal Surveillance System. Severe maternal morbidity in Canada, 1991–2001. *CMAJ* 2005; 173: 759–64. [II-2; population database, *n* = 11,066]
16. Joseph KS, Liu S, Rouleau J et al. Severe maternal morbidity in Canada, 2003–2007: Surveillance including routine hospitalization data and ICD-9 codes. *J Obstet Gynaecol Can* 2010; 32: 837–46. [II-2; administrative database of 1.3 million]
17. Liu S, Joseph KS, Bartholomew S et al. Temporal trends and regional variations in severe maternal morbidity in Canada, 2003 to 2007. *J Obstet Gynaecol Can* 2010; 32: 847–55. [II-2; administrative database]
18. Zwart JJ, Dupuis JRO, Richters A et al. Obstetric intensive care unit admission: A 2-year nationwide population-based cohort study. *Intensive Care Med* 2010; 36: 256–61. [II-2; cohort study, *n* = 847]
19. Callaghan WM, MacKay AP, Berg CJ. Identification of severe maternal morbidity during delivery hospitalizations, United States, 1991–2003. *Am J Obstet Gynecol* 2008; 199: 133.e1–8. [II-2; administrative database, 423,480 records with 2235 qualifying cases]
20. Callagan WM, Creanga AA, Kuklina EV. Severe maternal morbidity among delivery and postpartum hospitalizations in the United States. *Obstet Gynecol* 2012; 120: 1029–36. [II-b; administrative database; 50 million records, 597,000 qualifying cases]
21. Martin JA, Hamilton BE, Osterman MJK, Curtin SC, Mathews TJ. Births: Final data for 2013. *National Vital Statistics Reports* 2015; 64(1). Online at http://www.cdc.gov/nchs/data/nvsr/nvsr64/nvsr64_01.pdf. Accessed 10/13/15. [Epidemiologic data]
22. Roberts CL, Ford JB, Algert CS et al. Trends in adverse maternal outcomes during childbirth: A population-based study of severe maternal morbidity. *BMC Pregnancy Childbirth* 2009; 9: 7. Available at http://www.biomedcentral.com/1471-2393/9/7. Accessed November 20, 2010. [II; administrative data set, *n* = 6242]
23. Knight M, Callaghan WS, Berg C et al. Trends in postpartum hemorrhage in high resource countries: A review and recommendations from the International Postpartum Hemorrhage Collaborative Group. *BMC Pregnancy Childbirth* 2009; 9: 55. Available at http://www.biomedcentral.com/1471-2393/9/55. Accessed November 20, 2010. [II-2; multiple data sets]
24. Plante LA. Public health consequences of cesarean on demand. *Obstet Gynecol Surv* 2006; 61: 807–15. [III; decision analysis]
25. Galyean AM, Lagrew DC, Bush MC et al. Previous cesarean section and the risk of postpartum maternal complications and adverse neonatal outcomes in future pregnancies. *J Perinatol* 2009; 29: 726–30. [II-3; database, *n* = 17,406]
26. Haupt MT, Bekes CE, Brilli RJ et al. Guidelines on critical care services and personnel: Recommendations based on a system of categorization of three levels of care. *Crit Care Med* 2003; 31: 2677–83. [III; expert opinion]
27. Nasrawat SA, Cohen IL, Dennis RC et al. Guidelines on admission and discharge for adult intermediate care units. *Crit Care Med* 1998; 26: 607–10. [III; expert opinion]
28. Zimmerman JE, Wagner DP, Sun X et al. Planning patient services for intermediate care units: Insights based on care for intensive care unit low-risk monitor admissions. *Crit Care Med* 1996; 24: 1626–32. [II-2; cohort study, *n* = 8040]

29. Seppelt I, for ANZIC writing committee. Critical illness due to 2009A/H1N1 influenza in pregnant and postpartum women: Population based cohort study. *BMJ* 2010; 340: c1279. [II-2; cohort study, *n* = 64]

30. Louie JK, Acosta M, Jamieson DJ et al., for the California Pandemic (H1N1) Working Group. Severe 2009 H1N1 influenza in pregnant and postpartum women in California. *N Engl J Med* 2010; 362: 27–35. [II-2; cohort, *n* = 102]

31. Siston AM, Rasmussen SA, Honein MA et al., for the Pandemic H1N1 Influenza in Pregnancy Working Group. Pandemic 2009 influenza A (H1N1) virus illness among pregnant women in the United States. *JAMA* 2010; 303: 1517–25. [II; public health surveillance data set, *n* = 788]

32. Intensive Care Society. Guidelines for the Provision of Intensive Care Services. http://www.ics.ac.uk/ics-homepage/guidelines -and-standards/. Accessed October 10, 2015. [Guideline]

33. Maternal Critical Care Working Group. The Royal College of Obstetricians and Gynaecologists, the Royal College of Anaesthetists, the Royal College of Midwives, the Intensive Care Society, the British Maternal and Fetal Medicine Society, the Obstetric Anaesthetists' Association, and the Department of Health. Providing equity of critical and maternity care for the critically ill pregnant or recently pregnant woman. July 2011. Online at https://www.rcog.org.uk/globalassets/documents /guidelines/prov_eq_matandcritcare.pdf. Accessed September 25, 2015. [Guideline]

34. Martin SR, Foley MR. Intensive care in obstetrics: An evidence-based review. *Am J Obstet Gynecol* 2006; 195: 673–89. [III; review]

35. Galvagno SM, Camann W. Sepsis and acute renal failure in pregnancy. *Anesth Analg* 2009; 108: 572–5. [III; review]

36. Afessa B, Green B, Delke I et al. Systemic inflammatory response syndrome, organ failure, and outcome in critically ill obstetric patients treated in an ICU. *Chest* 2001; 120: 1271–7. [II-3; case series, *n* = 74]

37. Bouvier-Colle M-H, Salanave B, Ancel P-Y et al. Obstetric patients treated in intensive care units and maternal mortality. *Eur J Obstet Gynecol Reprod Biol* 1996; 65: 121–5. [III; population-based survey, *n* = 435]

38. Collop NA, Sahn SA. Critical illness in pregnancy: An analysis of 20 patients admitted to a medical intensive care unit. *Chest* 1993; 103: 1548–52. [II-3; case series, *n* = 20]

39. Gilbert TT, Smulian JC, Martin AA et al. Obstetric admissions to the intensive care unit: Outcomes and severity of illness. *Obstet Gynecol* 2003; 102: 897–903. [II-3; case series, *n* = 233]

40. Graham SG, Luxton MC. The requirement for intensive care support for the pregnant population. *Anaesthesia* 1989; 44: 581–4. [II-3; case series, *n* = 23]

41. Karnad D, Guntupalli KK. Critical illness and pregnancy: Review of a global problem. *Crit Care Clin* 2004; 20: 555–76. [III; review]

42. Kilpatrick SJ, Matthay MA. Obstetric patients requiring critical care: A five-year review. *Chest* 1992; 101: 1407–12. [II-3; case series, *n* = 32]

43. Kwee A, Bots ML, Visser GHA et al. Emergency peripartum hysterectomy: A prospective study in the Netherlands. *Eur J Obstet Gynecol Reprod Biol* 2006; 124: 187–92. [III; survey; 48 reports]

44. Mabie WC, Sibai BM. Treatment in an obstetric intensive care unit. *Am J Obstet Gynecol* 1990; 162: 1–4. [II-3; case series]

45. Mahutte NG, Murphy-Kaulbeck L, Le Q et al. Obstetric admissions to the intensive care unit. *Obstet Gynecol* 1999; 94: 263–6. [II-3; case series, *n* = 131]

46. Monaco TK, Spielman FJ, Katz VL. Pregnant patients in the intensive care unit: A descriptive analysis. *South Med J* 1993; 86: 414–7. [II-3; case series, *n* = 38]

47. Say L, Pattinson RC, Gulmezoglu AM. WHO systematic review of maternal morbidity and mortality: The prevalence of severe acute maternal morbidity (near miss). *BMC Reproductive Health* 2004; 1: 3. Available at: http://www.reproductive-health-journal .com/content/1/1/3. Accessed August 8, 2006. [Systematic review, 30 studies]

48. Soubra SH, Guntupalli KK. Critical illness in pregnancy: An overview. *Crit Care Med* 2005; 33(Suppl.): S248–55. [III; review]

49. Sriram S, Robertson MS. Critically ill obstetrics patients in Australia: A retrospective audit of 8 years' experience in a tertiary intensive care unit. *Crit Care Resusc* 2008; 10: 120–4. [II-3; case series, *n* = 56]

50. Zhang W-H, Alexander S, Bouvier-Colle M-H et al. Incidence of severe preeclampsia, postpartum haemorrhage and sepsis as a surrogate marker for severe maternal morbidity in a European population-based study: The MOMS-B survey. *BJOG* 2005; 112: 89–96. [III; survey, 1734 responses]

51. Crozier TM, Wallace EM. Obstetric admissions to an integrated general intensive care unit in a quaternary maternity facility. *Aust NZ J Obstet Gynaecol* 2011; 51: 233–8. [Case series, *n* = 60]

52. Paxton JL, Presneill J, Aitken L. Characteristics of obstetric patients referred to intensive care in an Australian tertiary hospital. *Aust NZ J Obstet Gynaecol* 2014; 54: 445–9. [Case series, *n* = 249]

53. Chantry AA, Deneux-Tharaux C, Bonnet M-P, Bouvier-Colle M-H. Pregnancy-related ICU admissions in France: Trends in rate and severity, 2006–2009. *Crit Care Med* 2015; 43: 78–86. [Administrative data, *n* = 11,824]

54. American College of Obstetricians and Gynecologists, Society for Maternal-Fetal Medicine. Obstetric Care Consensus. Levels of maternal care. 2015; 2. http://www.acog.org/-/media /Obstetric-Care-Consensus-Series/oc002.pdf?dmc=1&ts= 20151013T2112541967. Accessed September 15, 2015. [Guideline]

55. Brilli RJ, Spevetz A, Branson RD et al., the members of the American College of Critical Care Medicine Task Force on Models of Critical Care Delivery, the members of the American College of Critical Care Medicine Guidelines for the Definition of an Intensivist and the Practice of Critical Care Medicine. Critical care delivery in the intensive care unit: Defining clinical roles and the best practice model. *Crit Care Med* 2001; 29: 2001–19. [III; task force, expert report]

56. D'Alton ME, Bonanno CA, Berkowitz RL, Brown HL et al. Putting the "M" back in maternal-fetal medicine. *Am J Obstet Gyn* 2013; 208: 442–8. [III]

57. Dorman T, Angood P, Angus DC et al. Guidelines for critical care medicine training and continuing medical education. *Crit Care Med* 2004; 32: 263–72. [III; task force, expert opinion]

58. Soylemez Weiner R, Welch HG. Trends in the use of the pulmonary artery catheter in the United States, 1993 to 2004. *JAMA* 2007; 298: 423–9. [II-3; administrative database]

59. The Critical Care Anesthesiology Milestone Project. A joint initiative of the Accreditation Council for Graduate Medical Education and the American Board of Anesthesiology. October, 2014. https://www.acgme.org/acgmeweb/Portals/0 /PDFs/Milestones/CriticalCareMedicine.pdf. Accessed October 4, 2015. [Guideline]

60. The Surgical Critical Care Milestone Project. A joint initiative of the Accreditation Council for Graduate Medical Education and the American Board of Surgery. July 2015. https://www .acgme.org/acgmeweb/Portals/0/PDFs/Milestones/Surgical CriticalCareMilestones.pdf. Accessed October 4, 2015. [Guideline]

61. Catanzarite V, Willms D, Wong D et al. Acute respiratory distress syndrome in pregnancy and the puerperium: Causes, courses, and outcomes. *Obstet Gynecol* 2001; 97: 760–4. [III; case series, *n* = 28]

62. Tomlinson MW, Caruthers TJ, Whitty JE. Does delivery improve maternal condition in the respiratory-compromised gravida? *Obstet Gynecol* 1998; 91: 92–6. [III; case series, *n* = 10]

63. Cartin-Ceba R, Gajic O, Iyer V et al. Fetal outcomes of critically ill pregnant women admitted to the intensive care unit for non-obstetric causes. *Crit Care Med* 2008; 36: 2746–51. [II-2; cohort study, *n* = 153]

64. Warren J, Fromm RE, Orr RA et al. Guidelines for the inter- and intrahospital transport of critically ill patients. *Crit Care Med* 2004; 32: 256–62. [III; expert opinion]

65. American Hospital Association. AHA Hospital Statistics 2008. Chicago IL: Health Forum LLC, 2008. [Epidemiologic data]

66. Egol AB, Fromm RE, Guntupalli KK et al. Guidelines for ICU admission, discharge, and triage. *Crit Care Med* 1999; 27: 633–8. [III; expert opinion]

67. American College of Obstetricians and Gynecologists. Critical care in pregnancy. ACOG Practice Bulletin No. 100, 2009. Washington DC: ACOG 2009 Compendium of Selected Publications. [III; expert opinion]

68. Zeeman GG. Obstetric critical care: A blueprint for improved outcomes. *Crit Care Med* 2006; 34(Suppl.): S208–14. [III; review]

69. Pronovost PJ, Angus DC, Dorman T et al. Physician staffing patterns and clinical outcomes in critically ill patients: A systematic review. *JAMA* 2002; 288: 2151–62. [Systematic review, 26 observational studies]

70. Jenkins TM, Troiano NH, Graves CR et al. Mechanical ventilation in an obstetric population: Characteristics and delivery rates. *Am J Obstet Gynecol* 2003; 188: 549–52. [III; case series]

71. Plante LA. Mechanical ventilation in an obstetric population [letter]. *Am J Obstet Gynecol* 2003; 189: 1516. [III]

72. Chang SY, Multz AS, Hall JB. Critical care organization. *Crit Care Clin* 2005; 21: 43–53. [III; review]

73. Barba CA. The intensive care unit as an operating room. *Surg Clin N Am* 2000; 80: 957–73. [III; review]

74. Kelly JJ, Puyana JC, Callery MP et al. The feasibility and accuracy of diagnostic laparoscopy in the septic ICU patient. *Surg Endosc* 2000; 14: 617–21. [II-3; case series, $n = 16$]

75. Pecoraro AP, Cacchione RN, Sayad P et al. The routine use of laparoscopy in the intensive care unit. *Surg Endosc* 2001; 15: 638–41. [II-3; case series, $n = 11$]

76. Jaramillo EJ, Trevino JM, Berghoff KR et al. Bedside diagnostic laparoscopy in the intensive care unit: A 13-year experience. *JSLS* 2006; 10: 155–9. [III; case series, $n = 13$]

77. Charalambous C, Zipitis CS, Keenan DJ. Chest reexploration in the intensive care unit after cardiac surgery: A safe alternative to returning to the operating theater. *Ann Thorac Surg* 2006; 81: 191–4. [II-2; cohort study, $n = 240$]

78. Schreiber J, Nierhaus A, Vettorazzi E, Braune SA et al. Rescue bedside laparotomy in the intensive care unit in patients too unstable for transport to the operating room. *Crit Care* 2014; 18(3): R123. doi:10.1186/cc13925. [II-3; case series, $n = 41$]

79. Weber DJ, Sickbert-Bennett EE, Brown V et al. Comparison on hospitalwide surveillance and targeted intensive care unit surveillance of healthcare-associated infections. *Infect Control Hosp Epidemiol* 2007; 28: 1361–6. [III; surveillance data]

80. Edwards JR, Peterson KD, Andrus ML et al. National Healthcare Safety Network (NHSN) Report, data summary for 2006. *Am J Infect Control* 2007; 35: 290–301. [III; surveillance data]

81. American College of Obstetricians and Gynecologists. Coping with the stress of medical professional liability litigation. ACOG Committee Opinion No. 309, 2005. Washington DC: ACOG 2008 Compendium of Selected Publications. [Review]

82. Sperling D. Do pregnant women have (living) will? *J Health Care Law Policy* 2005; 8(2): 331–42. [III; review]

83. Bernard GR, Artigas A, Brigham KL et al. Report of the American-European consensus conference on ARDS: Definitions, mechanisms, relevant outcomes and clinical trial coordination. *Intensive Care Med* 1994; 20: 225–32. [III; expert opinion, consensus]

84. The ARDS Definition Task Force. Acute respiratory distress syndrome: The Berlin definition. *JAMA* 2012; 307: 2526–33. [Consensus guideline]

85. Mabie WC, Barton JR, Sibai BM. Adult respiratory distress syndrome in pregnancy. *Am J Obstet Gynecol* 1992; 167: 950–7. [III; case series, $n = 16$]

86. Callaghan WM, Creanga AA, Kuklina EV. Severe maternal morbidity among delivery and postpartum hospitalizations in the United States. *Obstet Gynecol* 2012; 120: 1029–36. [II-2]

87. Joseph KS, Liu S, Rouleau J, Kirby RS et al., for the Maternal Health Study Group of the Canadian Perinatal Surveillance System. Severe maternal morbidity in Canada, 2003 to 2007: Surveillance using routing hospitalization data and ICD-10CA codes. *J Obstet Gynaecol Can* 2010; 32: 837–46. [Administrative data set, 1.3 million records]

88. Creanga AA, Johnson TF, Graitcer SB et al. Severity of 2009 pandemic influenza A (H1N1) virus infection in pregnant women. *Obstet Gynecol* 2010; 115: 717–26. [II-3; case series, $n = 62$]

89. Davies AR, Jones D, Bailey M et al., for the Australia and New Zealand Extracorporeal Membrane Oxygenation (ANZ ECMO) Influenza Investigators. Extracorporeal membrane oxygenation for 2009 influenza A (H1N1) acute respiratory distress syndrome. *JAMA* 2009; 302: 1888–95. [II-3; case series, $n = 68$]

90. Smith JL, Thomas F, Orne JF et al. Adult respiratory distress syndrome during pregnancy and the puerperium. *West Med J* 1990; 153: 508–10. [II-3; case series, $n = 14$]

91. Perry KG, Martin RW, Blake PG et al. Maternal mortality associated with adult respiratory distress syndrome. *South Med J* 1998; 91: 441–5. [II-3; case series, $n = 41$]

92. Vasquez DN, Estenssoro E, Canales HS et al. Clinical characteristics and outcomes of obstetric patients requiring ICU admission. *Chest* 2007; 131: 718–24. [II-3; cohort study, $n = 161$]

93. Rubenfeld GD, Caldwell E, Peabody E et al. Incidence and outcomes of acute lung injury. *N Engl J Med* 2005; 353: 1685–93. [II-2; cohort study, $n = 1113$]

94. Nicolaides KH, Economides DL, Soothill PW. Blood gases, pH, and lactate in appropriate- and small-for-gestational-age fetuses. *Am J Obstet Gynecol* 1989; 161: 996–1001. [II-3; cross-sectional study, $n = 404$]

95. Erkkola R, Pirhonen J, Polvi H. The fetal cardiovascular function in chronic placental insufficiency is different from experimental hypoxia. *Ann Chir Gynaecol Suppl* 1994; 208: 76–9. [III; experimental trial, $n = 10$]

96. The Acute Respiratory Distress Syndrome Network (ARDSNet). Ventilation with lower tidal volumes as compared with traditional tidal volumes for acute lung injury and the acute respiratory distress syndrome. *N Engl J Med* 2000; 342: 1301–8. [I; RCT, $n = 861$]

97. Fraser D, Jensen D, Wolfe LA et al. Fetal heart rate response to maternal hypocapnia and hypercapnia in late gestation. *J Obstet Gynaecol Can* 2008; 30(4): 312–6. [III; experimental trial, $n = 35$]

98. Siddiqi AK, Gouda H, Multz AS et al. Ventilator strategy for status asthmaticus in pregnancy: A case-based review. *J Asthma* 2005; 42: 159–62. [II-3; case series, $n = 2$]

99. Elsayegh D, Shapiro JM. Management of the obstetric patient with status asthmaticus. *J Intensive Care Med* 2008; 23(6): 396–402. [II-3; case series, $n = 5$]

100. Hirani A, Marik PE, Plante LA. Airway pressure release ventilation in pregnant patients with acute respiratory distress syndrome: A novel strategy. *Respir Care* 2009; 54: 1405–9. [II-3; case series, $n = 2$]

101. Grisaru-Granovsky S, Ioscovich A, Hersch M et al. Temporizing treatment for the respiratory-compromised gravida: An observational study of maternal and neonatal outcome. *Int J Obstet Anesthesia* 2007; 16: 261–4. [II-3; case series, $n = 3$]

102. Knight M, Kenyon S, Brocklehurst P, Neilson J, Shakespeare J, Kurinczuk JJ (Eds.) on behalf of MBRRACE-UK. Saving Lives, Improving Mothers' Care—Lessons learned to inform future maternity care from the UK and Ireland Confidential Enquiries into Maternal Deaths and Morbidity 2009–12. Oxford: National Perinatal Epidemiology Unit, University of Oxford, 2014. [II-3]

103. Singer M, Deutschman CJ, Seymour CW, Shankar-Hari M et al., for the Sepsis Definitions Task Force. The Third International Consensus Definitions for Sepsis and Septic Shock (Sepsis-3). *JAMA* 2016; 315(8): 801–10.

104. Seymour CW, Liu VX, Iwashyna TJ, Brunkhorst FM et al. Assessment of clinical criteria for sepsis. For the Third International Consensus Definitions for Sepsis and Septic Shock (Sepsis-3). *JAMA* 2016; 315(8): 762–74.

105. Shankar-Hari M, Phillips GS, Levey MM, Seymour CW et al., for the Sepsis Definitions Task Force. Developing a new definition and assessing new clinical criteria for septic shock. For the Third International Consensus Definitions for Sepsis and Septic Shock (Sepsis-3). *JAMA* 2016; 315(8): 775–87.

106. Acosta CD, Kurinczuk JJ, Lucas DN, Tuffnell DJ, Sellers S, Knight M, on behalf of the United Kingdom Obstetric Surveillance System. Severe maternal sepsis in the UK, 2011–2012: A national case-control study. *PLoS Med* 2014; 11(7): e1001672. doi:10.1371/journal.pmed.1001672. [II-3, case control, *n* = 365]

107. Bauer ME, Bateman BT, Bauer ST, Shanks AM, Mhyre JM. Maternal sepsis mortality and morbidity during hospitalization for delivery: Temporal trends and independent associations for severe sepsis. *Anesth Analg* 2013; 117: 944–50. [II-3, case series, *n* = 22]

108. Al-Ostad G, Kezouh A, Spence AR, Abenhaim HA. Incidence and risk factors of sepsis mortality in labor, delivery and after birth: Population-based study in the USA. *J Obstet Gynaecol Res* 2015; 41: 1201–6. [II-2, cohort study, *n* = 5 million]

109. Acosta CD, Knight M, Lee HC, Kurinczuk JJ, Gould JB, Lyndon A. The continuum of maternal sepsis severity: Incidence and risk factors in a population-based cohort study. *PLoS ONE* 2013; 8(7): e67175. doi:10.1371/journal.pone.0067175. [II-2, cohort study, *n* = 1.6 million]

110. Kramer HMC, Schutte JM, Zwart JJ, Schuitemaker NEW, Steegers EAP, van Roosmalen J. Maternal mortality and severe morbidity from sepsis in the Netherlands. *Acta Obstet Gynecol* 2009; 88: 647–53. [II-2, cohort, *n* = 78]

111. Stevenson EK, Rubenstein AR, Radin GT, Soylemez Wiener R, Walkey AJ. Two decades of mortality trends among patients with severe sepsis: A comparative meta-analysis. *Crit Care Med* 2014; 42: 625–31. [Ia, meta-analysis, 36 trials]

112. Finkielman JD, De Feo FD, Heller PG et al. The clinical course of patients with septic abortion admitted to an intensive care unit. *Intensive Care Med* 2004; 30: 1097–102. [II-3; case series, *n* = 63]

113. Albright CM, Ali TN, Lopes V, Rouse DJ, Anderson BL. The Sepsis in Obstetrics Score: A model to identify risk of morbidity from sepsis in pregnancy. *Am J Obstet Gynecol* 2014; 211(1): 39.e1–8. [Scoring system drawn from single-center cohort]

114. Bauer ME, Lorenz RP, Bauer ST, Rao S, Anderson FWJ. Maternal deaths due to sepsis in the state of Michigan, 1999–2006. *Obstet Gynecol* 2015; 126: 747–52. [III]

115. Gaieski DF, Mikkelsen ME, Band RA, Pines JM et al. Impact of time to antibiotics on survival in patients with severe sepsis or septic shock in whom early goal-directed therapy was initiated in the emergency department. *Crit Care Med* 2010; 38: 1045–53. [II-2, cohort, *n* = 261]

116. Dellinger RP, Levy MM, Rhodes A, Annane D et al., for the Surviving Sepsis Campaign Guidelines Committee. Surviving Sepsis Campaign: International guidelines for management of severe sepsis and septic shock: 2012. *Crit Care Med* 2013; 41: 580–637. [Guideline]

117. Lefrant JY, Muller L, Raillard A et al. Reduction of the severe sepsis or septic shock associated mortality by reinforcement of the recommendations bundle: A multicenter study. *Ann Fr Anesth Reanim* 2010; 29: 621–8. [II-3; time series, *n* = 445]

118. Kumar A, Roberts D, Wood KE, Light B et al. Duration of hypotension before initiation of effective antimicrobial therapy is the critical determinant of survival in human septic shock. *Crit Care Med* 2006; 34: 1589–96.

119. Gaieski DF, Mikkelsen ME, Band RA, Pines JM et al. Impact of time to antibiotics on survival in patients with severe sepsis or septic shock in whom early goal-directed therapy was initiated in the emergency department. *Crit Care Med* 2010; 38: 1045–53.

120. Ferrer R, Martin-Loeches I, Phillips G, Osborn TM et al. Empiric antibiotic treatment reduces mortality in severe sepsis and septic shock from the first hour: Results from a guideline-based performance improvement program. *Crit Care Med* 2014; 42: 1749–55.

121. Kankuri E, Kurki T, Hiilesma V. Incidence, treatment and outcome of peripartum sepsis. *Acta Obstet Gynecol Scand* 2003; 82: 730–5. [II-2; cohort study]

122. Zhou P, Qian Y, Xu J et al. Occurrence of congenital syphilis after maternal treatment with azithromycin during pregnancy. *Sex Transm Dis* 2007; 34: 472–4. [II-3; case series, *n* = 5]

123. Mabie WC, Barton JR, Sibai BM. Septic shock in pregnancy. *Obstet Gynecol* 1997; 90(4 Pt. 1): 553–61. [II-3; case series, *n* = 18]

124. Miyazaki K, Furuhashi M, Matsuo K et al. Impact of subclinical chorioamnionitis on maternal and neonatal outcomes. *Acta Obstet Gynecol Scand* 2007; 86: 191–7. [II-2; cohort study, *n* = 100]

125. Rivers E, Nguyen B, Havstad S et al. Early goal-directed therapy in the treatment of sepsis and septic shock. *N Engl J Med* 2001; 345: 1368–77. [I; RCT, *n* = 263]

126. Guinn DA, Abel DE, Tomlinson MW. Early goal directed therapy for sepsis during pregnancy. *Obstet Gynecol* 2007; 34: 459–79. [III; review]

127. Barton JR, Sibai BM. Severe sepsis and septic shock in pregnancy. *Obstet Gynecol* 2012; 120: 689–706.

128. Pacheco LD, Saade GR, Hankins GDV. Severe sepsis during pregnancy. *Clinical Obstet Gynecol* 2014; 57: 827–34.

129. Yealy DM, Kellum JA, Huang DT, Barnato AE et al., for the ProCESS Investigators. A randomized trial of protocol-based care for early septic shock. *NEJM* 2014; 370: 1683–93.

130. Peake SL, Delaney A, Bailey M, Bellomo R et al., for the ARISE Investigators and the ANZICS Clinical Trials Group. *NEJM* 2014; 371: 1496–1506.

131. Mouncey PR, Osborn TM, Power S, Harrison DA et al, for the ProMISe Trial Investigators. Trial of early, goal-directed resuscitation for septic shock. *NEJM* 2015; 372: 1301–11.

132. Clark SL, Cotton DB, Lee W et al. Central hemodynamic assessment of normal term pregnancy. *Am J Obstet Gynecol* 1989; 161: 1439–42. [II-3; cross-sectional study, *n* = 10]

133. Marik P, Bellomo R. A rational approach to fluid therapy in sepsis. *Br J Anaesthesia* 2016; 116(3): 339–49.

134. Lee CWC, Kory PD, Arntfield RT. Development of a fluid resuscitation protocol using inferior vena cava and lung ultrasound. *J Crit Care* 2016; 31: 96–100.

135. Monnet X, Marik P, Teboul J-L. Passive leg raising for predicting fluid responsiveness: A systematic review and meta-analysis. *Intens Care Med* 2016 Jan 29 [Epub ahead of print]. doi:10.1007/s00134-015-4134-1.

136. Macedo ML, Luminoso D, Savvidou MD et al. Maternal wave reflections and arterial stiffness in normal pregnancy as assessed by applanation tonometry. *Hypertension* 2008; 51: 1047–51. [II-3; cross-sectional study, *n* = 193]

137. Ngan Kee WD, Lee SWY, Ng FF, Tan PE, Khaw KS. Randomized double-blinded comparison of norepinephrine and phenylephrine for maintenance of blood pressure during spinal anesthesia for cesarean delivery. *Anesthesiology* 2015; 122: 736–45. [I, RCT, *n* = 104]

138. Mintzer BH, Johnson RF, Paschall RL et al. The diverse effects of vasopressors on the fetoplacental circulation of the perfused human placenta. *Anesth Analg* 2010; 110: 857–62. [II-1; controlled trial]

139. Fishburne JI, Meis PJ, Urban RB et al. Vascular and uterine responses to dobutamine and dopamine in the gravid ewe. *Am J Obstet Gynecol* 1980; 137: 944–52. [III; experimental trial, *n* = 6]

140. Hinton L, Locock L, Knight M. Maternal critical care: What can we learn from patient experience? A qualitative study. *BMJ Open* 2015; 5: e006676. doi:10.1136/bmjopen-2014-006676. [III, qualitative; *n* = 46]

41

Amniotic fluid embolism

Antonio F. Saad and Luis D. Pacheco

KEY POINTS

- Amniotic fluid embolism (AFE) classically presents as a triad of **sudden hypoxia, hypotension, and coagulopathy**.
- Management of AFE is mainly supportive.
- In the case of a viable pregnancy, immediate delivery is advised.
- Early high-quality cardiopulmonary resuscitation and adherence to advanced cardiac life support guidelines are recommended.
- The initial phase is defined by right ventricular failure physiology. Bedside transthoracic echocardiography is a valuable tool in identifying this phase early.
- Later phase is predominated by left ventricular failure, and treatment should be tailored accordingly.
- Early management of AFE-related coagulopathy should be initiated as soon as possible with transfusion of blood products and with adjuvant agents.
- A multidisciplinary team of maternal-fetal medicine physicians, intensivists, and anesthesiologists should be involved in the management of such critically ill patients.

Background

Amniotic fluid embolism (AFE) is a rare, often lethal disease that occurs in pregnancy or in the puerperium period. In the developed world, it is one of the most common etiologies of maternal mortality. It is estimated that up to 10% of maternal deaths are caused by AFE [1]. According to a recent United States national registry review of around 1.5 million deliveries, AFE, second only to preeclampsia, was the most common disease leading to maternal death [2]. Historically, AFE patients have a poor prognosis. Based on a 1995 national registry, mortality rate after an AFE event was reported to be 61% and neurological intact maternal survival rate to be only 15% [3]. Recent data has reported better outcomes with maternal mortality rates as low as 26% and neurological intact survival rates up to 93% [4,5]. Perinatal mortality has been described to be as high as 25%.

Incidence

The incidence of AFE ranges between 1/8000 and 1/80,000 [3]. This large discrepancy can be explained by differences in study methodology and by unclear or inconsistent definitions of AFE. Absence of validated case identification that excludes false positives can lead to overestimation and even doubling of its incidence [6]. In population analysis estimates or administrative databases that use case validation, the description of disease outcomes and incidence are more accurate because fewer false positives (non-AFE cases have better outcomes) are included. By accounting for false positive cases, the true incidence of AFE can be elucidated [6,7].

Emphasis on developing a clear case definition and diagnostic criteria of AFE is of utmost importance.

Pathophysiology

The pathophysiology of AFE remains to be elucidated. Historically, it was thought to occur secondary to travelling of acellular fragments and squamous cells from the amniotic fluid to the pulmonary system with vessel obstruction leading to acute right ventricular failure and eventually to death. Examples of inciting factors that promote the travelling of amniotic fluid into the maternal side include pelvic lacerations, placental abruption, and cesarean section. **The embolism hypothesis has been recently discredited by studies that failed to reproduce the syndrome after direct injection of amniotic fluid into the pulmonary vascular space [3,8,9]** in animal models. Moreover, despite fetal or amniotic-derived tissue being found in the pulmonary vascular system of pregnant women, patients did not develop AFE [10]. Because the presence of these histologic landmarks are neither sensitive nor specific and are not necessary for the development of AFE, genetic predisposition may explain why some women develop the syndrome of AFE and others do not.

Recently AFE has been linked to a **massive inflammatory response secondary to activation of maternal immunity by fetal antigens/epitopes**. Amniotic fluid consists of a milieu rich in potent mediators that can explain the different clinical manifestations of AFE. Examples include platelet activator factor, cytokines, bradykinin, histamine, arachidonic acid, leukotrienes, prostaglandins, tissue factor, and endothelin [11,12].

Endothelin has been suggested as a major mediator in the pathogenesis of AFE. It is a potent constrictor that can cause **prominent pulmonary vascular spasm** and acute elevation of the pulmonary vascular resistances. Within the first minutes of AFE (**first phase**), the resulting **surge in afterload leads to acute core pulmonale** in the absence of anatomical occlusion of the pulmonary vasculature [13]. Two major detrimental events result from acute right ventricular failure and chamber dilation: **massive ventricular ischemia from compressive occlusion of the feeding right coronary vessels within the myocardium, leading to a right ventricular infarction, and displacement of the inter-ventricular septum toward the left ventricle, decreasing left ventricular preload and cardiac output secondary to diastolic dysfunction.**

Left ventricular failure, cardiogenic pulmonary edema, and hypotension define the second phase of the disease. During this time, the mainstream of management is comprised of vasopressors and inotropes [14]. The observed left ventricular dysfunction is due to a amalgamation of cardiac stunning from hypoxia that occurred in the first phase of the disease and to cytokine-induced myocardial depression from inflammatory proteins, such as tumor necrosis factor-α, nitric oxide, platelet activating factor, and interleukin 1 [15]. The physiologic consequence of decreased left heart function is cardiogenic pulmonary edema.

Disseminated intravascular coagulation (DIC) is another feature of AFE, occurring in up to 83% of reported cases [3]. Amniotic fluid tissue factor binds to maternal serum factor VII activating the extrinsic pathway of the clotting cascade. Amniotic fluid alone has also been reported to directly activate factor X and platelets. Other important stimulators of the clotting cascade include major inflammatory proteins from tissue factor released from activated monocytes and neutrophils. DIC in AFE is mainly a consumptive coagulopathy manifested as hemorrhage.

For those that survive the first two phases, a third phase of AFE ensues. It is characterized by slow and delayed improvement in left ventricular function secondary to prolonged severe inflammation coupled with the need for prolonged critical care (risk factor for nosocomial infections such as ventilator-associated pneumonia, line bacteremia, urinary tract infections, sinusitis) and by distributive shock with inflammation induced noncardiogenic pulmonary edema [14].

Some have suggested a common link between AFE and anaphylaxis [3]. In addition, up to 41% of patients with AFE have reported previous history of atopy [3]. The proposed similarity is justified because all three conditions, AFE, anaphylaxis, and sepsis, involve significant inflammatory responses. This relationship has been challenged as severe biventricular heart failure and profound coagulopathy, the defining pillars of AFE, are not found in anaphylaxis.

Risk Factors for Amniotic Fluid Embolus

There are modifiable and nonmodifiable risk factors for AFE [13]. Modifiable risk factors include medical induction of labor, instrumental vaginal delivery (forceps and vacuum-assisted deliveries), cervical lacerations, uterine rupture, and cesarean section. Nonmodifiable risk factors include advanced maternal age (more than 30 years old), African American race, eclampsia, polyhydramnios, male fetus, placenta previa, placental abruption, and multiple pregnancies [6,7,16–18].

The association between AFE and oxytocin administration or prolonged protracted labor has been inconsistent [3]. The common use of oxytocin in contrast to the paucity of AFE makes this causative link extremely unlikely [19]. Another misconception is that uterine tone anomalies (hypo- or hypertonous) may play a role in AFE development; instead, it appears that uterine hypoperfusion due to maternal hypoxia and shock with massive adrenergic surge is responsible for the tone anomalies [3].

Currently, evidence is lacking to determine if cesarean or operative vaginal deliveries are associated with AFE. Most publications lack information on the temporal relationship between operative delivery and AFE. It is unclear if the interventions indeed preceded AFE events or they were performed after the AFE to improve fetal outcomes [6].

Despite identifiable risk factors, AFE remains unpredictable and unpreventable. The inability for the described risk factors to predict AFE may be secondary to their nonspecificity along with the rarity of the disease. Modifying obstetrical practice for the sole purpose to prevent AFE is not recommended.

DIAGNOSIS
Clinical Presentation of Amniotic Fluid Embolism

Based on the national registry data, AFE cases have occurred 70% during labor, 11% after a vaginal delivery, and 19% during a cesarean delivery [3].

AFE classically presents as a triad of sudden hypoxia, hypotension, and coagulopathy. It seldom happens in the second or third trimester or at the time of amniocentesis or pregnancy termination [20]. It may be preceded by a period of anxiety, altered mental status, agitation, and sensation of "doom" [21]. AFE should be considered in the differential workup in any woman that is pregnant or recently delivered with acute cardiovascular collapse, seizures, severe respiratory difficulty/arrest, or coagulopathy unexplained by other etiologies.

Arterial pulmonary vasculature constriction leading to ventilation perfusion mismatch and right ventricular heart failure account for the observed hypoxia. Decreased arterial pressure results from right ventricular dilation and impingement of the interventricular septum into the left ventricular chamber, decreasing cavity size and end-diastolic volume, ultimately diminishing cardiac output. The subsequent hypoxemia increases the hazard of seizures, left heart failure, and uterine atony [14].

Cardiac arrest may occur suddenly, with asystole, ventricular fibrillation, pulseless electrical activity (PEA), or pulseless ventricular tachycardia. If arrest occurs while pregnant, common fetal heart tracings include fetal tachycardia, decelerations, loss of variability, bradycardia, and terminal decelerations.

DIC is a common finding in up to 83% of AFE cases [3]. It is secondary to consumptive activation of the clotting cascade by either amniotic fluid constituents (e.g., tissue factor) or by the systemic inflammatory response that is triggered during the event. Coagulopathy can be the only manifestation in AFE, but it can also manifest with unstable hemodynamics or even after completion of initial resuscitative maneuvers [22–24]. AFE patients with DIC are at risk for the following serious hemorrhagic complications: venipuncture bleeding, gastrointestinal hemorrhage, hematuria, pelvic laceration bleeding, and uterine bleeding.

Differential Diagnosis of AFE

Despite being long, one should narrow the differential diagnosis to clinically relevant diseases that have specific treatment strategies. More importantly, one should initiate treatment for suspected AFE even before an exact diagnosis is determined. This is especially true because management mainly involves life-supporting interventions (i.e., cardiorespiratory resuscitation). Common medical conditions that need to be considered when ruling out AFE include **myocardial infarction, thromboembolism, high spinal anesthesia, air embolism, eclampsia, and anaphylactic shock**.

Bedside echocardiography with evidence of right ventricular dysfunction favors the diagnosis of AFE over anaphylaxis and most of the other conditions that mimic AFE.

Patients with risk factors, such as diabetes, smoking, obesity, advanced maternal age, chronic hypertension, dyslipidemia, and previous history of coronary artery disease, should be ruled out for acute myocardial infarction. Workup should include **cardiac troponins** and a **12-lead electrocardiograph** as soon as possible. A bedside echocardiograph is a useful tool in assisting in the diagnosis of cardiogenic shock secondary to myocardial ischemia or to rare causes, such as a peripartum dilated cardiomyopathy [25].

Pulmonary embolism from a pelvic clot needs to be considered high on the differential list. Findings of acute right ventricular dilation and hypocontractility in a bedside transthoracic echocardiograph during the acute event may be helpful. **Once the patient is stabilized, confirmatory testing, such as a computed tomography angiography or ventilation perfusion scan, should be considered.** The possibility of thromboembolism is unlikely in cases with profuse bleeding.

In the absence of cardiac decompensation and hemorrhage, high spinal anesthesia leading to apnea should be considered in the differential diagnosis. Local anesthetic toxicity secondary to inadvertent intravascular injection can manifest by seizures and cardiovascular collapse [26]. Timing between injection and onset of symptoms is of utmost importance. If suspicion is high, cardiopulmonary resuscitation should be initiated as soon as possible, and administration of intravenous lipids (20% Intralipid) should be started [27].

Acute cardiorespiratory compromise can also be seen with air embolism. The initial management of this condition is identical to that of AFE. In addition, normobaric 100% oxygen should be administered if highly suspected. The patient should also be placed in the left lateral decubitus position to avoid air from travelling to the pulmonary vasculature. If a central venous catheter is in place, blood aspiration of air bubbles can be attempted. Hyperbaric oxygen therapy should be used in cases of arterial air embolism.

In the absence of profound coagulopathy and cardiopulmonary decompensation, eclampsia should be high in the differential diagnosis of patients presenting with new onset of seizures.

Anaphylactic shock is a known imitator of AFE, and it should be considered when AFE is suspected. Important clues that favor anaphylaxis versus AFE include development of urticarial rash, laryngospasm, and bronchospasm. The latter is only present in 15% of cases of AFE. Coagulopathy and cardiac dysfunction are seldom seen in anaphylaxis. The observed hypotension is secondary to vasodilation and increased vascular permeability rather than ventricular failure. Treatment of anaphylactic shock involves prompt administration of epinephrine, steroids, and inhaled bronchodilators.

Diagnostic Laboratory Testing

AFE is not diagnosed based on a specific laboratory test but rather based on exclusion. Historically, the presence of acellular fetal debris or fetal squamous cells in the maternal circulation was believed to be pathognomonic of the disease. This has been challenged because the same pathologic findings have been described in normal asymptomatic pregnant women and are not always present in women with AFE [10,28].

Recent data has proposed a novel serum biomarker for AFE: insulin like growth factor binding protein 1 (IGFBP-1) [29]. Further evidence is needed before it reaches the confirmatory stage.

Investigators have proposed renaming AFE to "anaphylactoid reaction of pregnancy" due to similarities in inflammatory biomarkers between anaphylaxis and AFE [3]. Of note, these biomarkers are not exclusive to either disease and are found in other nonspecific inflammatory responses. Although in anaphylaxis the enzyme serum tryptase is commonly elevated, this is not found in cases with AFE and cannot be used to rebut or confirm diagnosis [30–32]. Moreover,

this evidence refutes the hypothesis that AFE and anaphylaxis have similar pathogenesis [33].

Activation of the complement pathway has also been shown in AFE [33]. Confirmation of the disease is not advised based on low serum complement levels due to poor sensitivity and specificity.

In summary, diagnosis of AFE is mainly based in clinical presentation, and there is no specific confirmatory laboratory testing.

Management of Cardiac Arrest

The main basis of initial management of cardiac arrest is supportive care with standard resuscitative efforts; immediate cardiopulmonary resuscitation (**CPR**) should be initiated as soon as possible. Because most events occur inpatient and are witnessed, blood oxygen content is initially normal; hence, high-quality chest compressions are recommended before administration of rescue breathing [34].

Chest compressions should be performed using a firm black board, the patient in a supine position, hands in center of chest (as in nonpregnant patient), compressions at a rate of at least 100 per minute at a depth of at least 2 in (5 cm), allowing full recoil before the next compression with minimal interruptions and at a compression–ventilation ratio of 30:2 [35]. If the patient is undelivered, continuous manual left uterine displacement should be implemented, with which the uterus is lifted up and displaced leftward off the maternal major vessels [35]. The use of vasopressors, anti-arrhythmics, and defibrillating doses should be no different than those utilized in nonpregnant individuals. There is no evidence that fetal monitors will result in electrical arcing; defibrillation may be performed with the monitors in place.

If the patient has a viable pregnancy at the time of the arrest, expeditious operative assisted vaginal delivery (forceps or vacuum) is recommended when the cervix is dilated and fetal head is at low station. If vaginal delivery is not possible and return of spontaneous circulation (ROSC) has not been achieved despite initial resuscitative interventions, a **perimortem cesarean delivery (PMCD)** should be considered.

The classical **indication for PMCD is failure to achieve ROSC after 4 minutes of CPR** [35]. In addition to obvious fetal benefits of delivering the fetus, improving chances of ROSC after CPR can be increased by relief of aortocaval compression from evacuation of the uterus [36]. With the goals of rapid fetus delivery and low bleeding complications, techniques such as a vertical skin incision and a classical cesarean are recommended by some.

Waiting for the full 4 minutes to initiate PMCD is not an absolute rule; patient care should be individualized based on fetal indications versus maternal well-being.

Post cardiac arrest management is of paramount importance [37]. After ROSC, patients are often hemodynamically unstable, and management is mainly based on fluids, vasopressors, and inotropes. Mean arterial blood pressure of 65 mmHg should be maintained [37]. To avoid ischemia–reperfusion injury, fever should be avoided and aggressively treated. Hyperoxia should be avoided for the same reason, and administration of 100% oxygen to patients after survival of cardiac arrest is not recommended. This is achieved by weaning the inspired fraction of oxygen to sustain pulse oxymetry values of 94%–98% [38]. As the standard of care in any critical ill patient, serum glucose levels should be maintained between 140 and 180 mg/dL with implementation of an insulin drip if needed.

Mild therapeutic hypothermia (TH) has been shown to benefit comatose adult nonpregnant survivors after outpatient cardiac arrest. It consists of bringing down the patient's body temperature to 32°C to 34°C (89.6°F–93.2°F) for 12 to 24 hours. The American Heart Association has recommended temperature management, and it has become the standard of care in this patient population [37,39]. A recent clinical trial has shown no difference in outcomes when comparing targeted temperatures of 33°C versus 36°C in patients that achieved ROSC after cardiac arrest [40]. Current guidelines recommend maintaining temperature between 33°C and 36°C after cardiac arrest.

Evidence on TH during pregnancy is scant and based on case reports, and its application should be considered on an individual basis [41,42]. Most survivors of AFE will not be pregnant anymore after successful resuscitation. One of the major adverse effects or complications of TH is the risk of hemorrhage. TH should be considered in patients whose bleeding risk is low. It is recommended to target a temperature of 36°C rather than lower temperatures to decrease the risk of bleeding.

Resuscitative efforts of suspected AFE are mainly supportive and focus on rapid maternal hemodynamic stabilization. A multidisciplinary team of maternal-fetal medicine and intensive care specialists should be involved in the management of these critically ill survivors. When possible, a transthoracic and/or transesophageal echocardiography should be performed. Pertinent findings include a severely dilated hypokinetic right ventricle with left sided deviation of the inter-ventricular septum. During the initial phase of right ventricular failure, acidosis, hypercapnia, and hypoxia should be avoided as they worsen the condition by increasing pulmonary vascular resistances [13]. Dobutamine and milrinone are the drugs of choice for right ventricular heart failure because, along with being ionotropes, they also are pulmonary vasodilators. Other specific agents that decrease the pulmonary vascular resistances include sildenafil, inhaled or intravenous prostacyclin, and inhaled nitric oxide. Common vasopressors used to treat hypotension include norepinephrine or vasopressin [43]. Table 41.1 contains commonly used dosages of the described agents.

Table 41.1   Common Drugs Used in Cases of Acute Right Ventricular Failure

Agent	Mechanism of Action	Contraindication/Adverse Effects	Dose
Sildenafil	Selective inhibitor of cGMP-phosphodiesterase type 5 (PDE5); vasodilator by relaxing the vascular smooth muscle. Selective pulmonary vasodilator in patients with pulmonary hypertension.	Hypotension risk in patients with severe aortic stenosis, left ventricular outflow tract obstruction, concomitant nitrates, or hypovolaemia.	20 mg tid PO or through nasogastric/orogastric tube
Dobutamine	Direct beta2-receptor agonist with chronotropic, arrhythmogenic, and vasodilative effects.	Avoid in idiopathic hypertrophic subaortic stenosis. Hypersensitivity Higher doses may compromise right ventricular filling time due to tachycardia.	2.5–5.0 micrograms/kg/minute
Milrinone	Selective inhibitor of peak III cAMP phosphodiesterase isozyme in cardiac and vascular smooth muscle.	Hypersensitivity Systemic hypotension	0.25–0.75 micrograms/kg/minute
Inhaled nitric oxide	Stimulates guanylate cyclase leading to increase in cGMP and protein phosphorylation leading to selective pulmonary vasodilator of those areas of the lung being ventilated.	Methemoglobinemia	5–40 ppm (parts per million). Follow methemoglobin levels every 6 hours and avoid abrupt discontinuation.
Inhaled prostacyclin	Inhibits platelet activation. Selective pulmonary vasodilator of those areas of the lung being ventilated. Anti-inflammatory properties.	Hypersensitivity	10–50 nanograms/kg/minute
Intravenous prostacyclin	Inhibits platelet activation. Nonselective pulmonary vasodilator	Avoid in severe left ventricular systolic dysfunction. Hypersensitivity Systemic hypotension Nausea/vomiting Headache Jaw pain Diarrhea	Start at 1–2 nanograms/kg/minute through a central line and titrate to desired effect.
Norepinephrine	Peripheral vasoconstrictor (alpha-adrenergic action) and inotropic stimulator of the heart and dilator of coronary arteries (beta-adrenergic action). Alpha action is greater than beta action.	None	0.05–3.3 micrograms/kg/minute
Vasopressin	Potent analog of the posterior pituitary hormone antidiuretic hormone. Effects are through the V1 vascular receptors.	Hypersensitivity Hyponatremia and water retention.	0.03–0.06 units/minute

In the setting of a massively dilated right ventricle (acute core pulmonale), fluid resuscitation should be administered judiciously. Fluid overload can lead to overdistention of the right ventricular chamber, raising the risk of a right-sided myocardial infarction and to left inter-ventricular septum shift, leading to left ventricular chamber obliteration, ultimately compromising left ventricular cardiac output.

Within hours of initial presentation, right ventricular dysfunction starts to recover, and left ventricular dysfunction predominates with resulting cardiogenic pulmonary edema [21]. Noninvasive mechanical ventilation or endotracheal intubation should be considered early in patients who are not intubated. The mainstay of therapy consists of fluid restriction, diuretics (in normotensive patients), vasopressors in cases of hypotension, and inotropes (dobutamine or milrinone) with the aim of maintaining coronary perfusion and optimizing left ventricular contractility. Persistent pulmonary congestion despite diuretic therapy may necessitate renal replacement therapy for fluid removal.

The role of steroids in the management of AFE remains controversial and is not indicated.

Prolonged care in the intensive care unit and persistent severe inflammation predispose survivors to develop nosocomial infections and distributive shock with noncardiogenic pulmonary edema secondary to endothelial injury from severe sepsis [14]. Figure 41.1 summarizes the main points in the management of AFE.

Management of Coagulopathy Associated with Amniotic Fluid Embolism

DIC is often present in AFE cases; its onset is variable, and it can occur in early or late phases of the syndrome. Therapy involves a medical and surgical approach.

Medical management involves administration of blood products to maintain a platelet count above 50,000/mm^3 to correct for prolonged activated partial thromboplastin time (aPTT), international normalized ratio (INR), and low fibrinogen levels (less than 150–200 mg/dL). In cases of massive hemorrhage, massive transfusion of blood products should be administered as soon as possible and not delayed just for the sake of waiting for laboratory results. Early aggressive hemostatic resuscitation with a 1:1:1 ratio of packed red blood cells, fresh-frozen plasma, and platelets is likely to result in improved outcomes [44]. Although administration of recombinant activated factor VII has been described in cases of AFE [45–47], some authors believe that excessive diffuse thrombosis and multiorgan failure can occur secondary to the combination of recombinant activated factor VII and elevated levels of tissue factor present in AFE. Hence, it is recommended to consider using this agent only as a last resort in cases of intractable hemorrhage despite massive blood component replacement and surgical interventions [46].

Amniotic fluid has been shown to contain both plasminogen activators and plasminogen activator inhibitors [48]. Hyperfibrinolysis has been involved in AFE-related coagulopathy and antifibrinolytics, such as tranexamic acid or epsilon amino caproic acid, and bedside thromboelastography should be considered in the management of AFE [49].

In the United States, most of the fibrinogen replacement is done in the form of cryoprecipitates (2 g of fibrinogen are found in 100 cc of cryoprecipitate). Each unit of cryoprecipitate will correct the serum fibrinogen by 10 mg/dL. An adult will require a usual dose of 10 units for expected fibrinogen correction of 100 mg/dL. Just like fresh frozen plasma, cryoprecipitate needs to be thawed before its use and carries the risk for virus transmission. Although not widely available in the United States, fibrinogen concentrates have emerged as another alternative to replenish serum fibrinogen levels without the risk of viral transmission or transfusion reactions like transfusion related acute lung injury (TRALI). It is stored at room temperature and available for immediate use. Fibrinogen concentrates contains high concentrations of fibrinogen (100 mL contains 2 g of fibrinogen).

Uterine atony, when present, should be managed aggressively with the use of uterotonics such as oxytocin, ergot derivatives, and prostaglandins [50]. If medical therapy fails, uterine tamponade with the use of packing or commercially available intrauterine balloons should be considered. Surgical approaches, such as bilateral uterine artery ligation, B-Lynch stitch, or even a hysterectomy, may be needed in extreme cases of uterine atony.

After vaginal delivery, thorough assessment of vaginal canal lacerations as potential sources of bleeding is strongly recommended. For patients undergoing a cesarean section with diffuse bleeding not amenable to surgical control, damage control surgery should be considered with packing the pelvis and transfer to the intensive care unit for further medical therapy with delayed closure/abdominal exploration.

PROGNOSIS OF PATIENTS WHO SURVIVE AN AFE EVENT

Prognosis AFE is very poor with mortality rates up to 61% and with only 15% ending up with intact neurologic status [3]. In-hospital cardiac arrest patients have an overall survival of 15%–20% [51]. Due to improvement in the health care system, **better outcomes have been reported with maternal mortality rates down to 26% and 93% of survivors neurologically intact [4,5]. Perinatal mortality has been reported to be as high as 25%.** Of note, when discussing outcomes of cases with suspected AFE, one should account for patients' characteristics because these can skew the data to either better or worse survival/mortality rates. For example, in patients with the full-blown syndrome of coagulopathy and cardiorespiratory arrest, mortality rates would be invariably higher than those with isolated coagulopathy alone [19].

Postpartum Counseling about Recurrence Rates of AFE

AFE is so rare that recurrence rates are difficult, if not impossible, to describe. In the literature, multiple cases of uneventful pregnancies after an episode of AFE have been reported [52,53]. **No recurrent cases have been published**, and no data exists to counsel AFE survivors about the possibility of recurrence.

SUMMARY

AFE is a rare but often lethal condition. In the past decade, better maternal and perinatal outcomes have been observed secondary to improvements in the management of the critically ill patient. Its pathophysiology remains largely unknown. Diagnosis is mainly clinical and one of exclusion because specific diagnostic tests are currently absent. Management consists mainly of supportive care. Core treatment principles include delivery of fetus when indicated, respiratory support

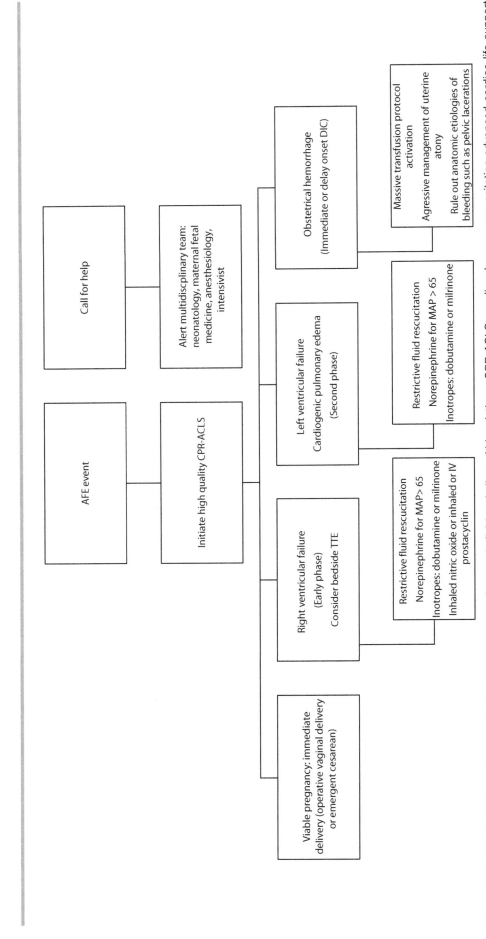

Figure 41.1 Pearls in the management of suspected cases of amniotic fluid embolism. *Abbreviations:* CPR-ACLS, cardiopulmonary resuscitation-advanced cardiac life support; DIC, disseminated intravascular coagulation; MAP, mean arterial pressure; TTE, transthoracic echocardiography.

(usually in the form of endotracheal intubation and mechanical ventilation), and hemodynamic support. Judicious use of fluids, vasopressors, inotropes, and pulmonary vasodilators are crucial in the therapy of the underlying cardiovascular dysfunction. High index of suspicion with prompt initiation of treatment is crucial to improve outcomes of this serious and lethal disease.

REFERENCES

1. Conde-Agudelo A, Romero R. Amniotic fluid embolism: An evidence-based review. *Am J Obstet Gynecol* 2009; 201: 445–13. [Review, 2 population-based cohort studies and 6 case control studies].
2. Clark SL, Belfort MA, Dildy GA et al. Maternal death in the 21st century: Causes, prevention, and relationship to cesarean delivery. *Am J Obstet Gynecol* 2008; 199: 36.e1–5. [II-2; Retrospective chart review, *n* = 95]
3. Clark SL, Hankins GDV, Dudley DA et al. Amniotic fluid embolism: Analysis of the national registry. *Am J Obstet Gynecol* 1995; 172: 1158–69. [II-2; Retrospective chart review, *n* = 46]
4. Gilbert WM, Danielsen B. Amniotic fluid embolism: Decreased mortality in a population-based study. *Obstet Gynecol* 1999; 93: 973–77. [II-2; Restrospective chart review, *n* = 53]
5. Tuffnell DJ. United Kingdom amniotic fluid embolism register. *BJOG* 2005; 112(12): 1625–9. [II-2; Retrospective chart review, *n* = 44]
6. Knight M, Berg C, Brocklehurst P et al. Amniotic fluid embolism incidence, risk factors and outcomes: A review and recommendations. *BMC Pregnancy and Childbirth* 2012; 12: 7. [II-2; Retrospective chart review, *n* = 2341]
7. Kramer MS, Rouleau J, Bartholomew S et al. Amniotic fluid embolism: Incidence, risk factors, and impact on perinatal outcome. *BJOG* 2012; 119: 874–9. [Review]
8. Petroianu GA, Altmannsberger SH, Maleck WH et al. Meconium and amniotic fluid embolism: Effects on coagulation in pregnant minipigs. *Crit Care Med* 1999; 27: 348–55. [Animal study]
9. Hankins GD, Snyder RR, Clark SL et al. Acute hemodynamic and respiratory effects of amniotic fluid embolism in the pregnant goat model. *Am J Obstet Gynecol* 1993; 168: 1113–29. [Animal study]
10. Lee W, Ginsburg KA, Cotton DB et al. Squamous and throphoblastic cells in the maternal pulmonary circulation identified by invasive hemodynamic monitoring during the peripartum period. *Am J Obstet Gynecol* 1986; 155: 999–1001. [II-2; cohort *n* = 14]
11. Tufnell DJ. Amniotic fluid embolism. *Curr Opin Obstet Gynecol* 2003; 15: 119–22. [III; Review]
12. Margarit L, Griffiths AN, Tsapanos V et al. Amniotic fluid endothelin levels and the incidence of premature rupture of membranes. *Int J Gynecol Obstet* 2006; 93: 18–21. [II-2; case control; *n* = 125]
13. Dean LS, Rogers RP, Harley RA et al. Case scenario: Amniotic fluid embolism. *Anesthesiology* 2012; 116(1): 186–92. [II-2; Population-based cohort study, *n* = 292]
14. Moore J, Baldisseri MR. Amniotic fluid embolism. *Crit Care Med* 2005; 33(10S): S279–285. [III; Review]
15. Hunter JD, Doddi M. Sepsis and the heart. *Br J Anesth* 2010; 104(1): 13–11. [III; Review]
16. Knight M, Tuffnell D, Brocklehurst P et al. Incidence and risk factors for amniotic fluid embolism. *Obstet Gynecol* 2010; 115(5): 910–7. [II-2; case control; *n* = 60]
17. Stein PD, Matta F, Yaekoub AY. Incidence of amniotic fluid embolism: Relation to cesarean section and to age. *J Womens Health (Larchmt)* 2009; 18(3): 327–9. [II-2; Retrospective chart review, *n* = 1200]
18. Kramer MS, Rouleau J, Baskett T et al. Amniotic fluid embolism and medical induction of labour: A retrospective, population based cohort study. *Lancet* 2006; 368: 1444–8. [II-2; Retrospective chart review, *n* = 180]
19. Clark SL. Amniotic fluid embolism. *Obstet Gynecol* 2014; 123(2): 337–48. [III; Review]
20. Cromley MG, Taylor PJ, Cumming DC. Probable amniotic fluid embolism after first trimester termination. A case report. *J Reprod Med* 1983; 28: 209–11. [III; Case report]
21. Ecker JL, Solt K, Fitzsimons MG et al. A 43 year old woman with cardiorespiratory arrest after a cesarean section. *N Eng J Med* 2012; 376(26): 2528–36. [III; Case report]
22. Awad IT, Shorten GD. Amniotic fluid embolism and isolated coagulopathy: Atypical presentation of amniotic fluid embolism. *Euro J Anesthesiol* 2001; 18: 410–3. [III; Case report]
23. Yang JI, Kim HS, Chang KH et al. Amniotic fluid embolism with isolated coagulopathy. *J Reprod Med* 2006; 51(1): 64–7. [III; Case report]
24. Laforga JBM. Amniotic fluid embolism: Report of two cases with coagulation dosrder. *Acta Obstet Gynecol Scand* 1997; 76: 805–6. [III; Case report]
25. Stafford I, Sheffield J. Amniotic fluid embolism. *Obstet Gynecol Clin N Am* 2007; 34: 545–53. [III; Review]
26. Marwick PC, Levin AI, Coetzee AR. Recurrence of cardiotoxicity after lipid rescue from bupivacaine induced cardiac arrest. *Anesth Analg* 2009; 108(4): 1344–6. [III; Case report]
27. Mazoit JX, Le Guen R, Beloeil H et al. Binding of long lasting local anesthetics to lipid emulsions. *Anesthesiology* 2009; 110(2): 380–6. [Nonclinical; basic science]
28. Hankins GDV, Snyder R, Dinh T et al. Documentation of amniotic fluid embolism via lung histopathology. Fact or fiction? *J Reprod Med* 2002; 47(12): 1021–4. [Animal study]
29. Legrand M, Rossignol M, Dreux S et al. Diagnostic accuracy of insulin like growth factor binding protein 1 for amniotic fluid embolism. *Crit Care Med* 2012; 40(7): 2059–63. [II-3, case control, *n* = 119]
30. Benson MD, Kobayashi H, Silver RK et al. Immunologic studies in presumed amniotic fluid embolism. *Obstet Gynecol* 2001; 97(4): 510–4. [II-3; case series, *n* = 31]
31. Farrar SC, Gherman RB. Serum tryptase analysis in a woman with amniotic fluid embolism: A case report. *J Reprod Med Obstet Gynecol* 2001; 46(10): 926–8. [III; Case report]
32. Marcus BJ, Collins KA, Harley RA. Ancillary studies in amniotic fluid embolism: A case report and review of the literature. *Am J Forens Med Pathol* 2005; 26(1): 92–5. [III; Case report, review]
33. Benson MD. Current concepts of immunology and diagnosis in amniotic fluid embolism. *Clin Dev Immunol* 2012; 2012: 946576. doi:10.1155/2012/946576. [III; Review]
34. Field JM, Hazinski MF, Sayre MR et al. Executive summary: 2010 American Heart Association Guidelines for cardiopulmonary resuscitation and emergency cardiovascular care. *Circulation* 2010; 122: S640–56. [Guidelines]
35. Jeejeebhoy FM, Zelop CM, Lipman S et al. Cardiac arrest in pregnancy: A scientific statement from the American Heart Association; American Heart Association Emergency Cardiovascular Care Committee, Council on Cardiopulmonary, Critical Care, Perioperative and Resuscitation, Council on Cardiovascular Diseases in the Young, and Council on Clinical Cardiology. *Circulation*. 2015; 132(18): 1747–73. [Guidelines]
36. Katz VL. Perimortem cesarean delivery: Its role in maternal mortality. *Semin Perinatol* 2012; 36: 68–72. [III; Review]
37. Peberdy MA, Callaway CW, Neumar RW et al. Post cardiac arrest care: 2010 American Heart Association Guidelines for cardio pulmonary resuscitation and emergency cardiovascular care. *Circulation* 2010; 122: S768–86. [Guidelines]
38. Nolan PN. Optimizing outcome after cardiac arrest. *Curr Opin Crit Care* 2011; 17(5): 520–6. [III; Review]
39. Weng Y, Sun S. Therapeutic hypothermia after cardiac arrest in adults: Mechanism of neuroprotection, phases of hypothermia, and methods of cooling. *Crit Care Clin* 2012; 28: 231–43. [III; Review]
40. Nielsen N, Wetterslev J, Cronberg T et al. Targeted temperature management at 33°C versus 36°C after cardiac arrest. *N Engl J Med* 2013; 369: 2197–206. [I; Randomized control trial, *n* = 939]

41. Chauhan A, Musunuru H, Donnino M et al. The use of therapeutic hypothermia after cardiac arrest in a pregnant patient. *Ann Emerg Med* 2012; 60(6): 786–9. [III; Case report]

42. Wible EF, Kass JS, Lopez GA. A report of fetal demise during therapeutic hypothermia after cardiac arrest. *Neurocrit Care* 2010; 13(2): 239–42. [III; Case report]

43. Duarte AG, Thomas S, Safdar Z et al. Management of pulmonary arterial hypertension during pregnancy: A retrospective, multicenter experience. *Chest* 2012. doi:10.1378. (epub ahead of print). [II-2; multicenter retrospective cohort, *n* = 18]

44. Pacheco LD, Saade GR, Gei AF et al. Cutting-edge advances in the medical management of obstetrical hemorrhage. *Am J Obstet Gynecol* 2011; 205(6): 526–32. [III; Review]

45. Franchini M, Manzato F, Salvagno GL et al. Potential role of recombinant activated factor VII for the treatment of severe bleeding associated with disseminated intravascular coagulation: A systematic review. *Blood Coagul Fibrinolysis* 2007; 18: 589–93. [II-3; systemic review, *n* = 99]

46. Leighton BL, Wall MH, Lockhart EM et al. Use of recombinant factor VII in patients with amniotic fluid embolism: A systematic review of case reports. *Anesthesiology* 2011; 11596: 1201–8. [II-3; systemic review, *n* = 13]

47. Lim Y, Loo CC, Chia V et al. Recombinant factor VII after amniotic fluid embolism and disseminated intravascular coagulopathy. *Intl J Gynecol Obstet* 2004; 87: 178–9. [III; Case report]

48. Uszynski M, Uszynski W. Coagulation and fibrinolysis in amniotic fluid: Physiology and observations on amniotic fluid embolism, preterm fetal membrane rupture, and preeclampsia. *Semin Thromb Hemost* 2011; 37(2): 165–74. [III; Review]

49. Collins NF, Bloor M, McDonell NJ. Hyperfibrinolysis diagnosed by rotational thromboelastometry in a case of suspected amniotic fluid embolism. *Intl J Obstet Anesth* 2012; 22(1): 71–6. [III; Case report]

50. Matsuda Y, Kamitomo M. Amniotic fluid embolism: A comparison between patients who survived and those who died. *J Intl Med Research* 2009; 37(5): 1515–21. [II-3; case series, *n* = 9]

51. Sandroni C, Nolan J, Cavallaro F et al. In-hospital cardiac arrest: incidence, prognosis, and possible measures to improve survival. *Intensive Care Med* 2007; 33(2): 237–45. [III; Review]

52. Clark SL. Successful pregnancy outcomes after amniotic fluid embolism. *Am J Obstet Gynecol* 1992; 167: 511–2. [III; Case report]

53. Stiller RJ, Siddiqui D, Laifer SA et al. Successful pregnancy after suspected anaphylactoid syndrome of pregnancy (amniotic fluid embolism): A case report. *J Reprod Med* 2000; 45: 1007–9. [III; Case report]

42

Cancer

Elyce Cardonick

KEY POINTS
Cancer Diagnosed in Pregnancy
- Avoid delay in diagnosis by performing necessary diagnostic studies in a timely and adequate fashion as in nonpregnant adults with rare exceptions.
- Postpone radiologic studies that will not alter cancer treatment or patient decisions during pregnancy.
- Avoid iatrogenic preterm deliveries.
- When choosing a particular chemotherapeutic regimen for a particular cancer, choose the one with the most experience of use and proven safety during pregnancy as long as it will offer a similar chance of cure for the patient. Administer the same doses of chemotherapy as given to nonpregnant women based on the actual height and weight of the patient during pregnancy. Prepregnancy weight or ideal body weight should not be used to calculate chemotherapy dosage during pregnancy.
- At least 3 weeks between a cycle of chemotherapy during pregnancy and delivery is recommended. Halt/complete chemotherapy regimens by 34/35 weeks gestation.
- Send placental pathology for all cancers, especially in cases of melanoma.
- Close multidisciplinary management with an oncologist and maternal-fetal specialist knowledgeable regarding the unique considerations of cancer during pregnancy is vital to optimize outcomes.

Cancer Diagnosed before Pregnancy
- Women who have been treated for childhood cancer with chemotherapy, radiation therapy, or both are not at increased risk of having children with congenital or chromosomal anomalies.
- The available data do not support an adverse effect of prior chemotherapy on the risk of miscarriage, fetal demise, or birth weight.
- Women who have received prior irradiation deliver infants with a statistically lower birth weight compared to survivors only treated with chemotherapy, and those with a history of pelvic irradiation specifically can have perinatal complications, such as miscarriage, preterm labor and delivery, low birth weight, and placenta accreta.
- Unless the cancer suffered by the patient was part of an inherited syndrome, such as retinoblastoma, the offspring of cancer survivors are not at increased risk for cancer.
- With the possible exception of gestational trophoblastic disease, pregnancy does not affect the risk of recurrence of any type of cancer.

- Women with a history of left-sided chest radiation therapy or anthracycline-based chemotherapy (daunorubicin, doxorubicin, idarubicin, epirubicin, and mitoxantrone) can have delayed cardiac toxicity and should undergo cardiac evaluation prior to pregnancy.

CANCER DIAGNOSED IN PREGNANCY
Incidence/Epidemiology
Cancer complicates approximately 1/1000 pregnancies, and 1 out of every 118 malignancies is associated with pregnancy [1]. There is no increased incidence of malignancy in pregnant women. The biggest risk for cancer during pregnancy is advanced maternal age as the incidence of cancer in women increases with age. The most common cancers that occur during pregnancy are breast, cervical, leukemia, lymphoma, thyroid, and melanoma [2].

General Considerations
Delays in diagnosis should be avoided. The necessary diagnostic studies to work up a concerning sign or symptom in a pregnant patient should proceed in the same timely and efficient matter as if the patient were not pregnant [3]. The safest diagnostic studies should be employed, for example, an MRI in place of CT if similar diagnostic information can be obtained. Staging procedures and radiologic studies should be limited during pregnancy to those that will determine the treatment course during pregnancy or affect patient decisions about continuing the pregnancy. Chemotherapy regimens should be comparable to those used in nonpregnant patients; however, using the newest agents is not recommended in absence of safety data even if favored for nonpregnant patients. For example, nonpregnant women may be treated for breast cancer with doxorubicin/cyclophosphamide (AC); idarubicin/cyclophosphamide, 5-fluorouracil/doxorubicin/cyclophosphamide, cyclophosphamide/methotrexate/r-fluoruracil, or epirubicin/cyclophosphamide. The latter may be better tolerated in nonpregnant patients, and data is accumulating outside of the United States with using epirubicin/cyclophosphamide during pregnancy; however, the first regimen (AC) has the most reported cases in the pregnancy literature and is usually the first line of treatment for breast cancer during pregnancy. The second regimen (idarubicin/cyclophosphamide) has been associated with transient cardiomyopathy in infants exposed in utero [4–6]. Different drugs in the same class of chemotherapy agents may have different properties that allow more placental transfer. Once the regimen is chosen, the pregnant woman should be given the same doses of chemotherapy as given to nonpregnant women with the same cancer type and stage. The woman's changing weight during pregnancy should be used,

not prepregnancy or ideal body weight, to determine the dose of chemotherapy. This recommendation may change if pharmacokinetic studies are performed in the future on pregnant women receiving chemotherapy as free drug levels may not be the same as in nonpregnant women due to the many physiologic changes during pregnancy that affect drug metabolism. **For most cancers, termination of pregnancy does not improve or affect outcome.** If the patient wishes to continue the pregnancy, cancer treatment is discussed if treatment cannot be delayed until postpartum without compromising the woman's disease-free or overall survival. This concept brings into conflict what is best for maternal survival yet not harmful to the developing fetus. Close multidisciplinary management, especially with oncologists and maternal-fetal specialists knowledgeable in cancer and pregnancy and the neonatal team is vital to optimize outcomes. Obstetrical management and mode of delivery (aside from cervical or vulvar cancers) rarely need to be altered, and evidence based interventions proven beneficial in pregnancy should be available to all pregnant women with cancer. Iatrogenic preterm deliveries prior to 34/35 weeks should be avoided. Placental pathology should be sent for all cancers, especially in cases of melanoma.

General Chemotherapy Considerations

Chemotherapy given during the first trimester has the highest chance of causing malformations as the majority of organogenesis occurs between three and eight weeks postconception. The literature supports the relative safety of fetal exposure to chemotherapy during the second and third trimesters [7–9]. **References for specific chemotherapy regimens are listed below by cancer type. If one controls for the gestational age at delivery, fetal growth restriction does not appear to be increased in most cases, especially with solid tumors.** Patients with systemic disease, such as leukemia, are at risk for increased perinatal morbidity and mortality including fetal growth restriction and intrauterine fetal demise.

Transplacental studies of chemotherapeutic drugs during pregnancy are scarce. Doxorubicin was not detectable in amniotic fluid, placental tissue, fetal brain, or GI tract but detectable in fetal liver, kidney, and lung 15 hours after IV administration [10]. Placental transfer of various chemotherapeutic agents can be modified by placenta proteins, such as P-glycoprotein, which act as efflux proteins to decrease fetal exposure [11]. Umbilical blood sampling two and five weeks post multiagent chemotherapy for maternal leukemia showed that fetal hematopoesis was normal [12].

Breast Cancer

Breast cancer is the most common cancer complicating pregnancy with more than 900 cases reported in the literature. Seven percent to 15% of premenopausal breast cancers occur during pregnancy. The histology of breast cancer diagnosed during pregnancy is no different from the nonpregnant patient population with invasive ductal carcinoma being the most common subtype. Beadle et al. evaluated the survival of 668 patients younger than 35 years of age with breast cancer: 51 diagnosed during pregnancy, 53 within 1 year postpartum, and 548 nonpregnant women. During the median follow-up of 114 months, patients with pregnancy-associated cases had no statistically significant differences in 10-year locoregional

recurrence, distant metastases, or overall survival. For patients diagnosed with breast cancer during pregnancy, any treatment intervention during pregnancy provided a trend toward improved overall survival compared to delaying evaluation and treatment until after delivery, 78.8% versus 44.6%, $p = 0.68$ [13]. Loibl, too, found that delaying treatment until after delivery did not afford a survival advantage [14]. Women diagnosed with and treated for breast cancer during pregnancy have comparable survival to age- and stage-matched nonpregnant women [13–15]. Pregnant women may be more likely to be diagnosed at stage II compared to nonpregnant women (74% vs. 37%) and less likely to be diagnosed with early-stage disease (21% vs. 54%) [16]. Pregnant and nonpregnant women younger than 40 are more likely to be diagnosed with stage-II disease compared to women older than 40. When matched for stage, women younger than 40 have a statistically worse five-year survival compared to women older than 40 years of age at diagnosis (55% vs. 75%). According to these data, it may be the age of reproductive-age women that has a stronger influence on survival than pregnancy [16].

Delay in Diagnosis

Studies show both patients and physicians follow a breast mass longer in pregnant women before performing a biopsy. This is not solely due to ascribing the palpable mass as "normal breast changes" of pregnancy. Pregnant women, therefore, are often diagnosed with larger tumors at later stages than nonpregnant women. A **delay in diagnosis obviously worsens prognosis and is inexcusable. During routine prenatal care, the examination of the breast all the way into and including the axillae should be included in all breast examinations as this can be the sole area of a breast cancer presentation during pregnancy.**

Diagnostic Tests and Safety in Pregnancy

The fetal exposure to mammography is not the deterrent to performing this as the first line for the workup of a mass in pregnancy as the exposure is only 0.4 rads. Mammography has less sensitivity for screening in pregnancy due to the increased overall density, vascularity, cellularity, and water content, which leads to less contrast during pregnancy. **During pregnancy, breast ultrasound has a better accuracy than mammography and should be performed for palpable masses.** The sensitivity and specificity of ultrasound to detect solid versus cystic breast masses is not altered by pregnancy. The biopsy of a solitary mass should continue as in nonpregnant women with **core needle biopsy preferred over fine needle aspiration during pregnancy.** False positive cytological findings can occur in pregnancy due to the highly proliferative state of the breast, and the pathologist should be aware that the patient is pregnant [17]. As in premenopausal nonpregnant women, most tumors in pregnant women are estrogen receptor negative [18]. HER2neu expression is comparable to nonpregnant premenopausal women [18]. Maternal age, rather than pregnancy, determine the biologic features of breast cancer.

Effects on the Pregnancy

Breast cancer itself (excluding therapy) does not directly affect perinatal outcome.

Termination of Pregnancy and Breast Cancer

Routine termination of pregnancy does not appear to offer a survival advantage for pregnant women diagnosed with breast cancer [16,19,20].

Staging during Pregnancy

Mammography is indicated once breast cancer is diagnosed during pregnancy to exclude multifocal disease in the affected breast or cancer in the contralateral breast. To detect metastases to lungs, liver, or bone, the most common sites of metastases in breast cancer, a chest X-ray (with abdominal shielding) is recommended and can be safely performed with fetal exposure of 0.06 mrad. Abdominal ultrasound can be performed to detect liver metastases, and liver function tests are not reliable for management decisions as alkaline phosphatase is physiologically increased in pregnancy. The risk of bony metastasis with stage I or II breast cancer is 3% to 7%. A bone scan can be safely deferred until after pregnancy for asymptomatic patients with early-stage disease. If a patient is symptomatic or has advanced-stage disease, a bone scan can be performed with a Foley catheter in place and intravenous hydration to promote washout of the excreted radiopharmaceutical from the patient's bladder. An exposure of 10 mCi rather than 20 mCi of Technitium-99m (Tc-99m) methylene diphosphonate (MDP) and doubling the imaging time can reduce fetal radiation exposure [21]. Alternatively, an MRI of the skeleton can detect 80% of metastatic deposits. Brain scan is of little yield unless the patient has neurologic symptoms and physical findings. Positron emission tomography (PET) scans are performed postpartum. Detecting spread to regional lymph nodes is discussed below.

Surgery during Pregnancy

Either modified radical mastectomy or breast conservation surgery with axillary or sentinel lymph node dissection can be safely performed at any gestational age during pregnancy with attention paid to avoid the supine position after 20 weeks gestation. Intraoperative fetal monitoring is performed during a procedure at or after 24 weeks gestation; otherwise fetal viability is documented before and after surgery. Pregnant patients should have the same discussion as nonpregnant women with breast cancer about the pros and cons of breast conservation surgery. There does not appear to be a survival advantage of mastectomy over breast conservation [22]. Patients choosing breast conservation and patients requiring radiation despite mastectomy will need to defer radiotherapy until postpartum. Depending on the gestational age at diagnosis and surgery, chemotherapy can be given during this time until postpartum radiation. Before prescribing taxanes in pregnancy, mastectomy was encouraged for patients diagnosed early in pregnancy as completing surgery and only four cycles of AC chemotherapy occurred too early in pregnancy to consider a preterm delivery. Recent evidence showing the safety of taxane treatment has given an alternative to this suggestion as up to four cycles of taxane treatment may be given every 2 weeks to fill that period of time between completing anthracycline-based therapy and postpartum radiation. Autologous breast reconstruction is delayed for the best cosmetic results to match the unaffected postpartum breast, but expanders/spacers can be placed. Surgeons should be advised of the safe use of narcotics in pregnancy for postoperative pain management.

Sentinel Node Biopsy

Sentinel node mapping and biopsy is commonly used for nonpregnant women to avoid the complications of lymphedema after complete axillary lymphadenectomy. **Sentinel node biopsy can be safely performed in pregnancy with Tc-99m sulfur colloid, which identifies the first draining node(s) relative to the site of the primary invasive tumor** [23]. For sentinel node imaging, only a minimal dose (500–600 mCi) of double-filtered Tc-99m sulfur colloid is injected at the site of the breast tumor. The entire radioisotope stays trapped at the sight of injection or within the lymphatics until decay occurs (half-life = six hours), not traveling throughout the body to expose the fetus [23]. There is limited information on the use of blue dyes such as lymphazurin for sentinel node mapping in pregnancy, and this carries a risk of anaphylaxis. The current recommendation is to use Tc-99 as a same-day procedure rather than any dye injection.

Treatment during Pregnancy (Figure 42.1)

Radiation therapy is usually postponed until postpartum. As the pregnancy advances, the fetus has increased proximity to the breast and radiation field increasing exposure risk. The majority of women reported in the literature are treated with cyclophosphamide, doxorubicin, or epirubicin, with or without 5-fluouracil (5FU). Currently doxorubicin is the preferred anthracycline to use during pregnancy and is commonly included in the regimens to treat various types of cancer during pregnancy. Data is accumulating, however, in Europe concerning epirubicin during pregnancy as it has lower myelotoxic and cardiotoxic properties and is better tolerated in nonpregnant patients. Transient neonatal cardiomyopathy has been reported after idarubicin exposure, and the use of this anthracycline is not recommended during pregnancy [4,5]. Taxanes, widely used as standard first-line treatment for high-risk early-stage and advanced/metastatic breast cancer in nonpregnant women, result in a better response rate and longer time to progression than standard anthracycline-based regimens. Nonpregnant women with positive nodes receive taxane therapy, simultaneously or after completing cyclophosphamide and an anthracycline with or without 5FU. Case reports of taxane use in human pregnancy are accumulating, and the placental transfer rate is suspected to be low [24–32]. An increased risk for growth restriction was noted in some reports. If taxane therapy is to be postponed until after delivery, giving one to two additional cycles of anthracycline-based chemotherapy can be considered. Herceptin/trastuzumab use is contraindicated in pregnancy as its use has been found to be associated with oligohydramnios and pulmonary hypoplasia [33–38]. Hormonal agents, such as tamoxifen, are also postponed until postpartum.

Hodgkin's Disease

The mean age of diagnosis for Hodgkin's disease (HD) is 32 years [39]. Pregnant women are not more likely to be diagnosed at a higher stage compared to nonpregnant women [40]. Pregnancy does not adversely affect survival rate. The safety of the doxorubicin bleomycin/vincristine/dacarbazine (ABVD) during pregnancy has been documented [8]. Chemotherapy during organogenesis in the first trimester will increase the risk for malformations (see treatment below). If patients require treatment during the first trimester, consider single-agent treatment with vinblastine followed by a complete regimen during second and third trimesters.

Presentation, Diagnostic Tests, and Safety in Pregnancy

The clinical behavior of HD during pregnancy does not appear to differ from nonpregnant women. Pregnant women can present with a cough, night sweats, and weight loss. A patient with such complaints should have a complete physical exam,

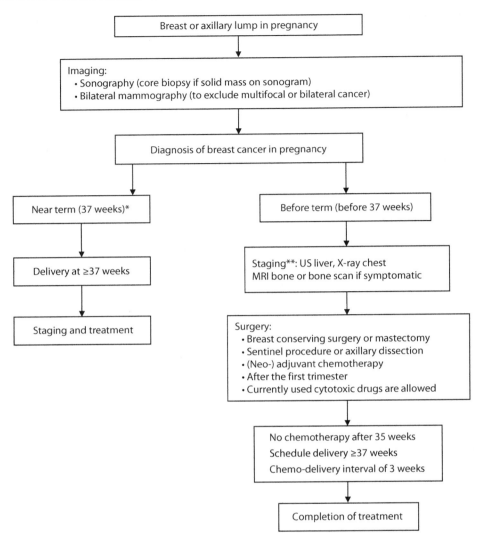

Figure 42.1 Algorithm for the treatment of breast cancer diagnosed during pregnancy. * a waiting policy of 2–4 weeks is allowed to attain fetal maturity. ** as far as this will change clinical practice. (Adapted from Amant F, Deckers S, Van Calsteren K, Loibl S, Halaska M, Brepoels L et al. *Eur J Cancer* 46, 3158–68, 2010.)

and clavicular adenopathy can be safely biopsied during pregnancy. A chest X-ray can be performed safely with minimal fetal exposure. An abdominal shield is indicated for all radiologic studies during pregnancy. A bone marrow biopsy can also be safely performed with appropriate analgesia.

Effects on Pregnancy
HD does not directly affect perinatal outcome. Infants born to women with HD do not have a higher risk for prematurity or intrauterine growth restriction [40].

Termination of Pregnancy
Therapeutic termination of a pregnancy does not improve the course of disease [41].

Surgery during Pregnancy
At times, histologic examination of a clavicular lymph node is inconclusive. In such cases, if mediastinal adenopathy is evident on X-ray or CT of the chest, a guided biopsy may be indicated to confirm a diagnosis.

Staging of Disease in Pregnancy
The staging of lymphoma is based on history and physical examination, hematologic and biochemical testing, bone marrow biopsy, and radiologic imaging. Gallium scanning, staging laparotomy, and splenectomy are no longer routinely performed in nonpregnant patients. Currently, women with stages I and II receive combination modality treatment, so full staging during pregnancy is unlikely to change the recommended treatment during the course of pregnancy and can be delayed to the postpartum period. Image staging in nonpregnant patients includes a chest X-ray and CT. In the pregnant woman, a two-view chest X-ray is suggested. Fetal exposure is negligible with abdominal shielding. A chest MRI can assess lymphadenopathy, and the information gained is comparable to a CT [42]. MRI can also evaluate the bone marrow and detect splenic involvement that may be undetectable with CT.

Treatment of HD during Pregnancy
The ABVD regimen for Hodgkin's lymphoma has been reported to be safe in pregnancy [8]. Similar doses should be

given to the pregnant patient with adjustment for weight gain during pregnancy.

Radiotherapy during Pregnancy

Radiotherapy for HD during pregnancy has been reported to be tolerable for the fetus at certain gestational ages [43]. Exposure of the fetus to radiation is determined by the internal scatter, leakage from the tube head, and scatter from the collimator. Internal scatter depends on the source of radiation, the distance of the fetus from the source, and the size of treatment fields. Blocks are not recommended in pregnancy because of the additional scatter they create. Exposure of the fetus can be estimated with simulated measurements, which have shown that treatment with a 6 MV linear accelerator exposes the fetus to less radiation than treatment with Cobalt 60 [43]. The highest risk of brain damage and mental retardation is between 8 and 15 weeks gestation [44]. Radiation for HD is usually reserved for cases progressing despite chemotherapy, lymphocyte predominant type, or if chemotherapy is not an option.

Non–Hodgkin's Lymphoma

Non–Hodgkin's lymphoma (NHL) is rarely reported during pregnancy as this generally occurs in an older age group (mean age at diagnosis is 42 years). Pregnant women present with an aggressive histology [39,45], but the response to treatment, failure, and progression rates are similar to nonpregnant patients. Symptoms can vary widely, with many complaints similar to symptoms in normal pregnancy, which can lead to a delay in diagnosis of NHL in pregnancy.

Avoid Delay in Diagnosis

Pregnant women with NHL can present with breast or ovarian masses, misleading the initial diagnosis to a gynecologic malignancy. When masses are *bilateral* and *massive in size*, one should suspect NHL.

Effects of Cancer on the Pregnancy and Vice Versa

NHL does not directly affect pregnancy. However, pregnancy can affect the presentation of NHL, and some authors report a progression of NHL postpartum [45,46]. In some cases, such as lymphoproliferative T-cell lymphoma, a component of Epstein–Barr virus in the etiology of NHL may explain, given the immunosuppression of pregnancy, why some cases of NHL seem to progress more rapidly in pregnant women. The number of cases, however, is too small to determine if termination of the pregnancy would improve prognosis. In addition to the typical presentation of lymphadenopathy, pregnant patients can have involvement of the breasts, ovaries, and uterus. A hormonal influence of pregnancy on the progression of NHL is suggested by the frequent and massive involvement of such organs during pregnancy, which are otherwise unusually involved with NHL in nonpregnant patients [45].

Treatment of NHL during Pregnancy

Breast or ovarian masses should *not* be surgically removed after biopsy confirms non-Hodgkin's lymphoma. The masses will respond to systemic chemotherapy. Thirty-five cases of NHL were treated during pregnancy with multiple regimens, most including doxorubicin, cyclophosphamide, and vincristine. No malformations occurred even with first trimester treatment in 11 cases. Rituximab is often used in nonpregnant patients in addition to chemotherapy. It is a chimeric IgG 1 antibody, which can cross the placenta and interact with fetal B-cells. It is unlikely that rituximab has any mutagenic potential. Infants exposed to rituximab in pregnancy initially had a period of low IgG, but B-cell counts normalized by four months after birth, and the period with low IgG might not have been longer than average [47].

Leukemia

Acute Leukemia

Acute leukemia is rarely diagnosed during pregnancy as affected women usually have amenorrhea.

Avoid Delay in Diagnosis. Pregnant women with leukemia can present with severe anemia, thrombocytopenia, infection or sepsis, fever, bone pain, or bleeding.

Diagnostic Tests and Safety in Pregnancy. Bone marrow biopsy can be safely performed during pregnancy.

Termination of Pregnancy Issues. Termination of pregnancy has not been shown to improve prognosis but may be a clinically relevant option for pregnant women diagnosed during the first trimester as chemotherapy cannot be delayed until after 12 weeks gestation. **Patients newly diagnosed with acute leukemia are too ill to safely undergo a dilatation and curettage procedure even when termination is elected without first undergoing induction chemotherapy. It is suggested to start therapy before termination to induce remission so that the procedure can be safely performed.** The patient is otherwise at too high a risk for the complications of D and E, such as infection and sepsis, uterine perforation and hemorrhage, and disseminated intravascular coagulation (DIC).

Effects of Cancer on the Pregnancy. Acute leukemia is one of the cancers that can affect perinatal outcome. The earlier the diagnosis is made in pregnancy, the higher the perinatal mortality. Pregnancies complicated by acute leukemia are at higher risk for miscarriage, intrauterine fetal demise, preterm labor, and fetal growth restriction, unrelated to cancer treatment [48,49]. Suspected etiologies include maternal anemia, DIC, or leukemic cells affecting blood flow and nutrient exchange in the intervillous spaces of the placenta, and decreased oxygen transport to the fetus [49]. When intensive chemotherapy is given in pregnancy, complete remission is achieved in 75% of patients [49].

Treatment of Cancer during Pregnancy: Chemotherapy, Radiation Therapy. Aggressive hematologic and obstetric management is advocated when acute leukemia is diagnosed. The prognosis for both mother and fetus is poor when acute leukemia is not treated during pregnancy. Without therapy, maternal death may occur within two months time [49]. Chemotherapy treatment during pregnancy is associated with higher maternal and fetal/neonatal survival compared to postponing chemotherapy until postpartum [49]. All cases with anomalies occurred with first-trimester exposure to cytarabine or 6-thioguanine, alone or in combination with an anthracycline. Cytarabine and 6-thioguanine should be avoided in the first trimester if possible. Combinations including vincristine, 6-MP, doxorubicin or daunorubicin, cyclophosphamide, prednisone, and methotrexate were used in all trimesters without anomalies. Transient myelosuppression can occur in neonates, especially if delivered within three to four weeks of chemotherapy [50]. More rarely, transient neonatal cardiomyopathy has been reported. Cardiomyopathy occurred mostly after use of idarubicin [4,5]. Iatrogenic preterm deliveries or elective inductions should be avoided before remission is attempted as the patient with acute leukemia is at risk for hemorrhage, DIC, and sepsis during labor and delivery if lacerations, uterine atony, or endometritis occurs.

Chronic Leukemia
Pregnancy does not alter the natural course of chronic leukemia, but there are potentially perinatal risks of placental insufficiency secondary to leukostasis as well as maternal risks if left untreated. Treatment of severe leukocytosis is necessary to reduce maternal risk of stroke hypoxia, DVT. There are case reports of observation alone during pregnancy in patients without splenomegaly. Leukophoresis can be a temporizing measure to reduce WBC and spleen size if necessary [51,52]. Tyrosine kinase inhibitors, such as Imatinib, the newest advance in the treatment of chronic leukemia in nonpregnant adults, has been shown to cause teratogenic effects in rats including exencephaly or encephalocele and absent or reduced frontal and absent parietal bones. Postimplantation loss occurred as well. No teratogenicity has been shown in rabbits. In humans, the majority of reports concerning Imatinib use during pregnancy are first trimester exposures in patients on maintenance therapy who conceive while taking this drug despite the recommendations to use contraception and to avoid unplanned pregnancies. Patients with CML who conceive while taking Gleevec are advised to discontinue use during pregnancy with the majority of patients able to regain remission status postpartum [53]. If a pregnant patient newly diagnosed with CML is symptomatic with splenomegaly with no clinical response to leukophoresis or other medications, **Imatinib would be preferred over second-generation tyrosine kinase inhibitors, such as desatinib or nolotinib.** Reports show imatinib is 95% bound to plasma proteins with a molecular weight of 590, which suggests low placental transfer. There are just a few case reports of tyrosine kinase inhibitor therapy during pregnancy beyond the first trimester. Four of seven exposed infants were small for gestational age but with no other abnormalities reported [54–58].

Melanoma

One third of women diagnosed with malignant melanoma are of childbearing age. When pregnant patients are matched to nonpregnant controls for prognostic factors such as tumor thickness, there is **no significant difference in survival rates** for pregnant women with stage-I melanoma [59,60]. Slingluff reported that pregnancy at diagnosis was significantly associated with **metastatic disease** when controlling for tumor site, thickness, and Clark level, still with survival not significantly decreased for pregnant patients [61].

Avoid Delay in Diagnosis
Pregnant women are diagnosed with **thicker tumors** compared to nonpregnant women. This (as well as the increase in metastatic disease) has been ascribed to a delay in biopsy leading to delayed diagnosis when changes in moles' appearances are ascribed to pregnancy or the surgeon is hesitant to perform a biopsy during pregnancy. Hyperpigmentation can occur secondary to an increased secretion of melanocyte-stimulating

hormone (MSH); however, the color of the mole should still be uniform, and benign moles should not cause itching. Maximum increases/decreases in the size of melanocytic nevi in pregnancy is 1 mm [62]. During pregnancy, one must still look for signs of melanoma, listed below, which should *not* be ascribed to normal changes in pregnancy. These include the ABCD signs: A for asymmetry; B for notched, irregular, or indistinct borders; C for an uneven color; D for diameter greater than 6 mm. Again, itching of a mole can be an early sign of malignant melanoma.

Effects of Cancer on the Pregnancy
Melanoma is one of the rare cancers that can **metastasize to the placenta**. Eighty-seven cases of placenta/fetal metastasis have been reported. The largest percentage (31%) was in cases of maternal melanoma [63]. Patients with placental metastases also had widespread disease. The placenta should be sent for pathologic evaluation in all cases of melanoma diagnosed during pregnancy. If melanoma is found in the placenta, the neonate should be followed closely for one year with frequent skin evaluations.

Termination of Pregnancy Issues
No advantage in prognosis or survival has been demonstrated with elective pregnancy termination in patients with stage-I melanoma.

Surgery during Pregnancy
Wide local excision is the only cure for melanoma and can be safely performed during pregnancy at any gestational age. Patients should be positioned with uterine displacement after 20 weeks gestation. See sentinel node biopsy below.

Staging and Sentinel Node Biopsy
Sentinel node mapping can be safely performed during pregnancy with Tc-99 sulfur colloid. Intradermal injection of Technitium-labeled sulfur colloid exposes the fetus to negligible ionizing radiation. The majority of the dose stays localized to the injection site or within the lymphatics until decay occurs. For stage I or II melanoma, a chest X-ray is indicated for staging if the melanoma is greater than 1.0 mm thick. No other staging radiologic studies are required. For stage III disease, an MRI of the chest and abdomen with or without the pelvis is additionally recommended for evaluation of lymphadenopathy or evidence of liver metastases. MRI of the brain and skeleton is also recommended.

Treatment of Melanoma during Pregnancy
Surgery is the only effective treatment for melanoma, and chemotherapy has not been shown to significantly prolong survival. Postpartum, patients with advanced disease can enroll in clinical trials using interferon or melanoma vaccinations (see also Chapter 42).

Invasive Cervical Cancer

Invasive carcinoma of the cervix occurs in approximately 1 out of 2200 pregnancies, but this incidence is declining due to widespread and improved Papanicolau screening [64]. Tumor characteristics and maternal survival are not adversely affected by pregnancy; in fact, pregnant women are more likely to be diagnosed with earlier stage disease as cervical screening is routine during prenatal care [64]. Unlike nonpregnant patients, presenting symptoms are more likely to be abnormal Papanicolau screens rather than bleeding. The predominant histologic type is squamous cell. Prognosis is comparable to nonpregnant patients [64–67]. (For noninvasive cervical cancer, see Chapter 33 in *Obstetric Evidence Based Guidelines*.)

Avoid Delay in Diagnosis
When pregnant patients complain of vaginal bleeding, the cervix should be visualized for lesions.

Diagnostic Tests and Safety in Pregnancy
The cytobrush can be safely used during pregnancy to obtain an adequate Papanicolau screen during prenatal care. Pregnant patients should be warned of the possibility of bleeding afterward.

Effects of Cancer on the Pregnancy
Cervical cancer does not adversely affect pregnancy directly; however, cancer treatment affects future fertility if hysterectomy is indicated.

Termination of Pregnancy Issues
A spontaneous loss of the pregnancy may occur when treatment for cervical cancer is initiated for patients diagnosed prior to 18 weeks gestation.

Considerations Regarding Therapy during Pregnancy for Cervical Cancer
The gestational age at diagnosis determines the management choices for the pregnant patient. For stages IB–IIA diagnosed before 18 weeks, immediate surgery or radiotherapy treatment is recommended with the fetus in situ. Often a spontaneous miscarriage will occur within a short time after radiotherapy. For patients with advanced-stage disease, external radiotherapy and chemotherapy with fetus in situ is suggested. Spontaneous abortion often follows radiotherapy; however, hysterotomy may be required to facilitate brachytherapy if this does not occur [66].

Staging of Cervical Cancer during Pregnancy
Evaluation of regional lymph node chains is an important component of staging as lymphadenopathy has prognostic and therapeutic implications. **MRI can identify enlarged lymph nodes. MRI can also detect depth of stromal invasion, involvement of the parametria, and a dilated collecting system.** A two-view chest X-ray with proper shielding can be performed if indicated clinically.

Treatment of Cancer during Pregnancy: Surgery, Chemotherapy, Radiation Therapy
Treatment for invasive cervical cancer involves either surgery, radiation, or both, depending on the stage at diagnosis. The safe use of neoadjuvent platinum-based chemotherapy has been reported [68,69]. See also Chapter 33 in *Obstetrics Evidence Based Guidelines*.

Surgery for Cervical Cancer Diagnosed during Pregnancy
Patients diagnosed after 18 weeks gestation can consider delaying surgical treatment of cervical cancer in order to improve fetal maturity and survival. Neoadjuvant chemotherapy for invasive cervical disease may be given during the second and third trimesters of pregnancy during this interval until postpartum surgical treatment. The survival outcomes for pregnant women and their children when surgical treatment for cervical cancer is intentionally delayed for 6 to 17 weeks is very good with fetal outcomes markedly improved and maternal survival not adversely affected [70–74].

Delivery for Patients with Invasive Cervical Cancer during Pregnancy
In the majority of cases, a cesarean section is advised with radical hysterectomy performed simultaneously. A classical cesarean delivery is recommended to avoid extension into the lower uterine segment [72,73]. At the time of cesarean section, pelvic and para-aortic nodes should be sampled, and an oophoropexy can be performed to move the ovaries out of the planned radiation field. Presurgical consultation with a radiation oncologist is suggested prior to delivery. Episiotomy site recurrences of cervical cancer have been reported for women diagnosed with invasive cervical cancer during pregnancy who delivered vaginally [75]. Microinvasion of the cervix is not a contraindication to vaginal delivery.

Thyroid Cancer

The mean age of diagnosis for thyroid cancer is between 30 and 34 years of age with most cases in pregnancy presenting as a solitary nodule [76]. There is no evidence that pregnancy changes the clinical course of the disease and no evidence that thyroid cancer adversely affects pregnancy outcome. The prognosis of differentiated thyroid cancer is the same in pregnant and nonpregnant women [77]. No endocrine association between maternal hormonal changes and thyroid cancer has been found. Treatment depends on histologic subtype, degree of differentiation, stage, and gestational age at diagnosis.

Avoid Delay in Diagnosis
The thyroid can enlarge during normal pregnancy, but solitary nodules should be evaluated.

Diagnostic Tests and Safety in Pregnancy
Biopsy of a solid nodule can be safely performed during pregnancy at any gestational age.

Termination of Pregnancy Issues
Elective termination of pregnancy for thyroid cancer is not associated with any survival advantage.

Surgery during Pregnancy
The histologic type of thyroid cancer and the gestational age at diagnosis determine if thyroidectomy is necessary during pregnancy or can be safely postponed until postpartum. See section titled "Treatment of Thyroid Cancer During Pregnancy."

Treatment of Thyroid Cancer during Pregnancy
Differentiated types of thyroid cancer, such as papillary, follicular, or mixed types, are slow growing, and surgery can be postponed until postpartum for patients diagnosed after 12 weeks gestation. Prior to 12 weeks, a subtotal thyroidectomy is recommended [78]. If a nodule is noted to enlarge during pregnancy, if the surrounding tissues are fixed, or lymphatic invasion is seen on the original biopsy, surgery should not be delayed to postpartum regardless of the gestational age at diagnosis. Patients who delay treatment due to pregnancy should be advised to undergo surgery within 1 year of diagnosis [78].

Medullary or anaplastic types of thyroid cancer are more aggressive, and surgery should not be postponed. A total thyroidectomy may be necessary. If the lesion is compromising the airway, radiotherapy may be necessary during pregnancy. During total thyroidectomy, parathyroid tissue is often inadvertently removed as well. For the remainder of the pregnancy and during deliveries, calcium balance should be watched carefully. When magnesium is given for preterm labor or preeclampsia, calcium levels should be followed as should symptoms of hypocalcemia.

FOR ALL CANCER TYPES DIAGNOSED DURING PREGNANCY
Complications of Cancer Therapy

During chemotherapy, side effects, such as nausea and vomiting, can occur and can compound the nausea related to the pregnancy. Odansetron, metoclopramide, kytril, and benadryl can be safely given for nausea. Decadron can also be given to enhance the effectiveness of antiemetics but should be given in the lowest effective dose (see section titled "Fetal Surveillance and Timing of Delivery"). A common complaint during or immediately after chemotherapy sessions is uterine contractions. Patients should be well hydrated before, during, and after chemotherapy sessions. Given the relative immunosuppression of pregnancy combined with the bone marrow suppression with chemotherapy, pregnant women are at risk for infection, and therefore, the fetuses are at risk for exposure as well. No studies have shown an adverse effect on the neonate due to in utero exposure to neupogen; however, during pregnancy, it is given once neutropenia is demonstrated rather than prophylactically as in the nonpregnant setting. Another complication can be poor maternal weight gain due to either nausea and vomiting or chemotherapy-induced stomatitis. Patients should increase caloric and protein intake in the weeks preceding and following chemotherapy. Nutritional supplementation is sometimes necessary. Theoretically, additional antioxidants should not be supplemented with the prenatal vitamin as free radicals are supposed to be created by the chemotherapy and this may impede its therapeutic effect.

Maternal Surveillance

An echocardiogram is preferred over a multigated equilibrium radionuclide cineangiography (MUGA) to evaluate baseline cardiac function prior to anthracycline therapy. This can provide the necessary information regarding cardiac function and valvular disease. Patients who have any fevers during chemotherapy require comprehensive evaluations for presence of infection, especially during the nadir period. Monitor weight gain throughout pregnancy.

Fetal Surveillance and Timing of Delivery

Often decadron is given with chemotherapy to enhance the effectiveness of antiemetics. This is the intravenous form of dexamethasone. If the patient requires tocolysis for preterm labor and has received IV decadron with chemotherapy after 24 weeks, steroids, such as dexamethasone/betamethasone, may not be necessary to stimulate fetal lung maturity. The fetal/neonatal safety of repeated doses of steroids has not been demonstrated, and repeated courses of steroids are not currently recommended (see Chapter 16 in *Obstetrics Evidence Based Guidelines*).

The preterm infant cannot metabolize the chemotherapy agents as well as the term infant; therefore, iatrogenic preterm deliveries should be avoided in patients receiving chemotherapy, and preterm labor should be treated aggressively. Chemotherapy may need to be temporarily withheld/delayed if the patient has preterm labor. Growth ultrasounds in the late second and third trimesters are suggested for women receiving chemotherapy during pregnancy, especially for patients diagnosed with acute leukemia, given the increased risk of intrauterine growth restriction.

Transient bone marrow suppression of the neonate can occur if delivery is within three to four weeks of treatment. Chemotherapy should not be given after 34 weeks as the patient could potentially go into spontaneous labor during the nadir period. If additional treatment is still required, one can consider a late preterm induction so that the interval between the last treatment in pregnancy and the postpartum treatment is not greater than six weeks (e.g., if treatment is 33 weeks, consider induction at 38 weeks so that 1 week afterward the patient can resume chemo with a 6-week interval between last treatment during pregnancy and postpartum treatment).

Fetal/Neonatal Evaluation after Chemotherapy during Pregnancy

A single case of malignancy has been diagnosed in a child exposed in utero to chemotherapy. Papillary thyroid cancer at age 11 and neuroblastoma at age 14 were diagnosed in a 14-year-old exposed in utero to multiple chemotherapeutic agents for maternal leukemia. His fraternal twin (exposed to the same agents) was healthy [79]. He was also born with congenital anomalies including esophageal atresia, abnormal IVC, and right-arm deformity.

Long-term follow-up of children exposed to chemotherapy is limited but accumulating. A case series of neurodevelopmental follow-up for a mean of 18 years on 84 children exposed in utero to various types of chemotherapy for maternal hematologic malignancy shows that their clinical health status is comparable to their unexposed siblings. All displayed normal growth, development, neurologic function, and school performance. Cytogenetic studies were normal. Neurological, intellectual and visual–motor assessments were no different for exposed children compared to their siblings and unrelated controls. No cancer has been diagnosed in any of the children, and 12 children exposed in utero have now had their own children. All second-generation children were normal in appearance but did not undergo the same rigorous testing as their parents [8]. Recently, Amant, Calsteren, Halaska et al. reported a prospective study on the developmental outcomes of 70 children exposed to cancer treatment in utero. Children were assessed for cognitive performance. The children showing delays in development were concentrated in the group delivered preterm, the majority of which were iatrogenically delivered prematurely [80]. In another prospective follow-up study of children exposed to chemotherapy in utero, no significant differences were noted in cognitive ability, school performance, or behavioral competence for children exposed to chemotherapy in utero compared with nonexposed controls (also born to women diagnosed with cancer during pregnancy). Ninety-five percent scored within normal limits on cognitive assessments; 71% and 79% of children demonstrated at or above age equivalency in mathematics and reading scores, respectively [81].

The **placenta should be sent for pathology examination in all cases** of women diagnosed with cancer during pregnancy regardless of cancer type or treatment. A complete blood count with differential is recommended on either the cord blood or the neonate when chemotherapy has been given during pregnancy. Additional long-term follow-up on the children exposed to cancer and its treatment in utero is ongoing. A Cancer and Pregnancy Registry is established to follow all children of women diagnosed with cancer during pregnancy. The women are also followed yearly. Information about cancer diagnosis, treatment, pregnancy outcomes, and long-term neonatal health and maternal survival is collected and kept confidential. Contact the **Cancer and Pregnancy Registry: 1-877-635-4499**; 856-757-7876, 856-342-2491, or **Cancerinpregnancy. com; Cancerandpregnancy.com**.

CANCER DIAGNOSED BEFORE PREGNANCY
General Principles
Pregnancy after Chemotherapy
The Childhood Cancer Survivor Study compared pregnancy outcome in five-year female cancer survivors who were less than 21 years old at diagnosis with pregnancy outcomes in their sibling controls [82]. The most frequently used agents were cyclophosphamide, doxorubicin, vincristine, dactinomycin, and daunorubicin. More than 1900 females reported 4029 pregnancies. There were no significant differences in pregnancy outcome between patients who had received chemotherapy and controls. The available data do **not support an adverse effect of prior chemotherapy on the risk of miscarriage, fetal growth, congenital malformations and development, fetal demise, or uterine function** [82–88].

Chemotherapy-Induced Cardiac Toxicity
We suggest that **women who received anthracyclines** (daunorubicin, doxorubicin, idarubicin, epirubicin, and mitoxantrone) **undergo cardiac evaluation prior to pregnancy** [89].

Pregnancy after Radiation
Pregnancy in women who have received **prior pelvic irradiation appears to be associated with complications, such as miscarriage, preterm labor and delivery, low birth weight, impaired fetal growth, placenta accreta, and stillbirth** [90–97]. Hypotheses for these complications include changes in the uterine vasculature and its response to cytotrophoblast invasion or decreased uterine elasticity and volume from radiation-induced myometrial fibrosis. These responses to radiation, especially if before puberty, can affect fetoplacental blood flow or result in a small uterine size leading to preterm labor and delivery. In addition, radiotherapy may injure the endometrium and prevent normal decidualization, resulting in disorders of placental attachment, such as placenta accreta or percreta [92,93].

In the Childhood Cancer Survivor Study, compared with the children of survivors who did not receive any radiotherapy, the children of survivors treated with high-dose radiotherapy to the uterus (>500 cGy) were at significantly increased risk of preterm birth (50.0% vs. 19.6%), low birth weight (36.2% vs. 7.6%), and small for gestational age (18.2% vs. 7.8%). These risks were also noted at lower uterine radiotherapy doses (starting at 50 cGy for preterm birth and at 250 cGy for low birth weight) [82].

Radiation-Induced Cardiac Toxicity Due to Fibrosis
The clinical spectrum of cardiac injury resulting from radiation includes delayed pericarditis that can present abruptly or as chronic pericardial effusion or constriction; pancarditis, which includes pericardial and myocardial fibrosis with or without endocardial fibroelastosis; cardiomyopathy; coronary artery disease; and functional valve injury and conduction defects [98]. Women with a history of **prior thoracic radiation therapy** (including left-sided breast cancer) **should undergo a baseline echocardiogram and electrocardiogram** prior to pregnancy to detect subclinical radiation-induced cardiac sequelae. Consultation with a cardiologist is advised if the echocardiogram is abnormal or an arrhythmia is noted.

Patients who have undergone mediastinal/mantle radiation, such as after Hodgkin's disease, may be at risk for hypothyroidism and should have thyroid function studies performed at initial prenatal visit.

Children of Cancer Survivors: No Increased Risk for Cancer
The offspring of cancer survivors are not at increased risk for cancer unless the tumor suffered by the parent was a component of an inherited syndrome, such as retinoblastoma [99,100].

Pregnancy after Cancer: Risk of Recurrence?
With the possible exception of gestational trophoblastic disease, **pregnancy does not affect the risk of recurrence of any type of cancer although the diagnosis may be delayed because of the pregnancy**. In particular, recurrence of melanoma [101,102] and breast cancer [103–105] appear to be unaffected by a subsequent pregnancy.

Pregnancy after Specific Cancers
Aside from a history of choriocarcinoma, a pregnancy subsequent to cancer treatment should not increase a woman's risk for cancer recurrence or death.

Pregnancy after Breast Cancer
Breast cancer, being hormonally driven, is the most common cancer for which women hesitate to have subsequent pregnancies. Some reports suggest that a subsequent pregnancy after treatment of early-stage breast cancer has a favorable impact on survival [106–109]. **Prognosis is determined by nodal status and stage, not subsequent pregnancy** [110]. In one series, 94 women with early-stage disease who became pregnant after breast cancer were compared to 188 breast cancer survivors without subsequent pregnancies matched for nodal status, tumor size, age, and year of diagnosis [108]. The risk ratio for death was significantly lower (0.44) for women who became pregnant subsequent to the diagnosis of breast cancer compared to women with breast cancer who did not have a subsequent pregnancy. Sankila (RR 0.2 [0.1–0.5]) and Mueller (RR 0.54 [0.41–0.71]) also showed a decreased risk of death for women with subsequent pregnancy after breast cancer compared to controls matched for age, stage, and year of diagnosis [99,111]. Even for women with a history of estrogen receptor positive breast cancer, a subsequent pregnancy was not deleterious for survival status. In this multicenter retrospective cohort study, 333 pregnant patients and 874 matched nonpregnant patients were analyzed of whom 686 patients had ER-positive disease. No difference in disease-free survival was observed between pregnant and nonpregnant patients in the ER-positive (HR 0.91; 95% CI, 0.67 to 1.24, p 0.55) or the ER-negative (HR 0.75; 95% CI, 0.51 to 1.08, p 0.12)

cohorts. This group did not demonstrate a protective effect from pregnancy subsequent to the diagnosis of breast cancer [112]. Breast cancer survivors on endocrine therapy, such as tamoxifen, may not wish to delay pregnancy for 5 years to complete the suggested course. Ongoing trials are attempting to answer the safe time interval for elective interruption of hormonal therapy to pursue pregnancy.

Birth control should be strongly advised when survivors are taking tamoxifen and trastuzumab. There have been case reports of ambiguous genitalia and Goldenhar syndrome in children exposed to tamoxifen in utero [113,114]. Animal studies show rib abnormalities, metaplastic and dysplastic changes in the epithelium of the uterus and reproductive tract similar to DES, growth restriction, and death [114–116]. Pregnancies exposed to Trastuzumab have been complicated by reversible oligohydramnios and fetal renal insufficiency [33–38,117–119]. For women who become accidentally pregnant while taking trastuzumab and wish to continue pregnancy, trastuzumab should be stopped, and pregnancy could be allowed to continue.

Aside from issues pertaining to estrogen receptor status and the role of 5–10 years of tamoxifen use for ER+ tumors (see previous section above), the issue is **how long should breast cancer survivors wait before pursuing a subsequent pregnancy.** One study linked data from three cancer registries to birth certificate data to evaluate survival of breast-cancer patients who had pregnancies subsequent to cancer treatment [111]. Women with a history of breast cancer should plan to delay subsequent pregnancy at least 10 months after completing cancer treatment (not after diagnosis), realizing that the first two years after diagnosis carries the highest risk for recurrence. A total of 438 women with invasive breast cancer were matched to 2775 controls for age at diagnosis, race, year of diagnosis, and stage. Among women who were lymph-node negative at diagnosis, younger than 35 years of age, or with only localized disease, pregnancy did not affect cancer mortality even if conception occurred within 10 months of diagnosis. Among women with positive lymph nodes at diagnosis, older than 35 years of age, or diagnosed with regional recurrence prior to pregnancy, there was a significant increase in cancer mortality if they conceived within 10 months of diagnosis. Women who conceived at least 10 months after diagnosis had lower mortality than women without births after breast cancer (RR 0.54, 95% CI 0.41–0.71). Decreased mortality was noted regardless of local/metastatic disease, maternal age, tumor size, or lymph-node status. For each year delay in conception after breast cancer, the relative risk of death was further decreased: two to three years after diagnosis, RR 0.49 (95% CI 0.27–0.86); three to four years after diagnosis, RR 0.30 (95% CI 0.12–0.71); and four to five years after diagnosis, RR 0.19 (95% CI 0.05–0.81).

The half-life of methotrexate (a commonly used agent in the CMF [cyclophosphamide, methotrexate, fluorouracil] regimen) is approximately 8 to 15 hours and it is retained for several weeks to months in the kidney and liver, respectively, leading this author to recommend delaying conception for at least 12 weeks after stopping methotrexate [120].

Breast-feeding after treatment for breast cancer. Most women who have undergone irradiation for breast cancer are able to produce milk on the affected side, but the amount of milk produced may be less than that in a nonirradiated breast, particularly if the lumpectomy site was close to the areolar complex or transected many ducts [121]. Even when breast milk is produced, **breast-feeding from the irradiated**

breast is not advised because mastitis will be difficult to treat if it occurs [122,123].

Pregnancy after Hodgkin's Lymphoma
After mantle/mediastinal radiation, patients may have undiagnosed hypothyroidism and should be screened with thyroid function studies at the beginning of pregnancy. Patients s/p treatment for HD also have a lifetime risk for secondary cancers, so during prenatal care, breast and skin examination is important.

Pregnancy after Chronic Leukemia
Patients with CML who conceive while taking Gleevec are advised to discontinue use during pregnancy with the majority of patients able to regain remission status postpartum [53].

Pregnancy after Melanoma
The highest risk for recurrence after an adequately excised melanoma is during the first 2 years, so women are often advised to avoid pregnancy during this time period, but having a pregnancy during this time period does not increase one's risk for recurrence. Placental pathology should be sent after delivery in women with a history of melanoma, and prenatal skin examination should be performed at the first prenatal visit and vigilantly by the patient. Moles may darken and even increase in size during pregnancy but should not become irregular or itch.

Pregnancy after Thyroid Carcinoma
After a total thyroidectomy, calcium balance may become an issue during the exertion of labor or if magnesium therapy is given for preterm labor or preeclampsia as parathyroid glands may have been inadvertently removed during thyroidectomy. Check calcium levels during magnesium treatment and labor.

REFERENCES
1. Donegan W. Cancer and pregnancy. *CA Cancer J Clin* 1983; 33(4): 194–214. [Review, III]
2. Weisz B, Meirow D, Schiff E, Impact and treatment of cancer during pregnancy. *Expert Rev Anticancer Ther* 2004; 4(5): 889–902. [II-2]
3. Barnavon Y, Wallack MK. Management of the pregnant patient with carcinoma of the breast. *Surg Gynecol Obstet* 1990; 171(4): 347–52. [Review, II-3]
4. Siu BL, Alonzo MR, Vargo TA et al. Transient dilated cardiomyopathy in a newborn exposed to idarubicin and all-transretinoic acid (ATRA) early in the second trimester of pregnancy. *Int J Gynecol Cancer* 2002; 12: 399–402. [II-3]
5. Achtari C, Hohlfeld P. Cardiotoxic transplacental effect of idarubicin administered during the second trimester of pregnancy. *Am J Obstet Gynecol* 2000; 183: 511–2. [II-3]
6. Reynoso EE, Hueta F. Acute leukemia and pregnancy—Fatal fetal outcome after exposure to idarubicin during the second trimester. *Acta Oncolog* 1994; 33: 703–16. [II-3]
7. Cardonick E, Iacobucci A. Use of chemotherapy during human pregnancy. *Lancet Oncol* 2004; 5(5): 283–91. [Review; II-3]
8. Aviles A, Neri N. Hematological malignancies and pregnancy: A final report of 84 children who received chemotherapy in utero. *Clin Lymph* 2001; 2(3): 173–7. [II-2]
9. Hahn KM, Johnson PH, Gordon N et al. Treatment of pregnant breast cancer patients and outcomes of children exposed to chemotherapy in utero. *Cancer* 2006; 107(6): 1219–26. [II-2]
10. D'Incalci M, Broggini M, Buscaglia M et al. Transplacental passage of doxorubicin. *Lancet* 1983; 75: 8314–5. [II-2]

11. Syme MR, Paxton JW, Keelan JA. Drug transfer and metabolism by the human placenta. *Clin Pharmacokinet* 2004: 43(8): 487–514. [II-3]

12. Morishita S, Imai A, Kawabata I et al. Acute myelogenous leukemia in pregnancy: Fetal blood sampling and early effects of chemotherapy. *Int J Gynaecol Obstet* 1994; 44(3): 273–7. [II-2]

13. Beadle BM, Woodward WA, Middleton LP et al. The impact of pregnancy on breast cancer outcomes in women. *Cancer* 2009; 115(6): 1174–84. [II-1]

14. Loibl S, von Minckwitz G, Gwyn K et al. Breast carcinoma during pregnancy. International recommendations from an expert meeting. *Cancer* 2006; 106(2): 237–46. [III]

15. Psyrri A, Burtness B. Pregnancy-associated breast cancer. *Cancer J* 2005; 11(2): 83–95. [II-2]

16. Nugent P, O'Connell TX. Breast cancer and pregnancy. *Arch Surg* 1985; 120: 1221–4. [Review; II-3]

17. Finley JL, Silverman JF, Lannin DR. Fine-needle aspiration cytology of breast masses in pregnant in lactating women. *Diag Cytopath* 1989; 5: 255–8. [II-3]

18. Middleton LP, Amin M, Gwyn K, Theriault R, Sahin A. Breast carcinoma in pregnant women: Assessment of clinicopathologic and immunohistochemical features. *Cancer* 2003; 98(5): 1055–60. [II-2]

19. Amant F, von Minckwitz G, Han SN et al. Prognosis of women with primary breast cancer diagnosed during pregnancy: Results from an international collaborative study. *J Clin Oncol* 2013; 31(20): 2532–9. [II-3]

20. Jacobs IA, Chang CK, Salti GI. Coexistence of pregnancy and cancer. *Am Surg* 2004; 70(11): 1025–9. [II-2]

21. Baker J, Ali A, Groch MW et al. Bone scanning in pregnant patients with breast carcinoma. *Clin Nucl Med* 1987; 12(7): 519–24. [II-3]

22. Kuerer HM, Gwyn K, Ames FC, Theriault RL. Conservative surgery and chemotherapy for breast carcinoma during pregnancy. *Surgery* 2002; 131(1): 108–10. [II-2]

23. Keleher A, Wendt R 3rd, Delpassand E et al. The safety of lymphatic mapping in pregnant breast cancer patients using Tc-99m sulfur colloid. *Breast J* 2004; 10(6): 492–5. [II-3]

24. De Laurentiis M, Cancello G, D'Agostino D et al. Taxane-based combinations as adjuvant chemotherapy of early breast cancer: A meta-analysis of randomized trials. *J Clin Oncol* 2008; 26(1): 44–53. [Meta-analysis; 13 studies, n = 22,903]

25. Mir O, Berveiller P, Goldwasser F et al. Emerging therapeutic options for breast cancer chemotherapy during pregnancy. *Ann Oncol* 2008; 19: 607–13. [II-3]

26. Potluri V, Lewis D, Burton G. Chemotherapy with Taxanes in breast cancer during pregnancy: Case report and review of literature. *Clin Breast Cancer* 2006; 7(2): 167–70. [II-3]

27. Gadducci A, Cosio S, Genazzani AR et al. Chemotherapy with epirubicin and paclitaxel for breast cancer during pregnancy: Case report and review of literature. *Anticancer Res* 2003; 23: 5225–30. [II-3]

28. Gonzalez-Angulo A, Walter RS, Carpenter RJ Jr et al. Paclitaxel chemotherapy in a pregnant patient with bilateral breast cancer. *Clin Breast Cancer* 2004; 5(4): 317–9. [II-3]

29. Gainford MC, Clemons M. Breast cancer in pregnancy: Are taxanes safe? *Clin Oncol (R Coll Radiol)* 2006; 18(2): 159. [II-3]

30. Nieto Y, Santisteban M, Aramendia JM et al. Docetaxel administered during pregnancy for inflammatory breast carcinoma. *Clin Breast Cancer* 2006; 6(6): 533–4. [II-3]

31. Cardonick E, Bhat A, Gilmandyar D, Somer R. Maternal and fetal outcomes of taxane chemotherapy in breast and ovarian cancer during pregnancy: Case series and review of the literature. *Ann Oncol* 2012; 23(12): 3016–23.

32. Amant F, Deckers S, Van Calsteren K, Loibl S, Halaska M, Brepoels L et al. Breast cancer in pregnancy: Recommendations of an international consensus meeting. *Eur J Cancer* 2010; 46: 3158–68. [III]

33. Sekar R, Stone PR. Trastuzumab use for metastatic breast cancer in pregnancy. *Obstet Gynecol* 2007; 110: 507–9. [II-3]

34. Fanale MA, Uyei AR, Theriault RL et al. Treatment of metastatic breast cancer with trastuzumab and vinorelbine during pregnancy. *Clin Breast Cancer* 2005; 6: 354–6. [II-3]

35. Watson W. Herceptin (Trastuzumab) therapy during pregnancy: Association with reversible anhydramnios. *Obstet Gynecol* 2005; 105: 642–3. [II-3]

36. Bader AA, Schlembach D, Tamussino KF et al. Anhydramnios associated with administration of trastuzumab and paclitaxel for metastatic breast cancer during pregnancy. *Lancet Oncol* 2007; 8: 79–81. [II-3]

37. Shrim A, Garcia-Bournissen F, Maxwell C et al. Favorable pregnancy outcome following trastuzumab use during pregnancy—Case report and updated literature review. *Reprod Toxicol* 2007; 23: 611–3. [II-3]

38. Waterston AM, Graham J. Effect of adjuvant trastuzumab on pregnancy. *J Clin Oncol* 2006; 24: 321. [II-3]

39. Ward FT, Weiss RB. Lymphoma and pregnancy. *Semin Oncol* 1989; 16: 397–409. [Review]

40. Lishner M, Zemlickis D, Degendorfer P et al. Maternal and foetal outcome following Hodgkin's disease in pregnancy. *Br J Cancer* 1992; 65(1): 114–7. [III]

41. Nisce LZ, Tome MA, He S et al. Management of coexisting Hodgkin's disease and pregnancy. *Am J Clin Oncol* 1986; 9(2): 146–51. [II-3]

42. Vermoolen MA, Kwee TC, Nievelstein RAJ. Whole-body MRI for staging Hodgkin lymphoma in a pregnant patient. *Amer J Hematol* 2010; 85(6): 443. [II-2]

43. Woo SY, Fuller LM, Cundiff JH et al. Radiotherapy during pregnancy for clinical stages IA-IIA Hodgkin's disease. *Int J Radiat Oncol Biol Phys* 1992; 23(2): 407–12. [II-3]

44. Dekaban AS. Abnormalities in children exposed to x-radiation during various stages of gestation: Tentative timetable of radiation injury to the human fetus. *J Nucl Med* 1968; 9: 471–7. [II-3]

45. Ioachim HL. Non-Hodgkin's lymphoma in pregnancy. *Arch Path Lab Med* 1985; 109: 803–9. [II-3]

46. Mavrommatis CG, Daskalakis GJ, Papageorgiou IS et al. Non-Hodgkin's lymphoma during pregnancy—Case report. *Eur J Obstet Gynecol Reprod Biol* 1998; 79(1): 95–7. [II-3]

47. Klink DT, van Elburg RM, Schreurs MW, van Well GT. Rituximab administration in third trimester of pregnancy suppresses neonatal B-cell development. *Clin Dev Immunol* 2008; 2008: 271363. [II-2]

48. Reynoso EE, Shepherd FA, Messner HA et al. Acute leukemia during pregnancy: The Toronto leukemia study group experience with long-term follow-up of children exposed in utero to chemotherapeutic agents. *J Clin Oncol* 1987; 5: 1098–106. [II-2]

49. Catanzarite VA, Ferguson JE 2nd. Acute leukemia and pregnancy: A review of management and outcomes, 1972–1982. *Obstet Gynecol Surv* 1984; 39(11): 663–77. [II-2]

50. Okun DB, Groncy PK, Sieger L et al. Acute leukemia in pregnancy: Transient neonatal myelosuppression after combination chemotherapy in the mother. *Med Pediatr Oncol* 1979; 7(4): 315–9. [II-3]

51. Strobl FJ, Voelkerding KV, Smith EP. Management of chronic myeloid leukemia during pregnancy with leukapheresis. *J Clin Apheresis* 1999; 14: 42–4. [II-3]

52. Fitzgerald D, Rowe JM, Heal J. Leukapheresis for control of chronic myelogenous leukemia during pregnancy. *Am J Hematol* 1986; 22: 213–8. [II-3]

53. Ali R, Ozkalemkas F, Ozcelik T, Ozkocaman V, Ozan U, Kimya Y et al. Pregnancy under treatment of imatinib and successful labor in a patient with chronic myelogenous leukemia (CML). Outcome of discontinuation of imatinib therapy after achieving a molecular remission. *Leuk Res* 2005; 29(8): 971–3. [II-2]

54. Alkindi S, Dennison D, Pathare A. Imatinib in Pregnancy. *Eur J Haematol* 2005; 74(6): 535–7. [II-2]

55. Hensely ML, Ford JM. Imatinib treatment: Specific issues related to safety, fertility, and pregnancy. *Semin Hematol* 2003; 40(2): 21–5. [II-2]

56. Yadav U, Solanki SL, Yadav R. Chronic myeloid leukemia with pregnancy: Successful management of pregnancy and delivery with hydroxyurea and imatinib continued till delivery *Cancer Res Ther* 2013; 9(3): 484–6. [II-2]

57. Russell MA, Carpenter MW, Akhtar MS, Lagattuta TF, Egorin MJ. Imatinib mesylate and metabolite concentrations in maternal blood, umbilical cord blood, placenta and breast milk. *J Perinatol* 2007; 27(4): 241. [II-2]

58. Eskander RN, Tarsa M, Herbst KD, Kelly TF. Chronic myelocytic leukemia in pregnancy: A case report describing successful treatment using multimodal therapy. *J Obstet Gynecol* 2011; 37(11): 1371–3. [II-2]

59. Colbourn DS, Nathanson L, Belilos E. Pregnancy and malignant melanoma. *Semin Oncol* 1989; 16: 377–87. [Review, II-3]

60. Lens MB, Rosdahl I, Farahmand BY et al. Effect of pregnancy on survival of women with cutaneous malignant melanoma. *J Clin Oncol* 2004; 22(21): 4369–75. [II-2]

61. Slingluff CL Jr, Reintgen D. Malignant melanoma and the prognostic implications of pregnancy, oral contraceptives, and exogenous hormones. *Semin Surg Oncol* 1993; 9: 228–31. [II-2]

62. Pennoyer JW, Grin CM, Driscoll MS et al. Changes in size of melanocytic nevi during pregnancy. *J Eur Acad Dermatol Venereol* 2003; 17(3): 349–51. [II-3]

63. Baergen RN, Johnson D, Moore T et al. Maternal melanoma metastatic to the placenta: A case report and review of the literature. *Arch Pathol Lab Med* 1997; 121: 508–11. [II-3]

64. Zemlickis D, Lishner M, Degendorfer P et al. Maternal and fetal outcome after invasive cervical cancer in pregnancy. *J Clin Oncol* 1991; 9(11): 1956–61. [II-2]

65. Germann N, Haie-Meder C, Morice P et al. Management and clinical outcomes of pregnant patients with invasive cervical cancer. *Ann Oncol* 2005; 16(3): 397–402. [II-2]

66. Hopkins MP, Morley GW. The prognosis and management of cervical cancer associated with pregnancy. *Obstet Gynecol* 1992; 80(1): 9–13. [II-2]

67. Method MW, Brost BC. Management of cervical cancer in pregnancy. *Semin Surg Oncol* 1999; 16(3): 251–60. [Review, II-3]

68. Van Calsteren K, Vergote I, Amant F. Cervical neoplasia during pregnancy: Diagnosis, management and prognosis. *Best Pract Res Clin Obstet Gynecol* 2005; 19(4): 611–30. [Review, II-3]

69. Marana HR, de Andrade JM, da Silva Mathes AC et al. Chemotherapy in the treatment of locally advanced cervical cancer and pregnancy. *Gynecol Oncol* 2001; 80(2): 272–4. [II-2]

70. Prem KA, Makowski EL, McKelvey JL. Carcinoma of the cervix associated with pregnancy. *Am J Obstet Gynecol* 1966; 95: 99–108. [II-2]

71. Greer BE, Easterling TR, McLennan DA et al. Fetal and maternal considerations in the management of stage I-B cervical cancer during pregnancy. *Gynecol Oncol* 1989; 34(1): 61–5. [II-2]

72. McDonald SD, Faught W, Gruslin A. Cervical cancer during pregnancy. *J Obstet Gynecol Canada* 2002; 24(6): 491–8. [Review, II-3]

73. Sood AK, Sorosky JI, Krogman S et al. Surgical management of cervical cancer complicating pregnancy: A case control study. *Gynecol Oncol* 1996; 63(3): 294–8. [II]

74. Duggan B, Muderspach LI, Roman LD et al. Cervical cancer in pregnancy: Reporting on planned delay in therapy. *Obstet Gynecol* 1993; 82: 598–602. [II-3]

75. Cliby WA, Dodson MK, Podratz KC. Cervical cancer complicated by pregnancy: Episiotomy site recurrences following vaginal delivery. *Obstet Gynecol* 1994; 84(2): 179–82. [II-3]

76. Morris PC. Thyroid cancer complicating pregnancy. *Obstet Gynecol Clin North Am* 1998; 25(2): 401–5. [Review]

77. Moosa M, Mazzaferri EL. Outcome of differentiated thyroid cancer diagnosed in pregnant women. *J Clin Endocrinol Metab* 1997; 82(9): 2862–6. [II-3]

78. Vini L, Hyer S, Pratt B et al. Management of differentiated thyroid cancer diagnosed during pregnancy. *Eur J Endocrinol* 1999; 140(5): 404–6. [II-3]

79. Zemlickis D, Lishner M, Erlich R et al. Teratogenicity and carcinogenicity in a twin exposed in utero to cyclophosphamide. *Terat Carcin Mutagenesis* 1993; 13: 139–43. [II-3]

80. Amant F, Van Calsteren K, Halaska MJ, Gziri MM, Hui W, Lagae L, Willemsen MA, Kapusta L, Van Calster B, Wouters H, Heyns L, Han SN, Tomek V, Mertens L, Ottevanger PB. Long-term cognitive and cardiac outcomes after prenatal exposure to chemotherapy in children aged 18 months or older: An observational study. *Lancet Oncol* 2012; 13(3): 256–64. [II-1]

81. Cardonick EH, Gringlas M, Hunter K, Greenspan J. Development of children born to mothers with cancer during pregnancy: Comparing in utero chemotherapy-exposed children with nonexposed controls. *Am J Obstet Gynecol* 2015; 212(5): 658.e1–8. [II-1]

82. Green DM, Whitton JA, Stovall M et al. Pregnancy outcome of female survivors of childhood cancer: A report from the Childhood Cancer Survivor Study. *Am J Obstet Gynecol* 2002; 187: 1070. [II-1]

83. Chiarelli AM, Marrett LD, Darlington GA. Pregnancy outcomes in females after treatment for childhood cancer. *Epidemiology* 2000; 11: 161. [II-3]

84. Reulen RC, Zeegers MP, Wallace WH et al. Pregnancy outcomes among adult survivors of childhood cancer in the British Childhood Cancer Survivor Study. *Cancer Epidemiol Biomarkers Prev* 2009; 18: 2239. [II-1]

85. Dodds L, Marrett LD, Tomkins DJ et al. Case-control study of congenital anomalies in children of cancer patients. *Br Med J* 1993; 307(6897): 164–8. [II-2]

86. Blatt J, Mulvihill JJ, Ziegler JL et al. Pregnancy outcome following cancer chemotherapy. *Am J Med* 1980; 69: 828–32. [II-3]

87. Byrne J, Rasmussen SA, Steinhorn SC et al. Genetic disease in offspring of long-term survivors of childhood and adolescent cancer. *Am J Hum Genet* 1998; 62(1): 45–52. [II-3]

88. Li FP, Fine W, Jaffe N et al. Offspring of patients treated for cancer in childhood. *J Natl Cancer Inst* 1979; 62(5): 1193–7. [II-3]

89. Bar J, Davidi O, Goshen Y et al. Pregnancy outcome in women treated with doxorubicin for childhood cancer. *Am J Obstet Gynecol* 2003; 189: 853. [II-3]

90. Hawkins MM, Smith RA. Pregnancy outcomes in childhood cancer survivors: Probable effects of abdominal irradiation. *Int J Cancer* 1989; 43: 399. [II-3]

91. Green DM, Peabody EM, Nan B et al. Pregnancy outcome after treatment for Wilms tumor: A report from the National Wilms Tumor Study Group. *J Clin Oncol* 2002; 20: 2506. [II-1]

92. Pridjian G, Rich NE, Montag AG. Pregnancy hemoperitoneum and placenta percreta in a patient with previous pelvic irradiation and ovarian failure. *Am J Obstet Gynecol* 1990; 162: 1205. [II-3]

93. Norwitz ER, Stern HM, Grier H et al. Placenta percreta and uterine rupture associated with prior whole body radiation therapy. *Obstet Gynecol* 2001; 98: 929. [II-3]

94. Holm K, Nysom K, Brocks V et al. Ultrasound B—Mode changes in the uterus and ovaries and Doppler changes in the uterus after total body irradiation and allogeneic bone marrow transplantation in childhood. *Bone Marrow Transpl* 1999; 23: 259. [II-3]

95. Signorello LB, Cohen SS, Bosetti C et al. Female survivors of childhood cancer: Preterm birth and low birth weight among their children. *J Natl Cancer Inst* 2006; 98: 1453. [II-3]

96. Lie Fong, S, van den Heuvel-Eibrink MM, Eijkemans MJ et al. Pregnancy outcome in female childhood cancer survivors. *Hum Reprod* 2010; 25: 1206. [II-3]

97. Signorello LB, Mulvihill JJ, Green DM et al. Stillbirth and neonatal death in relation to radiation exposure before conception: A retrospective cohort study. *Lancet* 2010; 376: 624. [II-3]

98. Stewart JR, Fajardo LF, Gillette SM et al. Radiation injury to the heart. *Int J Radiat Oncol Biol Phys* 1995; 31: 1205. [II-3]

99. Sankila R, Olsen JH, Anderson H et al. Risk of cancer among offspring of childhood-cancer survivors. Association of the Nordic Cancer Registries and the Nordic Society of Paediatric Haematology and Oncology. *N Engl J Med* 1998; 338: 1339. [III]

100. Mulvihill JJ, Myers MH, Connelly RR et al. Cancer in offspring of long-term survivors of childhood and adolescent cancer. *Lancet* 1987; 2: 813. [III]

101. Reintgen DS, McCarty KS Jr, Vollmer R et al. Malignant melanoma and pregnancy. *Cancer* 1985; 55: 1340. [II-3]

102. Grin CM, Driscoll MS, Grant-Kels JM. The relationship of pregnancy, hormones, and melanoma. *Semin Cutan Med Surg* 1998; 17: 167. [II-3]

103. Azim HA Jr, Santoro L, Pavlidis N et al. Safety of pregnancy following breast cancer diagnosis: A meta-analysis of 14 studies. *Eur J Cancer* 2011; 47: 74–83. [Meta-analysis; 14 studies]

104. Velentgas P, Daling JR, Malone KE et al. Pregnancy after breast carcinoma: Outcomes and influence on mortality. *Cancer* 1999; 85: 2424. [II-2]

105. Danforth DN Jr. How subsequent pregnancy affects outcome in women with a prior breast cancer. *Oncology (Williston Park)* 1991; 5: 23. [II-3]

106. Cooper DR, Butterfield J. Pregnancy subsequent to mastectomy for cancer of the breast. *Ann Surg* 1970; 171: 429. [II-3]

107. von Schoultz E, Johansson H, Wilking N et al. Influence of prior and subsequent pregnancy on breast cancer prognosis. *J Clin Oncol* 1995; 13: 430. [II-2]

108. Kroman N, Jensen MB, Melbye M et al. Should women be advised against pregnancy after breast-cancer treatment? *Lancet* 1997; 350: 319. [II-2]

109. Gelber S, Coates AS, Goldhirsch A et al. Effect of pregnancy on overall survival after the diagnosis of early-stage breast cancer. *J Clin Oncol* 2001; 19: 1671. [II-2]

110. Ariel IM, Kempner R. The prognosis of patients who become pregnant after mastectomy for breast cancer. *Int Surg* 1989; 74(3): 185–7. [II-3]

111. Mueller BA, Simon MS, Deapen D et al. Childbearing and survival after breast carcinoma in young women. *Cancer* 2003; 98: 1131. [II-1]

112. Azim HA, Kroman N, Paesmans M, Gelber S, Rotmensz N, Ameye et al. Prognostic impact of pregnancy after breast cancer according to estrogen receptor status: A multicenter retrospective study. *J Clin Oncol* 2013; 31(1): 73. [II-2]

113. Tewari K, Bonebrake RG, Asrat T et al. Ambiguous genitalia in infant exposed to tamoxifen in utero. *Lancet* 1997; 350: 183. [II-3]

114. Cullins SL, Pridjian G, Sutherland CM. Goldenhar's syndrome associated with tamoxifen given to the mother during gestation. *J Am Med Assoc* 1994; 271: 1905–6. [II-3]

115. Wisel MS, Datta JK, Saxena RN. Effects of anti-estrogens on early pregnancy in guinea pigs. *Int J Fertil Menopausal Stud* 1994; 39: 156–63. [II-3]

116. Diwan BA, Anderson LM, Ward JM. Proliferative lesions of oviduct and uterus in CD-1 mice exposed prenatally to tamoxifen. *Carcinogenesis* 1997; 18: 2009–14. [II-3]

117. Gottschalk I, Berg C, Harbeck N et al. Fetal renal insufficiency following trastuzumab treatment for breast cancer in pregnancy: Case report und review of the current literature. *Breast Care (Basel)* 2011; 6: 475–8. [II-3]

118. Witzel ID, Müller V, Harps E et al. Trastuzumab in pregnancy associated with poor fetal outcome. *Ann Oncol* 2008; 19:191–2. [II-3]

119. Azim HA Jr, Peccatori FA, Liptrott SJ et al. Breast cancer and pregnancy: How safe is trastuzumab? *Nat Rev Clin Oncol* 2009; 6: 367–70. [II-3]

120. Donnenfeld AE, Pastuszak A, Noah JS et al. Methotrexate exposure prior to and during pregnancy. *Teratology* 1994; 49: 79. [III]

121. Wobbes T. Effect of a breast saving procedure on lactation. *Eur J Surg* 1996; 162: 419. [II-3]

122. Findlay PA, Gorrell CR, d'Angelo T et al. Lactation after breast radiation. *Int J Radiat Oncol Biol Phys* 1988; 15: 511. [III]

123. Higgins S, Haffty BG. Pregnancy and lactation after breast-conserving therapy for early stage breast cancer. *Cancer* 1994; 73: 2175. [III]

43

Dermatoses of pregnancy

Dana Correale, Joya Sahu, and Jason B. Lee

BACKGROUND

Polymorphic eruption of pregnancy (PEP) comprises the only pregnancy-specific dermatosis. All other dermatoses mentioned herein may be encountered outside of pregnancy, but they have been traditionally grouped and discussed as dermatoses of pregnancy as they represent common and uncommon dermatoses encountered during pregnancy.

Stretch marks are the only dermatologic condition for which there are trials for interventions. Dermatoses of pregnancy as well as melanoma in pregnancy are not well studied with no specific trials regarding treatment. Most evidence regarding pathogenesis and etiology as well as typical disease presentation is based on case reports and case series. Dermatoses of pregnancy have been plagued by disagreements about their nomenclature and classification. Although likely to be reworked and reclassified in the future, the current widely accepted classification, based on the largest series to date, consists of four major categories: 1) polymorphic eruption of pregnancy (PEP), 2) atopic eruption of pregnancy (AEP), 3) pemphigoid gestationis (PG), and 4) intrahepatic cholestasis of pregnancy (ICP). Under this classification, AEP has subsumed atopic dermatitis (eczema) of pregnancy, prurigo of pregnancy (PP), and pruritic folliculitis of pregnancy (PFP). Intrahepatic cholestasis of pregnancy, although not associated with any primary skin lesions, is currently accepted as one of the dermatoses of pregnancy. The most common skin disorder in pregnancy is atopic dermatitis (eczema) of pregnancy. As pruritus represents a significant symptom in all four dermatoses, differentiating one from the other, especially in their early stages, may pose a significant diagnostic challenge, requiring excluding each of the dermatoses methodically. Although not included in the current classification, impetigo herpetiformis (IH), a variant of pustular psoriasis, is frequently discussed together with dermatoses of pregnancy, considered by some as the fifth dermatosis of pregnancy. Table 43.1 provides a summary and classification of the dermatoses of pregnancy. Multidisciplinary management involving a dermatologist expert in dermatologic conditions in pregnancy is of paramount importance.

STRIAE GRAVIDARUM
Key Points

- The **exact cause** of striae gravidarum (SG) is **unknown**, but the strongest associated risk factors for their development are presence of preexisting breast and thigh striae and a family history.
- **There is no widely available product that has been shown to prevent the formation of SG.** Massage with either **Trofolastin cream** or **Verum ointment** is associated with a **decrease in the development of SG**.
- **Topical tretinoin and various types of laser therapy have been shown to be helpful in the treatment of SG.**

Diagnosis/Definition

Striae distensae (SD), or stretch marks, do not represent a disease but rather they are a cosmetic problem for many people. They often occur for the first time during pregnancy and are referred to as SG. SD initially appear as linear patches that are red to purple in color and lack noticeable surface change (striae rubra). With time, their color fades to lighter than normal skin tone. They become atrophic or depressed with a fine, wrinkled surface (striae alba).

Symptoms

SD are largely asymptomatic. They may be slightly pruritic in their early stages.

Epidemiology/Incidence

The prevalence of SG ranges from 50% to 90% [1]. The mean gestational age for the onset of SG is 25 weeks [1].

Genetics

There is no known clear genetic cause of SG; however, there may be a familial tendency to develop them [1].

Etiology/Basic Pathology

Many theories exist regarding the etiology of SG. Rapid weight gain, baseline weight, hormonal changes, and greater change in abdominal and hip girth during pregnancy have been associated in the past with SG [1,2]. None of these theories have been supported by any recent studies. It is known, however, that elastin and fibrillin fibers, components of the dermal extracellular matrix, are reduced in SD [3].

Risk Factors/Associations

The factors most strongly associated with the development of SG are the **presence of breast or thigh striae**, having a **mother with SG**, having **additional family members with SG**, and belonging to a nonwhite race. In contrast, prepregnancy body mass index (BMI), mean weight gain during pregnancy, mean percentage of weight gain, and mean change in BMI seem not to be associated with the development of SG [1].

Table 43.1 A Summary and Classification of the Dermatoses of Pregnancy

Dermatosis	Course	Skin Findings	Fetal Risks	Treatment
PEP	Third trimester. Resolution postpartum.	Urticarial lesions on the abdomen, often within striae with sparing of the periumbilical area. Extension to upper thighs and buttocks.	None	High-potency topical steroids
AEP	*ADP* First to third trimesters. Can persist postpartum.	Hyperpigmented, lichenified, excoriated patches and plaques on flexural surfaces in 80% and papules and/or prurigo nodules in 20%.	None	Mid- to high-potency topical steroids, emollients, and antihistamines; oral corticosteroids in severe cases
	PFP Second or third trimester. Resolution within 1–2 months postpartum.	Follicular papules and pustules	None	Mid- to high-potency topical corticosteroids
	PP Second or third trimester. Resolution postpartum.	Excoriated papules over extremities and occasionally abdomen	None	Mid- to high-potency topical steroids
ICP	See Chapter 10			
PG	Second or third trimester. Resolution postpartum after weeks to months.	Ranges from annular and polycyclic urticarial papules and plaques to grouped blisters on the abdomen and extremities involving the periumbilical and umbilical skin	Prematurity and small gestational age at birth	Topical steroid for mild cases and systemic steroid for more severe cases
IH	Third trimester. Persists after delivery if untreated.	Symmetric, erythematous patches with peripheral superficial sterile pustules on flexural skin	Placental insufficiency and fetal loss	Systemic corticosteroids

Abbreviations: ADP, atopic dermatitis of pregnancy; AEP, atopic eruption of pregnancy; ICP, intrahepatic cholestasis of pregnancy; IH, impetigo herpetiformis; PEP, polymorphic eruption of pregnancy; PFP, pruritic folliculitis of pregnancy; PG, pemphigoid gestationis; PP, prurigo of pregnancy.

Management

Prevention

Massage with Trofolastin cream containing *Centella asiatica* extract, alpha tocopherol, and collagen-elastin hydrolysates applied daily is associated with a 59% **decrease in the development of SG** compared to massage with placebo [4]. Overall, 56% of the placebo group developed SG compared with 34% of the Trofolastin group. **Massage with Verum ointment** containing tocopherol, essential fatty acids, panthenol, hyaluronic acid, elastin, and menthol is also associated with a 74% **decrease in the development of SG** compared to no treatment, so it is unclear in this study if the massage or the Verum ointment or the combination of the two were beneficial [4]. In women with stretch marks from a previous pregnancy, there is no benefit. It should be noted that neither of these compounds are widely available, nor is it known what their active ingredient, if any, might be. There is the suggestion from the second study that bland emollients and massage alone may be of benefit in preventing the formation of SG. Cocoa butter lotion is not associated with reduction in the likelihood of developing SG [5].

Therapy

Once SG have formed, there are treatment options. *Topical tretinoin* 0.1% cream has been shown to reduce the appearance of SG/SD when used *on early lesions* (striae rubra) [6]. It is important to note that once striae have become white and atrophic, topical tretinoin was shown to have no benefit in a double-blind, placebo-controlled study [7]. Topical tretinoin (Retin A) works by binding to cytoplasmic proteins and nuclear receptors of keratinocytes and altering downstream gene transcription. The end biologic effect is

to regulate the growth and differentiation of keratinocytes [8]. In addition to regulating keratinocyte proliferation, topical retinoids have been shown to decrease fine wrinkling, increase dermal collagen, and repair elastin fiber formation [9]. Improvement in the appearance of SD/SG is most likely the result of this particular biologic effect. Tretinoin is pregnancy category C. Its use is contraindicated during breast-feeding, which makes it difficult to use during the early stages of SG. The side effects of tretinoin therapy are erythema, desquamation, and photosensitivity limited to the application site.

In addition to tretinoin therapy, improvement in the appearance of SD/SG can be achieved with laser therapy. **Laser therapy** is a rapidly evolving field with new lasers and applications emerging on a regular basis. Two large, blinded studies using an objective grading system evaluating the treatment of SD using a 585-nm pulsed dye laser have shown improvement in their appearance [10]. Both increases and decreases in collagen production have been shown post-treatment depending on the wavelength and energy density of laser used. An increase in dermal elastin content has also been shown in biopsies obtained after laser therapy [10]. Again, newer, more erythematous striae respond more favorably to pulsed dye laser treatment. This may be a more reasonable treatment option during the postpartum period as laser therapy is believed to be safe in breast-feeding women. A more recent study evaluating the effects of a XeCl excimer ultraviolet B (UVB) laser and a UVB light device showed repigmentation of striae alba [2]. Repigmentation was associated with an increase in melanin content, hypertrophy of melanocytes, and an increase in number of melanocytes 6 months after treatment.

POLYMORPHIC ERUPTION OF PREGNANCY (PRURITIC URTICARIAL PAPULES AND PLAQUES OF PREGNANCY)
Key Points

- Polymorphic eruption of pregnancy (pruritic urticarial papules and plaques of pregnancy [PUPPP]) is an extremely pruritic urticarial eruption occurring during the third trimester of pregnancy.
- There is no associated fetal morbidity or mortality.
- The mainstay of **treatment** is **topical steroids**.

Historic Notes

This entity was originally described by Lawley and colleagues in 1979 in a series of seven patients [11].

Diagnosis/Definition

PEP is characterized by urticarial lesions that **begin on the abdomen**, often within abdominal striae, and spare the periumbilical area (Figure 43.1). Lesions frequently spread to the **upper thighs and buttocks and occasionally may affect the arms**. The face, palms, and soles are usually spared. Despite the severe pruritus, there is notable lack of excoriation. As its name implies, PEP is polymorphous. Clinical lesions may appear vesicular, targetoid, or purpuric. This eruption is seen mostly in primigravidas with onset in the third trimester of pregnancy. It resolves shortly after delivery, but there have been a few cases reported in which onset of the disease has occurred in the postpartum period [12–14]. The diagnosis is primarily clinical. Histopathologic examination of affected skin most often yields nonspecific findings.

Symptoms

The eruption is accompanied by extreme pruritus. The itching is often so severe that it may interfere with sleep.

Epidemiology/Incidence

PEP is one of the most common dermatoses of pregnancy. It occurs in approximately 0.5% of pregnancies [15].

Genetics

There are no known genetic factors in PEP. In fact, some studies have looked for but failed to document a human leukocyte antigen (HLA) association [16,17].

Etiology/Basic Pathology

To date, there are no widely accepted theories to explain the etiology of this disease. Associated factors include increased abdominal distension secondary to excessive maternal weight gain and fetal birth weight [13,17,18], increased incidence of multiple pregnancies [12,15,17,19], not autoimmune mechanisms [20], but decreased serum cortisol levels [21,22], and fetal DNA migration in PEP skin lesions [23].

Complications

There have been no consistent maternal or fetal complications associated with PEP with newborns not affected with any related skin disease [14,17,21].

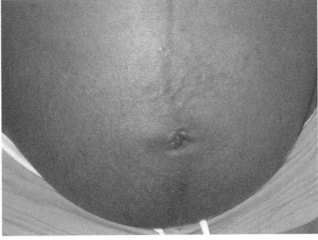

(a)

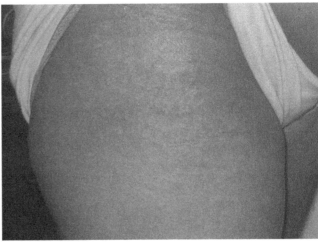

(b)

Figure 43.1 Polymorphous eruption of pregnancy (PEP). A 28-year-old primigravida with abrupt onset of extremely pruritic urticarial papules on the abdomen (a) and thighs (b) during her 39th week of pregnancy. Note the predilection for the abdominal striae with periumbilical sparing.

Management

Workup

The most important disease to exclude when diagnosing PEP is PG, which can present with urticarial lesions in the absence of more prototypical blisters. PG is usually a widespread eruption that begins on the abdomen but does not show a predilection for striae nor spares the periumbilical area. PG is rare, but it is associated with significant maternal and fetal morbidity and mortality [11,24]. Exclusion of PG relies on the clinical presentation, but direct immunofluorescence (DIF) of affected skin may be required in equivocal cases. There are no consistent DIF findings in PEP [13,14,17,21,25]. When positive DIF findings have been reported in PEP, they have been considered nondiagnostic for any particular disease [14,25]. In contrast, PG is associated with very consistent and reliable DIF findings [24].

Preconception Counseling

The vast majority of cases of PEP do not recur with subsequent pregnancies [11,17,21] or oral contraceptive use [1,7].

A few women affected by PEP have been reported to have episodes of transient hives while breast-feeding after the initial eruption resolved [11].

Therapy

The majority of cases of PEP can be effectively managed with **high-potency topical steroids** [11,17,21]. This class of medication does not cause any known fetal complications when used properly. In rare cases of prolonged and widespread use, significant systemic absorption could occur. In severe and widespread cases, short courses of oral corticosteroids have been used effectively [11,17,21]. The reader is referred to the guideline for impetigo herpetiformis for more detailed information on the use and safety of steroids in pregnancy. There is one reported case of severe PEP that required delivery by cesarean section at 35 weeks gestation for intractable pruritus uncontrolled by topical and oral corticosteroids [26]. In this case, the patient's symptoms were significantly improved within 12 hours of delivery.

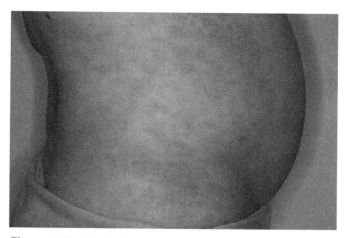

Figure 43.2 Atopic dermatitis (Eczema) of pregnancy. A 42-year-old G1P0 with multiple, lichenified, hyperpigmented patches and plaques on the abdomen and extremities.

ATOPIC DERMATITIS (ECZEMA) OF PREGNANCY
Key Points

- Atopic dermatitis of pregnancy (ADP) is an intensely pruritic eruption characterized by eczematous plaques or papular lesions involving the trunk and extremities.
- The mainstay of **therapy** is **topical steroids and emollients**.
- There is no associated maternal or fetal morbidity or mortality.

Diagnosis/Definition

ADP is characterized by intense itch accompanied by lichenified plaques or papular lesions in patients with a personal or family history of atopy and/or elevated IgE levels. The eruption most commonly presents before the third trimester of pregnancy in 75% of patients with onset occurring in all three trimesters and is a diagnosis of exclusion [27]. Recurrence in subsequent pregnancies is expected due to the background of atopy. The eruption consists of atopic dermatitis-like plaques and/or prurigo-like nodules accompanied by excoriations and secondary skin infections (Figure 43.2). ADP classically involves the trunk and extremities in typical atopic sites, such as the neck, décolletage, or flexural surfaces of extremities. Atopic dermatitis (eczema) of pregnancy, PFP, and PP have been grouped into one category, AEP [28,29]. Characteristic atopic clinical findings are key for diagnosis as histopathologic findings are nonspecific and DIF reveals no immunoreactive deposition [30].

Symptoms

ADP is accompanied by intense pruritus, which can lead to excoriations and secondary skin infections.

Epidemiology/Incidence

ADP is the most frequent dermatosis in pregnancy [22,27,31].

Etiology/Basic Pathology

Although causally linked to a personal or family history of atopy, there is no definitive evidence currently. One theory reflects a deterioration of existing atopic dermatitis or an exacerbation of a quiescent atopic state due to a TH2 shift in cytokine expression during pregnancy [22,31].

Pregnancy Considerations

There are no reports of adverse maternal or fetal outcomes in ADP. There is inadequate evidence to prescribe specific dietary intake for pregnant women to prevent atopic dermatitis in the newborn [32,33].

Management

Workup

The diagnosis of ADP is made clinically due to the characteristic clinical atopic presentation. Other specific dermatoses of pregnancy must first be ruled out. Sparing of striae and time of onset differentiate from PEP. Elevated IgE levels may be present in 20% to 70% of cases but are not diagnostic [27]. Total serum bile acid levels must be in the normal range. The relative nonspecific histopathologic changes of ADP do not discriminate among other pruritic dermatoses of pregnancy [34]. If PG is a diagnostic consideration, histopathologic exam and DIF testing may be performed in equivocal cases.

Therapy

Treatment strategies vary depending on the severity of the patient's clinical findings and symptoms. The mainstay of therapy for ADP is **mid- to high-potency topical steroids** accompanied by liberal use of emollients with or without antihistamines [27,30]. Topical calcineurin inhibitors—tacrolimus and pimecroliums—are relative safe (FDA category C) alternatives to topical steroids [35]. If necessary, first-generation antihistamines can safely be used in the first trimester of pregnancy, and second-generation antihistamines can be used in the second or third trimester of pregnancy [8]. In severe cases, a tapered course of systemic corticosteroids (CS) may be required in addition to treatment with phototherapy (UVB) [30]. In recalcitrant cases, systemic immunosuppressives, such as cyclosporine and azathioprine, may be considered while avoiding methotrexate and mycophenolate mofetil [35].

PRURITIC FOLLICULITIS OF PREGNANCY
Key Points

- PFP is a **benign** eruption presenting in the second or third trimester.
- There is no underlying infectious etiology.
- There are no adverse maternal or fetal outcomes.
- The mainstay of **therapy** is **topical corticosteroids**.

Historic Notes

PFP was originally described by Zoberman and Farmer in 1981 in a series of six pregnant patients [36]. It is now considered to be a part of the broad category of AEP [27,30].

Diagnosis/Definition

PFP is characterized by pruritic, follicular papules with some discrete pustules in a primarily truncal distribution (Figure 43.3). The eruption occurs anywhere from the fourth to ninth month of gestation and resolves by one to two months postpartum. The rash may recur with subsequent pregnancies. Histopathological examination of affected skin shows a sterile folliculitis [36]. Immunoreactive deposit is not detected in DIF in PFP [22,36,37].

Symptoms

PFP is usually accompanied by mild-to-moderate pruritus.

Epidemiology/Incidence

There are no formal data available that document the incidence of PFP, but estimated incidence ranges from 1:9 to 1:3000 pregnancies [22,38]. This entity may be underreported because of frequent mistaken diagnoses of bacterial folliculitis [37,39,40].

Etiology/Basic Pathology

The underlying etiology of PFP is unknown. The vast majority of case reports fail to reveal any causative organism by special staining during histopathological examination or by culture [19,30,36,37,39,41]. Some have proposed a hormone-related etiology based on the similarity of PFP to steroid acne [19,42], but a recent controlled, prospective study did not show any change in androgen levels in patients with PFP [22].

Pregnancy Considerations

There is one case report of premature delivery secondary to placental abruption at 32 weeks [41]. There is a reported increase in the male-to-female birth ratio [22]. Otherwise, there are no reports of adverse maternal or fetal outcomes in PFP.

Management

Workup

The diagnosis of PFP relies mostly on its clinical features. When follicular lesions are present, they need to be differentiated from exacerbation of acne vulgaris and bacterial folliculitis.

Therapy

The mainstay of therapy is **mid- to high-potency topical corticosteroids** [22,30,36,39]. The reader is referred to the guideline for PEP for a discussion on the use of topical corticosteroids during pregnancy. Narrow-band UVB phototherapy, which depresses certain components of the cell-mediated immune system, is a safe and effective alternative treatment [43].

PRURIGO OF PREGNANCY
Key Points

- PP is an intensely pruritic eruption confined mostly to the extremities.
- The mainstay of **therapy** is **topical steroids**.
- There is no associated maternal or fetal morbidity or mortality.

Historic Notes

PP was first described by Nurse in 1968 [44]. His case series of 31 patients is the largest group of women with PP to be described to date. A synonym for this skin disease is prurigo gestationis of Besnier. It is now considered to be part of AEP [27,30].

Diagnosis/Definition

PP is diagnosed by its clinical features. The eruption consists of pruritic papules occurring on the extensor surface of the extremities and occasionally the abdomen (Figure 43.4). Excoriation is often present. The lesions appear between the 25th and 30th weeks of gestation. In the original description of this disease, there was no tendency toward recurrence in subsequent pregnancies. However, others have found that this is not the case [34]. The eruption resolves in the postpartum period, but there have been a few patients in which lesions have persisted for as long as three months after delivery [44]. A skin biopsy shows nonspecific histopathological changes.

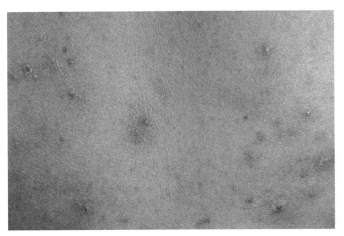

Figure 43.3 Pruritic folliculitis of pregnancy. A 28-year-old woman with erythematous, follicular papules on the abdomen.

Symptoms

The papules are intensely pruritic.

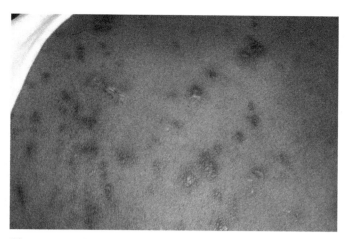

Figure 43.4 Prurigo of pregnancy. Grouped excoriated papules on the thigh of a 24-year-old primigravida with a prior history of asthma and seasonal allergies.

Epidemiology/Incidence

In Nurse's original report, the incidence was calculated as 1 in 300 pregnancies. A more recent prospective analysis of pruritic eruptions during pregnancy yielded an incidence of PP of 1 in 450 pregnancies [38].

Etiology/Basic Pathology

There is no definitive evidence regarding the etiology of PP. One theory is that women who are affected have an underlying predisposition to atopy either by personal history or family history and that this predisposition is unmasked during pregnancy [45]. Evidence to support this theory is that some women with PP have elevated serum IgE levels [22,45]. Evidence for atopy by personal and/or family history has been present in some series [22,45] and absent in others [38]. There have not been any significant changes detected in levels of beta-HCG, estradiol, or cortisol in women with PP versus controls [22,38].

Risk Factors/Associations

There may be an association between PP and a personal or family history of an atopic diathesis (atopic dermatitis, allergic rhinitis, asthma) [22,45].

Complications

There are no large-scale epidemiologic studies investigating maternal or fetal morbidity. No case series has ever reported any associated fetal or maternal complications [22,44,45] except for one patient who exhibited intrauterine growth restriction [38].

Management

Workup

The diagnosis of PP rests on the clinical features of the eruption. In all cases, DIF has been negative [22,38,45] and therefore is not indicated.

Therapy

Therapeutic options for PP are similar to that of ADP. The mainstay of therapy for PP is **mid- to high-potency topical steroids** [22,30,38,42,44,45].

PEMPHIGOID GESTATIONIS (HERPES GESTATIONIS)
Key Points

- Pemphigoid gestationis (PG) is a very rare autoimmune blistering disease in which patients develop autoantibodies against components of collagen XVII—primarily BP180, a transmembrane protein found in the basement membrane zone of the skin
- Patients develop extremely pruritic urticarial and blistering lesions, involving the periumbilical and umbilical skin, typically in the second and third trimesters that usually resolve after several weeks or months after parturition
- Circulating autoantibodies are detectable in more than 92% of the cases using a commercially available ELISA test

Historic Notes

This entity was originally described by English dermatologist John Laws Milton, the founder of London's St John's Hospital for Diseases of the Skin, in 1872 [46]. The designation pemphigoid gestationis has become more in favor over herpes gestationis recently to highlight its close resemblance to bullous pemphigoid with respect to its clinical, histologic, serologic, and immunofluorescent findings.

Diagnosis/Definition

Skin lesions range from urticarial and edematous papules and plaques that may be annular or polycyclic to grouped (i.e., herpetiform) frank tense subepidermal blisters (Figure 43.5).

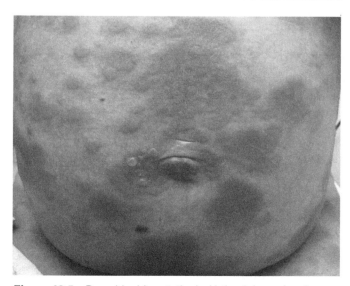

Figure 43.5 Pemphigoid gestationis. Urticarial annular plaques on the abdomen of a 31-year-old primigravida with no prior history of blistering disease. Note the involvement of the periumbilical skin with grouped tense blisters. (Courtesy of Sylvia Hsu, MD, Baylor College of Medicine.)

Typically, lesions begin on the abdomen involving the peri-umbilical and umbilical skin in contrast to PEP, spreading centripetally to the extremities, including the palms and soles. As a rule, face and mucosae are spared. PG usually appears in the second and third trimesters with a mean gestational age of onset that ranges from 21 to 28 weeks [47]. Although clinical course varies, there is a trend for improvement of the disease near parturition and exacerbation immediately after corresponding to the hormonal fluctuation during this period. The disease usually remits within weeks to months after parturition, but a small percentage of patients have an unremitting chronic course. The disease usually recurs during subsequent pregnancies, typically earlier in onset with more severity. The diagnosis is based on clinical, histologic, serologic, and/or immunofluorescent studies. As circulating autoantibodies are detectable in more than 92% of the cases, a commercially available ELISA test is becoming the confirmatory test of choice [48].

Symptoms
Similar to other dermatoses of pregnancy and classic bullous pemphigoid, severe pruritus is a significant symptom for patients with PG. The subepidermal blisters may also cause pain.

Epidemiology/Incidence
PG is a very rare autoimmune blistering disease with an approximate incidence of 1 in 50,000 births. There is no racial predilection of the disease.

Genetics
Although there is no known genetic basis for the disease, expression of major histocompatibility complex (MHC) II HLA-DR3 or HLA-DR4 are highly associated with developing PG as most patients express either of the two MHC [47].

Etiology/Basic Pathology
In contrast to other dermatoses of pregnancy, the pathomechanism of PG has been well delineated. Patients with PG develop autoantibodies against components of collagen XVII in the basement membrane zone of the skin, primarily against a 180 kDa transmembrane protein (BP180) and to a lesser extent 230 kDa intracellular protein (BP230). Once the autoantibodies bind to these antigens, complement cascade is triggered that recruits additional inflammatory mediators, resulting in local tissue injury and subsequent blisters. Characteristic histopathologic findings consist of a subepidermal blister accompanied by numerous eosinophils. On perilesional skin, linear deposition of C3 is uniformly detected, and linear deposition of IgG is detected in about half of the cases [47,48].

Complications
PG is associated with prematurity in about 20% of the cases and small gestational age weight at birth. Passive transfer of antibodies to the infant occurs in about 5% to 10% of the cases that result in transient neonatal disease with no adverse sequelae [47,48].

Management
Workup
A patient suspected of having PG should undergo lesional and perilesional skin biopsies for routine histologic examination and direct immunofluorescence study, respectively. Alternatively, because the sensitivity of serologic testing is relatively high, ELISA can be ordered as an additional confirmatory test or in lieu of the immunofluorescent studies.

Therapy
In mild cases, topical **steroid** may suffice to control the symptoms and skin lesions. In most cases, however, systemic steroid is required to sufficiently control the disease (e.g., prednisolone 20 to 40 mg daily or 1–2 mg/kg/day). In recalcitrant unremitting cases, other systemic agents used in autoimmune diseases may be considered such as azathioprine, rituximab, intravenous immunoglobulin, and plasmapheresis [49].

IMPETIGO HERPETIFORMIS (PUSTULAR PSORIASIS OF PREGNANCY)
Key Points

- Impetigo herpetiformis (IH) represents **pustular psoriasis** that occurs during pregnancy.
- Most patients have no prior history of psoriasis.
- There is an **increased risk of placental insufficiency and fetal loss**.
- Patients are at risk for recurrence of disease with subsequent pregnancies.
- The mainstay of **therapy** is **oral corticosteroids**.

Historic Notes
This disease was first described in 1872 by Von Hebra in a series of five pregnant women, 40 years before the first description of generalized pustular psoriasis [50].

Diagnosis/Definition
IH is characterized by symmetric, erythematous patches with peripheral superficial sterile pustules (Figure 43.6). There is **no underlying infectious etiology** despite the name this disorder was given. The eruption begins over the intertriginous and flexural skin and expands outward. Older lesions may become crusted or secondarily infected.

Symptoms
Patients may report very mild pruritus or burning at the sites of the lesions; however, most are asymptomatic. There may be accompanying fever, malaise, diarrhea, and vomiting.

Epidemiology/Incidence
There are no formal epidemiological data. IH is very rare with only about 100 cases being reported in the literature. The eruption most often occurs in the third trimester but can occur as early as the first trimester. Most women do not have a prior history of psoriasis.

Genetics
Generalized pustular psoriasis is associated with HLA types B17 and Cw6 [2].

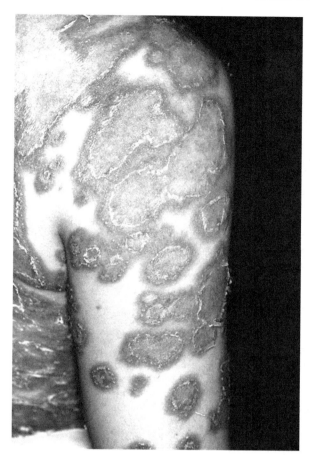

Figure 43.6 Impetigo herpetiformis. A 26-year-old pregnant woman with erythematous plaques bordered by tiny pustules on the trunk and extremities. There was no prior history of psoriasis. (From Semkova K, Black M. *Eur J Obstet Gynecol Reprod Biol*, 145, 138–44, 2009. With permission.)

Etiology/Basic Pathology

IH is considered a **variant of pustular psoriasis** that occurs during pregnancy [24,51,52]. The basic underlying etiology is unknown. Many theories exist including hormonal dysregulation and electrolyte imbalance, but these are based on a few case reports. Histopathology of the skin shows a characteristic sterile pustule containing polymorphonuclear neutrophils in the epidermis referred to as a spongiform pustule of Kogoj, which is indistinguishable from findings that are seen in pustular psoriasis. There may also be elongation of the rete ridges and overlying parakeratosis.

Risk Factors/Associations

Patients usually do not have a prior history of psoriasis, and there is no evidence that having such a history increases the risk of IH in pregnancy [24].

Complications

The most important complication is **placental insufficiency and fetal death**, the etiology of which is unknown [24,51]. There may be hypocalcemia or decreased vitamin D levels as a result of hypoparathyroidism or hypoalbuminemia [24,51,53]. If severe, these changes may lead to tetany or seizure.

Management

Principles
Pregnancy is speculated to be a trigger for IH [24]. The effect of the disease on the pregnancy is discussed above.

Workup
Workup includes **skin biopsy** for routine histopathology as well as a second specimen for DIF in order to rule out other pregnancy-specific dermatoses, such as HG. When the presentation is accompanied by systemic symptoms, systemic infection must be ruled out with blood cultures as well as bacterial and viral cultures of one or more pustules. Serum calcium, vitamin D, and hypoparathyroid levels should be monitored. The patient should be questioned regarding the history of skin eruptions during any previous pregnancies.

Prevention
None.

Preconception Counseling
Any patient with a history of IH should be counseled that it might recur with subsequent pregnancies.

Therapy
The mainstay of therapy of IH is **corticosteroids**, usually in the form of prednisone at a dose of 15 to 30 mg/day. Doses as high as 60 to 80 mg/day may be required [24]. Evidence for varying levels of effectiveness is based on case reports [50–52,54]. Once the disease is under control, steroids may be tapered very slowly. Disease rebound is common with rapid tapering.

When IH is insufficiently controlled with CS alone, the next therapeutic option is cyclosporine A (CsA). Doses of 3 to 10 mg/kg/day have been reported in the treatment of IH [54–56]. Again, medication should be tapered to the lowest possible dose that results in control of the disease. The mechanism of action is inhibition of calcineurin with resultant decrease in interleukin 2 production by CD4+ T-cells. CsA also inhibits interferon-γ production by T-cells. CsA is pregnancy category C. The most serious adverse effects are renal dysfunction and hypertension [8]. Renal function and blood pressure should be monitored during therapy. In a study of transplant recipients treated with CsA during pregnancy there was no evidence of teratogenicity [57]. However, 44.5% of infants were born at less than 37 weeks gestation, and 44.3% weighed less than 2500 g at birth [57]. CsA is excreted in human breast milk and breast-feeding should be avoided during therapy. Biologic therapies may be considered as an alternative to cyclosporine or next-in-line therapy. Tumor necrosis factor (TNF)-α inhibitors and ustekinumab are pregnancy category B drugs. As no significant pregnancy adverse outcomes have been observed, TNF-α inhibitors, such as infliximab, may be considered even as the first-line therapy [58]. No data are available on treatment safety during pregnancy for newer biologic agents, such as brodalumab, ixekizumab, tofcitinib, and apremilast.

Antepartum Testing
Patients must be monitored closely with fetal ultrasound and fetal testing because of the risk of placental insufficiency [50].

CUTANEOUS MELANOMA

See Chapter 42, "Cancer."

Key Points

- **Pregnancy** at the time of diagnosis or subsequent to the diagnosis of melanoma has **no impact on overall survival, tumor thickness, or disease-free survival**.
- Pregnant women who are diagnosed with melanoma should not be counseled or managed any differently than a nonpregnant woman with a similar stage of disease.

Diagnosis/Definition

Cutaneous melanoma is a malignant neoplasm of melanocytes that arises in the skin. Melanomas often display irregularities in color, border, and symmetry although these observations are neither sensitive nor specific (Figure 43.7). Even the most experienced dermatologist may have difficulty differentiating a benign pigmented lesion from a malignant one. The gold standard for the **diagnosis** of melanoma is **excisional biopsy of the entire lesion** for tissue pathology. Biopsy specimens of all clinically pigmented lesions should be evaluated by an experienced dermatopathologist.

Symptoms

Melanomas are usually asymptomatic. They may rarely itch or bleed spontaneously.

Epidemiology/Incidence

In the United States, the lifetime risk of developing melanoma is about 2.4% (1 in 40) for Caucasians, 0.5% (1 in 200) for Hispanics, and 0.1% (1 in 1000) for African-Americans [59]. Although the overall incidence is low for all cancers during pregnancy, melanoma is the most common cancer observed during pregnancy, followed by cervical and breast carcinoma [60,61]. The estimated incidence of melanoma during pregnancy is between 2.8 and 5 in 100,000 [62].

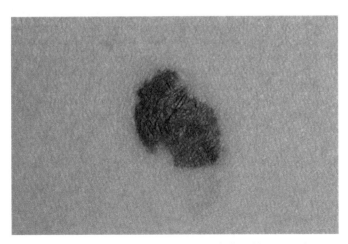

Figure 43.7   Melanoma. A 25-year-old G₂P₁ with a new, irregularly pigmented, asymmetric lesion on her back that had been gradually expanding over the past several months. Note the irregular borders.

Genetics

A rare group of patients with a family history of melanoma and many moles may carry germline mutations in CDKN2A and CDK4. An individual who carries one of these mutations has a 60% to 90% lifetime risk of melanoma [63]. BRAF and c-KIT represent known somatic mutations for which systemic therapies have been developed, interfering with the signaling pathway these mutations turn on.

Classification

There are four main clinical types of melanoma. They are superficial spreading, acral lentiginous, lentigo maligna, and nodular melanoma. The clinical type bears no significance on the prognosis in melanoma. Rather, the **Breslow depth, which is a measure of tumor thickness, and ulceration** are the two major factors that have been shown to **impact prognosis** [64]. In addition to Breslow depth, which is a measure of tumor thickness, ulceration, mitotic rate in thin melanomas, and although still controversial, sentinel lymph node status, are the major factors that have been shown more recently to impact prognosis [65,66].

Risk Factors

The major risk factors are fair skin, blue or green eyes, blond or red hair, inability to tan, intense intermittent sun exposure (especially during childhood), use of tanning beds, and inherited mutations in CDKN2A or CDK4 [63].

Complications

Melanoma is a malignant neoplasm that can metastasize to regional lymph nodes as well as viscera. In general, the thicker the primary cutaneous melanoma, the higher the likelihood for metastasis at the time of diagnosis.

Pregnancy Considerations

For many years, it was believed that pregnancy had an adverse impact on survival in patients diagnosed with malignant melanoma (MM). This belief was based on case reports and uncontrolled series in which confounding variables were not accounted for, namely, tumor thickness at the time of diagnosis [62,66]. Several large, retrospective, controlled cohort studies of women who were diagnosed with melanoma during their pregnancy have confirmed that this is *not* the case [52,57–59]. In fact, these recent large cohort studies have shown that there is **no difference in overall survival or tumor thickness between pregnant and nonpregnant age- and disease stage-matched patients** [62,67–69]. The **disease-free survival rate** is the **same** in pregnant and nonpregnant women [68,69]. **Pregnancy in women who have been previously diagnosed with melanoma does not affect overall survival** [52,59,70]. An important point related to pregnancy and melanoma is the concept that benign nevi may darken and change during pregnancy. There has been debate in recent years regarding this belief. In fact, there has been no study to date that has documented a significant change in size or color of benign nevi during pregnancy in normal, healthy women. The clinical lesions that are reported by patients to darken or change during pregnancy are usually nonpigmented lesions, such as dermatofibromas or skin tags [71]. Photographic documentation and blinded comparison by physicians do not show any change in size of nevi between the first and third trimesters of pregnancy [72]. Women with the *dysplastic nevus syndrome* (DNS) may have an increased rate of change in clinically dysplastic nevi with pregnancy [73], but women with DNS represent only a very small portion of the population. Histopathologic study of nevi removed during pregnancy fails to detect a statistically significant difference in criteria for atypia [71]. Therefore, **any nevus that changes during pregnancy should be considered suspect and be carefully considered for excisional biopsy**, not observation. The belief that nevi may normally darken and change during pregnancy may lead to a false sense of security and a delay in the diagnosis of melanoma [66,71,72].

Management
Pregnancy Management
There is no difference in pregnancy outcomes, including cesarean delivery, length of stay, risk of low birth weight, prematurity, or neonatal death [66]. Pregnant women who are diagnosed with melanoma **should not be counseled any differently than nonpregnant women** with a similar stage of disease with respect to both pregnancy outcomes and their overall prognosis [66,69]. There are approximately 22 cases of placental metastases of melanoma reported in the literature. Indeed, of all malignancies that tend to metastasize to the placenta, melanoma is the most common [66]. However, metastasis to the fetus and/or placenta is an extremely rare event and has occurred exclusively in the setting of hematogenous dissemination of metastatic disease in the mother [74–76]. **Placental involvement** implies a fatal prognosis for the mother and approximately 22% risk of metastasis to the fetus [76].

Workup
The extensiveness of the workup of primary cutaneous melanoma is primarily based on tumor thickness at the time of diagnosis. Initial diagnosis is made by tissue pathology. It is strongly recommended that all suspicious lesions be removed by **excisional biopsy with narrow margins** for diagnostic purposes [77]. Once the diagnosis of melanoma is made, all patients should have a thorough review of systems and physical exam with special attention given to the lymph nodes. There is no evidence that routine laboratory tests and imaging studies detect occult metastases in asymptomatic patients with tumors less than 4.0 mm in thickness [63,66]. Therefore, **CXR, serum lactate dehydrogenase, and hemoglobin are reserved for patients who are symptomatic or have tumors that are thicker than 4.0 mm at the time of initial diagnosis**. Patients should be taught to give themselves monthly self-exams and should be seen one to four times per year for the first two years after the initial diagnosis and then one to two times yearly thereafter [77]. The goal of follow-up is to detect recurrence or a new primary lesion. Screening tests should be ordered based on history and physical examination findings during follow-up care. **Sentinel lymph node biopsy** in melanoma is used as a staging procedure. It is used to detect occult nodal metastases at the time of diagnosis and is generally reserved for patients **with tumors that are 1.0 mm or greater in thickness** and for lesions that are less than 1.0 mm but are associated with presence of an ulcer and/or mitotic figures greater than 1 mm^2 [63]. Sentinel lymph node biopsy is typically performed at the time of definitive excision. This procedure

is considered safe to perform during pregnancy [66]. For patients with microscopic or clinically apparent nodal disease, a full metastatic work up is indicated [3], including blood work and CT or MRI of the chest, abdomen, and pelvis. MRI is preferable in pregnant patients because it is the safer alternative [66].

Prevention
General preventative measures include the use of sun protection via sunscreens and protective clothing, especially during childhood and adolescence. Regular skin examination by a physician is recommended. Melanomas that are detected by a physician are diagnosed at an earlier stage than those detected by patients; however, a direct reduction in mortality has not been documented [64].

Preconception Counseling
Because melanomas tend to recur within the first two years after diagnosis, women should be counseled to wait this length of time before conceiving [66]. Again, there is no evidence that pregnancy results in a higher rate of recurrence, but it seems unwise to conceive if there is *any* risk for recurrence of a potentially fatal disease. Additionally, in patients diagnosed with melanoma, future use of oral contraceptives and hormone replacement therapy has not been shown to enhance the risk for developing melanoma [69].

Therapy
The treatment of melanoma is primarily surgical. After the initial diagnostic biopsy, **excision of the primary lesion with 0.5 to 2 cm margins** depending on tumor thickness is recommended [53,66]. Patients with evidence of metastasis had limited therapeutic options historically, but significant advances in targeted molecular therapy have resulted in several FDA-approved systemic agents BRAF and MEK inhibitors, such as vemurafenib and trametinib, with more expected to be approved [78]. Data on treatment safety of these new targeted therapies during pregnancies are not known. One case of successful delivery of a premature healthy baby exposed to vemurafenib has been reported [79].

REFERENCES
1. Chang ALS, Agredano YZ, Kimball AB. Risk factors associated with striae gravidarum. *J Am Acad Dermatol* 2004; 51: 881–5. [III]
2. Goldberg DJ, Marmur ES, Schmults C et al. Histologic and ultrastructural analysis of ultraviolet B laser and light source treatment of leukoderma in striae distensae. *Dermatol Surg* 2005; 31: 385–7. [II-3]
3. Watson REB, Parry EJ, Humphries JD et al. Fibrillin microfibrils are reduced in skin exhibiting striae distensae. *Br J Dermatol* 1998; 138: 931–7. [II-3]
4. Young GL, Jewell D. Creams for preventing stretch marks in pregnancy. *Cochrane Database Syst Rev* 2005; 3. [Meta-analysis; 2 RCTs, n = 130]
5. Osman H, Usta IM, Rubeiz N et al. Cocoa butter lotion for prevention of striae gravidarum: A double-blind, randomized and placebo-controlled trial. *Br J Obstet Gynecol* 2008; 115: 1138–42. [RCT, n = 175]
6. Kang S, Kim KJ, Griffiths CEM et al. Topical tretinoin (retinoic acid) improves early stretch marks. *Arch Dermatol* 1996; 132: 519–26. [I]
7. Pribanich S, Simpson FG, Held B et al. Low-dose tretinoin does not improve striae distensae: A double-blind, placebo-controlled study. *Cutis* 1994; 54: 121–4. [I]

8. Wolverton SE. *Comprehensive Dermatologic Drug Therapy.* Philadelphia: W. B. Saunders Company, 2007: 625–41, 127–61. [III]

9. Kligman AM, Grove GL, Hirose R et al. Topical tretinoin for photodamaged skin. *J Am Acad Dermatol* 1986; 15: 836–59. [II-1]

10. McDaniel DH. Laser therapy of stretch marks. *Dermatol Clin* 2002; 20: 67–76. [III]

11. Lawley TJ, Hertz KC, Wade TR et al. Pruritic urticarial papules and plaques of pregnancy. *J Am Med Assoc* 1979; 241: 1696–9. [III]

12. Roger D, Vaillant L, Lorette G. Pruritic urticarial papules and plaques of pregnancy are not related to maternal or fetal weight gain. *Arch Dermatol* 1990; 126: 1517. [III]

13. Cohen LM, Capeless EL, Krusinski PA et al. Pruritic urticarial papules and plaques of pregnancy and its relationship to maternal-fetal weight gain and twin pregnancy. *Arch Dermatol* 1989; 125: 1534–6. [III]

14. Aronson IK, Bond S, Fiedler VC et al. Pruritic urticarial papules and plaques of pregnancy: Clinical and immunopathologic observations in 57 patients. *J Am Acad Dermatol* 1998; 39: 933–9. [II-3]

15. Powell FC. Pruritic urticarial papules and plaques of pregnancy and multiple pregnancies. *J Am Acad Dermatol* 2000; 43: 730–1. [II-3]

16. Weiss R, Hull P. Familial occurrence of pruritic urticarial papules and plaques of pregnancy. *J Am Acad Dermatol* 1992; 26: 715–7. [III]

17. Yancey KB, Hall RP, Lawley TJ. Pruritic urticarial papules and plaques of pregnancy. *J Am Acad Dermatol* 1984; 10: 473–80. [II-3]

18. Beckett MA, Goldberg NS. Pruritic urticarial papules and plaques of pregnancy and skin distension. *Arch Dermatol* 1991; 127: 125–6. [III]

19. Kroumpouzos G, Cohen LM. Specific dermatoses of pregnancy: An evidence-based systematic review. *Am J Obstet Gynecol* 2003; 188: 1083–92. [Meta-analysis, *n* = 282]

20. Alcalay J, Ingber A, Kafri B et al. Hormonal evaluation and autoimmune background in pruritic urticarial papules and plaques of pregnancy. *Am J Obstet Gynecol* 1988; 158: 417–20. [II-3]

21. Callen JP, Hanno R. Pruritic urticarial papules and plaques of pregnancy (PEP). *J Am Acad Dermatol* 1981; 5: 401–5. [II-3]

22. Vaughan Jones SA, Hern S, Nelson-Piercy C et al. A prospective study of 200 women with dermatoses of pregnancy correlating clinical findings with hormonal and immunopathological profiles. *Br J Dermatol* 1999; 141: 71–81. [II-2; *n* = 44]

23. Aractingi S, Berkane P, LeGoue' C et al. Fetal DNA in skin of polymorphic eruptions of pregnancy. *Lancet* 1998; 352: 1898–901. [II-2]

24. Kroumpouzos GK, Cohen LM. Dermatoses of pregnancy. *J Am Acad Dermatol* 2001; 45: 1–19. [III]

25. Alcalay J, Ingber A, David M et al. Pruritic urticarial papules and plaques of pregnancy. *J Reprod Med* 1987; 32: 315–6. [II-3]

26. Beltrani VP, Beltrani VS. Pruritic urticarial papules and plaques of pregnancy: A severe case requiring early delivery for relief of symptoms. *J Am Acad Dermatol* 1991; 26: 266–7. [III]

27. Ambros-Rudolph CM, Müllegger RR, Vaughan-Jones S et al. The specific dermatoses of pregnancy revisited and reclassified: Results of a retrospective two-center study on 505 pregnant patients. *J Am Acad Dermatol* 2006; 54: 395–404. [II-2]

28. Cohen LM, Kroumpouzos G. Pruritic dermatoses of pregnancy: To lump or to split? *J Am Acad Dermatol* 2007; 56: 708–9. [II-2]

29. Ambros-Rudolph CM, Jones SV, Black MM. Best serving the pregnant patient with pruritus. *J Am Acad Dermatol* 2008; 59: 530–1. [II-2]

30. Roth MM. Pregnancy dermatoses: Diagnosis, management, and controversies. *Am J Clin Dermatol* 2011; 1: 25–41. [Review]

31. Ambros-Rudolph CM. Dermatoses of pregnancy. *J Dtsch Dermatol Ges* 2006; 9: 748–59. [Review]

32. Kramer MS, Kakuma R. Maternal dietary antigen avoidance during pregnancy or lactation, or both, for preventing or treating atopic disease in the child. *Evid Based Child Health* 2014; 9: 447–8. [Review; I]

33. Netting MJ, Middleton PF, Makrides M. Does maternal diet during pregnancy and lactation affect outcomes in offspring? A systematic review of food-based approaches. *Nutrition* 2014; 30: 1225–41. [Review; I]

34. Massone C, Cerroni L, Heidrun N et al. Histopathological diagnosis of atopic eruption of pregnancy and polymorphic eruption of pregnancy: A study on 41 cases. *Am J Dermatopathol* 2014; 36: 812–21. [Review; II-3]

35. Babalola O, Strober BE. Treatment of atopic dermatitis in pregnancy. *Dermatol Ther* 2013; 26: 293–301. [III]

36. Zoberman E, Farmer ER. Pruritic folliculitis of pregnancy. *Arch Dermatol* 1981; 117: 20–2. [III]

37. Kroumpouzos G, Cohen LM. Pruritic folliculitis of pregnancy. *J Am Acad Dermatol* 2000; 43: 132–4. [III]

38. Roger D, Vaillant L, Fignon A et al. Specific pruritic diseases of pregnancy. A prospective study of 3192 pregnant women. *Arch Dermatol* 1994; 130: 734–9. [II-2]

39. Fox GN. Pruritic folliculitis of pregnancy. *Am Fam Physician* 1989; 39: 189–93. [III]

40. Kroumpouzos G, Cohen LM. Specific dermatoses of pregnancy: An evidence-based review. *Am J Obstet Gynecol* 2003; 188: 1083–92. [III]

41. Reed J. Pruritic folliculitis of pregnancy treated with narrowband (TL-01) ultraviolet B phototherapy. *Br J Dermatol* 1999; 141: 177–9. [III]

42. Black MM. Prurigo of pregnancy, papular dermatitis of pregnancy, and pruritic folliculitis of pregnancy. *Semin Dermatol* 1989; 8: 23–5. [III]

43. British Photodermatology Group. An appraisal of narrowband (TL-01) UVB phototherapy. British photodermatology group workshop report. *Br J Dermatol* 1997; 137: 327–30. [III]

44. Nurse DS. Prurigo of pregnancy. *Australas J Dermatol* 1968; 9: 258–67. [III]

45. Holmes RC, Black MM. The specific dermatoses of pregnancy. *J Am Acad Dermatol* 1983; 3: 405–12. [II-3]

46. Al-Fouzan AS, Galadari I, Oumeish I et al. Herpes gestationis (Pemphigoid gestationis). *Clin Dermatol* 2006; 24: 109–12. [Review; II-3]

47. Semkova K, Black M. Pemphigoid gestationis: Current insights into pathogenesis and treatment. *Eur J Obstet Gynecol Reprod Biol* 2009; 145: 138–44. [Review; II-3]

48. Tani N, Kimura Y, Kawakami KT et al. Clinical and immunological profiles of 25 patients with pemphigoid gestationis. *Br J Dermatol* 2015; 172: 120–9. [II-3]

49. Lehrhoff S, Pomeranz M. Specific dermatoses of pregnancy and their treatment. *Dermatol Ther* 2013; 26: 274–84. [Review; III]

50. Lotem M, Katzenelson V, Rotem A et al. Impetigo herpetiformis: A variant of pustular psoriasis or a separate entity? *J Am Acad Dermatol* 1989; 20: 338–41. [III]

51. Breier-Maly J, Ortel B, Breier F et al. Generalized pustular psoriasis of pregnancy (impetigo herpetiformis). *Dermatology* 1999; 198: 61–4. [III]

52. Chang SE. Impetigo herpetiformis followed by generalized pustular psoriasis: More evidence of the same disease entity. *Int J Soc Dermatol* 2003; 42: 754–5. [III]

53. Ott F, Krakowski A, Tur E et al. Impetigo herpetiformis with lowered serum level of vitamin D and its diminished intestinal absorption. *Dermatologica* 1982; 164: 360–5. [III]

54. Imai N, Watanabe R, Fujiwara H et al. Successful treatment of impetigo herpetiformis with oral cyclosporine during pregnancy. *Arch Dermatol* 2002; 138: 128–9. [III]

55. Raddadi AA, Damanhoury ZB. Cyclosporin and pregnancy. *Br J Dermatol* 1999; 140: 1197–8. [III]

56. Finch TM, Tan CY. Pustular psoriasis exacerbated by pregnancy and controlled by cyclosporine A. *Br J Dermatol* 2000; 142: 582–4. [III]

57. Lamarque V, Leleu MF, Monka C et al. Analysis of 629 pregnancy outcomes in transplant recipients treated with sandimmun. *Transpl Proc* 1997; 29: 2480. [II-3; *n* = 629]

58. Bae YC, Van Voorhees AS, Hsu S et al. Review of treatment options for psoriasis in pregnant or lactating women: From the Medical Board of the National Psoriasis Foundation. *J Amer Acad Dermatol* 2012; 67: 459–77. [Review; III]

59. American Cancer Society. Melanoma skin cancer overview. Revised March 15, 2015. http://www.cancer.org/acs/groups /cid/documents/webcontent/003120-pdf. (September 20, 2015). [III]

60. Andersson TM, Johansson AL, Fredriksson I et al. Cancer during pregnancy and the postpartum period: A population-based study. *Cancer* 2015; 121: 2072–7. [II-2]

61. Eibye S, Kjær SK, Mellemkjær L. Incidence of pregnancy-associated cancer in Denmark, 1977–2006. *Obstet Gynecol* 2013; 122: 608–17. [II-2]

62. Lens MB, Rosdahl I, Ahlbom A et al. Effect of pregnancy on survival in women with cutaneous malignant melanoma. *J Clin Oncol* 2004; 22: 4369–75. [II-2]

63. Tsao H, Atkins MB, Sober AJ. Management of cutaneous melanoma. *N Engl J Med* 2004; 351: 998–1012. [III]

64. Thompson JA. The revised American joint committee on cancer staging system for melanoma. *Semin Oncol* 2002; 29: 361–9. [III]

65. Stebbins WG, Garibyan L, Sober AJ. Sentinel lymph node biopsy and melanoma: 2010 update Part I. *J Am Acad Dermatol* 2010; 62: 723–34. [Review]

66. Katz VL, Farmer RM, Dotters D. From nevus to neoplasm: Myths of melanoma in pregnancy. *Obstet Gynecol Surv* 2002; 57: 112–9. [III]

67. O'Meara AT, Cress R, Xing G et al. Malignant melanoma in pregnancy. A population-based evaluation. *Cancer* 2005; 103: 1217–26. [II-2]

68. Daryanani D, Plukker JT, De Hullu JA et al. Pregnancy and early-stage melanoma. *Cancer* 2003; 97: 2248–53. [II-2]

69. Gupta A, Driscoll MS. Do hormones influence melanoma? Facts and controversies. *Clin Dermatol* 2010; 28: 287–92. [III]

70. Johhannsson AL, Andersson TML, Plym A et al. Mortality in women with pregnancy-associated malignant melanoma. *J Am Acad Dermatol* 2014; 71: 1093–101. [III]

71. Foucar E, Bentley TJ, Laube DW et al. A histopathologic evaluation of nevocellular nevi in pregnancy. *Arch Dermatol* 1985; 121: 350–4. [II-2]

72. Pennoyer JW, Grin CM, Driscoll MS et al. Changes in size of melanocytic nevi during pregnancy. *J Am Acad Dermatol* 1997; 36: 378–82. [II-2]

73. Ellis DL. Pregnancy and sex steroid hormone effects on nevi of patients with the dysplasctic nevus syndrome. *J Am Acad Dermatol* 1991; 25: 467–82. [II-3]

74. Borden EC. Melanoma and pregnancy. *Semin Oncol* 2000; 27: 654–6. [III]

75. Altman JF, Lowe L, Redman B et al. Placental metastasis of maternal melanoma. *J Am Acad Dermatol* 2003; 49: 1150–4. [III]

76. Alexander A, Harris RM, Grossman D et al. Vulvar melanoma: Diffuse melanosis and metastasis to the placenta. *J Am Acad Dermatol* 2004; 50: 293–8. [III]

77. Sober AJ, Chuang T, Duvic M et al. Guidelines of care for primary cutaneous melanoma. *J Am Acad Dermatol* 2001; 45: 579–86. [III]

78. Long GV, Stroyakovskiy D, Gogas H et al. Combined BRAF and MEK inhibition versus BRAF inhibition alone in melanoma. *N Engl J Med* 2014; 371: 1877–88. [I]

79. Maleka A, Enblad G, Sjörs G, Lindqvist A, Ullenhag GJ. Treatment of metastatic malignant melanoma with vemurafenib during pregnancy. *J Clin Oncol* 2013; 21: e192–3. [III]

44

Multiple gestations

Edward J. Hayes and Michelle R. Hayes

KEY POINTS

- **Determination of chorionicity by early (preferably first trimester) ultrasound** is of paramount importance for appropriate management of multiple gestations.
- **Preterm delivery** is the largest reason for the **increased morbidity and mortality associated with multiples**.
- No intervention has been consistently shown to prevent **preterm birth in multiple gestations**. Although tests have been developed to determine twin gestation's risk for early delivery, because there is no proven intervention, screening cannot be recommended. The most promising therapy at this point is vaginal progesterone for short cervical length with insufficient data for a recommendation.
- **Multifetal pregnancy reduction** should be offered in higher-order gestations (quadruplets or higher) **to decrease the likelihood of a very premature delivery**.
- For noninvasive aneuploidy screening, nuchal translucency (NT) testing can be used in any multifetal gestation. Sequential screening (NT and serum analytes) can be used in twin gestations. Cell-free DNA screening is not recommended for women with multiple gestations.
- Discordant growth between multiples may be a marker for genetic or structural anomalies, infection, twin-twin transfusion, or placental issues; however, evidence of **FGR, not discordance, best predicts adverse neonatal outcome**.
- Multiples have **higher rates of preeclampsia**. Although the United States Preventative Services Task Force recommends starting all patients with multiple gestations on aspirin, 81 mg per day, starting at 16 weeks, to decrease the likelihood of developing preeclampsia, this recommendation is not uniformly accepted given limited data specific to aspirin in multiple gestations.
- A **single fetal death in multiple gestations** should **not mandate immediate delivery**; the risk of disseminated intravascular coagulation (DIC) is theoretical, and if they are monochorionic, adverse effects on the remaining fetus have already occurred.
- Routine antepartum testing has not been proven to be advantageous in multiple gestations without coexisting morbidity.
- Chorionicity and amnionicity of otherwise uncomplicated twin gestations determine timing of delivery. **Monoamniotic twins (MA/MC) should be delivered at around 32 to 34 weeks. Monochorionic/diamniotic twins (MC/DA) should be delivered at around 34 to 37 weeks. Dichorionic/diamniotic twins (DC/DA) should be delivered around 37 0/7–37 6/7 weeks.**
- **Twin-twin transfusion syndrome** has significant mortality (>70%) if left untreated, particularly if diagnosed in the second trimester. Laser coagulation is the treatment of choice for stages II–IV between 16 and 24 weeks gestation in the United States.

DEFINITION

Multiple gestation is a gestation carrying >1 fetus. The overwhelming majority are twins. There are two types of twins:

- Monozygotic (MZ) twins are formed when a single fertilized ovum splits into two individuals who are almost always genetically identical unless after their division there is a spontaneous mutation.
- Dizygotic (DZ) twins are formed when two separate ovaries are fertilized by two different sperm resulting in genetically different individuals.

EPIDEMIOLOGY/INCIDENCE

It is important to differentiate the natural from the actual incidence of multiple gestations. Natural incidence of multiple gestations (Figure 44.1):

- MZ twinning occurs at a constant rate of about 4 per 1000 (1/250).
- DZ twinning rates vary with the individual's characteristics, such as race (low in Asians, high in blacks), age (increases with advanced maternal age), parity (increases with parity), and family history (especially on maternal side). The "natural" incidence of twins and triplets in the United States as reported in 1973 was 1 in 80 and 1 in 800, respectively [1].

Actual incidence of multiple gestations has been heavily influenced by use of **assisted reproductive technologies (ART)** since the 1980s. Currently >50% of multiple gestations in developed countries are from ART. The proportion of live births that are multiple gestations in the United States has increased significantly over the last three decades in association with the increase use of ART treatments with a 65% increase in twins and a 500% increase in triplets and higher-order births, which peaked in 1998 [2]. Understanding the significant morbidity and mortality associated with higher order multiples, there has been a 70% reduction in the transfer of three or more embryos during an IVF cycle. This has resulted in a 33% decrease in the proportion of triplets and higher-order births attributable to IVF [3] from 193.5 per 100,000 births in 1998 to 119.5 in 2013. In contrast, the **twin birth rate has continued to increase to 33.7 per 1000 births** in 2013, a U.S. record [4]. Although the vast majority of these pregnancies are DZ, MZ twin rates increase with ART to 3%–5% [5], stressing the importance of determining chorionicity even when multiples were conceived via ART.

ETIOLOGY (TABLE 44.1)

DZ twins are formed by two distinct fertilized ova and always have separate chorion and amnion (dichorionic/diamniotic, DC/DA).

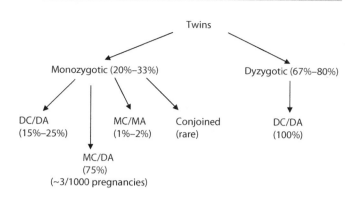

Figure 44.1   Natural incidence of twin gestations.

MZ twins are formed from the division of one fertilized egg. The type is determined by the timing of the fertilized ovum division.

DIAGNOSIS

The clinical signs for suspecting multiple gestations are a uterus larger than dates and pregnancy that has resulted from ART. The accuracy of diagnosing twins on clinical criteria is poor as 37% of women who do not undergo routine ultrasound screening will not have their twins diagnosed by 26 weeks, and 13% of multiples will only be diagnosed at the time of admission for delivery [6].

Ultrasound is 100% accurate in diagnosing multiple gestations [6]. The best time for accurate diagnosis is the **first trimester** as this is the **optimum time to determine** not only fetal number, but especially **chorionicity and amnionicity**.

Table 44.1   Timing of Zygote Division and Types of Twins

Timing of Division	Type of Twins	Characteristics	Picture
Day 1–3	Dichorionic diamniotic (DC/DA)	Two placentas with two chorions and two amnions	Dichorionic diamniotic (fused placentae) Dichorioinic diamniotic (separated placentae)
Day 3–8	Monochorionic diamnionic (MC/DA)	Monochorionic placenta with two amnions	Monochorionic diamniotic
Day 8–13	Monochorionic monoamniotic (MC/MA)	Monochorionic placenta with a single amniotic sac	Monochorionic monoamniotic
Day 13–15	Conjoined twins	Fused twins	

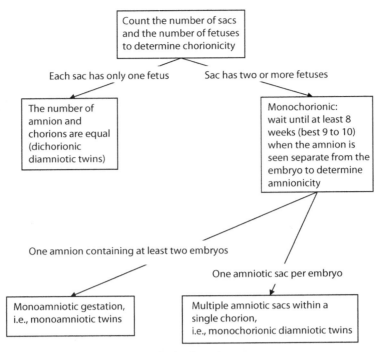

Figure 44.2   Determination of chorionicity and amnionicity in the first trimester.

Determination of chorionicity and zygocity is paramount for correct risk assessment, counseling, and management of complications (e.g., TTTS, FGR, single fetal death). In addition, this determination will help future medical care of the babies for genetic component of diseases and organ transplantation compatibility.

Determination of chorionicity and amnionicity in the first trimester is shown in Figure 44.2. **Determination of chorionicity and amnionicity status after first trimester is shown** in Figures 44.3 and 44.4. In the 30%–40% of cases in which there are clearly two placentas or differing fetal sex, the pregnancy is DC/DA and dizygotic. In the majority of cases, the best ultrasound characteristic to distinguish chorio- and amnionicity is the **twin peak sign**. Twin peak sign (also called lambda or delta sign) is a triangular projection of tissue with the same echogenicity as the placenta extending beyond the chorionic surface of the placenta [7] (Figure 44.4). DNA fingerprinting through polymorphisms or other means can also determine zygocity, but it is invasive and therefore associated with complications.

COMPLICATIONS

The incidence and severity of complications is related to chorionicity and amnionicity. ART multiple pregnancies are associated with a higher incidence of fetal/neonatal and maternal complications. Complications more common in all types of multiple gestations compared to singleton gestations include the following:

Fetal

Spontaneous Pregnancy Loss
A significant number of multiple gestations diagnosed in the first trimester undergo spontaneous reduction of one sac in the first trimester, referred to as the "vanishing twin." The rates of wastage of at least one gestation is increased compared to singletons both in the first and even the second trimester and is directly correlated with the initial number of gestational sacs, i.e., about 20%–50% of twins, 53% of triplets, and 65% of quadruplets [8]. Because the MSAFP is elevated in pregnancies with vanishing twins, this test is not accurate for screening and should not be performed subsequently. The

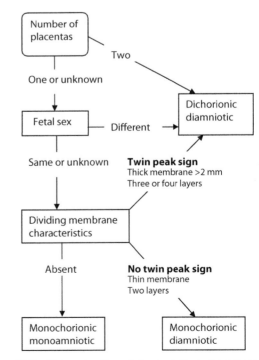

Figure 44.3   Determination of chorionicity and amnionicity after the first trimester.

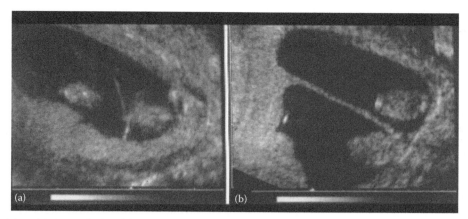

Figure 44.4 T-sign (a) and twin-peak sign (b).

risk of miscarriage of the whole pregnancy, especially in the first but also in the second trimester, is increased.

Higher Rates of Chromosomal and Congenital Anomalies
Due to the increased number of fetuses, particularly dizygotic, the risk of having one fetus affected by a trisomy is increased above the baseline risk of a singleton [9]. Therefore, the Downs syndrome risk of a 35-year-old singleton mother is obtained in twins at about age 31 to 33 [10], and for triplets, this risk is obtained at about age 28 [11]. Structural defects occur two to three times more commonly in live-born MZ twins than in DZ twins or singletons [12]. Only in 5% to 20% are both MZ twins affected.

Fetal Growth Restriction and Discordant Growth
Discordant growth of multiples is usually defined as a 20%–25% reduction in EFW of the smaller compared to the larger fetus (difference of larger minus smaller EFW, divided by larger EFW). Approximately 14% of DCDA twins have 20% discordance [13]. Discordance may be a marker for structural or genetic anomalies, infection, twin-twin transfusion syndrome, or placental issues. However, it is not the discordance per se, but evidence of **FGR of one fetus** that **predicts adverse neonatal outcome** [14]. The risk of mortality or neonatal morbidity is higher among neonates in SGA-discordant twins than in AGA-discordant twins (20% vs. 6%) [15].

Single Fetal Demise in Multiple Gestations
Up to 5% of twins and 17% of triplets in the second or third trimester undergo spontaneous loss of one or more fetuses [16]. This has been associated with a slight increase in risks of preterm birth and growth restriction in the remaining fetus. Other impacts on the remaining fetuses is dependent on chorionicity:

- Dichorionic twins: No significant neurologic morbidity in the remaining fetus after the death of one twin [17].
- Monochorionic twins: Due to vascular anastomoses, the remaining fetus is at significant risk of morbidity (about 25% neurologic) and mortality (about 10% perinatal) due to significant hypotension that occurs at the time of the demise.

Complications Specific to Monochorionic Gestations
Twin-twin transfusion syndrome (TTTS), acardiac twins, monoamniotic twins, and conjoined twins are all complications associated with monochorionicity. They are described below.

Preterm Birth (PTB)
PTB is the main reason for the increased morbidity and mortality associated with multiples. Increasing numbers of fetuses are inversely associated with gestational age at birth, so that about 50% of twins deliver preterm, and most of pregnancies carrying >4 fetuses do not even reach viability. Also, the way the multiples were conceived plays a role in determining the gestational age of delivery because twins conceived after in vitro fertilization are more likely delivered prior to 32 weeks than spontaneously conceived twins (OR 1.52 (1.18–1.97) [18]. Earlier delivery explains why multiples are 10 times as likely to be very low birth weight than singletons (11.6% vs. 1.1%) [19]. However, the earlier gestational age at delivery does not solely explain the higher rates of morbidity [20] and mortality in multiples for twins may have a higher rate of RDS when matched with gestational-age matched singletons [21] (Table 44.2).

Maternal
In addition to above: **heartburn, hemorrhoids, tiredness, anxiety, hyperemesis gravidarum, anemia, postpartum hemorrhage, postpartum depression, death,** as well as the following:

Preeclampsia
Multiples have a higher rate of preeclampsia, whose incidence is inversely proportional to the total fetal number. Increasing incidence of preeclampsia with twins (8%), triplets (10%), and quadruplets (12%) has been reported [22]. Multiples, besides having a higher rate of preeclampsia, are more likely to manifest this disease in an atypical fashion [23]. Multiple gestations that are a result of ART are at greater risk of developing hypertensive complications than spontaneous multiple gestations (relative risk, 2.1) [24].

Abruptio Placentae
It is more common in multiples and exhibits a correlation to the number of fetuses (1.2% of twins; 1.6% of triplets) [19].

Thrombocytopenia
Up to one third of triplet gestations can be complicated by thrombocytopenia, and unlike singletons with which the

Table 44.2   Delivery and Infant Outcomes per Number of Fetuses

Characteristic	Singleton	Twins	Triplets	Quadruplets
Mean birth weight[a]	3296 g	2336 g	1660 g	1291 g
Mean gestational age at delivery[a]	38.7 wk	35.3 wk	31.9 wk	29.5 wk
Rate of cerebral palsy per 1000 live births[b]	1.6	7	28	N/A
Infant mortality rate[c]	5.36	23.62	52.49	96.29[d]

[a]Martin JA, Hamilton BE, Ventura SJ, Osterman MJ, Kirmeyer S, Mathews TJ, Wilson EC. *Natl. Vital Stat. Rep.* 60, 1, 1–70, United States, 2011.
[b]Petterson B, Nelson KB, Watson L, Stanley F. *BMJ*, 307, 1239–43, 1993.
[c]Luke B, Brown M. *Pediatrics*, 118, 2488–97, 2006.
[d]Quadruplets and quintuplets combined

number one cause of thrombocytopenia is gestational, severe preeclampsia is the most common cause in triplets [25].

Acute Fatty Liver
In contrast to singleton gestations in which the rate of fatty liver is 1 in 10,000, the rate in triplets is up to 7% [26].

Gestational Diabetes
There is a mild correlation between twins and gestational diabetes when compared to singletons although insulin requirements between these two groups are not significantly different [27]. A significant association is demonstrated with triplets with a gestational diabetes rate of 22% [28].

Peripartum Hysterectomy
There is **a** significantly increased risk of emergent peripartum hysterectomy compared to singletons [29].

Pregnancy Considerations
Compared to singleton gestations, physiologic changes in twins include a 50%–60% increase in maternal blood volume (40%–50% in singletons) leading to higher incidence of anemia, higher increase in cardiac output, slightly lower diastolic blood pressure, and more discomfort, such as pressure, difficulty in ambulation, etc.

Pregnancy Management
Nutrition
The recommended weight gain for twin pregnancies starting with normal BMI is about 35–40 lbs. Diet should include an increase in caloric intake by 300 kcal above singletons (600 kcal above nonpregnant state), or caloric intake for twins is 40–45 kcal/kg each day. Extra supplementation above that supplied by a prenatal vitamin has been suggested for folic acid (1 mg/day) and iron (60 mg/day) as well as possibly magnesium and zinc. Less data for a recommendation is available for omega-3 fatty acids and vitamin D [30].

Low-Dose Aspirin
The United States Preventive Services Task Force recommends low dose aspirin initiated between 12 and 28 weeks in women with multiple gestations. They surmise that there is a substantial net benefit with reduced risk of preeclampsia, preterm birth, and fetal growth restriction without increasing the risk for placental abruption, postpartum hemorrhage, or fetal intracranial bleeding [31]. Other societies, such as ACOG and SMFM, also now recommend low-dose aspirin for multiple gestations.

Prenatal Diagnosis
First trimester: Nuchal translucency and maternal age identify about 75%–85% of trisomy 21 and 66.7% of trisomy 18 pregnancies with a 5% false positive rate in twin gestations [32–34]. However, only nuchal translucency alone has been validated for the detection of these disorders in higher order gestations [35]. In a recent meta-analysis, a first trimester combined test in twins had a pooled sensitivity of 0.893 [95% confidence interval (CI) 0.797–0.947] and a pooled specificity of 0.946 (95% CI 0.933–0.957). The performance of the test was good (summary receiver operating characteristic area under the curve: 0.817). In dichorionic twins, sensitivity and specificity were 0.862 (95% CI 0.728–0.936) and 0.952 (95% CI 0.942–0.96), respectively. In monochorionic twins, the sensitivity and specificity were 0.874% (95% CI 0.526–0.977) and 0.954% (95% CI 0.943–0.963), respectively [36]. Cell-free DNA screening is not recommended for women with multiple gestations [37]. **Chorionic villus sampling** can be performed between 10 and 12 weeks. It has the same risks as amniocentesis in multiples [38] and has a 1.1 rate of twin-twin contamination [39].

Second Trimester: Serum screening for neural tube defects with **MSAFP** using a cutoff of 4.5 MoM has a detection rate of 50% to 85% with a 5% false positive rate. Maternal **serum marker screening** for Trisomy 21 is 63% sensitive in twin gestations (71% when both twins were affected and 60% when one was affected) with false positive rates of 10.8% [40]. Genetic **amniocentesis** has been reported to have a loss rate with multiples similar to singletons [41]. At sampling of the first sac, indigo carmine (not available in the United States) or Evan's blue can be injected; a clear sample obtained from the second sac ensures that two different sacs have been sampled. Methylene blue dye should not be used because of the risks of fetal hemolytic anemia, small intestinal atresia, and fetal demise. If gestation is MC, sampling of one sac is suggested for karyotype.

Prediction of PTB
Transvaginal ultrasound (TVU) cervical length (CL) performed between 18 and 24 weeks gestation is a strong predictor of preterm delivery in asymptomatic women with twin gestations. A CL ≤20 mm increases the pretest probability of preterm birth prior to 32 weeks from 6.8% to 42.4% whereas a CL >20 mm decreased the risk to 4.5% [42]. However, because there is currently no beneficial intervention if this screening test is positive, **routine TVU CL screening of multiples at risk for preterm delivery cannot be currently recommended**, but this recommendation may soon change. Several other tests for prediction of PTB have been investigated in twin gestations, and none have been so far shown to be helpful in preventing preterm delivery [43].

PREVENTION AND MANAGEMENT OF COMPLICATIONS

Selective Termination of an Anomalous Fetus

Selective termination of an anomalous fetus is usually performed in the second trimester due to the time of diagnosis of the fetal anomaly.

In DC pregnancies, the procedure consists of injection of potassium chloride into the fetal heart transabdominally. The loss rate of the entire pregnancy is about 4% of those performed prior to 24 weeks with a difference if twins were reduced vs. higher order multiples (2.4% vs. 11.1%) and if more than one fetus is terminated (2.6% loss if one fetus vs. 42.9% if two) [44]. In a recent review of twin dichorionic pregnancies discordant for fetal anencephaly, there was no difference in survival of the nonaffected twin between those who elected selective termination versus expectant management; however, there was a statistically significant difference between both groups in mean gestational age at delivery (38.0 weeks vs. 34.9 weeks) [45].

In MC pregnancies, potassium chloride should not be used as it crosses to the other fetus through the placental anastomoses and causes fetal death therefore of both fetuses. Cord ligation or occlusion with clips, diathermy, or other means have been used with insufficient data for effective comparison.

Preterm birth (see also Chapter 17 in *Obstetric Evidence Based Guidelines*).

Prevention of Multiple Gestations

The incidence of multiple gestation is increased with both ovulation induction, which represent the majority of ART multiples, and IVF. Unfortunately, it is difficult to prevent multiple gestations with ovarian stimulation. Excessive stimulation and insemination in the presence of excessive number of ripe follicles should be avoided. Transfer of one embryo almost guarantees avoidance of multiple gestation and is associated with rates of successful pregnancy similar to transfer of >1 embryos with modern techniques. Many developed countries have laws that allow the transfer of only one or a maximum of two embryos. No more than three embryos should ever be transferred even in the woman with poor prognosis (i.e., >40 years old). The successful outcome of ART should be based on the rate of healthy term singleton per cycle.

Weight Gain

There have been several observational studies that suggest improved perinatal outcomes, decreased preterm birth rates, and larger birth weights in women with twin pregnancies who meet the Institute of Medicine weight gain guidelines [46,47].

Multifetal Pregnancy Reduction

The goal of first-trimester fetal reduction is to decrease the number of fetuses in higher order gestations, thereby lessening the likelihood of a premature delivery and the associated morbidity and mortality. A review of nonrandomized trials in the *Cochrane* database concluded that **pregnancy reduction from triplets to twins versus expectant management appears to be associated with reduction in pregnancy loss, birth before 36 weeks, cesarean birth, low birth weight infants, and neonatal deaths, similar to spontaneously conceived twins** [48]. Maternal morbidity has also been shown to be decreased: 14% of twin pregnancies

remaining after multifetal reduction developed preeclampsia compared with 30% of unreduced triplet pregnancies [49]. As reduction involves termination of one triplet fetus, overall perinatal survival is not different and might actually be slightly decreased, but improvements in morbidity and mortality are seen in "remaining" twin fetuses compared to nonreduced triplets and yield a **higher rate of "intact" normal babies** in the reduced-to-twins compared to the nonreduced triplets. In light of both improvement in maternal morbidity and fetal and neonatal morbidity and mortality, it is **reasonable to offer reduction to all patients with higher order (triplets or higher) multiples**. More than 90% of women who underwent pregnancy reduction would opt for the procedure again.

Triplets with a MC twin pair present a unique situation. Reduction of the MC twin pair is associated with significantly decreased early preterm birth and its associated long-term morbidity. On the other hand, miscarriage rate is lowest with expectant management and affords the parents the highest chance of a live born infant [50]. Again, parents should be informed of their options and allowed to decide regarding reduction according to their own personal wishes and priorities.

Bed Rest

Either prophylactic (before symptoms) or therapeutic (with symptoms of PTL) bed rest does not prevent PTB in multiple gestations [51]. Compared to normal activity, **prophylactic bed rest in the hospital increases the rate of delivery before 34 weeks by 84%** [44,52] in uncomplicated twin pregnancies. **There is no reduction in low birth weight or perinatal mortality**.

Progesterone

In a meta-analysis of the randomized trials, **neither 17–hydroxyprogesterone caproate or vaginally administered natural progesterone reduced the incidence of adverse perinatal outcome in unselected uncomplicated asymptomatic twin pregnancies**. In the subgroup of women with a **TVU CL ≤25 mm** at time of randomization or less than 24 weeks, **vaginal progesterone reduced the incidence of adverse perinatal outcome** [53]. However, the numbers were small, and further research is needed to confirm benefit in this subgroup of twins. In higher order multiples, progesterone use was associated with a significant increased rate of midtrimester fetal loss [54].

Cerclage

Cerclage, either history-indicated [55] or ultrasound-indicated for short TVU CL [56] does not prevent PTB in twins and triplet [57] gestations.

Home Uterine Activity Monitoring

Home uterine activity monitoring has not been proven to decrease the incidence of preterm birth in multiple gestations [58], and therefore, this costly screening intervention should not be undertaken.

Prophylactic Tocolysis

Prophylactic tocolysis has no proven effect on the incidence of preterm birth, low birth weight, or neonatal mortality (all similar incidences with placebo) in twin gestations, and therefore this practice should be avoided [59].

Preterm Labor (PTL)

Women with multiple gestations and PTL should be delivered if any of the following are present: ≥34 weeks gestation, PPROM, chorioamnionitis, or nonreassuring testing. If <34 weeks and none of the above criteria are present, management of multiples presenting <34 weeks in threatened PTL should be based on TVU CL because this directly correlates with delivery within 7 days in women with regular painful contractions at 24–36 weeks [60]:

    a. >25 mm: 0%
    b. 21–25 mm: 7%
    c. 16–20 mm: 21%
    d. 11–15 mm: 29%
    e. 6–10 mm: 46%
    f. 1–5 mm: 80%

Administration of one course of **antenatal corticosteroids** to women with singleton gestations at risk for delivering between 24 and 34 weeks gestation has been shown to decrease the incidence of neonatal death, respiratory distress syndrome, intraventricular hemorrhage, and necrotizing enterocolitis [61]. Although the data in multiples is limited, ACOG recommends one course of betamethasone (12 mg q24h × 2 doses) be administered to all patients who are between 24 and 33 6/7 weeks and at high risk (e.g., CL ≤20 mm) of delivery within 7 days [62].

In light of recent meta-analysis of randomized trials showing that prenatal administration of magnesium sulfate reduced the occurrence of cerebral palsy [63–65], it is reasonable to **offer magnesium for neuroprotection for those multiples at risk to deliver at 23 0/7 to 31 6/7 weeks** within the next 30 minutes to 24 hours in an ACOG-endorsed protocol [66]. Tocolytics have not been sufficiently studied in multiple gestations (no specific trials) with PTL to assess their efficacy in PTB prevention. They should be used judiciously due to higher incidence of side effects in multiple, i.e., pulmonary edema, compared to singleton gestations.

Preterm Premature Rupture of Membranes (PPROM)

Women with multiple gestations and PPROM should be delivered if any of the following are present: ≥34 weeks gestation, PTL, chorioamnionitis, or nonreassuring testing. If less than 34 weeks and none of the above criteria are present, then expectant management with antibiotics, usually ampicillin and a macrolide, together with **corticosteroid**s and **magnesium sulfate** for neuroprotection as above. Tocolysis should not be used in PPROM patients.

Subsequent Pregnancy Outcomes after Preterm Delivery of Twins

Prior spontaneous PTB of twins is a risk factor for PTB if the woman is now carrying a singleton only if the prior birth of twins occurred before 34 weeks [67].

FGR/Discordant Twins

If neither fetus of a DC/DA pregnancy is growth restricted (EFW <10% for GA), no significant change in management needs to be done as there is no increased risk in adverse perinatal outcomes [68]. If one fetus is growth restricted, then review all prenatal exposures, perform specialized ultrasound examination for anomalies, consider amniocentesis for karyotype [43], and consider twice weekly NSTs and weekly umbilical artery Doppler velocimetry. See also Chapter 45. Consider delivery of twins if one twin has REDF of UA at

>30–32 weeks, AEDF of UA at 32–34 weeks, or abnormal (but not REDF or AEDF) UA Doppler at 34–36 weeks.

Single Fetal Death

Single fetal death is associated with significant complications for the remaining twins in DC and even more MC pregnancies (Table 44.3) [69]. Management therefore depends on chorionicity and gestational age.

Dichorionic gestation:
  <12 weeks: Usually no consequences, so no intervention needed.
  >12 weeks: Immediate delivery has no benefit for the remaining fetus and the often-quoted maternal risk has not been demonstrated.
Monochorionic gestation:
  <12 weeks: Associated with high risk of loss of other twin with no intervention studied.
  >12 weeks: Associated with about 10% risk of intrauterine death and additional 25% risk of neurologic complications in other twin. This risk results from the spontaneous transfer of blood from the viable twin to the demised twin, which results in profound hypotension in the survivor. At the time the demise is discovered, the greatest harm has most likely already occurred in the remaining fetus, and there seems to be no benefit in immediate delivery, especially if the surviving fetus(es) are very preterm and otherwise healthy. In such cases, allowing the pregnancy to continue may provide the most benefit. The coagulopathy risk for the mother is minimal, probably <2%.

Twin-Twin Transfusion Syndrome (TTTS)

Incidence

TTTS occurs in about 10% of MC/DA pregnancies and therefore in about 1/2500 pregnancies. Rare cases have been reported in MA/MC pregnancies.

Etiology

All monochorionic pregnancies have one placenta only, all with **anastomoses of artery-to-artery (AA), vein-to-vein (VV), and artery-to-vein (AV) of the two twins**. TTTS may not occur in MC/MA gestations because of more AA and less AV anastomoses than in MC/DA gestations. An **imbalance** of arterial circulation of one twin (donor) to the venous circulation of another (recipient) probably through an AV anastomosis can lead to TTTS. More than 50% of TTTS placentas have ≥1 **velamentous cord insertion**, possibly associated with this imbalance. The donor twin develops anemia and resultant effects (e.g., IUGR, oligohydramnios), and the recipient twin has polyhydramnios, becomes polycythemic, and can develop heart failure.

Table 44.3 Consequences of Single Fetal Death in Twin Pregnancies, according to Chorionicity

	DC	MC
Co-twin death	3%	15%
PTB	54%	68%
Abnormal postnatal cranial imaging	16%	34%
Neurodevelopmental impairment	2%	26%

Source: Adapted from Hillman SC, Morris RK, Kilby MD. *Obstet Gynecol*, 1118, 928–40, 2011.

Diagnosis

The antepartum diagnosis requires ultrasound. The criteria are **MC/DA gestation** (see above) with **oligohydramnios** (maximum vertical pocket (MVP) <2 cm) in one sac and **polyhydramnios** (MVP >8 cm) in the other. Supporting (but NOT diagnostic) criteria can be the presence of same sex twins with a single placenta and significant discordance in fetal growth. It is important to rule out other etiologies for similar findings, such as FGR of just one twin with a normal other twin, chromosomal or structural abnormalities, infection, etc.

Screening

All MC/DA twin gestations should have serial sonographic evaluation of MVP every 2 weeks from 16 weeks until delivery to monitor for development of TTTS (Figure 44.5) [70]. Screening for congenital heart disease is warranted in all monochorionic twins, in particular those complicated by TTTS.

Staging

Staging is described in Table 44.4 [71].

Prognosis and Counseling

The natural history of TTTS is associated with poor prognosis and depends mostly on gestational age at diagnosis and stage of disease. About 5% of TTTS, especially in early stages, can regress. **Survival with diagnosis at less than 26 weeks without treatment is 30%** [72]. Survival can often be with severe

Table 44.4 Staging for TTTS

Quintero Staging	Ultrasound Findings
Stage 1	MC/DA gestation with oligo (MVP <2 cm) and polyhydramnios (MVP >8 cm)
Stage 2	Absent (empty) bladder (in donor)
Stage 3	Abnormal Doppler[a]
Stage 4	Hydrops
Stage 5	Death of one twin

Source: Adapted from Quintero RA, Morales WJ, Allen MH, Bornick PW, Johnson PK, Kruger M. *J Perinatol*,19, 550–5, 1999.
[a]Defined as either umbilical artery absent or reversed diastolic flow, ductus venosus absent or reversed diastolic flow, or umbilical vein pulsatile flow.

morbidity, including neurologic, cardiac, ischemia/necrosis of extremities, renal cortical necrosis, etc. Extensive counseling is necessary in cases of TTS given the gravity of the condition and the paucity of level 1 data on best management.

Therapy

Therapy for TTTS depends on the stage (Figure 44.6).

STAGE I

The natural history of stage 1 TTTS is that more than 75% of cases regress or remain stable without intervention with a

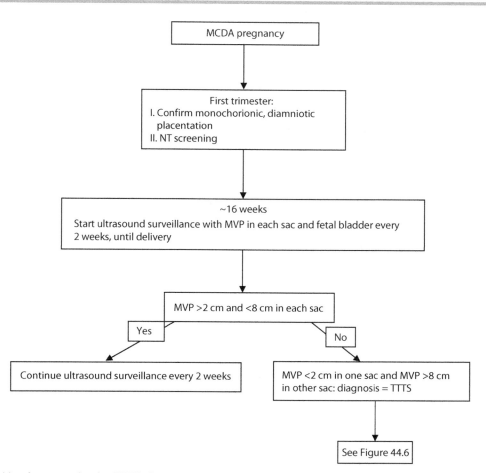

Figure 44.5 Algorithm for screening for TTTS. See text for details. MVP, maximum vertical pocket; TTTS, twin-twin transfusion syndrome. (Adapted from Simpson L, for the Society for Maternal-Fetal Medicine. *Am J Obstet and Gynecol*, 3–17, 2013.)

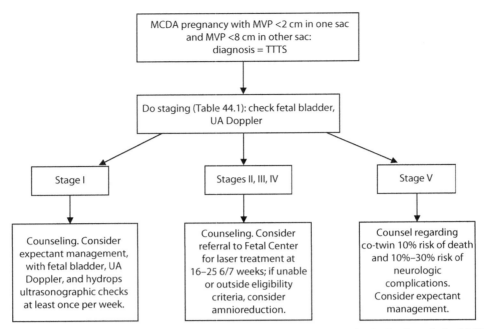

Figure 44.6 Algorithm for management of TTTS. See text for details. MCDA, monochorionic diamniotic; MVP, maximum vertical pocket; TTTS, twin-twin transfusion syndrome; UA, umbilical artery. (Adapted from Simpson L, for the Society for Maternal-Fetal Medicine. Twin-Twin transfusion syndrome. *Am J Obstet and Gynecol*, 3–17, 2013.)

perinatal survival rate of 86%. Therefore, **expectant management** with close follow-up at least weekly is the treatment of choice [73].

STAGES II, III, and IV

Most experts consider **fetoscopic laser coagulation** to be the best approach to treating advanced disease in continuing pregnancies less than 26 weeks. **Laser** therapy involves coagulation of the placental vessels transferring blood from the donor to the recipient twin. This can be done selectively, treating only those vessels visualized on the placental surface or by laser coagulation of the entire vascular equator. However, **a meta-analysis of the two RCTs showed no significant survival benefit, and the long-term neurologic outcomes in the Eurofetus trial were not different than in nonlaser treated (amnioreduction) group**. Of note, there were 12 voluntary terminations in the laser group of the largest trial, which, if eliminated, would result in no benefit from laser compared to amnioreduction [74]. It is important to counsel the patient that laser treated TTTS has a **30%–50% chance of perinatal death and a 5%–20% risk of long-term neurologic handicap**. This procedure should be undertaken for Quintero Stage II–IV disease between 16 0/7 weeks and 24 weeks in the United States (the upper threshold for gestational age has been set by the FDA), and 25 6/7 elsewhere based on data [75]. Laser **coagulation of the entire vascular equator** has been shown to be superior to selective vessel coagulation when examining the outcomes of overall survival rate and recurrent TTTS [76]. **Steroids for fetal maturation** should be considered at 24 0/7 to 33 6/7 weeks, particularly in pregnancies complicated by stage ≥III TTTS and those undergoing invasive interventions.

STAGE V

The woman should be counseled regarding cotwin 10% risk of death and 10%–30% risk of neurologic complications. Expectant management is usually considered unless gestational age is near-term or term.

Other possible interventions have been studied for women with TTTS. **Amnioreduction** involves removing with a 20- to 22-gauge needle excess fluid from the polyhydramniotic sac so to restore MVP <8. Although in 20% of cases one amnioreduction is sufficient to resolve TTTS, in the other cases, it might need to be performed serially as often fluid quickly reaccumulates. The theory behind its efficacy is that it prevents preterm delivery due to polyhydramnios and also helps to stabilize the flow in arterial–venous connections and thereby slows the rate of blood transfer and fluid reaccumulation [77]. The meta-analysis of the RCTs that compared amnioreduction to laser showed similar results as shown above, so amnioreduction can be considered, especially in cases in which laser therapy is not available.

Septostomy involves purposefully perforating the intertwine membrane under ultrasound guidance with a 22-gauge needle, thus allowing equalization of pressure in the two sacs. One RCT did not find it superior to amnioreduction [78].

Selective fetocide via bipolar diathermy can allow the survival of one twin without neurologic complications [79]. The most common indication for selective fetocide in twintwin is one of the twins has an anomaly or hydrops with impending fetal death. There are no trials available. The rate of loss or PPROM within 2–3 weeks of the procedure of the remaining twin is about 20%.

There is insufficient evidence to evaluate the efficacy of other interventions reported for TTTS, such as transfusion therapy, indomethacin, digoxin, etc. Cerclage placement for short cervix at the time of laser therapy has not been shown to be beneficial in limited data [80].

MONOAMNIOTIC TWINS

The incidence of MA twins is 1 in 10,000 pregnancies, but it is more common with IVF using zona manipulation affecting up to 17% of multiples using this technique [81]. Diagnosis is by ultrasound: Prior to 8 weeks, one yolk sac and two fetal poles is diagnostic [82]. If after 8 weeks, then same sex, single placenta, and single amniotic sac with no dividing amniotic membrane allow diagnosis. Fetuses must be of the same sex. Demonstration of umbilical cord entanglement is also diagnostic of monoamniotic twins.

The rate of loss due especially to cord accidents in utero but also to congenital anomalies and very preterm birth in pregnancies beyond 22 weeks is up to 32% despite intensive care and monitoring at tertiary care centers [83]. Perinatal mortality with aggressive inpatient monitoring (see below) and delivery at 32 weeks has recently been reported to be as low as 10% with later delivery probably associated with continuing risk of mortality [84].

Due to rarity of the condition, there are no randomized trials available. Several nonrandomized but controlled series have suggested offering first trimester screening with NT measurement, fetal echocardiography at 22–24 weeks, and ultrasound every 3 weeks to assess fetal biometry and cord entanglement. Admission at 24–26 weeks with very frequent fetal monitoring can be offered as well as steroids for fetal maturity at this point, but there is no level 1 data to support these interventions. The largest retrospective of 193 monoamniotic twin pregnancies determined that the risk of "potentially preventable death" was not significantly different in patients admitted to the hospital when compared with those managed as outpatients (2.1% compared with 4.7%, respectively). Although these patients were outpatient, they were watched very closely with both cardiotocograms (on average four times per week) and ultrasonograms (once to twice per week), and 56% of these pregnancies were admitted for surveillance at some point, and approximately 20% were delivered for suspected fetal nonreassuring status. They also concluded planned preterm delivery at approximately 33 weeks of gestation should be considered because the in utero risk of a monoamniotic twin fetus exceeds the risk of a postnatal nonrespiratory complication at this gestation [85].

It is difficult to give management recommendations in the rare cases in which only one twin of a MA pair dies. If gestational age is less than 30 weeks, expectant management can continue with close monitoring. This can be considered even up to 32 weeks.

Cesarean section at around 32–34 weeks is the preferred mode of delivery due to the risk of fetal interlocking and cord entanglement and to avoid the risk of inadvertently clamping and dividing the cord of the second twin during the delivery of the first twin, premature placental separation, and cord prolapse [86].

ACARDIAC TWIN

Acardiac twin (also called twin reversal arterial perfusion—TRAP—syndrome) is a MZ, MC pregnancy characterized by a **fetus lacking a normal developed heart and usually a head ("acardiac twin")**. It occurs in 1% of MC twins or about

1/35,000 pregnancies. This acardiac fetus survives in utero due to placental anastomoses shunting blood flow from the "pump twin." Diagnosis needs ultrasound Doppler confirmation of blood being pumped in from the "pump" twin. **The "pump twin" can develop a high cardiac output state and subsequent failure**, resulting in intrauterine or neonatal death of this normal twin in about 35%–50% of cases [87].

Due to the rarity of the condition, there are no trials available. As cardiac failure is more common when the EFW of the acardiac twin is >70% of the EFW of the pump twin, interventions to "terminate" in utero the acardiac twin have been proposed for EFW of acardiac >70% together with "pump" twin compromise. Of all the proposed techniques, **ultrasound-guided laser coagulation or radiofrequency ablation of intrafetal vessels** seems to be the first line of treatment in centers experienced with these techniques. Cord ligation and occlusion have also been reported with some success [88].

CONJOINED TWINS

Conjoined twins are an anomaly linked to MZ twinning with incidence of 1 in 50,000 to 1 in 10,000 births [89]. Classification is based on the site of connection with the suffix *pagus* added. Of those diagnosed in utero, 28% will die prior to delivery, 54% die immediately after birth with only an 18% survival rate [90]. Diagnosis of shared anatomy is imperative to management and prognosis [31]. Due to rarity of the condition, there are no trials available. Voluntary termination would be considered if cardiac (thoracopagus) or cerebral (craniopagus) fusion due to poor outcome [32] or if the pregnancy outcome due to the level of deformity is unacceptable to the parents. If pregnancy is continued, planned cesarean at term is recommended.

ANTEPARTUM TESTING
Ultrasounds

An ultrasound should be performed in the **first trimester** assessing viability, gestational age, and chorionicity. An ultrasound should be performed between **18 and 20 weeks** assessing gestational age, chorionicity (if not done previously), placental cord insertion sites, fetal anatomic surveys, and fetal gender. Twins grow at the same rate as singletons up to 28–32 weeks, and then the growth of twins slows so that fetal twin charts are best used for management. No uniform frequency of fetal growth scans. **Sonographic assessment for twin growth can be performed every 4 weeks from 18 to 20 weeks until delivery**. If discordance or IUGR is diagnosed, then frequency is increased to every 3 weeks. Multiple methods to access amniotic fluid by ultrasound in multiples has been described, including subjective assessment, total AFI, individual AFI, maximum vertical pocket (MVP), two-diameter pocket, and others. The **MVP technique**, using <2 cm for polyhydramnios and >8 cm for polyhydramnios, is accurate in assessing amniotic fluid volume.

Fetal Surveillance

Routine antepartum testing has not been proven to be valuable in the management of multiple gestations; therefore, antepartum fetal surveillance in multiple gestations is recommended in all situations in which surveillance would ordinarily be performed in a singleton pregnancy (e.g., FGR, maternal disease, decreased fetal movement, etc.) [43]. **Some** start NSTs in all twin gestations at around 32–34 weeks, but there is no firm evidence for or against this intervention. Doppler flow studies are not routinely beneficial [91] but probably have the same benefit in fetal morbidity and mortality in cases of twin FGR as in cases of singleton FGR.

DELIVERY
Timing of Delivery
Timing of delivery is about **37 0/7–37 6/7 weeks** for uncomplicated DCDA twin pregnancies as it is associated with similar maternal outcomes and lower incidence of serious adverse infant outcomes compared to expectant management until 38 weeks. Although there are no RCTs to suggest the best timing of delivery for other twins or higher order multiple gestations, Table 44.5 offers some guidance based on non-RCT data [92–94]. Timing of delivery should not be based on fetal lung maturity testing. If this is done nonetheless, as disparity in lung maturity occurs usually in only 5% of twins, just one gestational sac may be sampled for assessment of lung maturity. In certain circumstances, such as diabetes or growth discordance, a bigger difference in maturity discordance may necessitate sampling both sacs.

Route of Delivery
Twins
There are no trials for **twins presenting vertex/vertex** (40% of twin pregnancies) with **trial of labor** usually suggested as this has been shown to be safe.

In twin pregnancy at 32 0/7 weeks and beyond with the **first twin in cephalic presentation**, there is **no benefit to planned cesarean section over trial at vaginal delivery in perinatal outcomes** [95]. Attempt at vaginal twin delivery has been supported especially for twins with EFW of >1500 g

Table 44.5 Delivery Timing for Twins

Type of Twin Pregnancy	Suggested Timing of Planned Delivery
DC/DA twins uncomplicated	37 0/7 to 37 6/7 weeks[a]
MC/DA with one growth restricted twin with normal UA Doppler	36 0/7 to 36 6/7 weeks[b]
DC/DA twins with one growth restricted twin with abnormal UA Doppler (but some forward diastolic flow)	34 0/7 to 34 6/7 weeks
MC/DA twins with one growth restricted twin with absent UA Doppler	32 0/7 to 33 6/7 weeks
DC/DA twins with one growth restricted twin with absent UA Doppler	30 0/7 to 31 6/7 weeks
DC/DA twins complicated by maternal comorbidity, such as preeclampsia	32 0/7 to 34 6/7 weeks[b]
MC/DA twins uncomplicated	34 0/7 to 37 6/7 weeks[b]
MC/DA with one growth restricted twin	32 0/7 to 34 6/7 weeks[b]
MC/MA twin gestation	32 0 days to 33 6/7 weeks[c]

[a]Saccone G, Berghella V. *J Matern Fetal Neonatal Med*, 1–5, 2015.
[b]Medically indicated later-preterm and early-term deliveries. Committee Opinion No 560. American College of Obstetricians and Gynecologists. *Obstet Gynecol* 201, 121, 908–10.
[c]Van Mieghem T, De Heus R, Lewi L, Karitsch P, Kollmann M, Baud D, et al. *Obstet Gynecol*, 124, 498–506, 2014.

and can only be performed with adequate experience of the obstetrician and continuous availability of expert anesthesia, usually in or very close to an operating room. Interval between first and second twin deliveries is not critical as long as the second twin is monitored continuously and accurately. Oxytocin may need to be (re)started as contractions often diminish, and amniotomy should be performed only when presenting part is engaged. Total breech extraction is associated with shorter maternal stay and lower neonatal pulmonary disease, infection, and ICN stay compared to podalic version in retrospective studies [96,97].

There are no trials for twins presenting with **first twin nonvertex** (about 26%) with recommendation for CD made based mostly on data from singleton gestations.

Triplets and Higher Order Multiples
Because vaginal delivery of triplets is usually associated with an increased risk for stillbirth, neonatal, and infant deaths as compared to caesarean delivery [98], **cesarean delivery is the route of choice**. Some centers have recently reported similar outcomes for trial of labor or CD for triplets, but these series are small and not RCTs.

Delayed Interval Delivery
Preterm labor or PPROM can result in the delivery of only one twin or other multiple gestation fetus(es). Delaying the delivery of the remaining fetus(es) may result in decreased morbidity and mortality of these remaining fetuses with no trials to fully assess the effect of this intervention. Delayed delivery should not be attempted if MC gestation, abruption, preeclampsia, chorioamnionitis, need of CD, or other indications for delivery are present, making only about 25% of multiple deliveries in the second trimester candidates for this attempt. Delayed delivery is not very successful and does not result in significant improvements at >28 weeks (delay <2 weeks even with success). Although tocolytics, antibiotics, and cerclage are often used, there is no firm evidence of their benefit. Delayed delivery is associated with decreases in perinatal and infant mortality with average gain of about 2–5 weeks if successful. The interval between delivery is inversely correlated with gestational age of first delivery [99].

NEONATAL
There is probably no significant difference between multiples and singletons in odds of death and long-term outcomes (intraventricular hemorrhage, retinopathy of prematurity, necrotizing enterocolitis) at a given gestational age in those unaffected by FGR [100].

REFERENCES
1. Benirschke, K, Kim CK. Multiple pregnancy. *N Engl J Med* 1973; 288(24): 1276–84. [II-3]
2. Martin JA, Hamilton BE, Sutton PD et al. Births: Final data for 2002. *Natl Vital Stat Rep* 2003; 52(10): 1–102. [II-3]
3. Kulkarni D, Jamieson D, Jones H et al. Fertility treatments and multiple births in the United States. *N Engl J Med* 369: 23: 2218–25. [II-2]
4. Martin JA, Hamilton BE, Osterman MJK et al. Births: Final data for 2013. *Nat Vital Statistics Rep* 2015; 64(1). Hyattsville, MD: National Center for Health Statistics. [Epidemiologic data]
5. Wenstrom KD, Syrop CH, Hammitt DG, van Voorhis BJ. Increased risk of monochorionic twinning associated with assisted reproduction. *Fertil Steril* 1993; 60: 510–4. [III]

6. LeFevre ML, Bain RP, Ewigman BG et al. A randomized trial of prenatal ultrasonographic screening: Impact on maternal management and outcome. RADIUS (Routine Antenatal Diagnostic Imaging with Ultrasound) Study Group. *Am J Obstet Gynecology* 1993; 169(3): 483–9. [I, RCT]

7. Finberg HJ. The "twin peak" sign: Reliable evidence of dichorionic twinning. *J Ultrasound Med* 1992; 11(11): 571–7. [II-3]

8. Dickey, RP, Taylor, SN, Lu, PY et al. Spontaneous reduction of multiple pregnancy: Incidence and effect on outcome. *Am J Obstet and Gynecol* 2002; 186(1): 77–83. [II-2]

9. Meyers C, Adam R, Dungan J, Prenger V. Aneuploidy in twin gestations: When is maternal age advanced? *Obstet Gynecol* 1997; 89: 248–51. [II-2]

10. Rodis, JF, Egan, JFX, Craffey, A et al. Calculated risks of chromosomal abnormalities in twin gestations. *Obstet Gynecol* 1990; 76(6): 1037–41. [II-2]

11. Malone, FD, D'Alton, ME. Multiple gestation clinical characteristics and management. *Maternal-Fetal Medicine Principles and Practice, 5th ed.* Saunders, Philadelphia, PA. 2004. [III]

12. Jones KL. *Smith's Recognizable Patterns of Human Malformation, 5th ed*, WB Saunders Philadelphia, PA. 1997: 654. [III]

13. Miller J, Chauhan SP, Abuhamad AZ. Discordant twins: Diagnosis, evaluation, and management. *Am J Obstet Gynecol* 206: 10–20. [II-2]

14. Harper LM, Weis MA, Odibo AO et al. Significance of growth discordance in appropriately grown twins. *AJOG* 2013; 208: 393:e1–5. [II-1]

15. Yinon, Y, Mazkereth, R, Rosentzweig, N et al. Growth restriction as a determinant of outcome in preterm discordant twins. *Obstet Gynecol* 2005; 105: 80–4. [II-3]

16. D'Alton ME, Simpson LL: Syndromes in twins. *Semin Perinatol* 1995; 19(5): 375–86. [Level II-3]

17. Malone, FD, D'Alton, ME. Multiple gestation clinical characteristics and management. *Maternal-Fetal Medicine Principles and Practice, 5th ed.* Saunders, Philadelphia, PA. 2004. [III]

18. Kallen B, Finnstrom O, Lindam A et al. Selected neonatal outcomes in dizygotic twins after IVF versus non-IVF pregnancies. *BJOG* 2010; 117: 676–82. [II-2]

19. Martin JA, Hamilton BE, Ventura SJ, Osterman MJ, Kirmeyer S, Mathews TJ, Wilson EC. Births: Final data for 2009 *Natl Vital Stat Rep* 2011; 60(1): 1–70. [II-2]

20. Luke B, Brown M. The changing risk of infant mortality by gestation, plurality, and race: 1989–1991 versus 1999–2001. *Pediatrics* 2006; 118: 2488–97. [II-2]

21. Chasen ST, Madden A, Chervenak FA. Cesarean delivery of twins and neonatal respiratory disorders. *Am J Obstet Gynecol* 1999; 181(5 Pt. 1): 1052–6. [II-2]

22. Wen, SW, Demissie, K, Yang, Q, Walker, MC. Maternal morbidity and obstetric complications in triplet pregnancies and quadruplet and higher-order multiple pregnancies. *Am J Obstet Gynecol* 2004; 191: 254–8. [II-2]

23. Sibai BM, Hauth J, Caritis S et al. Hypertensive disorders in twin versus singleton gestations. National Institute of Child Health and Human Development Network of Maternal-Fetal Medicine Units. *Am J Obstet Gynecol* 2000; 182: 938–42. [I]

24. Lynch A, McDuffie R Jr, Murphy J, Faber K, Orleans M. Preeclampsia in multiple gestation: The role of assisted reproductive technologies. *Obstet Gynecol* 2002; 99(3): 445–51. [II-2]

25. Al-Kouatly HB, Chasen ST, Kalish RB, Chervenak, FA. Causes of thrombocytopenia in triplet gestations. *Am J Obstet Gynecol* 2003; 189(1): 177–80. [II-2]

26. Malone FD, Kaufman GE, Chelmow D et al. Maternal morbidity associated with triplet pregnancy. *Am J Perinatol* 1998; 15: 73–7. [II-3]

27. Schwartz DB, Daoud Y, Zazula P et al. Gestational diabetes mellitus: Metabolic and blood glucose parameters in singleton versus twin pregnancies. *Am J Obstet Gynecol* 1999; 181(4): 912–4. [II-2]

28. Silvan E, Maman E, Homko CJ et al. Impact of fetal reduction on the incidence of gestational diabetes. *Obstet Gynecol* 2002; 99: 91–4. [II-3]

29. Francois K, Ortiz J, Harris C et al. Is peripartum hysterectomy more common in multiple gestations? *Obstet Gynecol* 2005; 105(6): 1369–72. [II-3]

30. Goodnight W, Newman R, SMFM. Optimal nutrition for improved twin pregnancy outcome. *Obstet Gynecol* 2009; 114: 1121–34. [II-2]

31. LeFevre, ML. Low-dose aspirin use for the prevention of morbidity and mortality from preeclampsia: U.S. Preventive Services Task Force recommendation Statement. *Ann Intern Med* 2014; 161: 819–26. [III]

32. Chasen ST, Perni SC, Kalish RB, Chervenak FA. First-trimester risk assessment for trisomies 21 and 18 in twin pregnancy. *Am J Obstet Gynecol* 2007; 197(4): 374.e1–3. [II-2]

33. Sebire NJ, Snijders RJ, Hughes K, Sepulveda W, Nicolaides KH. Screening for trisomy 21 in twin pregnancies by maternal age and fetal nuchal translucency thickness at 10-14 weeks of gestation. *Br J Obstet Gynaecol* 1996; 103(10): 999–1003. [II-2]

34. Bush MC, Malone FD. Down syndrome screening in twins. *Clin Perinatol* 2005; 32(2): 373–86, vi. [Review]

35. Sepulveda W, Wong AE, Casasbuenas A. Nuchal translucency and nasal bone in first-trimester ultrasound screening for aneuploidy in multiple pregnancies. *Ultrasound Obstet Gynecol* 2009; 33(2): 152–6. [II-2]

36. Prats P, Rodríguez I, Comas C, Puerto B. Systematic review of screening for trisomy 21 in twin pregnancies in first trimester combining nuchal translucency and biochemical markers: A meta-analysis. *Prenat Diagn* 2014; 34(11): 1077. [Meta-analysis 12,974 with 69 Trisomy 21]

37. Cell-free DNA screening for fetal aneuploidy. Committee Opinion No. 640. American College of Obstetricians and Gynecologists. *Obstet Gynecol* 2015; 126: e31–7. [Review]

38. Wapner RJ, Johnson A, Davis G. Prenatal diagnosis in twin gestations: A comparison between second trimester amniocentesis and first trimester chorionic villus sampling. *Obstet Gynecol* 1993; 82(1): 49–56. [II-2]

39. Eddleman KA, Stone JL, Lynch L, Berkowitz RL. Chorionic villus sampling before multifetal pregnancy reduction. *Am J Obstet Gynecol* 2000; 183(5): 1078–81. [II-3]

40. Garchet-Beaudron A, Dreux S, Leporrier N, Oury JF, Muller F, ABA Study Group et al. Second-trimester Down syndrome maternal serum marker screening: A prospective study of 11,040 twin pregnancies. *Prenat Diagn* 2008; 28(12): 1105–9. [II-2]

41. Ghidini A, Lynch, L, Hicks, C et al. The risk of second-trimester amniocentesis in twin gestations: A case-control study. *Am J Obstet Gynecol* 1993; 169(4): 1013–6. [II-2]

42. Conde-Agudelo A, Romero R, Hassan SS et al. Transvaginal sonographic cervical length for the prediction of spontaneous preterm birth in twin pregnancies: A systematic review and metaanalysis. *Am J Obstet Gynecol* 2010; 203: 128.e1–12. [Meta-analysis]

43. Conde-Agudelo A, Romero R. Prediction of preterm birth in twin gestations using biophysical and biochemical tests. *Am J Obstet Gynecol* 2014; 211(6): 583–95. [Review]

44. Eddleman KA, Stone JL, Lynch L, Berkowitz RL. Selective termination of anomalous fetuses in multifetal pregnancies: Two hundred cases at a single center. *Am J Obstet Gynecol* 2002; 187: 1168–72. [II-3]

45. Lust A, De Catt L, Lewi L et al. Monochorionic and dichorionic twin pregnancies discordant for fetal anencephaly: A systematic review of management options. *Prenat Diagn* 2008; 28: 275–9. [II-2]

46. Gonzalez-Quintero VH, Kathiresan AS, Tudela FJ, Rhea D, Desch C, Istwan N. The association of gestational weight gain per institute of medicine guidelines and prepregnancy body mass index on outcomes of twin pregnancies. *Am J Perinatol* 2012; 29(6): 435–40. [II-2]

47. Goodnight W, Newman R, Society of Maternal-Fetal Medicine. Optimal nutrition for improved twin pregnancy outcome. *Obstet Gynecol* 2009; 114(5): 1121–34. [Review]

48. Dodd JM, Crowther CA. Reduction of the number of fetuses for women with triplet and higher order multiple pregnancies. *Cochrane Database Syst Rev* 2003; 2(2): CD003932. [Review/Meta-analysis]

49. Smith-Levitin M, Kowalik A, Birnholz J, Skupski DW, Hutson JM, Chervenak FA et al. Selective reduction of multifetal pregnancies to twins improves outcome over nonreduced triplet gestations. *Am J Obstet Gynecol* 1996; 175(4 Pt. 1): 878–82. [II-3]

50. Morlando M, Ferrara L, Lawin-O'Brien A et al. Dichorionic triplet pregnancies: Risk of miscarriage and severe preterm delivery with fetal reduction versus expectant management. Outcomes of a cohort study and systematic review. *BJOG* 2015; 122: 1053–60. [II-2, systematic review]

51. Crowther CA. Hospitalization and bed rest for multiple pregnancies. *Cochrane* 2005; 1. [meta-analysis; 4 RCTs, >1000 women. Mostly in Harare, Zimbabwe]

52. Crowther CA, Neilson JP, Verkuyl DAA, Bannerman C, Ashurst HM. Preterm labour in twin pregnancies: Can it be prevented by hospital admission? *BJOG* 1989; 96: 850–3. [RCT, *n* = 139]

53. Schuit E, Stock S, Rode L et al. A Global Obstetrics Network collaboration. Effectiveness of progestogens to improve perinatal outcome in twin pregnancies: An individual participant data meta-analysis. *BJOG* 2015; 122: 27–37. [meta-analysis; 13 RCTs, *n* = 3768 women, 7536 babies]

54. Combs CA, Garite T, Maurel K, Das A, Porto M, Obstetrix Collaborative Research Network. Failure of 17-hydroxyprogesterone to reduce neonatal morbidity or prolong triplet pregnancy: a double-blind, randomized clinical trial. *Obstet Gynecol* 2010; 203(3): 248.e1–9. [RCT]

55. Dor, J, Shalev, J, Mashiach, S et al. Elective cervical suture of twins pregnancies diagnosed ultrasonically in the first trimester following induced ovulation. *Gynecol Obstet Invest* 1982; 13(1): 55–60. [RCT, *n* = 50]

56. Berghella V, Odibo AO, To MS, Rust OA, Althuisius SM. Cerclage for short cervix on ultrasonography: Meta-analysis of trials using individual patient-level data. *Obstet Gynecol* 2005; 106(1): 181–9. [meta-analysis; 4 RCTs, *n* = 49 twin gestations]

57. Rebarber A, Roman AS, Istwan N, Rhea D, Stanziano G. Prophylactic cerclage in the management of triplet gestations. *Am J Obstet Gynecol* 2005; 193: 1193–6. [II-2]

58. Reichmann J. Home uterine activity monitoring: An evidence review of its utility in multiple gestations. *J Reprod Med* 2009; 54: 559–62. [Review/meta-analysis]

59. Yamasmit W, Chaithongwongwatthana S, Tolosa JE, Limpongsanurak S, Pereira L, Lumbiganon P. Prophylactic oral betamimetics for reducing preterm birth in women with a twin pregnancy. *Cochrane Database System Rev* 2005: 4. [meta-analysis; 5 RCTs, *n* = 344]

60. Fuchs I, Tsoi E, Henrich W et al. Sonographic measurement of cervical length in twin pregnancies in threatened preterm labor. *Ultrasound Obstet Gynecol* 2004; 23: 42–5. [Level II-3]

61. Roberts D, Dalziel S. Antenatal corticosteroids for accelerating fetal lung maturation for women at risk of preterm birth. *Cochrane Database Syst Rev* 2006; 3: 004454. [Review/meta-analysis]

62. Effect of corticosteroids for fetal maturation on perinatal outcomes. *NIH Consensus Statement* 1994; 12: 1–24. [III]

63. Doyle LW, Crowther CA, Middleton P, Marret S, Rouse D. Magnesium sulphate for women at risk of preterm birth for neuroprotection of the fetus. *Cochrane Database Syst Rev* 2009; 1(1): CD004661. [Review/meta-analysis]

64. Conde-Agudelo A, Romero R. Antenatal magnesium sulfate for the prevention of cerebral palsy in preterm infants less than 34 weeks' gestation: A systematic review and metaanalysis. *Am J Obstet Gynecol* 2009; 200(6): 595–609. [Review/meta-analysis]

65. Costantine MM, Weiner SJ, Eunice Kennedy Shriver National Institute of Child Health and Human Development Maternal-Fetal Medicine Units Network. Effects of antenatal exposure to magnesium sulfate on neuroprotection and mortality in preterm infants: A meta-analysis. *Obstet Gynecol* 2009; 114(2 Pt. 1): 354–64. [Meta-analysis]

66. Patient safety checklist no. 7: Magnesium sulfate before anticipated preterm birth for neuroprotection. Obstet Gynecol 2012 Aug;120(2 Pt 1):432-433. [Guideline]

67. Rafael TJ, Hoffman MK, Leiby BE, Berghella V. Gestational age of previous twin preterm birth as a predictor for subsequent singleton preterm birth. *AJOG* 2012; 206: 156.e1–6. [II-1]

68. Harper LM, Weis MA, Odibo AO et al. Significance of growth discordance in appropriately grown twins. *AJOG* 2013; 208: 393:e1–5. [II-1]

69. Hillman SC, Morris RK, Kilby MD. Co-twin prognosis after single fetal death. A systematic review and meta-analysis. *Obstet Gynecol* 2011; 1118: 928–40. [II-1]

70. Society for Maternal-Fetal Medicine, Simpson LL. Twin-twin transfusion syndrome. *Am J Obstet Gynecol* 2013; 208(1): 3–18. [Review]

71. Quintero RA, Morales WJ, Allen MH, Bornick PW, Johnson PK, Kruger M. Staging of twin-twin transfusion syndrome. *J Perinatol* 1999; 19: 550–5. [II-2]

72. Berghella V, Kaufmann M. Natural history of twin-twin transfusion syndrome. *J Reprod Med* 2001; 46(5): 480–4. [II-3]

73. Simpson L, for the Society for Maternal-Fetal Medicine. Twin-twin transfusion syndrome. *Am J Obstet and Gynecol* 2013: 3–17. [Review]

74. Senat MV, Deprest J, Boulvain M, Paupe A, Winer N, Ville Y. Endoscopic laser surgery versus serial amnioreduction for severe twin-to-twin transfusion syndrome. *N Engl J Med* 2004; 351(2): 136–44. Epub 2004 Jul 6. [RCT]

75. Emery SP, Bahtiyar MO, Moise KJ. The North American fetal therapy network consensus statement. Management of complicated monochorionic gestations. *Obstet Gynecol* 2015; 126: 575–84. [Review]

76. Slaghekke F, Lopriore E, Lewi L et al. Fetoscopic laser coagulation of the vascular equator versus selective coagulation for twin-to-twin transfusion syndrome: An open-labeled randomized controlled trial. *Lancet* 2014; 383: 2144–51. [RCT, *n* = 274]

77. Bower SJ, Flack NJ, Sepulveda W et al. Uterine artery blood flow response to correction of amniotic fluid volume. *Am J Obstet Gynecol* 1995; 173: 502–7. [II-3]

78. Moise KJ Jr, Dorman K, Lamvu G et al. A randomized trial of amnioreduction versus septostomy in the treatment of twin-twin transfusion syndrome. *Am J Obstet Gynecol* 2005; 193: 701–7. [RCT, *n* = 71]

79. Taylor MJ, Shalev E, Tanawattanacharoen S et al. Ultrasound guided umbilical chord occlusion using bipolar diathery for stage III/IV twin-twin transfusion syndrome. *Prenat Diagn* 2002; 22: 70–6. [Level II-3]

80. Papanna R, Habli M, Baschat AA et al. Cerclage for cervical shortening at fetoscopic laser photocoagulation in twin-twin transfusion syndrome. *AJOG* 2012; 206: 425.e1–7. [II-2]

81. Slotnick RN, Ortega JE. Monoamniotic twining and zona manipulation: A survey of U.S. IVF centers correlating zona manipulation procedures and high-risk twinning frequency. *J Assist Reprod Genet* 1996; 13: 381–5. [II-3]

82. Bromley B, Benacerraf B. Using the number of yolk sacs to determine amniocity in early first trimester monochorionic twins. *J Ultrasound Med* 1995; 14: 415–9. [II-2]

83. Demaria F, Goffinet F, Kayem G et al. Monoamniotic twin pregnancies: antenatal management and perinatal results of 19 consecutive cases. *BJOG* 2004; 111(1): 22–6. [II-3]

84. Roque H, Young BK, Lockwood CJ. Perinatal outcomes in monoamniotic gestations. *J Matern Fetal Neonatal Med* 2003; 13(6): 414–21. [II-3]

85. Van Mieghem T, De Heus R, Lewi L et al. Prenatal management of monoamniotic twin pregnancies. *Obstet Gynecol* 2014; 124(3): 498. [II-2]

86. Lee YM. Delivery of twins. *Semin Perinatol* 2012; 36(3): 195–200. [Review]

87. Van Gemert MJ, Umur A, van den Wijngaard JP et al. Increasing cardiac output and decreasing oxygenation sequence in pump twins of acardiac twin pregnancies. *Phys Med Biol* 2005; 50(3): N33–42. [II-3]

88. Wong AE, Sepulveda W. Acardiac anomaly: Current issues in prenatal assessment and treatment. *Prenat Diagn* 2005; 25: 796–806. [II-3]

89. Spitz L, Kiely EM. Conjoined twins. *JAMA* 2003; 289(10): 1307–10. [Level II-3]

90. Mackenzie TC, Crombleholme TM, Johnson MP et al. The natural history of prenatally diagnosed conjoined twins. *J Pediatr Surg* 2002; 37(3): 303–9. [II-3]

91. Giles W, Bisits A, O'Callaghan S, Gill A. The Doppler assessment in multiple pregnancy randomized controlled trial of ultrasound biometry versus umbilical artery Doppler ultrasound and biometry in twin pregnancy. *BJOG* 2003; 110(6): 593–7. [I]

92. Saccone G, Berghella V. Planned delivery at 37 weeks in twins: A systematic review and meta-analysis of randomized trials. *J Matern Fetal Neonatal Med* 2015; 1–5. [Meta-analysis; 2 RCTs, n = 271]

93. Medically indicated later-preterm and early-term deliveries. Committee Opinion No 560. American College of Obstetricians and Gynecologists. *Obstet Gynecol* 201; 121: 908–10. [III]

94. Van Mieghem T, De Heus R, Lewi L, Karitsch P, Kollmann M, Baud D et al. Prenatal management of monoamniotic twin pregnancies. *Obstet Gynecol* 2014; 124: 498–506. [II-3]

95. Barrett JF, Hannah ME, Hutton EK et al. A randomized trial of planned cesarean or vaginal delivery for twin pregnancy. *N Engl J Med* 2013; 369: 1295–305. [RCT, n = 2795]

96. Hogle KL, Hutton EK, McBrien KA, Barrett JFR, Hannah ME. Cesarean delivery for twins: A systematic review and meta-analysis. *Am J Obstet Gynecol* 2003; 188: 220–7. [meta-analysis; 4 studies; only 1 RCT, ref. 65; n = 1932]

97. Maudin JG, Newman RB, Mauldin PD. Cost-effective delivery management of the vertex and non-vertex twin gestation. *Am J Obstet Gynecol* 1998; 179: 864–9. [II-2]

98. Vintzileos AM, Ananth CV, Kontopoulos E, Smulian JC. Mode of delivery and risk of stillbirth and infant mortality in triplet gestations: United States, 1995 through 1998. *Am J Obstet Gynecol* 2005; 192: 464–9. [II-3]

99. Oyelese Y, Ananth CV, Smulian JC, Vintzileos AM. Delayed interval delivery in twin pregnancies in the United States: Impact on perinatal mortality and morbidity. *Am J Obstet Gynecol* 2005; 192: 439–44. [II-3]

100. Garite TJ, Clark RH, Elliot JP, and Thorp, JA. Twins and triplets: The effect of plurality and growth on neonatal outcome compared with singleton infants. *Am J Obstet Gynecology* 2004; 191: 700–7. [II-2]

45

Fetal growth restriction

Shane Reeves and Henry L. Galan

KEY POINTS

- **Fetal growth restriction (FGR) is defined as a sonographic estimated fetal weight (EFW) <10th percentile for gestational age.** Screening and diagnosis of FGR are based on ultrasound biometry that is dependent on accurate dating by an early ultrasound (preferably first trimester).
- FGR may be due to normal genetic (constitutional) reasons in about 70% of the cases and to pathologic reasons in about 30% of the cases.
- **Umbilical artery (UA) Doppler ultrasound is effective in differentiating between pathologic FGR (abnormal UA Doppler) and a constitutionally small fetus but not effective as a general screening modality.**
- **Risk factors associated with FGR are numerous and include maternal, fetal, and placental factors** (Table 45.1).
- **Complications of FGR occur in utero and in later life** (Table 45.2):
  - Fetus: **oligohydramnios, nonreassuring fetal heart testing (NRFHR), and death.**
  - Neonate: **preterm birth and its consequences:** respiratory distress syndrome (RDS), intraventricular hemorrhage (IVH), necrotizing enterocolitis (NEC), sepsis, hypoglycemia, electrolyte disturbances, hyperviscosity syndrome, neurodevelopmental delay, and death.
  - Infant and child (as well as later in life): impaired gross motor development, cerebral palsy, lower intelligence quotient, mental retardation, speech/reading disabilities, learning deficits, poor academic achievement, and suicide.
  - Adult: hypertension, coronary artery disease, diabetes, obesity, social and financial problems.
- **Maternal complications:**
  - FGR may precede the onset of **preeclampsia** in 50% of cases.
  - Risk of **cesarean delivery** when necessitating delivery before 32 weeks is as high as 90%.
  - Loss of time from work for increased fetal surveillance.
- **Effective prevention strategies for FGR include the following:**
  - **Early (<20 weeks) ultrasound.**
  - **Identification and treatment of modifiable risk factors** (e.g., smoking and other toxic exposures, medical disorders, etc.).
  - **Recurrence risk of FGR in sequential singleton pregnancies approaches 25%. A low-dose aspirin reduces the incidence of recurrent FGR by 10%, especially (decrease up to 56%) if >75 mg and started before 16 weeks.**

- Avoidance of a short interpregnancy (e.g., <12 months).
- **Workup of FGR should include the following:**
  - **Review of risk factors** (Table 45.1).
  - **Evaluation of fetal anatomy, placenta, amniotic fluid ultrasound.**
  - **Assessment of the UA by Doppler.**
- **Workup of FGR may also include the following:**
  - Infectious workup, including maternal serum IgG and IgM of cytomegalovirus (CMV), toxoplasmosis, and possibly herpes simplex virus (HSV). Rubella immunity should be ascertained.
  - **Amniocentesis to rule out aneuploidy (karyotype) and infection (PCR for CMV, toxoplasmosis, and possibly HSV).**
  - Antiphospholipid antibodies may be checked, but if positive, there is no intervention proven to alter outcome.
  - Maternal workup for preeclampsia should be performed or evaluation for any disease possibly associated with FGR should be done.
- **FGR Management:**
  - Fetal therapy is limited. Intervention studies have not shown benefit.
  - **Control or elimination of risk factors is recommended (e.g., stop drug abuse or smoking, avoid physically strenuous activity, control maternal disease).**
  - **UA Doppler velocimetry is the cornerstone of FGR follow-up and management as it is associated with a significant reduction in labor inductions, cesarean delivery, and perinatal mortality.**
  - In early severe FGR, delivery based on an absent or reversed a-wave in the ductus venosus may reduce neurodevelopmental delay.
  - If delivery is anticipated within a 7-day period and between 24 and 34 weeks gestation, maternal **steroid administration** is recommended for fetal benefit.
- **Timing delivery of the FGR fetus** should be individualized on the basis of gestational age, Doppler velocimetry, growth, and biophysical testing.
  - **Gestational age is the most important determinant of survival until approximately 30–32 weeks.**
  - Abnormal biophysical testing, such as electronic fetal heart rate monitoring **(EFM), showing absent variability with a biophysical profile score (BPS) ≤4 or recurrent late decelerations** is consistent with a hypoxemic and academic fetus at risk for impending death. These are usually the only findings warranting delivery before 30–32 weeks. Such findings warrant consideration of delivery based on gestational

Table 45.1 Risk Factors Associated with FGR

Maternal
   Hypertension (20%–30%)
     Preeclampsia
     Chronic hypertension
     Secondary hypertension
   Pregestational diabetes
   Autoimmune disease
   Antiphospholipid syndrome
   Lupus
   Maternal cardiac disease
   Congenital heart disease
   Heart failure
   Pulmonary disorders
     Cystic fibrosis
     COPD
     Uncontrolled asthma
   Renal disease
     Chronic renal insufficiency
     Nephrotic syndrome
     Chronic renal failure
   Gastrointestinal disease
     Ulcerative colitis
     Crohn's disease
     Malabsorptive disorders
     Gastric bypass
   Toxic exposure
     Smoking
     Alcohol
     Cocaine
     Stimulants
   Malnutrition
   Living at high altitudes
   Low socioeconomic status
   Race
   Extremes of maternal age
Fetal
   Genetic diseases[a]
   Aneuploidy[a]
   Fetal malformations (1%–2%)
   Multiple gestation (3%)
   Fetal infection (5%–10%)
     CMV
     Toxoplasmosis
     Rubella
     Malaria
     HSV
Placental
Abruption
   Placental mosaicism
   Placenta accreta
   Chorioangioma
   Implantation abnormalities with abnormal analytes on serum
     screening

Abbreviations: CMV, cytomegalovirus; COPD, chronic obstructive pulmonary disease; FGR, fetal growth restriction; HSV, herpes simplex virus.
[a]Incidence of genetic diseases or aneuploidy is about 5% to 20%.

Table 45.2 Complications Associated with FGR

Fetal
- Oligohydramnios
- Nonreassuring fetal heart rate testing (NRFHR)
- Fetal death

Neonate
- Iatrogenic or spontaneous preterm birth
- Its consequences (RDS, IVH, NEC, sepsis, etc.)
- Low Apgar score
- Hypoglycemia
- Electrolyte disturbances, acidosis
- Hyperviscosity syndrome
- Seizures
- Death

Child
- Neurodevelopmental and cognitive delay
- Cerebral palsy, impaired gross motor development
- Lower intelligence quotient
- Speech/reading disabilities
- Learning deficits
- Poor academic achievement
- Short stature

Adult
- Hypertension
- Coronary artery disease
- Stroke
- Type II diabetes mellitus
- Obesity
- Low socioeconomic status
- Suicide
- Financial problems

Mother
- Preeclampsia
- Cesarean delivery
- Lost time at work

Abbreviations: IVH, intraventricular hemorrhage; NEC, necrotizing enterocolitis; RDS, respiratory distress syndrome.

- In the presence of NST reactivity and/or BPS of 8 or 10, a FGR fetus with UA absent end-diastolic flow (**AEDF**) should be delivered at approximately **34 weeks**.
- Delivery of the early and severe FGR pregnancy based on development of absent or reversal of flow in the a-wave of the ductus venosus (DV) at ≥29–30 weeks reduces risk of neurodevelopmental delay.
- Although evidence shows that abnormal MCA Doppler waveforms, which suggest a brain-sparing effect, identifies a group of FGR fetuses at greater risk for perinatal morbidity and death, its routine use for management is not recommended due to a lack of data showing improvement in outcomes.

DEFINITIONS/DIAGNOSIS

FGR is diagnosed when the sonographic EFW is <10th percentile for gestational age on a standardized population growth curve. So both screening and diagnosis of FGR are based on ultrasound biometry, and they rely on accurate dating by an early ultrasound (preferably first trimester). The terms FGR, intrauterine growth restriction (IUGR), and small for gestational age (**SGA**) are often used interchangeably. However, FGR is the preferred term by the American College of Obstetricians and Gynecologists (ACOG), and it is used in the chapter. Small for gestational age (**SGA**) is a term used for the neonate [1] and is defined as a birth weight

age and patient desires and supersedes any Doppler velocimetry findings.
- In the presence of NST reactivity and/or BPS of 8 or 10, a FGR fetus with UA reverse end-diastolic flow (**REDF**) should be delivered at approximately **32 weeks**. Delivering <32 weeks for hypothetical avoidance of fetal hypoxia (e.g., in presence of abnormal fetal Doppler studies) has not been associated with improved perinatal outcomes.

<10th percentile for a given gestational age. **Low birth weight** (LBW) is defined as <2500 g. For FGR in a multiple gestation, please refer to Chapter 44.

The categorization of FGR as <10th percentile has often been criticized secondary to the inclusion of many fetuses that are constitutionally small and not at risk for poor perinatal outcome [2]. In fact, the majority of fetuses (up to 70%) with an EFW of <10th percentile are normally grown and not at risk for adverse perinatal outcome, and the remaining 30% truly have pathologic FGR, and these fetuses (and neonates) are most at risk [3,4]. It is also possible to have a fetus that is above the 10th percentile on a population growth curve who is still at risk for poor perinatal outcome secondary to not meeting its individualized growth potential [5]. **Severe FGR** can be defined as that associated with **EFW <3rd percentile**; the majority of these cases are associated with pathologic reasons for FGR. **UA Doppler ultrasound** is not helpful for screening but most effective in differentiating between pathologic FGR (abnormal UA Doppler) and a constitutionally small fetus [6].

EPIDEMIOLOGY/INCIDENCE

By definition, 10% of fetuses will be diagnosed as FGR by population growth charts. FGR complicates about 4% to 8% of pregnancies in developed countries and up to 25% of pregnancies in undeveloped countries [7]. Birth weight <3rd percentile carries the highest risk for perinatal morbidity [UA blood pH <7.0, grade 3 or 4 IVH, respiratory distress, NEC, and sepsis] and mortality when compared against other cutoffs [8].

Approximately 35% of infants identified as FGR have abnormal UA Doppler evaluation [9], and this was recently confirmed in the large PORTO trial showing 400 of 1119 FGR fetuses to have an abnormal UA waveform [4]. An additional percentage (about 20%) will have only an abnormal middle cerebral artery (MCA) Doppler, but normal UA Doppler flow. These fetuses are also at an increased risk of poor perinatal outcome [10]. So >30%, and possibly up to 50%, of FGR cases are at risk for poor perinatal outcome.

GENETICS/INHERITANCE/RECURRENCE

Because there are multiple risk factors associated with IUGR (Table 45.1), the recurrence risk is largely linked to the underlying etiology in the affected pregnancy. When looking at unselected pregnancies affected by LBW, the recurrence risk of another small child is increased [11–15]. When the prior neonate was SGA, **the risk of SGA in a subsequent singleton pregnancy is about 24%,** and it is about 17% if the subsequent pregnancy is a twin gestation [15,16]. Recurrence of FGR in cases associated with aneuploidy is low, but the risk of aneuploidy in subsequent pregnancies is higher than the risk of maternal age alone. In fact, the risk of aneuploidy recurrence is approximately 1% in women who have aneuploidy in the first pregnancy at a maternal age of <30 years [17–19]. The majority of FGR fetuses do not have a genetic change that can help predict inheritance and recurrence, but if a genetic syndrome is discovered as the cause, proper counseling regarding recurrence is indicated. When the cause of FGR is an intrauterine infection from a viral source, the recurrence risk is low, as the patient will have attained immunity prior to her subsequent pregnancies. In summary, the risk of recurrence is situation-dependent, and counseling regarding future risks will need to be based on the individual circumstances for each case.

CLASSIFICATION

FGR has been classified as asymmetric or symmetric. Asymmetric FGR refers to a reduction in abdominal circumference (AC) relative to other measures, such as head circumference (HC). Often, an HC/AC ratio >95th percentile is used as a cutoff. Symmetric FGR is characterized by a similar reduction in all biometric measurements. Usually, the etiology is present from the beginning of the pregnancy, and it can include aneuploid or euploid genetic diseases, viral infection, drug/toxic exposure, and/or placental causes.

This classification has been traditionally used as a tool to distinguish between etiologies with asymmetry pointing to a placental cause; however, early onset of placental disease may also lead to symmetric FGR, making the classification less helpful. The classification system has been predictive of outcome as asymmetric FGR has a stronger association with major anomalies, hypertensive disorders of pregnancy, cesarean delivery, lower birth weight, perinatal mortality, earlier gestational age at delivery, and poor postnatal outcome compared to symmetric FGR [20,21]. However, the value of the classification system is often criticized because both types are at risk for poor perinatal outcome, and Doppler velocimetry and antenatal monitoring are better predictors of pregnancy outcome in either form of FGR [21]. Although the segregation into asymmetric and symmetric FGR may help to stratify risk, **the clinical use of such a classification system has yet to be determined**.

ETIOLOGY/BASIC PATHOPHYSIOLOGY

There are two scenarios that can lead to an FGR fetus, and it is very important to distinguish between them. The so-called **"constitutional"** FGR fetus is the one with an EFW below the 10th percentile for gestational age but otherwise healthy. This baby characteristically grows at a constant velocity that usually parallels a specific percentile throughout the pregnancy. More importantly, this baby is not prone to develop any fetal or perinatal complications, has a normal postnatal outcome, and does not need therapy. Ultrasound shows normal amniotic fluid and UA Doppler patterns. Some ethnic groups are more likely to show FGR babies if race-adjusted charts are not used.

Some FGR fetuses are **not healthy** because of one or more disorders (Table 45.1) contributing to the FGR weight. Although the causes of FGR are diverse, many of them lead to a common pathway: **compromise of the uteroplacental perfusion**. Over time, the supply of nutrients and oxygen mismatch the fetal requirements that the normal process of growth entails. Then, the normal accretion of tissue decreases, and components of fetal structure and physiology are removed from the tissue to undertake abnormal biochemical paths (proteolysis, gluconeogenesis, and beta-oxidation), which are the results of an adaptive attempt to maintain a supply of energy substrates to support vital functions in an adverse environment, giving up on fetal growth. Placental apoptosis is increased. Such biochemical phenomena translate into sonographically recognizable traits, such as decreased growth. Often altered fetal proportion is evident because places of normal fat accretion, such as the abdominal wall, will show lack of it with the resultant small AC at ultrasound. At the same time, in an attempt to maintain blood supply to critical tissues (brain, heart, adrenals), the fetal circulation decreases in some not-so-critical organs, such as the splanchnic circulation and fetal kidneys, often generating oligohydramnios. This pattern of redistribution of the fetal blood flow is detected by Doppler analysis showing less diastolic flow (increased impedance) in the UA. At times, increased diastolic flow in the MCA develops as "brain-sparing" changes try to maintain adequate oxygenation and nutrition to the fetal brain circulation. Compared to an appropriate for gestational age (AGA) fetus, metabolic changes associated with the FGR fetus are **lower pH, pO$_2$, glucose, LDH, cholesterol, fatty acids, triglycerides, growth factors (e.g., insulin-like GF), insulin, most amino acids, and increased pCO$_2$, lactic acid, and bilirubin**. Finally, the process may be so severe that **heart failure** ensues and the fetus can die in utero.

The causes of FGR can be divided into three basic categories: **maternal factors, fetal factors, and placental factors** (Table 45.1). Although the pathophysiology of each factor is different, maternal factors (e.g., maternal medical disease) and placental factors may have a common final pathway of decreased placental perfusion and transfer of nutrients across the placenta to the fetus. Fetal factors describe scenarios in which growth is reduced secondary to genetic, chromosomal, or infectious causes. Details of how each of these contributes to FGR are outlined below.

Maternal Factors

Several maternal characteristics, including age, weight, height, race, and parity contribute to fetal growth [22]. These factors would largely be considered constitutional determinants of growth, and fetuses that are labeled FGR secondary to normal inheritable maternal characteristics would not be at risk for adverse pregnancy outcome. However, multiple other maternal factors have been associated with pathological growth inhibition. These include factors listed in Table 45.1 [1].

Many maternal medical conditions can lead to FGR with one of the leading causes being maternal hypertension in pregnancy (chronic hypertension, preeclampsia, and chronic hypertension with superimposed preeclampsia) [23,24]. In a recent randomized trial of delivery timing in FGR, the rate of maternal hypertensive disease complicating pregnancy was 70% [24]. Autoimmune disorders, chronic renal disease, pregestational diabetes, and chronic lung disease are other maternal factors that have been associated with FGR [25–27]. Thrombophilia due to antiphospholipid antibody syndrome has been associated with FGR in retrospective but not prospective studies (see Chapter 27), but hereditary thrombophilias (Factor V Leiden, Prothrombin gene mutation, and MTHFR mutations) have not [28–31].

In addition to maternal medical disorders, substance abuse, malnutrition, and pharmacotherapy have been associated with FGR. **The leading cause of preventable FGR is tobacco consumption**, and approximately 13% of growth restriction can be attributed to this drug [32]. Other illicit drug use, such as alcohol, cocaine, and narcotics, has been associated with FGR [33–36]. Not only is substance abuse associated with FGR, but poor nutritional status can inhibit growth. Longitudinal data from women who conceived and gave birth during times of famine suggests an association between FGR and maternal malnutrition [37,38]. Additionally, factors generally associated with poor nutritional status, such as low

maternal weight, severe caloric restriction, poor weight gain, and obesity, can all lead to pathological growth of the fetus [39,40]. Also, multiple medications have been associated with growth restriction, and a complete list would be out of the scope of this chapter. However, antineoplastic medications, antiepileptic drugs, and repeat courses of glucocorticosteroids that can cross the placenta have all been implicated as agents that increase the risk of FGR [41].

Fetal Factors

Multiple fetal factors affect growth. Between **4% and 25%** of fetuses with FGR will have an **abnormal karyotype** [42,43]. Trisomy 18 is particularly at risk for FGR as 35% of these fetuses will measure <10th percentile [44]. Other chromosomal anomalies, particularly trisomies, triploidy, translocations, and sex chromosome abnormalities, are also at high risk for FGR. Other than chromosomal aberrations, genetic disorders, such as uniparental disomy, and imprinting disorders are rare causes of FGR [41]. Many genetic disorders can lead to major structural malformations, and the findings of these on ultrasound will increase the risk of growth abnormalities to 22% [45]. **Fetal infection** has been associated with FGR, but data on the exact incidence of fetal infection in FGR are scant. Known infections that have been associated include cytomegalovirus, varicella, herpes simplex virus, malaria, human immunodeficiency virus, rubella, and syphilis [1]. Malaria is the most common cause of FGR worldwide.

Placental Factors

Placental risk factors for FGR include placental abruption, maternal floor infarct, placental mosaicism, velamentous cord insertion, and placenta accreta [1].

COMPLICATIONS

FGR is associated with morbidity and mortality to the fetus and infant (Table 45.2) [20,46–49]. FGR is the largest category associated with **stillbirth** accounting for up to 43% of stillbirths and has also been found in the majority of stillbirths considered "unexplained" [50]. Pregnancies complicated by SGA have a fivefold increased risk of stillbirth beyond 37 weeks. Furthermore, using cumulative risk analyses, there is a significant risk of stillbirth for each week of gestation >37 weeks [51]. Using delivery and birth weight data to estimate the risk of stillbirth overestimates the contribution of SGA as a fetus may be dead for several days. When SGA-associated stillbirth risk was studied on the basis of population, ultrasound, and individualized norms, population norms had the lowest adjusted OR (9.2; 95% CI 6.33–13.39) compared to ultrasound (10.79; 95% CI 8.11–14.35) and individualized groups (11.27; 95% CI 8.4–15.12) [52]. Perinatal death may be increased up to 100 times compared to normally grown babies. Additionally, **intrapartum asphyxia** has been reported to complicate 50% of pregnancies with FGR [53]. In addition to stillbirth, FGR increases the risk of **preterm birth, NEC, and RDS** [54,55]. Preterm infants with birth weight <3rd percentile carry the highest perinatal morbidity and mortality risk. When matched for gestational age at both term and preterm gestations, the smallest infants are at the highest risk for **low Apgar score, acidosis, intubation, seizures, and death in the first 28 days of life** [8].

The impact of FGR goes beyond the neonatal period. Children who were born with growth restriction have a higher risk of **cerebral palsy, short stature, and cognitive delay** [56]. In later life, adults who had FGR have a higher incidence of **hypertension, coronary artery disease, stroke, Type II diabetes mellitus, and obesity** [57]. Other than medical diseases, there is an increased risk of **low socioeconomic status, suicide, and financial distress in later life** [46]. Clearly, the implications of IUGR are grand, and rather than having complications limited to the peripartum period, the effects of IUGR may be lifelong.

The primary risk to the mother is **cesarean section** with a reported cesarean section rate of 43% if induction is performed in fetuses that have an EFW <5th percentile [58]. Rates as high as 90% were reported in the GRIT study [59]. Maternal **hypertensive disease** complicates up to 70% of early severe FGR (<32 weeks) with preeclampsia complicating 50% of all FGR cases [24].

The risk of recurrence for FGR in a subsequent pregnancy approaches 25%. This was recently evaluated in a large population-based study of pregnant women who delivered two sequential singleton pregnancies with a population incidence of FGR of 5% (FGR defined as birth weight of <5th percentile). If the first pregnancy was AGA, the recurrence risk was 3.4%. In contrast, a diagnosis of FGR in the first pregnancy carried a recurrence risk of 23% [16].

MANAGEMENT

Regarding the majority of recommendations for FGR management and delivery, it is important to recognize that these are based primarily on retrospective studies and expert opinion, rather than from level 1 data from RCTs.

Prevention

Gestational Age Determination

Because gestational age is the primary component dictating whether a fetus is measuring small, **accurate determination of an estimated date of confinement (EDC) is paramount. First-trimester ultrasound <13 weeks and 6 days** is the most precise method to determine the EDC. For precise estimation of gestational age by ultrasound, see Table 2 in Chapter 4 of *Obstetric Evidence Based Guidelines*.

Pregnancy Interval

A short interpregnancy interval has been associated with FGR. If conception occurs less than six months from a delivery, there is a 30% increase in FGR [60,61]. The **optimal timing to decrease rates of FGR is an interpregnancy interval of 18 to 23 months** [61].

Substance Cessation

Cessation of maternal substance abuse should be strongly encouraged. Women who quit smoking prior to 16 weeks will have the risk of FGR similar to women who never smoked at all [62]. **Smoking cessation interventions reduce LBW** (RR 0.83, 95% CI 0.73–0.95) and preterm birth (RR 0.86, 95% CI 0.74–0.98) [63]. Cessation of other substances in pregnancy or prior to conception also helps to reduce the risk of pathological FGR.

Nutrition

In low-risk women, significant dietary management does not prevent FGR. In this population, ineffective methods include individualized nutritional advice [64]; increased fish,

low-fat meats, grains, fruits, and vegetables [65]; low-salt diet [66]; iron supplementation [67]; and calcium supplementation [68]. Dietary supplements that may be beneficial include magnesium [69] and vitamin D [70]. Vitamin D levels have recently been reported to be low in patients with SGA in early onset severe preeclampsia, but supplement trials showing benefit are lacking [71]. In general, evidence is still limited for the use of dietary supplements to specifically reduce the risk of FGR, and they cannot be recommended for clinical use at this time.

In high-risk women with nutritional deficiencies, increasing caloric intake with low-protein supplementation reduces the risk of FGR by 32%. In the absence of nutritional deficiency, high-protein supplementation may lead to higher rates of FGR and should be avoided [72].

Control of Maternal Medical Disorders

Modification of maternal risk factors for FGR can be performed as a primary preventative factor. Hypertension has been associated with an increased risk of FGR, but **placing women on antihypertensive medication when the blood pressure is between 140–169/90–109 has not been shown to improve the rate of preeclampsia, FGR, preterm birth, or stillbirth** [73]. However, it does decrease the rates of severe hypertension. The recently published Control of Hypertension in Pregnancy Study (CHIPS trial) was a RCT trial to test if less-tight control (target diastolic blood pressure, 100 mmHg) or tight control (target diastolic blood pressure, 85 mmHg) of chronic hypertension in pregnancy demonstrated differences in maternal and fetal outcomes. No differences were seen between groups for birth weight <10th or <3rd percentiles or any other maternal or fetal outcomes although less-tight control was associated with a significantly higher frequency of severe maternal hypertension [74]. Current Task Force on Hypertension in Pregnancy (ACOG) recommendations are to continue with existing guidelines for management of women with mild-to-moderate hypertension (defined as systolic BP ≥140 mmHg but <160 mmHg or diastolic BP ≥90 mmHg but <110 mmHg), i.e., no need to lower BP further if SBP <160 and DBP <105; and this is endorsed by the Society of Maternal-Fetal Medicine [75]. For women with persistent chronic hypertension with systolic BP ≥160 mmHg or diastolic BP >105 mmHg, antihypertensive therapy is recommended. Controlling diabetes, autoimmune disorders, and other medical illnesses is important for both maternal and fetal health.

Aspirin

Aspirin therapy has been shown to be effective for reducing the risk of FGR in women determined to be at moderate-to-high risk for this disorder (e.g., those with hypertensive disorders or prior FGR). The benefit of aspirin seems to be largest in early gestational ages. Low-dose (e.g., 81–150 mg) aspirin is associated with a 56% decrease (RR 0.44, 95% CI 0.30–0.65) in FGR when initiated prior to 16 weeks, and it has no effect (RR 0.98, 95% CI 0.87–1.10) when initiated after this gestational age [76]. A dose of >75 mg is associated with the largest benefit [77]. Aspirin prophylaxis reduced the recurrence of FGR in subsequent pregnancies in mothers who have had a prior FGR pregnancy [76].

Screening for FGR

Serum Analytes

Abnormalities of trophoblastic invasion have also been suggested by many to be involved in abnormal fetal growth, and clues to aberrant placental cellular processes may be elucidated through investigating maternal serum screening for aneuploidy. First-trimester analytes have been shown to be associated with abnormal fetal growth and abnormal pregnancy outcomes as **low PAPP-A** levels significantly increase the risk of FGR [78,79]. If the PAPP-A level is below the fifth percentile, the sensitivity of detecting birth weight <10th percentile is only 10.4%, and the positive predictive value is only 18.7%. The negative predictive value is at 91.3% [79,80]. Second-trimester quadruple screen analytes associated with FGR include **AFP > 2.0 multiple of the medians (MoMs), uE3 < 0.5 MoMs, and an inhibin A > 2.0 MoMs** [81]. The risk of birth weight <10th percentile increases as the number of abnormal markers increases [82]. However, like PAPP-A, the sensitivity and positive predictive value of combining second-trimester markers to screen for FGR is low, questioning its clinical use as a screening test.

Fundal Height
Fundal height measurement is commonly used to screen for FGR, but data of effectiveness is mixed [83,84]. Maternal central adiposity and leiomyomata uteri are factors that affect the use of fundal height as a screening tool. A recent *Cochrane* systematic review concluded that there is insufficient evidence to determine if fundal height is effective in detecting FGR and that they could not recommend change in practice [85]. Fundal height measurement is an inexpensive and easy tool to use during prenatal visits (see also Chapter 2 of *Obstetric Evidence Based Guidelines*). When the risk of FGR is high, **ultrasound should be the primary modality used to screen for fetal growth abnormalities**.

Ultrasonographic Growth Curve
The identification of a population at risk for poor perinatal outcome depends largely upon the screening tool used. The tool most often used to determine if a fetus has FGR is the **ultrasonographic growth curve**. Standardized population growth curves can be created in a multitude of ways. Ideally, the optimal growth standard will be able to identify fetuses that are at the highest risk for adverse neonatal and fetal outcome. Data exist showing that race and regional differences affect mean birth weight [86–89]. In fact, individual regional differences in birth weight parallel the nadir of newborn mortality in those regions. In other words, one region in Europe will have a modal birth weight of 3446 g with the lowest perinatal mortality occurring at 3888 g. Another region will have a modal birth weight of 3622 g with a perinatal mortality nadir at 4305 g [90]. This suggests that an "ideal birth weight" exists, and this weight is dependent upon unique population characteristics. **Creating a growth standard that is population-specific will better identify fetuses that fall out of the range of "normal" for that population**.

A birth weight standard is created using cross-sectional data of newborn birth weight per gestational age strata. This has been criticized secondary to the known association between FGR and preterm gestations [91]. Fetal weight can be determined using mathematical modeling of measurable parameters, and this has been used to generate multiple in utero fetal weight standards [92–95]. Studies indicate that using birth weight data, rather than EFW data, to generate fetal growth standards will underestimate the amount of FGR fetuses and overestimate the number of large for gestational age (LGA) fetuses [96–98]. Additionally, fetal weight standards have been shown to better predict perinatal

outcomes of PTB, RDS, bronchopulmonary dysplasia, IVH, and retinopathy of prematurity [54,99]. However, a birth weight-derived growth curve is more predictive of neonatal mortality [99]. The difference in predictive ability for each standard probably lies in the fact that the fetuses identified as FGR by a birth weight standard are the smallest neonates using either schema, and these would be the ones at highest risk for demise and adverse perinatal outcome. However, a growth curve created from birth weight alone will miss a significant portion of infants at risk for poor outcome, and **evidence supports using a standardized growth curve generated from EFW by ultrasound**.

The creation of a **customized growth curve** using factors that are known to affect birth weight including **maternal height, weight in early pregnancy, parity, and ethnic group** has been proposed [5]. Using coefficients of variation, and a log polynomial equation, a growth curve is generated for each individual pregnancy, and deviation from this curve identifies fetuses with abnormal growth. In European populations, when comparing this growth standard to ones created using birth weight data, the customized growth model is better able to predict poor perinatal outcome including stillbirth, neonatal death, Apgar score of less than four at five minutes, cesarean section, admission to the neonatal intensive care unit, and neurologic morbidity [100–102]. However, in a U.S. population study, if the birth weight standard is customized to race, the birth weight standard is superior to the customized model in predicting poor perinatal outcome [103]. The mixed data in different populations suggest that **individual populations need more study to determine the optimal growth chart for predicting adverse outcomes**.

The effect of the use of these personal customized growth charts, with the diagnosis of FGR based on a change in an already established preexisting growth pattern, has not been assessed in any trial. Race/gender-specific nomograms of weight for gestational age make the diagnosis of FGR more accurate, but there are no trials to show change in outcome. The Royal College of Obstetricians and Gynecologists have adopted the customized standard to identify fetuses at risk for poor perinatal outcome [104]. However, **comparing an in utero standard to the customized growth model showed that they were similar in their ability to predict stillbirth and neonatal death**, and both were better at predicting these outcomes than a birth weight standard [105]. **There is no RCT to assess the benefits and harms of using population-based growth charts compared with customized growth charts as a screening tool for detection of fetal growth restriction in pregnant women** [106]. **Evidence supports the use of either the customized growth model or an in utero EFW standard by ultrasound** to identify fetuses at risk for poor perinatal outcome secondary to FGR.

Table 56.9 describes suggested ultrasound frequency for different conditions for monitoring for FGR and fetal condition in general.

In low risk women, ultrasound examinations at 28–32 weeks and at 36–37 weeks significantly increase the detection of FGR fetuses and decrease the likelihood of newborns with growth restriction although they do increase the rate of antenatal intervention [107,108]. Performing a growth ultrasound at 36 vs. 32 weeks is more sensitive (61% vs. 32%) in detecting severe FGR but not associated with significant differences in perinatal outcomes [109] (see Chapter 4 in *Obstetric Evidence Based Guidelines*).

Uterine Artery Doppler

Uterine artery Doppler interrogation has been used to stratify the risk of subsequent growth abnormalities in pregnancies at high and low risk for the development of FGR. Measurement of the uterine artery blood flow is determined through interrogation of uterine vessels bilaterally at the bifurcation from the internal iliac artery. There is a progressive decrease in uterine artery vascular impedance with advancing gestational age felt to be secondary to progressive trophoblast invasion and induction of uterine artery vascular remodeling (loss of muscularis layer) [110]. The presence of a protodiastolic notch or an elevated index of resistance (systolic/diastolic [S/D] ratio, pulsatility index [PI], or resistive index [RI]) has been used to predict the onset of FGR.

Abnormal first-trimester uterine artery Doppler waveforms have shown a correlation with aberrant growth. In the first trimester, notching is seen in the majority of all patients with 55% to 63% having bilateral notching and an additional 18% with unilateral notching [111–113]. Therefore, this characteristic pattern is not as helpful. When using an abnormal PI in the first trimester, the sensitivity for FGR is only 12% [111], and the sensitivity for severe FGR requiring delivery at <34 weeks is only 24% [111,112]. Despite its poor performance as a screening tool in the first trimester, using the information to initiate preventative measures may be beneficial. In women with abnormal uterine artery Doppler evaluation, giving low-dose aspirin prior to 16 weeks significantly reduced the incidence of FGR. Similar to data without using uterine artery Doppler, the benefit was not seen after this gestational age [76]. This is obviously not clinically effective if one already offers low-dose aspirin to women based on risk factors such as hypertension, prior preeclampsia, or prior FRG as discussed above.

Screening at a later gestational age improves the test characteristics. When comparing first- and second-trimester results, uterine artery Doppler notching or elevated PI was more predictive of FGR in the second trimester [114]. Timing in the second trimester is also important as investigators have shown that the test characteristics are better at 22 weeks than at 18 weeks [115]. When the uterine artery Doppler PI is >1.55 between 22 and 24 weeks, 47% of these pregnancies will develop preeclampsia, FGR, or fetal death [116]. When using Doppler as a screening tool in a population with abnormal serum analytes (AFP >3.5 MoMs, or HCG >5.3 MoMs), the sensitivity increases to 94% with a positive predictive value of 67% [117]. However, it is rare for patients to have these abnormal AFP or HCG values, and the use of combining serum markers and uterine artery Doppler has been less predictive in other studies [118,119]. There certainly is a relationship between abnormal uterine artery Doppler blood flow and FGR. **The test performs best at gestational ages between 22 and 24 weeks in populations determined to be at high risk for preeclampsia and FGR.** However, **the sensitivity, negative predictive value, and positive predictive value for predicting FGR may be too low to be clinically useful** and presently is **not recommended for routine screening** in the clinical setting [120].

Additionally, **no therapeutic measure has been shown to be useful at this gestational age.** An argument can be made to initiate low-dose aspirin therapy prior to 16 weeks in all women at high risk for the development of preeclampsia and FGR. Use of uterine artery Doppler to determine the optimal management of surveillance of growth has yet to be determined.

UA Doppler

UA Doppler is predictive of FGR in the second trimester, and abnormal values in a high-risk population will increase the development of FGR later in pregnancy [6]. Nonetheless, UA Doppler cannot be used for screening for FGR due to its poor sensitivity and positive predictive value as well as lack of standardization for gestational age at screening, technique and abnormal screening criteria [120].

Diagnosis

When using ultrasound as a screening tool, **the diagnosis of FGR is made when the EFW is <10% for gestational age** (see section titled "Definitions/Diagnoses").

Workup

For all fetuses presenting as FGR, **the first step is to confirm the gestational age and ensure that the fetus is truly measuring small.** As knowing the appropriate gestational age is key in making the diagnosis, it is particularly difficult when a patient presents for her first ultrasound later in pregnancy and is found to have a fetus measuring small for the proposed gestational age. In these instances, the cerebellar diameter can be used to assist in stratifying risk. In both FGR and LGA fetuses, the cerebellar diameter is largely conserved, and this can help identify a fetus that is measuring small when gestational age is uncertain [121]. For biometry, particular attention should be paid to the AC and to the HC/AC ratio. Asymmetric growth with a lagging AC (<5th percentile) should increase the suspicion for early growth abnormalities as this is often the first clue to pathological growth inhibition [122].

Identification of risk factors, especially modifiable risk factors, can be obtained by review of the medical history (Table 45.1). Maternal blood pressure can be obtained and, if abnormal, exclusion of preeclampsia is warranted. Any substance abuse should be discussed, and cessation of these substances should be encouraged. The identification of maternal diseases that increase the risk for FGR is helpful because optimal management of those disorders may improve growth in the fetus for the remainder of the pregnancy.

Detailed ultrasound evaluation should be performed by a center skilled in such assessments with special attention paid to identify fetal anomalies. Additionally, evaluation of the fetus for evidence of chromosomal abnormalities and intrauterine infection should be performed. The placenta, placental umbilical cord insertion, amniotic fluid, and biometry should be scrutinized. **UA Doppler evaluation should be performed.** Depending on these results, Doppler assessment of other vessels including the MCA, ductus venosus (DV), and umbilical vein may be considered, but there is not enough information to justify routine use of these Doppler studies. A fetal echocardiogram should be considered if inadequate heart views (four chamber and outflow tracts) are obtained [123].

Amniocentesis should be offered to rule out aneuploidy (karyotype) and infection (PCR for CMV, toxoplasmosis, and HSV), especially if no other causes are identifiable and the **FGR is severe (e.g., EFW <5%), diagnosed at early gestational age such as <24 weeks**, and/or **associated with fetal anomalies or hydramnios**. If the placental image on ultrasound is abnormal, placental biopsy (late CVS) may be considered to evaluate for placental mosaicism, which is present in up to 15% of placentas in cases of FGR [124].

An **infectious workup** including maternal serum IgG and IgM for CMV, toxoplasmosis, and HSV may be offered. Rubella immunity should be ascertained by checking IgG from earlier prenatal care or new testing if this is unavailable. If amniotic fluid is available, PCR for CMV, toxoplasmosis, and HSV can be performed. History should dictate any other further infectious workup for agents associated with FGR.

There is insufficient evidence to recommend an inherited thrombophilia workup because an association between inherited thrombophilia is not proven in the better studies, and there is no intervention proven to be beneficial [28,29] (see "Maternal Factors" above and see Chapter 27). Antiphospholipid antibodies (anticardiolipin IgG and IgM, lupus anticoagulant, and beta-2 microprotein IgM and IgG) may be checked, especially for counseling regarding etiology and a future pregnancy.

Counseling

When first sharing the diagnosis of FGR with a family, it is useful to begin with the fact that **the majority of fetuses less than the 10th percentile are going to be small but normal (constitutionally small) and not at significant risk for adverse outcomes** [3,4]. This provides some comfort following the initial patient anxiety that develops after they have been told that their fetus is growth-restricted. The clinician should discuss prognosis, complications, options regarding pregnancy termination, thresholds for delivery, timing of administration of antenatal corticosteroids, and the planned frequency and type of antenatal surveillance. Recommendations resulting from these discussions should be documented in the patient's chart [123]. Prognosis depends largely upon the underlying etiology. **Aneuploidy, fetal malformations, and intrauterine infection are associated with a worse prognosis.** In instances in which these factors are absent, gestational age at delivery, amniotic fluid volume, absent/reversed end-diastolic flow of the UA, and birth weight are independent predictors of adverse neonatal outcome [47]. More specifically, **gestational age is one of the best predictors of outcome**, and prior to 29 weeks and 2 days, it is the leading predictor of intact survival. Beyond this age, birth weight above 600 g, DV Doppler, and cord artery pH were the strongest predictors of intact survival and neonatal mortality in one study [125].

Complications of FGR include PTB, and in the newborn that was born small, the risk of the diseases of prematurity are higher than in age-matched controls [126]. Additionally, birth weight has been linked to fetal and newborn mortality and multiple neonatal morbidities [8]. Counseling should include a detailed discussion regarding weighing the **risks of prematurity secondary to an iatrogenic delivery against the risks of stillbirth while remaining in utero.** Multiple tools are available to help distinguish when the risk of remaining in utero is higher than the risk of delivery or vice versa, and these are discussed below.

Interventions for FGR Pregnancies

Avoidance of Toxins
Discontinuation of toxins known to be associated with FGR should be stressed. When the toxins are the result of substance abuse, such as in smoking, strong counseling should be performed to **encourage cessation of the substance** associated with FGR (Table 45.1). Very rarely, if the toxin is a pharmacotherapy,

weighing the potential risks of cessation of the medication with continued exposure to the fetus should be performed. Discussion of alternative therapies should be considered. However, once the fetus is identified as FGR, data is lacking on whether cessation of the offending agent will improve growth during the remainder of pregnancy, but biological plausibility exists, and cessation should still be encouraged.

Therapy for Medical Conditions
Proper treatment of chronic hypertension, preeclampsia, diabetes, or other medical condition is important, but there are no trials to prove a beneficial effect on FGR.

Bed Rest
Bed rest has long been used by obstetricians as a tool for improving pregnancy outcome even though data is lacking to support its use. The only RCT showed **no difference** in birth weight (RR 0.43, 95% CI 0.15–1.27) or neonatal outcomes when bed rest was compared to ambulation in patients with FGR [127]. In a recent summary of *Cochrane* reviews of bed rest in which six RCTs were identified, there was no support found for "therapeutic" bed rest for threatened abortion, hypertension, preeclampsia, preterm birth, multiple gestations, or impaired fetal growth [128]. Therefore, there is insufficient evidence to support the use of bed rest to treat patients with FGR. Hospitalization for bed rest is **possibly dangerous** (e.g., associated with venous thromboembolism), expensive, and inconvenient for the pregnant woman.

Nutrient Therapy
Improving nutrient delivery to the fetus by increasing maternal intake of these nutrients has been widely studied. Some nutrient supplementation may be beneficial in preventing FGR, and others are not. Docosahexenoic acid has been shown in a large RCT to result in larger birth weights if patients continue with the supplementation in pregnancy [129]. Maternal micronutrient therapy with the UNICEF/WHO/UNO international multiple micronutrient preparation has been shown to increase birth weight in regions where nutritional supplementation is rare [130]. Long-chain polyunsaturated fatty acid supplementation has not been shown to improve birth weight [131]. Although supplementation may improve birth weight prior to the development of FGR, **once there is FGR, there is insufficient evidence that supplementing the mother** with amino acids, minerals, vitamins, glucose, or energy supplements improves birth weight [132].

Betamimetics
The theoretical basis for using betamimetic therapy for impaired fetal growth is promoting fetal growth by increasing the availability of nutrients and by decreasing vascular resistance. In fetuses diagnosed with FGR, the administration of betamimetics is not associated with improvement in birth weight or neonatal morbidity and mortality [133]. Betamimetics are associated with several complications and therefore **should not be used for this indication**.

Calcium Channel Blockers
There is currently **insufficient evidence** to promote the use of calcium channel blockers for FGR. Calcium channel blockers may theoretically increase uteroplacental perfusion and, therefore, improve nutrient and oxygen delivery to a fetus that is at risk or currently growth-restricted. Only one study has been published which 100 smoking women were randomized

to either flunarizine or placebo. The treatment group had a higher mean birth weight, but no other significant differences were seen [134].

Aspirin

In high-risk populations, such as in women with a first-trimester uterine artery Doppler PI that is abnormal, low-dose aspirin has been shown to decrease the incidence of FGR when initiated prior to 16 weeks [76,77]. After this gestational age, and once FGR is established, aspirin has no proven benefit.

Heparin

There is insufficient evidence to assess the effect of heparin therapy in FGR pregnancies. In an RCT with heterogenous inclusion criteria for FGR including fundal height <10%, heparin was associated with better growth and almost a week-later gestational age at delivery compared to a Chinese root called Dan-shen [135].

Oxygen

There is **insufficient evidence** to evaluate the benefits and risks of maternal oxygen therapy for suspected impaired fetal growth. A *Cochrane* analysis showed that oxygen administration to pregnancies with suspected FGR **decreased the rates of perinatal mortality (33% vs. 65%; a 50% reduction) compared to no oxygenation** [136]. In all studies, birth weights were higher in the oxygen group, despite similar (average range: 10–20 days) intervals to delivery. No significant side effects or adverse outcomes have been reported. Higher gestational age in the oxygenation groups may have accounted for the difference in mortality rates. Also, two of the studies did not use placebos, there was no blinding, and the small number of patients does not allow a thorough assessment of effect [136].

Plasma Volume Expansion

There is **insufficient evidence** to assess the effect of increase in maternal fluid intake (either IV or orally) on FGR. In pregnancies complicated by FGR, maternal volume expansion is lower than in pregnancies with normally grown fetuses [137]. Expanding maternal plasma volume once FGR has been identified was evaluated in only one very small trial in patients with AEDF of the UA. Compared to no volume expansion, volume expansion in women with FGR fetuses with AEDF of UA was associated with a decrease (2/7 vs. 6/7) in perinatal mortality. There was no difference in the gestational age at delivery and mean birth weight [138].

Abdominal Decompression

There is **insufficient evidence** to assess the effect of this intervention as all trials are old, and they contain serious bias. Abdominal decompression consists of a rigid dome placed about the abdomen and covered with an airtight suit with the space around the abdomen decompressed to −50 to −100 mmHg for 15 to 30 seconds out of each minute for 30 minutes once to thrice daily or with uterine contractions during labor. This is thought to "pump" blood through the intervillous space. Therapeutic abdominal decompression is associated with reductions in persistent preeclampsia, "fetal distress" in labor, low birth weight, Apgar scores less than six at one minute, and perinatal mortality (7% vs. 40%) [139].

Nitric Oxide Donors

There is **insufficient evidence** to recommend the use of nitric oxide donors to fetuses with FGR. L-Arginine is a precursor to nitric oxide and may play a role in placental blood flow. In one randomized study evaluating pregnancies with FGR, administration of this compound did not increase mean birth weight or duration of pregnancy [140]. Alternatively, two other nonrandomized studies showed improvement in fetal growth when L-arginine was given, either orally or intravenously, to pregnancies with suspected FGR [141,142].

ANTEPARTUM TESTING

See also Chapter 56, "Antepartum testing."

Ultrasound

Intervals of Growth Assessment

Repeated in utero growth assessments through ultrasound have been used to monitor pregnancies complicated by FGR. Most growth curves are derived from cross-sectional data on large populations, and this gives the appearance of a continuous, smooth pattern of fetal growth. In truth, fetuses do not demonstrate growth in this fashion. Data on child growth through 22 months of age shows that infants will have long periods of stasis punctuated by short bursts of growth [143]. Fetuses show a similar saltatory pattern of growth in which EFW and anthropometric measures will show no demonstrable change over multiple intervals of assessment. In fact, when assessing growth every two to three days in normal fetuses, measures of femur length, AC, and biparietal diameter will show no growth for periods greater than two weeks, and all measures will have some growth by four weeks [144]. **Absence of growth in two weeks is therefore a normal phenomenon.** Additionally, mathematical modeling has shown that due to the error inherent to ultrasound, the false positive rate of diagnosing FGR when assessing a fetus at two-week intervals is significantly higher than at three-week intervals. The error rate is also gestational age-dependent. As gestational age advances, when assessing every 2 weeks, the false positive rate increases from 12% at 28 weeks to 24% at 38 weeks [145]. The optimal timing for repeat assessment of fetal growth has yet to be determined, but based on available data, **repeat assessment should be performed no earlier than every three weeks and only rarely every two weeks.** Table 56.9 describes suggested ultrasound frequency for measuring biometry in pregnancies with FGR.

Doppler Velocimetry

Ultrasound evaluation of fetal blood vessels using pulsed-wave (PW) Doppler velocimetry is the cornerstone of management and follow-up of FGR. PW Doppler velocimetry of any given larger conduit vessel provides information about the downstream vascular bed impedance to blood flow. **In FGR, the UA is the most commonly interrogated fetal vessel.** The flow velocity waveform in the umbilical artery demonstrates a progressive increase in diastolic flow across gestation, and after 15–16 weeks, forward diastolic flow should always be present. Nomograms of umbilical artery indices of resistance have been published and are available online at no cost (http://perinatology.com/calculators/umbilical artery.htm). The middle cerebral artery (MCA) vessel is the next most commonly interrogated vessel, reflecting changes in the cerebral vascular bed. A third vessel becoming more commonly interrogated over the past decade is the ductus venosus (DV). The inferior and superior vena cava (IVC, SVC) and hepatic veins (right, middle, and left) constitute the central venous structures in the fetus. These vascular structures are characterized by a triphasic Doppler waveform (systolic, diastolic, and atrial kick) that reflects changes in the central venous pressures as they relate to function of the right side of the fetal heart as well as fetal breathing. Doppler waveforms in these three vessels (UA, MCA, and DV) and the clinical implications are discussed further below.

UA Doppler Velocimetry. The UA Doppler flow patterns are predictive of fetal outcome. A decrease in UA end-diastolic velocity with elevated resistance indices but with forward end-diastolic flow (EDF) is associated with abnormalities in 30% of fetal vessels [146]. If the disease process continues with an increase in placental vascular resistance, this may first lead to absent (AEDF) and then to reversed end-diastolic flow (REDF) [147]. By the time fetuses reach AEDF/REDF, 60%–70% of villous vessels are abnormal, and 50% or more of fetuses will be hypoxemic [148,149]. Fetuses with absent or reversed end-diastolic flow (AREDF) of the UA have higher incidences of preterm delivery, stillbirth, neonatal mortality, low arterial pH, bronchopulmonary dysplasia, NEC, and severe neurologic morbidity [150–153]. Thus, UA Doppler surveillance of the FGR fetus will help to identify the fetus that has FGR and is at risk rather than one that is constitutionally small. In women with normal Doppler studies and AF volume, twice weekly nonstress tests (NSTs) are associated with higher incidence of labor induction at an earlier gestational age with no difference in infant morbidity or composite perinatal outcome compared to UA Doppler fortnightly in a small RCT [154]. **UA Doppler assessment of pregnancies at high risk for placental insufficiency (such as those with FGR) reduces the incidence of perinatal death** (1.2% vs. 1.7%, a 29% decrease), **induction of labor** (11% decrease), **and cesarean delivery** (10% decrease) compared to no Doppler or other mode of testing (e.g., CTG and/or biophysical profile, BPS) [155].

Limitations of UA Doppler: Although there is level 1 evidence for use of UA in FGR management, none of the studies provide specific guidance on the optimal frequency of UA interrogation (e.g., weekly, twice weekly, every two weeks) or a specified intervention protocol and there is no guidance on the type or frequency of concomitant biophysical testing (e.g., NST, BPS).

MCA Doppler Velocimetry. During instances of placental dysfunction that leads to fetal hypoxia, blood flow resistance in the fetal brain decreases, a phenomenon called "brain-sparing." **MCA** Doppler evaluation has been used as an adjunct to UA blood flow assessment, in which fetuses that show evidence of decreased resistance to flow in the brain are at higher risk of poor perinatal outcome. In fact, prior to 34 weeks, the prediction of poor perinatal outcome is improved over UA Doppler assessment alone when the MCA PI is decreased [156,157]. This helps to further identify fetuses at risk and separate them from fetuses that are constitutionally small. The **cerebroplacental ratio (CPR), calculated as CPR = MCA PI/UA PI,** has an improved adverse outcome predictive capacity compared to MCA Doppler alone [158,159].

One limitation of the UA Doppler assessment is that after 34 weeks, the UA in FGR may not become abnormal and the only fetal vessel that may show a Doppler waveform abnormality is the MCA. Several studies have now shown that late preterm/early term FGR fetuses with a normal UA waveform but an abnormal MCA waveform demonstrate higher rates of neurodevelopmental compromise, later behavioral problems, and a higher rate of nonreassuring EFM patterns leading more frequently to cesarean delivery (58% vs. 24%) [160–162].

Limitations of MCA Doppler: Although use of the MCA can change counseling in FGR pregnancies in terms of risk of adverse outcomes, unlike the UA Doppler, **there is insufficient evidence (no RCT) to recommend routine use of MCA for management** (e.g., timing of delivery) of FGR due to a lack of data showing improvement in outcomes.

Venous Doppler (DV) Velocimetry and Sequential Changes. Doppler assessment of the **fetal venous system** can also help to identify fetuses at risk for poor perinatal outcome. In FGR, when the NST is nonreactive, absent a-wave flow in the DV has better predictive ability for acidemia and significant neonatal morbidity than a contraction stress test [163]. Interest in the venous system expanded with demonstration that venous back flow during the atrial contraction in precordial venous structure (e.g., ductus venosus and IVC) is reflective of fetal metabolic acidemia [164,165]. In the presence of A/REDF of the UA, pulsations of the umbilical vein or absent/reversed flow of the a-wave of the DV increase the risk of acidemia, IVH, neonatal death, stillbirth, and neonatal death [166–169].

Subsequent studies were published to address the relationship between various longitudinal Doppler changes in multiple vessels (e.g., elevated UA PI, UA AEDF, UA REDF, elevated MCA PI, elevated DV, DV A/R a-wave, cardiac outflows) and biophysical testing (NST and BPS) in severe and early FGR fetuses (delivered <32 weeks) in order to better understand the progressive nature of the FGR pathologic process [170–172]. Collectively, these studies demonstrated two specific findings: 1) Doppler waveforms in the different vessels tended to become abnormal in sequential fashion with UA and MCA Doppler abnormalities consistently preceding DV changes, and 2) Abnormal venous Doppler changes (especially the DV) occurred in up to 70% of FGR 7 days to 24 hours prior to biophysical profile or FHR tracing abnormalities. Furthermore, there is a striking relationship between the ductus venosus and short-term variability [172]. **As the DV systolic-to-atrial ratio became abnormal, so did the STV in a nearly mirror image fashion (inverse relationship).** This may represent perhaps the first clear link between an abnormal Doppler vessel and the fetal heart rate parameter of short-term variability (balance between the parasympathetic and sympathetic autonomic nervous system) in the fetus and contributed to the impetus to conduct a RCT in Europe (TRUFFLE trial; see below). The more recently published PORTO study showed evidence that **there is no particular dominant pattern of sequential changes in the FGR fetus,** including no evidence that the DV becomes abnormal just prior to an abnormal CTG [173]. The PORTO study was a large, seven-center, observational study in which data was prospectively collected, a major strength. However, a limitation of this study, as cited the authors, is that the majority of their FGR fetuses were enrolled late (30 weeks) and delivered in the early term period on average (37 weeks). Thus, this cohort may behave differently in terms of Doppler patterns than the severe, early FGR fetuses described in the above studies.

The Trial of Umbilical Fetal Flow in Europe (**TRUFFLE study**) is the only RCT so far to **assess the effect of using venous Doppler for clinical management in FGR** [24]. Severe and early FGR pregnancies enrolled at <32 weeks were randomized to one of three groups for timing of delivery: 1) Reduced cardiotocographic FHR STV (CTG STV), 2) Early DV changes (DV PI >95th percentile but with forward atrial-wave flow), and 3) Late DV changes (a-wave at [absent] or below [reversed] baseline). The primary end point of the study was survival without cerebral palsy or neurosensory impairment or a Bayley III developmental score <85 at 2 years of age. The mean gestational age at delivery of 30.7 weeks and the mean birth weight of 1019 g with an overall survival of nearly 70% in each group confirms the early and severe nature of the FGR in the study subjects. **There was no difference among the three groups overall for survival without neuroimpairment.** However, when addressing the individual components of neurological outcomes among survivors, those infants randomized to the late DV changes group demonstrated improved Bayley III scores at 2 years of age (5% neuroimpairment) compared to the CTG STV group (15% neuroimpairment). There was no difference between the early and late DV groups [24].

Limitations of Venous and DV Doppler Velocimetry. There were several limitations of the TRUFFLE study including the following: 1) The survival and outcomes were much better than anticipated and, thus, the sample size for detecting differences may have been underestimated. 2) Monitoring frequency among centers varied. The frequency of monitoring (UA Doppler and CTG) was set at a minimum of once per week but left to local protocols. 3) Delivery criteria after 32 weeks varied among centers. After 32 weeks, delivery was based on local policy and could be based on CTG STV, elevated PI, or A/REDF in UA or DV changes. Perhaps the group delivered <32 weeks should have been assessed separately rather than including outcomes of those delivering after 32 weeks. 4) All study groups had UA Doppler performed; however, it was specifically stated that the CTG STV group did not have DV Doppler performed. This is a major limitation because it results in a blending of study groups rather than a true comparison of different delivery criteria. For example, an abnormality in the DV has been shown to occur in 50%–70% of cases prior to an abnormal CTG or BPS and these should have been eliminated from the TRUFFLE CTG STV group in order to allow for a true comparison of CTG versus DV. 5) Finally, there is limitation of generalizability of this study to the U.S. population in which computerized CTG and assessment of STV is not nearly universally performed.

In summary, **UA Doppler assessment is beneficial in managing pregnancies that have FGR** [155]. Most data suggest that **once FGR is diagnosed, weekly UA Doppler surveillance should be performed.** However, the exact UA Doppler flow pattern that should initiate timing of delivery has yet to be fully elucidated in the literature (Figure 45.1). MCA Doppler can be used as an adjunct to identify fetuses at risk for poor outcome, but the optimal timing of delivery when the MCA PI is abnormal has yet to be determined. Using venous Doppler abnormalities (specifically absent or reversed a-wave flow) in pregnancies with early and severe FGR as an indicator for delivery reduces neuroimpairment at 2 years of age. However, given the above limitations of the TRUFFLE study, applying the DV to determine the timing of delivery across the broad range of 24–32 weeks requires further research. It is reasonable to apply DV Doppler for timing of delivery beyond 29 weeks as combined European and U.S. data show that the most important predictor for intact survival prior to 29 weeks is gestational age [174].

Fetal Kick Counts

Although there are **no RCTs to assess the efficacy of fetal kick counts specifically in FGR pregnancies**, they are still commonly recommended in guidelines (e.g., RCOG, ACOG). Although several methods have been described for maternal assessment of fetal activity, a simple technique is for the mother to lay on her side and record any distinct fetal movements once or twice daily. Although most fetuses will achieve this degree of movement within the first 5–10 minutes, failure to achieve 10 movements within a two-hour period warrants further evaluation of the fetus with nonstress testing (see also Chapter 56).

NST/Cardiotocography

Monitoring of the fetal heart rate is commonly referred to as NST or as cardiotocography (CTG). CTG has not been well evaluated with high-quality studies in FGR. When comparing CTG with no CTG, there is no difference in the prediction of perinatal mortality, preventable deaths, or cesarean sections [175]. There is limited evidence from randomized controlled trials to inform best practice for fetal surveillance regimens and even their frequency when caring for women with pregnancies affected by FGR [176]. Computerized CTG may improve perinatal mortality when compared to traditional CTG [175]. However, this analysis was not limited to FGR fetuses, and the benefit of antenatal CTG has yet to be fully investigated in this population. In many management schemas, CTG has been cited as a standard monitoring tool, despite the lack of rigorous studies proving its efficacy [1]. Nonreactive and abnormal CTG has been associated with acidosis and hypoxemia [177,178], and this justifies its use as a screening tool for fetal well being.

Biophysical Profile Score

Evidence from RCTs does not support the use of BPS as a test of fetal well being in high-risk pregnancies [179]. In high-risk pregnancies (including FGR, post-term pregnancies, hypertensive disorders, or other conditions), when comparing a BPS to other tests of fetal well being, there is no difference in perinatal deaths or low Apgar scores [179]. Although the overall incidence of adverse outcomes was low, there are no significant differences between the groups in perinatal deaths (RR 1.33, 95% CI 0.60–2.98) or in Apgar score <7 at five minutes (RR 1.27, 95% CI 0.85–1.92). Combined data from the two high-quality RCTs suggest an increased risk of cesarean section in the BPS group (RR 1.60, 95% CI 1.05 to 2.44) [179]. The impact of the BPS on other interventions, length of hospitalization, serious short-term and long-term neonatal morbidity, and parental satisfaction requires further evaluation. In FGR alone, **RCTs are lacking to prove the value of the BPS**, but it is still mentioned as a surveillance tool in these pregnancies [1]. This is justified in that fetal death within one week of a normal score on BPS testing is rare, estimated at about <0.1% in one study [180]. Furthermore, in severe and early FGR, STV, accelerations (reactive NSTs) are delayed and additional testing with the BPS that does not rely on external fetal monitoring may be useful.

Amniotic Fluid Volume

Assessment of amniotic fluid (AF) volume is an essential component of antepartum testing with either the NST or the BPS (see Chapter 56). AF is an indirect measure of fetal

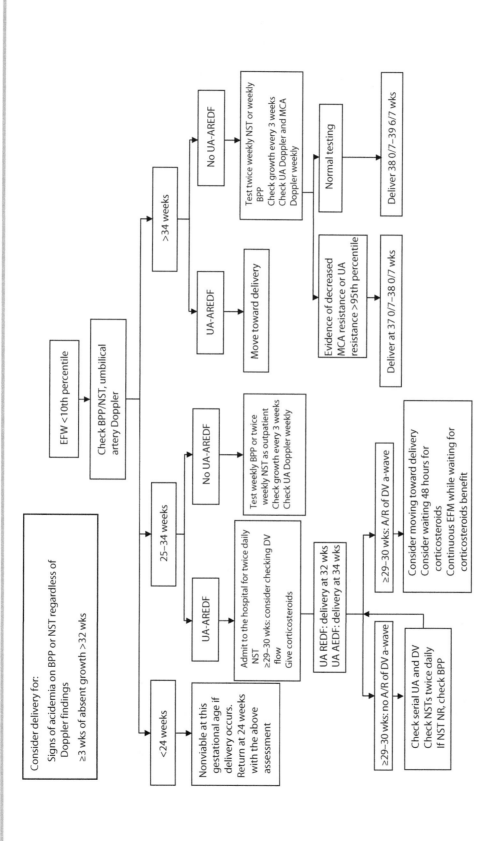

Figure 45.1 Algorithm of the management of FGR based on gestational age and surveillance. Normal Testing is defined as normal UA Doppler studies and reactive NST or BPP of 6/8 or 8/10 or higher. Signs consistent with fetal acidemia on the NST are defined as persistent absent variability and/or repetitive FHR decelerations (category III FHR tracing), or a persistent biophysical profile of <6. *Abbreviations*: AEDF, absent end-diastolic flow; A/R, absent or reversed; AREDF, absent or reversed end-diastolic flow; BPP, biophysical profile; DV, ductus venosus; EFW, estimated fetal weight; MCA, middle cerebral artery; NST, non-stress test; REDF, reversed end-diastolic flow; UA, umbilical artery.

vascular status and reflects the degree of fetal renal perfusion. Although low AF (anhydramnios or oligohydramnios) itself is a poor screening tool for FGR, it may be the first sign detected in a growth-restricted fetus. Up to 96% of fetuses with an AF MVP less than 1 cm in depth may be FGR [181]. The reduction in AF results from the progressive redistribution of blood flow toward the fetal heart, brain, and adrenal glands and away from lungs, digestive tract, kidneys, and torso. This has been well described in lambs with induced hypoxia and also in FGR in humans [182–184]. Further, the relationship of oligohydramnios and progressive worsening of both arterial and venous Doppler velocimetry findings has been previously described in the human FGR fetus [171].

Estriol Levels
Compared to concealed levels, knowledge of plasma estriol levels does not affect perinatal mortality (3% in each group) in women with FGR, hypertension, or adverse obstetric history [185].

Interval of Fetal Testing
Testing should start usually on the diagnosis of FGR. On the basis of the evidence above, **UA Doppler evaluation is recommended, usually initially on a weekly basis** with the option of increased Doppler frequency in the presence of abnormal UA Doppler flow.

   The other testing modalities and their testing interval are not supported by level 1 evidence. Some experts suggest monitoring with **NSTs twice a week with once weekly amniotic fluid assessment**, or BPSs weekly in pregnancies with FGR and normal UA Doppler. In the presence of abnormal UA Doppler, more frequent testing with NST/AFV and/or BPS can be considered. The NST will not show reactivity usually before 32 weeks, so a category III tracing may be used as criteria for delivery. The data on BPS screening are mostly from term pregnancies with very little data on the effectiveness of BPS monitoring on very preterm (e.g., <28 weeks) FGR.

DELIVERY
Preparation: Steroids and Magnesium Sulfate
When fetal testing in the FGR fetus suggests need for delivery at 24 to 34 weeks, several strategies should be considered. **If delivery is anticipated within seven days, steroids for fetal maturity should be administered to the mother.** Either betamethasone or dexamethasone can be used. Betamethasone 12 mg IM q24h × 2 doses (one course) is associated with decrease in RDS, IVH, NEC, and perinatal mortality [186]. A single "rescue" course can be considered >14 days from the first course if pregnancy is still <32 weeks [187,188]. Steroids can temporarily affect NST, BPS, and Doppler testing (see also Chapter 17 in *Obstetric Evidence Based Guidelines*). The evidence for safety and effectiveness of steroids specifically in FGR pregnancies is limited [189]. One recent, relatively small, retrospective study comparing steroids to no steroids in severe and early FGR pregnancies (delivered <32 weeks gestation) failed to show any immediate neonatal benefit of steroids (except for improved cord pH and 5-minute Apgar score) or long-term infant benefit (no improvement in Griffith's score at 2 years of age) [190]. Thus, further investigation of steroid benefit in FGR is needed in this early severe FGR group. However, in contrast to this study, an older and larger (n = 19,759 VLBW

cases) study from the Vermont Oxford Database of FGR fetuses between 501 and 1500 g, antenatal steroids were associated with significant reductions in RDS, IVH, and severe IVH but not in necrotizing enterocolitis [191].

   Although no study has addressed the benefit of **magnesium sulfate** and neuroprotection in FGR pregnancies alone, this medication should be administered for neuroprotection based on published protocols [192–194]. Lastly, **delivery should be accomplished at a facility that has neonatal intensive care unit capabilities** [1].

Timing
The timing of delivery of the FGR fetus should be **based mostly on gestational age** and **all antepartum testing factors** and in general not just one test. A possible management algorithm is shown in Figure 45.1. Given the current state of the literature and absence of strong data that specifically delineates the optimal timing of delivery, this proposed strategy for managing pregnancies complicated by FGR is largely based on Level II evidence and expert opinion and subject to change as new evidence accumulates. Retrospectively, the largest predictors of perinatal outcome are gestational age at delivery, birth weight, AREDF of the UA, abnormal DV blood flow, nonreassuring CTG or BPS, and placental villitis [195,196].

   Delivery timing is optimally determined by RCTs testing different strategies. To date, there have been two RCTs of timing delivery in the early FGR pregnancy (GRIT and TRUFFLE studies) and one RCT in the late preterm/early term FGR pregnancy (DIGITAT study).

   Growth Restriction Trial (GRIT study): In the GRIT study, 548 patients with FGR (>90% singletons, >70% with abnormal UA Doppler) at 24 to 36 weeks were randomized to delivery after 48 hours of steroid administration versus expectant management [59,196]. In the group randomized to expectant management, delivery criteria and surveillance strategies were not based on a protocol or described in detail. Patients moved toward delivery when the clinicians managing the pregnancy felt that pregnancy prolongation was no longer safe.

   Immediate delivery after 48 hours of steroids **was associated with similar incidence of perinatal death** (10%) **compared to delayed delivery** (9%) (delay in delivery was an average of only four days later). Incidence of fetal (0.7% vs. 3.1%) and neonatal (7.7% vs. 4.1%) deaths as well as death and disability at two years of age (19% vs. 16%) were similar in the two groups (59,196). Trends for ventilation >24 hours, IVH and NEC tended to favor delayed delivery. **Disability in babies younger than 31 weeks was higher in those delivered immediately** (13%) compared to those in the delayed group (5%) [196]. **At age 6 to 13 years, there was not a clinically significant difference between groups in standardized school-based evaluations of cognition, language, motor performance, and behavior** [197].

   Limitations of the GRIT Study: This trial has been criticized for several reasons, including the following: 1) There was no clearly defined surveillance strategy or explicit delivery indications described in the expectantly managed group; 2) the expectant management group only gained an average of four days, which may explain the lack in differences shown; and 3) the immediate delivery group average time to delivery was 0.9 days (range of 0.4–1.3 days), and thus fetuses did not likely benefit from steroid administration. However, the trial suggests that **early delivery does not necessarily prevent neurodevelopmental damage from fetal metabolic deterioration inherent to FGR**. Also, as no specific protocol based on fetal testing (either Doppler, CTG, or other) was followed, specific recommendations cannot be made from this important RCT except that delivering early for hypothetical avoidance of fetal hypoxia might not improve outcome with the authors recommending that the **"obstetrician should delay."**

TRUFFLE Study: The TRUFFLE study details, findings, and limitations are described in detail above. This study provides some evidence in support of delivery of the FGR fetus prior to 32 weeks based on either an absent or reversed a-wave in the DV. More specifically, there may be a reduction in neurodevelopmental delay at 2 years of age compared to delivery based on CTG alone.

DIGITAT study: The DIGITAT study is a multicenter RCT of induction of labor (IOL) versus expectant management (EM) of FGR fetuses (defined as an EFW <10th percentile) greater than 36 weeks gestation with the primary outcome being a composite adverse neonatal outcome. IOL infants delivered 10 days earlier and weighed 130 g less [198]. There were no differences in the composite neonatal outcomes between the IOL and EM groups (5.3% vs. 6.1%; 95%CI −4.3 to 3.2). Although there were no differences for any maternal outcomes between the two groups, including no difference in cesarean delivery, there was a significantly higher rate of preeclampsia in the expectant management group with a rate of 3.7% in the IOL and 7.9% in the EM group (difference in percentage −4.2 with 95%CI of −7.7 to 0.6). A two-year follow-up study did not reveal any differences in neurodevelopmental outcomes [199].

Limitations of the DIGITAT trial. There were several limitations of the DIGITAT study. Although UA Doppler studies were performed and rates of abnormal UA Doppler in each group reported, the outcome data were not analyzed (or at least reported) in the subgroup of patients with an abnormal UA Doppler. This would have helped separate which FGR fetuses were pathologically small from those constitutionally small. In addition, had MCA Doppler studies been performed, this could have further identified constitutionally small from pathologically small fetuses. Oligohydramnios was defined as an AFI of <5 cm, which has been shown to result in a greater number of interventions with no improvement in outcomes. As a result, the oligohydramnios rates were quite high in each group (IOL 31% and EM 34%). The report did not indicate what was done with oligohydramnios and, in the expectant management group, delivery indications were left to the local standard of each center. Finally, there was no report of neonatal outcomes by birth weight percentile. For example, there was a significantly lower rate of birth weight <3rd percentile in the IOL group (13%) compared to the EM group (31%), and it would be useful to know if outcomes were different between those groups.

The following recommendations are based primarily on nontrial evidence (Level II and Level III).

At **<24 weeks**, FGR is associated with poor outcome, and counseling regarding termination can be offered in some states. Transfer to a tertiary care center is recommended if pregnancy is continued. Delivery of a severe FGR fetus at <25 weeks is associated with a dismal prognosis [174], and delivery for nonreassuring FHR (NRFHR) testing at this gestational age is unlikely to improve survival.

At **any gestational age**, in particular after 23 to 24 weeks, **NRFHR** consistent with category III patterns (e.g., recurrent late decelerations or bradycardia with absent variability) on monitoring should prompt decision for delivery. Absent/minimal (<5 beats) variability ≥32 weeks in the presence of FGR should also be an indication for considering delivery. If BPS testing is employed, a **BPS <6** is an indication for delivery. **If the managing physician is not willing to deliver the fetus for a BPS of 4 or less (e.g., in cases of FGR <28 weeks), a BPS should not be performed.** In a FGR pregnancy in which the fetus has normal UA Doppler, the fetus may be constitutionally small, and UA Doppler could be performed every 1–2 weeks with continued weekly biophysical assessment (BPS or NSTs; see below). Otherwise, if UA Doppler is abnormal, but with forward end-diastolic flow, weekly UA Doppler with continued biweekly NSTs and/or BPs are suggested.

At **24 to 31 6/7 weeks**, the FHR tracing may not show accelerations or more than minimal variability even in normal fetuses, but delivery is always indicated for recurrent late decelerations or bradycardia on monitoring. It is unclear when in the progression of pathologic changes is delivery best indicated at this gestational age because **a very preterm delivery could prevent in utero deterioration or death but be associated with the morbidity and mortality of extreme prematurity. Whenever possible** (in the absence of recurrent late decelerations or bradycardia), **delivery should be postponed after 48 hours of steroids for fetal maturity.** At <30 weeks, gestational age and birth weight are the largest predictors of outcome, and antenatal surveillance tools may not contribute significantly to survival [174,200,201].

Between 24 and 34 weeks, weekly UA Doppler evaluation will be the mainstay of surveillance with either twice weekly NSTs with weekly amniotic fluid assessment or weekly BPSs. MCA Doppler velocimetry can help to identify fetuses that are pathologically FGR and the patient with an abnormal fetal MCA blood flow should be counseled about the increased risks in pregnancy and the newborn period. However, **MCA Doppler should not be used to time delivery** as this has not been tested in clinical trials. If there is evidence of AREDF of the UA, DV Doppler evaluation can be performed, and the patient should be hospitalized for corticosteroid administration and daily monitoring. Delivery for an absent or reversed a-wave in the DV can be considered at ≥29–30 weeks as this has been shown to improve 2-year neurodevelopmental outcomes compared to abnormal CTG STV alone. Prior to this time, gestational age has been shown to be the most important factor for intact survival [174].

At **32 to 33 6/7 weeks, REDF in the UA and BPS <6 are indications for delivery** 48 hours after steroids have been given [123] with continuous EFM showing no evidence of decelerations. With UA AEDF, reversed flow of the a-wave of the DV is a strong predictor of fetal acidemia and poor perinatal outcome [166–168], and delivery should also be considered when ≥29–30 weeks. Usually tocolysis should not be used for PTL or PPROM in the presence of FGR unless FHR tracing is reassuring and 48 hours are needed to obtain the benefit of steroid administration.

At **≥34 weeks, FGR should be delivered if there is a BPS <6, oligohydramnios with SDP <2, AEDF or REDF in UA, or absent/reversed flow of the a-wave in the DV** [123].

If the UA S/D, PI, or RI are at or above the 95th percentile, but flow during diastole is still present, delivery should

be considered at around 37 weeks. In singleton gestations with FGR at 36 to 41 weeks, induction at around 37 weeks was associated with similar maternal outcomes, incidences of cesarean delivery, and neonatal morbidity and mortality compared to expectant management [198]. The incidence of birth weight <3rd percentile is decreased from 31% with expectant monitoring to 13% with induction. **If the CTG and/or BPS remain reassuring, delivery at approximately 38 0/7 to 9 6/7 weeks can be performed for the remainder of FGR fetuses.** Some recommend delivery at 39 weeks (by EDC) of the FGR fetus with otherwise normal testing if dating is accurate (i.e., based on first-trimester ultrasound) and this is supported in a practice bulletin by the ACOG, which shows that perinatal mortality and infant mortality at 1 year of age, in general, is lowest for those infants born between 39 and 40 weeks [202].

Multiple Gestation and FGR

There are no trials of timing delivery in either monochorionic/diamniotic or dichorionic/diamniotic twin gestations affected by one or two FGR cotwins. Assuming that fetal surveillance has continued to be reassuring, recommendations based on expert opinion are provided by a committee opinion document from the ACOG [203]. In DC/DA twin gestations with isolated FGR, delivery in the late preterm (36 0/7 to 36 6/7 weeks) is suggested. If DC/DA twins have concurrent conditions, such as abnormal Doppler studies or maternal comorbidities (e.g., preeclampsia or chronic hypertension), delivery in the late preterm period is suggested (32 0/7–34 6/7 weeks). Because of the higher rate of fetal demise in the third trimester, even without FGR, in monochorionic/diamniotic twins, delivery in the late preterm period is recommended. Consider delivery of twins if one twin has REDF of UA at >32 weeks, AEDF of UA at 32–34 weeks, or abnormal (but not REDF or AEDF) UA Doppler at 34–36 weeks. For more details, see Table 45.3 and also Chapters 44 and 56.

Mode of Delivery

There is insufficient evidence to assess the mode of delivery associated with the best outcomes for the FGR fetus. The TRUFFLE and GRIT studies of early and severe FGR showed cesarean delivery rates that were quite high (90% or greater). However, some evidence exists showing that **pregnancies with suspected FGR that require delivery can be safely induced if there is a reassuring fetal tracing**, normal oxytocin contraction test (OCT), and normal BPS [204]. Fetuses with abnormal UA Doppler velocimetry are more likely to fail the OCT and require a cesarean section, but vaginal delivery is possible in 40% to 60% of these patients with FGR [58,205]. When induction of labor is performed, especially at or after 36 weeks, the rate of cesarean section does not increase [198]. The decision for either induction of labor or planned cesarean delivery should account for numerous variables like fetal hemodynamic status, monitoring, cervical ripening, and parent desires. A trial of labor for the vertex FGR fetus can only be attempted if fetal monitoring is reassuring. The placenta should be sent for pathologic evaluation after delivery of an FGR fetus.

NEONATOLOGY MANAGEMENT

FGR neonates frequently require assistance with ventilation and feeding, especially if born preterm. FGR neonates <32 weeks or <1500 g require special care, usually in a tertiary care center. Workup of the etiology of FGR should be completed if not already done prenatally. Hypoglycemia, polycythemia, and coagulopathies are common, and may need treatment. Involvement of the neonatology team on counseling the patient prior to delivery on expectations in the intensive care unit may be helpful for families.

FUTURE PREGNANCY PRECONCEPTION COUNSELING

Recurrence risks are dependent upon the etiology, but when the etiology is uncertain, the rate of recurrence is increased to as high as 24% [13,15,16]. The next pregnancy is also at increased risk for fetal death if FGR necessitated PTB [206]. When the first pregnancy had FGR, several interventions are available to prevent recurrence of FGR (Table 45.4) [207]. The subsequent pregnancy should have initiation of low-dose aspirin prior to 16 weeks (unless the cause has been identified and is either nonrecurrent or treatable otherwise) [76]. In the subsequent pregnancy, screening for FGR with ultrasound surveillance of fetal growth should be performed at regular intervals.

Table 45.3 Intervention to Prevent Recurrent FGR

Preconception
- Adequate spacing of pregnancies (e.g., 18–24 months between last delivery and next conception)
- Optimization of maternal medical conditions, such as diabetes and rheumatologic disease, smoking cessation

Prenatal
- Accurate dating by first trimester sonography
- Low-dose aspirin (81–150 mg) started at <16 wk
- Women with nutritional deficiencies, especially in developing countries.
  - Supplementation of 500 to 1000 calories with low (<25%) protein content
- Women living in areas endemic for malaria.
  - Antimalarial prophylaxis

Source: Modified from Berghella V. *Obstet Gynecol*, 110, 4, 904–12, 2007.

Table 45.4 Timing of Delivery in Twin Pregnancy Complicated by FGR

	Monochorionic/Diamniotic Twins	Dichorionic Twins
Twins with isolated FGR, normal NST, normal MVP and normal UA Doppler	36 0/7–36 6/7	36 0/7–37 6/7
Twins with isolated FGR, normal NST, normal MVP and elevated PI >95th % or elevated S/D ratio >95th % of the UA Doppler	34 0/7–36 6/7	34 0/7–36 6/7
Twins with concurrent findings including oligohydramnios, abnormal UA Doppler results (either AEDV or REDV)	32 0/7–34 6/7 weeks	32 0/7–34 6/7 weeks

REFERENCES

1. American College of Obstetricians and Gynecologists. *Practice Bulletin. No 134: Fetal Growth Restriction.* May 2013. [Level III]
2. Favre R, Nisand G, Bettahar K et al. Measurement of limb circumferences with three-dimensional ultrasound for fetal weight estimation. *Ultrasound Obstet Gynecol* 1993; 3: 176–9. [III]
3. Ott WJ. The diagnosis of altered fetal growth. *Obstet Gynecol Clin North Am* 1988; 15: 237. [II-2]
4. Unterscheider J, Daly S, Geary MP et al. Optimizing the definition of intrauterine growth restriction: The multicenter prospective PORTO Study. *Am J Obstet Gynecol* 2013; 208: 290.e1–6. [Level II]
5. Gardosi J. New definition of small for gestational age based on fetal growth potential. *Horm Res* 2006; 65(Suppl. 3): 15–8. [II-2]
6. Morris RK, Malin G, Robson SC et al. Fetal umbilical artery Doppler to predict compromise of fetal/neonatal wellbeing in a high-risk population: Systematic review and bivariate meta-analysis. *Ultrasound Obstet Gynecol* 2011; 37: 135–42. [II-1]
7. De Onis M, Blossner M, Villar J. Levels and patterns of intra-uterine growth retardation in developing countries. *Eur J Clin Nutr* 1998; 52(Suppl. 1): S5–15. [II-3]
8. McIntire D, Bloom S, Casey B et al. Birth weight in relation to morbidity and mortality among newborn infants. *N Engl J Med* 1999; 340(16): 1234–8. [II-2]
9. McCowan LM, Harding JE, Stewart AW. Umbilical artery Doppler studies in small for gestational age babies reflect disease severity. *Br J Obstet Gynecol* 2000; 107: 916–25. [II-2]
10. Hata T, Aoki S, Manabe A et al. Subclassification of small-for-gestational-age fetus using fetal Doppler velocimetry. *Gynecol Obstet Invest* 2000; 49(4): 236–9. [II-2]
11. Bakewell J, Stockbauer J, Schramm W. Factors associated with repetition of low birth weight: Missouri longitudinal study. *Paediatr Perinat Epidemiol* 1997; 11(Suppl. 1): 119–29. [II-2]
12. Bakketeig L, Bjerkedal T, Hoffman H. Small for gestational age births and successive pregnancy outcomes: Results form a longitudinal study of births in Norway. *Early Hum Dev* 1986; 14(3–4): 187–200. [II-3]
13. Bratton S, Shoultz D, Williams M. Recurrence risk of low birth weight deliveries among women with a prior very low birth weight delivery. *Am J Perinatol* 1996; 13(3): 147–50. [II-3]
14. Wang X, Zuckerman B, Coffman G et al. Familial aggregation of low birth weight among whites and blacks in the United States. *N Engl J Med* 1995; 333(26): 1772–4. [II-3]
15. Ananth C, Kaminsky L, Getahun D et al. Recurrence of fetal growth restriction in singleton and twin gestations. *J Matern Fetal Med* 2009; 22(8): 654–61. [II-2]
16. Voskamp BJ, Kazemier BM, Ravelli ACJ et al. Recurrence of small-for gestational-age pregnancy: Analysis of first and subsequent singleton pregnancies in The Netherlands. *Am J Obstet Gynecol* 2013; 208: 374.e1–6. [Level II; n = 259,481]
17. Warburton D, Dallaire L, Thangavelu M et al. Trisomy recurrence: A reconsideration based on North American data. *Am J Genet* 2004; 75: 376–85. [II-2]
18. DeSouza E, Halliday J, Chan A et al. Recurrence risks for trisomies 13, 18, and 21. *Am J Med Genet A* 2009; 149A: 2716–22. [II-2]
19. Morris JK, Mutton DE, Alberman E. Recurrences of free trisomy 21: Analysis of data from the national Down dyndrome cytogenetic register. *Prenat Diagn* 2005; 25: 1120–8. [II-2]
20. Dashe J, McIntire D, Lucas M et al. Effects of symmetric and asymmetric fetal growth on pregnancy outcomes. *Obstet Gynecol* 2000; 1996(3): 321–7. [II-2]
21. David C, Gabriellie S, Pilu G et al. The head-to-abdomen circumference ratio: A reappraisal. *Ultrasound Obstet Gynecol* 1995; 5(4): 256–9. [II-2]
22. Bukowski R, Uchida T, Smith G et al. Individualized norms of optimal fetal growth: Fetal growth potential. *Obstet Gynecol* 2008; 111: 1065–76. [II-2]
23. Ounsted M, Moar V, Scott A. Risk factors associated with small-for-dates and large-for-dates infants. *Br J Obstet Gynaecol* 1987; 92: 226–32. [II-2]
24. Lees CC, Marlow N, van Wassenaer-Leemhuis A et al. 2 year neurodevelopmental and intermediate perinatal outcomes in infants with very preterm growth restriction (TRUFFLE): A randomized trial. *Lancet* 2015; 385: 2162–72. [Level I]
25. Cunningham F, Cox S, Harstad T et al. Chronic renal disease and pregnancy outcome. *Am J Obstet Gynecol* 1990; 163: 453–9. [II-3]
26. Duvekot J, Cheriex E, Pieters F et al. Maternal volume homeostasis in early pregnancy in relation to fetal growth restriction. *Obstet Gynecol* 1995; 85: 361–7. [III]
27. Duvecott J, Cheriex E, Pieters F et al. Severely impaired fetal growth is preceded by maternal hemodynamic maladaptation in very early pregnancy. *Acta Obstet Gynecol Scand* 1995; 74: 693–7. [III]
28. American College of Obstetrics and Gynecology *Practice Bulletin No. 132: Antiphospholipid syndrome.* 2012. [Level III]
29. Facco F, You W, Grobman W. Genetic thrombophilias and iutrauterine growth restriction: A meta-analysis. *Obstet Gynecol* 2009; 113: 1206–16. [Level III]
30. Said JM, Higgins JR, Moses EK et al. Inherited thrombophilia polymorphisms and pregnancy outcomes in nulliparous women. *Obstet Gynecol* 2010; 115: 5–13. [Level II-2]
31. Silver RM, Zhao Y, Spong CY et al. Prothrombin gene G20210A mutation and obstetric complications. Eunice Kennedy Shriver National Institute of Child Health and Human Development Maternal–Fetal Medicine Units (NICHD MFMU) Network. *Obstet Gynecol* 2010; 115: 14–20. [Level II-2]
32. Bada H, Das A, Bauer C et al. Low birth weight and preterm births: Etiologic fraction attributable to prenatal drug exposure. *J Perinatol* 2005; 25(10): 631–7. [II-2]
33. Shu X, Hatch M, Mills J et al. Maternal smoking, alcohol drinking, caffeine consumption, and fetal growth: Results from a prospective study. *Epidemiology* 1995; 6: 115–20. [II-2]
34. Virji S. The relationship between alcohol consumption during pregnancy and infant birth weight. An epidemiologic study. *Acta Obstet Gynecol Scand* 1991; 70: 303–8. [II-3]
35. Naeye R, Blanc W, Leblanc W et al. Fetal complications of maternal heroin addiction: Abnormal growth, infections and episodes of stress. *J Pediatr* 1973; 83: 1055–61. [III]
36. Fulroth R, Phillips B, Durand D. Perinatal outcome of infants exposed to cocaine and/or heroin in utero. *Am J Dis Child* 1989; 143: 905–10. [III]
37. Anatov A. Children born during the siege of Leningrad in 1942. *J Pediatr* 1947; 30: 250. [III]
38. Smith C. Effect of maternal undernutrition upon newborn infant in Holland. *J Pediatr* 1947; 30: 29–243. [III]
39. World Health Organization. A WHO collaborative study of maternal anthropometry and pregnancy outcomes. *Int J Gynecol Obstet* 1997; 57: 1–15. [II-2]
40. Nieto A, Matorras R, Serra M et al. Multivariate analysis of determinants of fetal growth retardation. *Eur J Obstet Gynecol Reprod Biol* 1994; 53: 107–13. [II-2]
41. Maulik D. Fetal growth restriction: The etiology. *Clin Obstet Gynecol* 2006; 49(2): 228–35. [III]
42. Gersak K, Verdenik I, Antolic ZN. Karyotyping in symmetrically growth-restricted fetuses. *Eur J Obstet Gynecol Reprod Biol* 2009; 145(1): 123. [II-3]
43. Snijders RJ, Sherrod C, Gosden CM et al. Fetal growth retardation: Associated malformations and chromosomal abnormalities. *Am J Obstet Gynecol* 1993; 168: 547–55. [II-2]
44. Viora E, Zamboni C, Mortara G et al. Trisomy 18: Fetal ultrasound findings at different gestational ages. *Am J Med Genet A* 2007; 143(6): 3–557. [III]
45. Khoury J, Erickson D, Cordero J et al. Congenital malformations and intrauterine growth retardation: A population study. *Pediatrics* 1988; 82: 83–90. [II-3]
46. Mittendorfer-Rutz E, Rasmusen F, Wassertman D. Restricted fetal growth and adverse maternal and psychosocial and socio-economic conditions as risk factor for suicidal behavior of offspring: A cohort study. *Lancet* 2004; 364: 1135–40. [II-2]

47. Craigo SD, Beach ML, Harvey-Wilkes KB et al. Ultrasound predictors of neonatal outcome in intrauterine growth restriction. *Am J Perinatol* 1996; 13: 465–71. [II-3]

48. Hack M, Taylor HG, Drotar D et al. Chronic conditions, functional limitations, and special needs of school-aged children born with extremely low birth weight in the 1990's. *J Am Med Assoc* 2005; 294(3): 318–25. [II-2]

49. Gembruch U, Gortner L. Perinatal aspects of preterm intrauterine growth restriction. *Ultrasound Obstet Gynecol* 1998; 11: 233–9. [II-3]

50. Reddy UM. Prediction and prevention of recurrent stillbirth. *Obstet Gynecol* 2007; 110: 1151–64. [Level III]

51. Trudell AS, Cahill AG, Tuuli et al. Risk of stillbirth after 37 weeks in pregnancies complicated by small-for-gestational-age fetuses. *Am J Obstet Gynecol* 2013; 208(5): 376.e1–7. [Level II]

52. Bukowski R, Hansen NI, Willinger M et al. Fetal growth and risk of stillbirth: A population-based case-control study. *PLoS Med* 2014; 11: e1001633. [Level II]

53. Hepburn M, Rosenburg K. An audit of the detection and management of small-for-gestational age babies. *Br J Obstet Gynaecol* 1986; 93: 212–6. [II-2]

54. Lackman F, Capewell V, Richardson B et al. The risks of spontaneous preterm delivery and perinatal mortality in relation to size at birth according to fetal versus neonatal growth standards. *Am J Obstet Gynecol* 2001; 184: 946–53. [II-2]

55. Bernstein I, Horbar J, Badger G et al. Morbidity and mortality among very-low-birth weight neonates with intrauterine growth restriction. *Am J Obstet Gynecol* 1999; 182(1): 198–206. [II-3]

56. Pallotto E, Kilbride H. Perinatal outcome and later implications of intrauterine growth restriction. *Clin Obstet Gynecol* 2006; 49(2): 257–69. [II-2]

57. Barker D. Adult consequences of fetal growth restriction. *Clin Obstet Gynecol* 2006; 49(2): 270–83. [III]

58. Maslovitz S, Shenhav M, Levin I et al. Outcome of induced deliveries in growth-restricted fetuses: Second thoughts about the vaginal option. *Arch Gynecol Obstet* 2009; 279: 139–43. [II-3]

59. The GRIT study group. A randomized trial of timed delivery for the compromised preterm fetus: Short term outcomes and Bayesian interpretation. *Br J Obstet Gynecol* 2003; 110: 27–32. [RCT; n = 588; Level I]

60. Smith G, Pell J, Dobbie R. Interpregnancy interval and risk of preterm birth and neonatal death: Retrospective cohort study. *Br Med J* 2003; 327: 313–9. [II-2]

61. Zhu B, Rolfs R, Nangle B et al. Effect of the interval between pregnancies on perinatal outcomes. *N Engl J Med* 1999; 340: 589–94. [II-2]

62. MacArthur C, Knox E. Smoking in pregnancy: Effects of stopping at different stages. *Br J Obstet Gynaecol* 1988; 95: 551–5. [II-2]

63. Lumley J, Chamberlain C, Dowswell T et al. Interventions for promoting smoking cessation during pregnancy. *Cochrane Database Syst Rev* 2009; 3: CD001055. [Meta-analysis; 72 trials, n = 25,000]

64. Kfatos A, Vlachonikolis I, Codrington C. Nutrition during pregnancy: The effects of an educational intervention program in Greece. *Am J Clin Nutr* 1989; 50: 970–9. [II-1]

65. Khoury J, Henriksen T, Christophersen B et al. Effect of a cholesterol-lowering diet on maternal, cord, and neonatal lipids, and pregnancy outcome: A randomized clinical trial. *Am J Obstet Gynecol* 2005; 193: 1292–301. [RCT; n = 290]

66. Steegers E, Van Lakwijk HP, Jongsma H et al. Pathophysiological implications of chronic dietary sodium restriction during pregnancy; a longitudinal prospective randomized study. *Br J Obstet Gynecol* 1991; 98: 980–7. [RCT; n = 42]

67. Mohomed K. Iron supplementation in pregnancy. *Cochrane Database Syst Rev* 2007; 3: CD000117. [Meta-analysis; 20 trials]

68. Hofmeyr G, Lawrie T, Atallah A et al. Calcium supplementation during pregnancy for preventing hypertensive disorders and related problems. *Cochrane Database Syst Rev* 2010; 9: CD001059. [Meta-analysis; n = 15,730]

69. Makrides M, Crowther C. Magnesium supplementation in pregnancy. *Cochrane Database Syst Rev* 2001; 4: CD000937. [Meta-analysis; 7 trials, n = 2689]

70. Mohomed K, Gulmezoglu A. Vitamin D supplementation in pregnancy. *Cochrane Database Syst Rev* 2000; 2: CD000228. [Meta-analysis; n = 232]

71. Robinson CJ, Wagner CL, Hollis BW et al. Maternal vitamin D and fetal growth in early-onset severe preeclampsia. *Am J Obstet Gynecol* 2011; 2004(6): 556:e1–4. [Level II]

72. Kramer MS, Kakuma R. Energy and protein intake in pregnancy. *Cochrane Database Syst Rev* 2003; 4: CD000032. [Meta-analysis; 5 trials, n = 1134]

73. Abalos E, Duley L, Steyn D et al. Antihypertensive drug therapy for mild to moderate hypertension during pregnancy. *Cochrane Database Syst Rev* 2007; 1: CD002252. [Meta-analysis; 19 trials, n = 2437; Level I]

74. Magee LA, von Dadelszen P, Rey E et al. Less-tight versus tight control of hypertension in pregnancy. *N Eng J Med* 2015; 372: 407–17. [RCT, n = 987]

75. SMFM Statement: Benefit of antihypertensive therapy for mild-to-moderate chronic hypertension during pregnancy remains uncertain. SMFM Publications Committee. *Am J Obstet Gynecol* 2015; 213(1): 3–4. [Level III]

76. Bujold E, Roberge S, Lacasse Y et al. Prevention of preeclampsia and intrauterine growth restriction with aspirin started in early pregnancy: A meta-analysis. *Obstet Gynecol* 2010; 116(2): 402–14. [Meta-analysis: RCT = 34, n = 11,348; Level I]

77. Knight M, Duley L, Henderson-Smart DJ et al. Antiplatelet agents for preventing and treating pre-eclampsia. *Cochrane Database Syst Rev* 2005; 4. [Meta-analysis; 25 RCTs, n > 20,000]

78. Spencer K, Cowans NJ, Avgidou K et al. First-trimester biochemical markers of aneuploidy and the prediction of small-for-gestational age fetuses. *Ultrasound Obstet Gynecol* 2008; 31: 15–9. [II-2]

79. Dugoff L, Hobbins JC, Malone FD et al. First-trimester maternal serum PAPP-A and free beta subunit human chorionic gonadotropin concentrations and nuchal translucency are associated with obstetric complications: A population-based screening study (The FASTER Trial). *Am J Obstet Gynecol* 2004; 191: 1446–51. [II-2]

80. Krantz D, Goetzl L, Simpson JL et al. Association of extreme first-trimester free human chorionic gonadotropin-beta, pregnancy-associated plasma protein A, and nuchal translucency with intrauterine growth restriction and other adverse pregnancy outcomes. *Am J Obstet Gynecol* 2004; 191: 1452–8. [II-2]

81. Dugoff L. First-and second-trimester maternal serum markers for aneuploidy and adverse obstetric outcomes. *Obstet Gynecol* 2010; 115: 1052–61. [III]

82. Dugoff L, Hobbins J, Malone F et al. Quad screen as a predictor of adverse pregnancy outcome. *Obstet Gynecol* 2005; 106(2): 260–7. [II-2]

83. Cnattingius S, Axelsson O, Lindmark G. Symphysis-fundus measurements and intrauterine growth retardation. *Acta Obstet Gynecol Scand* 1984; 63(4): 335–40. [II-2]

84. Lindhard A, Nielsen PV, Mouritsen LA et al. The implications of introducing the symphyseal-fundal height-measurement: A prospective randomized controlled trial. *Br J Obstet Gynaecol* 1990; 97: 675–80. [Level I]

85. Robert PJ, Ho JJ, Villiapan J, Sivasangari S. Symphysial fundal height (SFH) measurement in pregnancy for detecting abnormal fetal growth. *Cochrane Database Syst Rev* 2012; 7: CD008136. [Level II]

86. Hulsey TC, Levkoff AH, Alexander GR et al. Differences in black and white infant birth weights. *South Med J* 1991; 84: 443–6. [II-2]

87. Goldenberg RL, Cliver SP, Cutter GR. Black white differences in newborn anthropometric measurements. *Obstet Gynecol* 1991; 78: 782–8. [II-2]

88. Yip R, Li Z, Chong WH. Race and birth weight: The Chinese example. *Pediatrics* 1991; 87: 688–93. [II-2]

89. Alver J, Brooke OG. Fetal growth in different racial groups. *Arch Dis Child* 1978; 53: 27–32. [II-2]

90. Graafmans WC, Richardus JH, Borsboom GJ et al. Birth weight and perinatal mortality: A comparison of "optimal" birth weight in seven Western European countries. *Epidemiology* 2002; 13: 569–74. [II-2]

91. Ott WJ. Intrauterine growth retardation and preterm delivery. *Am J Obstet Gynecol* 1993; 168: 1710–5. [II-2]

92. Warsof SL, Gohari P, Berkowitz RL et al. The estimation of fetal weight by computer assisted analysis. *Am J Obstet Gynecol* 1977; 128: 881–92. [II-3]

93. Hadlock FP, Harrist RB, Martinez-Poyer J. In utero analysis of fetal growth: A sonographic weight standard. *Radiology* 1991; 181: 129–33. [II-3]

94. Shepard MJ, Richards VA, Berkowitz RL et al. An evaluation of two equations for predicting fetal weight by ultrasound. *Am J Obstet Gynecol* 1982; 142: 47–54. [II-3]

95. Persson P-H, Weldner B-M. Intra-uterine weight curves obtained by ultrasound. *Acta Obstet Gynecol Scand* 1986; 65: 169–73. [II-2]

96. Bernstein IM, Meyer M, Capeless E. Fetal growth charts: Comparison of cross-sectional ultrasound examinations with birth weight. *J Matern Fetal Med* 1994; 3: 182–6. [II-2]

97. Bernstein IM, Mohs G, Rucquoi M et al. Case for hybrid "fetal growth curves": A population-based estimation of normal fetal size across gestational age. *J Matern Fetal Med* 1996; 5: 124–7. [II-3]

98. Salomon LJ, Bernard JP, Ville Y. Estimation of fetal weight: Reference range at 20–36 weeks' gestation and comparison with actual birth weight reference range. *Ultrasound Obstet Gynecol* 2007; 29: 550–5. [II-2]

99. Zaw W, Gagnon R, da Silva O. The risks of adverse neonatal outcome among preterm small for gestational age infants according to neonatal versus fetal growth standards. *Pediatrics* 2003; 111: 1273–7. [II-2]

100. Gardosi J. Customized fetal growth standards: Rationale and clinical application. *Semin Perinatol* 2004; 28: 33–40. [II-2]

101. Clausson B, Gardosi J, Francis A et al. Perinatal outcome in SGA births defined by customized versus population–based birth weight standards. *Br J Obstet Gynaecol* 2001; 108: 830–4. [II-2]

102. Figueras F, Figueras J, Meler E et al. Customised birth weight standards accurately predict perinatal morbidity. *Arch Dis Child Fetal Neonatal Ed* 2007; 92: F277–80. [II-2]

103. Constantine M, Lai Y, Bloom S et al. Population versus customized fetal growth norms and adverse outcomes in an intrapartum cohort. *Am J Perinatol* 2013; 30(4): 335–42. [II-2]

104. Royal College of Obstetricians and Gynaecologists. *The Investigation and Management of the small-for-Gestational-Age Fetus.* Green Top Guideline No. 31. Second Edition. London: RCOG, 2013. [III]

105. Hutcheon JA, Zhang X, Cnattingius S et al. Customized birth weight percentiles: Does adjusting for maternal characteristics matter? *BJOG* 2008; 115: 1397–404. [II-2]

106. Carberry AE, Gordon A, Bond DM, Hyett J, Raynes-Greenow CH, Jeffery HE. Customised versus *population-based growth charts as a screening tool for detecting small for gestational age infants in* low-risk pregnant women. *Cochrane Database System Rev* 2014; 5: CD008549. doi:10.1002/14651858.CD008549.pub3. [meta-analysis; no RCTs included]

107. McKenna D, Tharmaratnam S, Mahsud S, Bailie C, Harper A, Doman J. A randomized trial using ultrasound to identify the high-risk fetus in a low-risk population. *Obstet Gynecol* 2003; 101(4): 626–32. [RCT, n = 1998]

108. Sovio U, White IR, Dacey A, Pasupathy D, Smith GCS. Screening for fetal growth restriction with universal third trimester ultrasonography in nulliparous women in the Pregnancy Outcome Prediction (POP) study: A prospective cohort study. *Lancet* 2015; 386: 2089–97. [II-1, n = 4512]

109. Roma E, Arnau A, Berdala R et al. Ultrasound screening for fetal growth restriction at 36 vs 32 weeks' gestation: A randomized trial (ROUTE). *Ultrasound Obstet Gynecol* 2015; 46: 391–7. [RCT, n = 2586]

110. Papageorghiou AT, Yu CKH, Nicolaides KH. The role of uterine artery Doppler in predicting adverse pregnancy outcome. *Best Pract Res Clin Obstet Gynecol* 2004; 18: 383–96. [Level III]

111. Martin A, Bindra R, Curcio P et al. Screening for pre-eclampsia and fetal growth restriction by uterine artery Doppler at 11-14 weeks of gestation. *Ultrasound Obstet Gynecol* 2001; 18: 583–6. [II-2]

112. Gomez O, Martinez J, Figueras F et al. Uterine artery Doppler at 11–14 weeks of gestation to screen for hypertensive disorders and associated complication in an unselected population. *Ultrasound Obstet Gynecol* 2005; 26: 490–4. [II-2]

113. Pilalis A, Souka P, Antsakalis P et al. Screening for preeclampsia and fetal growth restriction by uterine artery Doppler and PAPP-A at 11–14 weeks' gestation. *Ultrasound Obstet Gynecol* 2007; 29: 135–40. [II-2]

114. Cnossen JS, Morris RK, ter Riet G et al. Use of uterine artery Doppler ultrasonography to predict pre-eclampsia and intrauterine growth restriction: A systematic review and bivariable meta-analysis. *Can Med Assoc J* 2008; 178: 701–11. [II-2]

115. Cooper S, Johnson J, Metcalfe A et al. The predictive value of 18 and 22 week uterine artery Doppler in patients with low first trimester serum PAPP-A. *Prenat Diagn* 2009; 29: 248–52. [II-2]

116. Palma-Dias RS, Fonseca MM, Brietzke E et al. Screening for placental insufficiency by transvaginal uterine artery Doppler at 22-24 weeks of gestation. *Fetal Diagn Ther* 2008; 24: 462–9. [II-2]

117. Alkazaleh F, Chaddha V, Viero S et al. Second trimester prediction of severe placental complications in women with combined elevations in alpha-fetoprotein and human chorionic gonadotriphin. *Am J Obstet Gynecol* 2006; 94(3): 821–7. [II-2]

118. Yu C, Khouri O, Onwudiwe N et al. Prediction of preeclampsia by uterine artery Doppler imaging: Relationship to gestational age at delivery and small-for-gestational-age. *Ultrasound Obstet Gynecol* 2008; 31: 310–3. [II-2]

119. Konchak P, Bernstein I, Capeless E. Uterine artery Doppler velocimetry in the detection of adverse obstetric outcomes in women with unexplained elevated maternal serum alpha-fetoprotein levels. *Am J Obstet Gynecol* 1995; 173: 1115–9. [II-2]

120. Berkely Chauhan, Abuhamad A. Doppler assessment of the fetus with intrauterine growth restriction. *Am J Obstet Gyencol* 2012; 206(4): 300–8. [Level III]

121. Chavez MR, Ananth CV, Smulian JC et al. Transcerebellar diameter measurement for prediction of gestational age at the extremes of fetal growth. *J Ultrasound Med* 2007; 26(9): 1167–71. [II-2]

122. Niknafs P, Sibbald J. Accuracy of single ultrasound parameters in detection of fetal growth restriction. *Am J Perinatol* 2001; 18(6): 325–34. [II-2]

123. Publication Committee, SMFM. Early severe fetal growth restriction: Evaluation and treatment. *Cont Ob-Gyn* 2011; 2: 32–5. [III]

124. Wilkins-Haug L, Quade B, Morton CC. Confined placental mosaicism as a risk factor among newborns with fetal growth restriction. *Prenat Diagn* 2006; 26(5): 428–32. [II-2]

125. Baschat A, Cosmi E, Bilardo C et al. Predictors of neonatal outcome in early-onset placental dysfunction. *Obstet Gynecol* 2007; 109(2 Pt. 1): 253–61. [II-2]

126. Engineer N, Kumar S. Perinatal variables and neonatal outcomes in severely growth restricted preterm fetuses. *Acta Obstet Gynecol Scand* 2010; 89(9): 1174–81. [II-2]

127. Laurin J, Persson P-H. The effect of bed rest in hospital on fetal outcome in pregnancies complicated by intra-uterine growth retardation. *Acta Obstet Gynecol Scand* 1987; 66: 407–11. [RCT, n = 107. Allocation of treatment was by odd or even birth date. Level I]

128. McCall CA, Grimes DA, Lyerly AD. "Therapeutic" bed rest in pregnancy. Unethical and unsupported by data. *Obstet Gynecol* 2013; 121: 1305–8. [Level III]

129. Ramakrishnan U, Stein A, Parra-Cabrera S et al. Effects of docosahexaenoic acid supplementation during pregnancy on gestational age and size at birth: Randomized, double-blind, placebo-controlled trial in Mexico. *Food Nutr Bull* 2010; 31(2 Suppl.): S108–16. [RCT, n = 1094]

130. Roberfroid D, Huybregts L, Lanou H et al. MISAME Study Group. Effects of maternal multiple micronutrient supplementation on fetal growth: A double-blind randomized controlled trial in rural Burkina Faso. *Am J Clin Nutr* 2008; 88(5): 1220–40. [RCT, n = 1426]

131. Horvath A, Koletzko B, Szajewska H. Effect of supplementation of women in high-risk pregnancies with long-chain polyunsaturated fatty acids on pregnancy outcomes and growth

measures at birth: A meta-analysis of randomized controlled trials. *Br J Nutr* 2007; 98(2): 253–9. [Meta-analysis; 2 RCTs, n = 291]

132. Say L, Gulmezoglu AM, Hofmeyr GJ. Maternal nutrient supplementation for suspected impaired fetal growth. *Cochrane Database Syst Rev* 2010; (7): 1–19. [4 RCTs, n = 165]

133. Say L, Gulmezoglu AM, Hofmeyr JG. Betamimetics for suspected impaired fetal growth. *Cochrane Database Syst Rev* 2009; (4): 1–13. [2 RCTs, n = 118]

134. Janssens D. Prevention of low birth weight by flunarizine given to smoking mothers. *Arch Gynecol* 1985; 237(Suppl. 1): 397. [RCT, n = 100]

135. Yu Y-H, Shen L-Y, Zou H et al. Heparin for patients with growth restricted fetus: A prospective randomized controlled trial. *JMFNM* 2010; 23(9): 980–7. [RCT, n = 73]

136. Say L, Gulmezoglu AM, Hofmeyr GJ. Maternal oxygen administration for suspected impaired fetal growth. *Cochrane Database Syst Rev* 2005; 4: 1–11. [I; 3 RCTs, n = 94]

137. Salas SP, Rosso P, Espinoza R et al. Maternal plasma volume expansion and hormonal changes in women with idiopathic fetal growth retardation. *Obstet Gynecol* 1993; 81(6): 1029–30. [II-2]

138. Karsdorp VHM, van Vugt JMG, Dekker GA et al. Reappearance of end-diastolic velocities in the umbilical artery following maternal volume expansion: A preliminary study. *Obstet Gynecol* 1992; 80: 679–83. [RCT, n = 14]

139. Hofmeyr GJ. Abdominal decompression for suspected fetal compromise/pre-eclampsia. *Cochrane Database Syst Rev* 2005; 4: 1–13. [3 RCTs, n = 367]

140. Winer N, Branger B, Azria E et al. L-Arginine treatment for severe vascular fetal intrauterine growth restriction: A randomized double-blind controlled trial. *Clin Nutr* 2009; 28(3): 243–8. [I: RCT n = 44]

141. Sieroszewski P, Suzin J, Karowicz-Bilinska A. Ultrasound evaluation of intrauterine growth restriction therapy by a nitric oxide donors (L-arginine). *J Matern Fetal Neonatal Med* 2003; 13: 115–8. [II-1]

142. Xiao XM, Li LP. L-Arginine treatment for asymmetric fetal growth restriction. *Int J Gynaecol Obstet* 2005; 88: 15–8. [II-1]

143. Lampl MD, Veldhuis JD, Johnson ML. Saltation and stasis: A model of human growth. *Science* 1992; 258: 801–3. [II-3]

144. Bernstein IM, Blake K, Wall B et al. Evidence that normal fetal growth can be noncontinuous. *J Matern Fetal Med* 1995; 4: 1997–2001. [II-3]

145. Mongelli M, Ek S, Tamyrajia R. Screening for fetal growth restriction: A mathematical model of the effect of time interval and ultrasound error. *Obstet Gynecol* 1998; 92(6): 908–12. [II-3]

146. Giles W, Trudinger B, Baird PJ. Fetal umbilical artery velocity waveforms and placental resistance: Pathological correlation. *Br J Obstet Gynaecol* 1985; 92: 31–8. [Level II]

147. Todros T, Sciarrone A, Piccoli E et al. Umbilical Doppler waveforms and placental villous angiongenesis in pregnancies complicated by fetal growth restriction. *Obstet Gynecol* 1999; 93: 499–503. [II-2]

148. Kingdom JC, Burrell SJ, Kaufmann P. Pathology and clinical implications of abnormal umbilical artery Doppler waveforms. *Ultrasound Obstet Gynecol* 1997; 9: 271–86. [Level II]

149. Morrow RJ, Adamson SL, Bull SB, Ritchie JW. Effect of placental embolizationon the umbilical arterial velocity waveform in fetal sheep. *Am J Obstet Gynecol* 1989; 161: 1055–60. [II-2]

150. Pardi G, Cetin I, Marconi AM. et al. Diagnostic value of blood sampling in fetuses with growth retardation. *N Eng J Med* 1993; 328: 692–6. [Level II]

151. Bilardo CM, Nicolaides KH, Campbel S. Doppler measurements of fetal and utero-placental circulations: Relationship with umbilical venous blood gases measured at cordocentesis. *Am J Obstet Gynecol* 1990; 162: 115–20. [Level II]

152. Hartung J, Kalache K, Heyna C et al. Outcome of 60 neonates who had ARED flow prenatally compared with a matched control group of appropriate-for gestational age preterm neonates. *Ultrasound Obstet Gynecol* 2005; 25: 566–72. [II-2]

153. Shand A, Hornbuckle J, Nathan E et al. Small for gestational age preterm infants and relationship of abnormal umbilical artery Doppler blood flow to perinatal mortality and neurodevelopmental outcomes. *Aust N Z J Obstet Gynaecol* 2009; 49: 52–8. [II-2]

154. McCowan L, Harding J, Roberts A et al. A pilot randomized controlled trial of two regimens of fetal surveillance for small-for-gestational age fetuses with normal results of umbilical artery Doppler velocimetry. *Am J Obstet Gynecol* 2000; 182(1): 81–6. [I: RCT n = 167]

155. Alfirevic Z, Stampalija T, Gyte G. Fetal and umbilical Doppler ultrasound in high-risk pregnancies. *Cochrane Database Syst Rev* 2010; 1: CD007529. [I, meta-analysis, 18 RCTs, n = 10,000]

156. Bahado-Singh R, Kovanci E, Jeffres A et al. The Doppler cerebroplacental ratio and perinatal outcome in intrauterine growth restriction. *Am J Obstet Gynecol* 1999; 180: 750–6. [II-2]

157. Odibo A, Riddick C, Are E et al. Cerebroplacental Doppler ratio and adverse perinatal outcomes in intrauterine growth restriction. *J Ultrasound Med* 2005; 24: 1223–8. [II-2]

158. Gramellini D, Folli MC, Raboni S et al. Cerebral-umbilical Doppler ratio as a predictor of adverse perinatal outcome. *Obstet Gynecol* 1992; 79: 416–20. [Level II]

159. Wladimiroff JW, van den Wiingaard JAGN, Degani S et al. Cerebral and umbilical arterial blood flow velocity waveforms in normal and growth retarded pregnancies: A comparative study *Obstet Gynecol* 1987; 69: 705–9. [Level II]

160. Oros D, Figueras F, Cruz-Martinez R et al. Middle versus anterior cerebral artery Doppler for the prediction of perinatal outcome and neonatal neurobehavior in term small-for-gestational-age fetuses with normal umbilical artery Doppler. *Ultrasound Obstet Gynecol* 2010; 35: 456–61. [Level II]

161. Eixarch E, Meler E, Iraola A et al. Neurodevelopmental outcome in 2-year-old infants who were small-for-gestational age term fetuses with cerebral blood flow redistribution. *Ultrasound Obstet Gynecol* 2008; 32: 894–9. [Level II]

162. Cruz-Martinez R, Figueras F, Hernandez-Andrade E et al. Fetal brain Doppler to predict cesarean delivery for non-reassuring fetal status in term small-for-gestational-age fetuses. *Obstet Gynecol* 2011: 117: 618–26. [Level II]

163. Figueras F, Martiniz J, Puerto B et al. Contraction stress test versus ductus venosus Doppler evaluation for the prediction of adverse perinatal outcome in growth-restricted fetuses with non-reassuring non-stress test. *Ultrasound Obstet Gynecol* 2003; 21: 250–5. [II-2]

164. Hecher K, Snijders R, Campbell S, Nicolaides K. Fetal venous, intracardiac, and arterial blood flow measurements in intrauterine growth retardation: Relationship with fetal blood gases. *Am J Obstet Gynecol* 1995; 173: 10–15. [Level II]

165. Rizzo G, Capponi A, Arduini D, Romanini C. The value of fetal arterial, cardiac and venous flows in predicting pH and blood gases measured in umbilical blood at cordocentesis in growth retarded fetuses. *Br J Obstet Gynaecol* 1995; 102: 963–9. [Level II]

166. Baschat A, Gembruch U, Weiner C et al. Qualitative venous Doppler waveform analysis improves prediction of critical outcomes in premature growth-restricted fetuses. *Ultrasound Obstet Gynecol* 2003; 22: 240–5. [II-2]

167. Schwarze A, Gembruch U, Krapp M et al. Qualitative venous Doppler flow waveform analysis in preterm intrauterine growth-restricted fetuses with ARED flow in the umbilical artery-correlation with short-term outcome. *Ultrasound Obstet Gynecol* 2005; 25: 573–9. [II-2]

168. Alves S, Francisco R, Miyadahira S et al. Ductus venosus Doppler and postnatal outcomes in fetuses with absent or reversed end-diastolic flow in the umbilical artery. *Eur J Obstet Gynecol Reprod Biol* 2008; 141: 100–3. [II-2]

169. Baschat AA. Doppler application in the delivery timing of preterm growth-restricted fetus: Another step in the right direction. *Ultrasound Obstet Gynecol* 2004; 23: 111–8. [LIII]

170. Ferrazzi E, Bozzo M, Rigano S et al. Temporal sequence of abnormal Doppler changes in the peripheral and central circulatory systems of the severely growth-restricted fetus. *Ultrasound Obstet Gynecol* 2002; 19: 140–9. [Level II]

171. Baschat AA, Gembruch U, Harman CR. The sequence of changes in Doppler and biophysical parameters as severe fetal growth restriction worsens. *Ultrasound Obstet Gynecol* 2001; 18: 571–7. [Level II]

172. Hecher K, Bilardo CM, Stigter RH et al. Monitoring of fetuses with intrauterine growth restriction: A longitudinal study. *Ultrasound Obstet Gynecol* 2001; 18: 564–70. [Level II]

173. Unterscheider J, Daly S, Geary MP et al. Predictable progressive Doppler deterioration in IUGR: Does it really exist? *Am J Obstet Gynecol* 2013; 209: 539.e1–7. [Level II]

174. Baschat AA, Cosmi E, Bilardo C et al. Predictors of neonatal outcome in early-onset placental dysfunction. *Obstet Gynecol* 2007; 109: 253–61. [II-2]

175. Grivell R, Alfirevec Z, Gyte G et al. Antenatal cardiotocography for fetal assessment. *Cochrane Database Syst Rev* 2015; 9: CD007863. [I, 6 studies, n = 2105]

176. Grivell RM, Wong L, Bhatia V. Regimens of fetal surveillance for impaired fetal growth. *Cochrane Database System Rev* 2012; 6: CD007113. doi:10.1002/14651858.CD007113.pub3. [meta-analysis; 1 RCT, n = 167]

177. Visser G, Sandovsky G, Nicolaides K. Antepartum fetal heart rate patterns in small-for-gestational-age third-trimester fetuses: Correlations with blood gas values obtained at cordocentesis. *Am J Obstet Gynecol* 1990; 162: 698–703. [II-2]

178. Donner C, Vermeylen D, Kirkpatrick C et al. Management of the growth-restricted fetus: The role of noninvasive tests and fetal blood sampling. *Obstet Gynecol* 1995; 85: 965–70. [II-3]

179. Lalor JG, Fawole B, Alfirevic Z et al. Biophysical profile for fetal assessment in high risk pregnancies. *Cochrane Database Syst Rev* 2008; 1: CD000038. [Meta-analysis; 5 RCTs; n = 2974]

180. Dayal A, Manning F, Berck D et al. Fetal death after normal biophysical profile score: An eighteen year experience. *Am J Obstet Gynecol* 1999; 181: 1231. [II-3]

181. Manning FA, Hill LM, Platt LD. Qualitative amniotic fluid volume determination by ultrasound: Antepartum detection of intrauterine growth retardation. *Am J Obstet Gynecol* 1981; 193: 254–8. [Level II]

182. Peeters JH, Sheldon RE, Jones MD et al. Blood flow to fetal organs as a function of arterial oxygen content. *Am J Obset Gynecol* 1979; 135: 637–46. [Level II]

183. Arabin B, Bergman PL, Saling E. Simultaneous assessment of blood flow velocity in uteroplacental vessels, the umbilical artery, the fetal aorta and the fetal common carotid artery. *Fetal Ther* 1987; 2: 17–26. [Level II]

184. Veille JC, Kanaan C. Duplex Doppler ultrasonography evaluation of the fetal renal artery in normal and abnormal fetuses. *Am J Obstet Gynecol* 1989; 161: 1502–7. [Level II]

185. Duenhoelter JH, Whalley PJ, MacDonald PC. An analysis of the utility of plasma immunoreactive estrogen measurements in determining delivery time of gravidas with a fetus considered at high risk. *Am J Obstet Gynecol* 1976; 125: 889–98. [I, RCT, n = 622 women with high risk pregnancies, including fetal growth restriction, hypertension, adverse obstetric history. RCT by hospital # to plasma estriol level either revealed or concealed]

186. Roberts D, Dalziel S. Antenatal corticosteroids for accelerating fetal lung maturation for woman at risk for preterm birth. *Cochrane Database Syst Rev* 2006; 3: CD004454. [Meta-analysis; 21 RCTs, n = 3885]

187. Garite T, Kurtzman J, Maurel K et al. Impact of a 'rescue course' of antenatal corticosteroids: A multicenter randomized placebo-controlled trial. *Am J Obstet Gynecol* 2009; 200: 248.e1–9. [RCT; n = 437]

188. McLaughlin K, Crowther C, Walker N et al. Effects of a single course of corticosteroids given more than 7 days before birth: A systematic review. *Aust N Z J Obstet Gynecol* 2003; 43: 101–6. [Meta-analysis; 7 trials; n = 862]

189. Vidaeff AC, Blackwell SC. Potential risks and benefits of antenatal corticosteroid therapy prior to preterm birth in pregnancies complicated by severe fetal growth restriction. *Obstet Gynecol Clin N Am* 2011; 38(2): 205–14. [III]

190. Mitsiakos G, Kovacs L, Papageorgiou A. Are antenatal steroids beneficial to severely growth restricted fetuses. *J Matern Fetal Neonatal Med* 2013; 26(15): 1496–9. [Level II]

191. Bernstein IM, Horbar JD, Badger GJ et al. Morbidity and mortality among very-low-birth-weight neonates with intrauterine growth restiction. The Vermont Oxford Network. *Am J Obstet Gynecol* 2000; 182: 198–206. [Level II]

192. Magnesium sulfate before anticipated preterm birth for neuroprotection. Committee Opinion No. 455. American College of Obstetricians and Gynecologists. *Obstet Gynecol* 2010; 115: 669–71. [Level III]

193. Marret S, Marpeau L, Zupan-Simunetk V et al. Magnesium sulphate given before very-preterm bith to protect infant brain: The randomized controlled PREMAG trial. PREMAG Trial Group. *BJOG* 2007; 114: 310–8. [Level I]

194. Rouse DJ, Hirtz DG, Thorn E et al. A randomized controlled trial of magnesium sulfate for the prevention of cerebral palsy. Eunice Kennedy Shriver NICHD Maternal–Fetal Medicine Units network. *N Engl J Med* 2008; 359: 895–905. [Level I]

195. Torrance H, Bloemen M, Mulde E et al. Predictors of outcome at 2 years of age after early intrauterine growth restriction. *Ultrasound Obstet Gynecol* 2010; 365: 171–7. [II-2]

196. The GRIT study group. Infant well being at 2 years of age in the Growth Restriction Intervention Trial (GRIT): Multicentered randomized controlled trial. *Lancet* 2004; 364: 513–20. [Level I; RCT follow-up, n = 588]

197. Walker D, Marlow N, Upstone L et al. The growth restriction intervention trial: Long-term outcomes in a randomized trial of delivery in fetal growth restriction. *Am J Obstet Gynecol* 2011; 204: 34e1–9. [RCT follow-up, n = 302]

198. Boers KE, Vijgen SMC, Bijlenga D et al. Induction versus expectant monitoring for intrauterine growth restriction at term: Randomized equivalence trail (DIGITAT). *Br Med J* 2010; 341: c7087. [Level I; RCT, n = 650]

199. van Wyk L, Boers KE, van der Post JAM et al. Effects on (neuro) developmental and behavioral outcome at 2 years of age of induced labor compared with expectant management in intrauterine growth-restricted infants: Long-term outcomes of the DIGITAT trial. *Am J Obstet Gynecol* 2012; 206: 406.e1–7. [Level I; RCT]

200. Sameshima H, Kodama Y, Kaneko M et al. Clinical factors that enhance morbidity and mortality in intrauterine growth restricted fetuses delivered between 23 and 30 weeks of gestation. *J Matern Fetal Neonatal Med* 2010; 23: 1218–24. [II-2]

201. Mari G, Hanif F, Treadwell M et al. Gestational age at delivery and Doppler waveforms in very preterm intrauterine growth-restricted fetuses as predictors of perinatal mortality. *J Ultrasound Med* 2007; 26: 55–9. [II-2]

202. American College of Obstetricians and Gynecologists. *Nonmedically indicated early-term deliveries.* Committee Opinion. No. 561, April 2013. [Level III]

203. American College of Obstetricians and Gynecologists. *Medically indicated late preterm and early-term deliveries.* Committee Opinion. No. 560, April 2013. [Level III]

204. Ben-Haroush A, Yogev Y, Glickman H et al. Mode of delivery in pregnancies with suspected fetal growth restriction following induction of labor with vaginal prostaglandin E2. *Acta Obstet Gynecol Scand* 2004; 83(1): 52–7. [II-1]

205. Li H, Gudmundsson S, Olofsson P. Prospect for vaginal delivery of growth restricted fetuses with abnormal umbilical artery blood flow. *Acta Obstet Gynecol Scan* 2003; 82: 828–33. [II-2]

206. Surkan PJ, Stephansson O, Dickman PW et al. Previous preterm and small-for-gestationalage births and the subsequent risk of still births. *N Engl J Med* 2004; 350: 777–85. [II-2]

207. Berghella V. Prevention of recurrent fetal growth restriction. *Obstet Gynecol* 2007; 110(4): 904–12. [III]

46

Fetal macrosomia

Oscar A. Viteri and Suneet P. Chauhan

KEY POINTS

- Although **clinical and sonographic estimated fetal weight (EFW)** can identify newborns with weight ≥4000 g (definition of fetal macrosomia), both methods **are poor at detecting neonates who will weigh ≥4500 g.**
- **Prevention of macrosomia** is obtained in women with gestational diabetes (GDM) with the following:
  - **Diet and glucose monitoring with insulin if needed** compared to no treatment or diet only.
  - **Postprandial blood glucose monitoring** compared to **preprandial in GDM requiring insulin therapy.**
  - **Strict glucose control with fasting blood sugar <90 and two hours postprandial <120.**
- Bariatric surgery prior to pregnancy is associated with decreased odds of macrosomia in obese women (body mass index >30 kg/m^2).
- Prenatal exercise reduces the odds of delivering a macrosomic newborn.
- Among uncomplicated pregnancies, **induction for suspected macrosomia is associated with a reduced risk for shoulder dystocia and increased risk of vaginal delivery without increasing the likelihood of cesarean delivery** when compared with expectant management. The likelihood of neonatal brachial plexus palsy (NBPP) is not influenced by induction for suspected macrosomia.
- There is insufficient evidence to recommend best management of suspected macrosomia among pregnancies complicated by diabetes mellitus, prior cesarean delivery, or shoulder dystocia because of the lack of randomized trials and the inaccuracy of predicting birth weight. The American College of Obstetricians and Gynecologists (ACOG) suggests a planned cesarean for women with no diabetes and an EFW of ≥5000 g, and for those with diabetes and an EFW of 4500 g, but these suggestions are not based on level 1 evidence.

DEFINITION

A fetus with EFW ≥4000 g can be presumed to be macrosomic. Macrosomic newborns can be classified as grades I (birth weight 4000–4499 g), II (4500–4999 g), and III (≥5000 g) [1]. This classification is clinically relevant because the grades are associated with different types of complications. Instead, a fetus is large for gestational age (LGA) when his/her EFW is estimated to be >95% for gestational age.

EPIDEMIOLOGY/INCIDENCE

The prevalence of macrosomia in developed countries has decreased significantly, affecting 1.3% to 1.5% of all pregnancies [2]; however, 5% to 10% of macrosomic fetuses are associated with maternal diabetes. The rate of neonates in the United States weighing ≥4000 g was 10.2% in 1996, 9.2% in 2002, and 8.0% in 2013, [3] continuing to decrease over 19 years. For newborns weighing ≥5000 g, the decrease in the prevalence has been notable as well (from 0.16% in 1996 to 0.13% in 2002 and 0.10% in 2008) [3,4]. In China, the prevalence of macrosomia increased from 6.6% in 1996 to 9.5% in 2000, then decreased to 7.0% in 2010 [5]. Similarly, in Korea, the frequency of macrosomia was reduced from 6.7% to 3.5% between 1993 and 2010 [6]. In some countries, such as Denmark, however, macrosomia is increasing. From 1998 to 2008, that country's rate of macrosomia (live births weighing >4000 g) has increased from 5.2% to 5.8% [7]. In developing countries, the prevalence of macrosomia is typically 1% to 5%, but ranges from 0.5% to 14.9% [8].

RISK FACTORS

Hispanic women, maternal obesity, maternal birth weight >8 lb, grand multiparity (≥5 deliveries), prior macrosomic fetus, abnormal 50-g glucose screen but normal three-hour glucose test, diabetes (pre- or gestational diabetes), gestational age ≥40 weeks, advanced maternal age, male infant sex, and excessive weight gain during pregnancy are well known risk factors [8,9]. Intrapartum hydramnios [10] and second stage of labor >120 minutes [11] are other risk factors for macrosomia. The majority of newborns with birth weights ≥4500 g do not have any known risk factors [9].

COMPLICATIONS

The *maternal* complications with macrosomic fetuses include **prolonged labor, operative vaginal delivery, cesarean delivery, postpartum hemorrhage, and vaginal lacerations** [9].

Compared to newborns with birth weights of 3000 to 3999 g, *neonatal* complications for grade I macrosomia include **breech presentation, induction, meconium staining, dysfunctional/prolonged labor, cephalopelvic disproportion, and cesarean delivery.** For grade II macrosomia, the complications are also Apgar scores ≤3 at 5 minutes, assisted ventilation >30 minutes, birth injuries, meconium aspiration, and hyaline membrane disease. For grade III macrosomia, there is **also a significantly higher likelihood of neonatal and infant mortality** [1].

MANAGEMENT
Prevention of Macrosomia

In diabetic women, a significant decrease in the rate of macrosomia can be obtained with the following:

- **Diet and glucose monitoring with insulin** if needed compared to no treatment or diet only [12].
- **Postprandial versus preprandial blood glucose monitoring in GDM requiring insulin therapy** [13].

- **Continuous glucose monitoring** compared to standard antenatal care with intermittent self-monitoring [14].
- **Management of GDM with fasting blood sugar <90 and 2-hour postprandial <120**, versus modified blood sugar goal based on whether the abdominal circumference is <75% versus ≥75% for gestational age (if abdominal circumference ≥75%, the fasting blood sugar should have been in this study <80 and 2-hour postprandial <100) [15].
- **Treatment, including nutrition instruction, diet, glucose testing, and insulin if necessary, of mild or borderline GDM, defined by abnormal one-hour glucose challenge test but normal two-hour glucose tolerance test** [16,17].

In nondiabetic women, rates of macrosomia were decreased with the following:

- **Bariatric surgery** in eligible obese women [18,19]. Compared to obese women who had not undergone bariatric surgery, those receiving the procedure had lower odds of macrosomia (OR 0.46; 95% CI 0.34–0.62).
- **Prenatal exercise** reduced the odds of having a macrosomic newborn by 31% (OR 0.69, 95% CI 0.55–0.86) [20].

In limited data, the rate of macrosomia was not significantly decreased with the following:

- Administering insulin twice daily versus four times daily in women with pre- and gestational diabetes [21]
- Use of insulin or glyburide in the management of GDM not controlled adequately on diet [22]
- Use of glyburide or metformin as alternatives to insulin therapy [23]

Screening

During labor, the detection of neonates weighing at least 4000 g is similar with clinical or sonographic EFWs although the likelihood ratio with clinicians' estimate was 15, and with **measurements of biometric parameters** it was 42 (i.e., **better**) [24]. Neither clinical nor sonographic EFW can accurately identify neonates that weigh 4500 g or more [25,26], systematically overestimating the actual birth weight. However, the overall proportion of clinically estimated fetal weights that are within 10% of the actual birth weight is significantly lower

than that for sonographic methods across all birth weights (35% vs. 68%, *p* < .001) and for macrosomic babies (76% vs. 100%, *p* = .009) [27]. Routine use of third trimester ultrasound provides a high detection of large-for-gestational age fetuses (sensitivity 70%, 95% CI 85%–795% and specificity 70%, 95% CI 68%–72%) [28].

Management of Suspected Macrosomia

Whenever macrosomia is suspected, the pregnancy should be classified into one of the following groups: 1) uncomplicated, 2) pregestational or gestational diabetes, 3) prior cesarean delivery, or 4) history of shoulder dystocia (Figure 46.1).

Uncomplicated

Induction of labor at 37 0/7 to 38 6/7 weeks for suspected fetal macrosomia (EFW ≥4000 g) in nondiabetic women has been **associated with a reduced risk for shoulder dystocia** (RR 0.32, 95% CI 0.12–0.85) **and associated morbidities** (RR 0.32, 95% CI 0.15–0.71) when compared to expectant management without increasing the risk for cesarean. In fact, induction of labor was associated with **increased likelihood of vaginal delivery** (RR 1.14, 95% CI 1.01–1.29) [29]. Thus, the number needed to treat to prevent one case of shoulder dystocia is 25 [30]. There were no cases of neonatal brachial plexus palsy (NBPP) in either group. Thus, there is no evidence that induction for suspected macrosomia influences the rate of NBPP.

Although the ACOG practice bulletin on fetal macrosomia [9] suggests that planned cesarean delivery should be considered if the EFW is at least 5000 g, there is insufficient evidence to assess this intervention, and there are insufficient reports on the peripartum outcomes when the fetus is suspected to have grade III macrosomia [4].

Diabetes

In insulin-requiring diabetic pregnancies, **induction at about 38 weeks**, compared to expectant management until 42 weeks, is associated with a significant decrease in the rate of macrosomic fetuses, but the limited sample size does not permit drawing "firm conclusions" [31,32].

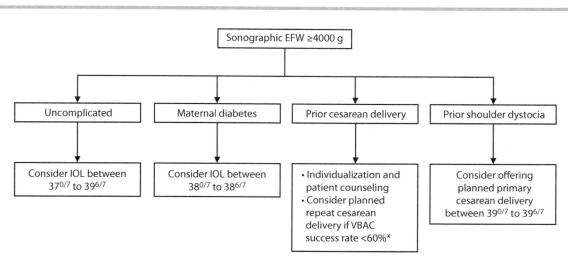

Figure 46.1 An algorithm for the management of suspected macrosomia.

A retrospective study concluded that a protocol involving induction for EFW ≥90% but <4250 g and cesarean delivery for sonographic weight ≥4250 g decreases the rate of shoulder dystocia by 50% but increases the rate of cesarean delivery by 16% [33]. Although the ACOG practice bulletin on fetal macrosomia [9] suggests that cesarean delivery among diabetics is indicated if the EFW is ≥4500 g, others have set the threshold at ≥4000 g [31,33] or at ≥4250 g [31] (see also Chapter 4).

Prior Cesarean Delivery

The majority of patients attempting vaginal birth after cesarean delivery (VBAC) can successfully deliver a macrosomic fetus [34–36]. The rate of uterine rupture may be higher (3.6%) for a macrosomic trial of labor with prior cesarean delivery, if the patient has not delivered vaginally before [37]. Thus, obstetric factors (prior deliveries, need for induction, etc.) should be considered when attempting VBAC with suspected macrosomia (see Chapter 14 in *Obstetric Evidence Based Guidelines*).

Prior Shoulder Dystocia

Women with prior shoulder dystocia are at much higher risk (about 12%–15%) of recurrence [38,39] (see Chapter 25 in *Obstetric Evidence Based Guidelines*). In the general obstetric population, the likelihood of brachial plexus injury is 1.4/1000 births, but among women who had prior shoulder dystocia and deliver vaginally, it is 13/1000 if there is no recurrent dystocia. If there is recurrent shoulder dystocia, the likelihood of brachial plexus injury is 45/1000 [39].

There are no randomized trials [4] on how to manage these pregnancies, but it is reasonable to discuss cesarean delivery at term when managing a patient with a prior shoulder dystocia because the likelihood of recurrent shoulder dystocia is quite high (about 12%–15% vs. 1% in general population) as is the risk of neurologic injury (see Chapter 25 in *Obstetric Evidence Based Guidelines*).

REFERENCES

1. Boulet SL, Alexander GR, Salihu HM, Pass M. Macrosomic births in the United States: Determinants, outcomes, and proposed grades of risk. *Am J Obstet Gynecol* 2003; 188(5): 1372–8. [Level II-1]
2. Campbell S. Fetal macrosomia: A problem in need of a policy. *Ultrasound Obstet Gynecol Off J Int Soc Ultrasound Obstet Gynecol* 2014; 43(1): 3–10. [Level III]
3. Hamilton BE, Martin JA, Osterman MH et al. National Vital Statistics Reports. Births: preliminary data for 2014. Available at: http://www.cdc.gov/nchs/data/nvsr/nvsr64/nvsr64_06.pdf. Accessed Nov. 02, 2015. [Epidemiologic data]
4. Chauhan SP, Grobman WA, Gherman RA, Chauhan VB, Chang G, Magann EF et al. Suspicion and treatment of the macrosomic fetus: A review. *Am J Obstet Gynecol* 2005; 193(2): 332–46. [Level III]
5. Shan X, Chen F, Wang W, Zhao J, Teng Y, Wu M et al. Secular trends of low birthweight and macrosomia and related maternal factors in Beijing, China: A longitudinal trend analysis. *BMC Pregnancy Childbirth* 2014; 14: 105. [Level II-2]
6. Kang B-H, Moon J-Y, Chung S-H, Choi Y-S, Lee K-S, Chang J-Y et al. Birth statistics of high birth weight infants (macrosomia) in Korea. *Korean J Pediatr* 2012; 55(8): 280–5. [Level III]
7. Statistics Denmark. Live births and stillbirths by weight of birth. 1998 and 2008 data. Available at: http://www.statbank.dk. [Epidemiologic data]
8. Koyanagi A, Zhang J, Dagvadorj A, Hirayama F, Shibuya K, Souza JP et al. Macrosomia in 23 developing countries: An analysis of a multicountry, facility-based, cross-sectional survey. *Lancet Lond Engl* 2013; 381(9865): 476–83. [Level II-2]
9. American College of Obstetricians and Gynecologists: Fetal macrosomia. ACOG Practice Bulletin No. 22. Washington DC: ACOG, 2000 (reaffirmed 2015). [Level III]
10. Chauhan SP, Martin RW, Morrison JC. Intrapartum hydramnios at term and perinatal outcome. *J Perinatol* 1993; 13: 186–9. [Level II-2]
11. Myles TD, Santolaya J. Maternal and neonatal outcomes in patients with a prolonged second stage of labor. *Obstet Gynecol* 2003; 102: 52–8. [Level II-2]
12. Crowther CA, Hiller JE, Moss JR et al. Effect of treatment of gestational diabetes mellitus on pregnancy outcomes. *N Engl J Med* 2005; 352: 2477–86. [RCT, n = 1000. Impaired glucose tolerance (defined following 75-g OGTT as fasting <7.0 mmol/L, 2 hours between 7.8 mmol/L and 11.0 mmol/L). Diet, glucose monitoring, and insulin as needed vs. routine care]
13. de Veciana M, Major CA, Morgan MA et al. Postprandial versus preprandial blood glucose monitoring in women with gestational diabetes mellitus requiring insulin therapy. *N Engl J Med* 1995; 333: 1237–41. [RCT, n = 66]
14. Murphy H, Rayman G, Lewis K et al. Effectiveness of continuous glucose monitoring in pregnant women with diabetes: Randomised clinical trial. *Br Med J* 2008; 337: a1680. [RCT, n = 71]
15. Bonomo M, Cetin I, Pisoni MP et al. Flexible treatment of gestational diabetes modulated on ultrasound evaluation of intrauterine growth: A controlled randomized clinical trial. *Diabetes Metab* 2004; 30: 237–44. [RCT n = 229]
16. Bonomo M, Corica D, Mion E et al. Evaluating the therapeutic approach in pregnancies complicated by borderline glucose intolerance: A randomized clinical trial. *Diabet Med* 2005; 1536–41. [RCT, n = 300]
17. Landon M, Sponge C, Thom E et al. A multicenter, randomized trial of treatment for mild gestational diabetes. *N Engl J Med* 2009; 361: 1339–48. [RCT, n = 958]
18. Galazis N, Docheva N, Smillis C, Nicolaides K. Maternal and neonatal outcomes in women undergoing bariatric surgery: A systematic review and meta-analysis. *Eur J Obstet Gynecol Reprod Biol* 2014; 181: 45–53. [Meta-analysis, 17 studies, n = 166,134]
19. Johanson K, Cnattingius, Näslund I et al. Outcomes of pregnancy after bariatric surgery. *NEJM* 2015; 372: 814–24. [Level II-1]
20. Wiebe H, Boulé N, Chari R. The effect of supervised prenatal exercise on fetal growth. *Obstet Gynecol* 2015; 125: 1185–94. [Meta-analysis, 36 studies, of which 28 were RCTs; n = 5322]
21. Nachum Z, Ben-Shlomo I, Weiner E et al. Twice daily versus four times daily insulin dose regimens for diabetes in pregnancy: Randomised controlled trial. *Br Med J* 1999; 319: 1223–7. [RCT, n = 392]
22. Langer O, Conway DL, Berkus MD et al. A comparison of glyburide and insulin in women with gestational diabetes mellitus. *N Engl J Med* 2000; 343: 1134–8. [RCT, n = 404]
23. Nicholson W, Bolen S, Witkop CT et al. Benefits and risks of oral diabetes agents compared with insulin in women with gestational diabetes: A systematic review. *Obstet Gynecol* 2009; 113: 193–205. [Meta-analysis; 9 studies of which 4 RCTs, n = 1229]
24. Hendrix NW, Grady CS, Chauhan SP. Clinical vs sonographic estimate of birth weight in term parturients: A randomized clinical trial. *J Reprod Med* 2000; 45: 317–22. [RCT, n = 758]
25. Gonen R, Spiegel D, Abend M. Is macrosomia predictable, and are shoulder dystocia and birth trauma preventable? *Obstet Gynecol* 1996; 88: 526–9. [Level II-1]
26. Gonen R, Bader D, Ajami M. Effects of a policy of elective cesarean delivery in cases of suspected fetal macrosomia on the incidence of brachial plexus injury and the rate of cesarean delivery. *Am J Obstet Gynecol* 2000; 183: 1296–300. [Level II-1]
27. Ugwu EO, Udealor PC, Dim CC, Obi SN, Ozumba BC, Okeke DO et al. Accuracy of clinical and ultrasound estimation of fetal weight in predicting actual birth weight in Enugu, Southeastern Nigeria. *Niger J Clin Pract* 2014; 17(3): 270–5. [Level II-1]

28. Skråstad RB, Eik-Nes SH, Sviggum O, Johansen OJ, Salvesen KÅ, Romundstad PR et al. A randomized controlled trial of third-trimester routine ultrasound in a non-selected population. *Acta Obstet Gynecol Scand* 2013; 92(12): 1353–60. [RCT, *n* = 6780]

29. Boulvain M, Senat M, Perrotin F et al. Induction of labour versus expectant management for large-for-date fetuses: A randomized controlled trial. *Lancet* 2015; 385: 2600–5. [RCT, *n* = 818]

30. Caughey A. Should pregnancies be induced for impending macrosomia? *Lancet* 2015; 385: 2557–9. [Level III]

31. Boulvain M, Stan C, Irion O. Elective delivery in diabetic pregnant women. *Cochrane Database Syst Rev* 2001; (2): CD001997. [Meta-analysis, *n* = 200]

32. Witkop C, Neale D, Wilson LM et al. Active compared with expectant delivery management in women with gestational diabetes: A systematic review. *Obstet Gynecol* 2009; 113(1): 206–17. [Meta-analysis; 5 studies of which 1 RCT, *n* = 200]

33. Conway DL, Langer O. Elective delivery of infants with macrosomia in diabetic women: Reduced shoulder dystocia versus increased cesarean deliveries. *Am J Obstet Gynecol* 1998; 178: 922–5. [Level II-1]

34. Phelan JP, Eglinton GS, Horenstein JM et al. Previous cesarean birth. Trial of labor in women with macrosomic infants. *J Reprod Med* 1984; 29: 36–40. [Level II-1]

35. Flamm BL, Goings JR. Vaginal birth after cesarean section: Is suspected fetal macrosomia a contraindication? *Obstet Gynecol* 1989; 74: 694–7. [Level II-1]

36. Zelop CM, Shipp TD, Repke JT et al. Outcomes of trial of labor following previous cesarean delivery among women with fetuses weighing > 4000 g. *Am J Obstet Gynecol* 2001; 185: 903–5. [Level II-1]

37. Elkousy MA, Sammel M, Stevens E et al. The effect of birth weight on vaginal birth after cesarean delivery success rates. *Am J Obstet Gynecol* 2003; 188: 824–30. [Level II-1]

38. Lewis DF, Raymond RC, Perkins MB et al. Recurrence rate of shoulder dystocia. *Am J Obstet Gynecol* 1995; 172: 1369–71. [Level II-2]

39. Bingham J, Chauhan SP, Hayes E et al. Recurrent shoulder dystocia: A review. *Obstet Gynecol Surv* 2010; 65: 183–8. [Level II-2]

47

Cytomegalovirus

Timothy J. Rafael

KEY POINTS

- Cytomegalovirus (CMV) is the most common cause of viral intrauterine infection, affecting **0.5% to 1.5% of all neonates.**
- In most of the cases, pregnant women acquire CMV by **exposure to children** in their home or from occupational exposure to children.
- Approximately **1%–4% of immunoglobulin G (IgG)-negative women acquire CMV infection during pregnancy.** Approximately **one third** (range 30%–65%) **of pregnant women with a primary infection transmit CMV infection to their fetus.** The rate of transmission increases with increase in gestational age (highest in the third trimester), but the severity of disease is instead inversely proportional to gestational age (the infant is most affected when maternal infection is in the first trimester). Overall, about **15% to 20% of infected infants develop sequelae** (so about 5%–8% of infants of infected mothers have sequelae).
- Complications of affected infants with congenital CMV infection include jaundice, petechiae ("blueberry muffin baby"), thrombocytopenia, hepatosplenomegaly, growth restriction, microcephaly, intracranial calcifications, nonimmune hydrops, and preterm birth as well as late complications, such as hearing loss, mental retardation, delay in psychomotor development, chorioretinitis, optic atrophy, seizures, expressive language delays, and learning disabilities. Long-term mortality for severely affected infants is about 5%.
- **Prevention (including avoiding intimate contact with children, frequent handwashing, and glove use) is associated with an 84% decrease in CMV seroconversion during pregnancy.**
- CMV screening in pregnancy is not routinely recommended in most countries until an appropriate fetal intervention is proven to decrease neonatal disease in cases of maternal CMV infection.
- **Maternal diagnosis of CMV infection is by serum IgM+.**
- **Fetal diagnosis of CMV infection is by detection of virus in amniotic fluid (AF) by polymerase chain reaction (PCR) testing.**
- **Presence or absence of fetal abnormalities on ultrasound can** help counseling (Table 47.2), but ultrasound is very insensitive and poorly predictive of an affected (symptomatic) child.
- **There is no in utero therapy for CMV supported by level 1 data.** Hyperimmune globulin has not been found to be effective at preventing vertical transmission of CMV in a randomized controlled trial. Gancyclovir has not been evaluated in an RCT. Gancyclovir and CMV-specific hyperimmune globulin are not supported by sufficient evidence for recommendation at this time, and should not be used outside of a research-type setting.

PATHOGEN

CMV is a double-stranded DNA virus of the herpes family [1].

INCIDENCE/EPIDEMIOLOGY

CMV is the most common cause of viral intrauterine infection, affecting **0.5% to 1.5% of all neonates** in different parts of the world [2,3]. The birth prevalence of symptomatic congenital CMV is about 1 in 1000 [4]. The prevalence of CMV infection varies according to socioeconomic background. Overall in the United States, the seropositivity rate is approximately 50%; by background, it is 40% to 50% for women of middle and high, and 60% to more than 80% for women of lower socioeconomic background. The overall age-adjusted seroprevalence of CMV did not change significantly from 1988–1994 to 1999–2004 [5].

TRANSMISSION/RISK FACTORS/ASSOCIATIONS

Transmission usually occurs from close contact with contamination from urine, saliva, blood, semen, and cervical secretions [4]. Risk factors are low socioeconomic status, exposure to infective individuals, multiple partners, extremes of age, multiparity, and blood transfusion. Only cellular blood products that contain leukocytes are capable of transmitting CMV, and the risk factor is 0.1% to 0.4% per unit in immunocompetent recipients [6]. The incidence of cases with congenital disease following maternal recurrent infection has been shown to be increased with immunodeficiency, hormonal exposure, nutritional deficiency, and genital tract infections [7]. Although sexual transmission of CMV can occur, **in most cases pregnant women acquire CMV by exposure to children in their home or from occupational exposure to children.** Data extrapolated to the U.S. population estimate that every two years between 31,000 and 168,000 susceptible pregnant women will be exposed to CMV by an infected child [8].

SYMPTOMS

CMV is **usually asymptomatic or with symptoms so mild that it goes undiagnosed.** The symptoms might include a mononucleosis-like or flu-like syndrome, malaise, fatigue, lymphadenopathy, or persistent fever, and abnormal laboratory values (lymphocytosis, or increased aminotransferase levels). Rarely, hepatosplenomegaly, cough, headache, rash, and gastrointestinal symptoms can occur [9]. The presence of symptoms or laboratory abnormalities is highly suggestive of primary infection [10].

PATHOPHYSIOLOGY/CLASSIFICATION
General
The CMV virus leads to infected large cells with intranuclear inclusions. It has a 4- to 8-week period of incubation

and 3- to 12-month-long viremia (infants can shed virus for up to 6 years). Serious disease occurs only in immunocompromised adults or fetuses. The transmission of the virus to the fetus can follow either a primary or recurrent infection. **Approximately 1%–4% of immunoglobulin G (IgG)-negative women acquire CMV infection during pregnancy** [11]. **Approximately one third (range 30%–65%) of pregnant women with a primary infection transmit CMV infection to their fetus** (Figure 47.1) [2,3]. Even periconception infection a week before or up to five weeks after the last menstrual period (LMP) is associated with this rate of transmission although these rates may not be as high as previously thought [12]. **The rate of transmission increases with increase in gestational age (highest in third trimester), but the severity of disease is instead inversely proportional to gestational age (infant is most affected when maternal infection is in first trimester)** (Table 47.1) [13]. In fact, one series reported no

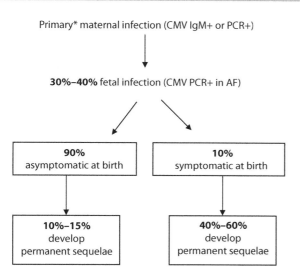

Figure 47.1 Natural history of CMV perinatal infection. *Abbreviations*: AF, amniotic fluid; CMV, cytomegalovirus; IgM, immunoglobulin M; PCR, polymerase chain reaction. *The prognosis is better for mothers with recurrent disease, with fetus having low risk of infection and low risk of developing sequelae. In fact, vertical transmission after recurrent infection is 0.5%–2%. (From Dollard SC, Grosse SD, Ross, DS. *Rev Med Virol*, 17, 5, 355–63, 2007; Kenneson A, Cannon MJ. *Rev Med Virol*, 17, 253–76, 2007.)

Table 47.1 Pooled Likelihood of Congenital Infection by Timing of Maternal Infection

Maternal Infection	Probability of Congenital Infection (%)
Preconception[a]	5.2
Periconception[a]	16.4
First trimester	36.5
Second trimester	40.1
Third trimester	65

Source: Modified from Picone O, Vauloup-Fellous C, Cordier AG et al. *Prenat Diagn*, 33, 751–8, 2013.

[a]In their cohort, Picone et al. define the "preconception" time period as 2 months to 3 weeks before the date of conception and "periconception" as 3 weeks before to 3 weeks after the date of conception. Please note that the above table represents their data combined with other existing literature, in which the definitions of pre- and periconception vary slightly.

affected neonates if fetuses were infected after 26 weeks if the ultrasound findings are normal [14]. The risk of congenital CMV disease at birth is mainly associated with maternal primary infection, but the presence of maternal antibodies before conception does not prevent transmission in all cases even if it is protective in most cases.

Primary Infection

Fetal infection generally (99.5%) occurs following maternal primary infection and rarely following recurrent CMV infection (Figure 47.1). Of the women who are not immune (IgG–, IgM–) for CMV at the beginning of pregnancy, about 2% acquire maternal infection. Transplacental transmission may occur weeks or months after primary maternal CMV infection and can be isolated from the AF by a PCR DNA technique to positively identify intrauterine transmission of CMV. **Overall, about 15% to 20% of infected infants develop sequelae (so about 5%–8% of infants of infected mothers have sequelae).**

Recurrent Infection

Recurrent infections can occur with immunosuppression and during pregnancy. Recurrent infections during pregnancy are most often asymptomatic and primarily caused by the reactivation of the endogenous virus but can also be caused by a low-grade chronic infection or reinfection by a different strain of CMV [15]. The risk of vertical transmission with recurrent infection is about 1.4% (range 0.5%–2%) [3]. Recurrent infection is responsible for only 0.5% of CMV congenital infections. Neonates infected from recurrent maternal infection have no symptoms at birth, do not have CMV in urine, and have a <10% risk of sequelae (hearing loss and chorioretinitis) [9].

Clinical Neonatal Findings and Complications

Clinical findings of symptomatic congenital CMV infection include **jaundice, petechiae (blueberry muffin baby), thrombocytopenia, hepatosplenomegaly, growth restriction, microcephaly, intracranial calcifications, nonimmune hydrops, and preterm birth** [1,16]. Primary and recurrent CMV has also been suggested as causes of isolated idiopathic IUGR [17]. CMV disease has late complications such as **hearing loss, mental retardation, delay in psychomotor development, chorioretinitis, optic atrophy, seizures, expressive language delays, and learning disabilities** [18]. CMV is the most common cause of congenital sensorineural hearing loss [19]. It appears that moderate or severe outcomes, when present, are identified by 1 year of age. Most impairment detected for the first time after 1 year of age appears to be milder in nature [20]. Long-term **mortality** for severely affected infants is about 5%.

PREGNANCY MANAGEMENT
Counseling/Prognosis

Counseling should include at least the natural history of the disease, the chances of vertical transmission, prognosis, and complications (Figure 47.1 and Table 47.2) [4,21]. A quantitative PCR count of $\geq 10^3$ genome equivalents/mL of AF is a certain sign of congenital infection, and $\geq 10^5$ genome equivalents/mL can predict symptomatic infection (Figure 47.2) [22]. In cases of severely injured fetuses on ultrasound, there is a high likelihood of sequelae, and pregnancy termination

Table 47.2 Chance of Affected (i.e., Symptomatic) Neonate Depending on Clinical Scenario of CMV Infection

Maternal	Fetal	Ultrasound	Affected Infant (reference)
Confirmed infection (e.g., seroconversion, with positive IgM)	Unknown	Normal	5%–7% [4]
	Unknown	Abnormal	35% [21]
	Confirmed infection (e.g., positive AF PCR)	Normal	14%–20% [4]
	Confirmed infection (e.g., positive AF PCR)	Abnormal	78% [21]

Abbreviations: AF, amniotic fluid; PCR, polymerase chain reaction.

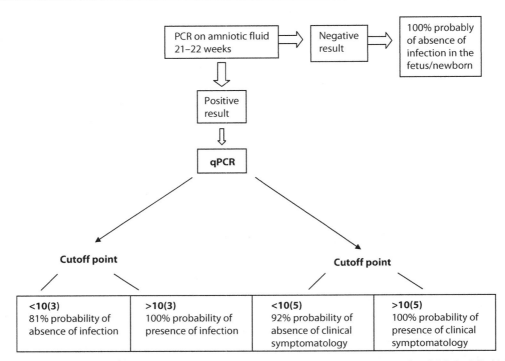

Figure 47.2 Assessment of chance of fetal infection and long-term complications by quantitative PCR in AF. *Abbreviations*: PCR, polymerase chain reaction; AF, amniotic fluid. (From Guerra B, Lazzarotto T, Quarta S et al. *Am J Ostet Gynecol*, 183, 476–82, 2000.)

can be offered as a management option [23]. When no ultrasonographic abnormalities are detected, the incidence of postnatal neurologic abnormalities is about 15% to 20% [24,25].

Prevention

Hygiene

Despite a higher prevalence of CMV-related childhood morbidity and mortality when compared with other infections, a recent survey study demonstrated only 13% of women being aware of congenital CMV. Most women practice behaviors that may place them at risk when interacting with children (e.g., kissing on lips, sharing utensils, sharing food, changing diapers, wiping child's nose, handling child's toys) [26]. Compared with no prevention, **prevention (including avoiding intimate contact with children, frequent hand washing, and glove use) is associated with an 84% decrease in CMV seroconversion during pregnancy,** especially in women in contact with children in day care facilities [27]. Following the administration of oral and written hygienic information to susceptible pregnant women, seroconversion rates during pregnancy have been reported to be as low as 0.26% [28].

Vaccine

A live-attenuated CMV vaccine is available but may be reactivated, and safety issues have not been resolved. In a trial including CMV-seronegative women of childbearing age, a **glycoprotein B vaccine demonstrated a 50% efficacy in preventing CMV infection**. One congenital infection occurred in the vaccine group, and three infections occurred in the placebo group although the sample size was not large enough to test the efficacy in reducing congenital infection [29]. Although this vaccine may have the potential to decrease incident cases of congenital CMV infection, it is likely that a CMV vaccine will not be available clinically for several years.

Screening

Serum

CMV screening in pregnancy is not routinely recommended in most countries even in women who are seronegative, mainly given the lack of proven intervention if seroconversion is detected [1].

If an appropriate fetal intervention is proven to decrease neonatal disease in cases of CMV, screening with IgM and IgG levels should be performed on all pregnant women between 8 and 12 weeks. IgM is 75% sensitive and persists for four to eight months. Seronegative women should be provided with basic information on how to avoid infection [28]. A second and possibly a third antibody control at 18 to 20 weeks and at 30 to 32 weeks could be recommended. IgG-positive and IgM-negative women with high IgG avidity index (e.g., >65%) could be assured of no risk of primary infection, which causes the majority of sequelae in the fetus [30]. No further controls would be necessary [18]. **Currently, however, there is no in utero therapy for CMV supported by level 1 data, and therefore routine CMV screening in pregnancy cannot be recommended** [11].

Ultrasound Fetal Findings

These findings are **growth restriction, ventriculomegaly, oligohydramnios, echogenic bowel, choroid plexus cyst (unilateral), pleural effusion, brain and liver calcification, and hydrops fetalis** [24]. Microcephaly, hydrocephaly, and intracranial calcifications are signs of high risk for neonatal sequelae [18]. A fetal cerebral periventricular "halo" seen on ultrasound examination is also suggestive of fetal infection and may be associated with white-matter lesions [31]. The limitations of ultrasound are well known. Fetal abnormalities may become evident late, change, or disappear during pregnancy, **and not all symptoms of congenital inclusion disease are detectable by ultrasound.** Ultrasound detects fetal abnormalities in only 8.5% of women with primary CMV infection and in 15% of congenitally CMV-infected fetuses. If fetal ultrasound abnormalities are detected, symptomatic CMV infection is present in 35% of neonates of primary-infected mothers and 78% of congenitally infected neonates (Table 47.2) [21].

Investigations/Diagnosis/Workup

Maternal primary CMV infection is diagnosed by IgM+ serum, which persists for four to eight months. Although seroconversion is a reliable method for diagnosing primary CMV infection, the diagnosis can be problematic. The rise in CMV-specific antibodies may be delayed for up to four weeks, and the presence of CMV-specific IgM can be found in up to 10% of women with recurrent disease. Of newly found IgM+ women, approximately 50% will be found on follow up immunoblot testing to be IgM negative with high CMV IgG avidity and can be provided some reassurance [32]. Although CMV can be transmitted to the fetus both by primary and secondary (recurrent) infection, invasive prenatal diagnosis should be offered to women with primary infection as they are at higher risk for fetal infection. In recurrent infection, the presence of maternal CMV IgG offers good protection, and fetal infection occurs only in 0.5% to 1% of cases [22].

At present, **detection of virus in AF by PCR testing is the most accurate means of diagnosis for CMV infection in the fetus** with sensitivities ranging from 80% to 100% [25]. Amniocentesis provides a direct method of diagnosing intrauterine CMV infection because the infected fetus excretes the virus via urine into AF. **The sensitivity of detecting a true infection by sampling the AF increases after 21 weeks gestation and after a minimum of 6 weeks interval following maternal primary infection, so that if an amniocentesis is performed before this interval, it should be repeated later** [7,25]. It does not appear that amniocentesis, in and of itself, is implicated in iatrogenic CMV infection of the fetus [33].

CMV DNA detected in AF reveals a history of viremia but it does not directly demonstrate the current fetal condition [19]. **Quantitative PCR in amniotic fluid can help predict infection and later sequelae** (Figure 47.2). Infected fetuses may also have abnormal ultrasound findings. Normal fetal ultrasound does not rule out severe neurological damage. Percutaneous umbilical blood sampling (PUBS) should be avoided and has been used in the past to diagnose the fetus with a high suspicion for CMV and negative PCR. The use of viral culture has decreased also because it takes 2 to 6 weeks to obtain final results.

Neonatal diagnosis is based on detection of PCR in body fluids, in particular in urine.

Therapy

CMV-Specific Hyperimmune Globulin

There is insufficient evidence to recommend CMV-specific hyperimmune globulin for prevention or treatment of CMV congenital infection. In a nonrandomized study, CMV hyper-immune globulin IV 100 U/kg every month until delivery to the mother for prevention of vertical transmission in primary maternal CMV infection was associated with a decrease in the incidence of infected neonates from 40% in controls to 16% [34]. Maternal CMV hyperimmune globulin 200 U/kg IV to the mother (with additional AF or umbilical cord infusions for persistent ultrasound findings) for therapy of known CMV DNA+ fetuses was associated with a decrease in the incidence of symptomatic CMV disease at birth from 50% in controls to 3% [34]. Follow-up to this study demonstrated a resolution of abnormal ultrasound findings in three treated fetuses, who subsequently had normal sensory, mental, and motor development at four to seven years of age [35]. In the original study, almost all these women were infected in the first or second trimester. A case of resolution of hydrops secondary to CMV fetal infection with CMV-specific hyperimmune globulin has been reported [36]. These findings were not validated in a **randomized, placebo-controlled, double-blind study** conducted in Italy [37]. This study randomized 124 pregnant women with primary CMV infection at 5–26 weeks to monthly hyperimmune globulin (100 U/kg) or placebo until 36 weeks gestation or until detection of CMV in amniotic fluid. The rate of congenital infection was 30% in the hyperimmune globulin group and 44% in the placebo group ($p = .13$). There was no significant difference between the two groups in viral DNA load in the amniotic fluid of infected fetuses or with respect to viral DNA in the urine or blood in infected newborns. Obstetrical complications (preterm birth, preeclampsia, and fetal growth restriction) occurred in 13% of the women in the hyperimmune globulin group compared with 2% in the placebo group ($p = .06$). Therefore, **at this time, the use of hyperimmune globulin for the prevention of vertical transmission of CMV is not recommended outside of a research setting** [11]. Two randomized, phase 3 studies for the prevention of congenital infection are currently underway, one sponsored by the NICHD in the United States (ClinicalTrials.gov NCT 01376778) and the other sponsored by Biotest in Europe. Further analyses will be forthcoming [38].

Ganciclovir and Valacyclovir

Ganciclovir inhibits viral DNA polymerase, and has been used successfully in adults, especially immunocompromised (AIDS, transplant, etc.) patients. **There are no randomized controlled trials evaluating fetal therapy with ganciclovir.** Ganciclovir administration into the umbilical vein and anti-CMV IgG injections into the fetal abdominal cavity have been reported in case reports [19] as has ganciclovir given orally to a pregnant woman with CMV DNA in the AF, but the evaluation of the prognosis is not well established; case reports have shown no teratogenicity of ganciclovir given in the early stages of pregnancy [39]. A small pediatric trial demonstrated reduction of hearing loss in neonates with proven congenital CMV infection with CNS involvement when treatment was begun within one month of birth [40].

There are no randomized controlled trials evaluating fetal therapy with valacyclovir. Valacyclovir (8 g/day orally for a median of 7 weeks) given to women with congenitally CMV-infected fetuses at about 30 weeks of gestations was associated with about a 50% normal child outcome at 1 to 5 years of age in one nonrandomized study [41]. A recent pediatric trial examining 6-week versus 6-month regimens of valganciclovir for the treatment of symptomatic congenital CMV infants found that the 6-month regimen did not improve hearing in the short term, but appeared to modestly improve hearing and developmental outcomes in the longer term, when compared to the 6-week regimen [42].

REFERENCES

1. ACOG Practice bulletin. *Cytomegalovirus, Parvovirus B19, Varicella Zoster, and Toxoplasmosis in Pregnancy.* No 151, June 2015. [Review]
2. Dollard SC, Grosse SD, Ross, DS. New estimates of the prevalence of neurological and sensory sequelae and mortality associated with congenital cytomegalovirus infection. *Rev Med Virol* 2007; 17(5): 355–63. [Review]
3. Kenneson A, Cannon MJ. Review and meta-analysis of the epidemiology of congenital cytomegalovirus (CMV) infection. *Rev Med Virol* 2007; 17: 253–76. [Review]
4. Bhide A, Papageoghiou AT. Managing primary CMV infection in pregnancy. *BJOG* 2008; 115: 805–7. [Review]
5. Lewis Bate S, Dollard SC, Cannon MJ. Cytomegalovirus seroprevalence in the United States: The national health and nutrition examination surveys, 1988–2004. *Clin Infect Dis* 2010; 50(11): 1439–47. [III]
6. Triulzi DJ. Transfusion transmitted cytomegalovirus. Available at: http://www.itxm.org/archive/tmu8-94.htm. [II-3; web document]
7. Henrich W, Meckies J, Dudenhausen JW et al. Recurrent CMV infection during pregnancy: Ultrasonographic diagnosis and fetal outcome. *Ultrasound Obstet Gynecol* 2002; 19: 608–11. [II-3]
8. Marshall BC, Adler SP. The frequency of pregnancy and exposure to cytomegalovirus infections among women with a young child in day care. *Am J Obstet Gynecol* 2009; 200: 163.e1–5. [III]
9. Nigro G. Maternal-fetal cytomegalovirus infection: From diagnosis to therapy. *J Matern Fetal Neonatal Med* 2009; 22(2): 169–74. [Review]
10. Nigro G, Anceschi MM, Cosmi EV. Clinical manifestations and abnormal laboratory findings in pregnant women with primary cytomegalovirus infection. *BJOG* 2003; 110: 572–7. [II-3]
11. Society for Maternal-Fetal Medicine (SMFM) Consult #39: Diagnosis and antenatal management of congenital cytomegalovirus (CMV) infection. *Am J Obstet Gynecol* 2016. pii:S0002-9378(16)00342-2. doi:10.1016/j.ajog.2016.02.042. [III; Guideline]
12. Hadar E, Yogev Y, Melamed N et al. Periconceptional cytomegalovirus infection: Pregnancy outcome and rate of vertical transmission. *Prenat Diagn* 2010; 30: 1213–6. [II-3]
13. Picone O, Vauloup-Fellous C, Cordier AG et al. A series of 238 cytomegalovirus primary infections during pregnancy: Description and outcome. *Prenat Diagn* 2013; 33: 751–8. [II-3]
14. Gindes L, Teperberg-Oikawa M, Sherman D et al. Congenital cytomegalovirus infection following primary maternal infection in the third trimester. *BJOG* 2008; 115: 830–5. [II-2]
15. Boppana SH, Rivera L, Fowler KB et al. Intrauterine transmission of CMV to infants of women with preconceptional immunity. *N Engl J Med* 2001; 344: 1366–71. [II-3]
16. Kylat RI, Kelly EN, Ford-Jones EL. Clinical findings and adverse outcome in neonates with symptomatic congenital cytomegalovirus (SCCMV) infection. *Eur J Pediatr* 2006; 165: 773–8. [II-3]
17. Pereira L, Petitt M, Fong A et al. Intrauterine growth restriction caused by underlying congenital cytomegalovirus infection. *J Infect Dis* 2014; 209: 1573–84. [II-3]
18. Azam A-Z, Vial Y, Fawer CL et al. Prenatal diagnosis of congenital CMV infection. *Obstet Gynecol* 2001; 97: 443–8. [II-2]
19. Matsuda H, Kawakami Y, Furaya K et al. Intrauterine therapy for a CMV infected symptomatic fetus. *BJOG* 2004; 111: 756–7. [II-3]
20. Townsend CL, Forsgren M, Ahlfors K et al. Long-term outcomes of congenital cytomegalovirus infection in Sweden and the United Kingdom. *Clin Infect Dis* 2013; 56(9): 1232–9. [II-2]
21. Guerra B, Simonazzi G, Puccetti C et al. Ultrasound prediction of symptomatic congenital cytomegalovirus infection. *Am J Obstet Gynecol* 2008; 198: 380.e1–7. [II-3]
22. Guerra B, Lazzarotto T, Quarta S et al. Prenatal diagnosis of symptomatic congenital CMV infection. *Am J Ostet Gynecol* 2000; 183: 476–82. [II-2]
23. Liesnard C, Donner C, Brancart F et al. Prenatal diagnosis of congenital CMV infection: Prospective study of 237 pregnancies at risk. *Obstet Gynecol* 2000; 95: 881–8. [II-2]
24. Lipitz S, Achiron R, Zalen Y et al. Outcome of pregnancies with vertical transmission of primary CMV infection. ACOG. *Obstet Gynecol* 2002; 100: 428–33. [II-3]
25. Oshiro BR. CMV infection in pregnancy. *Contemp Obstet Gynecol* 1999; 11: 16–24. [Review]
26. Cannon MJ, Westbrook K, Levis D et al. Awareness of and behavior related to child-to-mother transmission of cytomegalovirus. *Prevent Med* 2012; 54: 351–7. [II-3]
27. Adler SP, Finney JW, Manganello AM et al. Prevention of child-to-mother transmission of cytomegalovirus among pregnant women. *J Pediatr* 2004; 145: 485–91. [I, RCT, n = 166]
28. Picone O, Vauloup-Fellous C, Cordier AG et al. A 2-year study on cytomegalovirus infection during pregnancy in a French hospital. *BJOG* 2009; 116: 818–23. [II-3]
29. Pass RF, Zhang C, Evans A et al. Vaccine prevention of maternal cytomegalovirus infection. *N Engl J Med* 2009; 360: 1191–9. [I, RCT, n = 464]
30. Kanengisser-Pines B, Hazan Y, Pines G et al. High cytomegalovirus IgG avidity is a reliable indicator of past infection in patients with positive IgM detected during the first trimester of pregnancy. *J Perinat Med* 2009; 37: 15–8. [II-3]
31. Simonazzi G, Guerra B, Bonasoni P et al. Fetal cerebral periventricular halo at midgestation: an ultrasound finding suggestive of fetal cytomegalovirus infection. *Am J Obstet Gynecol* 2010; 202: 599.e1–5. [II-3]
32. Lazzarotto T, Guerra B, Lanari M et al. New advances in the diagnosis of congenital cytomegalovirus infection. *J Clin Virol* 2008; 41(3): 192–7. [Review]

33. Revello MG, Furione M, Zavattoni M et al. Human cytomegalovirus (HCMV) DNAemia in the mother at amniocentesis as a risk factor for iatrogenic HCMV infection of the fetus. *J Infect Dis* 2008; 197: 593–6. [II-3]

34. Nigro G, Adler SP, La Torre R et al. Passive immunization during pregnancy for Congenital CMV infection. *N Engl J Med* 2005; 353: 1350–62. [II-1]

35. Nigro G, La Torre R, Pentimalli H et al. Regression of fetal cerebral abnormalities by primary cytomegalovirus infection following hyperimmunoglobulin therapy. *Prenat Diagn* 2008; 28: 512–7. [II-3]

36. Moxley K, Knudson EJ. Resolution of hydrops secondary to cytomegalovirus after maternal and fetal treatment with human cytomegalovirus hyperimmune globulin. *Obstet Gynecol* 2008; 111: 524–6. [Case report; III]

37. Revello MG, Lazzarotto T, Guerra B et al. A randomized trial of hyperimmune globulin to prevent congenital cytomegalovirus. *N Engl J Med* 2014; 370: 1316–26. [I, RCT, *n* = 124]

38. McCarthy FP, Giles ML, Rowlands S et al. Antenatal interventions for preventing the transmission of cytomegalovirus (CMV) from the mother to fetus during pregnancy and adverse outcomes in the congenitally infected infant. *Cochrane Database Syst Rev* 2011; (3): CD008371. doi:10.1002/14651858.CD008371. [Meta-analysis]

39. Adler SP, Nigro G, Pereira L. Recent advances in the prevention and treatment of congenital cytomegalovirus infections. *Semin Perinatol* 2007; 31(1): 10–8. [Review]

40. Kimberlin DW, Lin C-Y, Sanchez PJ et al. Effect of ganciclovir therapy on hearing in symptomatic congenital cytomegalovirus disease involving the central nervous system: A randomized, controlled trial. *J Pediatr* 2003; 143: 16–25. [I, RCT, *n* = 42]

41. Jacquemard F, Yamamoto M, Costa J-M et al. Maternal administration of valacyclovir in symptomatic intrauterine cytomegalovirus infection. *BJOG* 2007; 114: 1113–21. [II-2]

42. Kimberlin DW, Jester PM, Sanchez PJ et al. Valganciclovir for symptomatic congenital cytomegalovirus disease. *N Engl J Med* 2015; 372: 933–43. [I, RCT, *n* = 96]

48

Toxoplasmosis

Corina N. Schoen and Timothy J. Rafael

KEY POINTS

- Maternal infection starts with ingestion (from food, water, hands, or insects) **of cysts from uncooked/ undercooked meat of infected animals *or* contact with oocysts from infected cats or contaminated soil.**
- Fetal/neonatal disease **is more severe if maternal infection occurs in the first trimester, and the incidence of maternal-fetal transmission is directly proportional to gestational age** (low in first trimester, high in third trimester).
- **Prevention by educating women to avoid exposures** has been shown to **decrease the incidence of the disease and remains the most important of interventions.**
- **Prenatal and/or neonatal screening** is controversial and is not adopted in most countries because of low incidence, concerns with poor/difficult diagnosis, availability of diagnostic and therapeutic services, population compliance, and high risk of terminating false-positive fetuses.
- The principle method used to diagnose and evaluate timing of congenital infection is based on detection of specific antibodies and by monitoring the immune response. *Maternal infection* **is diagnosed by sending maternal serology to a reference laboratory. *Fetal congenital infection* is diagnosed by amniotic fluid (AF) polymerase chain reaction (PCR).**
- **Correct interpretation of serologic testing carried out in a reference laboratory decreases unnecessary anxiety and even terminations.**
- **If maternal infection is confirmed by a reference laboratory, start spiramycin 3 to 4 g/day.**
- **If AF PCR is positive, start sulfadiazine, pyrimethamine, and folinic acid.**

PATHOGEN

Toxoplasma gondii (TG) is an obligate intracellular protozoan (parasite).

INCIDENCE/EPIDEMIOLOGY

The incidence of *primary acute maternal infection* is 0.01% to 0.1% in the United States and United Kingdom. The prevalence of past infection is approximately 22% in the United States [1,2] and as high as 44% in France/Europe [3]; 50% to 70% in Latin American countries; and 5% to 35% in Asia, China, and Korea. Once immune, immunity lasts for life [4].

The incidence of *congenital infection* is approximately 1.5 cases per 1000 live births worldwide, 0.5 to 1.5 per 1000 live births in France/Europe [5,6], and 0.7 per 1000 live births in the United States [6,7].

SYMPTOMS

There are *almost* never maternal symptoms; occasionally flu/ mononucleosis-like fever, fatigue, rash, and lymphadenopathy (around head and neck) can be associated with maternal infection. Rarely pregnant women will present with visual changes due to chorioretinitis from recently acquired infection or reactivation of chronic infection [8].

PATHOPHYSIOLOGY

TG can infect any mammal, which serves as an intermediate host. The definitive host is the cat (only one that can support both sexual and asexual reproduction). The parasite can exist as

1. Trophozoite (invasive form)
2. Cyst (latent form)
3. Oocyst (only in cats)

Sexual reproduction occurs in the small intestine of the cat that has eaten tissue cysts containing TG. Only during this first exposure is the cat infectious as these oocysts are produced for two weeks and contain infectious sporozoites. The oocysts require one to five days to become infected, and after two weeks, the cat is not infectious and becomes immune. Oocysts can remain infectious for years in soil. Human infection starts with **ingestion** (from food, water, hands, or insects) **of cysts from uncooked/undercooked meat of infected animals** (e.g., lamb and mutton) *or* **contact with oocysts from infected cats** (who get it from infected mice, etc.) **or contaminated soil**. The infected oocysts become infective inside the pregnant woman in 4 to 10 (average 7) days, leading to parasitemia. Eventually, TG can infect and live forever in striated muscle or brain. Only a very few cases of congenital toxoplasmosis transmitted by mothers who were infected prior to conception have been reported; they can be attributed to either reinfection with a different strain or to reactivation of chronic disease. This reactivation is very rare but can occur, especially in an immunocompromised woman. Immunocompetent women with prior toxoplasmosis can be reassured that the risks to the subsequent fetus/neonate are miniscule, especially >9 months after infection [4].

MATERNAL-FETAL TRANSMISSION

Primary maternal TG infection in pregnancy can lead to fetal infection with this rate highly dependent on gestational age of maternal infection [4] (Table 48.1) (Figure 48.1). Overall, the **vertical transmission rate ranges from approximately 20% to 50%** [9,10]. A recent meta-analysis based on 20 cohorts worldwide reports transmission rates of approximately 20% [10]. This analysis did not include many European cohorts included in an individual patient data meta-analysis by the SYROCOT study group, which reports much higher transmission rates ranging from 16% to 52% [9].

Table 48.1 Likelihood of Congenital Infection by Timing
of Maternal Infection

Maternal Infection	Probability of Congenital Infection (%)
Preconception[a]	1
First trimester	10–25
Second trimester	30–55
Third trimester	60–80

Source: Modified from Rorman E, Zamir CS, Rilkis I et al. *Reprod
Toxicol*, 21, 4, 458–72, 2006.
[a]Usually within nine months of conception.

Of congenitally infected fetuses who are PCR positive
by amniocentesis, 74% to 81% manifest only subclinical infection (only serologically positive) whereas 19% to 26% have fetal/
childhood illness even if they received treatment [9,11]. Overall,
about 7% of fetuses of primary infected mothers are affected.
**Fetal/neonatal disease is more severe if maternal infection
occurs in the first trimester**, but more common if maternal
infection occurs in the third trimester. A fetus has a <1/1000 risk
of being affected if infected at less than 4 weeks gestational age.

COMPLICATIONS

Fetal/neonatal complications are present in **36%** of cases in
one series and include ventriculomegaly, increased placental
thickness, hepatomegaly, ascites, intracranial calcifications,
hydrocephalus, microcephaly, and hepatosplenomegaly [12].
In the neonate, TG congenital infection is associated with neonatal **chorioretinitis** [11] (most prevalent consequence of TG),
deafness, decreased IQ, and subsequent blindness, seizure
disorders, and delay in neuropsychomotor development [4].

Congenital infection may also be associated with an
increased risk of preterm birth (PTB) (OR 3.49, 95% CI 1.91–
6.37), abortion (OR 6.63, 95% CI 4.56–9.65), stillbirth (OR 4.63,
95% CI 2.72–7.90), and intrauterine growth restriction (IUGR)
(OR 4.49, 95% CI 2.10–9.57) compared to uninfected controls.
Neonatal death is rare [10].

PREGNANCY MANAGEMENT
Principles

Counseling regarding basic pathophysiology, maternal-fetal
transmission, complications, and preventive/therapeutic

Table 48.2 Prevention of Congenital Toxoplasmosis

- Avoid raw or undercooked meat or eggs of any origin
- Use gloves when in contact with soil
- Wash fruits and vegetables before eating
- Avoid changing cat litter, wash hands after handling cats/litter
- Keep pet cats indoors and use commercial pet food

management should be done. Termination can be offered,
especially if the fetus is definitively positive (PCR-positive
AF) and the infection occurred in the first trimester (worse
prognosis).

Prevention

**Prevention has been shown to decrease the incidence of the
disease and remains the most important of interventions**
(Table 48.2). Although many U.S. obstetricians are counseling
adequately regarding avoidance of cat litter, more information needs to be provided to patients regarding avoidance of
raw or undercooked meat, gardening, and washing fruits and
vegetables [13]. **Prenatal education** can effectively change
pregnant women's behavior as it increases pet, personal, and
food hygiene [14]. Observational studies suggest prenatal
education may have a positive effect on the congenital toxoplasmosis rate, but there is limited evidence from RCTs supporting this [15].

Screening
Serum

Routine toxoplasmosis screening programs for pregnant
women have been established in some European countries,
such as France and Austria. **In the United Kingdom and the
United States, no prenatal or neonatal screening for TG is
formally recommended** by appropriate medical societies but
not without controversy [16,17]. Prenatal maternal screening has not been recommended in the United States because
of low incidence, concerns with poor/difficult diagnosis,
availability of diagnostic and therapeutic services, population compliance, and high risk of terminating false positive
fetuses. If prenatal screening is implemented, it should start

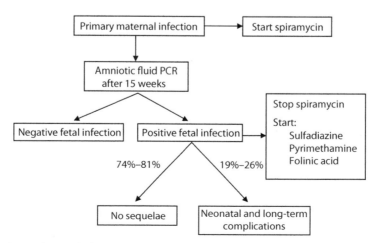

Figure 48.1 Natural history of toxoplasmosis in pregnancy.

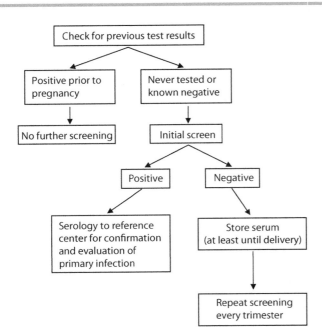

Figure 48.2 Laboratory diagnosis of congenital toxoplasmosis. (Modified from Rorman E, Zamir CS, Rilkis I et al. *Reprod Toxicol*, 21, 4, 458–72, 2006.)

preconception or at least in the first trimester and be repeated every month (or at least every trimester) in all IgG-negative mothers (Figure 48.2). Neonatal screening in the United States would detect about one positive neonate for every 12,000 screened mothers. The infected woman could receive treatment that may prevent severe sequelae, but this would probably not be cost-effective. In a decision analysis applying the French prenatal screening protocol to a U.S. population, monthly maternal screening was predicted to have a cost savings of $620 per child screened. Although accounting for low prevalence of maternal toxoplasmosis in the United States, the study did not account for a high false positive antibody screen likely to be encountered in this population [18]. Further study should be performed before clinical guidelines on screening are changed from the current recommendations against screening, at least in the United States.

Ultrasound
Ultrasound findings associated with TG congenital infection can include intracranial calcifications, microcephaly, ventricular dilatation and hydrocephalus, ascites, hepatosplenomegaly, and increased placental thickness [19].

Workup/Diagnosis

The principle method used to diagnose and evaluate the timing of congenital infection is based on detection of specific antibodies and monitoring the immune response (Figure 48.2). *IgG antibodies* usually appear within two weeks of infection and persist in the body indefinitely. *IgM antibodies* are considered to be a sign of recent infection and can be detected by enzyme immunoassays (EIAs) or an immunosorbent agglutination assay test (IAAT) within two weeks of infection. They often remain positive for up to one to two years. **A positive IgM antibody test result** at any time **does**

not necessarily mean the infection was acquired recently; this needs to be confirmed at a reference laboratory. Only approximately 22%–40% of positive IgM results obtained at nonreference laboratories in the United States are deemed to have had a recent acute infection [8,20]. *IgA antibodies* may also persist for more than one year, and their detection is informative mainly for the diagnosis of congenital toxoplasmosis. *IgE antibodies* increase rapidly and remain detectable for less than four months after infection, which is a very short time to use them for a diagnostic test.

The Sabin–Feldman dye test (SFDT) is still considered the "gold standard" [4]. It detects the presence of anti-TG-specific antibodies (total Ig). The absolute antibody titer is also important: values over 250 IU/mL are considered highly suggestive of recent infection. IgG avidity testing is based on the increase in functional affinity (avidity) between TG-specific IgG and antigen over time as the host immune response evolves. Pregnant women with high avidity antibodies are those who have been infected at least three to five months earlier [21]. In a prospective cohort of 139 women, an avidity index above 30% was not associated with any positive amniocentesis or congenital infection [22]. Current testing cannot define which specific strain of TG caused the antibody response, so that reinfection with the same or different strains cannot be determined.

Maternal infection **is diagnosed by sending maternal serology to a reference laboratory** (in the United States: Jack Remington, Palo Alto: 650-853-4828; FAX 650-614-3292; http://www.pamf.org/serology/clinicianguide.html). It is best to make the diagnosis based on two different serum specimens collected at least four weeks apart. Usually, the reference laboratory reports serologic results with a high possibility of infection if there is the following:

- Seroconversion during pregnancy
- Increase in both specific IgG titer (>3-fold) and dye test titer (>3-fold)
- Presence of specific IgM and dye test ≥300 IU/mL

Correct interpretation of serologic testing done in a reference laboratory decreases unnecessary anxiety and even terminations [23].

Fetal congenital infection is diagnosed by AF PCR. The specificity and positive predictive value on AF samples are close to 100%. Sensitivity is around 70% to 80% but is best when maternal infection occurs between 17 and 21 weeks of pregnancy. Real-time PCR appears to have a sensitivity of 92%, negative predictive value of 98%, and may not be as gestational-age dependent as conventional PCR [24]. However, a negative AF PCR does not always completely rule out congenital infection. AF PCR should obviously be done after 15 weeks. Ultrasound can also aid in diagnosis of fetal infection (see section titled "Complications"), but it has very poor sensitivity and specificity.

Therapy

If maternal infection is detected, counsel regarding the risks along with possibility of termination (especially in first trimester) and management.

If maternal infection is confirmed by a reference laboratory, start spiramycin 3 to 4 g/day (1 g every eight hours). This is available in the United States only by the Food and Drug Administration (FDA) when Palo Alto serology is positive. Spiramycin concentrates in the placenta and therefore may not be reliable for treatment of infection in the fetus [8].

If AF PCR is positive, start **sulfadiazine** (initial dose of 75 mg/kg, followed by 50 mg/kg every 12 hours with a maximum of 4 g/day), **pyrimethamine** (50 mg every 12 hours for two days followed by 50 mg daily) and **folinic acid** (leucovorin) 10 to 20 mg with each dose of pyrimethamine (decreases bone marrow toxicity) and one week after completion of pyrimethamine therapy [8]. Length of therapy is controversial and has varied for a minimum of 28 days (with ½ dose until term) versus continuing therapy as is until term. Treatment with pyrimethamine and sulfadiazine to prevent fetal infection is contraindicated during the first trimester (pyrimethamine is teratogenic), but at this time, sulfadiazine can be used alone [25,26]. This treatment should be stopped in the last few weeks of pregnancy. This is the basic treatment protocol recommended by the WHO and CDC [4]. Other drugs, such as spiramycin (3–4 g/day × 3–4 weeks), are recommended in certain circumstances. It is important to note that, at this time, treatment with sulfadiazine–pyrimethamine has not yet been shown to be superior to spiramycin alone for treatment of congenital TG. Spiramycin is used to prevent placental infection; it is used in European countries, but in the United States, it is not approved by the FDA. Mode of delivery should not be influenced by maternal infection as cesarean delivery does not reduce the risk of congenital infection [27].

Treatment decreases complications of TG, but possibly not fetal infection. In a meta-analysis of 7055 women with toxoplasmosis acquired during pregnancy, the pooled rate of congenital TG who received treatment was 16%. The rate of vertical transmission was similar for both spiramycin-only and spiramycin + sulfadiazine regimens (13%) [10]. It is estimated that for every three congenitally infected fetuses that are treated, one case of serious neurological sequela is prevented [28]. In one study, fetuses/neonates treated and subsequently followed for 12 to 250 months had a 17% rate of congenital TG with 74% of the children asymptomatic, 26% developing chorioretinitis (72% peripheral and unilateral), and all except one child having age-appropriate neurological and intellectual development [11]. In another prospective trial following treated children for a median of 10.5 years, **although 30% had at least one ocular lesion, the majority of lesions caused little or no visual impairment** [19]. Other long-term follow up of ante- and postnatally treated individuals suggests that **in the majority of cases, congenital TG may actually have little effect on overall quality of life and visual function** [29,30]. Despite these encouraging findings, well-designed randomized controlled trials are needed to elucidate the optimal treatment regimen and duration in affected pregnancies, optimally taking into account gestational age at seroconversion.

REFERENCES

1. Jones JL, Kruszon-Moran D, Sanders-Lewis K et al. *Toxoplasma gondii* infection in the United States, 1999–2004, decline from the prior decade. *Am J Trop Med Hyg* 2007; 77: 405–10. [III]
2. The Centers for Disease Control and Prevention. Parasites–Toxoplasmosis Web site. http://www.cdc.gov/parasites/toxoplasmosis/. Updated 2015. Accessed September 28, 2015. [Epidemiological data, III]
3. Berger F, Goulet V, Le Strat Y et al. Toxoplasmosis among pregnant women in France: Risk factors and change of prevalence between 1995 and 2003. *Rev Epidemiol Sante Publique* 2009; 57(4): 241–8. [III]
4. Rorman E, Zamir CS, Rilkis I et al. Congenital toxoplasmosis—Prenatal aspects of *Toxoplasma gondii* infection. *Reprod Toxicol* 2006; 21(4): 458–72. Epub 2005. [Review]
5. Villena I, Ancelle T, Delmas C et al. Toxosurv network and National Reference Centre for Toxoplasmosis. Congenital toxoplasmosis in France in 2007: First results from a national surveillance system. *Euro Surveill* 2010; 15(25): 1–6. [III]
6. Torgerson PR, Mastroiacovo P. The global burden of congenital toxoplasmosis: A systematic review. *Bull World Health Organ* 2013; 91(7): 501–8. [Epidemiological report, III]
7. Feldman DM, Timms D, Borgida AF. Toxoplasmosis, parvovirus, and cytomegalovirus in pregnancy. *Clin Lab Med* 2010; 30: 709–20. [Review]
8. Montoya JG, Remington JS. Management of *Toxoplasma gondii* infection during pregnancy. *Clin Infect Dis* 2008; 47: 554–66. [Review]
9. SYROCOT (Systematic Review on Congenital Toxoplasmosis) study group, Thiébaut R, Leproust S, Chêne G et al. Effectiveness of prenatal treatment for congenital toxoplasmosis: A meta-analysis of individual patients' data. *Lancet* 2007; 369: 115–22. [Meta-analysis: No RCTs, 26 cohorts, n = 691 infected live born infants]
10. Li XL, Wei HX, Zhang H et al. A meta-analysis on risks of adverse pregnancy outcomes in toxoplasma gondii infection. *PLoS One* 2014; 9(5): e97775. [Meta-analysis, no RCT, 53 case-control and cohort studies, II-2]
11. Berrébi MD, Assouline C, Bessiéres M-H et al. Long-term outcome of children with congenital toxoplasmosis. *Am J Obstet Gynecol* 2010; 203: 552.e1–6. [II-3]
12. Hohlfeld P, MacAleese J, Capella-Pavlovski M, Giovangrandi Y, Thulliez P, Forestier F, Daffos F. Fetal toxoplasmosis: Ultrasonographic signs. *Ultrasound Obstet Gynecol* 1991; 1(4): 241–4. [III]
13. Jones JL, Krueger A, Schulkin J et al. Toxoplasmosis prevention and testing in pregnancy, survey of obstetrician-gynaecologists. *Zoonoses Public Health* 2010; 57(1): 27–33. [III]
14. Carter AO, Gelmon SB, Wells GA et al. The effectiveness of a prenatal education programme for the prevention of congenital toxoplasmosis. *Epidemiol Infect* 1989; 103: 539–45. [Cluster RCT, n = 432]
15. Di Mario S, Basevi V, Gagliotti C et al. Prenatal education for congenital toxoplasmosis. *Cochrane Database Syst Rev* 2013; (2): CD006171. [Meta-analysis, two cluster RCTs, n = 5455]
16. Neto EC. Newborn screening for congenital infectious diseases. *Emerg Infect Dis* 2004; 10: 1068–73. [II-3]
17. American College of Obstetricians and Gynecologists. Practice bulletin no. 151: Cytomegalovirus, parvovirus B19, varicella zoster, and toxoplasmosis in pregnancy. *Obstet Gynecol* 2015; 125(6): 1510–25. [III]
18. Stillwaggon E, Carrier CS, Sautter M, McLeod R. Maternal serologic screening to prevent congenital toxoplasmosis: A decision-analytic economic model. *PLoS Negl Trop Dis* 2011; 5(9): e1333. [Decision-analysis, III]
19. El Ayoubi M, de Bethmann O, Monset-Couchard M. Lenticulostriate echogenic vessels: Clinical and sonographic study of 70 neonatal cases. *Pediatr Radiol* 2003; 33: 697–703. [II-3]
20. Dhakal R, Gajurel K, Pomares C et al. Significance of a positive toxoplasma immunoglobulin M test result in the United States. *J Clin Microbiol* 2015 [Epub ahead of print]. [III]
21. Montoya JG, Liesenfeld O, Kinney S et al. VIDAS test avidity of Toxoplasma specific immunoglobulin G for confirmatory testing of pregnant women. *J Clin Microbial* 2002; 40: 2505–8. [II-3]
22. Tanimura K, Nishikawa A, Tairaku S et al. The IgG avidity value for the prediction of toxoplasma gondii infection in the amniotic fluid. *J Infect Chemother* 2015; 21(9): 668–71. [III]
23. Liesenfeld O, Montoya JC, Tathinemi NJ et al. Confirmatory serologic testing for acute toxoplasmosis and rate of induced abortions among women reported to have positive Toxoplasma immunoglobulin M antibody titers. *Am J Obstet Gynecol* 2001; 184: 140–5. [II-2]
24. Wallon M, Franck J, Thulliez P et al. Accuracy of real-time polymerase chain reaction for *Toxoplasma gondii* in amniotic fluid. *Obstet Gynecol* 2010; 115: 727–33. [III]

25. WHO Model Prescribing Information. *Drugs Used in Parasitic Diseases, 2nd ed.* Geneva: World Health Organization, 1995. [Review]

26. Chin J. Toxoplasmosis. In: *Control of Communicable Disease Manual, 17th ed.* Washington DC: American Public Health Association, 2000: 500–3. [Review]

27. Wallon M, Kieffer F, Huissoud C, Peyron F. Cesarean delivery or induction of labor does not prevent vertical transmission of toxoplasmosis in late pregnancy. *Int J Gynaecol Obstet* 2015; 129(2): 176–7. [III]

28. Cortina-Borja M, Tan HK, Wallon M et al. Prenatal treatment for serious neurological sequelae of congenital toxoplasmosis: An observational prospective cohort study. *PLoS Med* 2010; 7(10): e1000351. [II-3]

29. Wallon M, Garweg JG, Abrahamowicz M et al. Ophthalmic outcomes of congenital toxoplasmosis followed until adolescence. *Pediatrics* 2014; 133(3): e601–8. [II-3]

30. Peyron F, Garweg JG, Wallon M et al. Long-term impact of treated congenital toxoplasmosis on quality of life and visual performance. *Pediatr Infect Dis J* 2011; 30(7): 597–600. [III]

49

Parvovirus

Timothy J. Rafael

KEY POINTS

- **The incidence of acute primary maternal parvovirus B19** infection during pregnancy is about **1% to 1.5%**.
- The major means of infection is by **contact with young infected children**. The infection is usually **asymptomatic** in the adult (and pregnant woman).
- About **25% to 30% of fetuses of mothers with primary parvovirus B19 infection become infected themselves by vertical transmission.**
- Perinatal complications of fetal infection occur in about 10% of fetuses and include **fetal anemia and myocarditis**, leading to **hydrops** (2%–6%) **and** occasionally **fetal death** if infection occurs <20 weeks.
- Screening is not recommended because 1/5000 screened women would be at risk for fetal hydrops from parvovirus B19.
- **Maternal infection is usually diagnosed by IgM+ or by IgG seroconversion.**
- **Fetal ultrasound** can screen for development of anemia and/or hydropic changes in the infected mother by increased **peak systolic velocity (PSV) of the middle cerebral artery (MCA)** using a **threshold of ≥1.50** multiples of the median **(MoM)**. If MCA PSV values are <1.50 MoM, it is suggested to **continue weekly ultrasound scans for 10 to 12 weeks after the exposure.**
- **If MCA PSV is ≥1.50 or fetal hydrops** is seen on ultrasound, **fetal transfusion is indicated** even though the incidence of spontaneous resolution of hydrops is about 30% because survival with transfusion is >75%–85%.
- In cases of fetuses transfused in utero for parvovirus B19-induced hydrops, there are differing data regarding long-term outcomes among survivors. There does not appear to be an increased risk of infant or childhood morbidity and mortality following parvovirus infection during pregnancy in general. In cases of fetal anemia or hydrops undergoing transfusion, however, there may be an increased risk of severe neurodevelopmental delay. **Patients need to be counseled regarding the overall uncertainty regarding long-term neurodevelopmental outcomes among survivors.**

PATHOGEN

Human parvovirus B19 is a single-stranded DNA virus. Parvovirus B19 is the only known parvovirus that is a human pathogen.

INCIDENCE/EPIDEMIOLOGY

The **incidence of acute primary maternal parvovirus B19** infection during pregnancy in susceptible women is about **1% to 1.5%** [1,2]. The parvovirus B19-specific immunoglobulin G (IgG) seroconversion incidence in susceptible pregnant women (primary infection) is about 1%–1.5% during endemic periods and about 13%–13.5% during epidemic periods [2]. Approximately 50% to 75% of women of reproductive age are IgG+ (immune) for parvovirus B19 with approximately 25% to 50% of women being susceptible to parvovirus B19 infection during pregnancy [1].

RISK FACTORS/ASSOCIATIONS

The infection is more common in the winter and spring. The risk of infection is associated with the level of **contact with young infected children**. The highest infection rates occur in schoolteachers, day care workers, and women with nursery or school-aged children in the home. Around 50% to 80% of susceptible household members and 20% to 30% of individuals exposed in a classroom acquire acute infection from an infected child. Adverse prognostic factors are older maternal age, maternal immunity and seroconversion, raised maternal serum alpha-fetoprotein (MSAFP), and ultrasound findings.

SYMPTOMS

In adults, at least half of the infections are **asymptomatic** [2]. About 30% may have flulike symptoms, arthralgias, and adenopathy. Parvovirus B19 causes a common exanthematous disease in children 5 to 14 years old, called fifth disease or erythema infectiosum. Children have symptoms such as low-grade fever and "slapped-cheeks" rash and are usually diagnosed just based on these symptoms.

PATHOPHYSIOLOGY

Parvovirus B19 is mainly transmitted by respiratory droplets. The incubation period for erythema infectiosum is 13 to 18 days, and infectivity is greatest 7 to 10 days before the onset of symptoms. The major target cells for parvovirus B19 are erythroid progenitors bearing the main cellular parvovirus B19 receptor P blood group antigen globoside on their surface (Figure 49.1). The virus is believed to cause arrest of maturation of red blood cell (RBC) precursors at the late normoblast stage and causes a decrease in the number of platelets. The virus causes infection and lysis of erythroid progenitor cells by apoptosis, leading to hemolysis and transient aplastic crisis. Subsequent fetal anemia is thought to be responsible for the development of skin edema and effusions. Hepatitis, placentitis, and myocarditis leading to heart failure may contribute to the development of fetal hydrops [2–4]. Parvovirus B19 has been demonstrated to carry an apoptosis-inducing factor and to induce cell-cycle arrest. Cells in the S-phase of DNA mitosis are particularly vulnerable to parvovirus B19, and the fetus is at risk because of the vast number of cells in active mitosis, shorter half-life of RBCs, and immature immune system.

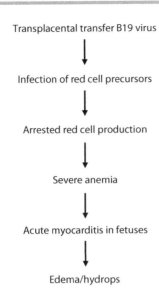

Figure 49.1 Pathophysiology of parvovirus B19 fetal infection.

MATERNAL-FETAL TRANSMISSION

About **25% to 30% of fetuses of mothers with primary parvovirus B19 infection become infected themselves by vertical transmission** (Figure 49.2). About 90% have no sequelae from this intrauterine infection [2]. Although it is not easy to determine the exact timing of transmission of parvovirus B19 infection to the fetus, it is likely that parvovirus B19 infects the fetus during or immediately after maternal viremia even in the early stages of gestation. Parvovirus B19 can persist until term or after birth even when infection occurs early in gestation.

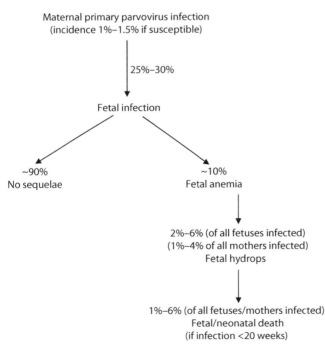

Figure 49.2 Natural history of parvovirus infection in pregnancy.

COMPLICATIONS

Of the infected fetuses, about 5% to 20% can develop **anemia**, of which 30% to 50% develop **hydrops fetalis** (about 2%–6% of all infected fetuses) with some series showing hydrops rates as high as 66% of anemic fetuses [5] (Figure 49.2). Overall, the data suggest a rate of 1% to 4% for fetal hydrops in infected mothers [3] with rates as high as 8%–10% with infections occurring between 9 and 20 weeks [6]. The risk of **fetal death** is 1% to 6% of all infected fetuses [7]. Fetal death occurs almost exclusively in hydropic cases diagnosed at <20 weeks [8], especially if cases >20 weeks are treated with timely transfusion (90% survival) [7]. Early embryonic/fetal death may manifest as miscarriage. A recent case-control study demonstrated an increased association of first trimester miscarriage with positive Parvovirus IgM women (OR 1.71, 95% CI 1.02–2.86) [9]. Overall for infected mothers <20 weeks, there is an approximate 10% risk for fetal loss. Although acute parvovirus infection may occur relatively commonly during pregnancy, an adverse fetal outcome is an uncommon complication [4,10,11]. Rarely, parvovirus has been detected in fetuses with hydrocephalus (possibly from vasculitis), but it is unclear if malformations seen with parvovirus are just coincidental and not related to the viral infection. Parvovirus B19 may be an important cause of fetal death not always associated with fetal hydrops. **All cases of fetal death, especially those associated with hydrops, should be considered for testing for parvovirus B19 by polymerase chain reaction (PCR)**. Maternal serology might be a less sensitive determinant for parvovirus B19-associated fetal death because immunoglobulin M (IgM) response generally lasts for two to four months, and parvovirus B19 infection can already be persistent in fetuses during the early stages of pregnancy, eventually leading to fetal death months later (see also Chapter 54). The more mature immune response in older fetuses could delay any pathogenic consequences of parvovirus B19 infection, resulting in a lower rate of hydrops than in younger fetuses [12,13].

ULTRASOUND FETAL FINDINGS

Sonographically detectable markers of fetal compromise include pericardial or pleural effusion, ascites, abdominal wall/skin edema, bilateral hydroceles, oligohydramnios or hydramnios, increased (>95th percentile) cardiac biventricular outer diameter, and, rarely, hydrocephalus, microcephaly, and intracranial and hepatic calcifications [3,4].

PREGNANCY MANAGEMENT
Counseling/Prognosis

Counseling should include the natural history of the disease, including vertical transmission, chances of fetal disease (anemia and hydrops), prognosis, and possible interventions. The long-term outcome of fetuses affected after 20 weeks is very good.

Prevention

Avoidance of contact with infected children—or (better) children in general—is the best prevention. This is not always feasible. No specific antiviral therapy or vaccine is available for parvovirus B19 infection. Frequent hand washing is effective in preventing disease transmission [2]. Intravenous immunoglobulin (IVIG) prophylaxis is reasonable to consider for documented exposures in immunocompromised patients although it is not currently recommended for prophylaxis in pregnancy.

Screening

Universal screening is not recommended as the risk of fetal hydrops from parvovirus infection is about 1/5000 screened pregnancies, making screening not warranted. Screening may be warranted in pregnant women who take care of young children, especially during epidemics [3].

Workup/Diagnosis

Workup includes determination of serum IgG and IgM. **Maternal infection is usually diagnosed by IgM+ or by IgG seroconversion.** IgM appears by 3 days of an acute infection, peaks at 25 to 30 days, and disappears by 4 months. Serum IgG appears a few days after IgM, and coincides with resolution of maternal symptoms. The detection of viral DNA by PCR is another means of diagnosis. Electron microscopy (EM) is also possible whereas virus culture usually fails. Increased MSAFP has also been used as a prognostic factor for poor outcome [14] although this has been questioned in recent studies [5].

Once maternal infection has been diagnosed, **fetal ultrasound** can screen for development of anemia and/or hydropic changes. Anemia can be detected by increased **PSV of the MCA** prior to the appearance of sonographically detectable markers of hydrops [15]. This is based on the observation (first in rhesus immunization, in which the mechanism leading to anemia is different) that with fetal anemia there is an increase of fetal cardiac output to maintain adequate oxygen delivery to tissues, leading to increased blood flow velocities also in anemic fetuses with hydrops from parvovirus B19. MCA PSV using a **threshold of ≥1.50 MoM** has a high sensitivity (100%) and specificity (100%) for detecting fetal anemia [15]. If MCA PSV values are <1.50 MoM, it is suggested to **continue weekly ultrasound scans for 10 to 12 weeks after the exposure** [16] to follow those fetuses that potentially are at high risk for anemia and hydrops (Figure 49.3). The peak incidence of hydrops is at about four to six weeks after maternal infection. Fetal surveillance should be initiated no later than four weeks after the onset of illness or estimate of seroconversion [2]. In cases of elevated MCA PSV but no hydrops, surveillance should be increased with ultrasound scans two to three per week to detect any sign of hydrops or umbilical cord sampling performed.

Fetal diagnosis is by amniotic fluid (AF) PCR+. There is at present no need for percutaneous umbilical blood sampling (PUBS) for diagnosis.

Therapy

There are **no trials** evaluating therapeutic interventions. **No antiviral therapy is available.**

Treatment should be directed at fetuses with abnormal MCA PSV and/or hydropic changes. In these fetuses, anemia and even hydrops can resolve spontaneously over four to six weeks (about **30% spontaneous resolution for hydrops**) [17]. Resolution is more common in older (>20 weeks) fetuses because of a more mature immune system.

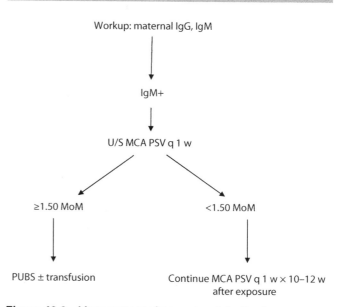

Figure 49.3 Management of parvovirus infection in pregnancy. *Abbreviations*: IgG, immunoglobulin G; IgM, immunoglobulin M; MCA, middle cerebral artery; MoM, multiples of the median; PSV, peak systolic velocity; PUBS, percutaneous umbilical blood sampling.

Intervention for anemic and/or hydropic fetuses is gestational-age dependent:

- Between 24 and 33 6/7 weeks, steroids for fetal lung maturity should be given. Fetal cordocentesis to document anemia and transfusion as necessary improve outcome in anemic and/or hydropic fetuses. Frequently, one transfusion is sufficient [2,5].
- Before 24 weeks, with severe hydrops, termination may be offered, but transfusion can be beneficial with apparently minimal to no significant sequelae if successful.
- After 34 weeks, delivery should be considered.

If cordocentesis is performed, anemia could be detected before a critical decrease of hemoglobin of <6 g/dL and before the development of severe hydrops. Blood sampling can allow testing for fetal hemoglobin/hematocrit and leukocyte and platelet counts. **Once sonographic signs of hydrops are present, transfusion is indicated using erythrocytes. Platelets should also be ready at the time of PUBS as multiple series have demonstrated a concomitantly high incidence of fetal thrombocytopenia at the time of transfusion** [18–20]. **An example of a step-by-step guide for both the set up and performance of fetal blood transfusion is described in detail elsewhere** [16]. Several nonrandomized but controlled studies suggest a significant benefit of transfusion of fetuses with anemia and/or hydrops from parvovirus infection compared with conservative treatment [4,7,21]. Overall, in cases of hydrops, although approximately 30% can resolve without treatment, death may occur in up to 50% of untreated fetuses compared with a 75%–85% survival rate with one or more transfusions [17,22]. Intracardiac transfusion is a last resort alternative to intraumbilical cord transfusion, particularly when intraumbilical cord transfusion is not possible because of risks of bradycardia and cardiac arrest of this procedure [23,24].

NEONATE AND LONG-TERM FOLLOW-UP

Infants born to IgM+ mothers are born IgG+ (mostly maternal), and 25% stay IgG+ at one year as they were infected and have become immune. Regarding long-term outcomes of children born to women infected with parvovirus during pregnancy, a recent large registry did not find an increased risk of infant or childhood morbidity and mortality [25]. Although the general health status of survivors is no different compared with the general population, there is conflicting evidence regarding incidences of developmental delay. Some trials illustrate an incidence of developmental delay similar to the general population even in cases of fetuses transfused in utero for parvovirus B19-induced hydrops [26,27]. More recent data of survivors aged six months to eight years demonstrated a **32% incidence of psychomotor developmental delay**, independent of pretransfusion hemoglobin, platelet, or blood pH values [28]. A related cohort of 28 children (all of whom had fetal hydrops and received one intrauterine transfusion) had an 11% incidence of severe developmental delay [29]. **Patients need to be counseled regarding the overall uncertainty regarding long-term neurodevelopmental outcome among survivors.** Two phases of the infantile infection are described: a first phase of viremia of two to three days, accompanied by fever and myalgia; a second phase that can last several weeks, with dermatological signs, such as erythema infectiosum, vasculitis, arthralgias, or arthritis. Long-term persistence of the virus in the neonate may be responsible for chronic manifestations.

REFERENCES

1. Mossong J, Hens N, Friederichs V et al. Parvovirus B19 infection in five European countries: Seroepidemiology, force of infection and maternal risk of infection. *Epidemiol Infect* 2008; 136: 1059–68. [II-3]
2. Lamont RF, Sobel JD, Vaisbuch E et al. Parvovirus B19 infection in human pregnancy. *BJOG* 2011; 118: 175–86. [Review]
3. Van Gessel PH, Gayvant MA, Vossen ACTM et al. Incidence of parvovirus B19 infection among an unselected population of pregnant women in the Netherlands: A prospective study. *Eur J Obstet Gynecol Reprod Biol* 2006; 128: 46–9. [II-3]
4. Von Kaisenberg CS, Jonat W. Fetal parvovirus B19. *Ultrasound Obstet Gynecol* 2001; 18: 280–8. [II-3]
5. Simms RA, Liebling RE, Patel RR et al. Management and outcome of pregnancies with parvovirus B19 infection over seven years in a tertiary fetal medicine unit. *Fetal Diagn Ther* 2009; 25: 373–8. [II-3]
6. Enders M, Klingel K, Weidner A et al. Risk of fetal hydrops and non-hydropic late intrauterine fetal death after gestational parvovirus B19 infection. *J Clin Virology* 2010; 49: 163–8. [II-3]
7. Enders M, Weidner A, Zoellner I et al. Fetal morbidity and mortality after acute human parvovirus B19 infection in pregnancy: Prospective evaluation of 108 cases. *Prenatal Diagn* 2004; 24: 513–8. [II-2]
8. Puccetti C, Contoli M, Bonvicini F et al. Parvovirus B19 in pregnancy: Possible consequences of vertical transmission. *Prenatal Diagn* 2012; 32: 897–902. [II-3]
9. Lassen J, Jensen AKV, Bager P et al. Parvovirus B19 infection in the first trimester of pregnancy and risk of fetal loss: A population-based case-control study. *Am J Epidemiol* 2012; 176(9): 803–7. [II-2]

10. Sarfraz AA, Samuelsen SO, Bruu AL et al. Maternal human parvovirus B19 infection and the risk of fetal death and low birthweight: A case-control study within 35,940 pregnant women. *BJOG* 2009; 116: 1492–8. [II-2]
11. Riipinen A, Väisänen E, Nuutila M et al. Parvovirus B19 infection in fetal deaths. *Clin Infect Dis* 2008; 47: 1519–25. [II-2]
12. Tolfvenstam T, Papadogiannakis N, Norbeck O et al. Frequency of human parvovirus B19 infection in intrauterine fetal death. *Lancet* 2001; 357: 1494–7. [II-2]
13. Skjöldebrand-Sparre L, Tolfvenstam T, Papadogiannakis N. Association with the third trimester intrauterine fetal death. *BJOG* 2000; 107: 476–80. [II-2]
14. Bernstein IM, Capeless IL. Elevated maternal serum alphafetoprotein and hydrops fetalis in association with fetal parvovirus B19 infection in the human fetus. *BJOG* 1989; 74: 456–7. [II-2]
15. Cosmi E, Mari G, Delle Chiaie L et al. Noninvasive diagnosis by Doppler ultrasonography of fetal anemia resulting from parvovirus infection. *Am J Obstet Gynecol* 2002; 187: 1290–3. [II-2]
16. Society for Maternal-Fetal Medicine (SMFM) Clinical Guideline #8: The fetus at risk for anemia—Diagnosis and management. *Am J Obstet Gynecol* 2015; 212(6): 697–710. [Guideline; III]
17. Rodis JF, Borgida AF, Wilson M et al. Management of parvovirus infection in pregnancy and outcomes of hydrops: A survey of members of the Society of Perinatal Obstetricians. *Am J Obstet Gynecol* 1998; 179: 985–8. [II-3]
18. Segata M, Chaoui R, Khalek N et al. Fetal thrombocytopenia secondary to parvovirus infection. *Am J Obstet Gynecol* 2007; 196: 61.e1–4. [II-3]
19. de Haan TR, van den Akker ESA, Porcelijn L et al. Thrombocytopenia in hydropic fetuses with parvovirus B19 infection: Incidence, treatment and correlation with fetal B19 viral load. *BJOG* 2008; 115: 76–81. [II-3]
20. Melamed N, Whittle W, Kelly EN et al. Fetal thrombocytopenia in pregnancies with fetal human parvovirus-B19 infection. *Am J Obstet Gynecol* 2015; 212: 793.e1–8. [II-3]
21. Schild RL, Bald R, Plath H et al. Intrauterine management of fetal parvovirus B19 infection. *Ultrasound Obstet Gynecol* 1999; 13: 161–6. [II-2]
22. Macé G, Sauvan M, Castaigne V et al. Clinical presentation and outcome of 20 fetuses with parvovirus B19 infection complicated by severe anemia and/or fetal hydrops. *Prenatal Diagn* 2014; 34: 1023–30. [II-3]
23. Galligan BR, Cairns R, Schifano JV et al. Preparation of packed red cells suitable for intravascular transfusion in utero. *Transfusion* 1989; 29(2): 179–81. [II-3]
24. Allaf MB, Matha S, Chavez MR, Vintzileos AM. Intracardiac fetal transfusion for Parvovirus-induced hydrops fetalis: A salvage procedure. *J Ultrasound Med* 2015; 34: 2107–9. [III]
25. Lassen J, Bager P, Wohlfahrt J, Böttiger B, Melbye M. Parvovirus B19 infection in pregnancy and subsequent morbidity and mortality in offspring. *Int J Epidemiol* 2013; 42: 1070–6. [II-2]
26. Dembinski J, Haverkamp F, Maara H et al. Neurodevelopmental outcome after intrauterine red cell transfusion for Parvovirus B19-induced fetal hydrops. *BJOG* 2002; 109: 1232–4. [II-2]
27. Rodis JF, Rodner C, Hansen AA et al. Long-term outcome of children following maternal human parvovirus B19 infection. *Obstet Gynecol* 1998; 91: 125–8. [II-2]
28. Nagel HT, de Haan TR, Vandenbussche FP et al. Long-term outcome after fetal transfusion for hydrops associated with parvovirus B19 infection. *Obstet Gynecol* 2007; 109: 42–7. [II-3]
29. De Jong EP, Lindenburg IT, van Klink JM et al. Intrauterine transfusion for parvovirus B19 infection: Long-term neurodevelopmental outcome. *Am J Obstet Gynecol* 2012; 206: 204.e1–5. [II-3]

50

Herpes

Timothy J. Rafael

KEY POINTS

- Around **20% to 30% of pregnant women have immunoglobulin G (IgG) for herpes simplex virus (HSV)-2 (prior infection) and are therefore infected with it with intermittent shedding from the vaginal mucosa.** About 2% to 4% of IgG-negative women seroconvert (acquire HSV and convert to IgM+) during pregnancy, and 90% of these women are undiagnosed because they are asymptomatic.
- Most neonatal infections result from contact with infected maternal genital secretions during delivery. Transplacental HSV vertical transmission is rare. **Primary first-episode infection,** defined as HSV confirmed in a person without prior HSV-1 or HSV-2 antibodies, **can lead to a 25% to 50% vertical transmission rate if delivery occurs vaginally** during this episode and therefore represents the most important clinical scenario to avoid. Vaginal delivery during recurrent infection is associated with a <1% incidence of neonatal HSV infection.
- **Prevention of maternal infection** is the most important management strategy.
  - Universal maternal screening with HSV-1 and HSV-2 specific serology has not been tested in a trial and is controversial.
  - If the woman is seronegative, the partner should be tested. If he is seropositive, avoidance of direct orogenital contact, use of condoms, the possibility of abstinence, and medical suppression of the partner should be discussed.
  - **If the woman is seropositive or has a history of HSV, education, suppression with acyclovir or valacyclovir from 36 weeks until delivery, examination for lesions in labor with cesarean delivery (CD) if they are present,** and avoidance (if possible) of artificial rupture of membranes (AROM), scalp electrodes, vacuum extractors, and forceps should be recommended.
- Diagnosis of genital herpes is most sensitive with polymerase chain reaction **(PCR) assay** of genital lesions (typed to determine whether HSV-1 or HSV-2 is the cause of the infection). Type-specific **(HSV-1 and HSV-2)** glycoprotein G-based **serologic testing** should also be sent.
- **Women with primary or first-episode genital HSV in pregnancy** should receive **acyclovir 400 mg po tid × 7–10 days or valacyclovir (Valtrex) 1 g po tid × 7–10 days (treatment can be extended in case of incomplete healing)** and receive suppression with acyclovir **400 mg po tid or valacyclovir 500 mg po bid at 36 weeks until delivery.**
- **Women with reactivation (recurrent) symptomatic HSV** should receive either **acyclovir 400 mg po tid × five days or valacyclovir (Valtrex) 500 mg po bid × three days**

and receive suppression with acyclovir or valacyclovir at 36 weeks until delivery.
- Regarding mode of delivery:
  - **If any genital lesion suspicious for HSV is seen at the time of labor, a CD should be performed.**
- Some clinicians advocate offering CD even for women with primary HSV within six weeks of delivery despite maternal therapy.
- An indicated CD for active genital HSV should be performed before membrane rupture or as soon as possible (ideally within 4–6 hours) following rupture of membranes. A CD may be of benefit regardless of duration of membrane rupture.
- Neonatal HSV causes **disseminated or CNS disease** (seizures, lethargy, irritability, tremors, poor feeding, temperature instability, and bulging fontanelles) **in approximately 55% of cases. Up to 30% of infants will die and more than 50% can have neurologic damage despite antiviral therapy.**

PATHOGENS

HSV-1 and HSV-2 are both DNA viruses.

INCIDENCE/EPIDEMIOLOGY

Genital herpes is an infection (HSV-1 or HSV-2) causing ulceration in the genital area. **In the United States, approximately 22% of pregnant women have IgG for HSV-2 [1] (prior infection) and are therefore infected with it with intermittent shedding from the vaginal mucosa**; 63% are HSV-1 seropositive, 13% have both HSV-1 and HSV-2, and 28% are seronegative [1]. These numbers are similar to more recent data from a single institution [2]. Approximately 12% to 20% of couples in early pregnancy are discordant for HSV status with the woman at risk to get primary infection from her partner [3]. **About 2% to 4% of IgG-negative women seroconvert (acquire HSV) during pregnancy [4], and 75% to 90% of HSV-2 infected people are not aware of having the infection [3].** Approximately 0.1% to 1% of pregnant women carry HSV in their genitalia. The incidence of neonatal herpes is 1/60,000 live births annually in the United Kingdom and 12–60/100,000 live births annually in the United States [3].

RISK FACTORS/ASSOCIATIONS

Risk factors for maternal HSV infection are immunocompromise, other sexually transmitted diseases (STDs), and risk factors for STDs. Risk factors for neonatal HSV infection are HSV in the genital tract at the time of delivery, primary HSV infection, and invasive obstetrical procedures [3].

SYMPTOMS

About 70% of newly acquired HSV infections among pregnant women are asymptomatic, and 30% of women have clinical presentations that range from minimal lesions to widespread genital lesions associated with severe local pain, dysuria, sacral paresthesia, tender regional lymph node enlargement, fever, malaise, and headache (rarely meningitis).

CLASSIFICATION/PATHOPHYSIOLOGY

HSV infection causes intranuclear inclusion bodies and multinucleated giant cells. Overall, HSV-1 causes about 90% of oral infections, and 10% of genital infections, and **HSV-2 causes 10% of oral and 90% of genital infections although among college-age populations, the majority of new cases of genital HSV are caused by HSV-1** [3]. Types of infection include the following:

Primary First Episode

Primary first episode infection is **defined as herpes simplex virus confirmed in a person without prior HSV-1 or HSV-2 antibodies**. About 2% to 4% of these seronegative women seroconvert to HSV-1 or HSV-2 during pregnancy (only 30% have symptoms—if symptoms are present, they are severe—and 50% have recurrence within 6 months), with no fetal consequences unless they convert shortly before labor and deliver vaginally; viral shedding is very high with primary infection with 50% to 80% of cases of neonatal HSV infection resulting from women who acquire genital HSV-1 or HSV-2 infection near term [5].

Nonprimary First Episode

Nonprimary first episode infection is HSV-2 confirmed in a person with prior findings of HSV-1 antibodies or vice versa. About 1.5% to 2% of HSV-1 IgG+ women seroconvert to HSV-2+ whereas the risk of conversion from HSV-2 IgG to HSV-1+ is <1%. If symptoms are present, they are usually milder than first episode primary infection.

Reactivation (Recurrent) Genital Herpes

Reactivation (recurrent) genital herpes is caused by **reactivation of latent HSV, usually HSV-2.** If symptoms are present, they last 7 to 10 days, are mild, with low viral load shedding for three to five days. Some clinicians distinguish another category within this one, called first-recognized recurrence, which is HSV-1 (or HSV-2) confirmed in a person with prior findings of HSV-1 (or HSV-2) antibodies, but this is not clinically different from reactivation disease.

More than 90% of HSV episodes in pregnancy are either recurrent or nonprimary first episode HSV. Intimate contact between a susceptible person (without antibodies against the virus) and an individual who is actively shedding the virus or with body fluids containing the virus is required for HSV infection to occur. Contact must involve mucous membranes or open or abraded skin. HSV invades and replicates in neurons as well as in epidermal and dermal cells. Virions travel from the initial site of infection on the skin or mucosa to the sensory dorsal root ganglion, where latency is established. Viral replication in the sensory ganglia leads to recurrent clinical outbreaks. These outbreaks can be induced by various stimuli, such as trauma, ultraviolet radiation, extremes in temperature, stress, immunosuppression, or hormonal fluctuations. Viral shedding, leading to possible transmission, occurs during primary infection, during subsequent recurrences, and during periods of asymptomatic viral shedding.

Maternal-Fetal Transmission

Maternal-fetal transmission of HSV usually occurs at delivery from contact with infected genital secretions. Women with a history of HSV can have viral shedding at the time of delivery. HSV-2 is detected in genital secretions at term by PCR assay in 8% to 15% of HSV-2 seropositive women, most of whom have no clinically detectable lesions at the time [5]. **Vaginal delivery during** *first episode primary infection* **is associated with a 25% to 50% incidence of neonatal HSV infection.** Vaginal delivery during *recurrent* **infection is associated with a <1% incidence of neonatal HSV infection** [3]. The infant of the mother with primary HSV in the third trimester lacks the protection of transplacental type-specific antibodies (which take 6 to 12 weeks to fully protect the infant) and is at risk of exposure during delivery when viral shedding could be of greatest load. The major sites of intrapartum viral entry are the neonatal eyes, nasopharynx, or a break in skin.

Transplacental infection is rare. First-episode primary infection during pregnancy can lead to microcephaly, ventriculomegaly, spasticity, echogenic bowel, hepatosplenomegaly, and flexed extremities [6].

COMPLICATIONS

In the mother, primary infection can lead to severe symptoms and occasionally to disseminated disease, hepatitis, and encephalitis.

Factors that influence the risk of fetal infection include primary maternal infection, gestational age, delivery mode, status of membranes, and maternal antibodies. Primary, rather than recurrent genital HSV, is the main risk factor for neonatal HSV. In the first episode, if genital herpes lesions are present at the time of delivery and the baby is delivered vaginally, the risk of **neonatal herpes** is 25% to 50%, calculated in different studies. The risk of neonatal infection in women with established infection and recurrence at term is <1% [5]. The risk of neonatal infection from postnatal transmission without prevention is 15% [7]. Neonatal HSV causes **disseminated or CNS disease (seizures, lethargy, irritability, tremors, poor feeding, temperature instability, and bulging fontanelles) in approximately 55% of cases. Up to 30% of infants will die and more than 50% can have neurologic damage despite antiviral therapy** [5]. Prenatal ultrasonography can detect **microcephaly, hydrocephaly, intracranial calcification, and placental calcifications** that result from a chronic fetal infection [6].

PREGNANCY MANAGEMENT
Pregnancy Considerations

The course of HSV infection in pregnancy is similar to that in nonpregnant women.

Counseling/Prognosis

Prevention, natural history, incidence of vertical transmission and sequelae, prognosis, and therapeutic options should all be reviewed with the pregnant woman with maternal HSV infection, especially if primary.

Prevention

Prevention of maternal infection includes avoidance of sexual contact with infected individuals. A **preventive strategy for maternal infection** involving universal screening has been proposed (Figure 50.1) [8]. Condoms can usually prevent infection from infected male partners if the condom covers the lesion(s). For prevention of fetal/neonatal infection, **avoidance of vaginal delivery at times of primary infection is most important. If any genital lesion suspicious for HSV is seen at time of labor, a CD should be performed**. About 46% of these lesions test positive by PCR. Clinical diagnosis by visual exam fails to identify all women with HSV in their genital secretions [9]. No scalp electrode, forceps, or vacuum should be used if viral shedding is possible. **Prevention of neonatal infection is critical as neonatal treatment is poorly effective at avoiding long-term CNS complications** (see also section titled "Therapy").

Screening

Universal screening is not generally offered to pregnant women but has been recently proposed (Figure 50.1). There has been no evidence that screening women to identify pregnancies at risk of new infections will effectively decrease incidence of infection at term as such a study would require thousands of women. Screening to identify pregnant women with asymptomatic herpes infections may have no value at present without any known safe and effective interventions to prevent an already unlikely neonatal transmission. **All pregnant women should be asked about their own and their partner's histories of genital (and oral) herpes and examined for evidence of active herpes at delivery.** Asymptomatic pregnant women with positive partners as well as HIV-positive pregnant women should be offered type-specific serologic testing.

Workup/Diagnosis

Diagnosis of genital herpes relies on laboratory confirmation with **HSV culture** or **PCR assay** of genital lesions (typed to determine whether HSV-1 or HSV-2 is the cause of the infection). Type-specific **(HSV-1 and HSV-2)** glycoprotein G-based **serologic testing** should also be sent. **PCR assays are more sensitive** and are now preferred, but lack of HSV detection by PCR does not indicate lack of HSV infection because viral shedding is intermittent. HSV culture should be done within 48 to 72 hours of appearance of the lesion. If the serology type-specific result is discrepant from the culture or PCR result, a new infection is diagnosed [3]. If a new infection is suspected and the virus is not isolated from the lesion, serologic testing should be repeated in six weeks. HSV antibodies appear during the first weeks after infection, and persist for life [8]. Tzanck smear (Wright's stain with material from the vesicle) is diagnostic with multinucleated giant cells and viral inclusions. An option exists for rapid HSV PCR at the time of delivery [10], but until this has been validated by prospective trials, it is not currently recommended.

Therapy

Antiviral Drugs

Acyclovir and the other HSV antivirals have, as a mechanism of action, the specific inhibition of viral thymidine kinase [11]. They cross the placenta but do not accumulate in the fetus. All these antivirals are safe for the fetus (category B) as exposure to acyclovir and valacyclovir do not appear to increase the overall risk of birth defects [12], although recent data raises the possibility of an association with first trimester exposure and gastroschisis [13].

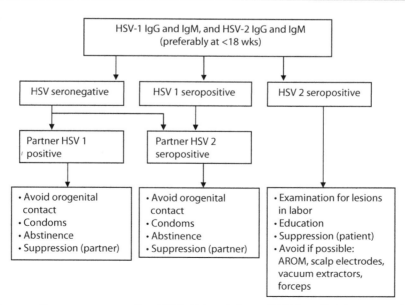

Figure 50.1 Testing and counseling women regarding HSV. *Abbreviations*: AROM, artificial rupture of membranes; HSV, herpes simplex virus; IgG, immunoglobulin G; IgM, immunoglobulin M. (Adapted from Brown ZA, Gardella C, Wald A et al. *Am Coll Obstet Gynecol*, 106, 845–56, 2005.)

Valacyclovir (Valtrex) is the prodrug of acyclovir and requires hepatic metabolism to become active. As for famciclovir, valacyclovir has better absorption, longer half-life, and decreased duration of pain and shedding compared to acyclovir.

Famciclovir is the prodrug of penciclovir and also requires hepatic metabolism to become active. As there are very limited studies in pregnant women taking famciclovir, **acyclovir and valacyclovir are preferred**.

Trials in nonpregnant adults show no differences in outcomes with any of these drugs for primary HSV.

Primary or First Episode HSV

Women with primary or first-episode genital HSV in pregnancy should be treated with the following:

- Analgesia (topical and systemic)
- Hygienic support to avoid secondary yeast and bacterial infection
- Antiviral therapy (hastens lesion healing and decreases viral shedding) with either of the following:
  - **Acyclovir 400 mg po tid × 7–10 days**
  - **Valacyclovir (Valtrex) 1 g po bid × 7–10 days**

Either regimen duration may be extended if healing is incomplete after 10 days.

These women should receive suppression with acyclovir 400 mg po tid or valacyclovir 500 mg po bid at 36 weeks until delivery. Suppression decreases the incidence of recurrent genital lesions at term, viral shedding, and therefore the need for CD. There is insufficient evidence to justify suppression based on neonatal HSV because this outcome is so rare. It is worth noting that suppression does not always eliminate all viral shedding as illustrated by a case series of eight neonates infected with HSV, in which five of the mothers were on suppressive therapy at the time of delivery [14].

Complicated HSV Infection

Women with **disseminated genital HSV, pneumonitis, hepatitis, or CNS complications** should receive the following:

- **IV acyclovir 5 to 10 mg/kg body weight q8h until clinical improvement, followed by oral antiviral therapy for 10 days of total therapy**

History of HSV

Women with a history of HSV with **reactivation (recurrent) symptomatic HSV** during pregnancy should be treated with the following:

- Analgesia (topical and systemic) as needed
- Hygienic support to avoid secondary yeast and bacterial infection as needed
- Antiviral therapy (hastens lesion healing, and decreases viral shedding) with either of the following:
  - **Acyclovir 400 mg po tid × five days**
  - **Valacyclovir (Valtrex) 500 mg po bid × three days, or 1 g po qd for five days**

These women should receive suppression (see dosages above) with acyclovir or valacyclovir at 36 weeks until delivery or starting even earlier if there are frequent recurrent episodes. **In women with recurrent genital herpes, antiviral suppressive medication initiated from 36 weeks until delivery reduces viral shedding and recurrences at delivery and reduces the need for CD.** There is insufficient evidence,

given the rarity of this outcome, to assess if antiviral prophylaxis reduces the incidence of neonatal HSV [15].

There is insufficient evidence to assess suppression in women with a **history of genital HSV and no recurrence during pregnancy**, but suppression might be a reasonable option after counseling [8]. Four out of seven RCTs evaluating suppression included women with a history of genital HSV but not necessarily a recurrence during the index pregnancy [15].

Mode of Delivery

- **With active genital lesions or prodromal symptoms of HSV (either primary or reactivation), especially in women presenting with first episode genital herpes lesions at the time of delivery, cesarean section is recommended [11]. Some clinicians advocate offering CD even for women with primary HSV within six weeks of delivery, despite maternal therapy** [3].
- For an indicated CD, it should be performed before membrane rupture or as soon as possible (ideally within 4–6 hours) following rupture of membranes. A CD may be of benefit regardless of duration of membrane rupture.
- A reactivation/**recurrent episode** of genital herpes occurring **during pregnancy** is not an indication for delivery by cesarean section. In women with a history of **genital HSV** but without active genital lesions or prodromal symptoms at the time of labor, CD is not indicated.

Postpartum/Neonate

Seventy percent of mothers of HSV-infected neonates are asymptomatic. Neonates with infection manifest symptoms at the end of the first week of life with skin lesions, cough, tachypnea, cyanosis, jaundice, seizures, and disseminated intravascular coagulation (DIC). The classic triad is skin lesions, chorioretinitis, and CNS abnormalities. Severe HSV neonatal infection can lead to a 30% incidence of death and more than 50% incidence of mental problems/neurologic damage in survivors despite antiviral therapy [5].

A neonate born to a mother with an active HSV lesion requires contact precautions, which should be maintained until all cultures are finalized. This information must be communicated with all members of the health care team, including obstetricians, pediatricians, and nurses. Mothers with HSV at the time of delivery should wash their hands and cover any lesions, but can handle their neonate. Acyclovir is compatible with breast-feeding.

REFERENCES

1. Xu F, Markowitz LE, Gottlieb SL et al. Seroprevalence of herpes simplex virus types 1 and 2 in pregnant women in the United States. *Am J Obstet Gynecol* 2007; 196: 43.e1–6. [III]
2. Delaney S, Gardella C, Saracino M, Magaret A, Wald A. Seroprevalence of herpes simplex virus type 1 and 2 among pregnant women, 1989–2010. *JAMA* 2014; 312: 746–8. [II-3]
3. Gardella C, Brown Z. Prevention of neonatal herpes. *Br J Obstet Gynecol* 2011; 118: 187–92. [Review]
4. Brown ZA, Selke SA, Zeh J et al. Acquisition of herpes simplex virus during pregnancy. *N Engl J Med* 1997; 337: 509–15. [II-2]
5. Corey L, Wald A. Maternal and neonatal herpes simplex virus infections. *N Engl J Med* 2009; 361: 1376–85. [Review]
6. Lanouette JM, Duquette DA, Jacques SM et al. Prenatal diagnosis of fetal herpes simplex infection. *Fetal Diagn Ther* 1996; 11: 414–6. [II-3]

7. Jungmann E. Genital herpes. Clinical evidence. *Br Med J* 2004; 11: 2073–88. [II-2]

8. Brown ZA, Gardella C, Wald A et al. Genital herpes complicating pregnancy. *Am Coll Obstet Gynecol* 2005; 106: 845–56. [Review]

9. Gardella C, Brown ZA, Wald A et al. Poor correlation between genital lesions and detection of herpes simplex virus in women in labor. *Obstet Gynecol* 2005; 106: 268–74. [II-2]

10. Gardella C, Huang ML, Wald A et al. Rapid polymerase chain reaction assay to detect herpes simplex virus in the genital tract of women in labor. *Obstet Gynecol* 2010; 115: 1209–16. [II-3]

11. ACOG Practice Bulletin. Clinical management guidelines for obstetrician-gynecologists. No. 82 June 2007. Management of herpes in pregnancy. *Obstet Gynecol* 2007, (Reaffirmed 2014); 109: 1489–98. [Review]

12. Pasternak B, Hviid A. Use of acyclovir, valacyclovir, and famciclovir in the first trimester of pregnancy and the risk of birth defects. *J Am Med Assoc* 2010; 304(8): 859–66. [II-2]

13. Ahrens KA, Anderka MT, Feldkamp ML et al. Antiherpetic medication use and the risk of gastroschisis: Findings from the National Birth Defects Prevention Study, 1997–2007. *Paediatr Perinat Epidemiol* 2013; 27(4): 340–5. [II-2]

14. Pinninti SG, Angara R, Feja KN et al. Neonatal herpes disease following maternal antenatal antiviral suppressive therapy: A multicenter case series. *J Pediatr* 2012; 161: 134–8. [II-3]

15. Hollier LM, Wendel GD. Third trimester antiviral prophylaxis for preventing maternal genital herpes simplex virus (HSV) recurrences and neonatal infection. *Cochrane Database Syst Rev* 2008; (1): CD004946. [Meta-analysis: 7 RCTs, *n* = 1249]

51

Varicella

Timothy J. Rafael

KEY POINTS

- As about 95% of pregnant women are immune (VZV IgG+) to varicella, **primary maternal varicella zoster virus (VZV) infection (chickenpox)** occurs in **about 0.5–3/1000 pregnancies.**
- **Pneumonia** can occur in up to **10% of pregnant women with chickenpox.**
- **Congenital varicella syndrome (CVS) occurs in 0.4% to 2% of all maternal infections, usually if maternal VZV infection occurs at <20 weeks of gestation.**
- CVS includes congenital limb hypoplasia, dermatomal skin scarring, rudimentary digits, intrauterine growth restriction (IUGR), and occasionally damage to the eyes (chorioretinitis, cataracts) and central nervous system (microcephaly, cortical atrophy, leading to mental retardation).
- All pregnant (and reproductive-age) women should be asked at their first prenatal visit if they have had a chickenpox infection. **All women who did not have chickenpox in the past, are unsure about their history, or had only one dose of the varicella vaccine, should have VZV IgG serology. VZV IgG-negative women should receive the vaccine postpartum.**
- Diagnosis of **maternal chickenpox** is usually made based on clinical findings alone, and confirmed by **VZV IgM.**
- **Ultrasound** can help in the diagnosis and estimation of the probability of CVS. **At least five weeks should be allowed between the onset of maternal symptoms and fetal ultrasound.** Fetal infection can be diagnosed by VZV DNA in amniotic fluid, but this does not predict risk of CVS.
- **VZV-seronegative pregnant women exposed to VZV** should receive **VZV IgG** (also known as **VariZIG™**).
- Pregnant women who develop **chickenpox** should receive oral (or intravenous [IV] if severe) **acyclovir** within 24 hours of rash and should avoid contact with susceptible individuals, such as other pregnant women or children. Varicella zoster immune globulin (VariZIG™) has no therapeutic effect once chickenpox has developed.
- **Delivery should be delayed until five days after the onset of maternal illness** to allow for passive transfer of maternal IgG. **Neonates born to women who develop chickenpox between five days before and two days after delivery should receive VZV IgG.** If neonatal infection occurs, the neonate should receive acyclovir.
- Pregnant women who develop **pulmonary chickenpox** should be immediately hospitalized in isolation and should receive **IV acyclovir.**
- **Maternal shingles (Herpes Zoster) is not a risk for the infant** who is protected from passively acquired maternal antibodies.
- **Nonimmune women should be offered postpartum varicella vaccination.** The vaccine is considered safe in breast-feeding women. Conception should be delayed until one month after the VZV vaccine was given (live attenuated vaccine).

PATHOGEN

VZV is a DNA virus of the herpes family.

INCIDENCE/EPIDEMIOLOGY

As about 95% of pregnant women are immune (VZV IgG+) to varicella, **primary maternal VZV infection (commonly called chickenpox or VZD)** is uncommon and estimated to **complicate about 0.5–3/1000 pregnancies.** Women from tropical areas are more susceptible (50% immunity only) to the development of chickenpox. VZV vaccine was licensed in 1995 and decreased the incidence of disease by 85% to 90% in the decade following licensure [1].

RISK FACTORS/ASSOCIATIONS

Maternal varicella infection is associated with contact with infected individuals, which usually are children if not immunized. Risk factors for varicella pneumonia are cigarette smoking, >100 skin lesions, advanced gestational age, history of chronic obstructive pulmonary disease (COPD), immunosuppression, and household contact.

SYMPTOMS

Pruritic rash with maculopapular skin lesions in crops, which become vesicles and pustules and later crust over, along with fever and malaise.

PATHOPHYSIOLOGY

VZV is highly contagious and transmitted by respiratory droplets and direct personal contact with vesicle fluid or indirectly via fomites. The incubation period is about 15 (10–21) days. The disease is infectious 48 hours before the rash appears and continues to be infectious until the vesicles crust over (Figure 51.1). The rash lasts 7 to 10 days. Chickenpox (or primary VZV infection) is a common childhood disease that usually causes a mild infection, leading to the 90% seropositivity of pregnant women. After the primary infection, the virus remains dormant in sensory nerve root ganglia and can be reactivated to cause a vesicular erythematous skin rash known as herpes zoster (commonly called shingles).

MATERNAL-FETAL TRANSMISSION

Primary maternal infection leads to an about **8% vertical transmission**, causing primary fetal infection. Of these,

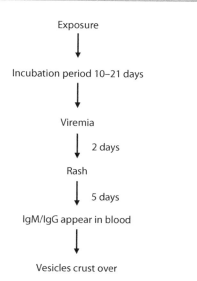

Exposure

↓

Incubation period 10–21 days

↓

Viremia

↓ 2 days

Rash

↓ 5 days

IgM/IgG appear in blood

↓

Vesicles crust over

Figure 51.1 VZV infectious sequence. *Abbreviation*: VZV, varicella zoster virus.

about 10% develop CVS **(0.4%–2% of all maternal infections) usually if maternal VZV occurs <20 weeks of gestation** [2].

COMPLICATIONS
Maternal

Although varicella infection is much less common in adults than in children, in adults it is more often associated with pneumonia, hepatitis, and encephalitis. Historically **pneumonia can occur in** up to 5% to 10% of pregnant women with chickenpox, and the severity seems increased in later gestation. More recent data points to a lower incidence of **2.5%** for varicella pneumonia during pregnancy [3]. Pulmonary symptoms start two to six days after the rash, with a mild cough leading to hemoptysis, chest pain, dyspnea, and cyanosis. The mortality rate with treatment for varicella pneumonia is now <1%.

Fetal

Sequelae are dependent on fetal age at the time of infection. In up to 98% of cases of maternal infection, the fetus remains healthy without clinical signs of illness, but when infection occurs, it can result in **CVS**, neonatal varicella, or asymptomatic seroconversion.

The overall rate for CVS **when maternal infection occurs** *in the first 20 weeks of gestation* has been demonstrated to be about **0.4% to 2%** [1,2,4–6]. CVS is characterized by **congenital limb hypoplasia, dermatomal skin scarring, rudimentary digits, IUGR, and occasionally damage to the eyes (chorioretinitis, cataracts) and central nervous system (microcephaly, cortical atrophy, leading to neurodevelopmental delay)**. It is hypothesized that CVS may reflect disseminated infection in utero or consequences of failure of virus–host interaction to result in establishment of latency as normally occurs in postnatal VZV infection [1]. **Prenatal ultrasound findings** can include limb deformity, microcephaly, hydrocephalus, soft tissue calcification, and IUGR [7].

CVS with **maternal infection >20** *weeks* is very rare as it has only been reported in <10 case reports (<1/1000

risk) [4]. Maternal infection after 20 weeks and up to 36 weeks may present as shingles in the first few years of infant life as a reactivation of the virus after a primary infection in utero.

If maternal infection occurs **one to four weeks before delivery,** up to 50% of babies are infected, and up to 23% of these develop clinical varicella. **Severe chickenpox occurs more often if the infant is born within seven days of onset of the mother's rash** when cord blood VZV IgG is low. Both intrauterine and peripartum VZV infection predispose to development of childhood zoster. Historically, neonates born to mothers who contract chickenpox between five days before delivery and two days after delivery have a 17% to 30% chance of developing **neonatal varicella** [8]. Before VZV immunoglobulin was available, the risk of death among these neonates was as high as 31% with current rates decreasing to 7% when the use of varicella immunoglobulin was introduced and neonatal intensive care improved [1]. Since the advent of routine varicella vaccination, the overall incidences of both CVS and neonatal varicella appear to be further decreasing [9]. There are no fetal consequences for herpes zoster because the viral load is very low, and the mother has already VZV IgGs that cross the placenta and protect the fetus.

PREGNANCY MANAGEMENT
Pregnancy Considerations

Chickenpox is a more severe disease in the adult than in the child. In pregnant women, frequency of VZV, frequency of pneumonia, and mortality are not increased compared to nonpregnant adults. Pneumonia may be more severe in pregnant women with up to an overall 5% risk of maternal death even with therapy although a more recent study reported no maternal deaths among 23 cases of VZV pneumonia diagnosed during pregnancy [3].

Counseling

Natural history, incidence of vertical transmission and sequelae (mostly occurring if maternal infection occurs <20 weeks), prognosis, and therapeutic options should all be reviewed with the pregnant woman with primary maternal VZV infection (Table 51.1).

Prevention

VZV-seronegative pregnant women should avoid exposure to individuals with chickenpox. A live attenuated varicella vaccine (Varivax®, Merck, New Jersey) has demonstrated to be safe in preventing chickenpox in adults. In the United States and in some European countries, seronegative women presenting for **preconception** counseling or women undergoing infertility treatment may be offered vaccination. The vaccine is not available in the United Kingdom for these indications. Varicella vaccine is contraindicated in pregnant women. If a woman accidentally receives VZV vaccine within a month of conception or in pregnancy, the incidence of fetal infection and complications does not appear to be increased from baseline, and termination should not be recommended. In one registry, among 131 live births to VZV-seronegative women, there was no evidence of CVS, and the major birth defect rate was not statistically increased [10]. Nonimmune health workers exposed to VZV should minimize patient contact from days 8 to 21 post contact.

Table 51.1   Counseling Advice for Pregnant Women at Risk

Maternal Rash Appears	Risk for Varicella Embryopathy	Counseling Advice
First 20 wks	0.5% to 2% above the baseline risk	VZV IgG ASAP or at most within 10 days after contact if the woman is seronegative. Ultrasound 5 wks after maternal rash appears to detect defects.
21–28 wks	Rare	VZV IgG ASAP or at most within 10 days after contact if the woman is seronegative. Ultrasound 5 wks after maternal rash appears to detect defects.
After 28 wks	None	VZV IgG ASAP, or at most within 10 days after contact if the woman is seronegative to prevent varicella complications. Explain baseline risk.
Five days before or two days after birth	None	If possible, delay the delivery until 5–7 days after the onset of maternal rash. Administer VZV IgG to neonate if exposed. IV Acyclovir is warranted for severe cases. IV Acyclovir 10–15 mg/kg every 8 hr for 5–10 days and antibiotics as needed.
Maternal varicella pneumonia		Blood gas, mechanical ventilation, and supportive therapy as needed.

Source: Centers for Disease Control and Prevention (CDC). Updated Recommendations for use of VariZIG-United States, 2013. *MMWR Morb Mortal Wkly Rep*, 62, 28, 574–6, 2013.
Abbreviations: ASAP, as soon as possible; VZV, varicella zoster virus.

Screening

Routine serologic screening of all pregnant women is currently not recommended. **All pregnant (and preconception reproductive-age) women should be asked at the first prenatal visit if they have had a prior chickenpox infection.** Over 97% of women who report a prior varicella infection with a typical presentation have VZV IgG and are therefore immune. **All women who did not have chickenpox in the past, are unsure about their history, or had only one dose of the varicella vaccine, should have VZV IgG serology.** In the United States, of women who are uncertain or give negative histories, approximately 80% to 90% have VZV IgG [11]. If testing is done in the preconception period, women can be offered two doses of the varicella vaccine at least one month apart. Pregnancy should be delayed one month after vaccination. Based on a decision model, the above prenatal screening (selective serotesting) with postpartum vaccination of susceptibles would seem cost-effective [12].

Workup/Diagnosis

Diagnosis of **maternal chickenpox** is usually made based on clinical findings alone. Diagnosis can be confirmed by **VZV IgM** newly positive by ELISA (enzyme-linked immunosorbent assay) or by VZV antigen (Ag) in skin/vesicular lesions by immunofluorescence antibody (Ab) to membrane Ag. **Fetal infection can be diagnosed by VZV DNA** detected by polymerase chain reaction (PCR) in amniotic fluid, but its presence has a poor positive predictive value for both fetal disease and disease severity [1]. The presence of fetal varicella-specific IgM, which remains in the blood for four to five weeks, is diagnostic [13]. **Ultrasound** can help in diagnosis and estimation of probability of CVS. **At least five weeks should be allowed between the onset of maternal symptoms and fetal ultrasound** to avoid false negative results. Initial PCR testing of amniotic fluid at 17 to 21 weeks may be negative with normal ultrasound findings, suggesting a low risk of CVS. Positive PCR at 17 to 21 weeks with normal ultrasound should lead to a repeat ultrasound at 22 to 26 weeks. A normal ultrasound at that stage makes CVS very unlikely. In contrast, an abnormal ultrasound suggests a high likelihood of CVS [14,15].

Therapy

Exposure

- **VZV-seronegative pregnant women exposed to VZV** should receive **VZV IgG (VariZIG™)** ideally as soon as possible (Table 51.1) and within 96 hours (4 days) of exposure up to a period of 10 days postexposure. In 2012, the Food and Drug Administration approved VariZIG™, a varicella zoster immune globulin preparation for use in the United States for postexposure prophylaxis for individuals at high risk for severe disease and subsequently extended the period for administration from 4 days to 10 days [16]. VariZIG can be obtained 24 hours a day from the sole authorized U.S. distributor (FFF Enterprises, Temecula, California, 1-800-843-7477 or online at http://www.fffenterprises.com). The recommended dose is 125 units/10 kg of body weight up to a maximum of 625 units IM (five vials) [17]. This may not prevent but may attenuate symptoms up to 10 days after exposure. It probably does not affect fetal infection, and it is expensive.

Chickenpox

- **Pregnant women who develop chickenpox** should receive oral **acyclovir** within 24 hours of rash. Oral acyclovir (800 mg, 5 times daily for 7 days) reduces the duration of fever and symptoms of varicella infection in immunocompetent adults if commenced within 24 hours of developing the onset of rash [18]. Administration of acyclovir does not appear to be teratogenic. Acyclovir is prescribed to treat extensive varicella at the high dose of 15 mg/kg of body weight or 500 mg/m² IV every 8 hours. Major side effects often include local tissue irritation, transient elevation of hepatic transaminases, CNS toxicity, and renal dysfunction. Transplacental passage of acyclovir is prompt and therapeutic levels reach the placenta and fetal blood [13]. **There is no information about whether giving acyclovir or valacyclovir to pregnant women with varicella reduces the already low risk for CVS** [1].

- **Pregnant women who develop chickenpox** should **avoid contact with susceptible individuals,** such as other pregnant women or children.
- **Pregnant women who develop chickenpox** should undergo symptomatic treatment and maintain hygiene to avoid bacterial superinfection.
- VZV IgG has no therapeutic effect once chickenpox has developed.
- If maternal infection occurs at term, there is a significant risk of varicella in the newborn. **Delivery should be delayed until five days after the onset of maternal illness** to allow for passive transfer of maternal IgG. Infants delivered when maternal symptoms develop five days prior to two days after delivery are at 17% to 30% risk of getting neonatal varicella, and of these, about 7% can die. **Neonates born to women who develop chickenpox between five days before and two days after delivery should receive VZV IgG.** If neonatal infection occurs, the neonate should receive acyclovir.
- If there is neonatal exposure in the first seven days of life (e.g., from an infected sibling), no intervention is required if the mother is immune; however, the neonate should be given VZV IgG if the mother is not immune to varicella. Neonates who develop chickenpox in the first 14 days of life should receive IV acyclovir.
- Pregnant women who develop **pulmonary chickenpox** should be immediately hospitalized in isolation. They should receive **IV acyclovir** 10 to 15 mg/kg every 8 hours × 7 days within 72 hours of symptoms (decreases severity and mortality).

Maternal Shingles (Herpes Zoster)

Despite maternal varicella being associated with the aforementioned fetal/neonatal risks, congenital varicella has never been documented in association with maternal herpes zoster infection. Should treatment be deemed necessary for zoster during pregnancy (e.g., moderate to severe rash, acute neuritis), PO acyclovir (800 mg 5 times daily for 7–10 days) or valacyclovir (1000 mg 3 times daily for 7 days) can be used [19]. Maternal shingles is **not a risk for the infant** who is protected from passively acquired maternal antibodies [5].

Nonimmune Women

Nonimmune women should be offered **postpartum varicella vaccination (two doses, one month apart)**. The vaccine is considered safe in breast-feeding women. Conception should be delayed until one month after the VZV vaccine was given (live attenuated vaccine).

Clinical Neonatal Findings of CVS [15]

- Skin scarring in a dermatomal distribution, 73%
- Neurological abnormalities (microcephaly, cortical atrophy, neurodevelopmental delay), 62%
- Eye defects (microphthalmia, chorioretinitis), 52%
- Hypoplasia of the limbs, 46%
- Muscle hypoplasia, 20%
- Gastrointestinal abnormalities, 19%
- Genitourinary abnormalities, 12%
- Internal organs effects, 13%
- Developmental delay, 12%

REFERENCES

1. Smith CK, Arvin AM. Varicella in the fetus and newborn. *Semin Fetal Neonatal Med* 2009; 14: 209–17. [Review]
2. Harger JH, Ernest JM, Thurnau GR et al. Frequency of congenital varicella syndrome in a prospective cohort of 347 pregnant women. *Obstet Gynecol* 2002; 100: 260–5. [II-3]
3. Zhang HJ, Patenaude V, Abenhaim HA. Maternal outcomes in pregnancies affected by varicella zoster virus infections: Population-based study on 7.7 million pregnancy admissions. *J Obstet Gynaecol Res* 2015; 41: 62–8. [II-2]
4. Tan MP, Koren G. Chickenpox in pregnancy: Revisited. *Reprod Toxicol* 2006; 21(4): 410–20. [Review]
5. Royal College of Obstet and Gynecol. Clinical Green Top Guideline: Chickenpox in pregnancy. January 17, 2005. [Guideline]
6. Sanchez MA, Bello-Munoz JC, Cebrecos I et al. The prevalence of congenital varicella syndrome after a maternal infection, but before 20 weeks of pregnancy: A prospective cohort study. *J Matern Fetal Neonatal Med* 2011; 24(2): 341–7. [II-3]
7. Pretorius DH, Hayward I, Jones KL et al. Sonographic evaluation of pregnancies with maternal varicella infection. *J Ultrasound Med* 1992; 11: 459–63. [II-3]
8. National Advisory Committee on Immunization update on varicella. *Can Common Dis Rep* 2004; 30: 1–26. [Review]
9. Khandaker G, Marshall H, Peadon E et al. Congenital and neonatal varicella: Impact of the national varicella vaccination programme in Australia. *Arch Dis Child* 2011; 96: 453–6. [II-3]
10. Wilson E, Goss MA, Marin M et al. Varicella vaccine exposure during pregnancy: Data from 10 years of the pregnancy registry. *J Infect Dis* 2008; 197: S178–84. [II-3]
11. Watson B, Civen R, Reynolds M et al. Validity of self-reported varicella disease history in pregnant women attending prenatal clinics. *Public Health Rep* 2007; 122: 499–506. [III]
12. De Moira AP, Edmunds WJ, Breuer J. The cost-effectiveness of antenatal varicella screening with post-partum vaccination of susceptibles. *Vaccine* 2006; 24: 1298–307. [III]
13. Mc Gregor JA. Varicella zoster infection in pregnancy. *Contemp Obstet Gynecol* 2002; 47–55. [Review]
14. Enders G, Miller E. *Varicella and Herpes Zoster in Pregnancy and in Newborn.* Cambridge: Cambridge University Press, 2000: 317–47. [Review]
15. Koren G. Congenital varicella syndrome in the third trimester. *Lancet* 2005; 366: 1591–2. [Review]
16. Centers for Disease Control and Prevention (CDC). Updated Recommendations for use of VariZIG-United States, 2013. *MMWR Morb Mortal Wkly Rep* 2013; 62(28): 574–6. [Guideline]
17. Centers for Disease Control and Prevention (CDC). A new product (VariZIG) for postexposure prophylaxis of varicella available under an investigational new drug application expanded access protocol. *MMWR Morb Mortal Wkly Rep* 2006; 55: 209–10. [Review]
18. Wallace MR, Bawler WA, Murray NB et al. Treatment of adult varicella with oral acyclovir. A randomized placebo-controlled trial. *Ann Intern Med* 1992; 117: 358–63. [RCT, nonpregnant adults]
19. Dworkin RH, Johnson RW, Breuer J et al. Recommendations for the management of herpes zoster. *Clin Infect Dis* 2007; 44: S1–26. [Review]

52

Fetal and neonatal alloimmune thrombocytopenia

Kelly M. Orzechowski

KEY POINTS

- Fetal and neonatal alloimmune thrombocytopenia (FNAIT) is a disorder resulting in **fetal platelet destruction (thrombocytopenia) from maternal antibodies against fetal human platelet antigens (HPAs) inherited from the father**.
- Diagnosis is usually made retrospectively after a first affected infant.
- The most serious complication is the **10%–30% risk of intracranial hemorrhage**, which usually occurs antepartum in the third trimester.
- The neonatal mortality from intracranial hemorrhage (ICH) is 5% to 13%.
- Only **HPA-1a antigen** and **past history of ICH** predict a more severe thrombocytopenia.
- **Goal** of management is to **prevent ICH** in the fetus and neonate. Keeping fetal/neonatal platelets >20,000/μL achieves this goal.
- Routine universal maternal screening is not cost-effective and is not recommended.
- **Intravenous immunoglobulin** (IVIG) is associated with a **75% response rate and a very rare risk of ICH** with half of the nonresponders showing improvement with the addition of a high dose of prednisone.
- **Fetal blood sampling (FBS)** with or without platelet transfusion is associated with a 1% to 2% risk of fetal loss per procedure with a cumulative pregnancy loss rate of 5%–10%.
- **Management is usually based on IVIG therapy with FBS as needed** as determined by prior history of ICH and associated risk (Figure 52.1).

DEFINITION

Fetal and neonatal alloimmune thrombocytopenia (FNAIT) is fetal/neonatal thrombocytopenia due to **platelet destruction** from **maternal antibodies against fetal human platelet antigens (HPAs) inherited from the father**. It is also called neonatal alloimmune thrombocytopenia (NAIT), alloimmune thrombocytopenia (AIT), or fetal maternal alloimmune thrombocytopenia (FMAIT).

EPIDEMIOLOGY/INCIDENCE

1/1000 to 1/1500 births [1]. NAIT is the most common reason for severe thrombocytopenia and/or ICH in term newborn.

ETIOLOGY/BASIC PATHOPHYSIOLOGY

The fetus inherits paternal human platelet antigens (HPAs) that are not present on maternal platelets. Maternally produced anti-HPA IgG antibodies can cross the placenta, resulting in destruction of fetal platelets and thrombocytopenia.

Maternal platelet count and function is normal (although 10% of women with NAIT may have gestational thrombocytopenia). **Most maternal-fetal HPA incompatibilities will not become sensitized** [1].

- **FNAIT is similar to RBC Rh disease:**
  - Like red blood cells, platelets have specific surface proteins called antigens.
  - Fetus inherits paternal antigens that the mother lacks (platelet antigen incompatibility).
  - Mother develops antibodies (becomes sensitized) to fetal platelet antigens during pregnancy.
  - Maternal IgG antiplatelet antibodies cross the placenta and coat fetal platelets, resulting in sequestration and destruction of platelets in the fetal reticuloendothelial system.
- **FNAIT differs from Rh disease:**
  - Antiplatelet IgG production can occur in first pregnancy.
  - **First born children are often affected** because antiplatelet IgG production can occur in a first pregnancy; nulliparous women account for 20%–60% of cases.
  - Maternal antibody titers do not predict pregnancy outcome.

GENETICS/INHERITANCE

- HPA-1b is due to a single base pair change of cytosine to thymine at position 196 (proline to leucine) in platelet glycoprotein IIIA [2].
- Platelet antigens are **inherited in the fetus in an autosomal codominant fashion**.

CLASSIFICATION

Alloantigens are antigens present in the majority of individuals in a population but absent in a some individuals. There are 24 recognized platelet-specific alloantigens numbered in the order in which they were discovered.

- 12 of the platelet alloantigens are grouped into biallelic systems (HPA 1, 2, 3, 4, 5, 15), which are further divided into subcategories "a" for high frequency and "b" for low frequency. The **old and new nomenclature** is described in **Table 52.1**.
  - 97%–98% of Caucasian women express HPA-1a: 68% are homozygotes (HPA-1a1a), and 29% are heterozygotes (HPA-1a/HPA-1b)
  - Only 2% of Caucasian women are HPA-1a negative (HPA-1b/1b) [3].
  - **Only 10% of HPA-1a negative pregnant women develop anti-HPA-1a IgG antibodies** [3].

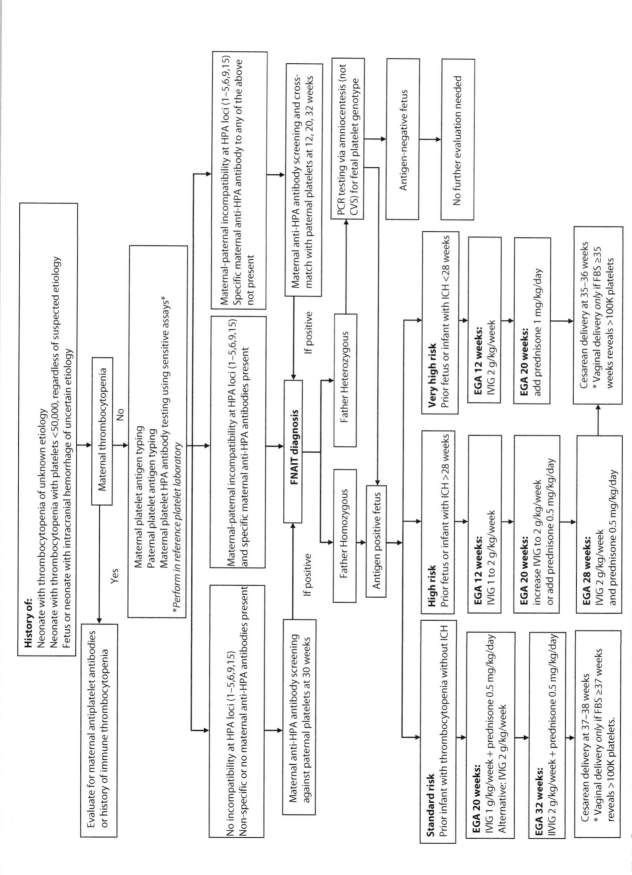

Figure 52.1 Suggested antenatal management for FNAIT. *Abbreviations:* FBS, fetal blood sampling; fetal and neonatal alloimmune thrombocytopenia; ICH, intracranial hemorrhage; IVIG, intravenous immunoglobulin therapy; EGA, estimated gestational age. (Adapted from Pacheco LD, Berkowitz RL, Moise KJ. *Obstet Gynecol*, 118, 1157–63, 2011.)

Table 52.1   Nomenclature for NAIT

Old Nomenclature	New Nomenclature (In Order of Discovery)	
PI^A1, PLA-1, ZW^A	**HPA-1a**	Most common (>75%) (2% whites, 0.4% blacks, <0.1% Asians are negative) Worse severity
PI^A2, PLA-2	**HPA-1b**	
Ko^b	**HPA-2a**	
Ko^a	**HPA-2b**	
Bak^a, Lek^a	**HPA-3a**	Second most common (15% whites are negative)
Bak^b, Lek^b, PLA-3	**HPA-3b**	
Pen^a, Yuk^b	**HPA-4a**	
Pen^b, Yuk^a	**HPA-4b**	More common in Asians
Br^b	**HPA-5a**	
Br^a, PLA-5	**HPA-5b**	Third most common (<1% whites are negative) Most common in Japan

Abbreviation: FNAIT, neonatal alloimmune thrombocytopenia.
aHigh-frequency antigen.
bLow-frequency antigen.

- Rarely, alloantibodies may also be made against **human leukocyte antigens (HLAs)**
  - Human leukocyte antigens (HLAs) are proteins located on white blood cells and other tissues, including platelets.
  - There are three HLA groups (HLA-A, HLA-B, and HLA-DR), each with many different proteins designated numerically (e.g., HLA-A1, HLA-A2, etc).
  - HLA is inherited as a "set" of the three HLA groups: A, B, DR.
  - Each HLA set is a haplotype, and a haplotype is inherited from each parent.
- **Of HPA-1a negative pregnant women who develop anti-HPA-1a IgG antibodies**, ~1/3 are positive for the **HLA-DR antigen B3*0101** (which is linked to HPA-1a). These women are at high risk to become immunized against HPA-1a when they carry an HPA-1a positive fetus [3].

The frequency of HPAs varies worldwide. In the Asian populations, HPA-5b incompatibility is the most common cause of FNAIT.

NATURAL HISTORY/COMPLICATIONS

The natural history of FNAIT ranges from mild asymptomatic fetal/neonatal thrombocytopenia to severe thrombocytopenia leading to intracranial hemorrhage with potentially severe perinatal morbidity and mortality.

- 90% affected neonates have diffuse petechiae.
- **10% to 30% ICH** [4,5].
  - **~50% occur antenatally, most often in the third trimester at around 30 to 35 weeks**, but as early as 20 weeks.
  - **Mostly intraparenchymal, leading to encephalomalacia.**
  - May result in porencephalic cysts (which may be seen by ultrasound).
  - Sometimes intraventricular hemorrhage (IVH), leading to arachnoiditis +/− hydrocephalus.
- 5% to 13% **neonatal mortality**.
- First case in family usually detected shortly after birth (due to petechiae, bleeding, or incidentally).

DIAGNOSIS

The diagnosis is **most often** made retrospectively **after delivery of an infant with thrombocytopenia or fetal/neonatal ICH**. Occasionally FNAIT may be diagnosed via family history if the mother's sister had an affected child or if prenatal screening was performed.

Indications for Testing

- Neonate with petechiae and ecchymosis, unexplained thrombocytopenia.
- Fetus with unexplained ICH, hydrocephalus, or porencephalic cyst.
- Woman incidentally found to be HPA-1a negative.
- Family history of NAIT.

Diagnostic Criteria: Fetal or neonatal thrombocytopenia (<150,000 platelets/μL) *plus* identification of a paternal, fetal, or neonatal platelet antigen with identification of maternal antibodies to that *specific* antigen.

- **Serologic Testing**
  - Test parents in reference laboratory (e.g., Blood Center of Southeastern Wisconsin).
  - **Initial testing: Maternal platelet antibody.**
    - If maternal antibody positive, perform maternal and paternal human platelet antigen testing simultaneously.
    - Reference laboratories vary in the number of platelet alloantigens screened. They typically test for HPA-1a and b, 3a and b, 4a and b, and 5a and b but cannot test for every platelet antigen.

Therefore, diagnosis is made if mother is **antibody positive** (specific to father and fetal platelet antigen) and **antigen negative**.

The **father's antigen zygosity** determines the risk of recurrence in subsequent pregnancies: 100% if father is homozygous, 50% if heterozygous. **This documentation of maternal, paternal, and neonatal serologic diagnosis should be always reviewed to guide management in the next pregnancy.**

PREVENTION AND SCREENING

Some have advocated routine universal maternal serologic screening for platelet antigens to identify pregnancies at risk for FNAIT before it happens in the first pregnancy without warning [6]. However, screening for HPA-1a alloimmunization detects about two cases in every 1000 pregnancies. Severe NAIT occurs in about 31% of these immunized pregnancies, and perinatal ICH in about 10% of pregnancies with severe NAIT. Therefore, nearly 15,000 pregnancies would need to be screened to identify one case of ICH for possible prevention [7].

Rationale Against Routine Maternal Serologic Screening

* 25% of FNAIT is NOT caused by the most common antigen.
* Maternal immune response is influenced by other factors (**e.g., HLA type**).
* Only a minority of infants of mothers negative for platelet antigen will develop significant thrombocytopenia.
* Three are many false negatives and false positives.
* No major organizations consider maternal HPA-1a typing an appropriate routine prenatal screening test.
* Screening by fetal ultrasound is not useful because fetal thrombocytopenia cannot be detected by ultrasound, and when it is so severe as to cause fetal ICH, it is too late for effective intervention.
* Screening is not cost-effective, given the low prevalence of NAIT (1/1000 births) and the inability to predict the risk of fetal ICH in pregnancies at risk but with no history of a previously affected neonate.
* A prospective epidemiologic study estimated that it would cost approximately $100,000 to detect one severe case of NAIT and approximately $2,000,000 to prevent a case of intracranial hemorrhage, assuming that early detection allowed successful intervention [8].

Since there is no consensus regarding utility of screening unaffected women for alloimmune antiplatelet antibodies, active **management of the disease is usually confined to women who have had a previously affected fetus**.

* Clinical history of affected sibling is the best indicator of risk in current/future pregnancy.
* **Recurrence** in subsequent pregnancy **is generally of greater severity, but newer data challenges this concept**. In a recent study, neonatal platelet counts in two of three subsequent pregnancies were not worse than the index pregnancy in the absence of treatment [9]. Thus, studies of increased platelets in subsequent pregnancies may not necessarily always be due to treatment effect. These findings support the current management strategies, which favor less invasive treatments.
* There is no correlation between platelet count at cordocentesis and degree of thrombocytopenia in a previously affected infant. How severe NAIT was in the last pregnancy is not as predictive.
* Only **HPA-1a** alloimmunization and **past history of ICH** predict a more severe thrombocytopenia.
* **Prior ICH**: greatest risk, only true predictor of severity.
* Fetal platelets in first-monitored pregnancy: **70% <50,000/µL** at first percutaneous umbilical blood sampling (PUBS); 50% <20,000/µL, 50% <24 weeks. If the count is >50,000/µL on first PUBS, it is still possible that it will decrease later (in HPA-1a, fetal platelets decrease as much as about 23,000/µL/week) [2].
* The **father's antigen zygosity** and **neonatal antigen** determines the risk of recurrence in subsequent pregnancies: 100% if father is homozygous, 50% if heterozygous.

MANAGEMENT

Optimal management of NAIT has not been determined, and no one therapy is proven to be 100% effective [5,10]. Studies on which to base treatment are largely observational or small RCTs due to the low incidence of FNAIT. There are some RCTs and several case series that can help guide management. The **current preferred approach recommends risk-stratified management with IVIG and prednisone without FBS** [5]. This is an empiric approach, which tries to avoid FBS, which is associated with significant complications and pregnancy loss. However, the debate between empiric treatment and treatment guided by measurement of the fetal platelet count using FBS is not yet resolved. Either approach is acceptable until the issue is resolved by further clinical trials.

Principles

* **Goal: prevent hemorrhage, specifically ICH, in fetus and neonate**.
* ICH is rare with platelets >20,000/µL; therefore, **the goal is to keep platelets >20,000/µL**. The normal platelet count of a fetus ≥18 weeks is ≥150,000/µL, as in an adult.
* FBS with direct measurement of fetal platelet count is the only method to assess disease severity, but given its risks, it's currently rarely used.

There are two antenatal treatment options:

1. **Intravenous immunoglobulin** with or without corticosteroids **(preferred option) (Figure 52.1)**.
   * >$1000/dose.
   * Most common initial therapy in North America.
   * Pooled blood product, but risks of hepatitis and HIV transmission are minuscule (donor screening and viral inactivation procedures decrease risk).
   * Usually given as **weekly infusion** over 6 to 12 hours.
   * IVIG has unclear mechanism of action, but is theorized to work via the following:
     * Fc-receptor **saturation in the placenta** with a reduction of antibody transfer across the placenta (most probable main mechanism).
     * Fc-receptor blockade on macrophages leading to inhibition of uptake of the antibody-coated platelets by fetal macrophages. Endothelial stabilization prevents damage by maternal platelet antibodies (low platelets not a cause of ICH).
     * Suppression of maternal IgG antibody production.
   * IVIG can not only prevent/improve thrombocytopenia in the majority of cases, but it also prevents ICH. **There are only very rare reports of IVIG failures to prevent ICH** [11].
   * Side effects: headaches and febrile reactions (pretreat with benadryl and acetaminophen).
   * Only way to monitor efficacy of IVIG treatment is via FBS.
   * **75% respond to weekly IVIG; half of the nonresponders improve with the addition of high-dose prednisone** (1 mg/kg = 60 mg/day) [12]. Dexamethasone has been associated with oligohydramnios and FGR [12].
   * IVIG is administered with or without steroid administration. Side effects of maternal steroid administration include osteoporosis, impaired glucose tolerance and gestational diabetes, depressed immunity, mood swings, and gastrointestinal irritation.

2. Repeated **intrauterine transfusion** of antigen-compatible platelets via FBS.

   • **FBS as the main treatment option has largely been abandoned due to significant procedure-related risk.**

   • In the past, weekly in utero transfusion of platelets via FBS was often required after 20 weeks.

   • Goal was to prevent undertreatment, which can result in risk of ICH in utero, and to avoid overtreatment, which is expensive and can cause adverse maternal side effects.

   • Empiric therapy has not been compared with fetal cordocentesis-indicated treatment in a randomized trial.

   • Risk of increasing sensitization due to fetomaternal hemorrhage.

   • **Risk of fetal hemorrhage** is at least 1% to 2% per procedure and 5% to 10% cumulative loss for each pregnancy [13–15]. Procedure-related fetal loss rates are higher when the first IUT occurs <20 weeks (5% versus 1%) [16].

   • FBS is now used primarily to assess response to IVIG therapy (typically performed around 32 weeks) or to determine **eligibility for vaginal delivery (at about 36–37 weeks)** [5].

   • If FBS is performed to guide IVIG (and/or steroid) therapy (usually between 20 and 35 weeks), the following principles are generally followed:

     ▪ If adequate (platelet count ≥50,000/µL), continue current regimen to term.

     ▪ If the first fetal platelet count is >20,000/µL while on IVIG, the chance of platelet count >20,000/µL at a later sampling is 89%, and if the first count is ≤20,000/µL, this chance is only 51% [17]. Therefore, if the response is adequate (>50,000 µL), continue current regimen [17].

     ▪ **If inadequate platelet count <50,000/µL, increase therapy depending on current treatment (up to maximum of IVIG 2 g/kg/week + prednisone 1 mg/kg/d).**

   • **FBS Technique:**

     ▪ Have platelets ready at any FBS with slow transfusion started after sampling even before platelet count (PC) is available to minimize risk fetal hemorrhage.

     ▪ Transfuse maternal platelets (antigen negative), packed, washed, and irradiated. Transfusion volume: aim for 200 to 400,000 platelets to avoid volume overload by using the equation in Table 52.2.

     ▪ Typical volume of platelet concentrate transfused is 5 to 15 mL.

     ▪ Goal: platelets >50,000/µL and usually 200,000 to 400,000/µL.

     ▪ Because of risk of emergent delivery, corticosteroids for fetal lung maturity before FBS are suggested at ≥24 weeks.

     ▪ In fetuses with platelets >80,000/µL at first FBS and not treated, follow-up FBS showed decreases of at least 10,000/µL/wk.

RISK-BASED FETAL THERAPY FOR PREGNANCIES AT RISK FOR FNAIT

There is insufficient data to assess different types of interventions for the pregnancy with NAIT. Current preferred

Table 52.2 Calculations for Fetal Platelet Transfusion for FNAIT Volume (in mL) to raise platelet count by 50,000

$$= \frac{\text{(fetal weight in grams)}(0.14)(50,000)(2)}{\text{Platelet count from lab expressed as per uL}^a}$$

Platelet Goal	Volume to Infuse
100,000	
150,000	
200,000	
250,000	
300,000	
350,000	
400,000	

Abbreviation: FNAIT, neonatal alloimmune thrombocytopenia

[a]If volume is given in milliliters, just divide by mL volume × 1000; that is, if given total platelets is 6 million in 55 mL, then (6,000,000/55,000) = platelet count from lab. The factor of "2" is used in the numerator of the equation to allow for possible platelet sequestration in the fetal spleen or liver. Then one can use the following chart to fill in, according to initial fetal platelet count obtained at PUBS.

management is based upon the risk of ICH. Fetuses at highest risk are those with a sibling affected by ICH [5,18]. The earlier the ICH occurred in the sibling, the greater the risk for intracranial hemorrhage in the currently affected fetus.

Risk is based on history of ICH in past pregnancy as defined below [5]:

1. **Standard risk** – Previous child had thrombocytopenia without intracranial hemorrhage.
2. **High risk** – Previous child had an intracranial hemorrhage in the third trimester or neonatal period.
3. **Extremely high risk** – Previous child had an intracranial hemorrhage in the second trimester.

Standard Risk = Criteria for NAIT is Met; Previous Siblings with Thrombocytopenia But NO In Utero ICH (Figure 52.1)

A. **At 20 weeks gestation, begin IVIG at 1 g/kg/week with prednisone 0.5 mg/kg/day.**

   • Alternative regimen: IVIG at 2 g/kg/week [18]; this option was shown to be comparable in a RCT [19].

   • Consider starting at the higher dose (2 g/kg/week) if the initial platelet count of the affected neonate was <20,000/µL at birth [17].

   • Some advocate using IVIG only as initial therapy due to the side effects of prednisone.

   • Treatment can be tailored to the patient after discussion of adverse effects of both arms.

B. **At 32 weeks, escalate therapy to IVIG at 2 g/kg/week with prednisone 0.5 mg/kg/day.**

   • Previous data recommended FBS to assess therapy at 32 weeks, but therapy prevented ICH in all 73 patients [19]. Additional expanded data from those authors showed only 3 cases of mild grade I ICH out of 100 cases, which is similar to group of normal term neonates [5,18].

   • Thus, current recommendation is **escalate therapy without FBS** [5].

C. Delivery at 37–38 weeks by cesarean section [5].
 • For those desiring vaginal delivery, perform FBS at 37 weeks (see *FBS technique* above). Vaginal delivery at 37–38 weeks only recommended if PUBS ≥37 weeks reveals >100K platelets.

High Risk = Previous Sibling Had In Utero ICH in the third trimester or neonatal period (Figure 52.1) [5,18]

A. **At 12 weeks gestation, begin IVIG at 1 to 2 g/kg/week** (Figure 52.1).
B. **At 20 weeks gestation, either add prednisone 0.5 mg/ kg/day OR increase the dose of IVIG to 2 g/kg/week.**
C. **At 28 weeks gestation, give IVIG 2 g/kg/week AND prednisone 0.5 mg/kg/day.**
D. **Deliver at 35–36 weeks by cesarean section.**
 • For those desiring vaginal delivery, perform FBS at 35 weeks (see *FBS technique* above). Vaginal delivery only recommended if PUBS ≥35 weeks reveals >100K platelets.

Very High Risk = Previous Sibling Had In Utero ICH <28 weeks (Figure 52.1) [5,18]

A. **At 12 weeks gestation, begin IVIG at 2 g/kg/week** (Figure 52.1).
B. **At 20 weeks gestation, add prednisone 1 mg/kg/day.**
C. **Deliver at 35–36 weeks by cesarean section.**
 • For those desiring vaginal delivery, perform FBS at 35 weeks (see *FBS technique* above). Vaginal delivery only recommended if PUBS ≥35 weeks reveals >100K platelets.

Other Clinical Concerns/Issues Regarding Therapy

• Patients should avoid activities (i.e., sports) that could result in potential trauma.
• External cephalic versions and NSAIDs are contraindicated.
• There are **reported cases of ICH while receiving IVIG treatment** [11,19], so that IVIG should be considered a highly effective but not a perfect therapy to prevent ICH (and in some situations FBS and possible transfusions may still be indicated).
• Women with prior IVIG administration should have their serum checked for HTLV I+II and HepC antibodies.

Other Clinical Scenarios (Figure 52.1)

1. *Personal history of fetal intracranial hemorrhage/neonatal thrombocytopenia and HPA incompatibility but no antibodies*: does NOT meet criteria for NAIT.
 • Perform serially testing of maternal serum for anti-HPA antibodies at 12, 24, and 32 weeks of gestation by both a panel of platelets expressing common HPA antigens and cross-matching against paternal platelets to detect alloimmunization to a rare antigen carried by the father [5]. If antibodies are detected, treatment is initiated.

2. *Personal history of fetal intracranial hemorrhage/neonatal thrombocytopenia, but no HPA incompatibility and no antibodies*: does NOT meet criteria for NAIT [5].
 • Consider maternal serum for anti-HPA antibodies at 30 weeks of gestation to check for development of previously undetected antibodies.
3. *No personal history of fetal intracranial hemorrhage or neonatal thrombocytopenia, but HPA incompatibility [5].*
 • Routine screening for HPA incompatibility is not recommended.

COUNSELING

Prognosis, natural history and complications, and management criteria should all be reviewed with the family. **All patients should be advised that the optimal management of NAIT has not been determined and that no one therapy has proven to be 100% effective.**

INVESTIGATIONS AND CONSULTATIONS

With heterozygous father, consider **amniocentesis to determine fetal antigen** status by PCR (CVS only if mother would terminate affected fetus). Multidisciplinary management should involve a hematologist and the blood bank.

FETAL MONITORING/TESTING

Serial ultrasounds may be performed every 4–6 weeks to evaluate for ICH, but if ICH is detected, it is too late for intervention to prevent severe sequelae.

ANESTHESIA

No special precautions, since maternal platelets are usually normal, but 10% of women with FNAIT have gestational thrombocytopenia.

DELIVERY

• Avoid fetal trauma: avoid maternal abdominal trauma, external cephalic version, fetal scalp lead, vacuum, or forceps.
• There is no evidence to prove that cesarean delivery prevents ICH.
• If platelet count >100,000/µL at the 35–37 weeks FBS and patient is compliant with the effective therapy, vaginal delivery can be allowed. Therefore, in cases with platelets >100,000/µL at 35–37 weeks, trial of labor and attempt at vaginal delivery can be considered [18].

NEONATOLOGY MANAGEMENT

• Maternal platelets (Ag negative, obtained by plasmaphoresis, plasma depleted, washed, irradiated, and packed) should always be available for transfusion after delivery.
• Neonatal treatment is with IVIG, IV steroids, and antigen-compatible platelets until platelet count recovers, usually by 7 to 10 days of age.
• The volume of platelets transfused can be calculated as blood volume × (desired platelet count – actual platelet count/platelet concentration). For a term neonate, this equates to 1 cc platelet = increase platelet count by 5000/µL

(10 cc = 50,000; 20 cc = 100,000). Often neonatologists choose to transfuse 10 cc of platelets per kg of neonatal weight.

FUTURE PREGNANCY PRECONCEPTION COUNSELING

Management, events, and outcome of the pregnancy should be reviewed with the family postpartum (after discharge of the neonate). As stated above, the natural history of NAIT is that, if it recurs (depending on father's zygocity), it is more severe than in the previous pregnancy.

- **Recurrence risk is close to 100% of antigen (+) fetuses/neonates.**
- For women with high-risk and extremely high-risk prior pregnancies, options include sperm donation using an HPA-1b/1b donor or in vitro fertilization (IVF) with preimplantation genetic diagnosis (PGD) if the partner is a HPA heterozygote (HPA-1a/1b).

REFERENCES

1. Davoren A, McParland P, Crowley J et al. Antenatal screening for human platelet antigen 1a: Results of a prospective study at a large maternity hospital in Ireland. *Br J Obstet Gynecol* 2003; 110: 492–6. [II-2]
2. Bussel JB, Zabusky MR, Berkowitz RL et al. Fetal alloimmune thrombocytopenia. *N Engl J Med* 1997; 337: 22–6. [II-3]
3. Peterson JA, McFarland JG, Curtis BR et al. Neonatal alloimmune thrombocytopenia: Pathogenesis, diagnosis and management. *Br J Haematol* 2013; 161: 3–14. [Literature Review]
4. Spencer JA, Burrows RF. Feto-maternal alloimmune thrombocytopenia: A literature review and statistical analysis. *Aust N Z J Obstet Gynaecol* 2002; 41: 45–5. [Literature Review]
5. Pacheco LD, Berkowitz RL, Moise KJ. Fetal and neonatal alloimmune thrombocytopenia: A management algorithm based on risk stratification. *Obstet Gynecol* 2011; 118: 1157–63. [Literature Review]
6. Tiller H, Killie MK, Skogen B et al. Neonatal alloimmune thrombocytopenia in Norway: Poor detection rate with non-screening versus a general screening programme. *Br J Obstet Gynecol* 2009; 116: 594–8. [II-3]
7. Kamphuis MM, Paridaans N, Porcelijn L et al. Screening in pregnancy for fetal or neonatal alloimmune thrombocytopenia: Systematic review. *Br J Obstet Gynecol* 2010; 117: 1335–43. [Systematic Review]
8. Turner ML, Bessos H, Fagge T et al. Prospective epidemiologic study of the outcome and cost-effectiveness of antenatal screening to detect neonatal alloimmune thrombocytopenia due to anti-HPA-1a. *Transfusion* 2005; 45: 1945. [II-2]
9. Tiller H, Husebekk A, Skiogen B et al. True risk of fetal/neonatal alloimmune thrombocytopenia in subsequent pregnancies: A prospective observational follow-up study. *Br J Obstet Gynecol* 2015. doi:10.1111/1471-0528.13343. [II-2]
10. Rayment R, Brunskill SJ, Soothill PW et al. Antenatal interventions for feto-maternal alloimmune thrombocytopenia. *Cochrane Database System Rev* 2011; 5: CD004226. doi:10.1002/14651858.CD004226.pub3. [Systematic Review]
11. Kroll H, Kiefel V, Giers G et al. Maternal intravenous immunoglobulin treatment does not prevent intracranial haemorrhage in fetal alloimmune thrombocytopenia. *Transfus Med* 1994; 4(4): 293–6. [II-2]
12. Bussel JB, Berkowitz RL, Lynch L et al. Antenatal management of alloimmune thrombocytopenia with intravenous gamma-globulin: A randomized trial of the addition of low dose steroid to intravenous gamma-globulin. *Am J Obstet Gynecol* 1996; 174(5): 1414–23. [RCT, *n* = 54]
13. Paidas MJ, Berkowitz RL, Lynch L et al. Alloimmune thrombocytopenia: Fetal and neonatal losses related to cordocentesis. *Am J Obstet Gynecol* 1995; 172: 475–9. [II-3]
14. Overton T, Duncan KR, Jolly M et al. Serial aggressive platelet transfusion for fetal alloimmune thrombocytopenia: Platelet dynamics and perinatal outcome. *Am J Obstet Gynecol* 2002; 186: 826–31. [II-2]
15. Berkowitz RL, Kolb EA, McFarland JG et al. Parallel randomized trials of risk-based therapy for fetal alloimmune thrombocytopenia. *Obstet Gynecol* 2006; 107: 91–6. [RCT, *n* = 79]
16. Lindenburg ITM, van Kamp IL, van Zwet EW et al. Increased perinatal loss after intrauterine transfusion for alloimmune anaemia before 20 weeks gestation. *Br J Obstet Gynecol* 2013: 847–52. [II-2]
17. Gaddipatti S, Berkowitz RL, Lembert AA et al. Initial fetal platelet counts predict the response to intravenous gammaglobulin therapy in fetuses that are affected by PLA1 incompatibility. *Am J Obstet Gynecol* 2001; 185: 976–80. [II-2]
18. Bussel JB, Berkowitz RL, Hung C. Intracranial hemorrhage in alloimmune thrombocytopenia: Stratified management to prevent recurrence in the subsequent affected fetus. *Am J Obstet Gynecol* 2010; 203: 135.e1. [I, based on 2 RCTs, *n* = 37 pregnancies]
19. Berkowitz RL, Lesser ML, McFarland JG et al. Antepartum treatment without early cordocentesis for standard-risk alloimmune thrombocytopenia. *Obstet Gynecol* 2007; 110: 249–55. [RCT, *n* = 73]

Hemolytic disease of the fetus/neonate

Danielle L. Tate, Jacques E. Samson, and Giancarlo Mari

KEY POINTS

- The formation of maternal antibodies to fetal red blood cell (RBC) antigens is called **RBC alloimmunization** and can lead to hemolytic disease and anemia of the fetus and neonate.
- The most common antigens causing alloimmunization in the United States today are **Rh(D)** and Kell. Rh(D) alloimmunization occurs when a pregnant woman develops an immunological response to a paternally derived Rh(D) antigen foreign to the mother and inherited by the fetus. The IgG antibodies cross the placenta, bind to the antigens on the fetal RBCs, and can lead to hemolysis. Kell alloimmunization is usually caused by previous blood transfusions but may also occur by maternal-fetal hemorrhage during pregnancy.
- **Anti-D immune globulin** prophylaxis prevents >99% of cases of Rh(D) alloimmunization if given **both antepartum and postpartum**. It should be given to all Rh(D)-negative women with a negative antibody screen at **28 weeks** and, if the neonate is Rh(D) positive, **within 72 hours after birth**. Anti-D immune globulin can be given as late as **28 days postpartum** if previously not given but indicated. Anti-D immunoglobulin prophylaxis used in the United States and other countries is **300 μg (1 μg = 5 IU)** at 28 weeks as well as after delivery if the neonate is Rh(D) positive. **A 100-μg dose** administered at 28 and 34 weeks is also used. However, there are no trials to directly compare the different regimens. Mothers who are weak D positive (formerly called Du) do not need anti-D prophylaxis. A **Kleihauer–Betke (KB) test** should be done to determine the number of fetal cells that has entered the maternal circulation and hence **the appropriate dose of anti-D immune globulin** in certain high-risk situations (abdominal trauma, abruption, manual extraction of the placenta, etc.), or when the 100-μg dose is used, after delivery of an Rh(D)-negative, nonalloimmunized woman.
- Currently, **there is no prophylactic immune globulin to prevent alloimmunization from Kell or other antigens except Rh(D)**.
- If Rh(D) antibodies are detected in the maternal circulation on the antibody screen, the patient is considered alloimmunized. Management of the alloimmunized pregnancy is shown in **Figure 53.1**. This is based initially on genotyping of the fetus' father and, if necessary, fetal Rh(D) status determination, usually by polymerase chain reaction (PCR) from amniocytes. Maternal blood for fetal DNA testing is also available. **The critical titer for Rh(D) antibody should be determined in each laboratory**.
- **Ultrasound using the middle cerebral artery peak systolic velocity (MCA-PSV)** has 100% sensitivity for detecting significant fetal anemia (95% CI: 0.86–1.00) and is the screening method of choice in RBC alloimmunized pregnancies if available and quality assurance can be confirmed. Compared with amniocentesis for delta OD450, the MCA-PSV assessment is associated with approximately 70% to 80% reduction in the number of invasive tests. Screening with MCA-PSV can be started as early as 15 weeks. If the **MCA-PSV is ≥1.5 multiple of the median (MoM), fetal blood sampling (FBS) is indicated**. When a cordocentesis is performed at >24 weeks gestation, corticosteroids for fetal lung maturation should be considered before the procedure. Blood transfusions should be initiated for fetal hemoglobin <5th percentile.
- If adequately trained sonographers are not available, screening for anemia should be done with amniocentesis using ΔOD_{450} values.
- In **Kell**-alloimmunized pregnancies, maternal titers do not correlate well with fetal disease. ΔOD_{450} levels also do not correlate with fetal anemia. However, MCA-PSV screening is predictive and accurate for the diagnosis of fetal anemia from Kell alloimmunization.

DEFINITION

RBC alloimmunization, formerly known as isoimmunization or erythroblastosis fetalis, is the formation of maternal antibodies to fetal RBC antigens [1]. Maternal RBC alloimmunization can cause hemolytic disease of the fetus and neonate.

EPIDEMIOLOGY/INCIDENCE

The most common antigen causing alloimmunization is Rh(D) followed closely by the Kell antigen [2,3]. The Rh(D)-negative blood group is found in about 15% of whites, 3% to 5% of black Africans, and is rare in Asians. Spontaneous fetomaternal hemorrhages occur in increasing frequency and volume with advancing age. In 3%, 12%, and 46% of women, 0.01 mL or more of fetal cells in each of the three successive trimesters have been noted using the Kleihauer assay [4]. The risk of Rh(D) alloimmunization during or immediately after a first pregnancy is about 0.7% to 1%. The risk of fetal anemia from RBC alloimmunization is about 0.35%, of which about 10% of cases require transfusion. Rh(D) alloimmunization affects 6.7 out of every 1000 live births [5].

The Kell (K1) antigen is found on red cells of 9% of Caucasians and 2% of people of African descent. Kell alloimmunization occurs in 1 to 3 per 1000 fetuses [6].

GENETICS

Rh(D)-negative pregnant women have a deletion of the sequence on both copies of the short arm of chromosome 1. The Kell glycoprotein is a type II membrane protein with homology to zinc endopeptidases (M13 family) [7].

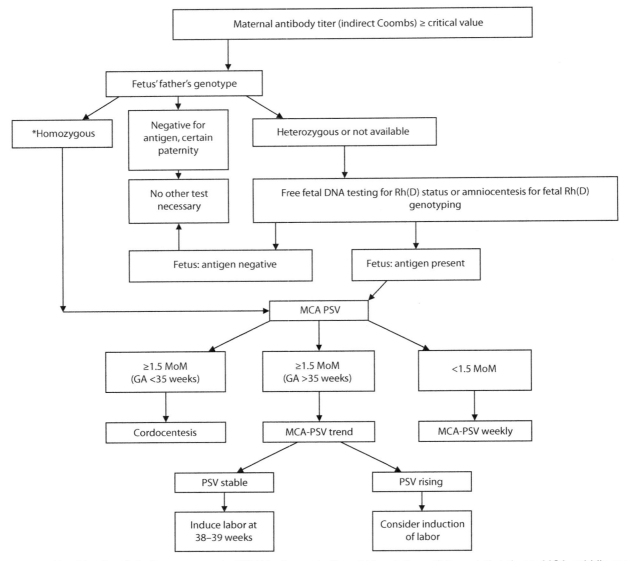

Figure 53.1   Algorithm for clinical management of RhD isoimmunization. *Abbreviations*: GA, gestational age; MCA, middle cerebral artery; MoM, multiples of the median; PSV, peak systolic velocity. (From Society for Maternal-Fetal Medicine (SMFM); Mari G; Norton ME; Stone J et al. Society for Maternal-Fetal Medicine (SMFM) Clinical Guideline #8: The fetus at risk for anemia—Diagnosis and management. *AJOG*, 212, 697–710, 2015.)

ETIOLOGY/BASIC PATHOPHYSIOLOGY

Maternal Rh(D) alloimmunization occurs when a pregnant woman develops an immunologic response to a paternally derived RBC antigen—for example, Rh(D), that is foreign to the mother and inherited by the fetus. The immunoglobulin G (IgG) antibodies cross the placenta, bind to the antigens present on the fetal RBCs, and can cause hemolysis. Hemolysis then causes anemia which, if severe, leads to fetal cardiac failure, edema, hydrops, and eventually fetal death. Other antigens ("irregular antigens") than Rh(D) can cause RBC alloimmunization.

Alloimmunization of the Kell antigen may be caused by previous blood transfusion or by maternal-fetal hemorrhage during the pregnancy with a fetus who is a Kell antigen carrier [8,9]. The Kell glycoprotein is expressed very early in erythropoiesis [10]. Antibody to Kell appears to inhibit

erythropoiesis, suggesting another functional role for Kell in addition to its endopeptidase activity [11].

NATURAL HISTORY

About 17% of Rh(D)-negative women who do not receive prophylaxis become immunized. Over 90% of this immunization occurs from fetomaternal hemorrhage at delivery, and the majority of the remaining 10% occurs in the third trimester. Most of this immunization is caused by <0.1 mL of fetomaternal hemorrhage. Before anti-D immune globulin prevention, hemolytic disease of the fetus/neonate affected 9% to 10% of pregnancies, and was a major cause of perinatal mortality. The risk of RBC alloimmunization from different clinical situations is shown in Table 53.1.

Table 53.1 Risk of RBC Alloimmunization in Different Clinical Situations

Clinical Situation	Risk of Red Blood Cell Alloimmunization (%)
Induced abortions	4–5
First-trimester losses	1–2
Chorionic villus sampling	14
Amniocentesis	7–15
External cephalic version	2–6
Threatened abortion	↑ (controversial)
Antepartum hemorrhage	↑↑
Placenta previa with bleeding	↑
Suspected abruption	↑
Blunt trauma to abdomen (including motor vehicle accidents)	↑
Fetal death	↑
Fetal blood sampling	↑
Fetal surgery	↑
Ectopic	↑
Partial molar pregnancy	↑

Anti-K1 is responsible for severe neonatal anemia in approximately 40% of K1-positive babies of women with anti-K1 [12].

PREVENTION (ANTI-D IMMUNOGLOBULIN)

The ABO type, the Rh(D) status, and the antibody screen should be determined in all pregnant women at the initial prenatal visit. If the woman is Rh-negative and the antibody screen is negative, the patient should receive Rh(D) immune globulin. Anti-D immunoglobulin prophylaxis properly given prevents >99% of cases of alloimmunization. The American Association of Blood Banks recommends a repeat antibody screen prior to administration of antenatal anti-D immune globulin as this second screening test has the advantage of detecting those rare cases in which immunization occurs early in pregnancy. However, given the low incidence (0.18%) of alloimmunization occurring prior to 28 weeks and the unknown cost-effectiveness of routine repeat screening, the practice of screening prior to administration of anti-D immune globulin remains controversial [13]. After delivery, if the neonate is Rh(D) positive, the patient should receive immune globulin. If the patient has never received immune globulin and the screening test is positive, the patient is at risk for having an anemic baby in the current pregnancy (if she has not delivered yet) or in a future pregnancy if she already has delivered. Usually, the effect of the immune globulin is not present 12 weeks after its administration.

Anti-D immune globulin prophylaxis properly given prevents the majority of cases of alloimmunization. Despite recommendations, 0.1% to 0.2% of susceptible women still become alloimmunized, largely due to either failure of implementation of immunoprophylaxis protocols or spontaneous immunization in the setting of these protocols [13]. Anti-D immune globulin is extracted by cold alcohol fractionation from plasma of individuals with high-titer D IgG antibodies. The risk of transmission of viral infections or side effects is minimal to absent and clinically not a significant factor. Unfortunately, there is no immune globulin available for prevention of RBC antigens other than Rh(D).

The accepted regimens of **anti-D immune globulin prophylaxis** are 1) 100 µg at 28 and 34 weeks and after delivery

if the neonate is Rh(D) positive, or 2) 300 µg at 28 weeks and after delivery if the neonate is Rh(D) positive and delivery occurs at least three weeks after the first administration. There are no trials to directly compare these two different regimens, but they probably both achieve >99% prevention of Rh(D) alloimmunization.

The half-life of anti-D immune globulin is 16 to 24 days. **When the 300 µg dose is used and delivery does not occur within 12 weeks of injection, a second 300 µg dose of anti-D immunoglobulin should be given.** The antibody titer obtained at term is occasionally still positive (1:1, 1:2 titer) after anti-D immunoglobulin at 28 weeks gestation.

When indicated, a second dose of immune globulin is administered after delivery, even in cases of preterm delivery.

Mothers who are **weak D** positive with D present in reduced quantities (formerly called Du) **do not need anti-D prophylaxis**. Mothers who are **partial D** positive (lacking some epitopes of D) should receive anti-D immunoglobulin, since they are at risk for hemolytic disease [14]. In those cases where the **father of the fetus/neonate is definitely known to be Rh(D) negative**, neither antepartum nor postpartum anti-D prophylaxis is administered.

Evidence for Dosing and Timing

After Birth (Postpartum)
Anti-D immune globulin given within 72 hours **after birth** is associated with a **96% decreased incidence** of Rh(D) alloimmunization six months after birth, and with a 88% **decreased incidence** of Rh(D) alloimmunization in a subsequent pregnancy in Rh(D)-negative women who have given birth to an Rh(D)-positive infant [15]. These benefits are seen regardless of the ABO status of the mother and baby. **Higher doses (up to 200 µg) are more effective than lower doses (up to 50 µg]** in preventing Rh(D) alloimmunization [15]. Anti-D immune globulin can be given **as late as 28 days postpartum** if indicated but not previously given. **Anti-D immune globulin is given to all Rh(D)-negative women after confirmation from cord blood of Rh(D)-positive status of the neonate.**

Even when immune globulin is correctly administered and with higher doses, alloimmunization can still occur (antepartum) in up to 2% of these women if only postpartum anti-D is administered.

Before Birth (Antepartum)
The addition of anti-D immune globulin 100 µg (500 IU) prophylaxis at 28 and 34 weeks **lowers this risk (about 1%–2%) to about 0.2%** without any adverse effects [16–18]. When women receive anti-D immune globulin at 28 and 34 weeks gestation, there is a trend for less immunization 1) for all women (RR: 0.42, 95% CI: 0.15–1.17); and 2) for women giving birth to an Rh-positive infant (RR: 0.41, 95% CI: 0.16–1.04), compared with no prophylaxis [16–18]. In trials that used a 100-µg dose of anti-D immune globulin, there was a nonsignificant reduction in immunization at 2 to 12 months following birth of an Rh-positive infant in women who had received anti-D (RR: 0.14, 95% CI: 0.02–1.15). However, women receiving anti-D were significantly less likely to have a positive KB test (which detects fetal cells in maternal blood) both in pregnancy (RR: 0.60, 95% CI: 0.41–0.88) and at the birth of an Rh-positive infant (RR: 0.60, 95% CI: 0.46–0.79) [17]. No data were available for the risk of Rh(D) alloimmunization in a subsequent pregnancy. No differences were seen for neonatal jaundice.

There are no trials using the 300-μg dose or trials comparing just 28-week versus both 28- and 34-week prophylaxis.

Even with antepartum and postpartum prophylaxis, the risk of Rh(D) alloimmunization remains because of inadvertent antepartum or postpartum omission, failure to use the drug for other antenatal complications, and insufficient dosing at delivery in cases of large fetomaternal hemorrhage. **Practice guidelines in the United States** recommend that anti-D immune globulin be administered early in the third trimester: **300 μg at 28 weeks.** This practice reduces the incidence of antenatal alloimmunization from 2% to 0.1% [2,3]. In the **United Kingdom,** 100 μg of anti-D immune globulin is given at 28 and 34 weeks [14]. **In Canada, 100 to 120 μg** is administered at 28 and 34 weeks. Studies have shown improved compliance with the single dose protocol over the two-dose protocol [19].

Special Clinical Situations
In addition to antepartum and postpartum prophylaxis, other indications for the use of anti-D immune globulin include those situations in which there is significant risk of fetomaternal hemorrhage. These indications are listed in Table 53.1. A repeat dose is unnecessary after prophylaxis if delivery occurs <3 weeks from the last dose.

Anti-D immune globulin 300 μg protects against 30 μL of fetal whole blood or 15 mL of fetal RBCs in the maternal circulation. In certain high-risk situations in which excessive fetomaternal bleeding may have occurred (e.g., abruption, manual removal of the placenta, abdominal trauma), this dose may be inadequate, and a **KB test** should be done **to determine** the amount of fetal cells that have entered the maternal circulation and, hence, **the appropriate dose of anti-D immune globulin** to be given. Some clinicians have advocated the KB test for all Rh(D)-negative women at delivery, since 50% of cases requiring more than the standard postpartum dose of anti-D immunoglobulin can be missed by high-risk situation screening only [20]. **The risk of fetomaternal hemorrhage >30 mL is about 0.1% to 0.2%.**

The anti-D immunoglobulin available in the United States and other countries (RhoGAM, Rhophylac, WinRho, and BabyRho-D) are all very effective with none shown to be significantly more effective in the prevention of hemolytic disease than the others. Thus cost and route of administration—intramuscular (IM) or intravenous (IV)—may be the only factors determining choice.

MANAGEMENT OF RBC ALLOIMMUNIZED PREGNANCIES
Counseling
If Rh(D) antibodies are detected in the maternal circulation, for example, positive indirect Coombs, the patient is considered alloimmunized. Among Rh(D) alloimmunized pregnancies, mild-to-moderate hemolytic anemia and hyperbilirubinemia occur in 25% to 30% of fetuses/neonates, and 25% of these can develop hydrops [21]. With correct management, the **perinatal survival rate in cases of anemia is >90%;** when fetal hydrops is present, the survival rate is >80%. There is no trial that has assessed the best management for RBC alloimmunized pregnancies; however, fetal transfusion is probably the most beneficial of all the available therapies. Although it is reported that the risk of fetal demise is between 1% and 2% for each FBS, there are situations in which the risk is much higher, such as when cordocenteses and transfusions

are performed at gestational ages (GAs), as early as 15 to 18 weeks.

Workup/Investigations Required
Management of the **alloimmunized** pregnancy is shown in Figure 53.1. In patients at risk for fetal anemia because of red cell alloimmunization, it is important to perform a first-trimester ultrasound to establish the GA. Assessment for risk of fetal anemia depends on history of previous Rh complications in pregnancies, titer of RBC antibodies, and MCA-PSV values [22,23].

The genotype of the fetus' father can be determined by zygosity testing. The most likely zygosity can also be predicted by evaluating the pattern of C, D, and E loci since they are inherited together and some combinations are more common than others, but this is not 100% exact and not very useful clinically. If the father is Rh(D) negative, no further testing or intervention is necessary. If the father is heterozygous for the Rh(D) antigen, fetal Rh(D) testing is indicated. If the father is Rh(D) homozygous, the fetus is assumed to be Rh(D) positive and no fetal Rh(D) testing is necessary. Of course, the paternity should be certain; otherwise, fetal testing is indicated.

Fetal Rh(D) status can be determined by **PCR from amniocytes** with >95% accuracy (sensitivity and specificity). This is available in the United States in several centers. One of them is the Blood Center of Southwestern Wisconsin (http://www.bloodcenter.com). This is also available for many other antigens, such as c, E, Kell, M, N, etc. Chorionic villus sampling (CVS) is not advised as it results in high risk of worsening alloimmunization from fetomaternal hemorrhage. Determination of fetal Rh(D) status can **also** be obtained **noninvasively** as early as 38 days gestation with fetal DNA analysis from maternal blood [24–26]. This can be done through the International Blood Group Reference Laboratory in Bristol, United Kingdom (Molecular.Diagnostics@nhsbt.nhs.uk; http://ibgrl.blood.co.uk/) or in the United States through laboratories.sequenom.com. Accuracy of noninvasive Rh(D) genotyping is >99.3% when testing is performed at 11 weeks gestation or greater [27]. Currently, the Rh(D) antigen is the only antigen available for testing through cell-free fetal DNA analysis from maternal blood in the United States. Kell, c, and E antigen testing is available in Europe [28].

Rh(D) antibody titers correlate somewhat with risk of anemia/hydrops, with 1:16 = 10%, 1:32 = 25%, 1:64 = 50%, and 1:128 = 75% risk of anemia. **The critical titer should be determined in each laboratory.** Unfortunately, large differences in titer can be seen in the same woman between laboratories. In most laboratories, the critical titer is ≥1:16 in albumin or ≥1:32 in indirect antiglobulin (indirect Coombs test). If the titer is less than 1:16, the fetus is not in jeopardy at that time. However, **serial titers should be obtained every four weeks.** If the patient has had a prior affected pregnancy, and the fetus is known to be Rh(D) positive, titers are not necessary. The MCA-PSV is used to detect those fetuses that are going to develop anemia [29]. The presence of additional antibody(ies) with anti-D increases the need for intrauterine fetal transfusions [30].

Ultrasound is the screening method of choice for fetal anemia. With fetal anemia, decreased blood viscosity leads to increased venous return and consequent increase in cardiac output with increased blood flow velocity in all vessels. Degrees of blood velocity (Table 53.2) correlate with

Table 53.2 Expected Peak Velocity of Systolic Blood Flow in the Middle Cerebral Artery as a Function of Gestational Age

Week of Gestation	Multiples of the Median			
	1.00	1.29	1.50	1.55
18	23.2[a]	29.9	34.8	36.0
20	25.5	32.8	38.2	39.5
22	27.9	36.0	41.9	43.3
24	30.7	39.5	46.0	47.5
26	33.6	43.3	50.4	52.1
28	36.9	47.9	55.4	57.2
30	40.5	52.2	60.7	62.8
32	44.4	57.3	66.6	68.9
34	48.7	62.9	73.1	75.6
36	53.5	69.0	80.2	82.9
38	58.7	75.7	88.0	91.0
40	64.4	83.0	96.6	99.8

Notes: Mild anemia: MCA-PSV between 1.29 and 1.49 MoM; moderate anemia: MCA-PSV between 1.50 and 1.54 MoM; severe anemia: MCA-PSV ≥1.55 MoM.
[a]Data shown are in cm/sec (median).

anemia (Table 53.3). The vessel to study is the **middle cerebral artery** (MCA). The main advantage of the MCA is that it is easy to measure at a 0° angle. In the biparietal diameter view, the MCA can be visualized with color Doppler. The MCA-PSV should be measured at its proximal point after the origin from the internal carotid artery at a 0° angle (avoiding angle correction). Measurement at this point allows the lowest intra- and interobserver variability as well as standardization of the measurement [31]. Multiples of the median for the hemoglobin concentration and MCA-PSV correct for the effect of GA on the measurement. The MCA-PSV had a sensitivity of 100% (95% CI: 0.86–1.0) for detection of significant fetal anemia with a false positive rate of 12% at 1.50 MoM in one study [23]. Other studies have reported lower sensitivity but, in general, above 85% to 90% [32]. The number of false positives increases following 35 weeks gestation [33]. The number of false positive cases after 35 weeks may be decreased by looking at the trend of the MCA-PSV [29].

Table 53.3 Reference Ranges for Fetal Hemoglobin Concentrations as a Function of Gestational Age

Week of Gestation	Multiples of the Median				
	1.16	1.00	0.84	0.65	0.55
18	12.3[a]	10.6	8.9	6.9	5.8
20	12.9	11.1	9.3	7.2	6.1
22	13.4	11.6	9.7	7.5	6.4
24	13.9	12.0	10.1	7.8	6.6
26	14.3	12.3	10.3	8.0	6.8
28	14.6	12.6	10.6	8.2	6.9
30	14.8	12.8	10.8	8.3	7.1
32	15.2	13.1	10.9	8.5	7.2
34	15.4	13.3	11.2	8.6	7.3
36	15.6	13.5	11.3	8.7	7.4
38	15.8	13.6	11.4	8.9	7.5
40	16.0	13.8	11.6	9.0	7.6

Notes: The values at 1.16 and 0.84 multiples of the median correspond to the 95th and 5th percentiles, respectively (the normal range). Mild anemia: hemoglobin concentration between 0.84 and 0.66 MoM; moderate anemia: hemoglobin concentration between 0.65 and 0.55 MoM; severe anemia: hemoglobin concentration <0.65 MoM.
[a]Data shown are in g/dL (median).

Compared with amniocentesis for ΔOD_{450}, the MCA-PSV assessment is associated with a 70% to 80% reduction in the number of invasive tests [23]. The MCA-PSV is more accurate than amniocentesis in detecting fetal anemia [32,34–36].

The correction of fetal anemia with intrauterine transfusion decreases significantly and normalizes the value of fetal MCA-PSV [37,38] because of an increased blood viscosity and an increased oxygen concentration in fetal blood. The MCA-PSV may be used in fetuses previously transfused [39,40].

Accuracy with the MCA-PSV can only be achieved with appropriate training and quality assurance. If adequately trained sonographers are not available, screening for anemia should be done with amniocentesis (see below). Screening with MCA-PSV can be started as early as 15 weeks [41]. The MCA-PSV can also be used for other causes of anemia, including parvovirus infection, nonimmune hydrops, fetal–maternal hemorrhage, and twin–twin transfusion syndrome.

The steps for the correct measurement of the MCA-PSV are the following: 1) An axial section of the head is obtained at the level of the sphenoid bones; 2) color Doppler evidences the circle of Willis; 3) the circle of Willis is enlarged; 4) the color box is placed around the MCA; 5) the MCA is zoomed; and 6) the MCA flow velocity waveforms are displayed and the highest point of the waveform (PSV) is measured. The waveforms should be all similar. The above sequence is repeated at least three times in each fetus.

There should be an absence of fetal movement or fetal breathing during measurement of the MCA-PSV.

Severe intrauterine growth restriction also shows an increased MCA-PSV [42]. Therefore, this should be taken into account when the MCA-PSV is used to diagnose fetal anemia. However, it is very unlikely that an anemic fetus is also a severe IUGR fetus.

Moderate-to-severe anemia may also be suggested by hydropic signs (at least two of pericardial or pleural effusion, ascites, or skin edema), an increase in the size of fetal liver or placental thickness, or tricuspid regurgitation.

Amniocentesis for ΔOD_{450} measurement is currently not used anymore unless accurate MCA screening is not available. The ΔOD_{450} measurement can be evaluated using either the Liley [43] or Queenan [44] charts. There is controversy over which one is best before 27 weeks, the "extended" Liley curve or the Queenan curve [45]. The guidelines for the amniocentesis are arbitrary and serial MCA-PSV measurements are superior in terms of sensitivity, specificity, and positive and negative predictive values to both the Liley and the Queenan curve [31].

If the MCA-PSV test cannot be done and the patient opts for an amniocentesis, the following are general guidelines for managing the Liley curve readings:

- Zone 1: repeat amniocentesis in two to four weeks. If zone 1, follow with ultrasound every one or two weeks until delivery.
- Zone 2 (low/middle third): repeat amniocentesis in about two weeks. If low zone 2, follow with ultrasound every week until delivery. If upper third zone 2, consider FBS.
- Zone 2 (upper third): consider FBS or repeat amniocentesis in 7 days. If again upper third zone 2 or higher, FBS.
- Zone 3: FBS.

The advantage of using Queenan's curve is that it can be used following 14 weeks gestation. Amniocentesis is associated with a 2% to 3% (up to 15%) risk of fetomaternal hemorrhage. Following fetal transfusions the maternal anti-body titer rises significantly.

Fetal Intervention

An IV fetal transfusion is indicated **when the MCA-PSV is ≥1.5 MoM** (Table 53.2). Other ultrasonographic signs of hydrops may also suggest fetal anemia, or if ΔOD_{450} is being used for screening instead of the MCA-PSV, a value in the upper third of zone 2 or zone 3 is an indication for FBS.

Fetal blood sampling (FBS) is the only procedure that allows for direct access to fetal circulation and is the procedure of choice when invasive testing is planned for suspected severe fetal anemia. There is an overall high success rate with blood samples obtained in >98% of patients in the setting of a fetal loss rate of approximately 1.3% [46]. Table 53.4 shows an example of FBS transfusion setup. Table 53.5 shows an example of a step-by-step guide to perform FBS [28]. Transfusion is performed usually at the umbilical vein either at the placental insertion or inside the abdomen. Intraperitoneal transfusion is rarely performed, and it is contraindicated in the hydropic fetus because of the poor absorption of blood. **Corticosteroids for fetal maturation should be considered before the procedure when FBS is performed at or after 24 weeks.** Type O, Rh(D) negative, cytomegalovirus negative, washed, leukoreduced, irradiated packed RBCs cross-matched against maternal blood should be used. The blood usually contains 75% to 85% RBCs to allow minimal blood volume for the transfusions [47].

The procedure is performed under continuous ultrasound guidance. Although some providers elect to use prophylactic antibiotics, no trial has evaluated optimal class, timing, or dosing of antibiotics to prove the efficacy of this practice. Therefore, there is no recommendation of prophylactic antibiotic use in these procedures. Following 24 weeks, the procedure should be performed in a location close to the OR and the anesthesiologist consulted should an emergency occur. Tubing and syringes should be heparinized. Maternal skin can be anesthetized with 1% lidocaine at the point of needle entry. A 20- (usually after 28 weeks) or 22-gauge (usually <28 weeks) needle is used for the procedure. After entering the umbilical vein, a sample of fetal blood is withdrawn and the hemoglobin immediately (within one or two minutes) determined. Fetal blood is confirmed by a mean corpuscular

Table 53.4 Sample Guide for Preparing for Fetal Blood Transfusion

- Obtain O negative, CMV-negative, irradiated packed red blood cells from the blood bank. O positive blood may be needed when antibodies to the c antigen are present because the rate of O negative and c negative blood is very rare (0.0001%).
- Under sterile conditions open.
  - Four drapes or single sterile drape
  - Towel clips as needed
  - Twenty- or 22-gauge spinal needle (22-gauge for transfusions <24–28 weeks of gestation or if thrombocytopenia is suspected) prepared with heparin to prevent clot formation
- Length of needle is determined ahead by measuring distance on ultrasound from maternal abdominal wall to cord insertion site.
  - Sterile ultrasound probe cover
  - Sterile ultrasound gel
  - A skin preparation solution (chlorhexidine-alcohol solution)
  - Eight to 10 1-mL syringes flushed with heparin to avoid clot formation
  - One 1-mL syringe for paralytic agent (atracurium or vecuronium)
  - Five to 10 20-mL syringes (for storing blood)
  - Four 12-mL syringes
  - One 3-mL syringe
  - Three needles 18 or 20 gauge for drawing blood from blood bank into 20-mL syringes
  - A 5.5-inch small bore extension set with t-connector and luer adaptor
  - Three-way stopcock
- Fill two 5-mL syringes with physiological saline solution.
- Flush 1-mL syringes with heparin, save one unflushed 1-mL syringe for vecuronium (or atracurium).
- Draw up normal saline to make 3 saline flushes, remove air bubbles by holding syringes upright and tapping to release bubbles to top, attach small bore connection tubing, and flush air through.
- Reconstitute vecuronium with 10 mL of normal saline.
  - Draw up 1 mL of vecuronium and 9 mL of normal saline in a 12 mL syringe.
  - Transfer 1 mL of vecuronium mixture to a unheparinized 1 mL syringe.
  - Mark both the 12 mL and 1 mL syringes with vecuronium to avoid confusion.
  - Usual dose of vecuronium is 0.1 mg/kg and atracurium is 0.4 mg/kg.
- Draw up 2% lidocaine in 3-mL syringe, attached to 22- or 25-gauge needle for injection at puncture site for maternal local anesthesia.
- Care should be taken to maintain sterility when drawing up solutions: either have an assistant holding saline, vecuronium, lidocaine, and blood from blood bank or use single operator technique keeping one hand sterile and one hand unsterile.
- Attach intravenous connection tubing to unit of packed red blood cells.
- Attach stopcock, taking care to maintain sterility on one end of the stopcock.
- Fill 20-mL syringes with blood by opening stopcock.
  - Remove any air bubbles that may be present by holding syringes upright and tapping side of syringe to release air bubbles.
- Have tubes available to send for laboratory studies.
  - Remember to include not only initial, midway, and final blood counts plus any additional tubes for genetic studies, liver function studies, or other tests.

Source: Adapted from Society for Maternal-Fetal Medicine (SMFM); Mari G; Norton ME; Stone J et al. Society for Maternal-Fetal Medicine (SMFM) Clinical Guideline #8: The fetus at risk for anemia—Diagnosis and management. *AJOG*, 212, 697–710, 2015.
Abbreviation: CMV, cytomegalovirus.

Table 53.5 Example of a Fetal Blood Sampling Procedure Steps

- Obtain maternal sample of blood.
- Precalculate amount of fetal transfusion needed based on different possible fetal hematocrit values (see text).
- Perform ultrasound to select site.
  - Placental cord insertion, free loop, umbilical cord insertion or intrahepatic vein.
  - Obtain measurement from maternal abdomen to umbilical vein site of puncture to ensure correct needle length.
  - Document fetal heart rate.
- Have sonographer and assistant ready in addition to main operator.
- Intravenous access and use of antibiotics is not always necessary and is at the preference of the operator.
- Under aseptic conditions prepare patient with antibacterial solute and place drapes leaving abdomen exposed.
- Cover ultrasound transducer with sterile cover.
- Identify site of puncture.
- Give local anesthesia to patient (mother).
- Inject fetus with intramuscular paralytic agent if necessary (vecuronium or atracurium).
- Use 20- or 22-gauge needle to enter umbilical vein.
- Remove stylet.
- If flow is immediate, obtain sample in 1-mL syringe and send to laboratory.
- If flow is not immediate and you think you are in Wharton's jelly, slowly and carefully reposition the needle to enter into the vein.
- Some operators document flow by injecting saline: if that is done prior to obtaining fetal blood sample, discard first 1-mL fetal blood because it may be diluted with saline.
- Document fetal blood sample by comparing maternal (previously drawn and analyzed) and fetal hematocrit and MCV. This may not be necessary if sampling a free loop or the intrahepatic vein or if document flow with saline.
- Attach tubing to transfuse slowly: assistant can push blood slowly; watch segment of umbilical cord to see if blood is flowing through umbilical vein. A small slow transfusion of blood may be performed prior to obtaining confirmatory results of fetal blood from the laboratory to prevent clot from forming.
- When the fetal hematocrit returns and a transfusion is needed, calculate the amount of blood needed to transfuse based on precalculations.
- Intermittently obtain fetal heart rate.
- When transfusion is complete, obtain final hematocrit, and draw any other blood needed for workup.
- After the transfusion is complete and the needle is removed, watch the puncture site for streaming and check fetal heart rate for bradycardia.
- Monitor the patient and fetus after transfusion for at least 1–2 hours.

Source: Adapted from Society for Maternal-Fetal Medicine (SMFM); Mari G; Norton ME; Stone J et al. Society for Maternal-Fetal Medicine (SMFM) Clinical Guideline #8: The fetus at risk for anemia—Diagnosis and management. *AJOG*, 212, 697–710, 2015.
Abbreviations: GA, gestational age; MCV, mean corpuscular volume.

volume (MCV) >110 μm^3. Then the fetus is given a paralytic agent (e.g., pavulon 0.1 mg/kg) to stop fetal movements [48].

If the hematocrit is below the fifth percentile (<0.84 MoM) for GA, blood is transfused in a sterile fashion. A computer program (e.g., http://www.perinatology.com/protocols/rhc.htm) can be used to estimate the amount of blood to transfuse based on the initial fetal hematocrit, the estimated fetal weight, and the concentration of the blood transfused [49,50]. The following formula is used:

$$V_{transfused(mL)} = \frac{V_{fetoplacental(mL)}(Hct_{final} - Hct_{initial})}{Hct_{transfused\ blood}}$$

The volume of the fetal placental unit is equal to the fetal weight in grams multiplied by 0.14. A final fetal blood sample is taken a few seconds after the transfusion has been completed. If the fetus is hydropic, it is better to transfuse the fetus only to about a hematocrit of 30% or so and then perform a second transfusion at a distance of three to five days to increase the hematocrit to the median hematocrit value for GA. At and after 24 weeks, the fetal heart rate should be monitored for the next two to three hours until fetal movements resume. The risk of fetal death per FBS procedure is 1% to 2% even with ultrasound guidance, expert operators, and accurate management.

Thrombocytopenia, even at levels <100,000/mm³, can be found in about 9% of Rh(D) alloimmunized fetuses at times of fetal sampling [51]. Thrombocytopenia is associated with fetal hydrops and with perinatal mortality [51].

If performing intraperitoneal transfusion, calculate amount of blood needed by the following formula: GA (weeks) – 20 × 10. For example, at 30 weeks, 30 – 20 = 10 × 10 = 100 mL blood.

Intravenous immunoglobulin in addition to fetal transfusion has been studied insufficiently and is not currently recommended [52].

Hematocrit decreases about 1 point per day posttransfusion in the anemic alloimmunized fetus, and this knowledge helps to assess when to repeat the transfusion. The timing of the second FBS can also be aided again by MCA PSV monitoring [39] while MCA PSV is not reliable after the second transfusion has been done. If the fetus is nonhydropic, the second transfusion is often necessary 14 days after the first, but after the second/third transfusion, longer intervals of three weeks or more may be possible as the fetal RBCs are replaced by adult RBCs. Following three transfusions, 99% of the fetal blood is represented by the adult transfused blood. Maternal phenobarbital 30 mg three times per day for 7 to 10 days to enhance fetal liver maturity and ability to conjugate bilirubin is still unconfirmed by large studies [53].

Fetal Monitoring/Testing

Fetal testing with nonstress tests (NSTs) or biophysical profiles (BPPs) at least weekly is started around 32 weeks or earlier if indicated. Its benefit has not been confirmed in a specific trial. Fetuses with very severe anemia (hemoglobin ≤2 g/dL) due to RBC alloimmunization may develop brain injury (e.g., intracerebellar hemorrhage). Therefore, some studies have advocated fetal neuroimaging by ultrasound and/or MRI [54].

The surfactant/albumin ratio for fetal lung maturity (FLM) cannot be used since high amniotic fluid bilirubin can affect this result. The other tests for FLM are reliable (see also Chapter 57).

Delivery

See Figure 53.1 for the timing of delivery [46]. The mode of delivery depends on obstetrical indications.

Anesthesia

There are no specific anesthesia precautions.

Neonatology Management

Anemic neonates are usually treated with transfusions or exchange transfusions as necessary. They often need light therapy for hyperbilirubinemia. Breast-feeding is not contraindicated. A hearing screening test is indicated during the neonatal period and at two years of age given that hyperbilirubinemia can cause sensorineural hearing loss.

Long-Term Outcomes

Children who survive severe hemolytic disease (even with hydrops and/or necessitating transfusions) often have a normal neurologic outcome [28,55]. In the largest series evaluating outcome at an average of eight years of age of survivors of hemolytic disease of the fetus/newborn, the incidence of neurodevelopmental impairment was 4.8%. The incidence of severe developmental delay (3.1%) was similar to the general population (2.3%). Smaller series have reported 8% and 10% incidences of neurological impairment [56]. Prevention of hydrops was the suggested management to avoid long-term handicap.

OTHER "ATYPICAL" ANTIBODIES

There are many atypical (irregular) blood group antibodies that are capable of producing hemolytic disease. Given their rarity, and the absence of large studies or any trial, the management of antibodies known to cause hemolytic disease other than Rh(D) is based on poor evidence. Many aspects of management are unknown or similar to Rh(D) alloimmunization except for the details below. It should be acknowledged that the critical titer for antibodies other than Rh(D) has not been well established.

Kell Alloimmunization

The incidence of Kell alloimmunization is about 0.1% to 0.3% in pregnant women. Kell alloimmunization is usually caused by prior transfusion. Over 90% of partners of Kell-immunized women are Kell negative. In the white population, only 9% of fathers are Kell positive, and only 0.2% are homozygous. **Maternal titers do not correlate well with fetal alloimmune disease.** Severe anemia can be diagnosed in fetuses whose mothers had a titer as low as 1:2. ΔOD_{450} **levels also do not correlate with fetal anemia.** This is because fetal anemia is not caused by hemolysis but by suppression of erythropoiesis

at the progenitor-cell level. Anti-Kell antibodies specifically inhibit the growth of Kell-positive erythroid burst-forming units and colony-forming units [11]. In fact, anti-Kell anemic fetuses have lower reticulocyte counts and bilirubin levels compared to anti-D anemic fetuses. The Kell blood group is complex, consisting of over two dozen antigens. Kell 1 (Kell or K1) and its allelic partner Kell 2 (Cellano or K2) are strong immunogens. Poor fetal outcome occurs in about 1.5% to 3% of Kell-alloimmunized pregnancies, an incidence that is possibly higher than that of other RBC antigens. The management of Kell sensitization is somewhat controversial. **Genotyping of the father of the baby (FOB) is extremely important.** Most will be Kell negative, and if paternity is certain, no further testing is necessary. The vast majority of Kell-positive FOBs are heterozygote, so the fetal Kell status needs to be determined, usually by amniocentesis PCR. **MCA-PSV screening is predictive and accurate for the diagnosis of fetal anemia from Kell alloimmunization** [23,57]. MCA-PSV monitoring should start at 15 weeks and be performed as suggested in Figure 53.1. ΔOD_{450} measurements from amniocentesis are inaccurate and should not be used.

Other CDE System Antigens

c (small): This antigen carries a 65% risk of hemolytic disease; 80% of FOBs are positive of which half are homozygous, half heterozygous.

C (big): This antigen is associated with a 32% risk of hemolytic disease.

E (big): E-positive individuals have a 31% risk of hemolytic disease. Maternal titers do not correlate well with fetal hemolytic disease.

MNS Antigen System

Only 1% of titers ever rise to ≥1:64. Fewer than 100 cases of severe anemia as a result of anti-M alloimmunization have been reported worldwide to date such that even if sensitized the incidence of severe anemia is probably <1%.

Others

Other rare, but potentially lethal, antigens are **Duffy (Fya, Fyb, Fy3, etc.), and Kidd as well as others.**

REFERENCES

1. Levine P, Katzin E, Burnham L. Isoimmunization in pregnancy: Its possible bearing on the etiology of erythroblastosis fetalis. *J Am Med Assoc* 1941; 116: 825–7. [II-3]
2. Landsteiner K, Weiner A. An agglutinable factor in human blood recognized by immune sera for Rhesus blood. *Proc Soc Exp Biol Med* 1940; 43: 223. [II-3]
3. van Wamelen D, Klumper F, de Haas M et al. Obstetric history and antibody titer in estimating severity of Kell alloimmunization in pregnancy. *Obstet Gynecol* 2007; 109(5): 1093–8. [II-3]
4. Bowman J, Pollock J, Penston L. Fetomaternal transplacental hemorrhage during pregnancy and after delivery. *Vox Sang* 1986; 51: 117–21. [II-3]
5. Martin J, Park M, Sutton P. Births: Preliminary data for 2001. *Natl Vital Stat Rep* 2002; 50(10): 1–20. [II-3]
6. Geifman-Holtzman O, Wojtowycz M, Kosmas E et al. Female alloimmunization with antibodies known to cause hemolytic disease. *Obstet Gynecol* 1997; 89: 272–5. [II-3]

7. Castilho L, Rios M, Rodrigues A et al. High frequency of partial Dilla and DAR alleles found in sickle cell patients suggests increased risk of alloimmunization to RhD. *Transfus Med* 2005; 15: 49–55. [II-3]

8. Mayne K, Bowell P, Pratt G. The significance of anti-Kell sensitization in pregnancy. *Clin Lab Haematol* 1990; 12(4): 379–85. [II-2]

9. Grant S, Kilby M, Meer L et al. The outcome of pregnancy in Kell alloimmunisation. *Br J Obstet Gynecol* 2000; 107(4): 481–5. [II-3]

10. Southcott M, Tanner M, Anstee D. The expression of human blood group antigens during erythropoiesis in a cell culture system. *Blood* 1999; 93(12): 4425–35. [II-2]

11. Vaughan J, Manning M, Warwick R et al. Inhibition of erythroid progenitor cells by anti-Kell antibodies in fetal alloimmune anemia. *N Engl J Med* 1998; 338: 798–803. [II-3]

12. Caine M, Mueller-Heubach E. Kell sensitization in pregnancy. *Am J Obstet Gynecol* 1986; 154: 85–90. [III]

13. ACOG practice bulletin. Prevention of Rh D alloimmunization. Number 4, May 1999 (replaces educational bulletin Number 147, October 1990). Clinical management guidelines for obstetrician-gynecologists. American College of Obstetrics and Gynecology. International Journal of Gynaecology and Obstetrics: The Official Organ of the International Federation of Gynaecology and Obstetrics. 1999; 66(1): 63–70. PubMed PMID:10458556. [Guideline]

14. Lurie S, Rotmensch S, Glezerman M. Prenatal management of women who have partial Rh (D) antigen. *Br J Obstet Gynecol* 2001; 108: 895–7. [Review]

15. Crowther C, Middleton P. Anti-D administration after childbirth for preventing Rhesus alloimmunisation. *Cochrane Database Syst Rev* 2000; (2): CD000021. PMID:10796089. [Meta-analysis]

16. Crowther C, Keirse MJ. Anti-D administration in pregnancy for preventing rhesus alloimmunisation. *Cochrane Database Syst Rev* 2000; (2): CD000020. PMID:10796088. [Meta-analysis]

17. Huchet J, Dallemagne S, Huchet C et al. The antepartum use of anti-D immunoglobulin in rhesus negative women. Parallel evaluation of fetal blood cells passing through the placenta. The results of a multicentre study carried out in the region of Paris. *Eur J Obstet Gynecol Reprod Biol* 1987; 16: 101–11. [RCT, n = 1882 primiparous Rh-D negative women. Administration of 100 mg (500 IU) anti-D immune globulin at 28 weeks and 34 weeks of pregnancy (n = 927). No placebo was given to the control group (n = 955)]

18. Lee D, Rawlinson V. Multicentre trial of antepartum low-dose anti-D immunoglobulin. *Transfus Med* 1995; 5: 15–9. [RCT, n = 2541 Rh-D negative primigravidae. 50 mg (250 IU) anti-D intramuscularly at 28 and 34 weeks gestation (n = 952). Control group had no placebo (n = 1068)]

19. MacKenzie IZ, Dutton S, Roseman F. Evidence to support the single-dose over the two-dose protocol for routine antenatal anti-D Rhesus prophylaxis: A prospective observational study. *Eur J Obstet Gynecol Reprod Biol* 2011; 158(1): 42–6. PubMed PMID:21641101. [II-1]

20. Ness P, Baldwin M, Niebyl J. Clinical high-risk designations does not predict excess fetal-maternal hemorrhage. *Am J Obstet Gynecol* 1987; 156: 154–8. [II-2]

21. ACOG. Prevention of Rh D alloimmunization. *Obstet Gynecol* 1999 (Practice Bulletin No. 4, May). [Review]

22. Mari G, Adrignolo A, Abuhamad A et al. Diagnosis of fetal anemia with Doppler ultrasound in the pregnancy complicated by maternal blood group immunization. *Ultrasound Obstet Gynecol* 1995; 5: 400–5. [II-2]

23. Mari G, Deter R, Carpenter R et al. Noninvasive diagnosis by Doppler ultrasonography of fetal anemia due to maternal red-cell alloimmunization. Collaborative Group for Doppler Assessment of the Blood Velocity in Anemic Fetuses. *N Engl J Med* 2000; 342: 9–14. [II-2]

24. Bianchi D, Avent N, Costa J et al. Noninvasive prenatal diagnosis of fetal Rhesus D. Ready for prime(r) time. *Obstet Gynecol* 2005; 106: 841–4. [Review]

25. Harper T, Finning K, Martin P et al. Use of maternal plasma for noninvasive determination of fetal RhD status. *Am J Obstet Gynecol* 2004; 191: 1730–2. [II-3]

26. Moise KJJ, Boring NH, O'Shaughenessy R, Simpson LL, Wolfe HM, Baxter JK, Polzin W, Eddleman KA, Hassan SS, Skupski D, McLennan G, Paladino T, Oeth P, Bombard A. Circulating cell-free DNA for the detection of RHD status and sex using reflex fetal identifiers. *Prenat Diagn* 2013; 33(1): 95–101. [II-2]

27. Chitty LS, Finning K, Wade A, Soothill P, Martin B, Oxenford K et al. Diagnostic accuracy of routine antenatal determination of fetal RHD status across gestation: Population based cohort study. *BMJ* 2014; 349: g5243. PubMed PMID:25190055. Pubmed Central PMCID:4154470. [II-1]

28. Society for Maternal-Fetal Medicine (SMFM); Mari G; Norton ME; Stone J et al. Society for Maternal-Fetal Medicine (SMFM) Clinical Guideline #8: The fetus at risk for anemia—Diagnosis and management. *AJOG* 2015; 212: 697–710. [Guideline]

29. Detti L, Mari G, Akiyama M et al. Longitudinal assessment of the middle cerebral artery peak systolic velocity in healthy fetuses and in fetuses at risk for anemia. *Am J Obstet Gynecol* 2002; 187: 937–9. [II-2].

30. Spong C, Porter A, Queenan J. Management of isoimmunization in the presence of multiple maternal antibodies. *Am J Obstet Gynecol* 2001; 185: 481–4. [II-2].

31. Mari G, Abuhamad A, Cosmi E et al. Middle cerebral artery peak systolic velocity—Technique and variability. *J Ultrasound Med* 2005; 24: 425–30. [II-2]

32. Oepkes D, Seaward P, Vandenbussche F et al. Doppler ultrasonography versus amniocentesis to predict fetal anemia. *N Engl J Med* 2006; 355: 156–64. [II-1]

33. Zimmermann R, Durig P, Carpenter RJ et al. Longitudinal measurement of peak systolic velocity in the fetal middle cerebral artery for monitoring pregnancies complicated by red cell alloimmunisation: A prospective multicentre trial with intention-to-treat. *Br J Obstet Gynaecol* 2002; 109: 746–52. [II-2]

34. Mari G, Penso C, Sbracia M et al. Delta OD 450 and Doppler velocimetry of the middle cerebral artery peak velocity in the evaluation for fetal alloimmune hemolytic disease. Which is the best? (1997, January) Proceedings, Society for Perinatal Obstetricians, Anaheim, CA. *Am J Obstet Gynecol* 1997; 176: S18. [II-3]

35. Nishie E, Brizot M, Liao A et al. A comparison between middle cerebral artery peak systolic velocity and amniotic fluid optical density at 450 nm in the prediction of fetal anemia. *Am J Obstet Gynecol* 2003; 188(1): 214–9. [II-2]

36. Pereira L, Jenkins T, Berghella V. Conventional management of maternal red cell alloimmunization compared with management by Doppler assessment of middle cerebral artery peak systolic velocity. *Am J Obstet Gynecol* 2003; 189(4): 1002–6. [II-3]

37. Mari G, Rahman F, Oloffson P et al. Increase of fetal hematocrit decreases the middle cerebral artery peak systolic velocity in pregnancies complicated by rhesus alloimmunization. *J Matern Fetal Med* 1997; 6: 206–8. [II-3]

38. Stefos T, Cosmi E, Detti L et al. Correction of fetal anemia and the middle cerebral artery peak systolic velocity. *Obstet Gynecol* 2002; 99: 211–5. [II-2]

39. Detti L, Oz U, Guney I et al. Doppler ultrasound velocimetry for timing the second intrauterine transfusion in fetuses with anemia from red cell alloimmunization. Collaborative Group for Doppler Assessment of the Blood Velocity in Anemic Fetuses. *Am J Obstet Gynecol* 2001; 185: 1048–51. [II-3]

40. Mari G, Zimmermann R, Moise KJ et al. Correlation between middle cerebral artery peak systolic velocity and fetal hemoglobin after 2 previous intrauterine transfusions. *Am J Obstet Gynecol* 2005; 193: 1117–20. [II-3]

41. ACOG. Management of alloimmunization. *Obstet Gynecol* 2006; 108 (Practice Bulletin No. 75): 457–64. [Review]

42. Mari G, Hanif F, Kruger M et al. Middle cerebral artery peak systolic velocity: A new Doppler parameter in the assessment of growth restricted fetuses. *Ultrasound Obstet Gynecol* 2007; 29: 310–6. [II-3]

43. Liley A. Liquor amnii analysis in the management of the pregnancy complicated by rhesus sensitization. *Am J Obstet Gynecol* 1961; 82: 1359–70. [II-2]

44. Queenan J, Tomai T, Ural S et al. Deviation in amniotic fluid optical density at a wavelength of 450 nm in Rh-immunized pregnancies from 14 to 40 weeks' gestation: A proposal for clinical management. *Am J Obstet Gynecol* 1993; 168: 1370–6. [II-2]

45. Sikkel E, Vandenbussche P, Oepkes D et al. Amniotic fluid Delta OD 450 values accurately predict severe fetal anemia in D-alloimmunization. *Obstet Gynecol* 2002; 100: 51–7. [II-3]

46. Society for Maternal-Fetal M, Berry SM, Stone J, Norton ME, Johnson D, Berghella V. Fetal blood sampling. *Am J Obstet Gynecol* 2013; 209(3): 170–80. PubMed PMID: 23978246. [Guideline]

47. El-Azeem S, Samuels P, Rose R et al. The effect of the source of transfused blood on the rate of consumption of transfused red blood cells in pregnancies affected by red blood cell allimmunization. *Am J Obstet Gynecol* 1997; 177: 753–7. [II-2]

48. Mouw R, Klumper F, Hermans J et al. Effect of atracurium or pancuronium on the anemic fetus during and directly after intravascular intrauterine transfusion. *Acta Obstet Gynecol Scand* 1999; 78: 763–7. [RCT, *n* = 24]

49. Nicolaides K, Soothill P, Clewell W et al. Fetal haemoglobin measurement in the assessment of red cell isoimmunisation. *Lancet* 1988; 1(8594): 1073–5. [II-3]

50. Mandelbrot L, Daffos F, Forestier F et al. Assessment of fetal blood volume for computer-assisted management of in utero transfusion. *Fetal Ther* 1988; 3: 60–6. [II-3]

51. van den Akker E, de Haan T, Lopriore E et al. Severe fetal thrombocytopenia in Rhesus D alloimmunized pregnancies. *Am J Obstet Gynecol* 2008; 199: 387.e1–4. [II-3]

52. Dooren M, van Kamp I, Scherpenisse J et al. No beneficial effect of low-dose fetal intravenous gammaglobulin administration in combination with intravascular transfusions in severe Rh D haemolytic disease. *Vox Sang* 1994; 66: 253–7. [RCT, *n* = 44]

53. Trevett T, Dorman K, Lamvu G et al. Does antenatal maternal administration of Phenobarbital prevent exchange transfusion in neonates with alloimmune hemolytic disease? *Am J Obstet Gynecol* 2003; 189: s214. [II-3]

54. Ghi T, Brodelli L, Simonazzi G et al. Sonographic demonstration of brain injury in fetuses with severe red blood cell alloimmunization undergoing intrauterine transfusions. *Ultrasound Obstet Gynecol* 2004; 23: 428–31. [II-3]

55. Hudon L, Moise K, Hegemier S et al. Long-term neurodevelopmental outcome after intrauterine transfusion for the treatment of fetal hemolytic disease. *Am J Obstet Gynecol* 1998; 179: 858–63. [II-3]

56. Lindenburg IT, Smits-Wintjens VE, van Klink JM et al. Long-term neurodevelopmental outcome after intrauterine transfusion for hemolytic deisease of the fetus/newborn: The LOTUS study. *AJOG* 2012; 206: 141.e1–8. [II-2]

57. Van Dongen H, Klumper F, Sikkel E et al. Non-invasive tests to predict fetal anemia in Kell-alloimmunized pregnancies. *Ultrasound Obstet Gynecol* 2005; 25: 341–5. [II-3]

54

Nonimmune hydrops fetalis

Katherine Connolly and Joanne Stone

KEY POINTS

- Fetal hydrops is defined as the **accumulation of fluid in two or more fetal extravascular compartments**, including ascites, pleural effusion, pericardial effusion, and skin edema. These findings are commonly accompanied by polyhydramnios and placentomegaly.
- Nonimmune hydrops fetalis (NIH) is defined by the **absence of maternal antibodies against fetal cells** (negative indirect Coombs test in maternal serum).
- Because of the wide use of anti-Rh prophylaxis, currently **most cases (90%) of fetal hydrops are nonimmune** in origin. The frequency of NIH has been estimated between 1/2000 and 1/3000 births.
- The prognosis is often dismal with an **overall perinatal mortality of 50% to 100%**, which is related to the etiology, gestational age at presentation, the presence of early and significant pleural effusions, and the availability of treatment for certain conditions (e.g., parvovirus B19–induced NIH). Current data indicate that, among those who survive the neonatal period, 50% are free of long-term sequels at one year of age.
- NIH is a condition associated with a **large number of causes**. In general, **etiology may be suspected or confirmed prenatally in 50% to 80% of cases**. Chromosomal abnormalities account for a significant fraction of cases of NIH before 24 weeks while structural abnormalities of the heart and infectious conditions are more frequently found after 24 weeks gestation. After delivery, 5% of newborns remain classified as idiopathic. Following is a **simplified etiologic summary**:
  - Cardiovascular anomalies: 20%
  - Noncardiovascular anomalies: 15%–25%
  - Chromosomal abnormalities: 15%–20%
  - Infection: 10%–15%
  - Hematologic disorders: 5%–15%
  - Complications of monochorionic twins: 5%
  - Genetic syndromes: 1%
  - Metabolic syndromes: 1%–5%
  - Overlapping of these conditions is frequent (e.g., a fetus with trisomy 21 and cardiac structural malformations)
- **Evaluation of cases with NIH** should be exercised according to local resources, and when required, cases must be transferred to a tertiary center where advanced diagnostic tests/procedures and potential treatments are available.
  - Always make sure that antibody screening (indirect Coombs) is negative (even in Rh-positive patients).
  - Because of the broad spectrum of the disease, efforts should be made to establish whether a treatable condition is present. Likewise, identification of recurrent causes of the disease is mandatory to provide appropriate counseling.
- Suggested evaluation may include the following:
  - Detailed **history** (recent flu-like symptoms, ethnic background, family history)
  - **Ultrasound** to evaluate fetal anatomy, amniotic fluid volume, placenta, umbilical cord, **echocardiogram** and middle cerebral artery peak systolic velocity to search for cardiac and extracardiac malformations, arrhythmias and fetal anemia.
  - Maternal **laboratory** tests:
    - Blood type and antibody screening to rule out immune-mediated anemia.
    - CBC with red blood cell indices and hemoglobin electrophoresis to look for thalassemias.
    - Serology for parvovirus, CMV, rubella.
    - Nontreponemal tests for syphilis (RPR).
    - Kleihauer–Betke to exclude fetal anemia for fetomaternal hemorrhage.
    - Other tests may be necessary if there is a suggestive history (e.g., HSV, *Listeria monocytogenes*) or the etiology of the condition remains elusive. On the other hand, the workup may be concise or stopped if the etiology arises soon after initial evaluation of the patient.
  - **Amniocentesis** to perform fetal **karyotype with microarray**, PCR for parvovirus B19, toxoplasmosis and CMV as needed. It is a good practice to freeze and store amniotic fluid with the aim to test for rare conditions such as lysosomal storage disease.
  - **In cases still idiopathic after the workup above has been completed, consideration should be given to testing for lysosomal storage disorders (LSD) as up to 30% of idiopathic cases may have LSD as etiology.**
- **Management of NIH is based on the etiology** and may include the following:
  - Treatment of conditions that benefit from maternal interventions (e.g., penicillin for syphilis-induced NIH) or fetal interventions (e.g., intrauterine blood transfusion for parvovirus B19–induced fetal anemia/thrombocytopenia).
  - Rarely, the mother may develop generalized edema, which could be life-threatening (mirror syndrome).
  - Termination of pregnancy in regions where this option is permitted.
  - Fetal monitoring: nonstress test, biophysical profile, Doppler studies of umbilical artery and middle cerebral artery as well as heart and venous system as feasible and necessary.
  - Antenatal steroids to reduce the likelihood of neonatal complications associated with preterm delivery.

- Delivery if there is evidence of fetal or maternal deterioration (e.g., mirror syndrome). Delivery may be preceded by interventions aimed to reduce the frequency of fetal cardiac failure, dystocia, and fetal trauma (e.g., aspiration of excessive pericardial, pleural or peritoneal fluid). NIH increases the risk of postpartum hemorrhage and retained placenta.

DIAGNOSIS/DEFINITION

Hydrops fetalis is the end stage of many different disorders, characterized by the pathologic accumulation of fluid in body cavities or tissues. The diagnosis of **NIH** is established if **at least two** of the following conditions are present: **hydrothorax, ascites, pericardial effusion, and skin edema** (>5 mm measured at the level of skull or chest wall) (Figure 54.1). These diagnostic findings can be associated with polyhydramnios (in 40%–75% of cases) and placentomegaly (placental thickness ≥4 cm in the second trimester or ≥6 cm in the third trimester) [1]. Immune hydrops is associated with isoimmunization to an RBC antigen (e.g., Rh disease) (see

Chapter 53) while nonimmune hydrops (**NIH**) includes all other etiologies.

EPIDEMIOLOGY/INCIDENCE

The incidence of NIH ranges between **1/1700 and 1/3000 at birth** [2,3] and as high as 0.5% in tertiary referral centers. The incidence may be as high as 1/150 on ultrasound since the high rate of intrauterine demise makes the hydrops incidence at birth an underestimation. NIH may account for up to 3% of perinatal mortality. When Potter described for the first time NIH in 1943, its incidence was very low compared to fetal hydrops for isoimmunization. After the introduction of anti-D prophylaxis, **however, the incidence of Rh(D) alloimmunization has significantly decreased. Thus, NIH now represents 90% of all hydrops cases** [1].

ETIOLOGY/BASIC PATHOPHYSIOLOGY

NIH is the final phenotype of hundreds of different disorders. The exact pathogenesis depends on the underlying

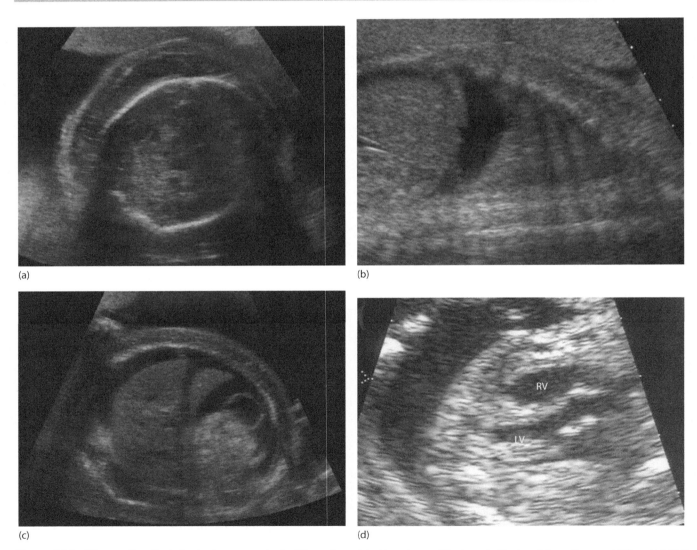

(a)

(b)

(c)

(d)

Figure 54.1   Diagnostic criteria for hydrops: need ≥2 of these four: (a) skin edema, (b) pleural effusion, (c) ascites, and (d) pericardial effusion.

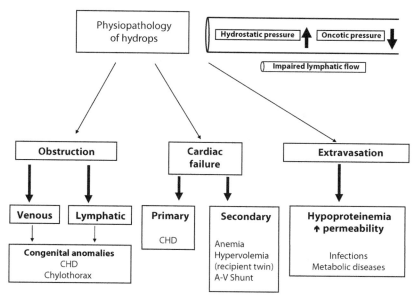

Figure 54.2 Possible pathophysiologic mechanisms for hydrops fetalis. *Abbreviations*: A-V, arterio-venous; CHD, congenital heart disease.

disorder, but the common disorder is an imbalance in the regulation of fluid movement between the vascular and interstitial spaces [1]. There are three basic mechanisms by which this occurs: impaired lymphatic flow, cardiac failure, and extravasation (either increased intravascular hydrostatic pressure, decreased intravascular osmotic pressure, or both) (Figure 54.2). These various etiologic factors and complex mechanisms lead to extra-accumulation of fluid in the fetal interstitial space with 10% to 20% of hydrops causes still undetermined after workup [4]. The complex physiopathology of hydrops makes it a challenge for the obstetrician to investigate its etiology and decide upon the management.

ASSOCIATIONS/POSSIBLE ETIOLOGIES/ DIFFERENTIAL DIAGNOSIS (TABLE 54.1) [2–4]
Cardiovascular Disorders (20%)
The main causal association of NIH is with fetal cardiovascular disease [5]. The most common disorders involved are tachyarrhythmias (40%), cardiac structural malformations (20%), high-output cardiac failure (15%), and bradyarrhythmias (6%) resulting from congenital heart malformation or maternal connective disorders (antibody mediated).

Fetal arrhythmias are the leading cause of cardiac disorders associated with NIH (40%) [6]. Most of them are secondary to tachyarrhythmias, and another fraction is the result of heart block. The most frequent tachyarrhythmia is supraventricular tachycardia, followed by atrial flutter and atrial fibrillation. Etiopathogenic disturbances induced by arrhythmias include reduction of the stroke volume, end-diastolic overload, and systemic venous congestion. These conditions are susceptible to in utero treatment with anti-arrhythmic drugs administered to the mother or the fetus, which improve survival. The first-line drug is digoxin. Alternatives are flecainide, amiodarone, verapamil, and adenosine. Maternal administration of these drugs is frequently hampered by difficulties associated to an enlarged placenta [7]. Therefore, direct administration to the fetus has been suggested as an alternative, particularly in cases where there is no fetal response to maternal oral administration of medications.

Bradyarrhythmias are most commonly the result of congenital heart block, either from an autoimmune cause or structural abnormalities affecting cardiac conduction. Transplacental passage of maternal antibodies associated with autoimmune diseases is seen in 30%–50% of these cases. They can be present in association with anti-Sjogren's-syndrome-related antigen A (anti Ro) or the combination or anti-Ro/SSA and anti-La/SSB antibodies (see Chapter 25) [1]. Structural abnormalities, such as endocardial cushion defects in the setting of a heterotaxy syndrome, can also interfere with cardiac conduction and lead to heart block. Complete fetal heart block yields to fetal hydrops when the fetal heart rate is below 60 beats per minute. There have been several case reports showing successful progression to hydrops after maternal administration of beta-sympathomimetics, such as terbutaline, although data are very limited [8,9]. Corticosteroids were studied as possible treatment for fetal heart block and were shown not to be effective in reversing third-degree block nor preventing progression from second- to third-degree block [10]. At this time, in utero treatment of fetal hydrops as a result of fetal bradyarrhythmia is not recommended [1].

Structural abnormalities leading to NIH are most commonly right heart defects but can also include atrioventricular septal defects (AV canal), hypoplastic left ventricle, large ventricular septal defects, atrial septal defects, Ebstein anomaly, and premature closure of the ductus arteriosus [2,11]. The pathophysiology underlying the NIH associated with these conditions is diverse and complex but is mainly attributable to an increase in the systemic venous pressure resulting from obstruction of right heart output as well as the transmission of systemic arterial pressure to the right heart by means of several pathologic shunts, including the primary

Table 54.1   Conditions Associated with Nonimmune Fetal Hydrops and Suggested Workup

Conditions Associated with NIHF	Suggested Workup
***Cardiovascular* (20%)**	Expert fetal **echocardiogram** for morphological and functional study, with 2D, M-mode, pulsed Doppler, color Doppler, including functional assessment of output tracts, ductus arteriosus and the fetal venous system (ductus venosus)
Fetal arrhythmias	
Supraventricular tachycardia, atrial flutter, heart block with bradyarrhythmia, Wolff-Parkinson-White, nonconducted premature atrial contractions, others	
Structural	**Accurate fetal anatomical ultrasound,** including the umbilical cord and placenta
Atrioventricular septal defects, hypoplastic left ventricle, hypoplastic right ventricle, large ventricular septal defects, atrial septal defects, Ebstein anomaly, premature closure of the ductus arteriosus, closure of the foramen ovale, tetralogy of Fallot and its variants, truncus, transposition of the great vessels, severe atrioventricular or arterial valve insufficiency, others	
Mass	Color and pulsed Doppler of peripheral vessels including umbilical cord, placenta, cranial venous system (especially the base of the skull, under the hemispheres), and middle cerebral artery peak systolic velocity
Cardiac rhabdomyoma, pericardial/intrapericardial/intracardiac teratoma	
High cardiac output failure	
Chorioangioma (>5 cm), aneurysmal malformation of the vein of Galen, large sacrococcygeal teratoma, umbilical cord aneurysms, neuroblastoma, vena cava obstruction	
Vascular disorders	
Cardiomyopathy, peripheral artery thrombosis	
***Extracardiac anomalies* (15%–25%)**	Accurate fetal anatomical ultrasound
Thorax	Consider thoracocentesis or paracentesis with biochemical, cytological, and microbiological analysis
Congenital pulmonary airway malformation (e.g., CCAM, pulmonary sequestration), congenital diaphragmatic hernia, pulmonary lymphangiectasia, chylothorax, bronchogenic cyst, any thoracic tumors	
Urinary	
Posterior urethral valves, urethral stenosis/atresia, prune-belly syndrome, congenital nephrosis	
Gastrointestinal	
Volvulus-atresia, malrotation, duplication, meconium, peritonitis, hepatic fibrosis, cholestasis, billiary atresia, cloacal dysgenesis, hemochromatosis	
Skeletal dysplasias	
Thanatophoric dysplasia, short rib-polydactyly, osteogenesis imperfecta, achondrogenesis, hypophosphatasia	
***Chromosomal abnormalities* (15%–20%)**	**Amniocentesis**
45x (or mosaic 45X/46XX), trisomy 21, trisomy 18, trisomy 13, triploidy, others	
***Infections* (10%–15%)**	**RPR, serology for parvovirus B19, CMV, toxoplasmosis, rubella**, and others if suspected
Parvovirus B19, CMV, syphilis, toxoplasmosis, rubella, lysteria, adenovirus, coxsackie B, others	Amniocentesis: PCR (or culture) of fluid
***Hematologic* (5%–15%)**	
Excessive red cells loss	
α-Thalassemia, G6PD-deficit, fetomaternal transfusion, TTTS, fetal hemorrhage, red cell enzyme deficiencies, congenital leukemia, others	
Underproduction	**Maternal testing**
Fetal liver and bone marrow replacement syndromes	• Indirect Coombs testing
Congenital leukemia	• Mean corpuscular volume
Parvovirus B19	• Hemoglobin electrophoresis
Red cell aplasia	• Maternal blood chemistry
	• Kleihauer–Betke
	Ultrasound: MCA peak systolic velocity PUBS (if indicated by other workup)
	• Fetal complete blood cell count
	• Hemoglobin electrophoresis
	• Fetal albumin
	Accurate fetal ultrasound with hemodynamic studies
***Monochorionic twin pregnancy* (5%)**	
Twin-twin transfusion syndrome (TTTS); TRAP sequence	

(Continued)

Table 54.1 (Continued) Conditions Associated with Nonimmune Fetal Hydrops and Suggested Workup

Conditions Associated with NIHF	Suggested Workup
Genetic syndromes (1%) Myotonic dystrophy, arthrogryposis, multiple pterygium, Noonan syndrome (congenital lymphedema), skeletal (see above)	Accurate fetal ultrasound, genetic and tissue studies from AF
Metabolic (1%–5%) Lysosomal storage disorders, Gaucher's disease, Niemann-Pick disease (types C and A), mucopolysaccharidosis (especially type VII), mucolipidosis, sialidosis, galactosialidosis, GM1-gangliosidosis, infantile sialic acid storage disease, others[a]	If indicated, **amniocentesis: enzymatic analysis of supernatant and cultivated amniocytes** (freeze AF if needed) **Maternal testing**

Abbreviations: AF, amniotic fluid; CCAM, congenital cystic adenomatoid malformation; NIHF, nonimmune hydrops fetalis.
[a]For complete detailed list, see Gimovsky AC, Luzi P, Berghella V. Am J Obstet Gynecol, 212, 3, 281–90, 2015.

or secondary closure of the foramen ovale. The presence of heart failure in the setting of structural heart abnormalities is poor with a combined fetal and neonatal mortality rate of 92% [12].

Chromosomal Abnormalities (15%–20%) [5,13,14]

The incidence of chromosome abnormalities is inversely proportional to GA at diagnosis of NIH, with 50% to 75% incidence when NIH is diagnosed <20 weeks [13]. Turner and Down syndromes account for 90% of all aneuploidies associated with hydrops although many other chromosomal abnormalities such as trisomy 18 and 13, 45X/46XX mosaicism, triploidy, and tetraploidy have been reported. The main features of Turner syndrome are cystic hygroma and tubular coartation of aorta, suggesting both lymphatic and cardiac etiology of hydrops [15]. The mere finding of a cystic hygroma in the first trimester strongly suggests aneuploidy (60% of risk) [15], but it needs to be differentiated from an increased nuchal translucency (NT) because of other etiologies (e.g., congenital heart defects). Due to the high incidence of aneuploidy in cases of NIH, prenatal diagnostic testing with karyotype, fluorescence in situ hybridization, and microarray analysis is recommended even in the setting of severe anemia [1].

Extracardiac Anomalies (15%–25%)

Thoracic (5%–10%) [16,17]

Congenital pulmonary airway malformation (CPAM) (previously also called congenital cystic adenomatoid malformation, CCAM), pulmonary sequestration, and congenital diaphragmatic hernia (CDH) are the most common causes of NIH in this category. Other less common causes in this category are lymphangiectasia, bronchogenic cyst, and other thoracic tumors.

Proposed pathophysiological mechanisms for these cases are the compression or deviation of the mediastinum due to the presence of a large lesion or effusion with resultant obstruction of lymphatic or venous return. This obstruction leads to cardiac failure. Compression of the esophagus may also lead to associated polydramnios. CDH produces compression of venous return especially when the liver is herniated in the chest and worse prognosis is expected when it is associated with hydrops. Not only are these fetuses at risk for NIH due to obstruction of cardiac output but those cases with substantial lung compression before 24 weeks are at risk for pulmonary hypoplasia.

Primary hydrothorax is the accumulation of lymphatic fluid in the pleural cavity without any other demonstrated anomaly (mass or chromosomal abnormality). The most common cause of primary hydrothorax in neonates is chylothorax, characterized by a milky pleural fluid for the high concentration of lymphocytes. This fluid may be sampled and the diagnosis is made by the presence of >80% lymphocytes in the absence of infection. With thoracoamniotic shunt placement, survival exceeds 50% in this setting [18].

Similar management has been proposed for fetuses with pulmonary sequestration and CPAM since the development of hydrops in this setting is associated with poor prognosis if untreated. Macrocystic lesions in fetuses with hydrops may be treated expectantly or with needle drainage or thoracoamniotic shunt placement. For microcystic lesions in fetuses with hydrops, management options include expectant management, steroid administration, or open fetal surgery. In a nonrandomized study comparing steroid treatment with fetal surgery, there was a statistically significant increase in resolution of hydrops in the steroid group although no difference in survival was seen [19]. Intrapleural injection of OK-432, a sclerosant product obtained from group A Streptococcus pyogenes, has been shown to have promising results in three studies reported so far [17]. The practice of serial thoracocentesis (e.g., every 48 hours) is discouraged.

Genitourinary (3%)

Urinary tract anomalies may be associated with ascites but rarely present generalized hydrops. Lower tract obstruction produces bladder overdistention that frequently leaks into the abdominal cavity. More rare causes of ascites are the rupture of a dilated renal pelvis or renal thrombosis. Congenital nephrotic syndrome of Finnish type, a rare fatal autosomal recessive disease, can be associated with fetal hydrops due to hypoproteinemia and diagnosed by serum or amniotic fluid α-fetoprotein.

Gastrointestinal (1%)

The primary gastrointestinal abnormalities that have been associated with NIH are diaphragmatic hernia, midgut volvulus, obstruction, jejunal atresia, malrotation of the intestines, and meconium peritonitis [2,12]. Gastrointestinal obstruction may lead to NIH due to decreased colloid osmotic pressure due to protein loss [12]. Intestinal perforation produces variable degrees of ascites (meconium peritonitis) not easy to differentiate from other kinds of intra-abdominal serum effusion. The presence of meconium seen as bright plaques or echo-poor cystic areas would lead to the diagnosis even in the absence of a dilated gut. When meconium peritonitis is not associated with generalized hydrops, the prognosis is good.

Meconium peritonitis may be associated with cystic fibrosis and a workup for this disorder is suggested. Prenatal causes of bowel obstructions are atresias ("apple peel" syndrome) and volvulus. Intra-abdominal masses may cause NIH due to obstruction of venous return. Hemangioma of the liver has also been associated with NIH, likely due to arteriovenous shunting leading to high output cardiac failure [1].

Skeletal Dysplasias (1%)
Many different skeletal dysplasias can be associated with hydrops with severe thoracic hypoplasia impairing venous return leading to hydrops and polyhydramnios. It has also been proposed that this is compounded also by hepatic enlargement that occurs secondary to intrahepatic proliferation of blood cell precursors in order to compensate for small bone marrow volume. It is thought that this hepatic enlargement causes decrease in venous return and resultant anasarca [1]. Conditions for which NIH has been described include, but are not limited to, thanatophoric dysplasia, short rib polydactily, osteogenesis imperfecta, achondrogenesis, and hypophosphatasia. The outcome is uniformly poor.

Vascular (<1%)
Vascular tumors or arteriovenous malformations can cause NIH due to high-output cardiac failure. Placental chorioangiomas occur in 1% of pregnancies and are usually clinically insignificant; however, lesions >5 cm can act as high volume arteriovenous shunts. Similarly, hemangiomas can lead to NIH due to severe anemia, hypoproteinemia, or extramedullary erythropoiesis [1]. Aneurysm of the great vein of Galen is a large cerebral arteriovenous malformation that can cause right-to-left shunting, causing congestive heart failure and hydrops.

Congenital Infections (10%–15%) [14,20]
Parvovirus B19 is the most common infective agent leading to severe anemia and NIH, representing about 5% of all cases of NIH. When congenital defects are excluded, parvovirus B19 infection accounts for about 25% to 50% of fetal hydrops. Approximately 30%–50% of pregnant women are nonimmune, and the incidence of acute Parvovirus infection during pregnancy is 1%–2% although it may be as high as 13% during epidemic periods. The risk of vertical transmission is 30% although in the majority of these cases the fetus is unaffected [14]. The risk of developing NIH after maternal infection with parvovirus is dependent on the gestational age at time of infection. In one study, the overall rate of development of NIH was 4.2% with a significantly higher rate seen in those patients infected at 9–20 weeks gestation (10.6%) [21].

Parvovirus is cytotoxic to bone marrow erythroid progenitor cells, and the destruction of these cells by the virus leads to transient aplastic crises in the fetus [22]. Fetal infection may lead to severe anemia, congestive heart failure, myocarditis, NIH, or death. Cardiac failure may either be the result of severe anemia or arrhythmias in the setting of myocarditis [14]. **The sonographic landmark of the disease is a NIH fetus with a significant increase in the middle cerebral artery peak systolic velocity (MCS PSV).** The process is often self-limited, but the degree of anemia frequently requires intrauterine fetal transfusions until the pathologic process finally remits. **Numerous studies have shown improved outcomes after fetal transfusion [14,23]. In one study, the rate of intrauterine death was significantly lower with transfusion than without treatment (6% vs. 30%)** [14,20,24]. Due to improved outcomes, transfusion is recommended in this setting unless the pregnancy is at a gestational age at which risks of delivery seem to be lower than continued pregnancy with transfusion [1] (Chapter 53).

Syphilis is a rare cause of fetal hydrops, which is the consequence of anemia and hepatic dysfunction resulting in hypoproteinemia and portal hypertension. Other infections such as toxoplasmosis, coxsackie virus, herpes simplex virus, rubella, and CMV have been shown to be occasionally associated with NIH. The pathophysiologic mechanisms involved in fetal hydrops because of infection are multiple and involve anemia (e.g., parvovirus B19, toxoplasmosis, and CMV), hepatitis with hypoproteinemia (e.g., CMV), and myocarditis (e.g., toxoplasmosis, rubella, and CMV). The diagnosis of these infections may be performed by demonstrating maternal seroconversion or through various specialized tests (mainly polymerase chain reaction, PCR). The treatment will vary according to the infectious agent involved. Infections because of CMV or toxoplasmosis have demonstrated to have little response to intrauterine treatment and the prognosis is poor (see Chapters 46 and 47). Sonographic landmarks of poor prognosis for NIH because of infections include fetal growth restriction (frequently early and severe), microcephaly, cerebral ventriculomegaly, and calcifications of various organs including the brain and the liver.

Hematological Disorders (5%–15%)
Anemia is the most frequent cause of NIH from hematologic disorders. Fetuses with anemia develop hydrops because of the combination of high-output heart failure and endothelial damage secondary to hypoxia, leakage of proteins, and reduction in the oncotic pressure. The diagnosis of fetal anemia can be determined noninvasively through Doppler evaluation of the cerebral circulation, which has proven to be valuable in identifying anemia of both immune and nonimmune origins. The mechanisms leading to fetal anemia can be classified as follows:

Reduced Red Blood Cell/Hemoglobin Production
α-Thalassemia is a common cause for fetal hydrops in Southeast Asia and European Mediterranean countries, where it accounts for 28%–55% of all cases of NIH [25,26]. This disease is characterized by a fetus that is unable to produce globin chains to form hemoglobin F in utero, leading to hypoxia and endothelial damage (see Chapter 14). A complete blood count can be used for screening as the mean cell volume will be <80 fL in carriers. Other causes are congenital medullar aplasia secondary to fetal leukemia or parvovirus B19 infection.

Hemolysis
This has been observed in some cases of glucose 6 phosphate dehydrogenase deficiency and infection (CMV and toxoplasmosis).

Hemorrhage
Fetomaternal hemorrhage may be significant enough to induce NIH and should be suspected after trauma or placental abruption. Even without a bleeding history, in one review, NIH was the presenting sign of fetomaternal hemorrhage greater than 50 mL in 7.5% of cases [27]. A Kleihauer–Betke test or flow cytometry may be used to aid in diagnosis and to assess the

magnitude of the transfusion. Management with delivery or intrauterine transfusion should be considered, depending on gestational age and results of fetal testing. If left untreated, fetuses subjected to severe anemia may develop cardiac failure, hydrops, hypovolemic shock, fetal or neonatal death, neurologic damage, cerebral palsy or persistent pulmonary hypertension [27].

Twin-to-Twin Transfusion Syndrome (TTTS) (1%–5%)
This complication of monochorionic twins leads to an imbalance in blood flow between the two fetuses. The pathophysiology is not clearly understood though it appears to be linked to disturbances in volume with a subsequent increase in central venous pressure [5]. This leads to hypoxia in the donor twin and vascular overload in the recipient twin. In some cases of twin-to-twin transfusion syndrome (TTTS) and TRAP sequence, invasive therapy with fetoscopy and laser coagulation or umbilical cord ligation have been associated in some studies with improved fetal survival (see Chapter 44).

Fetal Tumors (1%–5%)

Fetal tumors, such as lymphangiomas, hemangiomas, sacrococcygeal, mediastinal, pharyngeal teratomas, and neuroblastomas, have been associated with NIH [12,28,29]. The likely mechanism in these cases is the development of high-output cardiac failure due to their vascular nature. In utero treatment has been offered in cases of sacrococcygeal teratoma and open surgery resulted in survival in 6/11 cases, and minimally invasive approaches resulted in survival in 6/20 cases [30]. Rhabdomyomas, cardiac tumors often associated with tuberous sclerosis, can obstruct outflow or filling and result in NIH. The associated liver fibrosis can also lead to hepatic failure and NIH.

Metabolic Diseases (1%–5%) [31,32]

Metabolic diseases have historically been reported to account for only 1%–2% of NIH. There have been 14 specific lysosomal storage diseases (LSD) identified that cause NIH. The likely mechanism is obstruction of venous return due to visceromegaly or decreased erythropoiesis leading to anemia [1]. In a recent review of 678 cases of NIH, the overall incidence of LSD was 5.2%. A diagnosis of LSD was made in 17.4% of the idiopathic cases overall and in 29.6% of those idiopathic NIH cases in which a more comprehensive LSD workup was done in a specialized laboratory [33].

Although diagnosis is expensive, investigation for metabolic diseases is justified after the initial workup has been completed and the most frequent causes have been ruled out [34,35]. Prenatal LSD diagnosis can be performed by enzyme analysis of fetal cells from chorionic villus sampling or amniocentesis specimen. This enzyme analysis can be done in specialized national laboratories. Although uncommon, the identification of these disorders is important also due to their recurrence risk. Further, identification of the exact mutation in the proband or in the heterozygous parent can be used to aid in preimplantation and prenatal diagnosis in future pregnancies.

MATERNAL COMPLICATIONS

"**Mirror syndrome**," also known as Ballantyne's syndrome, is a rare complication of NIH in which edema develops in the mother that mirrors the hydropic fetus. The exact underlying pathogenesis is unknown, but this condition is characterized by edema and preeclampsia-like symptoms, such as hypertension (61% of cases), anemia/hemodilution (46.4%), proteinuria (42%), transaminitis (20%), and oliguria (16%) [36]. The incidence of mirror syndrome is so low that distinction between Mirror syndrome and preeclampsia has been difficult to assess. In a review of 56 cases from 1956 to 2009, the average age of diagnosis was 22.5–27.8 weeks. Major maternal morbidity was seen in 21% of all cases with pulmonary edema the most common. Resolution of maternal symptoms was seen an average of 8–9 days after delivery or successful treatment of the fetal hydrops. The average rate of intrauterine fetal demise was 36%. There are currently no management studies on expectant management in the case of Mirror syndrome. In some cases of NIH with a potentially treatable etiology, resolution of maternal symptoms has been seen after fetal treatment. Caution is advised in these situations, and delivery should not be delayed in the case of worsening maternal status. In most cases of Mirror syndrome, delivery is recommended [1].

There are other obstetric complications associated with NIH. Polyhydramnios is seen in 29% of cases, which can lead to maternal respiratory symptoms, preterm delivery, placental abruption or postpartum hemorrhage. The increased rates of postpartum hemorrhage seen in cases of NIH are likely a combination of uterine atony secondary to polyhydramnios and the presence of large edematous placentas, which may have greater uterine adherence [37].

MANAGEMENT
Counseling/Prognosis

NIH is the end stage of many severe diseases whose outcome is related to the etiology, the severity, and the time of onset. **In general, perinatal mortality in pregnancies complicated by NIH ranges between 50% and 100%, depending on the etiology** [38]. Outcomes are best in cases with potentially treatable etiology, such as Parvovirus or fetal cardiac arrhythmias. In those cases of live birth, there is a 64% survival. In those infants born alive, 40% will have associated morbidity [38]. The most significant factors associated with neonatal death are the underlying cause of NIH, gestational age at delivery, and lower serum albumin level at birth [39]. There is limited data regarding long-term follow-up in these children, however, in 2 studies with follow-up at a year, 16% of children were seen to have severe psychomotor developmental delay, and 16% had mild mental retardation.

The worst prognosis is expected in cases diagnosed before 24 weeks gestation, cases in which a cystic hygroma is present, or cases with chromosomal abnormalities. Half of cases diagnosed prior to 24 weeks are associated with aneuploidy and have very poor survival. Even in those cases diagnosed prior to 24 weeks without aneuploidy, survival is less than 50% [40]. Counseling should include the option of termination in regions where this is available. After 24 weeks of gestation, the survival rate in euploid fetuses is nearly 50% when effective treatments are performed. Fetal anemia and fetal arrhythmia are two of the etiologies of NIH associated with >70% to 90% survival rate, if appropriate treatment is instituted [1]. Consideration should also be given to transfer the patient to a tertiary care center for management and delivery where possible.

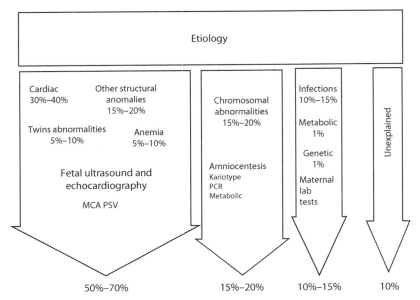

Figure 54.3   Etiology and basic work-up of hydrops. *Abbreviations*: MCA PSV, middle cerebral artery peak systolic velocity; PCR, polymerase chain reaction.

Workup/Diagnosis (Figures 54.3 and 54.4 and Table 54.1)

After the finding of hydrops by ultrasound, a systematic workup is mandatory. A thorough evaluation of cases with fetal hydrops allows determination of their cause in up to 80% of cases. This is important to determine the therapeutic strategies that should be mounted as well as providing appropriate genetic counseling for future pregnancies.

Basic Workup

Demographic and clinical history. Ethnicity and race, consanguinity, work exposure to infections, genetic/metabolic diseases, congenital anomalies, autoimmune diseases, and events of the pregnancy, including previous infection screening and ultrasound findings.

Laboratory. Rule out Rh disease or any other cause of immune fetal anemia. Identifications of infectious diseases, such as syphilis, parvovirus B19, toxoplasmosis, cytomegalovirus, rubella, coxsackie, HSV-1 and HSV-2, and *Listeria*. Perform the Kleihauer–Betke test and SSA and SSB antibody tests if patient has lupus.

Ultrasound. Include assessment of the following:

* Abdomen for ascites, thorax for pleural/pericardial effusion, and skin for edema
* Complete anatomy survey to look for anomalies of the fetus, placenta, and umbilical cord
* Assessment of amniotic fluid volume
* Fetal heart: arrhythmias (M-mode), structural anomalies, function (Doppler)
* Doppler analysis of umbilical artery, MCA PSV, ductus venosus, and possibly other arteries and veins
* Liver length, spleen size
* Placental thickness, malformations

Hydrothorax is an easily observable collection of fluid in the pleural space. It can be unilateral or bilateral and, when severe and presenting early in pregnancy, can lead to pulmonary hypoplasia. In the presence of severe-moderate *ascites,* liquid is evident all around the abdominal circumference, and a thorough observation is necessary to differentiate real ascites from the hypoechogenic rime produced by dorsal and abdominal musculature just beneath the abdominal wall. Pericardial effusion distends the pericardium without any motion during cardiac activity. Placental edema is diagnosed when its thickness is >6 cm, and polyhydramnios is conventionally defined as an amniotic fluid index above the 95th percentile for gestational age or a maximal pocket of amniotic fluid >8 cm.

A detailed sonographic examination is important to determine anatomical defects associated to fetal hydrops. A systematic analysis should be performed to evaluate cardiac anatomy, fetal heart rate and rhythm, and signs of heart failure that can be secondary to extracardiac anomalies, such as placental or fetal tumors (e.g., chorioangioma and teratoma), as well as arteriovenous shunts, such as those of vein of Galen aneurysm and hepatic hemangioendothelioma. Also, signs of intrauterine infection should be evaluated, including the presence of brain or hepatic calcifications, ventriculomegaly or hydrocephalus, hyperechogenic bowel, and fetal growth restriction. Magnetic resonance imaging can be employed to aid in diagnosis of anomalies.

An accurate **fetal echocardiography** aims first to examine position, size, function, and rhythm of the heart. The systematic observation of a four-chambers view, outflow tracts, great arteries, and arches can rule out the majority of CHD associated to hydrops. The addition of color and pulse Doppler allows a more complete evaluation of heart function and flow across atrioventricular valves and arterial valves while M-mode allows a more accurate study of heart squeezing, recording of wall thickness and rhythm. Color Doppler investigation can demonstrate atrioventricular valve regurgitation, and insonation of peripheral vessels can show venous abnormal pulsatility in ductus venosus or hepatic veins as signs of cardiac failure or provide information on right atrium pressure and heart function.

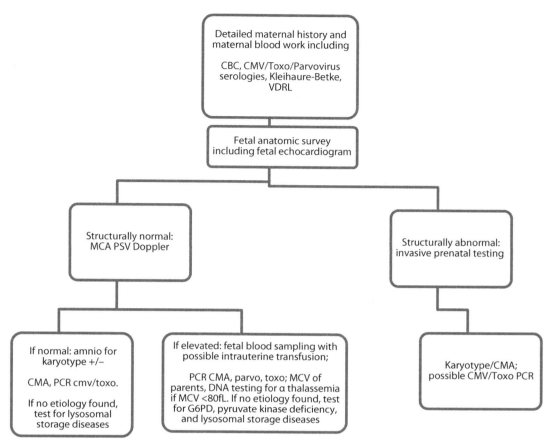

Figure 54.4 Workup of nonimmune hydrops: Amnio, amniocentesis; CBC, complete blood count; CMA, chromosomal microarray; CMV, cytomegalovirus; DNA, deoxyribonucelic acid; G6PD, glucose-6-phosphate dehydrogenase deficiency; MCA, middle cerebral artery; MCV, mean corpuscular volume; PSV, peak systolic velocity; PCR, polymerase chain reaction; Toxo, toxoplasmosis; VDRL, venereal disease research laboratory test.

Fetal Doppler velocimetry, M-mode, and color mapping can be useful to diagnose and evaluate cases of fetal arrhythmia as well as fetal anemia by evaluating the MCA PSV. MCA PSV is >90% sensitive and specific for fetal anemia, using MoM >1.50 [41,42]. The most likely explanation for the observed increase in MCA PSV is the reduction of blood viscosity, leading to enhanced venous return and preload with consequent increase in cardiac output. Fetal Doppler studies are useful for the evaluation of the venous circulation (ductus venosus and inferior vena cava) to determine the prognosis of fetal hydrops of cardiovascular origin and to evaluate fetal response to treatment. Along with other modalities to monitor fetal well being, it plays an important role in defining the appropriate moment for a timely delivery.

Amniocentesis. Different analyses in amniotic fluid permit the investigation of fetal karyotype, congenital infections, and metabolic diseases. Fluorescence in situ hybridization (FISH) and quantitative fluorescent polymerase chain reaction (QF-PCR) can provide a rapid assessment of chromosome 13, 18, 21, X and Y, assessing about 70% of chromosomal anomalies. A full karyotype from culture of amniocytes rules out all chromosome anomalies.

For the investigation of infectious etiology, PCR in the amniotic fluid is the most sensitive test although a negative result does not exclude the presence of the disease. Parvovirus B19, CMV, and toxoplasmosis are the most common infectious etiologies of NIH. Biochemical testing of enzymatic activity in cultured amniotic fluid allows the investigation of inborn errors of metabolism. Consider freezing amniotic fluid/extra fetal serum for future tests to study additional conditions when etiology remains unclear.

Cordocentesis and other invasive procedures. Cordocentesis should not be considered a routine procedure in the workup of NIH, but is strongly recommended when fetal anemia is suspected (i.e., MCA PSV >1.5 MoM). The fragile hemodynamic condition of the fetus with NIH suggests exercising caution when the procedure is performed, especially in severely compromised fetuses with functional cardiac involvement. When performed, fetal blood tests should include full blood count, blood group and Coombs test, and serum biochemistry. In special cases, thalassemia screening, total IgM, and G6PD in male fetuses can be investigated. PCR for infectious etiologies and testing for lysosomal storage disease can also be done with fetal blood sampling. Peritoneal fluid, pleural fluid, and urine can be obtained with diagnostic and sometimes therapeutic purposes. Cytological and biochemical analysis of these fluids may incline toward a final etiology of NIH. Likewise, karyotype and microorganisms can be searched from these fluids.

Therapeutic Approach

Management, including fetal monitoring, treatment, and delivery, should follow the **appropriate guidelines for the specific etiology of the NIH**.

Fetal Monitoring/Testing

There are no studies on the utility of antenatal fetal testing in the setting of NIH [43]. Testing is reasonable if the etiology of the NIH is nonlethal, the fetus is at a potentially viable gestational age, and if the findings of fetal testing would aid in guiding delivery timing [1]. Doppler studies (especially umbilical artery and MCA Doppler interrogation), NSTs, and BPPs (at ≥28 weeks) can be performed at weekly intervals in the hydropic fetus to assess fetal status and determine the appropriate time for delivery.

Treatment

Therapeutic approach depends on the differential diagnosis of the etiology of NIH. Careful assessment of the risks, benefits, and alternatives to each therapy should be considered and discussed with parents. These cases should be referred to tertiary care centers with physicians experienced with providing the appropriate treatment.

For parvovirus B19 and arrhythmias, treatment is feasible and effective. Intrauterine transfusion of fetuses with severe hydrops because of parvovirus B19 infection reduces the risk of fetal death. When heart failure and hydrops are associated with supraventricular tachycardia, the first-line drug is digoxin. Alternatives are flecainide, amiodarone, verapamil, and adenosine. Difficulties derived from placental enlargement may render maternal administration erratic and direct administration to the umbilical cord is an alternative.

In severe pleural effusions, pulmonary compression may lead to lung hypoplasia and polyhydramnios because of mediastinal compression and obstruction of fetal swelling, increasing the risk of preterm labor. These conditions as well as low output cardiac failure may explain the poor prognosis of severe hydrothorax. In these cases, thoracoamniotic shunting may be indicated. Several series including the last 20 years suggest that this procedure may improve fetal and neonatal outcome.

In cases of macrocystic CPAM, drainage and maternal corticosteroid administration is recommended. Cases of twin-to-twin transfusion syndrome should be referred to specialized centers for possible fetoscopic laser photocoagulation <26 weeks [1].

Amniodrainage may be considered in the case of severe polyhydramnios to reduce maternal respiratory dysfunction and provide the patient with comfort as well as potentially decreasing the risk of preterm delivery.

Obstetric Management

There are no studies assessing benefit with a course of corticosteroids prior to delivery in the setting of NIH. In two retrospective studies, there was no improvement in neonatal survival after steroids [44,45]. Based on expert opinion, it is reasonable to administer a course of corticosteroids if an intervention or delivery is planned between 24 and 34 weeks.

Tocolysis for preterm labor may not be advisable in all cases. Preeclampsia may develop in up to 50% of cases, adding another factor to consider when defining the time of delivery. Again, delivery at a tertiary care center is recommended.

Delivery Timing

There are no trials assessing the ideal timing of delivery in the setting of NIH. It has been suggested that prognosis is worse in cases of delivery <34 weeks [39]. Each case needs to be considered individually, given the spectrum of etiologies and severity. Based on expert opinion, **delivery is reasonable after 34 weeks if evidence of worsening fetal status and by 37–38 weeks if status has remained stable and delivery was not otherwise indicated earlier** [1].

Delivery/Anesthesia

The delivery route will depend on the obstetrical conditions. However, the unique cardiovascular derangements usually present in hydropic fetuses, leading to nonreassuring fetal testing, may necessitate a cesarean section. Hemodynamically stable fetuses may be offered a vaginal delivery. Aspiration of excessive fluid from the pericardium, pleural, and peritoneal cavities may be beneficial to facilitate delivery, minimize trauma, and improve neonatal resuscitative efforts. At all times, the patient should be informed about the diagnosis, prognosis, and management of NIH in general and the specific characteristics of her case. Fetal monitoring results, size of effusions, and need for procedures before delivery should all be taken into consideration. Written consent is mandatory, emphasizing the paucity of information about NIH. In cases where the decision has been made by the mother not to intervene for fetal indications, vaginal delivery is preferred, unless contraindicated [1].

NEONATOLOGY MANAGEMENT

In cases where fetal survival may potentially be improved with neonatal intervention, delivery should occur at a center with a level III neonatal intensive care unit [1]. These neonates require expert, intensive, and multidisciplinary management. In cases of fetal or neonatal death, an autopsy should be performed to determine the cause of NIH and death. Long-term follow-up shows that the majority of hydropic neonates who are born and discharged alive have intact long-term survival [46].

MATERNAL POSTPARTUM

A separate outpatient visit should be set up to discuss a postpartum review of the possible etiology of the NIH, including recurrence risks. Recurrent NIH is very rare and mostly due to inborn errors of metabolism (e.g., lysosomal storage disorders, rare hemoglobinopathies, or other genetic disorders).

REFERENCES

1. Society for Maternal-Fetal Medicine (SMFM), Norton ME, Chauhan SP, Dashe JS. Society for maternal-fetal medicine (SMFM) clinical guideline #7: Nonimmune hydrops fetalis. *Am J Obstet Gynecol* 2015; 212(2): 127–39. [Review]
2. Machin GA. Hydrops revisited: Literature review of 1,414 cases published in the 1980s. *Am J Med Genet* 1989; 34(3): 366–90. [Review]
3. Heinonen S, Ryynanen M, Kirkinen P. Etiology and outcome of second trimester non-immunologic fetal hydrops. *Acta Obstet Gynecol Scand* 2000; 79(1): 15–8. [II-2]
4. Sohan K et al. Analysis of outcome in hydrops fetalis in relation to gestational age at diagnosis, cause and treatment. *Acta Obstet Gynecol Scand* 2001; 80(8): 726–30. [II-3]

5. Bellini C et al. Etiology of nonimmune hydrops fetalis: A systematic review. *Am J Med Genet A* 2009; 149A(5): 844–51. [I]

6. Fukushima K et al. Short-term and long-term outcomes of 214 cases of non-immune hydrops fetalis. *Early Hum Dev* 2011; 87(8): 571–5. [II-3]

7. Hahurij ND et al. Perinatal management and long-term cardiac outcome in fetal arrhythmia. *Early Hum Dev* 2011; 87(2): 83–7. [II-3]

8. Cuneo BF et al. Atrial and ventricular rate response and patterns of heart rate acceleration during maternal-fetal terbutaline treatment of fetal complete heart block. *Am J Cardiol* 2007; 100(4): 661–5. [II-1]

9. Yoshida H et al. Treatment of fetal congenital complete heart block with maternal administration of beta-sympathomimetics (terbutaline): A case report. *Gynecol Obstet Invest* 2001; 52(2): 142–4. [III]

10. Friedman DM et al. Prospective evaluation of fetuses with autoimmune-associated congenital heart block followed in the PR Interval and Dexamethasone Evaluation (PRIDE) Study. *Am J Cardiol* 2009; 103(8): 1102–6. [II-1]

11. Abrams ME et al. Hydrops fetalis: A retrospective review of cases reported to a large national database and identification of risk factors associated with death. *Pediatrics* 2007; 120(1): 84–9. [II-2]

12. Randenberg AL. Nonimmune hydrops fetalis part II: Does etiology influence mortality? *Neonatal Netw* 2010; 29(6): 367–80. [III]

13. Iskaros J, Jauniaux E, Rodeck C. Outcome of nonimmune hydrops fetalis diagnosed during the first half of pregnancy. *Obstet Gynecol* 1997; 90(3): 321–5. [II-3]

14. Lamont RF et al. Parvovirus B19 infection in human pregnancy. *BJOG* 2011; 118(2): 175–86. [Review]

15. Ganapathy R et al. Natural history and outcome of prenatally diagnosed cystic hygroma. *Prenat Diagn* 2004; 24(12): 965–8. [II-2]

16. Aubard Y et al. Primary fetal hydrothorax: A literature review and proposed antenatal clinical strategy. *Fetal Diagn Ther* 1998; 13(6): 325–33. [Review]

17. Yinon Y, Kelly E, Ryan G. Fetal pleural effusions. *Best Pract Res Clin Obstet Gynaecol* 2008; 22(1): 77–96. [Review]

18. Yinon Y et al. Perinatal outcome following fetal chest shunt insertion for pleural effusion. *Ultrasound Obstet Gynecol* 2010; 36(1): 58–64. [II-2]

19. Loh KC et al. Microcystic congenital pulmonary airway malformation with hydrops fetalis: Steroids vs open fetal resection. *J Pediatr Surg* 2012; 47(1): 36–9. [II-2]

20. Tolfvenstam T, Broliden K. Parvovirus B19 infection. *Semin Fetal Neonatal Med* 2009; 14(4): 218–21. [Review]

21. Enders M et al. Risk of fetal hydrops and non-hydropic late intrauterine fetal death after gestational parvovirus B19 infection. *J Clin Virol* 2010; 49(3): 163–8. [II-2]

22. Young N et al. Direct demonstration of the human parvovirus in erythroid progenitor cells infected in vitro. *J Clin Invest* 1984; 74(6): 2024–32. [III]

23. Enders M et al. Fetal morbidity and mortality after acute human parvovirus B19 infection in pregnancy: Prospective evaluation of 1018 cases. *Prenat Diagn* 2004; 24(7): 513–8. [II-2]

24. Rodis JF et al. Management of parvovirus infection in pregnancy and outcomes of hydrops: A survey of members of the Society of Perinatal Obstetricians. *Am J Obstet Gynecol* 1998; 179(4): 985–8. [III]

25. Liao C et al. Nonimmune hydrops fetalis diagnosed during the second half of pregnancy in Southern China. *Fetal Diagn Ther* 2007; 22(4): 302–5. [II-2]

26. Suwanrath-Kengpol C et al. Etiology and outcome of non-immune hydrops fetalis in southern Thailand. *Gynecol Obstet Invest* 2005; 59(3): 134–7. [II-2]

27. Wylie BJ, D'Alton ME. Fetomaternal hemorrhage. *Obstet Gynecol* 2010; 115(5): 1039–51. [III]

28. Noreen S, Heller DS, Faye-Petersen O. Mediastinal teratoma as a rare cause of hydrops fetalis and death: report of 3 cases. *J Reprod Med* 2008; 53(9): 708–10. [III]

29. Isaacs H Jr. Fetal hydrops associated with tumors. *Am J Perinatol* 2008; 25(1): 43–68. [III]

30. Van Mieghem T et al. Minimally invasive therapy for fetal sacrococcygeal teratoma: Case series and systematic review of the literature. *Ultrasound Obstet Gynecol* 2014; 43(6): 611–9. [III]

31. Stone DL, Sidransky E. Hydrops fetalis: Lysosomal storage disorders in extremis. *Adv Pediatr* 1999; 46: 409–40. [II-3]

32. Burin MG et al. Investigation of lysosomal storage diseases in nonimmune hydrops fetalis. *Prenat Diagn* 2004; 24(8): 653–7. [II-3]

33. Gimovsky AC, Luzi P, Berghella V. Lysosomal storage disease as an etiology of nonimmune hydrops. *Am J Obstet Gynecol* 2015; 212(3): 281–90. [I]

34. Laneri GG, Claassen DL, Scher MS. Brain lesions of fetal onset in encephalopathic infants with nonimmune hydrops fetalis. *Pediatr Neurol* 1994; 11(1): 18–22. [III]

35. Larroche JC, Aubry MC, Narcy F. Intrauterine brain damage in nonimmune hydrops fetalis. *Biol Neonate* 1992; 61(5): 273–80. [III]

36. Braun T et al. Mirror syndrome: A systematic review of fetal associated conditions, maternal presentation and perinatal outcome. *Fetal Diagn Ther* 2010; 27(4): 191–203. [III]

37. Hutchison AA et al. Nonimmunologic hydrops fetalis: A review of 61 cases. *Obstet Gynecol* 1982; 59(3): 347–52. [III]

38. Santo S et al. Prenatal diagnosis of non-immune hydrops fetalis: What do we tell the parents? *Prenat Diagn* 2011; 31(2): 186–95. [Review]

39. Huang HR et al. Prognostic factors and clinical features in liveborn neonates with hydrops fetalis. *Am J Perinatol* 2007; 24(1): 33–8. [II-2]

40. Santolaya J et al. Antenatal classification of hydrops fetalis. *Obstet Gynecol* 1992; 79(2): 256–9. [III]

41. Hernandez-Andrade E et al. Fetal middle cerebral artery peak systolic velocity in the investigation of non-immune hydrops. *Ultrasound Obstet Gynecol* 2004; 23(5): 442–5. [II-3]

42. Cosmi E et al. Middle cerebral artery peak systolic and ductus venosus velocity waveforms in the hydropic fetus. *J Ultrasound Med* 2005; 24(2): 209–13. [II-3]

43. Practice bulletin no. 145: antepartum fetal surveillance. *Obstet Gynecol* 2014; 124(1): 182–92. [III]

44. Wy CA et al. Outcome of infants with a diagnosis of hydrops fetalis in the 1990s. *Am J Perinatol* 1999; 16(10): 561–7. [III]

45. Simpson JH et al. Severity of non-immune hydrops fetalis at birth continues to predict survival despite advances in perinatal care. *Fetal Diagn Ther* 2006; 21(4): 380–2. [III]

46. Haverkamp F et al. Good prognosis for psychomotor development in survivors with nonimmune hydrops fetalis. *BJOG* 2000; 107(2): 282–4. [II-3]

55

Fetal death

Nahida Chakhtoura and Uma M. Reddy

KEY POINTS

- **Ultrasound examination should be performed for confirmation of fetal death.**
- Most informative exams **to find the etiology** of fetal death are **autopsy; examination of the placenta, cord, and membranes; and chromosomal analysis.**
- **Induction of labor** in patients with fetal death is recommended unless patient is already in labor.
- **For fetal death at about 14 to 28 weeks, misoprostol** (200–**400** mcg vaginally **every 4 hours,** 400 mcg orally every 4 hours, 200 mcg buccal, or 600 mcg vaginally every 12 hours) is the **most cost-effective method of delivery with acceptable side effects.** After 28 weeks of gestation, drugs, such as oxytocin and/or prostaglandins administered for induction of labor, can be usually given according to standard obstetric protocols (see Chapter 21 in *Obstetric Evidence Based Guidelines*).

DEFINITIONS

Fetal death is defined by the U.S. National Center for Health Statistics (NCHS), a division of the Centers for Disease Control and Prevention, as

> **death prior to the complete expulsion or extraction from the mother of a product of human conception,** irrespective of the duration of pregnancy and which is not an induced termination of pregnancy. The death is indicated by the fact that after such expulsion or extraction, the fetus does not breathe or show any other evidence of life such as beating of the heart, pulsation of the umbilical cord, or definite movements of voluntary muscles. Heartbeats are to be distinguished from transient cardiac contractions; respirations are to be distinguished from fleeting respiratory efforts or gasps [1].

The WHO definition of fetal death does not exclude spontaneous abortion at <12 weeks, which has different etiologies and management than fetal death occurring in the second or third trimester. There is not complete uniformity even among U.S. states regarding the birth weight and gestational age criteria for reporting fetal deaths. However, **NCHS** has recommended the reporting of **fetal deaths** at ≥**20 weeks** of gestation with known gestational age or weight ≥**350 g** if the gestational age is unknown [2]. 350 g is the 50th percentile for weight at 20 weeks of gestation. Fetal losses because of terminations of pregnancy for lethal fetal anomalies and inductions of labor for previable premature rupture of membranes are excluded from these statistics and are classified separately as terminations of pregnancy. **Embryonic death** is defined as death occurring at ≤12 weeks. **Early fetal death** is defined as death occurring at 13 to 19 6/7 weeks of gestation. **Intermediate fetal death** is defined as death occurring at 20 to 27 weeks of gestation. **Late fetal death** is defined as death occurring at greater than 28 weeks of gestation.

Stillbirth is the term preferred by parent groups and therefore has been increasingly used by the research community and by ACOG for fetal deaths ≥20 weeks of gestation or weight >350 g [3] and can be used as a synonym for fetal death. **Fetal demise** (often abbreviated **IUFD** or intrauterine fetal demise) is often also used interchangeably with fetal death. **Unexplained fetal death** is defined as death before delivery with no identifiable cause after complete evaluation is performed.

DIAGNOSIS

The diagnosis of fetal death should be **confirmed by ultrasound** with absence of heart movement.

EPIDEMIOLOGY/INCIDENCE

An estimated 3.2 million stillbirths occur annually worldwide; 98% of all stillbirths occur in low- and middle-income countries with two thirds of stillbirths occurring in Southeast Asia and Sub-Saharan Africa [4,5]. In the United States, in 2013, there were 23,595 reported fetal deaths at 20 weeks of gestation or more, resulting in a fetal death rate of 5.96/1000 live births plus fetal deaths [3]. Close to one half of these deaths occur in the third trimester. U.S. fetal mortality rates have been stable since 2006 with some minor fluctuations [1,6].

ASSOCIATIONS/RISK FACTORS/ POSSIBLE ETIOLOGIES

There are many maternal and fetal factors that have been associated with fetal death (Table 55.1). About 25% of fetal deaths are not associated with any of these risks and are called "unexplained." Many classification schemes for assigning cause of stillbirth are currently used throughout the world. There are at least 35 different classification systems reported in the medical literature since 1954, and each system was created with a specific purpose by the investigators. The Stillbirth Collaborative Research Network (SCRN) Initial Causes of Fetal Death was devised for research purposes to provide a structured system so that the definitions used to assign the most likely cause of stillbirth are uniform and those reviewing the potential causes of stillbirth can communicate using a common language. An important goal of this system was to use the best available evidence and rigorous definitions determined before case review when assigning a cause of death [7]. **Fetal death rate is an important marker of quality of health care.** Other factors associated with fetal death are advanced maternal age, non-Hispanic black race, nulliparity or multiparity (>5), maternal medical disease, unmarried status, low socioeconomic status, low education, multiple gestation, assisted reproductive technology, and past obstetric history (previous stillbirth, preterm delivery, postdates, or growth restriction) [8–18]. **Obesity, smoking, and**

Table 55.1 Associations/Risk Factors/Possible Etiologies of Fetal Death

Maternal Risk Factors	Fetal Risk Factors
Chronic hypertension	**Congenital malformations**
Preeclampsia	(15%–20%)
Diabetes mellitus,	**Chromosomal/genetic**
thyroid disorders	**abnormalities** (8%–13%):
Renal disease	monosomy X, trisomy 21,
Systemic lupus	trisomy 18, and trisomy 13
erythematosus	**Single gene disorders:**
Autoimmune disease	hemoglobinopathies (e.g.,
Antiphospholipid	alpha-thalassemia); metabolic
syndrome	diseases (e.g., Smith–Lemli–Opitz
Cholestasis of pregnancy	syndrome)
Alloimmunization	Missense mutations leading to long
Obesity	QT syndrome
Substance abuse	Glycogen storage diseases
(especially cocaine,	Peroxisomal disorders amino acid
alcohol, coffee: >3 cups/	disorders
day, etc.)	Confined placental mosaicism
Smoking	(aneuploidy in placenta with a
Viral infections:	euploid fetus)
Parvovirus B19	Placental abruption, placenta, and
Cytomegalovirus	vasa previa
Enteroviruses (e.g.,	Placental pathology
coxsackie virus)	Chronic villitis
Echoviruses	Massive chorionic intervillositis
HSV-1, HSV-2	Complications of multifetal
HIV	gestation (e.g., twin–twin
Bacterial infections:	transfusion, twin
Listeria	reversed arterial perfusion
monocytogenes	syndrome, and discordant growth)
Escherichia coli	Umbilical cord complications,
Group B streptococci	fetomaternal hemorrhage
Ureaplasma	Fetal growth restriction
urealyticum	Uteroplacental insufficiency
Treponema pallidum	Intrauterine asphyxia
Parasitic infections:	Preterm labor or rupture of
Toxoplasma gondii	membranes
Uterine malformations	Postterm
Abdominal trauma	

Note: In bold, most common associations.

drug and alcohol abuse are common modifiable risk factors for fetal death. Pesticides, radiation, and fertility drugs have also been associated with fetal death [19]. In developing countries, the most common causes of stillbirths are complications of labor and infection.

PREVENTION

Some of the **risk factors** listed in Table 55.1, in particular obesity, smoking, and drug and alcohol abuse, are **modifiable** and should be avoided. Basic emergency obstetric care, births in adequate facilities with option for safe cesarean delivery (CD), improvement in nutrition, and prevention and treatment of syphilis, tuberculosis, and malaria are the most feasible and cost-effective interventions in developing countries to decrease the incidence of stillbirth [20].

As the vast majority of fetal deaths occur in developing countries, interventions should be focused on prevention in these settings and include [21] the following:

- Improving maternal nutritional status, such as micronutrient supplementation
- Periconception folate fortification [22]

- Insecticide-treated bed nets or intermittent preventative treatment for malaria
- Syphilis detection and treatment
- Detection and treatment of hypertensive disorders
- Detection and management of diabetes in pregnancy
- Smoking cessation
- Detection and management of FGR
- Induction at 41 weeks (prevention of postterm pregnancy)
- Skilled care at birth
- Basic and comprehensive emergency obstetric care

PREGNANCY MANAGEMENT
Counseling

Counseling should include review of possible etiologies (Table 55.1), workup (Table 55.2), and delivery options as well as possible complications. Grief counseling should be included in addition to the option for referral to grieving help groups. Understanding the cause of stillbirth is important to parents and management of future pregnancies. However, obtaining consent for autopsies, surgical investigations, imaging and other investigations is difficult for both parents and health care providers. Investigating the best possible way to support decision-making is important [23]. Review of risk of recurrence, prevention of recurrence, and best management for a future pregnancy (Table 55.3) should be done postpartum.

Workup

Evaluation of the etiology of fetal death is essential to counsel regarding recurrence risks, facilitate the grieving process, and improve understanding to facilitate therapeutic measures (Table 55.2) [3,24,25]. The evaluation can be emotionally difficult and should be multidisciplinary (obstetrician, maternal-fetal specialist, pathologist, geneticist, radiologist, and neonatologist). Communication between all these

Table 55.2 Maternal and Fetal Investigation for Fetal Death

Predelivery
- Amniotic fluid for cytogenetics
- Screen for coagulopathy (only if fetal death >4 wk from delivery)
- CBC, antibody screen, urine drug screen
- Kleihauer-Betke testing or flow cytometry
- Lupus anticoagulant, anticardiolipin antibodies (IgM, IgG) and anti-β_2-glycoprotein antibodies (IgM, IgG)
- Parvovirus B19 titers (IgM and IgG)[a]
- Syphilis testing (RPR or VDRL)
- Thyroid-stimulating hormone
- Glucose screening (oral glucose tolerance test, hemoglobin A1c) (if glucose screening not done in pregnancy)
- Thrombophilia workup only to be considered in cases of severe placental infarcts, fetal growth restriction, or in the setting of a personal history of thrombosis (factor V Leiden mutation; G20210A prothrombin gene mutation; antithrombin III)

Postdelivery
- Cord blood for cytogenetics
- **Autopsy and placental examination**
- Protein C, protein S activity (in selected cases as described above for other thrombophilia workup)
  - MRI

[a]Consider workup for parvovirus especially in cases with fetal hydrops or other signs of this viral infection.

Table 55.3 Management of Subsequent Pregnancy after Stillbirth

Preconception or initial prenatal visit
- Detailed medical and obstetrical history
- Evaluation/workup of previous stillbirth
- Determination of recurrence risk
- Discussion of increased risk of other obstetrical complications
- Smoking cessation
- Weight loss (back to normal BMI) in obese women
- Genetic counseling if family genetic condition exists
- Support and reassurance

First trimester
- Dating ultrasound by crown–rump length (first trimester)
- First-trimester screen-PAPP-A, hCG, and nuchal translucency
- Diabetes screen
- Antiphospholipid antibodies
- Thrombophilia workup only if stillbirth associated with severe placental infarcts, fetal growth restriction, or in the setting of a personal history of thrombosis. Support and reassurance

Second trimester
- Fetal anatomic survey at 18 to 20 wk
- Quadruple screen-MSAFP, hCG, estriol, and inhibin-A
- Uterine artery Doppler studies at 22 to 24 wk
- Support and reassurance

Third trimester
- Serial ultrasounds about every 4 wk to rule out fetal growth restriction, starting at 28 wk
- Fetal movement counting starting at 28 wk
- Antepartum fetal surveillance (e.g., nonstress tests or biophysical profiles) starting at 32 wk or 1 to 2 wk earlier prior to gestational age of previous stillbirth if occurred prior to 32 wk
- Support and reassurance

Delivery
- Planned induction at 39 wk or before 39 wk if desired by the couple and lung maturity documented by amniocentesis

Source: Adapted from Horey D, Flenady V, Haezell AEP et al. *Cochrane Database System Rev*, 2, CD009932, 2013.

members is important. Staff interacting with the family should refer to the stillborn baby by name if one was given. Parents should be informed about the reasons for autopsy, procedures, and potential cost. **The most important components of the evaluation of a stillbirth are fetal autopsy; examination of the placenta, cord, and membranes; and karyotype analysis.** A complete evaluation [3] identifies a probable cause in >60% of fetal deaths [26] and should include the following:

1. Review all relevant **maternal, perinatal, family history, and risk factors** to help identify specific possibilities (Table 55.1). See specific guideline if a specific risk factor is identified as probable cause. In family history, particular attention should be paid to pregnancy losses, consanguinity, mental retardation, diabetes, congenital anomalies with a three-generation pedigree. **All records** should be reviewed for any possible association.

2. Before delivery, **detailed ultrasound**, fetal echocardiogram, 3-D ultrasound, and whole-body X-rays and/or MRI can be considered. These exams should be recommended especially if a detailed autopsy will not be available. Karyotypic analysis is not possible in 50% of cases because of cell culture failure. To increase the yield of

cell culture, an **amniocentesis** (and/or CVS) should be offered for karyotype [27] and fetal infection workup. Even if 5% to 10% of cells from amniotic fluid of fetal deaths fail to grow, this yield is much higher than that obtained from postnatal study of karyotype [28].

3. Before delivery, **obtain consent for fetal autopsy**. If consent is not given for a full autopsy, ask the parents to consider a limited autopsy, such as external examination by pathologist/clinical geneticist or internal examination limited to brain and/or spinal cord, chest organs, or abdominal organs as appropriate, or an MRI [29].

4. At delivery, **examine baby and placenta carefully.** General exam immediately after delivery should include noting any dysmorphology/congenital abnormalities as well as obtaining weight, length, and head circumference. Foot length may be especially useful for earlier stillbirths that may have a few weeks lag between death and delivery to pinpoint gestational age at death. Photographs of the entire body; frontal and profile views of the face, extremities, and palms; and close-up photographs of specific abnormalities should be obtained [3]. The placenta should be weighed and compared to the norms for gestational age. Clinical geneticist evaluation if available is often helpful.

5. Prior to autopsy, **karyotypic analyses should be performed on all stillbirths** after parental consent is obtained. Yield for abnormalities is higher if the following is present: fetus with growth restriction, anomalies, or hydrops or the parent is a balanced translocation carrier or has a mosaic karyotype [3]. The most viable tissue for **cytogenetic and molecular genetic studies** is usually the **placenta** (1 × 1 cm block) taken from below the cord insertion site on the unfixed placenta or umbilical cord closest to the placenta, followed by fetal cartilage obtained from the costochondral junction or patella [3,30]. **Placental tissue can be sent for karyotype to check for confined placental mosaicism.** Skin surface should be cleansed with betadine or hibiclens prior to obtaining specimen. Tissue should be placed in Hanks solution (pink) or normal saline if Hanks solution is not available, not in formalin. Cytogenetic form should be completed with pertinent details. Attempts at cell culture, however, fail in half of the cases. If culture is unsuccessful, **fluorescent in situ hybridization** to detect most common aneuploidies or **comparative genomic hybridization (cGH)**, which detects small deletions or duplications, and termed copy number changes not detectable by karyotype may be useful since both technologies do not require live cells [31]. Testing for rarer causes of stillbirth such as single gene disorders or mutations in Long QT genes should be guided by clinical suspicion or family history [32].

6. **Autopsy** is the **most useful** test in identifying the cause of fetal death. Not only are gross birth defects and morphologic abnormalities identified, but subtle findings of the autopsy may confirm infection, anemia, hypoxia, and metabolic abnormalities as the cause of death. Autopsy reduces the number of unexplained fetal deaths by at least 10% [33]. Autopsy findings altered counseling and recurrence risks autopsy in 26% of all cases at one institution [34]. The addition of autopsy to clinical and laboratory data and placental examination resulted in improved identification of probable cause of death to 74% in a cohort study at a tertiary care center [35]. Autopsy should

include X-rays of the fetus and photographs and follow College of American Pathologists guidelines (http://www .cap.org). Whole-body X-ray with anterior–posterior and lateral views may reveal an unrecognized skeletal abnormality or further define an already visible abnormality. Estimation of the interval between intrauterine death and delivery should be performed. Clinical information, all records including ultrasound reports regarding the case, and any specific requests, should be made available to the pathologist. **It is suggested for the obstetrician to call the pathology resident/attending assigned to autopsy for discussion.** A perinatal pathologist with experience in fetal death cases should perform the autopsy. Examination by a physician experienced in genetics and dysmorphology may increase the yield of autopsy. If autopsy is declined, it is important to consider a head-sparing autopsy or at least **MRI** of the stillborn child [36]. If a complete autopsy is not feasible, minimal invasive autopsy, which includes postnatal MRI, blood sampling from the dead fetus at autopsy, clinical history review, and external evaluation can be performed [37]. Ultrasound of the brain may also be considered for confirmation or refining the diagnosis of genetic syndromes and chromosomal abnormalities in addition to autopsy [38].

7. Send **placenta, membranes, and umbilical cord for gross and microscopic pathologic examination.** Conditions causing or contributing to stillbirth may be diagnosed, such as abruption, placental infarcts, umbilical cord thrombosis, velamentous cord insertion, and vasa previa. Placental evaluation can also yield important information regarding infection, genetic abnormalities, anemia, and thrombophilia. Umbilical cord knots and tangling should be noted but interpreted carefully as cord entanglement occurs in 30% of normal pregnancies [3,39]. Examination of the placenta vasculature and membranes is particularly useful in multifetal gestations by establishing chorionicity and vascular anastomoses.

8. If autopsy, placental pathology, or history is suggestive of an infectious etiology, maternal or neonatal serology, special tissue stains, and/or testing for bacterial or viral nucleic acids may be undertaken. If clinical or histologic evidence is lacking, then routine testing for infection is of questionable benefit.

9. Maternal labs [3] (Table 55.2):
   a. Kleihauer–Betke testing or flow cytometry are sent to evaluate for fetal–maternal hemorrhage (prior to delivery is optimal).
   b. Lupus anticoagulant, anticardiolipin antibodies (IgM, IgG), and anti-β_2-glycoprotein antibodies (IgM, IgG) can be sent to test for antiphospholipid syndrome. Presence of lupus anticoagulant or anticardiolipin antibodies of moderate to high titer (>40 immunoglobulin M (IgM) binding/immunoglobulin G (IgG) binding or >99th percentile) or anti-β_2-glycoprotein antibody titer (>99th percentile) are all considered positive but should be confirmed with repeat testing 12 weeks later [40] (see also Chapter 26).
   c. Parvovirus B19 titers (IgM and IgG) can be considered, especially in cases in which there is suspicion for this infection, such as those with fetal hydrops or fetal anemia [41]. CMV, toxoplasmosis, and other viruses and/or bacteria are not suggested for workup, unless clinical history or other factors (pathology findings) point to these infections.

   d. Syphilis testing can be sent with RPR or VDRL.
   e. Glucose screening (oral glucose tolerance test, hemoglobin A1c) (if glucose screening not done in pregnancy).
   f. Thrombophilia workup should be sent only in cases of severe placental pathology, fetal growth restriction, or in the setting of a personal history or history in a first-degree relative (e.g., parent or sibling) of thrombosis (factor V Leiden mutation; G20210A prothrombin gene mutation; deficiencies of antithrombin III, protein C, protein S) (see Chapter 27). Routine testing is controversial and may lead to unnecessary interventions [3].

10. Consider any other workup, depending on risk factor identified in Table 55.1. For fetal demise before 20 weeks, consider individualized workup and refer to chapter on pregnancy loss (Chapter 15 in *Obstetric Evidence Based Guidelines*).

DELIVERY/ANESTHESIA

Once diagnosis is confirmed and counseling and workup initiated, options for delivery should be discussed. **Options include expectant management, induction, or dilation and evacuation (D&E).**

Expectant Management

Between 80% and 90% of women with fetal death will spontaneously enter labor within two weeks of fetal demise [42]. Duration of labor is shorter in patients with spontaneous labor [43]. However, **endomyometritis** rate is higher in the spontaneous labor group (6% vs. 1%) compared to induction. There is no difference in the frequency of postpartum hemorrhage, retained placenta, or need for blood transfusion. Retention of a dead fetus can cause chronic consumptive coagulopathy because of gradual release of thromboplastin from the placenta into the maternal circulation [30]. This usually occurs after four weeks but may occur earlier. **Coagulation abnormalities** occur in about 3% to 4% of patients with uncomplicated fetal deaths over the next four to eight weeks, and this number rises in the presence of abruption or uterine perforation [30]. Another disadvantage of expectant management is a long interval between fetal death and spontaneous labor, limiting the amount of information that can be obtained about the cause of death from a postmortem examination or autopsy of the baby. Moreover, women with fetal death find it **difficult psychologically** to continue a pregnancy with a known fetal death [44]. In patients opting for spontaneous labor (especially **with greater than four-week interval between fetal death and time of delivery**), a **screen for coagulopathy** (fibrinogen level, platelet count, prothrombin time, and activated partial thromboplastin measurement) should be obtained prior to administration of neuraxial anesthesia as well as other invasive procedures [30].

Dilation and Evacuation

Comparing complication rates of patients who undergo D&E or medical induction **between 14 and 24 weeks of gestation,** D&E is a **safe** method in this time frame, especially **if done by experienced operators under continuous ultrasound guidance** [45]. Surgical termination of pregnancy between 14 and 24 weeks of gestation has a lower overall rate of complications (4%) as compared to 29% in women undergoing labor induction [45]. Patients undergoing D&E are less likely to have failure of the initial method for delivery and retained products of conception. However, both groups are similar in the need for blood transfusion, infection, cervical laceration, maternal organ damage, or hospital readmission. Placement of **laminaria** is associated with a lower risk of complications from D&E, and **misoprostol** is associated with a lower complication rate in women undergoing medical termination [45]. A *Cochrane* review [46] concluded that D&E is superior to instillation of prostaglandin F2a and may be favored over mifepristone and misoprostol although larger randomized studies are needed. Using decision analysis, a cost-effectiveness analysis concluded that D&E is less expensive and more effective than misoprostol induction of labor for second-trimester pregnancy termination [47]. Studies do not show an increased rate of complications in subsequent pregnancies after D&E although data are limited [48,49]. Both methods for delivery are considered reasonably safe. Thus, **mode of delivery should usually be based on the patient's wishes.** However, patients should be counseled that **efficacy of autopsy is very limited with D&E** [3]. In addition, **the availability of D&E may be limited by provider experience or gestational age.**

Induction

Induction of labor in women with fetal death is **usually recommended** unless the patient is already in labor given the problems mentioned with expectant management. Induction of labor is typically **initiated soon after diagnosis of fetal death**. Most of the data for management of fetal death is from randomized trials of second-trimester pregnancy termination.

Up to 28 Weeks
Options for induction of labor for fetal death at about 16 to 28 weeks include misoprostol (prostaglandin E1, PGE1), prostaglandins E2 (PGE2), high-dose oxytocin, and hypertonic saline. **Misoprostol (preferred) and high-dose oxytocin are the two modalities with the best safety and effectiveness evidence.**

Available evidence from randomized trials do support the use of **vaginal misoprostol** as a medical treatment to terminate nonviable pregnancies before 24 weeks of gestation [50,51]. On the basis of the limited data, the use of misoprostol between 24 to 28 weeks of gestation also appears to be safe and effective [50]. **Therefore, for gestations less than 28 weeks, misoprostol is the most efficient method of induction** regardless of Bishop score although high-dose oxytocin infusion is an acceptable alternative [3]. Typical dosages for misoprostol use are 200 to 400 mcg vaginally, orally, or 200 mcg buccal every 4 to 12 hours [3]. Examples of regimens for misoprostol dosing are **200 mcg vaginally every 4 hours, 400 mcg orally every 4 hours, 200 mcg buccal, or 600 mcg vaginally every 12 hours. These result in successful expulsion (mostly within 24 hours) in 80% to 100% of cases** [3,52–54]. **Misoprostol 400 mcg given orally every 4 hours is more effective than misoprostol 200 mcg given vaginally every 12 hours for the induction of second- and third-trimester pregnancy with intrauterine fetal death within 24 hours** but is associated with more gastrointestinal side effects [52,55]. Misoprostol 600 mcg administered vaginally at 12-hour intervals is associated with fewer adverse effects and is as effective as dosing at 6-hour intervals [53].

High-dose oxytocin (200 units in 500 mL saline at 50 mL/hour) also may be used for induction of labor remote from term [56]. **The mother should be observed for signs of water intoxication, and maternal electrolyte concentrations should be monitored at least every 24 hours.** Nausea and malaise are the earliest findings of hyponatremia and may be seen when the plasma sodium concentration falls below 125 to 130 mEq/L. This may be followed by headache, lethargy, obtundation, and eventually seizures, coma, and respiratory arrest. Misoprostol 50 µg with dose doubled every 6 hours until effective contractions is associated with a success rate within 48 hours of induction of 100% compared to 96.7% to oxytocin infusion titrated on the basis of patient response with **mean induction to delivery time significantly longer (almost double) in the oxytocin group compared with the misoprostol group (23.3 vs. 12.4 hours). Misoprostol is also cheaper (1/10th the price of oxytocin)** [57].

Historically, **PGE2 suppositories** with a dose of 20 mg inserted vaginally every four hours were also utilized for labor induction before 28 weeks. Pretreatment with acetaminophen, compazine, and diphenoxylate is useful to minimize fever, nausea, vomiting, and diarrhea, which invariably occur. The PGE2 dose should be reduced to 5 to 10 mg if used at a more advanced gestation (off-label use) as uterine sensitivity and the risk of uterine rupture increase with gestational age [58]. High-dose PGE2 suppositories are contraindicated >28 weeks gestation [59]. Misoprostol is more efficacious and at least as safe and cheaper than PGE2, and so the use of PGE2 for induction of fetal death before 28 weeks is not recommended and of mostly historic importance only.

The efficacy and tolerance of **mifepristone** (RU 486), a progesterone antagonist, was investigated in a double-blind controlled multicenter study involving 94 patients with an intrauterine fetal death [60]. Success of treatment was defined as the occurrence of fetal expulsion within 72 hours after the first drug intake. Mifepristone treatment (600 mg/day for two days) was considered to be effective in 29 of 46 patients (63%). There were only eight successes in 48 patients (17.4%) in the placebo group (*p* = .001). Tolerance was good in the mifepristone group. In the placebo group, disseminated intravascular coagulation occurred in one woman for whom the investigator waited several weeks for spontaneous expulsion. Another RCT compared high-concentration oxytocin to misoprostol given 36 hours after initial mifepristone 200 mg in second trimester abortion for either IUFD or voluntary termination. The mifepristone–oxytocin regimen had longer time until expulsion but fewer side effects [61]. Mifepristone is of interest in the management of intrauterine fetal death **with more studies needed to compare the above methods, in particular misoprostol with mifepristone.**

To date, there are no studies evaluating **laminaria** for ripening of the cervix in conjunction with other methods of induction for cases of fetal death.

After 28 Weeks
After 28 weeks of gestation, **drugs such as oxytocin and/or prostaglandins administered for induction of labor can be given according to standard obstetric protocols** [3] (see Chapter 21 in *Obstetric Evidence Based Guidelines*). Cesarean delivery for stillbirth is reserved for unusual circumstances (maternal indications) because it is associated with maternal morbidity without fetal benefit [3].

Women with Prior Uterine Scar
Women with a **prior uterine scar** represent a special group and treatment should be individualized. **For women with**

a previous low transverse incision and a uterus less than 28 weeks size, the usual protocols for misoprostol induction at less than 28 weeks may be used [3,50]. Several studies have evaluated the use of misoprostol at a dosage of 400 mcg every six hours in women with a stillbirth up to 28 weeks of gestation and a prior uterine scar [62,63]. There does not appear to be an increase in complications in those women. The risk of uterine rupture is about 0.4% with one prior low transverse CD, up to 9% with ≥2 prior CD, and up to 50% with prior vertical CD [64]. Further research is required to assess effectiveness and safety, optimal route of administration, and dose [50].

For women with a previous low transverse incision, after 28 weeks of gestation, oxytocin protocols may be utilized and cervical ripening with Foley bulb may be considered [3,50]. Patients may elect for a repeat CD in the setting of a stillbirth, but the risks and benefits should be discussed with the patient. Ideally, a cesarean should be avoided. Therefore, on the basis of limited data in patients with a prior low transverse CD, trial of labor remains a favorable option [3,50]. There are limited data for patients with a prior classical uterine incision or prior myomectomy; therefore, the delivery plan should be individualized [3,50].

POSTPARTUM

Prior to discharge, the family needs to be counseled that results of all investigations may take two or three months for completion and that despite extensive evaluation a cause of death may not be found. Patients should be offered the **opportunity to see and hold their infant and be offered keepsake items such as photos, hand/footprints, or special blankets or clothing. Grief counseling** should be initiated prior to discharge from hospital. Referral to a bereavement counselor, religious leader, peer support group, or mental health professional is advisable for management of grief and depression.

Fetal death causes "very much" grief also in the majority of obstetricians, who can experience self-doubt, depression, and self-blame in relation to their patient's loss [65].

PREVENTION OF RECURRENCE AND MANAGEMENT IN A FUTURE PREGNANCY

A **special outpatient visit** should be set up to review the results of the complete workup and discuss possible etiology and future management (Table 55.3). If a particular medical problem is identified in the mother, it should be addressed prior to next conception (see specific guidelines). For example, tight control of blood glucose prior to conception can substantially reduce the risk of congenital anomalies in the fetus. Preconception counseling is helpful if congenital anomalies or genetic abnormalities are found. In the future, comparative genomic hybridization, FISH, and other novel genetic techniques will provide better ways to workup the myriad genetic causes of fetal death. A woman with a prior fetal loss and either factor V or prothrombin heterozygocity or protein S deficiency might benefit from enoxaparin 40 mg SQ daily starting at eight weeks [53]. Compared with low-dose aspirin, in women who had had a previous fetal loss after the 10th week and had a thrombophilic defect (heterozygous factor V Leiden, prothrombin G20210, or protein S deficiency), enoxaparin 40 mg daily treatment is associated with a tenfold increased live birth rate as compared with low-dose aspirin in only one trial [66]. In some cases, such as cord occlusion,

the patient can be assured that recurrence is unlikely [39,67]. Overall, there is an increased incidence of pregnancy complications, such as stillbirth (2.5- to 10-fold increase depending on the study) [17,68], preterm birth (OR 2.8, 95% CI 1.9–4.2), preeclampsia (OR 3.1, 95% CI 1.7–5.7), and placental abruption (OR 9.4, 95% CI 4.5–19.7) [80] in subsequent pregnancies [69]. Most patients find increased fetal surveillance with the next pregnancy reassuring. **Fetal growth ultrasounds and kick counts starting at 28 weeks and antepartum surveillance starting at 32 weeks may be implemented** [3]. In a woman with a prior IUFD, planned induction can be discussed with the patient in terms of risks and benefits [3]. If any of the surveillance demonstrates no maternal or fetal issues complicating the pregnancy, consideration for 38 0/7–39 6/7 week induction should be considered [70].

REFERENCES

1. MacDorman MF, Kirmeyer S. Fetal and perinatal mortality, United States, 2005. *Natl Vital Stat Rep* 2009; 57: 1–19. [II-2]
2. National Center for Health Statistics. Model state vital statistics act and regulations. 1992 revision. Hyattsville (MD): NCHS; 1994. Available at http://www.cdc.gov/nchs/data/misc/mvsact92b.pdf. Retrieved January 16, 2011. [Level III]
3. ACOG. Management of stillbirth. ACOG Practice Bulletin No. 102. *Obstet Gynecol* 2009; 113(3): 748–61. [Level III]
4. www.who.int/reproductive health/topics/maternal_perinatal/stillbirth. Accessed August 29, 2015. [II-2]
5. Lawn JE, Blencowe H, Pattison R et al. Stillbirths: Where? when? why? how to make the data count? *Lancet* 2011; 377(9775): 1448–63. [II-2]
6. McDorman MF, Gregory ECW. Fetal and Perinatal Mortality: United States, 2013. *National Vital Statistics Reports* 2015; 64(8). [II-2]
7. Dudley DJ, Goldenberg R, Conway D et al. Stillbirth Research Collaborative Network. A new system for determining the causes of stillbirth. *Obstet Gynecol* 2010; 116(2 Pt. 1): 254–60. [Level III]
8. Reddy UM, Ko CW, Willinger M. Maternal age and the risk of stillbirth throughout pregnancy in the United States. *Am J Obstet Gynecol* 2006; 195: 764–70. [II-2]
9. Sharma PP, Salihu HM, Oyelese Y et al. Is race a determinant of stillbirth recurrence? *Obstet Gynecol* 2006; 107: 391–7. [II-2]
10. Vintzileos AM, Ananth CV, Smulian et al. Prenatal care black–white fetal death disparity in the United States: Heterogeneity by high-risk conditions. *Obstet Gynecol* 2002; 99(3): 483–9. [II-3]
11. Arias E, Anderson RN, Kung HC et al. Deaths: Final data for 2001. *National Vital Statistics Reports*; 52(3). Hyattsville, MD: National Center for Health Statistics. 2003. [Data review]
12. Froen JF, Arnestad M, Frey K et al. Risk factors for sudden intrauterine unexplained death: Epidemiologic characteristics of singleton cases in Oslo, Norway, 1986–1995. *Am J Obstet Gynecol* 2001; 184: 694–702. [II-2]
13. Oron T, Sheiner E, Shoham-Vardi I et al. Risk factors for antepartum fetal death. *J Reprod Med* 2001; 46(9): 825–30. [II-2]
14. Nohr EA, Bech BH, Davies MJ et al. Prepregnancy obesity and fetal death: A study within the Danish National Birth Cohort. *Obstet Gynecol* 2005; 106: 250–9. [II-2]
15. Raymond EG, Cnattingius S, Kiely JL. Effects of maternal age, parity, and smoking on the risk of stillbirth. *BJOG* 1994; 101: 301–6. [II-2]
16. Wisborg K, Ingerslev HJ, Henriksen TB. IVF and stillbirth: A prospective follow-up study. *Hum Reprod* 2010; 25: 1312–6. [II-2]
17. Surkan PJ, Stephansson O, Dickman PW et al. Previous preterm and small-for-gestational-age births and the subsequent risk of stillbirth. *N Engl J Med* 2004; 350: 777–85. [II-2]
18. Gardosi J, Kady SM, McGeown P et al. Classification of stillbirth by relevant condition at death (ReCoDe): Population based cohort study. *BMJ* 2005; 331: 1113–7. [II-2]

19. Signorello LB, Mulvihill JJ, Green DM et al. Stillbirth and neonatal death in relation to radiation exposure before conception: A retrospective cohort study. *Lancet* 2010 376(9741): 624–30. doi:10.1016/S0140-6736(10)60752-0. [II-2]

20. Mullan Z, Horton R. Bringing stillbirth out of the shadow. *Lancet* 2011; 377: 1291–2. [III]

21. Bhutta ZA, Yakoob MY, Lawn JE et al. Stillbirths: What difference can we make and at what cost? *Lancet* 2011; 377: 1523–38. [II-2]

22. Gaskins AJ, Rich-Edwards JW, Hauser R et al. maternal Prepregnancy folate intake and risk of spontaneous abortion and stillbirth. *Obstet Gynecol* 2014; 124: 23–31. [II-2]

23. Horey D, Flenady V, Haezell AEP et al. Interventions for supporting parents' decision about autopsy after stillbirth (Review). *Cochrane Database System Rev* 2013; 2: CD009932. doi:10.1002/14651858.CD009932.pub2. [Review]

24. Reddy UM. Prediction and prevention of recurrent stillbirth. *Obstet Gynecol* 2007; 110: 1151–64. [Review]

25. Silver RM, Varner MW, Reddy U et al. Work-up of stillbirth: A review of the evidence. *Am J Obstet Gynecol* 2007; 196(5): 433–44. [Review]

26. The Stillbirth Collaborative Research Network Writing Group. Causes of death among stillbirths. *JAMA* 2011; 306: 2459–68. [II-1]

27. Korteweg FJ, Bouman K, Erwich JJ et al. Cytogenetic analysis after evaluation of 750 fetal deaths: Proposal for diagnostic workup. *Obstet Gynecol* 2008; 111(4): 865–74. [II-2]

28. Khare M, Howarth E, Sandler J et al. A comparison of prenatal versus postnatal karyotyping for the investigation of intrauterine fetal death after the first trimester of pregnancy. *Prenat Diagn* 2005; 25: 1192–5. [II-2]

29. Woodward PJ, Sohaey R, Harris DP et al. Postmortem fetal MR imaging: Comparison with findings at autopsy. *AJR Am J Roentgenol* 1997; 168(1): 41–6. [II-2]

30. Maslow AD, Breen TW, Sarna MC et al. Prevalence of coagulation abnormalities associated with intrauterine fetal death. *Can J Anaesth* 1996; 43(12): 1237–43. [II-3]

31. Reddy UM, Goldenberg R, Silver R et al. Stillbirth classification—Developing an international consensus for research: Executive summary of a National Institute of Child Health and Human Development workshop. *Obstet Gynecol* 2009; 114(4): 901–14. [III]

32. Crotti L, Tester DJ, White WM et al. Long QT syndrome-associated mutations in intrauterine fetal death. *JAMA* 2013; 309(14). doi:10.1001.jama.2013.3219. [II-3]

33. ACOG. Evaluation of stillbirths and neonatal deaths. ACOG Committee Opinion No. 383. *Obstet Gynecol* 2007; 110(4): 963–6. [III]

34. Faye-Petersen OM, Guinn DA, Wenstrom KD. Value of perinatal autopsy. *Obstet Gynecol* 1999; 94(6): 915–20. [II-3]

35. Miller ES, Minturn L, Linn R, Weese-Mayer DE, Ernst LM. Stillbirth evaluation: A stepwise assessment of placental pathology and autopsy. *Am J Obstet Gynecol* 2015; doi:10.1016/j.ajog.2015.08.049. [II-3]

36. Thayyil S, Cleary JO, Sebire NJ et al. Post-mortem examination of human fetuses: A comparison of whole body high-field MRI at 9.4 T with conventional MRI and invasive autopsy. *Lancet* 2009; 374: 467–75. [II-2]

37. Thayyil S, Sebire NJ, Chitty LS et al. Post-mortem MRI versus conventional autopsy in fetuses and children: A prospective validation study. *Lancet* 2013; 382: 223–33. [II-2]

38. Cain MA, Guidi CB, Steffensen T et al. Postmortem ultrasonography of the macerated fetus complements Autopsy following in utero fetal demise. *Ped Dev Path* 2014; 17: 217–20. [II-3]

39. Carey JC, Rayburn WF. Nuchal cord encirclements and risk of stillbirth. *Int J Gynaecol Obstet* 2000; 69(2): 173–4. [II-2]

40. ACOG. Antiphospholipid syndrome. ACOG Practice Bulletin No. 118. *Obstet Gynecol* 2011; 117(1): 192–9. [III]

41. Sarfraz AA, Samuelsen SO, Bruu AL et al. Maternal human parvovirus B19 infection and the risk of fetal death and low birthweight: A case-control study with 35,940 pregnant women. *BJOG* 2009; 116: 1492–8. [II-2, plus commentary]

42. Goldstein DP, Reid DE. Circulating fibrinolytic activity—A precursor of hypofibrinogenemia following fetal death in utero. *Obstet Gynecol* 1963; 22: 174–80. [III]

43. Salamat SM, Landy HJ, O'Sullivan MJ. Labor induction after fetal death. A retrospective analysis. *J Reprod Med* 2002; 47(1): 23–6. [II-2]

44. Erlandsson K, Lindgren H, Malm MC et al. Mother's experiences of the time after the diagnosis of an intrauterine death until the induction of the delivery: A qualitative Internet-based study. *J Obstet Gynacol Res* 2011; 37(11): 1677–84. [II-3]

45. Autry AM, Hayes EC, Jacobson GF et al. A comparison of medical induction and dilation and evacuation for second-trimester abortion. *Am J Obstet Gynecol* 2002; 187(2): 393–7. [RCT; n = 297]

46. Lohr PA, Hayes JL, Gemzell-Danielsson K. Surgical versus medical methods for second trimester induced abortion. *Cochrane Database Syst Rev* 2008; 1: CD006714. [Meta-analysis]

47. Cowett AA, Golub RM, Grobman WA. Cost-effectiveness of dilation and evacuation versus the induction of labor for second trimester pregnancy termination. *Am J Obstet Gynecol* 2006; 194: 768–73. [II-3]

48. Jackson JE, Grobman WA, Haney E et al. Mid-trimester dilation and evacuation with laminaria does not increase the risk for severe subsequent pregnancy complications. *Int J Gynaecol Obstet* 2007; 96: 12–5. [II-2]

49. Schneider D, Halperin R, Langer R et al. Abortion at 18–22 weeks by laminaria dilation and evacuation. *Obstet Gynecol* 1996; 88: 412–4. [II-2]

50. ACOG. Induction of labor. ACOG Practice Bulletin No. 107. *Obstet Gynecol* 2009; 114(2 Pt. 1): 386–97. [Review, III]

51. Neilson JP, Hickey M, Vazquez J. Medical treatment for early fetal death (less than 24 weeks). *Cochrane Database Syst Rev* 2006; 3: CD002253. [Review, III]

52. Bugalho A, Bique C, Machungo F et al. Vaginal misoprostol as an alternative to oxytocin for induction of labor in women with late fetal death. *Acta Obstet Gynecol Scand* 1995; 74: 194. [II-2]

53. Herabutya Y, Chanrachakul B, Punyavachira P. A randomized controlled trial of 6 and 12 hourly administration of vaginal misoprostol for second trimester pregnancy termination. *BJOG* 2005; 112(9): 1297–301. [RCT, n = 279, I]

54. Bracken H, Ngoc NTN, Banks E et al. Buccal misoprostol for treatment of fetal death at 14–28 weeks of pregnancy: A double-blind randomized controlled trial. *Contraception* 2014; 89: 187–92. [1, RCT, n = 153]

55. Ponce de Leon RG, Wing D. Misoprostol for termination of pregnancy in intrauterine fetal demise in the second and third trimester of pregnancy–a systematic review. *Contraception* 2000; 79: 259–71. [Review]

56. Toaff R, Ayalon D, Gogol G. Clinical use of high concentration drip. *Obstet Gynecol* 1971; 37: 112. [II-3]

57. Nakintu N. A comparative study of vaginal misoprostol and intravenous oxytocin for induction of labour in women with intra uterine fetal death in Mulago Hospital, Uganda. *Afr Health Sci* 2001; 1(2): 55–9. [RCT, n = 120, I]

58. Kent DR, Goldstein AI, Linzey EM. Safety and efficacy of vaginal prostaglandin E2 suppositories in the management of third-trimester fetal demise. *J Reprod Med* 1984; 29: 101. [II-2]

59. PROSTIN E2® Vaginal Suppository package insert. [III]

60. Cabrol D, Dubois C, Cronje H et al. Induction of labor with mifepristone (RU 486) in intrauterine fetal death. *Am J Obstet Gynecol* 1990; 163(2): 540–2. [II-2]

61. Elami-Suzin M, Freeman MD, Porat N et al. Mifepristone followed by misoprostol or oxytocin for second trimester abortion. A randomized trial. *Obstet Gynecol* 2013; 122: 815–20. [RCT, n = 145]

62. Dickinson JE. Misoprostol for second-trimester pregnancy termination in women with a prior cesarean delivery. *Obstet Gynecol* 2005; 105: 352–6. [Level II-2]

63. Daskalakis GJ, Mesogitis SA, Papantoniou NE et al. Misoprostol for second trimester pregnancy termination in women with prior caesarean section. *BJOG* 2005; 112: 97–9. [II-2]

64. Berghella V, Airoldi J, O'Neill AM et al. Misoprostol for second trimester pregnancy termination in women with prior caesarean: A systematic review. *BJOG* 2009; 116(9): 1151–7. [II-2]

65. Farrow VA, Goldenberg RL, Fretts R et al. Psychological impact of still births on obstetricians. *JMFNM* 2013; 26: 748–52. [II-2]

66. Gris JC, Mercier E, Quere I et al. Low-molecular-weight heparin versus low-dose aspirin in women with one fetal loss and a constitutional thrombophilic disorder. *Blood* 2004; 103(10): 3695–9. [RCT, *n* = 160]

67. Verdel MJ, Exalto N. Tight nuchal coiling of the umbilical cord causing fetal death. *J Clin Ultrasound* 1994; 22(1): 64–6. [II-2]

68. Samueloff A, Xenakis EM, Berkus MD et al. Recurrent stillbirth. Significance and characteristics. *J Reprod Med* 1993; 38(11): 883–6. [II-3]

69. Black M, Shetty A, Bhattacharya S. Obstetric outcomes subsequent to intrauterine death in the first pregnancy. *BJOG* 2008; 115(2): 269–74. [II-2]

70. Medically indicated late-preterm and early-term deliveries. Committee Opinion No. 560. American College of Obstetricians and Gynecologists. *Obstet Gynecol* 2013; 121: 908–10. [Guideline; III]

56

Antepartum testing

Nora Graham and Christopher R. Harman

KEY POINTS

- **There are no randomized trial data proving that antepartum testing reduces long-term neurologic deficits.**
- Although entrenched in high-risk pregnancy management, most antenatal testing schemes are not supported by high-level evidence. Recommendations regarding which pregnancies to test and at what gestational age testing should start cannot be made given lack of sufficient evidence.
- Multiple parameter testing schemes have better correlation with fetal condition than do single-parameter tests.
- Antenatal NST results appear to have no significant effect on perinatal mortality (PNM) or potentially preventable deaths. The NST used alone is not adequate to exclude several important sources of perinatal injury. **Computerized cardiotocography** may have benefit over standard NST in high-risk cases.
- Biophysical profile score (BPS) surveillance may be beneficial in reducing cerebral palsy with insufficient trial evidence. **Compared to other fetal testing (usually NST), biophysical profile increases the incidence of induction and cesarean delivery but not admission to ICN or perinatal mortality.** Individual components have been compared in some trials, but the value of that evidence is limited.
- **Umbilical artery (UA) Doppler decreases perinatal mortality in antenatal management of fetal growth restriction (FGR) fetuses** and should be routinely used in these pregnancies but not in normal pregnancies. Compared to no Doppler ultrasound, UA Doppler ultrasound in high-risk pregnancy (especially those complicated by hypertension or presumed FGR) is associated with a reduction in perinatal deaths with fewer inductions of labor and fewer admissions to the hospital.
- There are few studies comparing Doppler versus BPS. There are no management trials. BPS may correlate better with perinatal results, but this has not been shown to improve long-term neurologic outcomes. The combination of Doppler and BPS may improve perinatal mortality in severe IUGR, with limited evidence.
- Ancillary tests, such as contraction stress test, oxytocin challenge test, and vibroacoustic stimulation, may have specific uses but limited applicability.
- Formal maternal counting of fetal movement has been associated with differing results in trials and has insufficient data to prove ability in preventing fetal death.
- Testing frequency and complexity should be adjusted to reflect the stability of the clinical situation.

BACKGROUND

The main motive underlying antepartum fetal assessment is to prevent stillbirth. Prevention of neurologic handicap, such as cerebral palsy, is another aim. **Preventing these outcomes by prompt intervention for proven fetal compromise is balanced by avoiding impacts of unnecessary intervention for both fetus (iatrogenic prematurity) and mother (surgical complications).** Extending the pregnancy to reduce prematurity may increase the risk of unexpected stillbirth but has measurable benefits in reduced long-term neurologic outcomes. Optimizing testing regimens means choosing methods, frequency, and disease-specific components while accounting for gestational-age influences, drug interactions, test variability, and even the interaction of test components. **If we want to choose the test that is best at reducing stillbirth, there is some limited high-level evidence to inform us.**

PRINCIPLES OF FETAL MONITORING

The ideal antenatal fetal testing regimen should do the following:

- Identify impending fetal injury with near-perfect sensitivity with warning advanced enough to allow effective intervention.
- Distinguish normal variation, benign abnormality, and degrees of significant abnormality, facilitating graded response.
- Identify normal fetal condition with near-perfect predictive value, reliably excluding stillbirth or injury for a clinically relevant interval.
- Exclude grievous fetal abnormality as the source of abnormal testing.
- Be applicable to a variety of common sources of fetal compromise, practicable in common prenatal settings, and reproducible between situations.
- Produce measurable benefits in reduction of perinatal death and long-term neurologic handicap.

FETAL-MONITORING METHODS
Fetal Movement Counting in Low-Risk Pregnancy

The largest randomized trial of maternal monitoring of fetal movement [1] failed to show any benefit over "informal inquiry about movement during standard antenatal care." This trial produced a noticeable effect on control subjects, whose experience in the trial led to improved perinatal performance compared to nontrial participants in the general population. It did not produce a benefit in treated patients with the same perinatal mortality in both study and control patients. Many women do report reduced fetal activity prior to stillbirth, so why did this trial demonstrate no effect? First, decreased movement was not reported promptly by many subjects. Second, the "rescue" method was simple cardiotocography, where false reassurance of a normal heart rate preceded a large proportion of fetal deaths. It may be that maternal awareness of fetal activity can be a useful adjunct in monitoring low-risk situations if reporting is immediate and if the rescue method is full BPS or even more complex assessment. While three additional small studies of movement counting provide some information, there are no apparent benefits in reduced adverse outcomes [2]. **The "count to 10" method (count to 10 movements then resume normal activity)** versus counting for a specified length of time (e.g., 30 minutes of counting every six to eight hours) **was associated with better patient compliance** [3]. Overall, data do not support reliance on fetal movement counting between episodes of formal fetal assessment in high-risk pregnancy [3].

Fetal Heart Rate Testing (Nonstress Test, NST, or Cardiotocography, CTG)

In this chapter, **we use nonstress test (NST, more used in the United States) and cardiotocography (CTG, more used everywhere else in the world) interchangeably.** The NST (or CTG) is defined as "reactive" when there **are two or more accelerations of at least 15 beats per minute (bpm) above the baseline that last for at least 15 seconds in a 20-minute period** of combined fetal heart rate (FHR) and uterine activity

monitoring (Figure 56.1). A CTG (or NST) without these characteristics is called "nonreactive." These criteria should only be used for fetuses ≥32 weeks.

Up to 50% of NSTs from 24–28 weeks and 15% of NSTs 28–32 weeks are nonreactive. Therefore, criteria were adapted to premature fetuses <32 weeks, assigning reactivity to accelerations of at least 10 bpm for at least 10 seconds [4–7]. These criteria based on accelerations have not been associated with any change in outcomes [8,9], so a fetus <32 weeks should not be delivered for a nonreactive NST but only for bradycardia or other similar nonreassuring fetal heart tracings. These criteria for interpretation <32 weeks have been endorsed in national guidelines [4,10–12].

In fetuses ≥32 weeks, the concordance between fetal movement and accelerations in FHR is good evidence of fetal well-being with a **negative predictive value against fetal demise within seven days of 99.5% to 99.8%** [13]. However, in specific circumstances, such as FGR with abnormal placental resistance, the NST may give a false-positive reassurance against acidosis as high as 15% [14]. Missed anomalies and missed oligohydramnios are major contributors to fetal complications in patients with reactive tracings when NST is used in isolation.

In practical monitoring terms, the false-alarming nonreactive NST is more problematic, occurring in up to 10% of

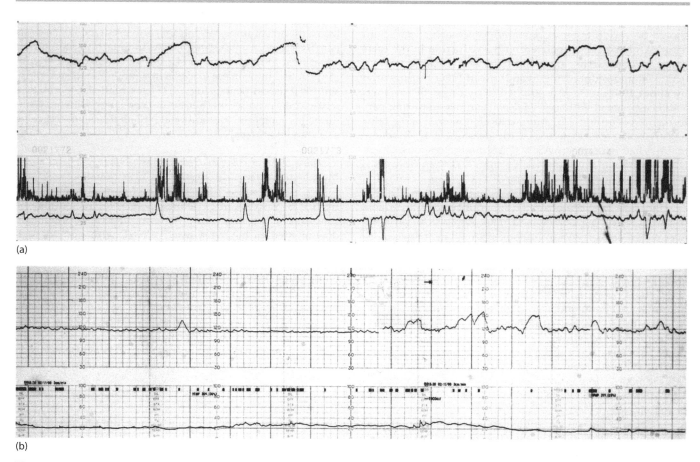

(a)

(b)

Figure 56.1 FHR monitoring. (a) A reactive nonstress test (NST) demonstrates multiple FHR accelerations associated with fetal movements. This external tracing, obtained at 37 weeks gestation, is highly reassuring of fetal health, the absence of hypoxemia, and the presence of a normal umbilical arterial pH. (b) Cyclic fetal behavior demonstrated by FHR tracing. For the first nine minutes, the fetus was virtually inactive with a nonreactive segment. When fetal movements resumed, an increase in variability and repetitive accelerations demonstrates conversion to active sleep (a "state change" from 1F on the left to 2F on the right).

tests at term [6] and up to 50% of the time at 24 to 28 weeks gestational age. Variable decelerations that are less than 30 seconds and nonrepetitive denote an "equivocal" NST and are not associated with fetal compromise [15]. Repetitive variable decelerations are associated with increased cesarean delivery [16] while decelerations lasting longer than one minute are associated with increased risk of cesarean delivery but also fetal demise [17–19]. When the subsequent confirmatory test (BPS, contraction stress test [CST], vibroacoustic stimulation [VAS], as examples) is performed after a nonreactive NST, up to 85% will be normal. If performed, the NST should be done in the **semi-Fowler ("sitting") position**—this decreases the need for prolonged monitoring compared to the supine position [20,21].

Modified CTG recording methods utilize **fetal stimulation to shorten the time to reach reactivity** to convert nonreactive FHR tracings to reactivity as a confirmatory test for nonreactive NST and in highest risk populations as a more precise test of fetal well being.

A type of stimulation is **VAS** [22]. The fetus is stimulated by external high-amplitude white noise applied to the maternal abdomen. This is capable of causing state change in most fetuses at term [23]. Occasional side effects include conversion to fixed fetal arrhythmia and serious concerns about delivery of high-pressure sound (up to 130 decibels) and effects on fetal hearing [23]. Since premature fetuses typically require more sound pressure to elicit responses and are more susceptible to hearing injury, use of VAS before 32 weeks should be very cautious. Compared to no such stimulation, fetal **VAS has been associated with a reduction in the incidence of nonreactive antenatal CTG test** (RR 0.62, 95% CI 0.52–0.74) and **reduced the overall mean CTG testing time by about 10 minutes** [24]. Applied to modified BPS testing, VAS is associated with a 67% false alarm rate requiring performance of full BPS [25]. More critical, however, is the false negative rate: 55% of fetuses with subsequent FHR abnormalities had reassuring VAS-NST [26]. Sound responsiveness is reduced in many high-risk groups (less than 32 weeks, hypertension, depression, severe IUGR, cocaine exposure, treatment with magnesium sulfate or antenatal steroids) [23]. Specific trials have demonstrated superiority of multivariable testing, including Doppler, NST, and biophysical variables over either CST or VAS in prolonged pregnancy and IUGR. Both trials concluded CST and VAS could be eliminated from fetal testing regimens [27,28]. The proven effect of VAS to provoke fetal neurologic state change seems outweighed by its ability to generate false reassurance. Routine application in high-risk fetal populations is not recommended.

Compared to no administration, **antenatal maternal glucose administration** (20–50 mg orally, e.g., as orange juice) **does not decrease the incidence of nonreactive antenatal CTG tests** regardless of prior fasting or nonfasting [29]. Compared to controls, neither orange juice nor chocolate decrease the incidence of nonreactive antenatal CTG tests [30].

Compared to no manipulation or to VAS, **manual fetal manipulation does not decrease the incidence of nonreactive antenatal CTG test** [31].

Shining a bright halogen light on the mother's abdomen shortens the time to first acceleration on NST [32].

Strong evidence, including randomized trial data, suggests that the NST should in general not be used as a solitary method of monitoring high-risk fetuses [33–36]. In a meta-analysis of randomized trials, compared to no NST or

concealment of information, **knowledge of antenatal NST results appears to have no significant effect on perinatal mortality (PNM) or potentially preventable deaths** with a worrying trend toward harm (RR 2.46, 95% CI 0.96–6.30). There is no significant impact on cesarean section rate or on the occurrence of various secondary outcomes [35].

Computerized interpretation of FHR monitoring has evolved as a more specific, objective means of maximizing the information obtained from the NST [37]. Computerized CTG (CCTG) analyzes digitized epochs of FHR for numerical criteria, out-putting objective data on short-term variability (mean of 4–8 milliseconds) and overall variability recorded as mean minute variation. Values for short-term variability below three milliseconds show strong correlation with fetal acidosis. The CCTG is not as limited by gestational age and does not require vigorous fetal activity to document a normal result, so it might be adopted as a better version of FHR analysis for a broader range of fetal indications. CCTG is superior to simple CTG in performance time, positive and negative predictive accuracies, and fewer equivocal test results [38]. **Computerized assessment is associated with lower PNM compared to traditional CTG interpretation** (9/1000 vs. 4.2/1000, RR 0.20, 95% CI 0.04–0.88), **but the clinical significance of this difference is elusive as there was no difference in potentially preventable deaths** [35].

Intrapartum FHR monitoring has advanced significantly because of advanced computerized analysis [39] (see Chapter 10 in *Obstetric Evidence Based Guidelines*). Access to computerized assessment improves intrapartum prediction of acidosis [40]. ST-segment analysis enhances intrapartum monitoring when fetal EKG is obtained [41] but has not led to a significant decline in neonatal acidosis in a randomized study [42]. *Antenatal* assessment using CCTG for high-risk premature fetuses may produce more accurate correlation with fetal condition (as compared to traditional NST) but has limited value as a standalone test [43].

Response to Abnormal CTG Test Results
Management depends heavily on gestational age. At ≥32 weeks, **a nonreactive NST should be followed immediately by full BPS**. In specific circumstances, intervention may be based on FHR testing alone. **At term, in a fetus previously documented as having a reactive NST with normal variability, delivery should be considered if the tracing shows minimal or absent variability and/or repetitive late decelerations.** In uncommon cases, an NST may detect a fetal arrhythmia, requiring prompt referral for fetal echocardiography and ultrasound examination. In other circumstances, (e.g., fetal growth restriction), umbilical artery Doppler testing is the main criteria that guides management, together with the CTG. **Before 32 weeks, a non-reactive CTG is often normal** as stated above and may only require outpatient follow-up.

Contraction Stress Test

The **CST (contraction stress test) and the OCT (oxytocin challenge test)** are fetal tests in which spontaneous and induced contractions, respectively, stress the fetoplacental unit either by placental compression or by cord compression, producing either decelerations in the abnormal test or no decelerations when the test is normal. These tests have higher negative predictive value than NST alone, similar to biophysical and Doppler methods (3–4 per 10,000 tests), but have high rates of equivocal results and a high rate of false alarming results. For example, when BPS is used as the backup test for positive (abnormal) CST, at least 50% of pregnancies can safely continue for at least a week [44]. High cost, requirement of hospital facilities, disagreement on fundamental interpretation of the test, and occasional complications resulting from the test methods have marginalized these techniques, which are **currently rarely used** if at all. The OCT may have a role in determining the route of delivery when the need for intervention has already been determined (e.g., a positive OCT means proceed to cesarean section), but the data available do not justify any firm conclusion.

Biophysical Profile Scoring

This ultrasound-based modality uses five parameters of fetal behavior in a protocol-driven format (Table 56.1) to manage high-risk pregnancies [45]. The parameters have different sensitivities for different fetal outcomes, but combining the variables gives a more accurate prediction of fetal status (Figure 56.2) [23,46,47]. Application of BPS has been shown to reduce PNM (historical controls, Table 56.2) [48–50], and long-term neurologic handicap; however, **randomized trials of BPS versus no monitoring have not been done**. One quasirandomized (odd vs. even numbers) nonblinded trial, done over 35 years ago, of BPS versus NST [51] concludes that BPS has a similar sensitivity of overall abnormal fetal outcomes, including perinatal mortality, compared to NST. Randomized trials comparing Doppler methods to BPS have been very small and unable to evaluate such infrequent outcomes [52–56]. In 315 high-risk pregnancies, BPS, umbilical Doppler, and uterine Doppler were performed in all subjects ≥36 weeks gestation [56]. In predicting nonreassuring fetal status, test sensitivity was 60% for BPS, 50% for UA Doppler, and 30% for uterine artery Doppler. Sensitivity was improved to 70% when BPS and umbilical Doppler were combined, reiterating the multivariable findings at earlier gestation [43]. **Compared to other fetal testing (usually NST), BPS may increase the incidence of cesarean section, but does not affect incidences of low Apgar scores, admission to ICN, or PNM** (2 trials) [57]. Further trials are needed to assess the utility of BPS in high-risk pregnancies.

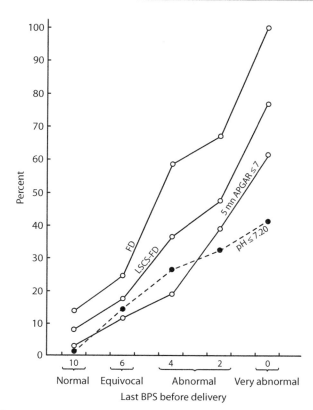

Figure 56.2 Biophysical profile score (BPS) has an exponential relationship to neonatal outcome. Declining scores strongly predict increasing frequency of fetal distress (FD), cesarean section for fetal distress (LSCS-FD), low five-minute Apgar score, and acidotic umbilical vein pH.

Fetal Breathing Movements

These are rhythmic contractions of the fetal diaphragms that demonstrate a maturational pattern. They are unrelated to fetal CO_2 levels but related to diurnal rhythms and fetal cortisol levels. Human fetuses are stimulated to breathe by maternal glucose levels; therefore, outpatient BPS can be done most

Table 56.1 Interpretation of BPS Variables

Fetal Variable	Normal Behavior (Score = 2)	Abnormal Behavior (Score = 0)
Fetal breathing movements	Intermittent, multiple episodes of more than 30-sec duration, within 30-min BPS time frame. Hiccups count. Continuous FBM for 30 min = R/O fetal acidosis	Continuous breathing without cessation. Completely absent breathing or no sustained episodes
Body or limb movements	At least four discrete body movements in 30 min. Includes fine motor movements, rolling movements, and so on, but not REM or mouthing movements	Three or fewer body/limb movements in a 30-min observation period
Fetal tone/posture	Demonstration of active extension with rapid return to flexion of fetal limbs and brisk repositioning/trunk rotation. Opening and closing of hand, mouth, kicking, and so on	Low-velocity movement only. Incomplete flexion, flaccid extremity positions, abnormal fetal posture. Must score = 0 when FM completely absent
Cardiotocogram	At least two episodes of fetal acceleration of >15 bpm and of >15 sec duration. Normal mean variation (computerized FHR interpretation), accelerations associated with maternal palpation FM (accelerations graded for gestation), 20-min CTG	Fetal movement and accelerations not coupled. Insufficient accelerations, absent accelerations, or decelerative trace. Mean variation <20 on numerical analysis of CTG
Amniotic fluid evaluation	At least one pocket ≥2 cm with no umbilical cord. Also consider criteria for subjectively reduced fluid	No cord-free pocket ≥2 cm or multiple elements of subjectively reduced amniotic fluid volume definite

Abbreviations: BPS, biophysical profile score; CTG, cardiotocogram; FBM, fetal breathing movements; FHR, fetal heart rate; FM, fetal movement; REM, rapid eye movement; R/O, rule-out.

Table 56.2 Perinatal Mortality Changes with BPS Application

Program	n	PNM with BPS	PNM without BPS
Ireland (44)	3200	4.1	10.7
Nova Scotia (45)	5000	3.1	6.6
Manitoba (19)	56,000	1.9	7.7
California (46)	15,000	1.3	8.8

Abbreviations: BPS, biophysical profile score; *n*, number tested; PNM, perinatal mortality/1000.

efficiently following mealtimes. Fetal breathing movements are very sensitive to hypoxemia, first illustrating longer periods of fetal apnea between bursts, then being lost altogether [58]. In BPS, fetal hiccups are treated equivalently.

Fetal Body Movements
Total fetal activity declines when hypoxemia begins, often associated with a gradual drop in amniotic fluid volume [59]. The frequency of fetal movements is a maturational variable—many term fetuses will move during only 10 to 15 minutes in an hour of observation while a 28-week fetus who only did that would frequently prove abnormal.

Fetal Tone
The fetus must move to demonstrate tone—it is not simply a flexed posture. The spasm of fetal activity during startle motions provoked by acoustic stimulation does not constitute normal muscle tone and may give a misleading impression of well being.

Amniotic Fluid Volume
This is discussed in detail in a separate guideline (see Chapter 57). In BPS, the maximum vertical pocket (MVP) is the standard [60,61]. MVP ≥2 cm meets criteria for a BPS score of 2 [23]. Reduced amniotic fluid volume is thought to represent reduced fetal urine production assuming normal fetal

swallowing. Hemodynamically mediated redistribution of fetal blood flow, not hypoxemic renal ischemia as once suggested, is the probable mechanism.

CTG
The FHR is a sensitive indicator of fetal compromise with serial loss of CTG reactivity, reduced variability, no variability, and appearance of late decelerations. However, fetuses show the first two of these during normal cyclic behavior, so a BPS of 8/8 is just as indicative of normal well being as a score of 10/10. **NST, therefore, should only be used in fetuses not demonstrating normal behavior in the ultrasound parameters done first [62].** When done in this order, only 2.7% require an NST. As noted above, BPS applies prematurity criteria to NST interpretation.

BPS Management
If biophysical profile testing is performed, the managing physician should be willing to act on the test results. Management by BPS follows a protocol that relates fetal condition, assumed perinatal risks, gestational age, and recommended action (Table 56.3). When BPS is persistently 8/10 on serial testing with the same variable missing, specific inquiry should be made about cause. In some cases, that is obvious from the clinical context (e.g., oligohydramnios in preterm premature rupture of membranes with normal fetal status). In other cases, it is not so clear. As suggested by Table 56.4, equivocal results in the preterm fetus call for repeated testing, transfer to appropriate neonatal resources, antenatal steroid administration, and so on, before moving to delivery. In high-risk fetuses, delivery can wait for valuable maturation time with normal BPS of 8/8 or 10/10 as proof that the fetus is not acidotic [63]. On the other hand, **a BPS of 0–2/10 or 4/10 repeatedly should justify delivery at local thresholds of viability in absence of a transient cause [64]. If very premature gestational age (e.g., <26 weeks) means delivery is not mandated by BPS no matter how low the score, then we advise not to utilize BPS for fetal monitoring.**

Table 56.3 Systematic Application of Biophysical Profile Scoring

BPS	Interpretation	Predicted PNM[a]	Recommended Management
10/10 8/8 8/10 (AFV—normal)	No evidence of fetal asphyxia present	Less than 1/1000	No acute intervention on fetal basis. Serial testing indicated by disorder-specific protocols
8/10-OLIGO	Chronic fetal compromise likely	89/1000	For absolute oligohydramnios, prove normal urinary tract and disprove asymptomatic rupture of membranes
6/10 (AFV—normal)	Equivocal test, fetal asphyxia is not excluded	Depends on progression (61/1000 on average)	Repeat testing in about 6 hr before assigning final value. If score is 6/10, then 10/10, in two continuous 30-min periods, manage as 10/10. For persistent 6/10, deliver the term fetus, repeat within 24 hr in the preterm fetus, then deliver if less than 6/10
4/10	Acute fetal asphyxia likely. If AFV-OLIGO, acute on chronic asphyxia very likely	91/1000	Deliver by obstetrically appropriate method, with continuous monitoring
2/10	Acute fetal asphyxia, most likely with chronic decompensation	125/1000	Deliver for fetal indications (usually needs cesarean section for intolerance to labor)
0/10	Severe, acute asphyxia virtually certain	600/1000	Deliver for fetal indications (usually needs cesarean section for intolerance to labor)

Abbreviations: AFV, amniotic fluid volume; OLIGO, oligohydramnios; PNM, perinatal mortality.
[a]Per 1000 live births, within one week of test result shown, without intervention. For scores of 0, 2, or 4, intervention should begin virtually immediately, provided the fetus is viable.

Table 56.4 Risks of Stillbirth vs. Neonatal Death due to Prematurity

BPS	Stillbirth Rate[a]	Equivalent Neonatal Death Rate (wk)
0	560	25.4
2	153	28.3
4	91	29.1
6	61	30.0
8	0.5	Full term
10	0.5	Full term

[a]Death (per 1,000 births) within one week if the fetus remains undelivered. These figures change with time and differ between centers, including differences between inborn and transported babies.

Modified Biophysical Profile Score

Many modifications have been proposed. The most popular combination suggested has been the amniotic fluid volume **(AFV)–NST combination** [65], including optional use of VAS [66,67] to shorten observation time. This combination uses AFV to reflect long-term uteroplacental function while the NST serves as an indicator of short-term function. Full BPS (all five variables) was the backup test, required in 15% to 30% of cases. MVP is used for AFV assessment. The simplified test reduced the time and complexity of BPS without altering the false negative rate, which is about 3 to 8 per 10,000 tests [66,68]. However, in assessing differences in the false positive rate, either the data are too few or the full BPS was superior to the restricted tests in avoiding unnecessary intervention.

The exceptions are trials of FGR management in which the modified BPS included Doppler information—in those cases, addition of Doppler assessment of umbilical arterial resistance both improved classification of fetal acidosis and reduced interference for false alarm BPS [65,66]. Shortening the BPS is not validated for high-risk fetuses with abnormal Doppler indices; preterm fetuses; postdate pregnancy; fetal anomalies; multiple gestation; or fetuses with arrhythmia, infection, anemia, or diabetic macrosomia.

Doppler of Fetal Vessels

The umbilical artery (UA) is the vessel most useful to screen by Doppler in clinical care, in particular for FGR fetuses. UA resistance progressively rises from tertiary stem villous deficiency and decreasing placental perfusion area and therefore is used as an indicator of placental function (Figure 56.3). UA Doppler assessment requires careful attention to technical detail and is usually done in the mid-portion of the free umbilical cord [69]. Although each mathematical expression of the Doppler arterial flow velocity waveform has some advantages, the **pulsatility index (PI)** has the advantage of infinite expression (remaining valid even when end-diastolic flow is reversed) and autocorrelation with the volume of the waveform itself. When UA PI reaches an individualized threshold, higher blood pressure leads to cardiac and systemic effects. Initial cardiac effects, including ejection fraction, wall velocity, and transvalvular velocity, are measurable with sophisticated techniques. The systemic effects are also measured as a shift toward more cerebral perfusion using the Doppler waveform of the **middle cerebral artery (MCA,** Figure 56.4). Initially there is a subtle change in the cerebroplacental ratio (CPR) called centralization. This is thought to be from resistance-mediated diversion of flow

away from an ailing placenta. Further deterioration in placental function may lead to a significant decline in the MCA PI as diastolic blood flow rises, which has been called brain sparing and may be mediated by hypoxemia-induced cerebral vasorelaxation [70]. Use of the CPR or MCA PI in monitoring FGR fetuses has an established relation to neurodevelopmental outcome [71], but CPR performs poorly as a screening test for adverse outcomes [72]. **As with all Doppler studies, the cerebroplacental ratio should not be used in isolation** if used at all. There is much recent enthusiasm, but no management trial data, to support use for the CPR to direct care [73].

As hemodynamic and respiratory declines continue to interact, oxygen-sensitive interfaces between nutrient rich and nonrich streams begin to dictate flow [74]. Diversion through an opening **ductus venosus (DV)** is readily depicted as progressive changes in waveform pattern (Figure 56.5). Deep reversal of the atrial contraction wave, a-wave, indicates both cardiac impairment (forward volume flow insufficiency forcing the waveform more retrograde) and hypoxemia (dilating the DV itself). DV contains the highest venous velocities in the fetal abdomen, but when the waveform is abnormal, it must be carefully differentiated from adjacent hepatic venous structures.

Functional aspects of the placenta, including placental volume flow, sequential placental flow distribution, and vascular responses to maternal hyperoxygenation are interesting from the physiologic point of view but too operator-dependent for clinical monitoring.

Doppler Application

Routine application of UA and/or uterine artery Doppler in normal pregnancy is of no proven benefit [75,76]. UA Doppler is instead beneficial in some high-risk pregnancies, especially those complicated by FGR. Worsening **UA Doppler** correlates well with declining placental function and the emergence of hypoxemia and acidosis (70). The UA Doppler will start to increase when the placenta is 60%–70% compromised [77]. Absent end-diastolic velocities denote an increasing risk of stillbirth, preterm delivery, birth weight below 10th percentile, and many neonatal complications (Table 56.5) [78]. UA Doppler is useful in directing care—small fetuses with normal Dopplers probably do not need the same level of surveillance as do those with abnormal umbilical flow [79]. Perinatal outcome is superior when UA Doppler is utilized in decision-making although interventions based on umbilical Doppler alone have a substantial risk of causing unnecessary prematurity [80,81]. Compared with no Doppler ultrasound, **Doppler (mostly UA) ultrasound in high-risk pregnancy (especially those complicated by hypertension or presumed FRG) is associated with a reduction in perinatal death** (1.2% vs. 1.7%, RR 0.71,95% CI 0.50–0.98). The use of Doppler ultrasound is also associated with **fewer inductions of labor** (RR 0.89) and **fewer cesarean sections** (RR 0.90) without reports of adverse effects. No difference is found for FHR abnormalities in labor or low Apgar scores [82] (see Chapter 45). **In cases of FGR, fetuses with absent end-diastolic UA Doppler flow should be delivered around 34 weeks, and those with reversed end-diastolic UA Doppler flow should be delivered around 32 weeks** [83]. Despite the strong correlations with fetal status, basing delivery decisions on UA Doppler alone, especially before 32 to 34 weeks and without the presence of absent or reversed diastolic flow, may lead to unnecessary mortality and morbidity due to extreme

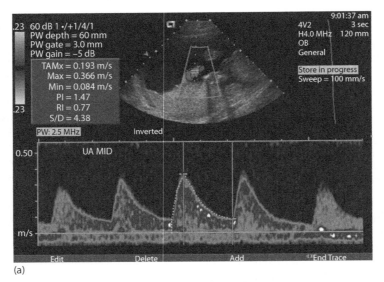

(a)

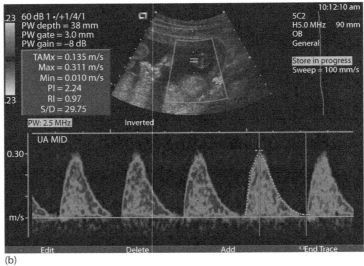

(b)

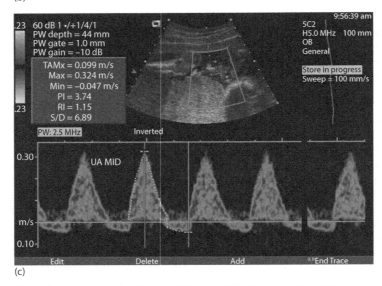

(c)

Figure 56.3 Abnormalities in Doppler velocity waveforms of the umbilical artery depict increasing placental resistance. These Doppler examinations are from the same patient as pregnancy progresses. (a) The umbilical artery resistance is modestly elevated at 18 weeks (PI 1.47). By 24 weeks (b), end-diastolic velocities are absent in most cardiac cycles. By 28 weeks (c), reversal of end-diastolic flow occupies nearly one quarter of the cardiac cycle. Cesarean section was carried out on the basis of oligohydramnios at 29+ weeks with umbilical venous pH 7.18. *Abbreviation*: PI, pulsatility index.

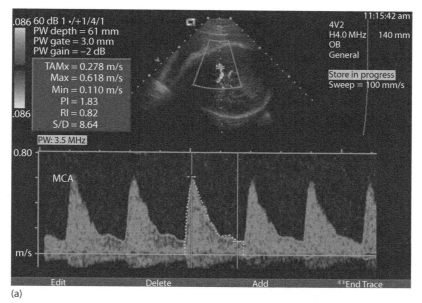

(a)

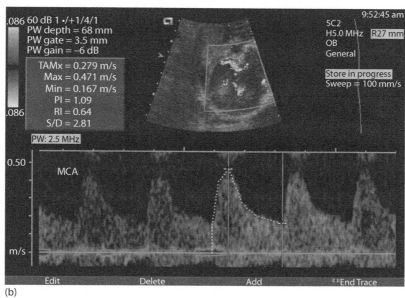

(b)

Figure 56.4 Serial MCA Dopplers demonstrate an increase in diastolic blood flow, termed centralization. Normally, the middle cerebral artery shows high resistance with low diastolic velocity (a, high PI 1.83). Diversion of blood flow toward the brain correlates with worsening umbilical artery depiction of increased placental resistance with falling cerebrovascular resistance, increased end-diastolic velocities, and PI falling to 1.09 (b). *Abbreviations*: MCA, middle cerebral artery; PI, pulsatility index.

prematurity [84–86]. This was shown also by the GRIT trial (Table 56.6) [87,88].

Evaluation of **venous Doppler waveforms** may be useful in prediction of morbidity and mortality in FGR. Ductus venosus (DV) abnormality is a strong predictor of adverse perinatal outcome, surpassing all other predictors [89,90]. However, the best outcomes occurred when BPS was used to maximize the safe prolongation of pregnancy [91]. Even in the most compromised pregnancy, gestational age was the most influential factor in determining outcome. These principles have been amplified further in nontrial observations. First, the most severe DV abnormality, absence or reversal of the a-wave (Figure 56.5), is an accurate predictor of stillbirth when it exists >7 days (in fetuses with the most severe UA patterns)

[92]. Second, however, **when severe DV abnormality is found** *without* **abnormal UA Doppler, outcome may well be normal.** A large randomized trial, the TRUFFLE trial, suggests that there is no difference in neuroimpairment of surviving infants even at 2 years if they are delivered based on CCTG short term variation, early DV changes (>95th percentile PI) or late DV changes (a-wave reversal) [93]. **There is no level-1 evidence that DV Doppler improves perinatal or infant outcomes, and therefore it should not be used routinely for clinical management in unselected patients.** Again, the principle is emphasized: Solitary Doppler abnormality, even reverse a-wave in the DV, is not sufficient for intervention [94].

In virtually all Doppler-outcome trials, the single most critical influence on outcome has been gestational

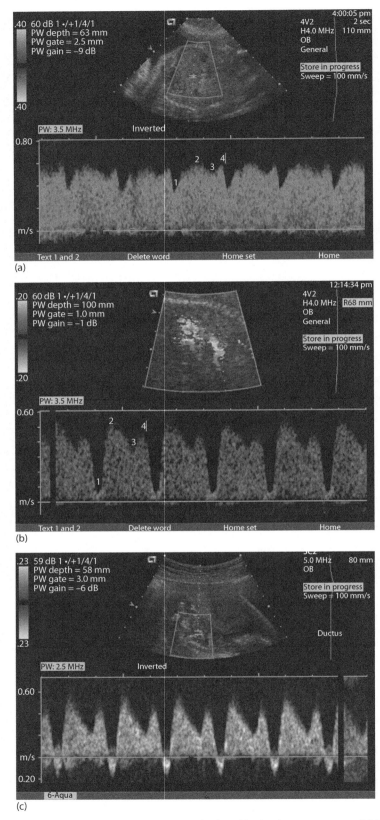

Figure 56.5 Progressive changes in venous return to the heart as depicted in the ductus venosus. (a) There are normally four phases in the waveform, consisting of 1) atrial contraction, 2) ventricular contraction, 3) restitution of the annulus, 4) diastole. Typically, the a-wave (1) shows the only significant downward deflection, a modest reduction in forward flow. (b) Increased afterload from placental resistance causes abnormal forward cardiac output with the a-wave nearly retrograde. (c) Further progression in placental insufficiency is associated with cardiac malfunction with severe retrograde a-waves as well as distorted cardiac function, producing midwave depression as the annulus rises against an overfilled circulation.

Table 56.5 Abnormal Umbilical Artery Doppler Correlates with Neonatal Compromise

Cesarean section for fetal nonreassuring testing
Acidosis
Hypoxemia
Low Apgar-5
Ventilator required
Long-term oxygen
Bronchopulmonary dysplasia
Anemia
Increased NRBC
Thrombocytopenia
Prolonged NRBC release
Neutropenia
Transfusions required
IVH
NEC
Perinatal mortality

Note: For all of these outcomes, their frequency rises exponentially from abnormal indices to absent end-diastolic velocities to reversed end-diastolic velocities.
Abbreviations: IVH, intraventricular hemorrhage; NEC, necrotizing enterocolitis; NRBC, nucleated red blood cells.

Table 56.6 GRIT Trial

End Point	Immediate Delivery	Delayed Delivery	Odds Ratio
C/S rate	91%	79%	2.7 (CI 1.6–4.5)
Early PNM	10%	9%	1.1 (CI 0.61–1.8)
Late PNM	2%	2%	1.0
Cerebral palsy	5%	1%	Not calculated
All disabilities	8%	4%	Not calculated
Death or disability	55/290	44/283	1.1 (CI 0.7–1.8)
at 2 years	19%	15.5%	

Sources: Modified from Thorton JG, Hornbuckle J, Vail A et al. *Lancet*, 364, 9433, 513–20, 2004; GRIT study group. *Br J Obstet Gynecol*, 110, 1, 27–32, 2003.
Abbreviations: C/S, cesarean section; CI, 95% confidence interval; PNM, perinatal mortality.

age at delivery and its determination of adverse impacts of prematurity. In general, no Doppler abnormality by itself warrants iatrogenic delivery before 32 weeks. At present, level 1 data suggests that **the only Doppler useful for timing of delivery and improving outcomes is the UA Doppler**. Other Doppler studies remain of limited clinical utility for fetal testing and timing of delivery (with the exception of MCA for fetal anemia). For management of FGR, see also Chapter 45.

An approach to sequential testing with Doppler establishing the appropriate level of intense surveillance and BPS indicating the timing of delivery has been proposed by several independent teams. An example is shown in Table 56.7.

Doppler Surveillance and BPS: Integrated Fetal Testing

Fetuses at risk for placental insufficiency are best assessed with UA Doppler. However, elevated UA resistance may persist for months, absent end-diastolic velocity for weeks, and a-wave reversal for days without fetal deterioration [95]. Especially in the critical gestational ages before 32

Table 56.7 Umbilical Artery Doppler Index Abnormality Suggests NST/MVP or BPS Surveillance

Abnormality[a]	NST/MVP or BPS Frequency[b]	Decision to Deliver (Fetal)[c]
Decreased but present diastolic flow	Weekly	Abnormal BPS[d] or ≥36–37 wk
AEDV	Twice weekly	Abnormal BPS[d] or ≥34 wk
REDV	Daily	Abnormal BPS[d] or ≥32 wk

Abbreviations: BPS, biophysical profile scoring; MVP, maximum vertical pocket; NST, nonstress test.
[a]Umbilical artery (UA) and precordial venous Doppler. MCA abnormalities confirm the elevated placental resistance, but do not directly alter management according to this scheme.
[b]*Minimum* frequency, increased on the basis of severity—maternal condition(s), degree of IUGR, gestational age.
[c]Neonatology consultation, maternal clinical factors, fetal blood sampling parameters, all will impact this collaborative decision.
[d]Any BPS ≤4/10.

weeks, such an interval may be crucial in reducing prematurity impacts. A nonrandomized study of 113 pregnancies managed by combined UA and DV Doppler with delivery triggered by BPS, concluded that gestational age and birth weight were "the predominant factors for poor neurodevelopment" assessed at age 2 [96]. The rationale underlying the multivessel Doppler and BPS approach is the relationship of deterioration in vascular indices to the (later) decline in BPS (Figure 56.6) [97]. **A high-level of evidence is now available, showing that waiting until the need for delivery is certain maximizes intrauterine time, optimizes reduction of prematurity, and at the same time does not add morbidity or mortality by "delaying" intervention [89–92,95,97–101]. A fetus, even if IUGR, should not be delivered based solely on Doppler flow studies before 32 weeks. Integrated fetal testing has not been studied in randomized trials, and so its real safety and effectiveness are unknown.**

Condition-Specific Testing

Many conditions have increased risks of fetal compromise but may not have identical patterns of fetal deterioration; it may be necessary/beneficial to modify testing to fit the disorder. **FGR, late-term pregnancy, and PPROM are the only conditions in which there is some evidence from RCTs regarding antenatal fetal testing.** Many other conditions have been proposed as necessitating antenatal fetal testing (Table 56.8) [102]. Table 56.9 summarizes our suggested management for antenatal fetal testing based on different conditions.

Preeclampsia
There are no randomized trials to determine type or frequency of fetal monitoring for preeclampsia. We recommend a fetal growth scan and MVP and UA Doppler at the time of diagnosis and twice weekly NSTs to evaluate for placental insufficiency if initial assessments are normal.

Diabetes
The critical issue is glycemic control—when this is good, antenatal testing is less critical. When diabetic control is

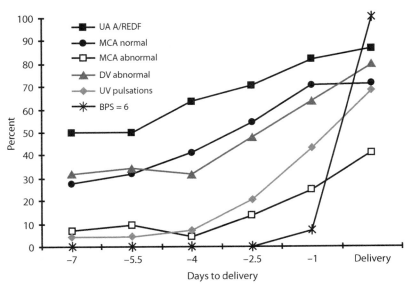

Figure 56.6 Progressive changes in multivessel Doppler occur in sequence before the BPS deteriorates, in many fetuses. Virtually all fetuses were delivered for abnormal BPS (asterisks). Most of these IUGR fetuses had reached the end of their Doppler progression before delivery. *Abbreviations*: A/REDV, absent or reversed diastolic velocity; BPS, biophysical profile score; DV, ductus venosus; MCA, middle cerebral artery; UA, umbilical artery; UV, umbilical vein.

Table 56.8 Examples of Possible Indications for Antenatal Surveillance[a]

Primarily Maternal Conditions	Primarily Placental Conditions	Primarily Fetal Conditions	Miscellaneous Conditions
Hyperthyroidism	Antiphospholipid syndrome	Decreased fetal movement	IVF pregnancy
Symptomatic hemoglobinopathy	Systemic lupus erythematosus	Oligohydramnios/polyhydramnios	Previous stillbirth
Cyanotic heart disease	Hypertensive disorders	Intrauterine growth restriction	Previous recurrent abruption
Chronic renal disease	Marked placental anomalies	Postdates pregnancy	Teratogen exposure
Type I diabetes	Umbilical artery Doppler abnormalities	Alloimmunization macrosomia	
Marked uterine anomalies	Gestational diabetes	Anomalies/aneuploidy	
Advanced maternal age		Multiple gestation	
Obesity		Preterm premature rupture of membranes	
Organ transplant		Fetal arrhythmia	

Source: Modified from Practice bulletin no. 145: antepartum fetal surveillance. *Obstet Gynecol*, 124, 1, 182–92, 2014.
[a]Not a complete list.

poor, identification and monitoring of the macrosomic fetus requires individualized care [103,104]. Poor glycemic control as judged by maternal blood sugars or as denoted by fetal macrosomia (estimated fetal weight >90th percentile) and polyhydramnios or both requires increased surveillance. Diabetic women with hypertension, cardiac, renal, and other vascular diabetopathy and fetuses with FGR have pregnancies with the highest risk of adverse outcome from elevated placental resistance. UA Doppler can detect this and is thought to correctly stratify the adverse outcomes better than BPS [105] although prospective randomized evaluation of management has not been reported. In the absence of Doppler abnormalities of placentation, management by BPS protocol using twice-weekly testing achieves the same or better outcome (cord vein pH, mortality, neonatal morbidity) than euglycemic controls [106]. Expert opinion generally recommends weekly NSTs starting at 32 weeks and

then twice-weekly NSTs starting around 36 weeks and serial growth ultrasounds for all women requiring medications to achieve glycemic control.

Fetal Growth Restriction

This issue is covered in more details in Chapter 45. **UA Doppler monitoring of the FRG fetus is associated with improved perinatal outcomes, including less perinatal death [107]. Therefore, weekly UA Dopplers should be performed after FGR is diagnosed. A FGR fetus should be delivered around 32 weeks for reversed UA end-diastolic flow or around 34 weeks if absent UA end-diastolic flow [83]** (Table 56.7). Doppler studies of other vessels have not been shown to be associated with perinatal benefits and remain, therefore, investigational [93]. In addition to UA Dopplers, CTG and amniotic fluid assessment should be performed regularly.

Table 56.9 Suggested Antenatal Surveillance for Specific Conditions

Condition	Initiation of Testing	Testing	Initiation of Growth Ultrasounds[f]	Delivery (Weeks)	
Chronic HTN	32 wk	Weekly NST[a]	24 wk (if on meds)	Q4 wk	No meds — 38 0/7–39 6/7; Controlled on meds — 37 0/7–39 6/7; Poorly controlled — 36 0/7–37 6/7
Gestational HTN	32 wk	Weekly NST	At diagnosis	Q4 wks	37 0/7–37 6/7
Preeclampsia	At diagnosis	Twice weekly NST	At diagnosis	Q4 wks	Without severe features — 37 0/7–37 6/7; With severe features — 34 0/7–34 6/7
GDMA1	None	None	30–32 wks	Once	Early delivery <39 weeks not indicated
GDMA2	32 wk / 36 wk	Weekly NST/MVP / Twice weekly NST/MVP	At diagnosis	Q4 wks	Late preterm or early term delivery might be indicated if poorly controlled
Pregestational DM	32 wk / 36 wk	Weekly NST / Twice weekly NST[c]	24 wk (if on meds)	Q4 wks	Well controlled — 39 0/7–39 6/7; Poorly controlled/complications — 37 0/7–38 6/7
Fetal growth restriction	At diagnosis	Weekly NST/MVP and dopplers	At diagnosis	Q3 wks	No other abnormalities — 38 0/7–39 6/7; Absent UA end diastolic flow — 34 0/7–34 6/7; Reversed UA end diastolic flow — 32 0/7–32 6/7
Maternal age at delivery ≥35 yrs	36 wk	Weekly NST	30–32 wks	Once	39 0/7–39 6/7
Obesity	32–36 wk	Weekly NST	–	–	Early delivery <39 weeks usually not indicated
Preterm premature ruptured membranes	At diagnosis	In patient management	At diagnosis	Q3 wks	34 0/7 (or later[g])
Late-term (≥41 weeks)	41 wk	Twice weekly NST	–	–	41 0/7–41 6/7
Concordant, non IUGR di/di twins	None	None[b]	24 wk	Q4 wks	37 0/7–38 6/7
Mono/di twins	34–36 wk	Weekly NST, q2 wk dopplers	18–20 wks	Q2 wks	34 0/7–37 6/7
Mono/mono twins	28 wk	Twice weekly NST, q2 wk dopplers	24 wk	Q3 wks	32 0/7–33 6/7
Prior unexplained IUFD	32 wk	Weekly NST	28 wk	Q4 wks	39 0/7–39 6/7
SLE or renal disease	32 wk	Weekly NST	24 wk	Q4 wks	39 0/7–39 6/7
Organ transplant	32 wk	Weekly NST	28 wk	Q4 wks	Early delivery <39 weeks usually not indicated
Hypothyroidism or hyperthyroidism	32 wk[d]	Weekly NST[d]	30–32 wk	Once	Early delivery <39 weeks usually not indicated
Maternal cardiac disease	Individualize	Comprehensive cardiovascular	28 wk	Q4 wks	Early delivery <39 weeks usually not indicated
Oligohydramnios (MVP <2 cm)	32 wk[e]	Weekly NST/MVP	At diagnosis	Q3–4 wks	37 0/7–37 6/7
Polyhydramnios (MVP >8 cm)	28 wk[e]	Weekly NST/MVP	At diagnosis	Q3–4 wks	37 0/7–37 6/7
Sickle cell disease	32 wk	Weekly NST	24 wk	Q4 wks	Early delivery <39 weeks usually not indicated
Fetal arrhythmia	Individualize	Comprehensive cardiovascular	At diagnosis	Q4 wks	Early delivery <39 weeks usually not indicated

Abbreviations: di/di, chorionic diamniotic; DM, diabetes mellitus; GDMA, gestational diabetes mellitus; HTN, hypertension; IUFD, intrauterine fetal demise; IUGR, intrauterine growth restriction; meds, mediations; mono/di, monochorionic diamniotic; mono/mono, monochorionic monoamniotic; MVP, maximum vertical pocket; NST, non stress test; q, every; SLE, systemic lupus erythematosus; wk, week; yrs, years; early term, 37 6/7–38 6/7 weeks; late preterm, 34 0/8–36 6/7 weeks.

[a]Instead of NSTs, some practitioners use biophysical profile score (BPS) or modified BPS (NST and MVP). There is no level 1 evidence to compare NST to BPS (or modified BPS) fetal testing.

[b]Some practitioners starts NSTs (or BPS) fetal testing in multiple gestations at 32–36 weeks, with very limited evidence.

[c]If poorly controlled, consider starting at 28 wks twice weekly.

[d]For hypothyroidism, only if poorly controlled.

[e]Or at diagnosis if diagnosed later.

[f]cHTN off meds, abnormal placentation, substance abuse in pregnancy, uterine fibroids >5 cm all indications for one growth scan at 30 wk.

[g]See Chapter 19 in *Obstetric Evidence Based Guidelines* for more details.

Advanced Maternal Age

The number of women delivering over the age of 35 years is rising. The risk of stillbirth increases with age with women over 40 years old at 39 weeks gestation having similar still-birth rates to women 25–29 years old at 41 weeks [108]. Many experts, therefore, recommend early delivery. To our knowledge, there are no large randomized controlled trials exploring antepartum testing in this population; however, there is one in progress in the United Kingdom randomizing women over 35 years to either delivery from 39 0/7 to 39 6/7 weeks or expectant management [109]. We recommend weekly NST/MVP starting at 36 weeks, as well as one growth ultrasound around 30 weeks.

Obesity

The exponential rise in obesity and morbid obesity in pregnancy is alarming in many respects, including accelerated fetal risks [110]. These associations include the effects of associated medical disorders, such as hypertension and diabetes, but obesity itself has an independent impact on fetal macrosomia, stillbirth, and intrapartum complications that mandates heightened monitoring [111]. Many experts now recommend at least weekly NSTs or BPS for women with BMI ≥30 (or ≥35), starting at either 32 or 36 weeks, based on the fact that the incidence of fetal death is increased in this population [112]. Early delivery is not recommended.

Preterm Premature Ruptured Membranes

NST or BPS management may be helpful in managing preterm premature ruptured membranes (PPROM), but the evidence for effectiveness is very limited. When the NST was nonreactive and fetal breathing was absent, delivery produced superior neonatal and maternal infectious outcomes in one study [113]. This finding has not been replicated in other studies. **Randomized comparison of BPS and NST alone in this setting showed that neither test has good sensitivity (25.0% and 39.1%, respectively) in predicting infectious morbidity, but both had good predictive accuracy when abnormal (66.7% and 52.9%, respectively)** [114]. Neither amniocentesis [115] nor endovaginal ultrasounds [116] decrease neonatal death. A recent Cochrane review reports that there is insufficient evidence to draw clear conclusions for antenatal testing in PPROM from the existing evidence [117]. **Expert opinion varies greatly between countries; in the United States inpatient antenatal fetal monitoring of women with PPROM between 23 and 33 6/7 weeks is recommended, including CTG two to three times daily. Delivery is indicated usually once 34 weeks is reached**, but newest evidence may allow longer expectant management (see Chapter 19 in *Obstetric Evidence Based Guidelines*).

Postdate Pregnancy

A policy of **labor induction at 41 completed weeks (41–41 6/7) or beyond is associated with significantly fewer perinatal deaths (1/2814 vs. 9/2785; RR 0.30, 95% CI 0.09–0.99)** compared with expectant management with induction not before 42 weeks [118]. There were **fewer cesarean sections** in the induction group (RR 0.89, 95% CI 0.81–0.97). **Labor induction at 41 weeks also significantly reduces the risk of perinatal meconium aspiration syndrome** compared with expectant management (RR 0.50, 95% CI 0.34–0.73).

Admission and delivery outcomes for pregnancies being monitored at 40 and 41 weeks gestation were the same indicating that fetal monitoring may need to start at 40 weeks

[119]. At present, the best recommendation is made with moderate confidence: **pregnancies at 41 0/7 weeks should receive weekly CTG/MVP and be delivered before 42 0/7 weeks.** When delivery before 42 weeks is not selected, twice-weekly monitoring should include amniotic fluid assessment using at least CTG and MVP [120] (see Chapter 27 in *Obstetric Evidence Based Guidelines*).

Fetal Anemia

MCA Doppler velocimetry is effective in determining the need for fetal transfusion, the timing between transfusions, and in differentiating degrees of fetal anemia [121]. However, since there is a 1% to 10% failure rate in detecting severe anemia and a higher rate of missing mild anemia (which may progress rapidly) [122], MCA should form the core of a comprehensive approach that also includes fetal blood sampling by cordocentesis and an experienced team familiar with fetal hematology [123,124] (see Chapter 53).

Nonobstetric Procedure Monitoring

Before the locally accepted viable gestational age (currently about 23 weeks in the United States), fetal heart tones should be obtained before and after the procedure. When the fetus is considered viable, the decision to monitor fetal heart tones continuously throughout the case should be made on a case-by-case basis. If continuous intraoperative CTG is to be performed, there should at least be a skilled obstetrical provider available to perform an emergent cesarean section and the nonobstetrical procedure taking place should be able to be stopped in order for delivery to be performed. Postoperative CTG should be considered in procedures that might increase the risk of preterm labor [125].

Practical Antenatal Testing: Who, When, How, and Why?

Table 56.9 summarizes our recommendations. **No trial has conclusively proven that antenatal testing lowers long-term adverse neurologic outcomes, so recommendations might be rated as Level B or even C (i.e., consensus, expert opinion, but no clear evidence).** The standard of care, accordingly, can only be a suggestion and probably varies considerably from region to region [126].

Thresholds for viability, knowledge of the disease process, severity of individual cases, past history—all may indicate starting monitoring earlier than recommended by general guidelines (32–34 weeks for most at-risk fetuses, according to ACOG) (Table 56.9). Routine application of testing methods such as NST or UA Doppler alone, pose substantial risk of iatrogenic prematurity in fetuses with abnormal testing—a blanket proposal of "testing early and testing often" is potentially more dangerous than helpful. Testing should be timed in recognition of the characteristics of the test and the fetus.

The choice of test is determined not only by specific condition-related advantages above, but also by available personnel and equipment, cost, availability of effective treatment for abnormal results, and evidence of outcome impact of the management protocol (Table 56.9). Testing interval will depend on severity (e.g., up to three times daily or even continuous in FGR fetuses with the worst UA Doppler pattern).

Last, one should remember that the goal of antenatal fetal testing is to decrease perinatal morbidity and mortality. Many other interventions (e.g., smoking cessation for smokers, euglycemia for diabetics) can help achieve the same goal of better perinatal health and should be implemented aggressively to complement antenatal fetal testing.

REFERENCES

1. Grant A, Chalmers I. Randomized trial of fetal movement counting. *Lancet* 1982; 2(8296): 501. [I; RCT, *n* = 68,000]
2. Mangesi L, Hofmeyr GJ. Fetal movement counting for assessment of fetal wellbeing. *Cochrane Database Syst Rev* 2007; (1): CD004909. [I; Meta-analysis; 4 RCTs, *n* = 71,370]
3. Olesen AG, AVare JA. Decreased fetal movements: Background, assessment, and clinical management. *Acta Obstet Gynecol Scand* 2004; 83(9): 818–26. [III; Review]
4. Liston R, Sawchuck D, Young D. Fetal health surveillance: Antepartum and intrapartum consensus guideline. *J Obstet Gynaecol Can* 2007; 29(Suppl. 4): S3–56. [III]
5. Bishop EH. Fetal acceleration test. *Am J Obstet Gynecol* 1981; 141: 905–9. [II]
6. Lavin JP Jr, Miodovnik M, Barden TP. Relationship of nonstress test reactivity and gestational age. *Obstet Gynecol* 1984; 63: 338–44. [II-3]
7. Druzin ML, Fox A, Kogut E, Carlson C. The relationship of the nonstress test to gestational age. *Am J Obstet Gynecol* 1985; 153: 386–9. [III]
8. Cousins LM, Poeltler DM, Faron S, Catanzarite V, Daneshmand S, Casele H. Nonstress testing at </= 32.0 weeks' gestation: A randomized trial comparing different assessment criteria. *Am J Obstet Gynecol* 2012; 207: 311. [I]
9. Glantz JC, Bertoia N. Preterm nonstress testing: 10-beat compared with 15-beat criteria. *Obstet Gynecol* 2011; 118: 87–93. [II-3]
10. Macones GA, Hankins GD, Spong CY et al. The 2008 national institute of child health and human development worksheet on electronic fetal monitoring: Update on definitions, interpretation, and research guidelines. *J Obstet Neonatal Nurs* 2008; 37(5): 510–5. [III]
11. Snijders RJ, McLaren R, Nicolaides KH. Computer-assisted analysis of fetal heart rate patterns at 20-41 week's gestation. *Fetal Diagn Ther* 1990; 5(2): 79–83. [II-2]
12. Park MI, Hwang JH, Cha KJ et al. Computerized analysis of fetal heart rate parameters by gestational age. *Int J Gynaecol Obstet* 2001; 74(2): 157–64. [II-2]
13. Manning FA. The fetal heart rate. In: *Fetal Medicine Principals and Practice*. Norwalk, CT: Appleton & Lange, 1995: 13–111. [III; Review]
14. Visser GH, Sadovsky G, Nicolaides KH. Antepartum heart rate patterns in small-for-gestational-age third-trimester fetuses: Correlations with blood gas values obtained at cordocentesis. *Am J Obstet Gynecol* 1990; 162(3): 698–702. [II-2; Case control study of fetal heart rate patterns correlated with cordocentesis-derived blood gas values]
15. Meis PH, Ureda JR, Swain M, Kelly RP, Penry M, Sharp P. Variable decelerations during nonstress tests are note a sign of fetal compromise. *Am J Obstet Gynecol* 1986; 154: 586–90. [II-3]
16. Anyaegbunam A, Brustman L, Divon M, Langer O. The significance of antepartum variable decelerations. *Am J Obstet Gynecol* 1986; 155: 707–10. [II-3]
17. Bourgeois FJ, Thiagarajah S, Harbert GM Jr. The significance of fetal heart rate decelerations during nonstress testing. *Am J Obstet Gynecol* 1984; 150: 213–6. [III]
18. Druzin ML, Gratacos J, Keegan KA, Paul RH. Antepartum fetal heart rate testing. VII. The significance of fetal bradycardia. *Am J Obstet Gynecol* 1981; 139: 194–8. [III]
19. Pazos R, Vuolo K, Aladjem S, Lueck J, Anderson C. Association of spontaneous fetal heart rate decelerations during antepartum nonstress testing and intrauterine growth retardation. *Am J Obstet Gynecol* 1982; 144: 574–7. [III]
20. Nathan EB, Haberman S, Burgess T et al. The relationship of maternal position to the results of brief nonstress tests: A randomized trial. *Am J Obstet Gynecol* 2000; 182: 1070–2. [I; RCT, *n* = 108]
21. Alus M, Okumus H, Mete S et al. The effects of different maternal positions on non-stress test: An experimental study. *J Clin Nurs* 2007; 16(3): 562–8. [II-3]
22. Gagnon R, Patrick J, Foreman J et al. Stimulation of human fetuses with sound and vibration. *Am J Obstet Gynecol* 1986; 155(4): 484–51. [II-3; Development of VAS]
23. Harman CR. Antenatal assessment of fetal status. In: Creasy R, Iams J, Resnik R, eds. *Maternal-Fetal Medicine. 6th ed.* Toronto: WB Saunders, 2010. [III; Review]
24. Tan KH, Smyth R. Fetal vibroacoustic stimulation for facilitation of tests of fetal wellbeing. *Cochrane Database Syst Rev* 2010, 1. [I; Meta-analysis; 9 RCTs, *n* = 4838]
25. Kamel HS, Makhlouf AM, Youssef AA. Simplified biophysical profile: An antepartum fetal screening test. *Gynecol Obstet Invest* 1999; 47(4): 223–8. [II-2; Although vibroacoustic stimulation shortened the testing time for normal results, 67% of the abnormal results were false-alarms]
26. Serafini P, Lindsay MP, Nagey DA et al. Antepartum fetal heart rate response to sound stimulation: The acoustic stimulation test. *Am J Obstet Gynecol* 1984; 148(1): 41–4. [II-2; Comparative study showed testing efficiency of VAS, but included 55% false negative results for prediction of fetal distress]
27. Arabin B, Becker R, Mohnhaupt A et al. Prediction of fetal distress and poor outcome in prolonged pregnancy using Doppler ultrasound and fetal heart rate monitoring combined with stress tests (II). *Fetal Diagn Ther* 1994; 9(1): 1–6. [II-2; CTG was the only reliable prediction of acidemia in post-term pregnancy. Doppler, CST, and OCT were all irrelevant to predicting acidemia, while none were effective in predicting low Apgar scores]
28. Arabin B, Becker R, Mohnhaupt A et al. Prediction of fetal distress and poor outcome in intrauterine-growth retardation—A comparison of fetal heart rate monitoring combined with stress tests and Doppler ultrasound. *Fetal Diagn Ther* 1993; 8(4): 234–40. [II-2; IUGR fetuses (*n* = 103) were studied with NST/CST, VAS, and Doppler. The passive tests—Doppler and NST—were better predictors of adverse outcome. The authors recommended abolishing the stress test]
29. Tan KH, Sabapathy A. Maternal glucose administration for facilitating tests of fetal wellbeing. *Cochrane Database Syst Rev* 2005; 4. [I; Meta-analysis; 2 RCTs, *n* = 708]
30. Esin S, Baser E, Cakir C et al. Chocolate or orange juice for non-reactive non-stress test (NST) patterns: A randomized prospective controlled study. *JMFNM* 2013; 26(9): 915–9. [I; RCT, *n* = 180]
31. Tan KH, Sabapathy A. Fetal manipulation for facilitating tests of fetal wellbeing. *Cochrane Database Syst Rev* 2005; 4. [I; Meta-analysis; 3 RCTs, *n* = 1100]
32. Caridi BJ, Bolnick JM, Fletcher BG et al. Effect of halogen light stimulation on nonstress testing. *Am J Obstet Gynecol* 2004; 190(5): 1470–2. [I; RCT fetal light perception shortens NST time]
33. Manning FA, Lange IR, Morrison I et al. Fetal biophysical profile score and the nonstress test: A comparative trial. *Obstet Gynecol* 1984; 326–31. [I; RCT]
34. Keane MW, Horger EO III, Vice L. Comparative study of stressed and nonstressed antepartum fetal heart rate testing. *Obstet Gynecol* 1981; 57(3): 320–4. [II-1; Sequential testing used each high-risk fetus (*n* = 566) as its own control. Only 24.8% of nonreactive NST had positive CST]
35. Grivell RM, Alfirevic Z, Gyte GM et al. Antenatal cardiotocography for fetal assessment. *Cochrane Database Syst Rev* 2010; 20(1): CD007863. [I; Meta-analysis; 6 RCTs, *n* = 2105]
36. Morrison I, Menticoglou S, Manning FA et al. Comparison of antepartum results to perinatal outcome. *J Matern Fetal Med* 1994; 3: 75–83. [II-2; All FGR fetuses underwent all tests: NST, BPS, umbilical artery Doppler and OCT. The best prediction of poor outcome used all tests. NST alone predicted only 32% of compromised fetuses]
37. Visser GH, Dawes GS, Redman CW. Numerical analysis of the normal human antenatal fetal heart rate. *Br J Obstet Gynaecol* 1981; 88(8): 792–802. [III; Original development of the system 8000, with 196 fetal heart records]

38. Bracero LA, Morgan S, Byrne DW. Comparison of visual and computerized interpretation of nonstress test results in a randomized controlled trial. *Am J Obstet Gynecol* 1999; 181 (5 Pt. 1): 1254–8. [I; RCT, *n* = 410; computerized evaluation of fetal heart rate testing is superior to standard visual interpretation]

39. Roemer VM, Walden R. Sensitivity, specificity, receiver-operating characteristic (ROC) curves and likelihood ratios for electronic foetal heart rate monitoring using new evaluation techniques. *Z Geburtshilfe Neonatal* 2010; 214(3): 108–18. [II-2]

40. Costa A, Santos C, Ayres-de-Campos D et al. Access to computerized analysis of intrapartum cardiotocographs improves clinicians' prediction of newborn umbilical artery blood pH. *Br J Ostet Gynecol* 2010; 117(10): 1288–93. [II-2]

41. Ross MG, Devoe LD, Rosen KG. ST-segment analysis of the fetal electrocadiogram improves fetal heart rate tracing interpretation and clinical decision-making. *J Matern Fetal Neonatal Med* 2004; 15(3): 181–5. [II-3]

42. Westerhuis ME, Visser GH, Moons KG et al. Cardiotocography plus ST analysis of fetal electocardiogram compared with cardiotocography only for intrapartum monitoring: A randomized controlled trial. *Obstet Gynecol* 2010; 115(6): 1173–80. [I; RCT]

43. Turan S, Turan OM, Berg C et al. Computerized fetal heart rate analysis, Doppler ultrasound and biophysical profile score in the prediction of acid-base status of growth-restricted fetuses. *Ultrasound Obstet Gynecol* 2007; 30(5): 750–6. [II-2]

44. Nageotte MP, Towers CV, Asrat T et al. The value of a negative antepartum test: Contraction stress test and modified biophysical profile. *Obstet Gynecol* 1994; 84(2): 231–4. [II-1; Controlled study, not randomized. New surveillance method, modified BPS was compared in a high-risk population to CST. The authors agreed that CST was no longer first line]

45. Manning FA, Platt LD, Sipos L. Antepartum fetal evaluation: Development of a fetal biophysical profile. *Am J Obstet Gynecol* 1980; 136(6): 787–95. [II-1; Blinded study of first clinical BPS application, *n* = 216]

46. Manning FA, Morrison I, Lange IR et al. Fetal assessment based on fetal biophysical profile scoring: Experience in 12,620 referred high-risk pregnancies. I. Perinatal mortality by frequency and etiology. *Am J Obstet Gynecol* 1985; 151(3): 343–50. [III-3; Combined variables provided best indication of perinatal mortality]

47. Manning FA, Morrison I, Harman CR et al. The abnormal fetal biophysical profile score. V. Predictive accuracy according to score composition. *Am J Obstet Gynecol* 1990; 162(4): 918–24. [III-3; Different adverse outcomes are predicted better by different combinations of variables. This study included only fetuses with abnormal scores 131—6/10, 258—4/10, 113—2/10]

48. Chamberlain PF. Later fetal death—Has ultrasound a role to play in its prevention? *Irish J Med Science* 1991; 160: 251–4. [II-3; Application of biophysical profile score in an Irish health care region dropped PNM by more than 60%. Historical/concurrent nonrandomized controls]

49. Baskett TG, Allen AC, Gray JH et al. Fetal biophysical profile and perinatal death. *Obstet Gynecol* 1987; 70: 357–60. [II-2; Concurrent controls had PNM more than double those managed by BPS]

50. Miller DA, Rabello YA, Paul RH. The modified biophysical profile: Antepartum testing in the 1990s. *Am J Obstet Gynecol* 1996; 174: 812–7. [II-2; Large comparative trial of biophysical methodology demonstrated significant difference in outcome of cases managed or not managed by BPS]

51. Platt LD, Walla CA, Paul RH et al. A prospective trial of the fetal biophysical profile versus the nonstress tests in the management of high-risk pregnancies. *Am J Obstet Gynecol* 1985; 153(6): 624–33. [I; RCT; *n* = 652]

52. Vintzileos AM, Campbell WA, Rodis JF et al. The relationship between fetal biophysical assessment, umbilical artery velocimetry and fetal acidosis. *Obstet Gynecol* 1991; 77: 622–6. [II-3; Clinical study showed BPS was superior and Doppler added nothing, in detection of fetal acidosis, *n* = 62]

53. Soothill PW, Ajayi RA, Campbell S et al. Prediction of morbidity in small and normally grown fetuses by fetal heart rate variability, biophysical profile score and umbilical artery Doppler studies. *Br J Obstet Gynaecol* 1993; 100: 742–5. [II-3; Prospective longitudinal study of 191 women studied with all three methods. Doppler discriminated small "sick" fetuses from small normal fetuses, while the other tests did not]

54. Shalev E, Zalel Y, Weiner E. A comparison of the nonstress test, oxytocin challenge test, Doppler velocimetry and biophysical profile in predicting umbilical vein pH in growth-retarded fetuses. *Int J Gynaecol Obstet* 1993; 43: 15–9. [II-3; Clinical series of 23 IUGR fetuses studied by all methods. NST, OCT, and BPS all had positive predictive values of 57% while Doppler was only 14%]

55. Yoon BH, Romero R, Roh CR et al. Relationship between the fetal biophysical profile score, umbilical artery Doppler velocimetry and fetal blood acid-base status determined by cordocentesis. *Am J Obstet Gynecol* 1993; 169: 1586–94. [II-2; Interventional cohort study. Doppler and BPS both had statistically significant association with acidemia and hypercarbia at cordocentesis, but Doppler scored higher in logistic regression, *n* = 24]

56. Bardakci M, Balci O, Acar A et al. Comparison of modified biophysical profile and Doppler ultrasound in predicting the perinatal outcome at or over 36 weeks of gestation. *Gynecol Obstet Invest* 2010; 69(4): 245–50. [II]

57. Lalor JG, Fawole B, Alfirevic Z et al. Biophysical profile for fetal assessment in high risk pregnancies. *Cochrane Database Syst Rev* 2008; 23(1): CD000038. [I; Meta-analysis]

58. Bocking AD, Harding R. Effects of reduced uterine blood flow in electrocortical activity, breathing and skeletal muscle activity in fetal sheep. *Am J Obstet Gynecol* 1986; 154(3): 655–62. [II-1; Controlled study of fetal sheep model showed increased sensitivity to hypoxia in abolishing FBM as gestation progresses]

59. Ribbert LS, Nicolaides KH, Visser GH. Prediction of fetal acidaemia in intrauterine growth retardation: Comparison of quantified fetal activity with biophysical profile score. *Br J Obstet Gynecol* 1993; 100(7): 653–6. [II-2; Comparative trial of multivariable testing methods]

60. Magann EF, Doherty D, Field K et al. Biophysical profile with amniotic fluid volume assessments. *Obstet Gynecol* 2004; 104(1): 5–10. [I; RCT demonstrates lower false positive cases, fewer iatrogenic interventions, more accurate depiction of fetal status with single pocket method compared to AFI]

61. Naghan AF, Abdelmoula YA. Amniotic fluid index versus single deepest vertical pocket: A meta-analysis of randomized controlled trials. *Int J Gynaecol Obstet* 2009; 104(3): 184–8. [I; Meta-analysis]

62. Manning FA, Morrison I, Lange IR et al. Fetal biophysical profile scoring: Selective use of the nonstress test. *Am J Obstet Gynecol* 1987; 156(3): 709–12. [II-3]

63. Manning FA, Snijders R, Harman CR et al. Fetal biophysical profile score. VI. Correlation with antepartum umbilical venous fetal pH. *Am J Obstet Gynecol* 1993; 169(4): 755–63. [II-2; Multicenter clinical trial demonstrates close relationship of multi-variable testing to fetal pH determined by antenatal cordocentesis, *n* = 493]

64. Manning FA, Harman CR, Morrison I et al. Fetal assessment based on fetal biophysical profile scoring. III. Positive predictive accuracy of the very abnormal test (biophysical profile score = 0). *Am J Obstet Gynecol* 1990; 162(2): 398–402. [II-2; A score of 0/10 is rare (9.2/10,000 tests), but has 100% positive predictive value for death or severe permanent handicap, justifying immediate delivery]

65. Nageotte MP, Towers CV, Asrat T et al. Perinatal outcome with the modified biophysical profile. *Am J Obstet Gynecol* 1994; 170(6): 1672–6. [I; RCT; clinical trial valuating BPS (NST plus AFI) with randomized back-up testing (full BPS or CST) for abnormal values. MBPS discrimination well between adverse outcome (RR 2.0) and IUGR (RR 2.2) and those without these outcomes. CST was without benefit and led to iatrogenic morbidity compared to BPS]

66. Phattanachindakun B, Boonyagulsrirung T, Chanprapaph P. The correlation in antepartum fetal test between full fetal biophysical profile (FBP) and rapid biophysical profile (rBPP). *J Med Assoc* 2010; 93(7): 759–64. [II-2]

67. Papadopoulos VG, Decavalas GO, Kondakis XG et al. Vibroacoustic stimulation in abnormal biophysical profile: Verification of facilitation of fetal well-being. *Early Hum Dev* 2007; 83(3): 191–7. [II-3]

68. Manning FA, Morrison I, Harman CR et al. Fetal assessment based on fetal biophysical profile scoring: Experience in 19,221 referred high-risk pregnancies. II. An analysis of false-negative fetal deaths. *Am J Obstet Gynecol* 1987; 157: 880. [II-2]

69. Harman CR, Baschat AA. Arterial and venous Dopplers in IUGR. *Clin Obstet Gynecol* 2003; 46(4): 931–46. [III; Review]

70. Baschat AA, Gembruch R, Reiss I et al. Relationship between arterial and venous Doppler and perinatal outcome in fetal growth restriction. *Ultrasound Obstet Gynecol* 2000; 16: 407–13. [II-3; Time sequence of Doppler in IUGR]

71. Meher S, Hernandez-Andrade E, Basheer SN, Lees C. Impact of cerebral redistribution on neurodevelopmental outcome in small-for-gestational-age or growth-restricted babies: A systematic review. *Ultrasound Obstet Gynecol* 2015; 46(4): 398–404. [III; Review]

72. Bakalis S, Akolekar R, Gallo DM, Poon LC, Nicolaides KH. Umbilical and fetal middle cerebral artery Doppler at 30-34 weeks' gestation in the prediction of adverse perinatal outcome. *Ultrasound Obstet Gynecol* 2015; 45(4): 409–20. [II-3]

73. DeVore GR. The importance of the cerebroplacental ratio in the evaluation of fetal well-being in SGA and AGA fetuses. *Am J Obstet Gynecol* 2015; 213(1): 5–15. [III]

74. Bellotti M, Pennati G, De Gasperi C et al. Simultaneous measurements of umbilical venous, fetal hepatic and ductus venosus blood flow in growth-restricted human fetuses. *Am J Obstet Gynecol* 2004; 190(5): 1347–58. [II-2; Case-control study depicting the progression of ductal opening and increased flow as condition deteriorated in 56 IUGR fetuses]

75. Alfirevic Z, Stampalija T, Gyte GM. Fetal and umbilical Doppler ultrasound in normal pregnancy. *Cochrane Database Syst Rev* 2010; 4(8): CD001450. [I; Meta-analysis; 5 RCTs, n = 14,185]

76. Stampalija T, Gyte GM, Alfirevic Z. Utero-placental Doppler ultrasound for improving pregnancy outcome. *Cochrane Database Syst Rev* 2010; 8(9): CD008363. [I; Meta-analysis, 2 RCTs, n = 4993]

77. Thompson RS, Trudinger BJ. Doppler waveform pulsatility index and resistance, pressure and flow in the umbilical placental circulation: An investigation using a mathematical model. *Ultrasound Med Biol* 1990; 16(5): 449. [III]

78. Maulik D, Mundy D, Heitmann E et al. Evidence-based approach to umbilical artery Doppler fetal surveillance in high-risk pregnancies: An update. *Clin Obstet Gynecol* 2010; 53(4): 869–78. [III]

79. Baschat AA, Weiner CP. Umbilical artery Doppler screening for the small for gestational age fetus in need of antenatal surveillance. *Am J Obstet Gynecol* 2000; 182: 154–8. [II-2; Case-control trial. Umbilical artery Doppler differentiates small fetuses that do not need intensive surveillance from those with serious IUGR]

80. Alfirevic Z, Neilson JP. Doppler ultrasonography in high-risk pregnancies: Systemic review with meta-analysis. *Am J Obstet Gynecol* 1995; 172(5): 1379–87. [I; Meta-analysis; umbilical artery Doppler application reduces perinatal mortality and critical neonatal impacts in IUGR and preeclampsia]

81. Divon MY. Randomized control trials of umbilical artery Doppler velocimetry: How many are too many? *Ultrasound Obstet Gynecol* 1995; 6: 377–9. [III; Review]

82. Alfirevic Z, Stampalija T, Gyte GM. Fetal and umbilical Doppler ultrasound in high-risk pregnancies. *Cochrane Database Syst Rev* 2010; 20(1): CD007529. [I; Meta-analysis; 18 RCTs, n > 10,000]

83. SMFM, Berkley, E et al. Doppler assessment of the fetus with intrauterine growth restriction. *Am J Obstet Gynecol* 2012; 206(4): 300–8. [III; Review]

84. Nelson KB. The epidemiology of cerebral palsy in term infants. *Ment Retard Dev Disabil Res Rev* 2002; 8(3): 146–50. [III; Review]

85. Goffinet F, Paril-Llado J, Nisand I et al. Umbilical artery Doppler velocimetry in unselected and low risk pregnancies: A review of randomized controlled trials. *Br J Obstet Gynaecol* 1997; 104: 425–30. [III; Review]

86. Divon MY, Girz BA, Lieblich R et al. Clinical management of the fetus with markedly diminished umbilical artery end-diastolic flow. *Am J Obstet Gynecol* 1989; 161(6 Pt. 1): 1523–7. [II-2; Case control study of 51 fetuses with severe elevation of umbilical artery resistance. Immediate delivery may not be necessary. Combined surveillance can safely prolong the pregnancy]

87. Thorton JG, Hornbuckle J, Vail A et al. Infant wellbeing at 2 years of age in the Growth Restriction Invervention Trial (GRIT): Multicentered randomized controlled trial. *Lancet* 2004; 364(9433): 513–20. [I]

88. GRIT study group. A randomized trial of timed delivery for the compromised preterm fetus: Short term outcomes and Bayesian interpretation. *Br J Obstet Gynecol* 2003; 110(1): 27–32. [I; Multicenter RCT]

89. Baschat AA, Gembruch U, Reiss I et al. Relationship between arterial and venous Doppler and perinatal outcome in fetal growth restriction. *Ultrasound Obstet Gynecol* 2000; 16(5): 407–13. [II-2; Multicenter cohort study using multivessel Doppler to evaluate severe IUGR. Abnormal venous patterns denoted the worst outcomes, while prematurity retains a critical role]

90. Baschat AA, Gembruch U, Weiner CP et al. Qualitative venous Doppler waveform analysis improves prediction of critical perinatal outcomes in premature growth-restricted fetuses. *Ultrasound Obstet Gynecol* 2003; 22(3): 240–5. [II-2; Cohort study demonstrates combined arterial and venous Doppler maximized prediction of critical outcomes, n = 224]

91. Baschat AA, Cosmi E, Bilardo CM et al. Predictors of neonatal outcome in early-onset placental dysfunction. *Obstet Gynecol* 2007; 109(2 Pt. 1): 253–61. [II-2]

92. Turan OM, Turan S, Berg C et al. The duration of persistent abnormal ductus venosus flow and its impact on perinatal outcome in fetal growth restriction. *Ultrasound Obstet Gynecol* 2011; 38: 295–302. [II-2 Multicenter Study of FGR. Secondary analysis of 175 FGR fetuses with DV abnormality demonstrates that the duration of a-wave reversal is the factor predictive of stillbirth]

93. Lees CC, Marlow N, van Wassenaer-Leemhuis et al. 2 year neurodevelopmental and intermediate perinatal outcomes in infants with very preterm fetal growth restriction (TRUFFLE): A randomised trial. *Lancet* 2015; 385(9983): 2162–72. [I]

94. Baschat AA, Harman CR. Discordance of arterial and venous flow velocity waveforms in severe placenta-based fetal growth restriction. *Ultrasound Obstet Gynecol* 2011; 37(3): 369–70. [II-3]

95. Baschat AA, Galan HL, Bhide A et al. Doppler and biophysical assessment in growth restricted fetuses: Distribution of test results. *Ultrasound Obstet Gynecol* 2006; 27(1): 41–7. [II-1; Multicenter study of combined Doppler and biophysical profile in IUGR suggests both should be used to maximize gestational age, n = 38]

96. Baschat AA, Viscardi RM, Hussey-Gardner B et al. Infant neurodevelopment following fetal growth restriction: Relationship with antepartum surveillance parameters. *Ultrasound Obstet Gynecol* 2009; 33(1): 44–50. [II-3]

97. Baschat AA, Gembruch U, Harman CR. The sequence of changes in Doppler and biophysical parameters as severe fetal growth restriction worsens. *Ultrasound Obstet Gynecol* 2001; 18: 571–7. [II-2]

98. Cosmi E, Ambrosini G, D'Antona D et al. Doppler, cardiotocography, and biophysical profile changes in growth-restricted fetuses. *Obstet Gynecol* 2005; 106(6): 1240–5. [II-2]

99. Tyrrel SN, Lilford RJ, MacDonald HN et al. Randomized comparison of routine vs. highly selective use of Doppler ultrasound and biophysical profile scoring to investigate high risk pregnancies. *Br J Obstet Gynaecol* 1990; 97(10): 909–16. [I; RCT

demonstrating combined Doppler and BPS reduced neonatal morbidity by directing intervention, but did not increase iatrogenic prematurity, n = 500]

100. Habek D, Hodek B, Herman R et al. Fetal biophysical profile and cerebro-umbilical ratio in assessment of perinatal outcome in growth-restricted fetuses. *Fetal Diagn Ther* 2003; 18(1): 12–6. [II-2; Clinical trial demonstrated the complimentary positive predictive values of biophysical profile and Doppler, n = 87 FGR fetuses]

101. Williams KP, Farwuharson DF, Bebbington M et al. Screening for fetal well-being in a high-risk pregnant population comparing the nonstress test with umbilical artery Doppler velocimetry: A randomized controlled clinical trial. *Am J Obstet Gynecol* 2003; 188(5): 1366–71. [I; RCT; Randomized "high-risk" patients, beyond 32 weeks, to umbilical artery Doppler or nonstress testing as primary monitoring, amniotic fluid volume as secondary test]

102. Practice bulletin no. 145: Antepartum fetal surveillance. *Obstet Gynecol* 2014; 124(1): 182–92. [III; Review]

103. Graves CR. Antepartum fetal surveillance and timing of delivery in the pregnancy complicated by diabetes mellitus. *Clin Obstet Gynecol* 2007; 50(4): 1007–13. [II-2]

104. Zisser HC, Biersmith MA, Jovanovic LB et al. Fetal risk assessment in pregnancies complicated by diabetes mellitus. *J Diabetes Sci Technol* 2010; 4(6): 1368–73. [II-3]

105. Maulik D, Lysikiewicz A, Sicuranaza G. Umbilical arterial Doppler sonography for fetal surveillance in pregnancies complicated by pregestational diabetes mellitus. *J Matern Fetal Neonatal Med* 2002; 12(6): 417–22. [III; Review]

106. Harman CR, Menticoglou SM. Fetal surveillance in diabetic pregnancy. *Curr Opin Obstet Gynecol* 1997; 9(2): 83–90. [III; Review]

107. Alfirevic Z, Stampalija T, Gyte GM. Fetal and umbilical Doppler ultrasound in high-risk pregnancies. *Cochrane Database Syst* 2013; 12(11): CD007529. [I; Meta-analysis; 18 studies, n = 10,156]

108. Rath W, Wolff F. Increased risk of stillbirth in older mothers— A rationale for induction of labour before term? *Z Geburtshife Neonatol* 2014; 218(5): 190–4. [III]

109. Walker KF, Bugg G, Macpherson M et al. Induction of labour versus expectant management for nulliparous woumen over 35 years of age: A multi-centre prospective, randomized controlled trial. *BMC Pregnancy Childbirth* 2012; 12: 145. [I]

110. Davies GA, Maxwell C, McLeod L et al. Obesity in pregnancy. *J Obstet Gynaecol Can* 2010; 32(2): 165–73. [II-3]

111. Ehrenberg HM, Mercer BM, Catalano PM. The influence of obesity and diabetes on the prevalence of macrosomia. *Am J Obstet Gynecol* 2004; 191(3): 964–8. [II-2]

112. Chu SY, Kim SY, Lau J et al. Maternal obesity and risk of stillbirth: A metaanalysis. *Am J Obstet Gynecol* 2007; 197(3): 223–8. [I; Meta-analysis]

113. Vintzileos AM, Bors-Koefoed R, Pelegano JF et al. The use of fetal biophysical profile improves pregnancy outcome in premature rupture of the membranes. *Am J Obstet Gynecol* 1987; 157(2): 236–40. [II-2]

114. Lewis DF, Adair CD, Weeks JW et al. A randomized clinical trial of daily nonstress testing versus biophysical profile in the management of preterm premature rupture of membranes. *Am J Obstet Gynecol* 1999; 181(6): 1495–9. [I; RCT of two schemes of monitoring patients after PPROM. Both NST and BPS had good specificity, but detected less than half the babies who developed infectious complications]

115. Cotton DB, Gonik B, Bottoms SF. Conservative vs aggressive management of preterm rupture of membranes. A randomized trial of amniocentesis. *Am J Perinatol* 1984; 1: 322–4. [I]

116. Carlan SJ, Richmond LB, O'Brien WF. Randomized trial of endovaginal ultrasound in preterm premature rupture of membranes. *Obstet Gynecol* 1997; 89(3): 458–61. [I]

117. Sharp GC, Stock SJ, Norman JE. Fetal assessment methods for improving neonatal and maternal outcomes in preterm prelabour rupture of membranes. *Cochrane Database Syst Rev* 2014; 3(10): CD010209. [I; Meta-analysis]

118. Sanchez-Ramos L, Olivier F, Delke I, Kaunitz A M. Labor induction versus expectant management for postterm pregnancies: A systematic review with meta-analysis. *Obstetrics and Gynecology* 2003; 101(6): 1312–8 [Meta-analysis; 16 RCTs, n = 6588]

119. Mackeen AD, Edelson PK, Wisch S et al. Antenatal testing in uncomplicated pregnancies: Should testing be initiated after 40 or 41 weeks? *J Perinat Med* 2015; 43(2): 233–7. [II-2]

120. Clinical Practice Obstetrics Committee; Maternal Fetal Medicine Committee, Delaney M, Roggensack A, Leduc DC et al. Guidelines for the management of pregnancy at 41 +0 to 42+0 weeks. *J Obstet Gynaecol Can* 2008; 30(9): 800–23. [III]

121. Mari G. Middle cerebral artery peak systemic velocity: Is it the standard of care for the diagnosis of fetal anemia? *J Ultrasound Med* 2005; 24(5): 697–702. [III; Review]

122. Divakaran TG, Waugh J, Clark TJ et al. Noninvasive techniques to detect fetal anemia due to red blood cell alloimmunization: A systemic review. *Obstet Gynecol* 2001; 98(3): 509–17. [I; Meta-analysis suggests MCA Doppler lacks precision and the studies are incomplete]

123. Illanes S, Soothill P. Management of red cell alloimmunisation in pregnancy: The non-invasive monitoring of the disease. *Prenat Diagn* 2010; 30(7): 668–73. [III; Review]

124. Mari G, Norton ME, Stone J et al. Society for Maternal-Fetal Medicine (SMFM) Clinical Guideline #8: The fetus at risk of anemia—Diagnosis and management. *Am J Obstet Gynecol* 2015; 212(6): 697–701. [III; Review]

125. ACOG Committee Opinion No. 474: Nonobstetric surgery during pregnancy. *Obstet Gynecol* 2011; 117: 420–1. [III; Review]

126. Unterscheider J, Daly S, Geary MP, Kennelly MM et al. Definition and management of fetal growth restriction: A survey of contemporary attitudes. *Eur J Obstet Gynecol Reprod Biol* 2014; 174: 41–5. [III]

57

Sonographic assessment of amniotic fluid: oligohydramnios and polyhydramnios

Ibrahim A. Hammad and Suneet P. Chauhan

AMNIOTIC FLUID ASSESSMENT IN SINGLETON PREGNANCIES
Key Points
- Ultrasound estimates of amniotic fluid volume (AFV) correlate poorly with dye-determined or directly measured oligohydramnios and polyhydramnios.
- **The single deepest pocket (SDP) is the best ultrasound technique to estimate AFV** in both singleton and twin gestations because the amniotic fluid index (AFI) overdiagnoses oligohydramnios.
- **AFI should be abandoned, and SDP should be used instead in most situations for clinical decisions because AFI use leads to unnecessary inductions and operative deliveries without concomitant neonatal benefit.**

Background
- Urine production: urethra patent at 8 to 9 weeks; 18 weeks: about 50 to 100 cc/day; term: 800 cc/day or 5 cc/kg/hr. The primary component of amniotic fluid (AF) in the second half of pregnancy is fetal urine.
- AF swallowing: half of AF/day (about 0.5 L/day at term).
- Lungs also produce and absorb AF. Other systems involved include skin, saliva/nasal, membranes/placenta/cord.
- The fetus with in utero placental insufficiency will shunt blood flow to the brain, heart, and adrenal glands at the expense of the rest of the organ systems including the kidneys. Inadequate renal perfusion will result in decreased urinary output and oligohydramnios.

Indications
AFV can help in the assessment of the following:

In the second trimester,
- o Evidence of **fetal anomalies** (e.g., urinary obstruction or dysfunction)
- o Severe **fetal growth restriction (FGR; associated** with fetal aneuploidy)
- o Assist in the confirmation of preterm premature rupture of the fetal membranes **(PPROM)**

In the late second and third trimesters of pregnancy, as above, plus
- o Used along with the nonstress test (NST) or with the other components of the biophysical profile (BPP) in the **assessment of fetal well being** in pregnancies at risk for an adverse outcome.

Techniques
AFV can be precisely measured antepartum by a dye-dilution technique (the dye marker is placed into the uterine cavity by amniocentesis) and directly at the time of cesarean delivery.

These measurement techniques are invasive, time-consuming, require laboratory support, and if measured at cesarean can only be done at the time of delivery. Because of these limitations, the AFV is estimated antepartum by ultrasound.

Following are three ultrasound methods of **estimating AFV** and identifying abnormalities of fluid:

- The subjective assessment evaluates the AFV without measurements and labels the observed volume as low, normal, or high. It is usually done at the time of the second trimester ultrasound between 16 and 24 weeks [1].
- The **AFI**, divides the abdomen into four quadrants and measures the SDP in each quadrant without fetal small parts or cord and sums the measurements [2]. AFI ≤5.0 is labeled as oligohydramnios, 5.1 to 20 as normal, and >20–25 as hydramnios [3]. The AFI can also be evaluated more accurately by gestational age (GA)-specific charts that label AFV as oligohydramnios (<5th percentile), normal (5th–95th percentile), and hydramnios (>95th percentile) [4,5].
- The **SDP** technique (also called **maximum vertical pocket, MVP**) identifies the deepest vertical pocket of fluid that has a horizontal measurement of at least 1 cm and is without cord or fetal small parts [6]. SDP ≤2 is consistent with oligohydramnios, 2 to 8 cm is normal, and >8 cm is hydramnios.

Originally, the pocket of fluid was measured if it did not have an aggregate of cord or small parts [3]. There is a significantly greater number of low dye-determined AFVs identified using the **"to the cord"** measurement technique rather than "through the cord" and without any difference for normal and high dye-determined volumes [7]. Therefore, the "to the cord" measurement is recommended.

Accuracy of Ultrasound to Identify Oligohydramnios
By direct measurements at the time of cesarean delivery or dye-determined fluid volumes, all three of the ultrasound techniques used to estimate AFV (subjective evaluation, AFI, SDP) can identify normal volumes but poorly identify oligohydramnios and hydramnios [8]. The cumulative world's literature shows that the association between ultrasound measurements and normal actual volume is good (sensitivity of 70%–98%), but in the clinically concerning area of oligohydramnios the association between an ultrasound-estimated AFV and the actual volume is poor (sensitivity of 6%–18%) [1,8–16]. A comparison of the third and fifth percentiles of the AFI and SDP adjusted for GA and the fixed cutoffs of

an AFI of ≤5 and the SDP of ≤2, all compared to actual AFVs [17], showed that the percentiles were no better predictors of actual oligohydramnios. Additionally, the normal values and percentiles for one specific patient population do not correlate with different patient populations, and, if percentiles are used, then normative values should be established for each patient population [4,5].

Despite the fact that subjective assessment of fluid is as accurate in identifying abnormalities of AFV as SDP or AFI, we recommend measurement of the deepest pocket (SDP) because it is linked with adverse outcome, and its use in BPP has been shown to decrease the rate of perinatal mortality and cerebral palsy.

Use of Color Doppler to Estimate AFV

Color Doppler has been suggested to increase the detection of oligohydramnios by identifying pockets of fluid containing the umbilical cord that would not be detected by grayscale. Both the measurements of the AFI and the SDP are decreased by approximately 20% with the use of color Doppler compared with grayscale [18,19]. In a study comparing color Doppler versus grayscale to determine if the color Doppler identified more dye-determined oligohydramnios than grayscale, color Doppler not only did not identify any more dye-determined oligohydramnios but labeled a number of normal pregnancies as having oligohydramnios [19]. Because of the overdiagnosis of oligohydramnios and because its use has not been to correlate with peripartum outcomes, **the use of color Doppler cannot be recommended in the ultrasound estimate of AFV.**

Accuracy of the Ultrasound Estimates of AF to Predict Pregnancy Outcomes

Although the subjective estimation of AFV is as accurate as the AFI and SDP in the identification of dye-determined low, normal, and high AFVs [1], nearly all ultrasound evaluation and studies use either the AFI or the SDP technique.

The role of the AFI in classifying a pregnancy as high risk on antenatal testing remains uncertain. An AFI of ≤5 is associated with an increased risk of nonreassuring fetal heart tracing (NRFHT) in labor, meconium-stained AF, cesarean delivery for NRFHT, and low Apgar scores at one and five minutes [3,20]. Some investigators have found no association with an AFI <5 and adverse pregnancy outcomes [21,22]. Among diabetic patients, AFI <5.0 cm is not associated with cesarean delivery for NRFHT [23]. In postdate pregnancies and other high-risk pregnancies screened **comparing the SDP with the AFI, the AFI labels more pregnancies as having oligohydramnios** (relative risk [RR] 2.39, 95% confidence intervals [CI] 1.73–3.28), **resulting in more labor inductions** (RR 1.92; 95% CI 1.50–2.46) **and subsequent cesarean deliveries for NRFHT** (RR 1.46; 95% CI 1.08–1.96) **without a concomitant decrease in the likelihood of admission to neonatal intensive care unit** (RR 1.04; 95% CI 0.85, 1.26) **or in umbilical arterial pH <7.10** (RR 1.10; 95% CI 0.74, 1.65) [24].

Cesarean deliveries for NRFHT and Apgar scores of <7 at five minutes occurs in a significantly greater number of women if the AFI is ≤5 compared to controls [25]. Both the Apgar score <7 at five minutes and cesarean delivery for NRFHT are subjective evaluations and can be influenced by a number of factors. The most objective assessment, umbilical arterial pH, has not been linked with an AFI ≤5.0 [25].

The above findings were confirmed in a meta-analysis that included 43 studies and over 244,490 fetuses [26].

Do We Estimate AFV with the SDP or the AFI?

Both the AFI as a component of the modified BPP (NST + AFV estimation) and the SDP as part of the BPP (fetal movement, fetal breathing, fetal tone, NST, AFV estimation) are used extensively to monitor at-risk preterm pregnancies. While both fluid estimations have been linked with fetal intolerance of labor, cesarean deliveries for NRFHT, and low Apgar scores, **only the SDP as a component of the BPP has been correlated with the umbilical cord pH** [27]. In addition **as a standalone test the SDP has been linked with perinatal morbidity and mortality** [28] while the AFI has never been evaluated as a standalone test for this outcome. No investigations have evaluated the AFI with the NST in the prediction of cerebral palsy. A low BPP is associated with antenatal asphyxial events, and may be of use in selected pregnancies to prevent poor pregnancy outcomes [29,30].

The AFI has been compared with the SDP as a component of the modified BPP (NST + AFI or SDP), the BPP (fetal movement, fetal tone, fetal breathing movement, NST, and AFI or SDP) in the antepartum evaluation of at-risk pregnancies and as a fetal admission test. In high-risk pregnancies monitored using the BPP [31], **the AFI and SDP are similar in their predictability of adverse antepartum or intrapartum outcomes; however, the AFI labels twice as many women with low fluid compared to the SDP, resulting in more interventions without any improvement in outcome.** In high-risk pregnancies undergoing *modified* BPP, more women are labeled as having low fluid by the AFI with more interventions without any improvement in outcome compared to the SDP [32]. As intrapartum screening tests, neither AFI nor SDP are found to be predictive of adverse intrapartum outcomes [33].

In summary, **both the AFI and the SDP poorly predict oligohydramnios.** The AFI + NST have been linked to perinatal morbidity and mortality but not to umbilical cord pH at delivery. The AFI as a standalone test has not been linked to perinatal morbidity or mortality. The SDP as a component of the BPP has been correlated to perinatal morbidity and mortality, umbilical cord pH at delivery, and cerebral palsy, and as a standalone test the SDP has been independently linked with perinatal mortality [34]. Directly compared, the AFI and SDP are similar in their prediction of outcomes, but the AFI overcalls the diagnosis of oligohydramnios leading to increased interventions and more operative deliveries without any improvement in perinatal outcomes. For these reasons, **the SDP appears to be the better ultrasound estimator of AFV to use with the NST or the BPP.**

Management

In pregnancies at-risk for an adverse pregnancy outcome, antenatal surveillance can be undertaken with either the **NST and SDP** technique or the **BPP using the SDP** technique to assess the AFV. If an estimation of the AFV is undertaken on admission to labor and delivery to identify those pregnancies that will have a greater risk of intrapartum complications, then the SDP techniques should also be used.

A *Cochrane* review (5 trials with 3226 pregnancies) **comparing AFI to SDP** showed that there was no improvement in peripartum outcomes, like operative vaginal or cesarean delivery, Apgar score <7 at 5 min, admission to NICU, and umbilical artery pH less than 7.1. **The diagnosis of oligohydramnios is more frequent (RR 2.39; 95% CI 1.73, 3.28) when AFI rather than SDP is used as well as induction of labor and rate of cesarean deliveries for fetal distress (RR 1.46; 95% CI 1.08, 1.96) [35].**

OLIGOHYDRAMNIOS
Key Points

- **Oligohydramnios** should be defined as **an SDP <2 cm. This definition correlates with abnormal neonatal outcome with the least false positive rate.** Using the AFI (e.g., <5th percentile for gestational age or <5.0 cm) is not recommended to define oligohydramnios.
- **Question** the woman concerning **(P)PROM.**
- **Document** by ultrasound **normal fetal kidneys, bladder, and fetal weight.**
- **Suggest hydration** with 2 L of water orally.

At 16 to 22 weeks

- Consider **amniocentesis**.
- Consider transabdominal amnioinfusion for better diagnostic visualization. The role of amnioinfusion as therapy for pregnancy prolongation and prevention of pulmonary hypoplasia has not been tested in a trial.

At 23 to 40 weeks

- Consider intervention as for 16 to 22 weeks if severe oligohydramnios and fetal karyotype and anatomy have not been checked before.
- At ≥23 weeks, perform NST and/or BPP to assure fetal well being. If reassuring, continue SDP/NST weekly/biweekly depending on fetal status.
- **At ≥36 weeks, consider induction/delivery if SDP <2.0 cm.**

At >40 weeks

- Deliver.
- Transcervical amnioinfusion can be discussed and offered to women at or near term with oligohydramnios, but data are limited regarding safety and efficacy.

Diagnosis/Definition
Oligohydramnios should be defined as low AFV that is linked with an adverse pregnancy outcome. Therefore, oligohydramnios can be defined as an **SDP of <2 cm** measured vertically.

Epidemiology/Incidence
The true incidence of oligohydramnios appears to be approximately 0.2% in the second trimester and 3% to 5% in the third trimester. The incidence depends on definition, being lower when defined as SDP <2 cm.

Etiology
ROM, renal hypofunction, urinary obstruction, placental insufficiency with/without FGR.

Complications
Fetal anomalies (up to 30% in second trimester, up to 50% if severe). Oligohydramnios, in particular SDP <2 cm, has been associated with FGR, NRFHT, CD for NRFHT, endometritis, etc., but the true natural history is not well-known since many intervene for oligohydramnios.

There is a significant association between oligohydramnios, small for gestational age, neonatal death, and perinatal mortality [26]. Isolated oligohydramnios at term by itself is not associated in some studies with increased obstetrical morbidity [36].

Management (Figure 57.1)
Question woman concerning **(P)PROM**, and perform clinical exam if (P)PROM suspected.

The ultrasound should document normal **fetal kidneys, bladder, stomach bubble and fetal weight**.

At 16 to 22 weeks: consider amniocentesis, if feasible. Also consider transabdominal amnioinfusion for better diagnostic visualization. The role of amnioinfusion as therapy for pregnancy prolongation and prevention of pulmonary hypoplasia has not been tested in a trial.

At 23 to 40 weeks, consider intervention as for 16 to 24 weeks if severe oligohydramnios and fetal karyotype and anatomy have not been checked before.

At ≥28 to <36 weeks, perform NST and/or BPP to assure fetal well being. If reassuring, continue SDP/NST weekly/biweekly depending on fetal status.

- a. If SDP is ≥2, follow with weekly NST/SDP.
- b. If SDP <2, manage individually (suggest at least twice weekly NST/AFIs).
    Consider delivery only if there are substantial signs of fetal compromise, such as abnormal BPP, UA Doppler flow, NST, etc.
- c. If SDP normalizes in the consecutive ultrasounds, these patients can be followed with routine care.
- d. **For any oligohydramnios, strongly encourage maternal hydration with 2 L water and reassess AFV.**

At ≥36 weeks, consider induction/delivery if SDP <2. If SDP ≥2, follow with NST/SDP.

Maternal Hydration
The effects of maternal hydration on the AFV as estimated by an increase in the AFI or an increase in fetal urine production, have been assessed in four randomized trials [37–40]. The meta-analysis [41] of these four trials with 122 women concluded that **hydration (by drinking water or by intravenous route) increases AF as assessed by pre- and post-hydration AFI.** For oral hydration, the women were asked to **drink 2 L of water** before having a repeat ultrasound examination. Maternal hydration in women with and without oligohydramnios was associated with an increase in amniotic volume (mean difference [MD] for women with oligohydramnios 2.01, 95% confidence interval [CI] 1.43 to 2.60; and MD for women with normal AFV 4.50, 95% CI 2.92 to 6.08).

Intravenous hypotonic hydration in women with oligohydramnios was associated with an increase in AFV (MD 1.35, 95% CI 0.61–2.10). Isotonic intravenous hydration had no measurable effect. These findings were confirmed by a fifth randomized trial in which **pregnancies complicated by third trimester idiopathic oligohydramnios**

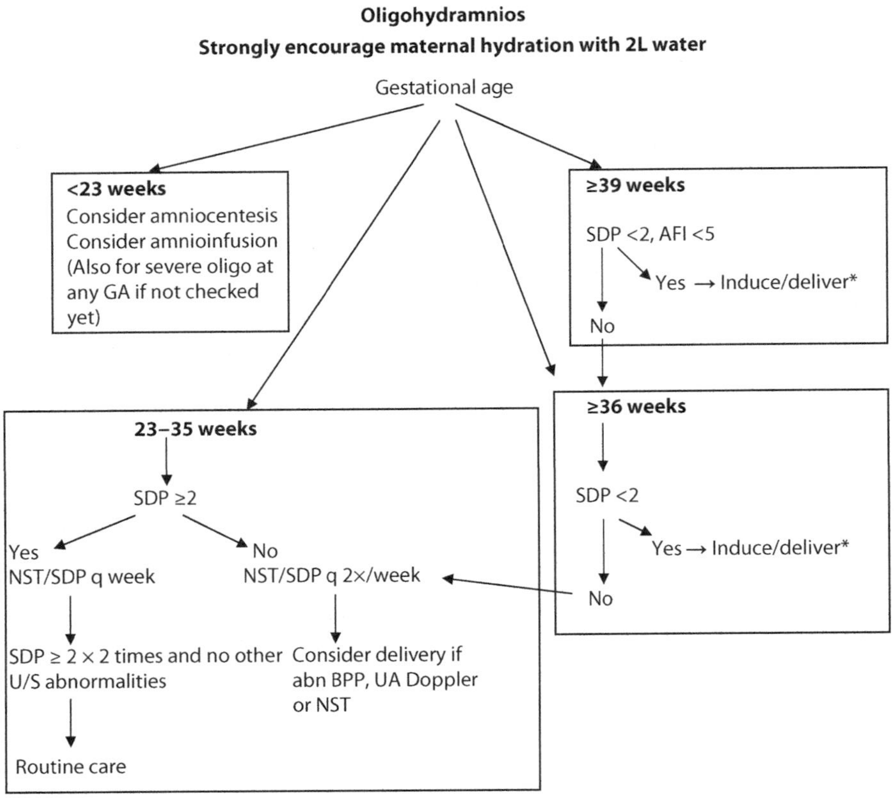

Oligohydramnios
Strongly encourage maternal hydration with 2L water

Figure 57.1 Management of oligohydramnios. *, Amnioinfusion for labor at ≥34 weeks: cesarean delivery for obstetrical indications; BPP, biophysical profile; GA, gestational age; NST, non-stress test; oligo, oligohydramnios; q, every; SDP, single deepest pocket; UA, umbilical artery; U/S, ultrasound.

found that **long-term hydration (six days) of intravenous isotonic infusion (1500 mL/day) increased the mean AFI from 39.7 to 77.7 mm**. Patients were then randomized to home oral hydration therapy of 1500 or 2500 mL/day and the higher volume group demonstrated significantly increased amniotic fluid at delivery compared to the lower volume group (112.45 ± 14.92 versus 86.21 ± 16.89 mm, respectively $p < .001$). [42] However, it is notable that, **no clinically important outcomes have been assessed** in these four trials [41]. Thus, while oral hydration seems safe and helpful, additional trials assessing clinical benefits are warranted before hydration is recommended in the setting of oligohydramnios [41].

Amnioinfusion
If oligohydramnios (without PROM) is detected just before or in **labor near or at term**:

- **Transabdominal amnioinfusion**: reduces NRFHT (from 42% to 5%) and CD for NRFHT (from 25% to 5%) [43].
- **Transcervical amnioinfusion**: In term women with oligo (usually AFI <5 cm), amnioinfusion of usually about 500 cc normal saline and more as needed decreases CD for NRFHT by 77%, overall CD by 48%, umbilical artery pH <7.20 by 60%, NRFHT by 76%, and low Apgar scores <7 at five minutes by 48%. The rate of endometritis tended to be lower with amnioinfusion [44–46]. There is

no difference in outcomes in one RCT between prophylactic vs. therapeutic amnioinfusion (47).

Given better results and a lot more data with this latter technique, prophylactic **transcervical amnioinfusion should be offered to women at or near term with oligohydramnios.**

POLYHYDRAMNIOS (AKA HYDRAMNIOS)
Key Points

- Polyhydramnios is defined as an **SDP ≥8 or AFI ≥95th percentile (AFI ≥24)** or ≥97.5 percentile (AFI >25) **for GA**. AFI >24 or subjective assessment of increased fluid volume are all labeled as polyhydramnios at any GA. Severe polyhydramnios is a SDP ≥15 cm or AFI of ≥35.1 cm.
- **Major associations are diabetes and fetal malformation, but up to 50% of mild polyhydramnios is of unknown cause (idiopathic).**
- **Risk of major anomaly at birth after normal ultrasound is 1% with AFI <30, 2% with AFI 30 to 34.9, 11% with AFI ≥35 cm.**
- Polyhydramnios is associated with higher rates of **macrosomia, malpresentation, cord prolapse, abruption, primary cesarean delivery, and uterine atony.**
- **Workup should include** (at least) a **glucose screening test**, antibody screen if not done in last four weeks, RPR,

and accurate fetal anatomy ultrasound. Parvovirus, toxoplasma, and CMV IgM and IgG can be included. Amniocentesis should be strongly considered if there is severe polyhydramnios, hydramnios with fetal anomaly on ultrasound, polyhydramnios associated with FGR or detected <24 weeks.

Diagnosis/Definition

SDP ≥8 or **AFI ≥95th percentile (AFI ≥24)** or ≥97.5 percentile (AFI >25) **for GA** or subjective assessment of increased AF. Any of these ultrasound measurements or if subjectively the AF is present then the AF would be labeled as polyhydramnios. Mild polyhydramnios AFI ≥25 to 30, moderate AFI 30.1 to 35, **severe polyhydramnios AFI ≥35.1** [48,49]. Severe polyhydramnios can also be defined as **SDP ≥12**.

Incidence/Epidemiology

1% to 5% of pregnancies depending on definition, but <1% severe polyhydramnios.

Etiology

Increased production (most commonly maternal diabetes) or decreased clearance (obstruction or poor swallowing). Most common causes are 1) maternal diabetes (20%–30%), [2] fetal malformations (10%–15%), [3] multiple gestations (5%), Rh or other isoimmunization, "Mirror syndrome," others; unknown cause (about 50%, especially for mild polyhydramnios). Severe polyhydramnios is usually pathologic, not idiopathic.

Complications

Fetal anomalies may be present (risk of major anomaly on prenatal ultrasound: 8% with AFI <30, 12% with AFI 30 to 34.9, 31% with AFI ≥35. **Risk of major anomaly at birth after normal ultrasound: 1% with AFI <30, 2% with AFI 30 to 34.9, 11% with AFI ≥35.** Fetus may have chromosomal abnormality (risk of aneuploidy: ≤1% if normal ultrasound, about 10% if major anomaly present). Detailed ultrasound should detect about 60% to 80% of major anomalies associated with polyhydramnios. Perinatal mortality for normal anatomy fetuses is <5%. For anomalous fetuses is 10% to 80% depending on anomaly [50]. There is an association between the frequencies of a variety of adverse pregnancy outcomes and the severity of polyhydramnios as reflected by the maximal AFI [51] Preterm birth (PTB) by preterm labor (PTL) or PPROM is increased especially with severe polyhydramnios. Polyhydramnios is associated with higher rates of **macrosomia, malpresentation, cord prolapse, abruption, primary cesarean delivery and uterine atony.** Idiopathic polyhydramnios is linked with fetal macrosomia, fetal labor intolerance, low five minute Apgar scores, greater risk for newborn intensive care unit admission, and **a two- to fivefold increase in perinatal mortality** [52,53]. In the Cochrane meta-analysis, there was no evidence of an association between polyhydramnios and birth weight <10th centile or <2500 g, Apgar score at 1 minute <7, fetal distress or neonatal death. There was a strong positive association with polyhydramnios and birthweight >90th centile and this corresponded to low sensitivity with high specificity [26].

Workup (Differential Diagnosis)

History: **Diabetes mellitus**. Rh isoimmunization and diabetes insipidus. Family history of myotonic dystrophy or inborn errors of metabolism. Ask regarding maternal discomfort.

Ultrasound: Multiple gestation (in particular TTTS).

CNS/Neuro: Anencephaly, holoprosencephaly, Dandy Walker malformation, lissencephaly, agenesis of corpus callosum, NTD, etc.

Neuromuscular: Arthrogryposis.

Cardiac: Septal defects, truncus arteriosus, aortic coartation, arch interruption, arrhythmias, etc.

Thoracic: CDH, CCAM, sequestration, chylothorax, tracheal atresia.

GI: Cleft lip/palate, TE fistula, esophageal or intestinal atresia, inperforate anus, abdominal wall defects, annular pancreas.

Skeletal: Achondroplasia, thanatophoric dysplasia, campomelic dysplasia, OI, hypophosphatasia, etc.

Other: Cystic hygroma, neck masses, goiter, SCT [54]. Rule out hydrops. Perform umbilical and middle cerebral artery (PI and PSV) Doppler.

Laboratory: One hour glucola and antibody screen if not done in last four weeks. Parvovirus IgM and IgG; Toxo IgM and IgG; CMV IgM and IgG; RPR (r/o syphilis).

Amniocentesis: *Strongly consider if* **severe polyhydramnios, hydramnios with fetal major or minor anomaly on ultrasound, polyhydramnios associated with IUGR or detected <24 weeks.** Some advocate offering amniocentesis to all women with polyhydramnios given the 0.5% to 1% incidence of aneuploidy. If *amniocentesis* is done:

1. Karyotype (T21, T18, 45X: most common) and/or microarray.
2. PCR for parvovirus, CMV, toxoplasmosis, syphilis.
3. Myotonic dystrophy study if positive family history or ultrasound evidence of hypotonia, for example, clubbed feet or positional abnormalities of the extremities [54].
4. Inborn errors of metabolism: Gaucher, gangliosidoses, mucopolysaccharidoses, etc. (consider especially if positive family history or above workup negative and severe polyhydramnios).

Labor Precautions

For appropriate management to decrease complications from polyhydramnios—associated macrosomia, malpresentation, cord prolapse, abruption, primary cesarean delivery and uterine atony, see appropriate chapters. Consider delaying or avoiding artificial ROM to avoid cord prolapse or at least "needling" the membranes.

Management

- Appropriate **counseling** regarding complications as above.
- **Workup** as above.
- Manage anomaly/aneuploidy/maternal or fetal disease if detected during workup.
- GA <23 weeks: consider amniocentesis.
- GA 23 to 38 6/7 weeks:
  - AFI <30 cm: AFI/SDP every two to three weeks.
  - AFIs ≥30 cm: AFI/SDP and evaluations to rule out fetal hydrops weekly. Consider weekly NSTs or BPP. Consider amniocentesis.

- AFI ≥35 cm, SDP ≥12, and/or maternal symptoms: as per severe polyhydramnios, plus consider the following options:
  - Amnioreduction: goal to normalize AFV; 1.5% complication rate, such as PPROM, chorioamnionitis, abruptio, membrane detachment. Associated with PTL/PPROM, and also abruptio if >2 L taken out at one time.
  - NSAID therapy.
    - Indomethacin: 75 to 200 mg/day (25–50 mg po q6–8h). Mechanism of action: decreases fetal urine production by increasing proximal tubular resorption of water and sodium. Side effects: Oligohydramnios and ductal closure (see Chapter 16 in *Obstetric Evidence Based Guidelines*). Only treat for 48 hours and <32 weeks to avoid/minimize side effects.
    - Sulindac: 200 mg q12h. Same mechanism of action and side effects as indomethacin.
  - For idiopathic hydramnios, consider antenatal testing beginning at diagnosis or 28 weeks.
- GA ≥39 weeks: induction/delivery for maternal discomfort in severe polyhydramnios. Cesarean delivery for obstetrical indications only. Induction and delivery for idiopathic polyhydramnios.

AMNIOTIC FLUID ASSESSMENT IN TWIN PREGNANCIES
Background
In twin pregnancies the AFV of each sac is about the same (slightly exceeds) that for normal singleton pregnancies of similar third-trimester GA [55].

Technique
The most consistent method of estimating AFV in twin pregnancies is the **SDP** technique. The dividing membrane is identified and the SDP of AF in each amniotic sac is measured. Since the AFVs of twin pregnancies are similar to single pregnancies, **the same categories of oligohydramnios (SDP <2), normal (2–8 cm) and hydramnios (>8 cm) can be used**.

The summated AFI technique [56,57], which measures sums the four SDPs as have been identified in singleton pregnancies and without regard to membrane placement or fetal position, is inaccurate. When correlated to known AFVs in twin pregnancies, it has low sensitivity for intertwin differences in AFV and cannot identify twin pairs with either oligohydramnios or hydramnios [58]. The subjective evaluation of the amount of AF surrounding each fetus, when correlated with dye-determined AFVs in diamniotic twins, has been found to be as accurate as the AFI and SDP in the identification of oligohydramnios (all of the ultrasound techniques poorly identify AFVs) [59].

Management of Oligohydramnios and/or Hydramnios
In dichorionic, diamniotic twin pregnancies, workup and management of either oligohydramnios or hydramnios is similar to singleton gestations. If SDP <2 in one sac and SDP >8 in the other sac are found in a monochorionic gestation,

the diagnosis of twin–twin transfusion syndrome should be considered with workup and management covered in Chapter 44.

REFERENCES

1. Magann EF, Perry KG, Chauhan SP et al. The accuracy of ultrasound evaluation of amniotic fluid volume in singleton pregnancies. The effect of operator experience and ultrasound interpretive technique. *J Clin Ultrasound* 1997; 25: 249–53. [II-2]
2. Phelan JP, Ahn MO, Smith CV. Amniotic fluid index measurements during pregnancy. *J Reprod Med* 1987; 32: 601–4. [II-3]
3. Rutherford SE, Smith CV, Phelan JP et al. The four quadrant assessment of amniotic fluid volume; an adjunct to antepartum fetal heart rate testing. *Obstet Gynecol* 1987; 87: 353–6. [II-3]
4. Moore TR, Cayle TE. The amniotic fluid index in normal human pregnancy. *Am J Obstet Gynecol* 1990; 162: 1168–73. [II-2]
5. Magann EF, Sanderson M, Martin JN Jr et al. The amniotic fluid index, single deepest pocket, and two-diameter pocket in normal human pregnancy. *Am J Obstet Gynecol* 2000; 182: 1581–8. [II-2]
6. Manning FA, Platt LD, Sipos L. Antepartum fetal evaluation: Development of a fetal biophysical profile. *Am J Obstet Gynecol* 1980; 136: 787–95. [II-3]
7. Magann EF, Chauhan SP, Washington W et al. Ultrasound estimation of amniotic fluid volume using the largest vertical pocket containing umbilical cord: Measure to or through the cord? *Ultrasound Obstet Gynecol* 2002; 20: 464–7. [II-2]
8. Magann EF, Nolan TE, Hess LW. Measurement of amniotic fluid volume: Accuracy of ultrasonography techniques. *Am J Obstet Gynecol* 1992; 167: 1533. [II-2]
9. Croom CS, Banias BB, Ramos-Santos E. Do semiquantitative amniotic fluid indexes reflect actual volume. *Am J Obstet Gynecol* 1992; 167: 995. [II-2]
10. Dildy GA, Lira N, Moise KJ. Amniotic fluid volume assessment: Comparison of ultrasonographic estimates versus direct measurement with a dye-dilution technique in human pregnancy. *Am J Obstet Gynecol* 1992; 167: 986. [II-2]
11. Horsager R, Nathan L, Leveno KJ. Correlation of measured amniotic fluid volume and sonographic predictions of oligohydramnios. *Am J Obstet Gynecol* 1994; 83: 955. [II-3]
12. Sepulveda W, Flack NJ, Fisk NM. Direct volume measurement at midtrimester amnioinfusion in relation to ultrasonographic indexes of amniotic fluid volume. *Am J Obstet Gynecol* 1994; 170: 1160–3. [II-3]
13. Magann EF, Morton ML, Nolan TE et al. Comparative efficacy of two sonographic measurements for the detection of aberrations in the amniotic fluid volume and the effect of amniotic fluid volume on pregnancy outcome. *Obstet Gynecol* 1994; 83: 959–62. [II-2]
14. Magann EF, Nevils BD, Chauhan SP et al. Low amniotic fluid volume is poorly identified in singleton and twin pregnancies using the 2 × 2 pocket technique of the biophysical profile. *South Med J* 1999; 92: 802–5. [II-2]
15. Chauhan SP, Magann EF, Morrison JC et al. Ultrasonographic assessment of amniotic fluid volume does not reflect actual volume. *Am J Obstet Gynecol* 1997; 177: 291–7. [II-2]
16. Magann EF, Chauhan SP, Martin JN Jr. Oligohydramnios at term and pregnancy outcome. *Fetal Matern Med Rev* 2001; 12: 209–27. [II-3]
17. Magann EF, Doherty DA, Chauhan SP et al. How well do the amniotic fluid index and single deepest pocket indices (below the 3rd and the 5th and above the 95th and 97th percentiles) predict oligohydramnios and hydramnios? *Am J Obstet Gynecol* 2004; 190: 164–9. [II-2]
18. Bianco A, Rosen T, Kuczynski E et al. Measurement of the amniotic fluid index with and without color Doppler. *J Perinat Med* 1999; 27: 245–9. [II-2]
19. Magann EF, Chauhan SP, Barrilleaux S et al. Ultrasound estimate of amniotic fluid volume: Color Doppler overdiagnosis of oligohydramnios. *Obstet Gynecol* 2001; 98: 71–4. [II-2]

20. Miller DA, Rabello YA, Paul RH. The modified biophysical profile: Antepartum testing in the 1990s. *Am J Obstet Gynecol* 1996; 174: 812–7. [II-3]

21. Magann EF, Chauhan SP, Kinsella MJ et al. Antenatal testing among 1001 high risk women: The role of the ultrasonographic estimate of amniotic fluid volume. *Am J Obstet Gynecol* 1999; 180: 1330–6. [II-3]

22. Garmel SH, Chelmow D, Sha SJ et al. Oligohydramnios and the appropriately grown fetus. *Am J Perinat* 1997; 14: 359–63. [II-3]

23. Kjos SL, Leung A, Henry OA et al. Antepartum surveillance in diabetic pregnancies: Predictors of fetal distress in labor. *Am J Obstet Gynecol* 1995; 173: 1532–9. [II-2]

24. Nabhan AF, Abdelmoula YA. Amniotic fluid index versus single deepest vertical pocket as a screening test for preventing adverse pregnancy outcome. *Cochrane Database Syst Rev* 2008; (3): CD006593. [Meta-analysis; 5 RCT; *n* = 3326]

25. Chauhan SP, Sanderson M, Hendrix NW et al. Perinatal outcome and amniotic fluid index in the antepartum and intrapartum periods: A meta-analysis. *Am J Obstet Gynecol* 1999; 181: 1473–8. [Meta-analysis; 18 studies, *n* = 10,551]

26. Morris RK, Meller CH, Tamblyn J, Malin GM, Riley RD, Kilby MD, Robson SC, Khan KS. Association and prediction of amniotic fluid measurements for adverse pregnancy outcome: Systematic review and meta-analysis. *BJOG* 2014; 121(6): 686–99. [Meta-analysis; 43 studies, *n* = 244,493]

27. Manning FA, Harman CR, Morrison I et al. Fetal assessment based on fetal biophysical profile scoring IV. An analysis of perinatal morbidity and mortality. *Am J Obstet Gynecol* 1990; 162: 703–9. [II-2]

28. Chamberlain PR, Manning FA, Morrison I et al. Ultrasound evaluation of amniotic fluid. I The relationship of marginal and decreased amniotic fluid volumes to perinatal outcomes. *Am J Obstet Gynecol* 1984; 150: 245–9. [II-3]

29. Manning FA, Bondaji N, Harman CR et al. Fetal assessment based on the fetal biophysical profile score: Relationship of the last BPS result to subsequent cerebral palsy. *J Gynecol Obstet Biol Reprod* 1997; 26: 720–9. [II-3]

30. Manning FA, Bondaji N, Harman CR et al. Fetal assessment based on fetal biophysical scoring VIII. The incidence of cerebral palsy in tested and untested perinates. *Am J Obstet Gynecol* 1998; 178: 696–706. [II-2]

31. Magann EF, Doherty DA, Field K et al. Biophysical profile with amniotic fluid volume assessments. *Obstet Gynecol* 2004; 104: 5–10. [II-3]

32. Chauhan SP, Doherty DA, Magann EF et al. Amniotic fluid index vs. single deepest pocket technique during modified biophysical profile: A randomized clinical trial. *Am J Obstet Gynecol* 2004; 191: 661–7. [RCT, *n* = 1080]

33. Moses J, Doherty DA, Magann EF et al. A randomized clinical trial of the intrapartum assessment of amniotic fluid volume: Amniotic fluid index versus the single deepest pocket. *Am J Obstet Gynecol* 2004; 190: 1564–9. [RCT, *n* = 1000]

34. Magann EF, Chauhan SP, Bofill JA et al. Comparability of the amniotic fluid index and single deepest pocket measurements in clinical practice. *Aust N Z J Obstet Gynaecol* 2003; 43: 75–7. [II-2]

35. Nabhan AF, Abdelmoula YA. Amniotic fluid index versus single deepest vertical pocket as a screening test for preventing adverse pregnancy outcome. *Cochrane Database Syst Rev* 2008; (3): CD006593. doi:10.1002/14651858.CD006593. [Meta-analysis]

36. Ashwal E, Hiersch L, Melamed N et al. The association between isolated oligohydramnios at term and pregnancy outcome. *Arch Gynecol Obstet* 2014; 290(5): 875–81. Epub 2014 Jun 13. [II-3]

37. Kilpatrick SJ, Safford SL. Maternal hydration increases the amniotic fluid index in women with normal amniotic fluid volume. *Obstet Gynecol* 1993; 81: 49–52. [RCT, *n* = 40]

38. Kilpatrick SJ, Safford SL, Pomeroy T et al. Maternal hydration increases the amniotic fluid index. *Obstet Gynecol* 1991; 78: 1098–102. [RCT, *n* = 36]

39. Doi S, Osada H, Seki K et al. Effect of maternal hydration on oligohydramnios. A comparison of three volume expansion methods. *Obstet Gynecol* 1998; 92: 525–9. [RCT, *n* = 84]

40. Yan-Rosenberg L, Burt B, Bombard AT et al. A randomized clinical trial comparing the effect of maternal intravenous hydration and placebo on the amniotic fluid index in oligohydramnios. *J Matern Fetal Neonatal Med* 2007; 20(10): 715–8. [RCT]

41. Hofmeyr GJ, Gülmezoglu AM, Novikova N. Maternal hydration for increasing amniotic fluid volume in oligohydramnios and normal amniotic fluid volume. *Cochrane Database Syst Rev* 2002; (1): CD000134. doi:10.1002/14651858.CD000134. [Meta-analysis]

42. Patrelli TS, Gizzo S, Cosmi E el al. Maternal hydration therapy improves the quantity of amniotic fluid and the pregnancy outcome in third-trimester isolated oligohydramnios: A controlled randomized institutional trial. *J Ultrasound Med* 2012; 31(2): 239–44. [RCT, *n* = 137]

43. Vergani P, Ceruti P, Strobelt N et al. Transabdominal amnioinfusion in oligohydramnios at term before induction of labor with intact membranes: A randomized clinical trial. *Am J Obstet Gynecol* 1996; 175: 465–70. [RCT; *n* = 79]

44. Pitt C, Sanchez-Ramos L, Kaunitz AM et al. Prophylactic amnioinfusion for intrapartum oligohydramnios: A meta-analysis of randomized controlled trials. *Obstet Gynecol* 2000; 96: 861–6. [Meta-analysis of 14 RCTs; *n* = 793/740]

45. Amin AF, Mohammed MS, Sayed GH et al. Prophylactic transcervical amnioinfusion in laboring women with oligohydramnios. *Int J Gynecol Obstet* 2003; 81: 183–9. [RCT; *n* = 160; not included in Ref. 41]

46. Hofmeyr GJ, Justus G. Amnioinfusion for potential or suspected umbilical cord compression in labour. *Cochrane Database System Rev* 2010; 8. [Meta-analysis; 14 RCTs, most with <200 women each—See also chapter 10 in *Obstetric Evidence Based Guidelines*]

47. Novikova N, Hofmeyr GJ, Essilfie-Appiah G. Prophylactic versus therapeutic amnioinfusion for oligohydramnios in labour. *Cochrane Database System Rev* 2012; 9: CD000176. doi:10.1002/14651858.CD000176.pub2. [Meta-analysis; 1 RCT, *n* = 116]

48. Lazebnik N, Many A. The severity of polyhydramnios, estimated fetal weight, and preterm delivery are independent risk factors for the presence of congenital anomalies. *Gynecol Obstet Invest* 1999; 48: 28–32. [II-2]

49. Reddy UM, Abuhamad AZ, Levine D et al. Fetal imaging: Executive summary of a joint Eunice Kennedy Shriver National Institute of Child Health and Human Development, Society for Maternal-Fetal Medicine, American Institute of Ultrasound in Medicine, American College of Obstetricians and Gynecologists, American College of Radiology, Society for Pediatric Radiology, and Society of Radiologists in Ultrasound Fetal Imaging workshop. *Obstet Gynecol* 2014; 123(5): 1070. [II-2]

50. Dashe JS, McIntire DD, Ramus RM et al. Hydramnios: Anomaly prevalence and sonographic detection. *Obstet Gynecol* 2002; 100: 134–9. [II-3, *n* = 672, largest series of hydramnios, II-2]

51. Pri-Paz S, Khalek N, Fuchs KM et al. Maximal amniotic fluid index as a prognostic factor in pregnancies complicated by polyhydramnios. *Ultrasound Obstet Gynecol* 2012; 39(6): 648–53.

52. Magann EF, Chauhan SP, Doherty DA et al. A review of idiopathic hydramnios and pregnancy outcomes. *Obstet Gynecol Surv* 2007; 62: 795–802. [II-2]

53. Magann EF, Doherty DA, Lutgendorf MA et al. Peripartum outcomes of high risk pregnancies complicated by oligo-and polyhydramnios. A longitudinal prospective study. *J Obstet Gynaecol Res* 2010; 36: 268–77. [II-2]

54. Esplin MS, Hallam S, Farrington PF et al. Myotonic dystrophy is a significant cause of idiopathic polyhydramnios. *Am J Obstet Gynecol* 1998; 179: 974–7. [II-3]

55. Magann EF, Whitworth NS, Bass JD et al. Amniotic fluid volume of third-trimester diamniotic twins. *Obstet Gynecol* 1995; 85: 857–60. [II-2]

56. Porter TF, Dildy GA, Blanchard JR et al. Normal values for amniotic fluid index during uncomplicated twin pregnancy. *Obstet Gynecol* 1996; 87: 699–702. [II-2]

57. Chau AC, Kjos SC, Kovacs BW. Ultrasonographic measurement of amniotic fluid volume in normal diamniotic twin pregnancies. *Am J Obstet Gynecol* 1996; 174: 1003–7. [II-2]

58. Magann EF, Chauhan SP, Whitworth NS et al. Accuracy of the summated AFI in evaluating amniotic fluid volume in diamniotic twin pregnancies. *Am J Obstet Gynecol* 1997; 177: 1041–5. [II-2]

59. Magann EF, Chauhan SP, Whitworth NS et al. Determination of amniotic fluid volume in twin pregnancies: Ultrasonic evaluation versus operator estimation. *Am J Obstet Gynecol* 2000; 182: 1606–9. [II-3].

58

Fetal maturity testing

Paniz Heidari and Sarah Poggi

KEY POINTS

- **The determination of fetal lung maturity (FLM) in well-dated pregnancies by amniocentesis generally is unnecessary and should not be used to guide the timing of delivery**. FLM testing is not necessary if delivery is indicated by accepted maternal and/or fetal obstetrical indications.
- Consideration for FLM testing is rarely indicated, such as in cases of **unsure gestational dating**.
- If FLM testing is done, the probability for respiratory distress syndrome (RDS) should be calculated as **a function of gestational age** and the specific FLM test.
- **Lamellar body count** or **surfactant/albumin ratio** can be used as **the initial and only FLM test** given their high negative predictive value, ease, and low cost. Lecithin/sphingomyelin **(L/S) ratio** can be used as a confirmatory test if necessary.
- For diabetic pregnancies, positive phosphatidylglycerol (PG), surfactant/albumin ratio ≥70 mg/g, L/S >3, or a combination of these tests have a high predictive value for maturity. Some experts, however, use the same threshold values of nondiabetic pregnancies for assessment of FLM in diabetic pregnancies.
- **Even with a "mature" fetal lung profile, neonates delivered at less than 39 weeks can demonstrate morbidity associated with prematurity.**

HISTORIC NOTES

The L/S ratio for assessment of FLM was first introduced by Gluck and colleagues in 1971, and this test is still the standard to which others are compared [1].

DEFINITIONS

Surfactant is a complex substance containing phospholipids and apoproteins produced by the type II alveolar cells. It reduces surface tension throughout the lung, contributing to its compliance, leading to alveolar stability, and reducing the likelihood of alveolar collapse. Surfactant is "packaged" in lamellar bodies.

Neonatal respiratory distress syndrome (RDS) occurs when the lungs fail to produce an adequate amount of surfactant. RDS is defined in many different ways but, in general, involves mechanical ventilation and oxygen requirement at ≥24 to 48 hours of life and radiographic chest findings (air bronchograms and reticulogranular appearance) without any other explanation for the respiratory insufficiency. The natural (without steroids) incidence of RDS depends on gestational age: about 80% to 90% at 25 to 27 weeks, 55% to 65% at 28 to 30 weeks, 30% to 40% at 31 to 33 weeks, 13% at 34 weeks, 6% at 35 weeks, 3% at 36 weeks, and 1% or less at ≥37 weeks. Therefore, **the probability for RDS should be calculated as a function of gestational age**. RDS affects approximately 1% of all live births. Complications of its treatment are associated with an increased risk of serious acute and long-term pulmonary and nonpulmonary morbidities. Although the frequency and severity of RDS are worse for delivery remote from term, the pulmonary system is the last organ systems to mature, and RDS can occur even near term.

INDICATIONS FOR ASSESSMENT OF FETAL PULMONARY MATURITY

The determination of FLM in well-dated pregnancies by amniocentesis generally is unnecessary and should not be used to guide the timing of delivery. FLM testing is not necessary if delivery is indicated by accepted maternal and/or fetal obstetrical indications. Therefore, **FLM testing is rarely indicated**. There are no absolute indications for assessment of FLM. If an evidence-based, clear indication for delivery is present, the use of amniocentesis to assess FLM would not assist in guiding management. For example, FLM testing is not indicated if delivery is indicated by accepted maternal (e.g., severe preeclampsia after 34 weeks) and/or fetal (e.g., category III fetal heart rate monitoring after viability) indications. Because of the risk for HIV infection, uterine rupture with prior uterine surgery with extensive myomectomy or vertical CD, and hemorrhage with placenta previa and/or accreta, proof of lung maturity before delivery is not necessary in these and other selected indications (see Chapter 21 in *Obstetric Evidence Based Guidelines*). Tests for FLM are not warranted before 33 weeks because they are rarely positive this early in gestation. FLM testing in well-dated (e.g., by first-trimester ultrasound) singletons at ≥39 weeks or twins at ≥37 to 38 weeks is not indicated. As the probability of RDS depends on gestational age, gestational age estimation should be as accurate as possible, preferably based on first-trimester ultrasound (see Chapter 4 in *Obstetric Evidence Based Guidelines*). Consideration for FLM testing may occur in rare cases, such as in a woman with **unsure gestational dating**.

The American College of Obstetricians and Gynecologists (ACOG) recommends that a mature fetal lung test before 39 weeks of gestation, in the absence of appropriate clinical circumstances, is not an indication for delivery [2]. It is also noted that although FLM testing may help identify fetuses at risk of RDS, **mature fetal pulmonary test results may not reliably predict adverse outcomes and should not justify a delivery without other indications** [3].

TECHNIQUES FOR OBTAINING AMNIOTIC FLUID
Amniocentesis

Third-trimester amniocentesis performed under ultrasonographic guidance in experienced hands is associated with low rates of failure or of bloody fluid collection and a <1%

risk of complication, such as emergent delivery [4]. The risk of complications (e.g., PTL, PROM, abruption, and fetomaternal hemorrhage) associated with amniocentesis for FLM performed under continuous ultrasound guidance has been estimated at about 0.7% [5,6].

Vaginal Pool Collection

The assessment of fetal pulmonary maturity can be obtained from vaginal pool specimens in the presence of premature rupture of membranes. Blood, meconium, and mucous can alter the results. In the absence of these contaminants, vaginally free-flowing collected fluid can be evaluated for determination of L/S ratio, surfactant/albumin ratio, PG, and lamellar body count yielding results similar to those observed with samples obtained with amniocentesis (Table 58.1). As obtaining a specimen via a sterile syringe is not always technically feasible, an alternative collection method using the commonly available "4 × 4" gauze sponge has been validated for both PG and TDx-FLM II analyses (see below). Essentially, the gauze is inserted into the vagina at the posterior fornix and then plunged into a 60-cc syringe to extract the vaginal pool specimen [7].

SPECIFIC TESTS FOR LUNG MATURITY (TABLE 58.1)
Lecithin/Sphingomyelin Ratio

The concentrations of these two substances are approximately equal until the mid-third trimester of gestation when the concentration of pulmonary lecithin (phosphatidylcholine, most common of surfactant compounds) increases significantly while the nonpulmonary sphingomyelin concentration remains unchanged.

Technique
Following amniocentesis, the sample should be kept on ice or refrigerated if transport to a laboratory is required. Thin-layer chromatography after centrifugation to remove the cellular component and organic solvent extraction is used.

Interpretation of Results
An L/S ratio of 2.0 or greater predicts absence of RDS in 98% of neonates. With a ratio of 1.5 to 1.9, approximately 50% of infants will develop RDS. Below 1.5, the risk of subsequent RDS increases to 73%.

Special Considerations
Maternal serum has an L/S ratio ranging from 1.3 to 1.9; thus, blood-tinged samples could falsely lower a mature result. The presence of meconium can interfere with test interpretation, increasing the L/S ratio by 0.1 to 0.5, thus leading to an increase in falsely mature results.

Phosphatidylglycerol

PG is a minor constituent of surfactant that becomes evident in amniotic fluid several weeks after the rise in lecithin [8]. Its presence indicates a more advanced state of fetal lung development and function as PG enhances the spread of phospholipids on the alveoli.

Technique
The original PG testing was performed by thin-layer chromatography and required time and expertise. More recently,

enzymatic assay or slide agglutinations have been used successfully to determine the presence of PG. Amniostat-FLM (Irvine Scientific, California) is one such test.

Interpretation
The results are typically reported qualitatively as positive or negative, where positive represents >3% of total phospholipids and an exceedingly low risk of RDS.

Special Considerations
PG determination is not generally affected by blood, meconium, or vaginal secretion.

Surfactant/Albumin Ratio

The fluorescence polarization assay uses polarized light to evaluate the competitive binding of a probe to both albumin and surfactant in amniotic fluid [9].

Technique
The TDx-FLM (Abbott, Illinois) analyzer provides a quantitative and automated measurement of the amniotic fluid surfactant/albumin ratio (SAR). The test is simple, rapid, objective, and reproducible and can be performed with equipment commonly available in clinical laboratories. A recent commercial modification of the assay (TDx-FlxFLM II) allows simple, automated, and rapid results.

Interpretation
An SAR of 55 mg/g has been proposed as the optimal threshold to indicate maturity [9]. Values of 35 to 55 are considered "borderline." As per other tests, **the probability for RDS should be calculated as a function of gestational age and the FLM test results** (Table 58.2) [11]. In other words, other pretest probabilities for maturity should be taken into account when interpreting these tests.

Special Considerations
As for L/S ratio, red blood cell phospholipids may falsely lower the TDx-FlxFLM II result, but a mature test can reliably predict pulmonary maturity.

Is a course of steroids indicated in the face of an immature result at >34 weeks? In a small RCT of patients over 34 weeks with "immature" TDX-FlxFLM II, results demonstrated a benefit to a single course of corticosteroids in terms of a progression to "mature" results with repeat amniocentesis one week later (50% vs. 27%, p = .002). However, as no actual neonatal outcomes were presented, this approach must be interpreted with some caution at this time [12].

Lamellar Body Counts

Lamellar bodies (LB) are produced by type II pneumocytes and are a direct measurement of surfactant production because they represent its storage form.

Technique
Lamellar bodies are quantified with a commercial blood cell analyzer, which takes advantage of the similar size between LB and platelets. The results can be obtained quickly with a small fluid volume, and the test is less expensive than traditional phospholipids analysis. Although initial studies employed centrifugation, it is now agreed that the sample should be processed without spinning as centrifugation reduces the number of LB.

Table 58.1 Characteristics of Fetal Lung Maturity Tests

Test	Technique	Threshold	Predictive Value Mature Test (%)	Predictive Value Immature Test	Accurate with Blood Contamination	Accurate with Meconium Contamination	Accurate in Vaginal Pool	Difficulty	Cost
L/S ratio	Thin-layer chromatography	2/1	95–100	33–50	No	No	No	High	High
PG	Thin-layer chromatography	Present (usually means >3% of total phospholipids)	95–100	23–53	Yes	Yes	Yes	High	High
	Slide agglutination	Positive (>2%)						Low	Low
Surfactant/ albumin ratio (TDx-FLM)	Fluorescence polarization	>55 mg (of surfactant)/g (of albumin)	96–100	47–61	No	No	Yes	Low	Moderate
LBC	Cell counter	30,000–50,000/iiL	97–98	29–35	No	Yes	Yes	Low	Low
FSI	Ethanol dilution	> 47	95	51	No	No	No	Moderate	Moderate

Abbreviations: FSI, foam stability index; LBC, lamellar body count; L/S, lecithin/sphingomyelin; PG, phosphatidylglycerol.

Table 58.2 Probability of RDS on the Basis of Gestational Age and Surfactant/Albumin (S/A) Ratio (TDx-FLM)

S/A	27	28	29	30	31	32	33	34	35	36	37	38	39	40
0	72%	66%	59%	51%	44%	37%	30%	24%	19%	15%	12%	9%	7%	5.1%
10	67%	60%	53%	46%	39%	32%	26%	20%	16%	12%	9.6%	7.3%	5.5%	4.2%
20	62%	55%	48%	40%	33%	27%	22%	17%	13%	10%	7.8%	6%	4.5%	3.4%
30	57%	50%	42%	35%	29%	23%	18%	14%	11%	8.4%	6.4%	4.8%	3.6%	2.7%
40	51%	44%	37%	30%	24%	19%	15%	12%	9%	6.8%	5.2%	4%	3%	2.2%
50	46%	39%	32%	26%	21%	16%	13%	10%	7.4%	5.6%	4.2%	3.2%	2.4%	1.8%
60	40%	34%	27%	22%	17%	13%	10%	8%	6%	4.5%	3.4%	2.5%	1.9%	1.4%
70	35%	29%	23%	18%	14%	11%	8.5%	6.4%	4.9%	3.7%	2.7%	2%	1.5%	1.1%
80	31%	25%	20%	15%	12%	9.1%	7%	5.2%	4%	3%	2.2%	1.7%	1.2%	0.9%
90	26%	21%	16%	13%	10%	7.4%	5.6%	4.2%	3.2%	2.4%	1.8%	1.3%	1%	0.7%
100	22%	17%	14%	10%	8%	6%	4.6%	3.4%	2.6%	2%	1.4%	1%	0.8%	0.6%
110	19%	14%	11%	9%	6.5%	4.9%	3.7%	2.8%	2.1%	1.5%	1.2%	0.9%	0.6%	0.5%
120	15%	12%	9%	7%	5.3%	4%	3%	2.2%	1.7%	1.2%	1%	0.7%	0.5%	0.4%
130	13%	9.8%	7.5%	6%	4.3%	3.2%	2.4%	1.8%	1.3%	1%	0.7%	0.6%	0.4%	0.3%
140	10%	8%	6.1%	4.6%	3.5%	2.6%	2%	1.4%	1.1%	0.8%	0.6%	0.5%	0.3%	0.25%
150	9%	6.6%	5%	3.7%	2.8%	2.1%	1.6%	1.2%	0.9%	0.6%	0.5%	0.4%	0.3%	0.2%
160	7%	5.3%	4%	3%	2.3%	1.7%	1.3%	1%	0.7%	0.5%	0.4%	0.3%	0.2%	0.2%
170	5.7%	4.3%	3.2%	2.4%	1.8%	1.4%	1%	0.8%	0.6%	0.4%	0.3%	0.2%	0.2%	0.1%
180	4.7%	3.5%	2.6%	2%	1.5%	1.1%	0.8%	0.6%	0.4%	0.3%	0.2%	0.2%	0.2%	0.1%
190	3.8%	2.8%	2.1%	1.6%	1.2%	0.9%	0.7%	0.5%	0.4%	0.3%	0.2%	0.1%	0.1%	0.1%
200	3%	2.3%	1.7%	1.3%	0.9%	0.7%	0.5%	0.4%	0.3%	0.2%	0.1%	0.1%	0.1%	0.1%

Source: Pinette MG, Blackstone J, Wax JR et al. *Am J Obstet Gynecol*, 187, 1721–2, 2002.

Interpretation
Values of 30,000 to 50,000/mL (least false positives) generally indicate pulmonary maturity [13,14]. Values of <15,000/µL are usually associated with immaturity. The test compares favorably with L/S and PG with a negative predictive value of a mature cutoff of 97.7% versus 96.8% and 94.7%, respectively [15]. A meta-analysis calculated receiver-operating characteristic curves based on data from six studies and showed the lamellar body count performed slightly better than the L/S ratio in predicting RDS [16].

Special Considerations
Meconium has a marginal impact on LB counts, increasing the count by 5000/µL. Bloody fluid can initially slightly increase the count because the platelets are counted as LB. Afterward, the procoagulant activity of AF produces an entrapment of both, platelets and LB, causing a decrease in LB counts. Because of variations in hematology analyzers, ideally laboratories should develop their own reference standards [17].

Foam Stability Index

The foam stability index (FSI) is a simple and rapid predictor of FLM based on the ability of surfactant to generate stable foam in the presence of ethanol.

Technique
After centrifugation, ethanol is added to a sample of amniotic fluid to eliminate the contributions of protein, bile salts, and salts of free fatty acids. The mixture is shaken for 30 seconds and will demonstrate generation of a stable ring of foam if surfactant is present in the amniotic fluid. Amniotic fluid samples should not be collected in silicone tubes as the silicone will produce "false foam."

Interpretation
The FSI is calculated by utilizing serial dilutions of ethanol to quantitate the amount of surfactant present. RDS is very unlikely with an FSI value of 47 or higher. A positive result virtually excludes the risk of RDS; however, a negative test often occurs in the presence of mature lung.

Special Considerations
Contamination of the amniotic fluid specimen by blood or meconium interferes with the FSI results.

SINGLE TEST, MULTIPLE TESTS, OR CASCADE?

Faced with different assays for FLM, some laboratories perform multiple tests simultaneously, leaving the clinician with the possibility of results discordant for pulmonary maturity from the same amniotic fluid specimen. In general, any mature test result is indicative of fetal pulmonic maturity given the high predictive value of any single test (5% or less of false mature rates). Conversely the use of a "cascade" approach has been proposed to minimize the risk of delivery of an infant with immature lungs while avoiding unnecessary delay in delivery and costs. According to this approach, a rapid and inexpensive test is performed first with follow-up tests performed only in the face of immaturity of the initial test (e.g., **lamellar body count or surfactant/albumin ratio as the initial and only test and L/S ratio as the confirmatory test as necessary**).

CLINICAL CONDITIONS AFFECTING RISK OF RDS AND PREDICTIVE VALUE OF PULMONARY MATURITY TESTS

Several maternal/fetal clinical or nonclinical circumstances can affect the risk of RDS and modify the predictive value of pulmonary maturity tests, including the following:

- African-American race is associated with FLM achieved at lower gestational ages and at lower L/S ratios (1.2 or greater) than in Caucasians.

- Female gender is associated with acceleration of lung maturation.
- Intrauterine growth restriction and preeclampsia are possibly associated with an acceleration of FLM.
- **Maternal diabetes** and Rh-isoimmunization are associated with a delay in fetal lung maturation. Some authors have recommended the use of higher thresholds of L/S ratio (e.g., a cutoff ratio of 3) to establish pulmonic maturity in these conditions. Presence of a lamellar body count 50,000/μL has similarly been recommended to indicate mature fetal lungs in diabetic women [18]. Presence of PG is commonly considered as gold standard for documentation of FLM with diabetes or Rh-isoimmunization. For diabetes, also a TDx-FLM value of ≥70 mg/g, or a L/S ≥3, or the combination of the two, have been associated with >95% predictive value for a mature test. Gestational age-stratified TDx-FLM ratios have been reported in risk tables [18,19].
- Hydramnios is associated with lower levels of L/S ratio, lamellar body count, and PG test.
- In twin gestations, it is commonly recommended that the sac of the male twin or the larger twin be sampled at amniocentesis. The reasoning is that if the sampled twin has mature pulmonic results, the co-twin is even more likely to be mature.

FINAL NOTE: FACTORS OTHER THAN LUNG MATURITY IMPACT FETAL OUTCOME

A retrospective cohort study compared the outcomes of neonates born between 36 and 38 6/7 weeks in the setting of mature fetal lung profile studies to those born at 39 0/7 to 40 6/7 weeks and found an increase in a composite adverse neonatal outcomes (RR = 2.4, 95% CI 1.7–3.5) with common complications including respiratory distress, hyperbilirubinemia, and hypoglycemia [21]. It is **important to remember that fetal maturation does not involve "just" the lungs. Given these data and considerations, the decision to proceed with FLM amniocentesis for the purposes of hastening delivery should always be carefully considered, and in the vast majority of cases, this test should not be performed** [3,21].

REFERENCES

1. Gluck L, Kulovich MV, Boerer RC Jr et al. Diagnosis of the respiratory distress syndrome by amniocentesis. *Am J Obstet Gynecol* 1971; 109: 440. [II-2]
2. American College of Obstetricians and Gynecologists. *Induction of Labor.* ACOG Practice Bulletin No. 107. Washington, DC: ACOG, 2009. [Review]
3. Nonmedically indicated early-term deliveries. Committee Opinion No. 561. American College of Obstetricians and Gynecologists. *Obstet Gynecol* 2013; 121: 911–5. [Guideline]
4. Hodor JG, Poggi SH, Spong CY et al. Risk of third-trimester amniocentesis: A case-control study. *Am J Perinatol* 2006; 23: 177–80. [II-2]
5. Gordon MC, Narula K, O'Shaughnssy R et al. Complications of third trimester amniocentesis using continuous ultrasound guidance. *Obstet Gynecol* 2002; 99: 255–9. [II-3]
6. Stark CM, Smith RS, Lagrandeur RM et al. Need for urgent delivery after third trimester amniocentesis. *Obstet Gynecol* 2000; 95: 48–50. [II-3]
7. Gleaton KD, White JC, Koklanaris N. A novel method for collecting vaginal pool for fetal lung maturity studies. *Am J Obstet Gynecol* 2009; 201: 408.e1–4. [II-3]
8. Hallman M, Kulovich M, Kirkpatrick E et al. Phosphatidylinositol and phosphatidylglycerol in amniotic fluid: Indices of lung maturity. *Am J Obstet Gynecol* 1976; 125: 613. [II-2]
9. Russell JC, Cooper CM, Ketchum CH et al. Multicenter evaluation of TDx test for assessing fetal lung maturity. *Clin Chem* 1989; 35: 1005. [II-2]
10. Kesselman EJ, Figueroa R, Garry D et al. The usefulness of the TDx/TDxFLx fetal lung maturity II assay in the initial evaluation of fetal lung maturity. *Am J Obstet Gynecol* 2003; 188: 1220–2. [II-2]
11. Pinette MG, Blackstone J, Wax JR et al. Fetal lung maturity indices—A plea for gestational age-specific interpretation: A case report and discussion. *Am J Obstet Gynecol* 2002; 187: 1721–2. [III]
12. Shanks A, Gross G, Shim T et al. Administration of steroids after 34 weeks of gestation enhances fetal lung maturity profiles. *Am J Obstet Gynecol* 2010; 203: 47.e1–5. [I]
13. Dubin, SB. The laboratory assessment of fetal lung maturity. *Am J Clin Pathol* 1992; 97: 836. [II-2]
14. Ghidini A, Poggi SH, Spong CY et al. Role of lamellar body count for the prediction of neonatal respiratory distress syndrome in non-diabetic pregnant women. *Arch Gynecol Obstet* 2005; 271: 325–8. [II-2]
15. Neerhof MG, Haney EI, Silver RK et al. Lamellar body counts compared with traditional phospholipid analysis as an assay for evaluating fetal lung maturity. *Obstet Gynecol* 2001; 97: 305–9. [II-2]
16. Wijnberger LD, Huisjes AJ, Voorbij HA et al. The accuracy of lamellar body count and lecithin/sphingomyelin ratio in the prediction of neonatal respiratory distress syndrome: A meta-analysis. *BJOG* 2001; 108: 585–8. [II-2]
17. Janicki MB, Dries LM, Egan JF et al. Determining a cutoff for fetal lung maturity with lamellar body count testing. *J Matern Fetal Neonatal Med* 2009; 22: 419–22. [II-2]
18. Ghidini A, Spong CY, Goodwin K et al. Optimal thresholds of lecithin/sphingomyelin ratio and lamellar body count for the prediction of the presence of phosphatidylglycerol in diabetic women. *J Matern Fetal Neonatal Med* 2002; 12: 95–8. [II-2]
19. McElrath TF, Colon I, Hecht J, Tanasijevic M, Norwitz ER. Neonatal respiratory distress syndrome as a function of gestational age and an assay for surfactant-to-albumin ratio. *Obstet Gynecol* 2004; 103: 463–8. [II-2]
20. Parvin CA, Kaplan LA, Chapman JF, McManamon TG, Gronowski AM. Predicting respiratory distress syndrome using gestational age and fetal lung maturity by fluorescent polarization. *Am J Obstet Gynecol* 2005; 192: 199–207. [II-2]
21. Bates E, Rouse DJ, Mann ML et al. Neonatal outcomes after demonstrated fetal lung maturity before 39 weeks gestation. *Obstet Gynecol* 2010; 116: 1288–95. [II-3]

Index

Page numbers followed f and t indicate figures and tables, respectively.

A

Abacavir, 300, 302t
Abdominal decompression, in FGR pregnancies, 420
Abilify® and Abilify Discmelt®, 186t
Abnormal blood chemistry, pregnancy after LTx, 128
Abnormal uterine Doppler ultrasound, CHTN and, 10
Abruptio placentae, 7, 9, 13, 16, 173, 340, 401
Absent end-diastolic flow (AEDF), UA, 404, 413, 421, 425, 426
Absent or reversed end-diastolic flow (AREDF), UA, 421, 425, 426
Acardiac twin, 407
Acesulfame-K, 53
Acetaminophen, 83, 162, 164, 164t, 165, 249t, 250, 492
Acetylcholinesterase, 167
ACOG, see American College of Obstetricians and Gynecologists (ACOG)
Acquired immune deficiency syndrome (AIDS), 297
ACS, see Acute chest syndrome (ACS)
Activated charcoal, 107
Activated partial thromboplastin time (aPTT), 369
Active tuberculosis infection, 241–242, 241t
Actual therapy, APS, 256–257, 257t
Acupressure
  auricular, 97
  wrist bands, 94, 97
Acupuncture, 97, 201
Acustimulation wrist bands, 97
Acute cellular rejection (ACR) rate, pregnancy after LTx, 127
Acute chest syndrome (ACS)
  complications, 143
  defined, 143
  incidence, 143
  pathophysiology, 143
  sickle cell disease and, 139, 140, 142
  symptoms, 143
  therapy, 143
  workup, 143
Acute cholecystitis
  classification, 120, 121t
  complications
    fetal, 121
    maternal, 121
  defined, 120
  diagnosis, 120, 120f
  epidemiology/incidence, 121
  ERCP, 121–122
  etiology/pathogenesis, 121
  labor and delivery considerations, 122
  management, 122
    laparoscopic vs. open cholecystectomy, 122
    surgery, 122
  MRCP, 121
  pregnancy considerations, 121–122
    imaging, 121

laboratory investigations, 121
    principles, 121
    workup, 121
  risk factors/associations, 121
  symptoms, 121
Acute fatty liver
  rate, in triplets, 402
  singleton gestations and, 402
Acute HIV infection, 303
Acute intoxication, opioids and, 210
Acute leukemia, 377–378
  delay in diagnosis, 377
  diagnostic tests and safety, 377
  effects, on pregnancy, 377
  termination of pregnancy, 377
  treatment, 377–378
Acute lung injury (ALI), 356
Acute renal disease, 158
Acute respiratory distress syndrome (ARDS), 349, 356–357, 356t
Acute retroviral syndrome, 303
Acyclovir, 451, 453, 454, 456, 458, 459
Adalimumab, 112t, 113
Addiction
  criminalization of, 209
  defined, 207
Adenosine, 479, 486
Adipokines, defined, 33
Adiponectin, 33
Admissions
  ICU, 349, 350t, 353, 354t
  preeclampsia, prevention, 12
  trauma, 340, 345
ADP, see Atopic dermatitis of pregnancy (ADP)
ADR, see Autonomic dysreflexia (ADR)
Adrenocorticoticotropic hormone (ACTH), 99
Advair (salmeterol), 226t, 232
Advanced maternal age, fetal monitoring and, 508
Adverse pregnancy outcome, inherited thrombophilias and, 262–263, 263t
Aerosolized pentamadine, 301t
AFE, see Amniotic fluid embolism (AFE)
β-agonists, for asthma, 232, 233
Agranulocytosis, 82
Air bags, 341
Air embolism, 366, 367
Airway
  CPAP, 35
  drug abuse and, 210, 211, 213
  in eclampsia, 7, 19
  edema, 343
  inflammation, 225
  maternal stabilization after trauma, 339, 342f, 343, 343t
  obstruction, asthma and, 225, 229
Airway pressure release ventilation (ARPV), 357
Alanine aminotransferase (ALT), 241
Albuterol, 227t, 233
Alcohols, 165, 209, 341, 488, 489
Aldomet (Methyldopa), 4, 5, 12, 19

Alloantibodies, 142
Allograft rejection, renal, 156
Alloimmune thrombocytopenia (AIT), defined, 460
Alloimmunization
  RBC, 467–474; see also Hemolytic disease
  sickle cell disease, 142
Alpha- and beta-blockers, labetalol, 1, 4, 5, 6t, 7, 13, 16, 208, 215
Alpha-fetoprotein (AFP)
  levels, for seizures, 167, 170
  screening, 55
Alphanate, 148
Alpha tocopherol, 387
Alternative treatments, smoking, 201
Amantadine, 238
American Academy of Neurology (AAN), 168
American Academy of Pediatrics (AAP), 188, 189, 190, 213, 217, 312
American Association for Study of Liver Diseases (AASLD), 289
American College of Critical Care Medicine (ACCM), 349, 350, 352
American College of Obstetricians and Gynecologists (ACOG)
  amphetamine, use, 217
  chlamydial infection, 310, 312
  critical care, 352, 353
  for fetal deaths, 488
  fetal macrosomia, 432, 433, 434
  fetal maturity testing, 521
  FGR, 413, 416
  GDM, diagnosis of, 60
  intimate partner violence, 341
  multiple gestations, 402, 404
  NAEPP program, 228
  NRT, use, 200
  screening for depression, 178
  syphilis, 318
  trauma, 341, 342
  weight gain in pregnancy, 39
American College of Radiology, 345
American College of Rheumatology (ACR), 246, 247t
American Heart Association (AHA), 10, 20, 346, 368
American Psychiatric Association (APA), 188
American Society of Regional Anesthesia, 278
American Stroke Association Women, 10
American Thoracic Society (ATS), 234, 235
Amikacin, 242
Aminoglycoside, 235
Aminosalicylates, 110, 112t, 113
Amiodarone, 479, 486
Amlodipine, 4
Amniocaproic acid, 145
Amniocentesis
  anemia, screening for, 467
  CMV-infected women, 439
  for ΔOD$_{450}$ measurement, 467, 471–472, 474
  FGR management, 412, 418

FLM, 522, 525
HCV-infected women, 293–294
HIV-infected women, 302
multiple gestations, 402, 404
NIH, management, 477, 485
polyhydramnios, 517
technique for obtaining AF, 521–522
Amnioinfusion, oligohydramnios and, 516
Amnionicity, multiple gestations, 398, 399, 400, 400f
Amniotic fluid (AF)
AF PCR, 444
CMV infection, diagnosis for, 439
NIH, diagnosis, 485
sonographic assessment, 513–518
accuracy of ultrasound, for oligohydramnios, 513–514
AFV, estimation with SDP/AFI, 514
background, 513
color Doppler for AFV, 514
indications, 513
key points, 513, 515, 516–517
management, 514–515
oligohydramnios, 515–516; *see also* Oligohydramnios
polyhydramnios (hydramnios), 516–518; *see also* Polyhydramnios (hydramnios)
in singleton pregnancies, 513–515
techniques, 513
in twin pregnancies, 518
ultrasound estimates, accuracy, 514
techniques for obtaining
amniocentesis, 521–522
vaginal pool collection, 522, 523t
Amniotic fluid embolism (AFE), 365–371
background, 365
diagnosis, 366–369
cardiac arrest, management, 367–369, 368t, 370f
clinical presentation, 366
differential, 366–367
laboratory testing, 367
management of coagulopathy with, 369
DIC in, 366, 369
incidence, 365
key points, 365
management, 369, 370f
oxytocin administration and, 366
pathophysiology, 365–366
postpartum counselling about recurrence rates, 369
risk factors, 366
survivors, prognosis, 369
Amniotic fluid index (AFI)
AFV, estimation, 514
maternal hydration on AFV, 515
NRFHT and, 514
oligohydramnios and, 513–514
Amniotic fluid volume (AFV)
accuracy of ultrasound, for oligohydramnios, 513–514
assessment in twin pregnancies
background, 518
management of oligohydramnios and/or hydramnios, 518
technique, 518
BPS, assessment, 500, 500t
color Doppler for, 514
estimation
with SDP or AFI, 514
ultrasound, accuracy of, 514
for FGR, 422, 424

NST and, 501
Amoxicillin, 156, 235, 242, 310, 312, 313t
Amphetamines, 216–217
anesthesia, 217
antepartum testing, 217
complications
congenital anomalies, 216–217
fetal/neonatal morphometrics, 217
long-term neurodevelopmental outcome, 217
neonatal withdrawal, 217
obstetrical and neonatal, 217
defined, 216
diagnosis, 216
epidemiology/incidence, 216
etiology/basic pathophysiology, 216
historic notes, 216
incidence, 206
postpartum/breast-feeding, 217
risk factors/associations, 216
symptoms, signs, and organ toxicity, 216
therapy, 217
urine drug screening for, 208, 208t
Amphotericin B, 155t
Ampicillin, 26–27, 157, 235, 325, 328t, 329
Amyl nitrate, 173, 174
Analgesics, 164–165, 164t, 454
Anaphylactic shock, 366, 367
Anatomy
clinical hypothyroidism, in pregnancy, 74
fetus, 128, 142, 302, 412, 477, 515, 517
oropharyngeal, 41
ultrasound, 5, 477, 517
Ancef, 157
Anemia
defined, 131
fetal, 142, 447, 448, 449, 467, 470–471, 472, 474, 477, 482, 483, 484, 485, 491, 505, 508
of fetus and neonate, 467–474
hemolytic; *see also* Hemolytic disease
APS and, 255
fetal, 402
inherited, 132
microangiopathic, 8
mild-to-moderate, 470
pruritus during pregnancy, 104f
sickle cell disease and, 139, 140
iron deficiency, 133
LTx, pregnancies after, 128
maternal, *see* Maternal anemia
multiple gestations, 401, 402, 404
NIH and, 481, 482, 483, 484, 485
renal diseases, 146, 150, 152, 154
SCI and, 173, 174
sickle cell, 139–144; *see also* Sickle cell disease
treatment, 112
women with leukemia, 377
Anencephaly, 181
Anesthesia
ADR, 174–175
amphetamines, use, 217
APS, 258
asthma, 233
cardiac disease and
epidural, 26
spinal, 26
CHTN, pregnancy with, 5
cocaine, use, 215
fetal death, 491–493
D&E, 491–492

expectant management, 491
induction, 492–493
FNAIT, 465
GDM, 67
HAV infections, 284
HBV infections, 289
HCV infection, 295
HELLP syndrome, 17
hemolytic disease, 474
marijuana (cannabis), 210
maternal anemia, 137
NIH, management, 486
obesity and, 40–41
pneumonia, 235
preeclampsia, pregnancy with, 13
pregestational diabetes, 55
prolactinoma, 90
SCI, 175
sickle cell disease, 143
trauma, 346
VTE, 278–279
vWD, 149
Aneuploidy screening, HIV infection, 302
Angina, stable/unstable, 29
Angiotensin-converting enzyme (ACE) inhibitors, 1, 3, 4, 6t
Angiotensin type II (AII) receptor antagonists, 3
Annual influenza vaccination, 237
Anomalous fetus, selective termination, 403–404
preterm birth, 403–404
bed rest, 403
cerclage, 403
home uterine activity monitoring, 403
multifetal pregnancy reduction, 403
PPROM, 404
prevention of multiple gestations, 403
progesterone, 403
prophylactic tocolysis, 403
PTL, 404
subsequent pregnancy outcomes, after delivery of twins, 404
weight gain, 403
Anorexia, 209
Antenatal management
GHTN, 5, 6
of preexisting SCI, 173
Antenatal testing
CRI, 152
sickle cell disease, 142
Antenatal visits, renal transplantation and, 155
Antepartum activity restriction, cardiac disease, 25, 26
Antepartum testing, 496–509
ADR, 174
amphetamines, 217
APS, 257–258
asthma, 233
background, 496
benzodiazepines, 218
cardiac disease, 25
CD, 114
CHTN, 5
clinical hypothyroidism, 76
cocaine, use, 215
eclampsia, 19
fetal monitoring, 40
BPS, 499–501, 499f, 499t, 500t, 501t
condition-specific testing, 505, 506–508, 506t, 507t
CST, 498–499

Doppler of fetal vessels, 501–505, 502f, 503f, 504f, 505t
Doppler surveillance and BPS, 505, 506f
FHR testing (NST or CTG), 497–498, 497f
methods, 496–509
modified BPS, 501
movement counting in low-risk pregnancy, 496–497
practical, 508–509
principles, 496
FGR, 420–424
AF volume, 422, 424
BPS, 422, 424
Doppler velocimetry, 420–421
estriol levels, 424
fetal kick counts, 422
growth assessment, intervals of, 420
interval of fetal testing, 424
MCA Doppler velocimetry, 421
NST/CTG, 422
ultrasound, 420–422
venous Doppler (DV) velocimetry, 421–422, 423f
GBS, 330
GDM, 67
hallucinogens, exposure, 220
HAV infections, pregnancy with, 284
HBV infections, 289
HCV infection, 294–295
HIV infection, 302
hyperthyroidism, 82–83
ICP, 107
IH (pustular psoriasis of pregnancy), 393
influenza, 238
key points, 496
LTx, pregnancy after, 128
marijuana (cannabis), 210
maternal anemia, 137
multiple gestation, 407–408
fetal surveillance, 407–408
ultrasounds, 407
opioids, heroin and prescription opioid analgesics, 213
PCP, 219
pneumonia, 235
preeclampsia, 13
pregestational diabetes, 55, 55t
prolactinoma, 90
sickle cell disease, 142
SLE, 250
trauma, 346
tuberculosis, 242
UC, 116
VTE, 278
vWD, 148
Anthracyclines, 375, 377, 380, 381
Anthrax vaccine, 335t
Antibiotics
ACS, 143
broad-spectrum, 122
cefazolin, 27, 41, 325, 328t, 329
dosing of, 472
erythromycin, see Erythromycin
IBD, 112t, 113
infective endocarditis, 26–27, 27t
metronidazole, 112t, 113, 212, 322, 324
penicillins, see Penicillins
pneumonia, 235
ristocetin, 145
for sepsis, 359
sickle cell disease, 142

traumatic brain injury, 344
vancomycin, 155t, 235, 325, 328t, 329
Antibodies
antiphospholipid, 151
antithyroid
thyroglobulin, 73, 75
TPO, 73, 74, 75, 76–77
TRAbs, 80
Anticardiolipin antibodies (ACAs), 254, 255t
Anti-chlamydia IgM, 312
Anticholinergics, 227t, 232–233
Anticoagulation
postpartum management of, 279
preventing thromboembolic risk, 27
VTE management, 272, 273, 274–276, 275t
Anticonvulsants
headache, 165
magnesium sulfate, 12
Antidepressants, 181–184
discontinuation, 178
effects of prenatal exposure to, 184
MAOIs, 184
mood disorders, management during lactation, 188–189
bupropion, 189
duloxetine, 189
MAOIs, 189
mirtazapine, 189
SSRIs, 188–189
TCAs, 189
trazodone, 189
venlafaxine, 189
neonatal toxicity, 181, 182t–183t
paroxetine, 181
SNRIs, 184
SSRIs, 181, 182t–183t
autism spectrum disorders, 184
neonatal toxicity, 181, 182t–183t
neurodevelopmental effects, 181, 184
teratogenicity, 181, 182t–183t
TCAs, 184
treatment resistance to, 180
Anti-D immunoglobulin prophylaxis, 467, 469–470
after birth (postpartum), 469
before birth (antepartum), 469–470
special clinical situations, 470
Antiemetics
for headache, 164t, 165
NVP and HG, 98
Antiepileptic drugs (AEDs)
during breast-feeding, 189
congenital malformations, 168
seizures, 167, 168, 169t, 170–171
syndrome, 187
Antifibrinolytic amino acids, 145
Antigens, defined, 460
Antihistamines, 95t, 97, 107, 233, 389
Antihypertensive drugs
for ADR, 174
alpha-2 adrenergic agonist, 99
CHTN, management, 4
common types, 4
effectiveness, 4–5
mild-to-moderate HTN, 4–5
severe HTN, 5
indications, 5
preeclampsia, 7, 12–13
SCI, 175
urgent blood pressure control in hospital, 6t
Anti-K1, for severe neonatal anemia, 469
Antioxidant(s)

for preeclampsia, 11
selenoproteins as, 74
with vitamin C, for preeclampsia, 7
Antiphospholipid antibodies (APAs)
lupus nephritis and, 151
SLE and, 247
testing, 254, 255t
VTE, risk of, 277–278
Antiphospholipid syndrome (APS), 254–258
anesthesia, 258
antepartum testing, 257–258
APA testing, 254, 255t
classification, 254
complications
fetal, 255
maternal, 254–255
defined, 270
diagnosis, 254, 255t
epidemiology/incidence, 254
etiology/basic pathophysiology, 254
historic notes, 254
management, 255–257
prevention, 256
principles, 255
screening, 255–256
postpartum/breast-feeding, 258
pregnancy considerations, 255
preparations for delivery, 258
SLE and, 246
symptoms, 254
testing, 491
therapy, 256–257
actual therapy, 256–257, 257t
evidence, 256
issues, 257
Antiplatelet agents, for preeclampsia, 13
Antipsychotics
lactation and, 189–190
during pregnancy, 187–188
Antiretroviral therapy (ART)
combination, 297
HIV infection, 300–301, 301t, 302t
Antithrombin III (ATIII) deficiency, 260, 262, 264, 265t, 266, 274, 277
Anti-TNF-alpha agents, 112t
Antiviral drugs, for herpes, 453, 454
Anti-Xa levels, 256, 257, 275, 276
Anxiety disorders, 41, 174, 177, 178, 209, 210, 211, 216, 217, 218, 355, 366, 401, 419, 442, 444
Aorta, coarctation of, 27
Aortic insufficiency, 28
Aortic stenosis, 28
Apgar score, 19, 34t, 35, 40, 206, 218, 236, 299, 360, 415, 417, 420, 422, 424, 432, 499, 501, 514, 515, 516, 517
Apixaban, 273
"Apple peel" syndrome, 482
Apremilast, 393
APS, see Antiphospholipid syndrome (APS)
Aptiom (Eslicarbazepine), 169t
ARDS (acute respiratory distress syndrome), 349, 356–357, 356t
ARDSNet trial, 357
Arfonad, 174
L-Arginine
in FGR pregnancies, 420
preeclampsia, 19
Aripiprazole, 186t, 190
Armour Thyroid, 76
Arrhythmias, 104, 206, 367, 479, 498
Arterial pulmonary vasculature, 366
Arteriovenous malformations, NIH and, 482

Arthritic pain, 41
Asenapine, 187
Aspart insulin, 53t, 54, 55, 62t, 65t, 66–67, 67f
Aspartame, 53
Aspirin
    APS, 256
    baby, 3
    FGR pregnancies, 420
    FGR, prevention, 416
    for headache, 164–165, 164t
    multiple gestation, 402
    preeclampsia, 7, 10, 152, 249
    prevention of recurrence, fetal death, 493
    sickle cell disease, 141
    thromboembolism, high risk of, 29
    VTE, management, 276, 278
Assault, during pregnancy, 340–341
Assessments
    antepartum fetal assessment, *see*
        Antepartum testing
    Brazelton Neonatal Assessment Scale,
        210
    fetal pulmonary maturity, indications,
        521
    growth, intervals of, 420
    inpatient, NVP and HG, 98–99
    intervention, smoking, 197t, 199
    5Rs, for smokers, 197t
    SOFA score, 357
    sonographic
        of AF, *see* Sonographic assessment
        for twin growth, 407
Assisted reproductive technologies (ART),
        use, 398
Associations
    acute cholecystitis, 121
    amphetamines, 216
    benzodiazepines, abuse, 218
    cholelithiasis, 119, 120t
    CHTN, 2
    CMV, 436
    cocaine, 214
    fetal death, 488–489, 489t
    GBS, 325, 326
    GDM, 60
    HAV infections, 283
    HBV infections, 286
    HCV infection, 293
    herpes, 451
    ICP, 104
    IH (pustular psoriasis of pregnancy), 393
    inherited thrombophilias, 262
    marijuana (cannabis), 209
    NIH, 479–483
    NVP and HG, 92, 93
    opioids, use, 211
    parvovirus, 447
    PCP, 219
    PP, 391
    preeclampsia, 9
    pregestational diabetes, 50
    seizures, 168
    SG, 386
    tuberculosis, 239
    VTE, 270, 272t
    VZV infection, 456
Asthma, 225–233
    acute treatment, 233
    anesthesia, 233
    antepartum testing, 233
    classification, 225–227, 226t, 227t
    delivery, 233
    diagnosis, 225

etiology and basic pathophysiology, 225
incidence, 225
key points, 225
management
    preconception care, 228
    prenatal care, 228
    prevention, 228, 228t
    principles, 228
    workup, 229
mild intermittent, 227
mild persistent, 227
moderate persistent, 227
postpartum/breast-feeding, 233
pregnancy
    complications, 227–228
    considerations, 228
severe persistent, 227
status asthmaticus, 233
symptoms, 225
therapy, 229–233
    anticholinergics, 232–233
    β-agonists, 232
    cromolyn, 232
    general, 229
    goals, 229
    inhaled corticosteroids and
        long-acting β-agonists
        (fixed-drug combination), 232
    inhaled steroids, 232
    LTRA, 232
    mild intermittent, 230, 232
    mild persistent, 232
    moderate persistent, 232
    oral corticosteroids, 233
    severe persistent, 232
    suggested medications, 229–230, 229f,
        230f, 231f
    theophylline, 232
Asymmetric FGR, 414
Asymptomatic bacteriuria, treatment, 143
Atazanavir, 302t
Atopic dermatitis of pregnancy (ADP)
    defined, 389
    diagnosis, 389, 389f
    epidemiology/incidence, 389
    etiology/basic pathology, 389
    key points, 389
    management
        therapy, 389
        workup, 389
    overview, 386, 387t
    pregnancy considerations, 389
    symptoms, 389
Atopic eruption of pregnancy (AEP), 386,
        387t
Atovaquone, 301t
Attention deficit hyperactivity disorder
        (ADHD), 178, 216
"Atypical" antibodies, hemolytic disease
    CDE system antigens, 474
    Kell alloimmunization, 474
    MNS antigen system, 474
Atypical antipsychotics, 186t, 190
Aura, defined, 168
Auricular acupressure, 97
Autism spectrum disorders, 184
Autoimmune hepatitis, 124
Autoimmune thrombocytopenia, 255
Autonomic dysreflexia (ADR)
    anesthesia, 174–175
    delivery, 175
    preeclampsia *vs.*, 174, 174t
    preventive management, 174

psychological challenges, 175
symptoms/sign of, 173, 174
treatment, 174–175
uterine palpation techniques, 175
Autopsy, fetal, 490–491
Azapropazon, 155t
Azasan, 249, 249t
Azathioprine, 112t, 113, 128, 129, 155, 155t,
        246, 248, 249, 249t, 389, 392
Azithromycin, 142, 235, 301t, 305, 306, 307,
        308, 308t, 310, 312, 313t, 319, 359

B

Bacille Calmette-Guerin (BCG) vaccine, 239,
        240, 241, 242, 302, 332, 336t
Bacterial endocarditis prophylaxis, 26–27, 27t
Ballantyne's syndrome, 483
Balloon valvuloplasty, percutaneous, 28
Balsalazide, 112t, 113
Banzel (Rufinamide), 169t
Bariatric surgery, 32, 38–39, 38t, 42, 134, 432,
        433
Baseline tests, 3
Bath salts, 216–217; *see also* Amphetamines
BCG (Bacille Calmette-Guerin) vaccine, 239,
        240, 241, 242, 302, 332, 336t
Beclomethasone, 226t, 232
Bed rest
    FGR pregnancies, 419
    hypertensive disorders
        CHTN, 3
        GHTN, 6
        preeclampsia, 7
    multiple gestation, 403
    preeclampsia, 11
Bedside echocardiography, 366–367
Behavior therapy, prepregnancy weight
        reduction, 38
Behavioral educational interventions, 188
Bejel, transmission, 318
Benadryl (Diphenhydramine), 95t, 97, 380
Bendectin, 97
Benzodiazepines, 217–219
    antepartum testing, 218
    complications
        congenital anomalies, 218
        long-term neonatal outcome, 218
        neonatal withdrawal, 218
        obstetrical and neonatal, 218
    defined, 217
    diagnosis, 217
    epidemiology/incidence, 218
    etiology/basic pathophysiology, 218
    historic notes, 217
    NVP and HG, 99
    postpartum/breast-feeding, 219
    during pregnancy, 206, 210, 215, 217
    risk factors/associations, 218
    symptoms/signs, 218
    therapy, 218
Benzoylmethylecognine, *see* Cocaine
Beta-adrenergic antagonist drug,
        for thyrotoxicosis, 77
Beta-blockers, 4, 29, 82
Betadine, 490
Betamethasone, 17, 249, 249t, 251, 356, 360,
        380, 404, 424
Betamimetics, for FGR, 419
Bile acids, cholesterol metabolism, 104
Bilirubin, 107, 128
Biomarkers
    AFE, 367

first-trimester serum levels of, 9
  testing, 9
Biophysical profile score (BPS)
  fetal monitoring, 499–501, 501t
    AF volume, 500, 500t
    body movements, 500
    breathing movements, 499, 500
    CTG, 500
    Doppler surveillance and, 505, 506f
    fetal tone, 500
    management, 500, 500t, 501t
    modified BPS, 501
    PNM with, 499, 500t
    prediction of fetal status, 499, 499f
    variables, 499, 499t
  for FGR, 422, 424, 425
    AF volume, 422, 424
  reducing cerebral palsy, 496
  VAS and, 498
Biopsy, sentinel node
  breast cancer, 375
  melanoma, 378, 395
Bipolar depression, 177, 178, 179–180
  complications, 180
  defined, 178
  epidemiology, 178
  markers, 180
  pregnancy considerations, 180
  risk factors, 179–180
  screening, 180
  SSRIs in, 180
Birth defects
  AED treatment, 168
  cardiac and neural tube defects, 55
  long-term follow-up of babies, 4
  metformin and, 66
  MMF and EC-MPS, 128
  risks
    immunosuppressive agents, 128
    PPIs, 98
Birth weight, low
  CRI and, 152
  IUGR and, 211
  pregnancy after LTx, 126t, 127
  smoking, complication, 198
Bitolterol, 227t
Bleeding, UFH therapy, 273
Bleomycin, 375
Blood chemistry, abnormal, 128
Blood cultures, for sepsis, 359
Blood plasma volume, 12
Blood sampling, FBS, 83, 460, 464–465, 467, 472–473, 472t, 473t
Blood tests, 9
Blood transfusions
  anemia, 131, 137, 482
  HBV-infection, 286
  HCV infection, 292t, 293
  hemolytic disease, 467, 468, 470, 471–473, 472t, 473t, 474
  HIV-infection, 299
  for sickle cell disease, 139, 140, 141, 142, 143
  syphilis, 315, 316
Blunt abdominal trauma, 343–344
Boceprevir, 294
Body mass index (BMI)
  calculation of, 32
  prepregnancy, 386
Body movements, fetal, 500
Body packing, 215
Bone scan, 375
BPS, *see* Biophysical profile score (BPS)

Bradyarrhythmias, 479
Brain-sparing, defined, 421, 501
Brazelton Neonatal Assessment Scale, 210
Breast cancer, during pregnancy, 374–375
  breast-feeding after treatment, 382
  diagnosis
    delay in, 374
    tests and safety, 374
  pregnancy after, 381–382
  sentinel node biopsy, 375
  staging, 375
  surgery, 375
  termination of pregnancy, 374
  treatment, 375, 376f
Breast-feeding
  after treatment for breast cancer, 382
  amphetamines, 217
  antidepressants and, 188–189
    bupropion, 189
    duloxetine, 189
    MAOIs, 189
    mirtazapine, 189
    SSRIs, 188–189
    TCAs, 189
    trazodone, 189
    venlafaxine, 189
  antipsychotics, 189–190
  APS, 258
  asthma, 233
  benzodiazepines, 219
  CD, 114
  CHTN, 5
  cocaine, use, 215
  CRI, 153
  CsA and, 393
  GDM, 68, 68f
  HAV infections, pregnancy with, 284
  HBV infections, 289
  HCV infection, 295
  HIV infection, 303
  influenza, 238
  LTx, pregnancy after, 129
  marijuana (cannabis), use, 210
  maternal anemia, 137
  obesity, 41
  opioids, use, 213–214
  PCP, 219
  pneumonia, 235
  pregestational diabetes, 55, 56
  prolactinoma, 90
  renal transplantation, 156
  SCI, 175
  seizures, 171
  SLE, 250
  smoking, 201
  stabilizers
    carbamazepine, 189
    lamotrigine, 189
    lithium, 189
    valproic acid, 189
  trauma, 346
  tuberculosis, 242
  UC, 116
  vWD, 149
Breathing
  CO$_2$ rebreathing, 357
  in eclampsia, 7, 19
  fetal, 197, 421, 471, 499–500, 499t, 508, 514
  maternal stabilization after trauma, 339, 342f, 343, 343t
  problems
    asthma, 225
    GBS, 325

Breathing movements, fetal, 499, 500
Breslow depth, 394
Broad-spectrum antimicrobial therapy, sepsis/septic shock, 359
Brodalumab, 393
Bromocriptine (Parlodel), 86, 87, 88, 89, 155t
Budesonide (Pulmacort), 232
Budesonide dry powder, 226t
Buprenorphine, 206, 210, 211, 212–213
Bupropion, 183t, 184, 189, 200–201
Bupropion HCl (Zyban®, Wellbutrin®), 201

C

Cabergoline, 86, 87, 88, 89
Caffeine, 164t, 165
Calcineurin inhibitors (CNI), 125, 250, 389
Calcitonin gene-related peptide (CGRP), 163
Calcium, for preeclampsia, 7, 10–11
Calcium carbonate, 75
Calcium channel blockers
  for CHTN, 4, 5
  FGR pregnancies, 419–420
  post-LTx pregnancy, 125
  stable angina, 29
  verapamil, 155t, 165, 479, 486
Calcium gluconate, 152
Cancer, during pregnancy, 373–382
  breast, 374–375
    breast-feeding after treatment, 382
    delay in diagnosis, 374
    pregnancy after, 381–382
    sentinel node biopsy, 375
    staging, 375
    surgery, 375
    termination of pregnancy, 374
    tests and safety, 374
    treatment, 375, 376f
  cervical cancer, invasive, 378–379
    delay in diagnosis, 379
    delivery for patients with, 379
    diagnostic tests and safety, 379
    effects, on pregnancy, 379
    staging, 379
    surgery, 379
    termination of pregnancy, 379
    therapy, 379
  chemotherapy
    acute leukemia, 377–378
    breast cancer, 375
    cervical cancer, 379
    complications, 380
    considerations, 374
    decadron with, 380
    dosage, 373, 374
    fetal/neonatal evaluation after, 380–381
    HD, 375, 377
    NHL, 377
    preterm labor, 380
  children of cancer survivors, 381
  complications, of therapy, 380
  diagnosis, 373–382
    chemotherapy, pregnancy after, 381
    chemotherapy-induced cardiac toxicity, 381
    general principles, 381–382
    before pregnancy, 381–382
    radiation, pregnancy after, 381
    radiation-induced cardiac toxicity due to fibrosis, 381
  epidemiology, 373

fetal surveillance and timing of delivery, 380
general considerations, 373–374
HD, 375, 376–377
  diagnosis, 375
  pregnancy after, 382
  presentation, diagnostic tests, and safety, 375–376
  radiotherapy, 377
  staging, 376
  surgery, 376
  termination of pregnancy, 376
  treatment, 376–377
incidence, 373
key points, 373
leukemia, 377–378
  acute, 377–378
  chronic, 378
  pregnancy after, 382
maternal surveillance, 380
melanoma
  delay in diagnosis, 378
  effects, on pregnancy, 378
  pregnancy after, 382
  staging and sentinel node biopsy, 378
  surgery, 378
  termination of pregnancy, 378
  treatment, 378
NHL
  delay in diagnosis, 377
  effects, on pregnancy, 377
  treatment, 377
risk of recurrence, 381
specific cancers, pregnancy after, 381
thyroid, 379–380
  delay in diagnosis, 379
  diagnostic tests and safety, 379
  pregnancy after, 382
  surgery, 379
  termination of pregnancy, 379
  treatment, 379–380
Cancer and Pregnancy Registry, 381
Cannabis sativa (cannabis), *see* Marijuana (cannabis)
Capreomycin, 242
Caproic acid, 369
Capsular polysaccharide (CPS)-based protein, GBS, 326
Carbamazepine, 75, 155t, 167, 169, 169t, 170, 171, 185t, 187, 189
Carbatrol®, 185t
Carbohydrate, counting, 54
Carbon monoxide, 196, 197
Carboxyhemoglobin, 197
Carcinogens, 197
Cardiac arrest, management, 367–369, 368t, 370f
Cardiac disease, 24–30
background, 24
classification, 25, 25t
complications, 25
epidemiology/incidence, 24
etiology/basic pathophysiology/ pregnancy considerations, 24–25
genetics, 24
key points, 24
management, 25, 26–30
  aortic stenosis, 28
  coarctation of aorta, 27
  coronary artery disease, 29–30
  dilated cardiomyopathy, 29
  general, 25, 26–27, 27t
  hypertrophic cardiomyopathy, 29

Marfan syndrome, 29
  mechanical heart valves, 28–29
  mitral and aortic insufficiency, 28
  mitral stenosis, 28
  palpitations, 27
  peripartum cardiomyopathy, 29
  preconception counseling, 25
  pregnancy management of specific diseases, 27–30
  prenatal care/antepartum testing, 25
  pulmonary hypertension, 27
  pulmonic stenosis (PS), 28
  tetralogy of fallot, 28
risk factors, 25, 26t
symptoms/signs, 24
Cardiac neonatal lupus (CNL), SLE, 250–251
counseling, 250–251
delivery, 251
etiology, 250
management, 251
prenatal care evaluation, 251
prevention, 251
therapy, 251
Cardiac toxicity
chemotherapy-induced, 381
radiation-induced, fibrosis and, 381
Cardiomyopathy
defined, 29
dilated, pregnancy management, 29
neonatal, 378
peripartum, 29
Cardiopulmonary complications, cocaine abuse, 214
Cardiopulmonary resuscitation (CPR), 345–346, 367
Cardiotocography (CTG), fetal surveillance
BPS, assessment, 500
for FGR, 422
heart rate testing, 497–498, 497f
preventing fetal death in ICP, 107
Cardiovascular disorders, NIH and, 479–481, 480t
Care and caring
critical, *see* Critical care
intrapartum
  HIV infection, 303
  obesity and, 40
postpartum
  HIV infection, 303
  SCI, 175
preconception
  asthma, 228
  obesity, 35–37, 36f, 36t, 37t
pregnant trauma patient, 341
prenatal
  after bariatric surgery, 38t
  asthma, 228
  cardiac disease, 25
  CD, 112
  CHTN, 3
  CRI, 152
  drug abuse, 208–209, 209t
  evaluation, CHB/CNL, 251
  HAV infections, pregnancy with, 283, 284
  HBV infections, 288
  HIV infection, 300
  NS, 153
  obesity, 39–40, 39t
  pregestational diabetes, 52, 53–54
  prolactinoma, 89–90, 90t
  renal transplantation, 155, 155t
  SCI, 173–174

seizures, 170
sickle cell disease, 140, 141–142
SLE, 248, 249
trauma, 346
UC, 115
vWD, 146
preventive, sickle cell disease, 140
Carpenter–Coustan stricter criteria, 60
CD, *see* Crohn's disease (CD)
CDE system antigens, 474
Cefazolin, 27, 41, 325, 328t, 329
Cefepime, 235
Cefixime, 307, 308, 308t
Cefpodoxime, 235
Ceftriaxone, 27, 156, 235, 306, 308, 308t, 319
Cefuroxime, 235
Celexa® (citalopram), 182t
Centella asiatica extract, 387
Centers for Disease Control and Prevention (CDC), 297, 305, 307, 310, 312, 315, 327, 488
Cephalexin, 156
Cephalosporins, 139, 142, 143, 307, 308
Cerclage, 403, 408
Cerebral palsy, 125, 404, 412, 416
Cerebroplacental ratio (CPR)
calculation, 421
change in, 501
Certolizumab, 112t, 113
Cervical cancer, during pregnancy, 378–379
delay in diagnosis, 379
delivery for patients with, 379
diagnostic tests and safety, 379
effects, on pregnancy, 379
staging, 379
surgery, 379
termination of pregnancy, 379
therapy, 379
Cervical length (CL) screening, 402
Cervical lymphadenopathy, 306
Cervicitis, symptoms, 311, 313t
Cesarean delivery
acute cholecystitis, 122
AFE, risk factors for, 365, 366, 367, 369
AFV, measurement, 513, 514
benzodiazepine exposure, 206
BPS and, 496, 499
cervical cancer during pregnancy, 379
CHTN, maternal complications of, 1, 2
epilepsy, women with, 168, 171
fetal death, 489, 492, 493
fetal macrosomia, 432, 433, 434
FGR and, 412, 414, 416, 417, 421, 422, 425, 426
FHR testing, 497–498, 497f
FNAIT, 465
gallstones, presence of, 120
GBS, 330
GDM, 59, 60, 67, 68
gonorrhea, 305
HCV-infected woman, 291, 294, 295
heart diseases, reserved for obstetric indications, 27
HIV-infected woman, 297, 299, 300, 303
HSV-infected woman, 451, 454
hydrocortisone and, 249
IBD, 110, 111, 114, 115
in ICU, 355, 360
LTx, pregnancy after, 129
magnesium, 7, 12
maternal substance abuse, 210, 213, 215, 416
multiple gestations, 403, 407, 408

NIH, management of, 486
for NRFHT, 19, 514
obesity and, 32, 33, 35, 40, 41
PEP and, 389
PMCD, 367
polyhydramnios and, 516, 516f, 517, 518
postdate pregnancy, 508
pregestational diabetics, 50, 54, 55
rate of, 13, 13t
renal diseases, 156, 158
retention sutures, 29
SCI patients, 175
sickle cell disease, 142, 143
SLE patients, 250
for stillbirth, 492
trauma during pregnancy, 340, 346
VBAC, 40, 434
von Willebrand disease, 149
VTE, 266, 270, 278, 279
women with HELLP syndrome, 17–18
Chamomile, 97
Chantix® (varenicline), 201
CHB, see Congenital heart block (CHB)
Chemical tests, for illicit substances, 208
Chemoprophylaxis, after exposure, 237
Chemotherapy
induced cardiac toxicity, 381
nausea and vomiting and, 209, 380
during pregnancy
acute leukemia, 377–378
breast cancer, 375
for cancer, 373, 374
cervical cancer, 379
complications, 380
decadron with, 380
dosage, 373, 374
fetal/neonatal evaluation after, 380–381
HD, 375, 377
NHL, 377
preterm labor, 380
pregnancy after, 381
sickle cell anemia, 141
Chest compressions, 367
CHEST Guidelines, 28
Chest X-ray, 240
Chickenpox, see Varicella zoster virus (VZV) (chickenpox)
Childhood Cancer Survivor Study, 381
Children, of cancer survivors, 381
Chitosin, 38
Chlamydia, 310–313
background, 310
complications/risks, 311
epidemiology/incidence, 310, 311t
key points, 310
management
diagnosis, 312
prevention, 311–312
screening, 312
pathophysiology/etiology, 311
symptoms, 310–311
cervicitis/urethritis, 311
chlamydial conjunctivitis, 311
LGV, 311
maternal genital infection, 311
proctitis/proctocolitis, 311
transmission, 311
treatment, 312–313, 313t
Chlamydial conjunctivitis, 311, 313t
Chlamydia pneumoniae, 143
Chlamydia trachomatis, 305, 306, 307, 308, 310–313, 322

Chlordiazepoxide, 218
Chlorhexidine, 330
Chlorpromazine (Thorazine), 19, 189–190
Cholecystectomy, for acute cholecystitis, 122
Choledocholithiasis, 121
Cholelithiasis, 119–120
complications
maternal, 119
defined, 119
diagnosis, 119
differential diagnosis, 119
epidemiology/incidence, 119
etiology/pathophysiology, 119
management
imaging, 120
labor and delivery issues, 120
laboratory investigations, 120
pregnancy considerations, 120
principles, 120
therapy, 120
workup, 120
risk factors/associations, 119, 120t
symptoms, 119
Cholestasis, ICP, see Intrahepatic cholestasis of pregnancy (ICP)
Cholestyramine, 107, 250
Chorioamnionitis, 33, 325, 359
Chorionicity, multiple gestations, 398, 399, 400, 400f, 401, 404, 404t, 407, 491
Chorionic villus sampling, 402
Chorioretinitis, neonatal, 443
Chromosomal abnormalities, NIH and, 480t, 481
Chromosomal anomalies, multiple gestation, 401
Chronic hypertension (CHTN), 1–5
anesthesia, 5
antepartum testing, 5
classification, 1, 2
complications, 2–3
fetal, 2–3
maternal, 2
defined, 1
delivery, 5
diagnosis/definition, 1, 2t
epidemiology/incidence, 1
etiology/basic pathophysiology, 1
key points, 1
management, 3–5
antihypertensive drugs, 4
initial evaluation/workup, 3
lifestyle changes and bed rest, 3
preconception counseling, 3
prenatal care, 3
prevention, 3
principles, 3
screening/diagnosis, 3
therapy, 3
postpartum/breast-feeding, 5
risk factors/associations, 2
superimposed preeclampsia with, 14
Chronic leukemia (CML), 378, 382
Chronic renal failure (CRF), 150
Chronic renal insufficiency (CRI)
antenatal testing, 152
complications, 151, 151t
defined, 150
delivery, 153
laboratory tests, 152
long-term renal prognosis, 153
management, 152
overview, 150, 151t

patient education, 152
postpartum/breast-feeding, 153
pregnancy considerations, 152
prenatal care, 152
prevention, 152
therapy
HTN, 152
preeclampsia, 152
preterm labor, 152
workup, 152
Chylothorax, 481
Cimetidine (Tagamet), 95t, 97, 155t
Ciprofloxacin, 235
Circulation
in eclampsia, 7, 19
fetal, 128, 197, 316
hyperdynamic pulmonary, 272
maternal, 9, 33, 197
maternal stabilization after trauma, 339, 342f, 343, 343t
ROSC, 367
cis-α-thalassemia, 131
Citalopram, 182t, 188
Clarithromycin, 235, 242, 301t
Classifications
acute cholecystitis, 120, 121t
APS, 254
asthma, 225–227, 226t, 227t
cardiac disease, 25, 25t
CHTN, 1, 2
CMV, 436–437, 437f, 437t
cutaneous melanoma, 394
FGR, 414
FNAIT, 460, 462, 462t
GBS, 325, 326t
HBV infections, 286, 286t
herpes
nonprimary first episode, 452
primary first episode, 452
reactivation (recurrent) genital herpes, 452
HIV, 299, 299t
ICP, 104
inherited thrombophilias
ATIII deficiency, 262
FVL, 261–262, 261t
MTHFR/homocysteinemia, 262
protein C, 262
protein S, 262
prothrombin G20210A gene, 262
NVP and HG, 92
obesity, 32, 33t
pneumonia, 233, 234
preeclampsia, 9
pregestational diabetes, 50
prolactinoma, 86
renal disease, 150, 151t
SCI, 173
seizures, 168
for sepsis, 357, 358t
syphilis, 316–317
incubation period, 316
late benign (tertiary) syphilis, 316–317
latent, 316
neurosyphilis, 317
primary, 316
secondary, 316
vWD, 145
Clavulanic acid, 242
Clindamycin, 27, 312, 325, 328t, 329
Clinical behavior, of HD, 375–376
Clinical concerns/issues, FNAIT, 465
Clinical hyperthyroidism, diagnosis, 81

Clinical hypothyroidism, 73–76
    antepartum management, 76
    complications, 74
    defined, 73, 74f
    incidence, 73
    management
        preconception, 74
        prevention, 74
    neonatal, 76
    pathophysiology, 73–74
    postpartum, 76
    pregnancy considerations, 74–75, 75t
        anatomy/radiology, 74
        fetal thyroid physiology, 74
        maternal physiology, 74, 75t
        placenta physiology, 74–75
    screening/diagnosis, 75, 75t
    signs/symptoms, 73
    treatment, 75–76
        dose, 75
        goal, 75
        iodine supplementation, 76
        new diagnosis, 75
        preexisting hypothyroidism, 75
        thyroxine replacement, 75–76
        type, 76
Clinical Laboratory Improvement
        Amendments (CLIA), 306, 318
Clinical neonatal findings
    CMV, 437
    CVS, 459
Clinical presentation, AFE, 366
Clinical remission, defined, 112
Clinical scenarios
    FNAIT, 465
    VTE management, 272, 273, 274–276, 275t
Clofazimine, 242
Clomiphene citrates, 124
Clonidine, 99, 201, 213
Clostridium difficile, 112
Clostridium spp., 112, 121
Clozapine, 186t, 187, 190
Clozaril®, 186t
CMV, see Cytomegalovirus (CMV)
Coagulation studies, trauma and, 344–345
Coagulopathy and AFE, management, 369
Coarctation of aorta, 27
Cobalt 60, treatment with, 377
Cocaethylene, 214
Cocaine abuse, 214–215
    anesthesia, 215
    antepartum testing, 215
    diagnosis/definition, 214
    epidemiology/incidence, 214
    etiology/basic pathophysiology, 214
    historic notes, 214
    maternal and perinatal complications,
        214–215
        congenital anomalies, 214
        fetal/neonatal morphometrics, 215
        long-term neonatal outcome, 215
        neonatal withdrawal, 215
        obstetrical complications, 215
    overview, 206
    postpartum/breast-feeding, 215
    risk factors/associations, 214
    symptoms, signs, and cardiopulmonary
        complications, 214
    therapy, 215
Cochrane systematic review, 4, 5, 97, 107, 181,
        188, 212, 213, 228
Cocoa butter lotion, 387
Cocooning, defined, 332

Codeine, 162, 164t, 165, 210, 211
Cognitive behavioral therapies
        headache, 165
        mood disorders, 188
Cognitive delay, 416
Colectomy, UC, 115
Collagen-elastin hydrolysates, 387
Colon cancer, risk of, 114
Color Doppler, for AFV, 514
Communicating and Relating Effectively
        (CARE), 188
Community-acquired pneumonia (CAP),
        see Pneumonia
Comorbidity
    LTx, pregnancy after, 125–127
        ACR rate, 127
        CMV acute infection, 125, 127
        diabetes, 125
        fetal and maternal outcomes, 125, 126t
        hepatitis virus reactivation, 125
        hypertension and renal insufficiency,
            125
        infrarenal aortic graft, 127
Comparative genomic hybridization (cGH),
        490
Compazine (prochlorperazine), 96t, 98, 162,
        164t, 165, 492
Competence, in core procedural skills, 352
Complications
    ACS, 143
    acute cholecystitis
        fetal, 121
        maternal, 121
    amphetamines
        congenital anomalies, 216–217
        fetal/neonatal morphometrics, 217
        long-term neurodevelopmental
            outcome, 217
        neonatal withdrawal, 217
        obstetrical and neonatal, 217
    anemia, 134
    APS
        fetal, 255
        maternal, 254–255
    benzodiazepines, abuse
        congenital anomalies, 218
        long-term neonatal outcome, 218
        neonatal withdrawal, 218
        obstetrical and neonatal, 218
    bipolar depression, 180
    cancer therapy, 380
    cardiac disease, 25
    CD
        fetal and neonatal, 111
        maternal, 111
    chlamydia, 311
    cholelithiasis
        fetal, 119
        maternal, 119
    CHTN, 2–3
        fetal, 2–3
        maternal, 2
    clinical hypothyroidism, 74
    CMV, 437
    cocaine, use, 214–215
        cardiopulmonary, 214
        congenital anomalies, 214
        obstetrical, 215
        perinatal, 214–215
    CRI, 151, 151t
    cutaneous melanoma, 394
    dialysis, 154
    eclampsia, 18

fetal macrosomia, 432
FGR, 415–416
FNAIT, 462
GBS, 326
GDM, 60–61
GHTN, 5
gonorrhea, 306
hallucinogens, exposure
    congenital anomalies, 220
    long-term neonatal outcome, 220
    obstetrical and neonatal, 220
HAV, 283
HBV, 286
HCV, 293
HELLP syndrome, 16, 17t
herpes, 452
HIV
    fetal, 299
    maternal, 299
HSV infection, 454
hyperthyroidism, 81
ICP, 104, 106
IH (pustular psoriasis of pregnancy), 393
influenza, 236–237
inherited thrombophilias, 262–263
    adverse pregnancy outcome, 262–263,
        263t
    VTE, 262
marijuana, use, 209–210
    congenital anomalies, 210
    fetal/neonatal morphometrics, 210
    long-term neonatal outcome, 210
    neonatal withdrawal, 210
    obstetrical, 210
maternal
    acute cholecystitis, 121
    anemia, 134
    APS, 254–255
    CD, 111
    cholelithiasis, 119
    CHTN, 2
    cocaine, 214–215
    HIV, 299
    NIH, 483
    NVP and HG, 93
    preeclampsia, 9
    prolactinoma, 86
    seizures, 168
    SLE, 246
    smoking, 198
    trauma, 340
    UC, 114
mood disorders, 178
multiple gestation, 400–402
    abruptio placentae, 401
    acute fatty liver, 402
    anomalous fetus, selective
        termination, 403–404; see also
        Anomalous fetus
    chromosomal and congenital
        anomalies, 401
    fetal, 400, 401
    FGR and discordant growth, 401
    FGR/discordant twins, 404
    gestational diabetes, 402
    low-dose aspirin, 402
    maternal, 401, 402
    monochorionic gestations, 401
    peripartum hysterectomy, 402
    preeclampsia, 401
    pregnancy considerations, 402
    pregnancy management, 402
    prenatal diagnosis, 402

prevention and management, 403–407
PTB, 401, 402t
PTB, prediction of, 402
single fetal death, 404, 404t
single fetal demise in, 401
spontaneous pregnancy loss, 400, 401
thrombocytopenia, 401–402
TTTS, 404, 405–407; *see also* Twin-twin
    transfusion syndrome (TTTS)
NS, 153
NVP and HG
    fetal/neonatal, 93
    maternal, 93
obesity, 33–35, 34t–35t, 41
oligohydramnios, 515
opioids
    congenital anomalies, 211
    fetal/neonatal morphometrics, 211
    long-term neonatal outcome, 211–212
    neonatal withdrawal, 211
    obstetrical, 211
parvovirus, 448
PCP
    congenital anomalies, 219
    fetal/neonatal morphometrics, 219
    long-term neonatal outcome, 219
    neonatal withdrawal, 219
    obstetrical, 219
PEP, 388
PG (herpes gestationis), 392
pneumonia, 234
polyhydramnios (hydramnios), 517
PP, 391
preeclampsia, 9, 14, 15–20
pregestational diabetes, 51
pregnancy
    asthma, 227–228
    PCP, 219
prolactinoma, 86–87
    fetus, 86–87
    mother, 86
renal transplantation, 154
seizures, 168–169
    fetal, 168–169
    maternal, 168
sickle cell disease, 140, 141t
SLE, 246–247
    fetal/neonatal, 246–247
    maternal, 246
smoking
    congenital anomalies, 198
    fetal death, 198
    LBW, 198
    maternal lifetime, 198
    placental abruption, 198
    placenta previa, 198
    postnatal morbidities, 198
    preeclampsia, 198
    pregnancy loss, 198
    preterm birth, 198
    PROM, 198
    smokeless tobacco, 198
syphilis, 317
toxoplasmosis, 443
trauma
    abruptio placentae, 340
    assault, hospitalization for, 340–341
    fetal death, 340
    fetal injury, 340
    fetal/neonatal outcomes, 340
    hospitalization, 340
    hysterectomy, 340
    maternal death, 340

neonatal death, 340
    transfusion, 340
trichomoniasis, 322–323
UC, 114–115
    fetal, 115
    maternal, 114
urinary nephrolithiasis, 157
UTI, 156
VTE, 270
vWD, 146
VZV infection
    fetal, 457
    maternal, 457
Computed tomography (CT)
    cancer, 373, 376
    CTPA, 272
    dermatoses, 395
    headache, 164
    prolactinoma, 87, 89
    renal disease, 157
    seizures, 168
    trauma and, 343, 343t, 344, 345
Condition-specific testing, fetal monitoring,
        505, 506–508
    advanced maternal age, 508
    antenatal surveillance
        indications for, 505, 506t
        suggested, 505, 507t
    diabetes, 505, 506
    fetal anemia, 508
    FGR, 506
    nonobstetric procedure monitoring, 508
    obesity, 508
    postdate pregnancy, 508
    PPROM, 508
Condoms, 175, 300, 303, 305, 306, 310, 311,
        322, 323, 451, 453
Condyloma lata, 316
Congenital anomalies
    amphetamines, complication, 216–217
    benzodiazepines, abuse, 218
    cocaine, 214
    hallucinogens, exposure, 220
    marijuana (cannabis), complication, 210
    multiple gestation, 401
    opioids, use, 211
    PCP, use, 219
    phencyclidine and, 206
    smoking, complication, 198
Congenital bleeding disorder, defined, 149
Congenital cystic adenomatoid
        malformation (CCAM), 481
Congenital diaphragmatic hernia (CDH), 481
Congenital heart block (CHB)
    risks, SSA/SSB antibodies, 246
    SLE, 250–251
        counseling, 250–251
        delivery, 251
        etiology, 250
        management, 251
        prenatal care evaluation, 251
        prevention, 251
        therapy, 251
Congenital heart defects (CHDs)
    antibiotics, 26–27
    genetics, 24
    risk factor for, 33
Congenital infections, NIH and, 482
Congenital malformations, 168–169
Congenital nephrotic syndrome, 481
Congenital pulmonary airway malformation
        (CPAM), 481
Congenital varicella syndrome (CVS)

clinical neonatal findings, 459
    VZV and, 456
Conjoined twins, 407
Conjunctivitis, chlamydial, 311, 313t
Consequences, smoking, 202
Constitutional FGR, 414
Consultations
    FNAIT, 465
    HG, diagnosis, 94
Continuous positive airway pressure
        (CPAP), 35
Continuous subcutaneous insulin infusion
        therapy (CSII), 54
Contraception, 25, 27, 42, 125, 143, 251, 279,
        459
Contraceptives, oral, 25, 27, 42, 125, 171, 175,
        251
Contraction monitoring, 344
Contraction stress test (CST), 498–499
Contraindications, to vaccination, 337
Control of Hypertension in Pregnancy Study
        (CHIPS trial), 416
Cordocentesis, workup of NIH, 485
Coronary artery disease, 25, 29–30, 50, 51,
        366, 381, 412, 416
Cortical spreading depression (CSD), 163
Corticosteroids
    administration, 12, 16
    asthma, 228, 232, 233
    benefit of, 302
    fetal heart block, 479
    HELLP syndrome, 16, 17
    HG, 98, 99
    IBD, 112t, 113
    in ICU setting, 356
    IH (pustular psoriasis of pregnancy), 393
    inhaled
        for asthma, 233
        long-acting β-agonists (fixed-drug
            combination) and, 232
    NIH, 486
    NPV, 99
    for PEP, 389
    in septic shock, 360
    SLE, 249, 249t
    women with singleton gestations, 404
Cost(s)
    CRI, pregnancy with, 152
    wet preparation, 323
Cotyledon, 238
Coumadin (warfarin), 29, 275–276
Counseling
    cardiac neonatal lupus/CHB, 250–251
    CMV, management, 437–438, 438f, 438t
    dialysis, 153
    dietary, for GDM, 61
    fetal death, 489, 489t, 490t
    FGR, management, 419
    FNAIT, 465
    HCV infection, 294
    hemolytic disease, 470
    herpes, 452–453
    HIV infection, 300
    long-term, preeclampsia, 20
    NIH, 483
    parvovirus, 448
    postpartum, recurrence rates of AFE, 369
    preconception, *see* Preconception
        counseling
    prenatal, seizures, 170
    smoking, 199–200
    sterilization, 25
    TTTS, 405

VZV infection, 457, 458t
Cranberry juice, 156
Craniosynostosis, 181
Creatinine
    clearance, calculation, 1, 3
    diabetic nephropathy, 51, 52
    LTx, pregnancy after, 124, 125, 127t
    preeclampsia, 6, 7, 8, 11, 15, 16
    renal diseases, 150, 151
    renal transplantation, 155
CRI, *see* Chronic renal insufficiency (CRI)
Criminalization, of addiction, 209
Critical care, 349–361
    background, 349
    considerations in transfer (interhospital),
        353
    ICU, admission to, 349, 350t, 353, 354t
    incidence, 349
    key points, 349
    levels of, 349–350, 350t, 351t
    logistics, 353, 354–355
    Ob-Gyn, role, 355–356
    obstetric critical care services,
        organization, 350, 351, 352–353
    requirement, specific conditions, 356–361
        ARDS and mechanical ventilation,
            356–357, 356t
        sepsis, 357–361, 358t, 359t
Crohn's disease (CD), 110–114
    antepartum testing, 114
    complications
        fetal and neonatal, 111
        maternal, 111
    defined, 110
    delivery, 114
    diagnosis, 110
    epidemiology/incidence, 110
    etiology/basic pathophysiology, 111
    HSV and, 451
    management, 111–114
        adalimumab, 112t, 113
        aminosalicylates, 112t, 113
        antibiotics, 112t, 113
        azathioprine/6-mercaptopurine, 112t,
            113
        certolizumab, 112t, 113
        corticosteroids, 112t, 113
        cyclosporine, 112t, 113
        differential diagnosis, 112
        immunomodulators/
            immunosuppressants, 112t, 113
        infliximab, 112t, 113
        medications in, 112–113, 112t
        methotrexate, 112t, 113
        naltrexone, 112t, 113–114
        natalizumab, 112t, 113
        preconception counseling, 112
        prenatal care, 112
        principles, 111
        thalidomide, 112t, 113
        workup, 112
    postpartum/breast-feeding, 114
    pregnancy considerations, 111
    signs/symptoms, 110, 111t
    UC *vs.*, 111t
Cromolyn, 226t, 232, 233
CT, *see* Computed tomography (CT)
CT pulmonary angiography (CTPA), 272
Cutaneous melanoma, 394–395
    classification, 394
    complications, 394
    defined, 394
    diagnosis, 394, 394f

epidemiology/incidence, 394
    genetics, 394
    key points, 394
    management
        preconception counseling, 395
        pregnancy, 395
        prevention, 395
        therapy, 395
        workup, 395
    pregnancy considerations, 394–395
    risk factors, 394
    symptoms, 394
Cyclophosphamide, 249t, 250, 373, 375, 377,
        378, 381, 382
Cycloserine, 242
Cyclosporine, 112t, 113, 125, 127, 128, 155,
        155t, 249t, 250, 389, 393
Cyclosporine A (CsA), for IH, 393
Cymbalta® (Duloxetine), 183t, 184, 189
Cytarabine, 377
Cytomegalovirus (CMV), 436–440
    acute infection, 125, 127
    associations, 436
    incidence/epidemiology, 436
    key points, 436
    pathogen, 436
    pathophysiology/classification
        clinical neonatal findings
            and complications, 437
        general, 436–437, 437f, 437t
        primary infection, 437
        recurrent infections, 437
    pregnancy management, 437–440
        CMV-specific hyperimmune
            globulin, 439–440
        counseling/prognosis, 437–438, 438f,
            438t
        ganciclovir and valacyclovir, 440
        hygiene, 438
        investigations/diagnosis/workup,
            439
        prevention, 438
        screening, 439
        serum, 439
        therapy, 439–440
        ultrasound fetal findings, 439
        vaccine, 438
    risk factors, 436
    symptoms, 436
    transmission, 436–437, 437f

D

Dacarbazine, 375
Daclatasvir, 291, 295
Dactinomycin, 381
Dalteparin, 256, 257, 266, 275
Danazol, 155t
Dapsone, 301t
Dark-field microscopy, for syphilis, 319
Darunavir, 302t
Dasabuvir, 291, 295
DASH diet, 61
Dating ultrasound, 5
Daunorubicin, 378, 381
1-Deamino-8-D-arginine vasopressin
        (DDAVP), 146, 148
Debendox, 97
Decadron, 380
Deep vein thrombosis (DVT)
    diagnosis, 269, 270, 271–272, 273f
    treatment of new onset DVT and PE,
        276–277, 276f

Delayed interval delivery, multiple
        gestation, 408
Delivery
    APS, 258
    asthma, 233
    CD, 114
    cesarean, *see* Cesarean delivery
    cesarean, obesity and, 41
    CHTN, 5
    eclampsia, 19
    fetal death, 491–493
        D&E, 491–492
        expectant management, 491
        induction, 492–493
    FGR pregnancies, 424–426
        DIGITAT study, 424, 425
        GRIT study, 424–425, 426
        mode of, 426
        multiple gestation and, 426, 426t
        preparation, steroids and magnesium
            sulfate, 424
        timing, 412, 423f, 424–426
        TRUFFLE study, 424, 425, 426
    FNAIT, 465
    GBS, 330
    GDM, 67
    GHTN, 6
    HAV infections, pregnancy with, 284
    HBV infections, 289
    HCV infection, 294–295
    HELLP syndrome, 17, 18
    hemolytic disease, 474
    HIV infection, 303
    ICP, 107–108
    in ICU, 355
    influenza, 238
    intrapartum glucose management
        GDM, 67, 68f
        pregestational diabetes, 55, 56f
    issues
        acute cholecystitis, 122
        cholelithiasis, 120
        sickle cell disease, 142
    LTx, pregnancy after, 129
    lung maturity, GDM, 67
    maternal anemia, 137
    mode
        CD, 114
        CRI, 153
        GDM, management, 67
        HELLP syndrome, 17, 18
        HSV infection, 454
        preeclampsia, 13
        pregestational diabetes, 55
        SCI, 175, 175t
        UC, 116
    multiple gestation
        delayed interval, 408
        route, 408
        timing of, 408, 408t
    patients with cervical cancer, 379
    pneumonia, 235
    preeclampsia, 13
        hemodynamic monitoring, 13
        severe, 16
    prolactinoma, 90
    SCI, 175
    seizures, 171
    sickle cell disease, 143
    SLE, 250, 251
    TB, 242
    timing
        cancer and, 380

GDM, 67
HELLP syndrome, 17
NIH, 486
preeclampsia, 13
pregestational diabetes, 55
severe preeclampsia, 16
trauma, 346
vaginal, *see* Vaginal delivery
VTE, 278–279
vWD, 149
Delta sign, defined, 400
Demerol (meperidine), 19, 164t, 165
Depakene (valproic acid), 165, 169, 169t, 185t
Depakote (valproic acid), 165, 169, 169t, 185t
Depakote®, Depakote ER®, and Depakote
    Sprinkles®, 185t
Department of Health and Human Services
    (DHHS), 298, 300
Depot medroxyprogesterone acetate
    (DMPA), 143
Depression
    amphetamine use, 216, 217
    benzodiazepines, use, 219
    bipolar, *see* Bipolar depression
    cocaine use, 214
    CSD, 163
    EPDS, 177, 178, 179f
    GDM, 59, 67
    HG and, 93
    marijuana, use, 210
    maternal, 177, 178
    maternal respiratory, 19
    MDD, 177, 180
    migraine and, 165
    myocardial, 27
    obesity and, 41
    opioids, use, 211, 212
    PCP, use, 219
    postpartum, 134, 177, 178, 179, 188
    postpartum thyroiditis, 77
    in pregnancy, 177
    psychological intervention for, 188
    risk factors, 178
    SCI and, 175
    screening for, 178
    smoking relapse, 201
    SSRIs for, 181, 182t–183t
    symptoms, 177
Dermatology, SCI and, 174
Dermatoses, of pregnancy, 386–395
    ADP (eczema)
        defined, 389
        diagnosis, 389, 389f
        epidemiology/incidence, 389
        etiology/basic pathology, 389
        key points, 389
        management, 389
        overview, 386, 387t
        pregnancy considerations, 389
        symptoms, 389
        therapy, 389
        workup, 389
    background, 386, 387t
    cutaneous melanoma, 394–395
        classification, 394
        complications, 394
        defined, 394
        diagnosis, 394, 394f
        epidemiology/incidence, 394
        genetics, 394
        key points, 394
        management, 395
        preconception counseling, 395

pregnancy considerations, 394–395
pregnancy management, 395
prevention, 395
risk factors, 394
symptoms, 394
therapy, 395
workup, 395
IH (pustular psoriasis of pregnancy)
    antepartum testing, 393
    complications, 393
    defined, 392
    diagnosis, 392, 393f
    epidemiology/incidence, 392
    etiology/basic pathology, 393
    genetics, 392
    historic notes, 392
    key points, 392
    management, 393
    overview, 386, 387t
    preconception counseling, 393
    prevention, 393
    principles, 393
    risk factors/associations, 393
    symptoms, 392
    therapy, 393
    workup, 393
PEP
    complications, 388
    defined, 388
    diagnosis, 388, 388f
    epidemiology/incidence, 388
    etiology/basic pathology, 388
    genetics, 388
    historic notes, 388
    key points, 388
    management, 388–389
    overview, 386, 387t
    preconception counseling, 388–389
    PUPPP, 388–389
    symptoms, 388
    therapy, 389
    workup, 388
PFP
    defined, 390
    diagnosis, 390, 390f
    epidemiology/incidence, 390
    etiology/basic pathology, 390
    historic notes, 390
    key points, 390
    management, 390
    overview, 386, 387t
    pregnancy considerations, 390
    symptoms, 390
    therapy, 390
    workup, 390
PG (herpes gestationis)
    complications, 392
    defined, 391–392
    diagnosis, 391–392, 392f
    epidemiology/incidence, 392
    etiology/basic pathology, 392
    exclusion of, 388
    genetics, 392
    historic notes, 391
    key points, 391
    management, 392
    overview, 386, 387t
    PEP and, 388
    symptoms, 392
    therapy, 392
    workup, 392
PP
    complications, 391

defined, 390
diagnosis, 390, 391f
epidemiology/incidence, 391
etiology/basic pathology, 391
historic notes, 390
key points, 390
management, 391
overview, 386, 387t
risk factors/associations, 391
symptoms, 390
therapy, 391
workup, 391
SG (stretch marks), 386, 387
    cause of, 386
    defined, 386
    diagnosis, 386
    epidemiology/incidence, 386
    etiology/basic pathology, 386
    genetics, 386
    key points, 386
    management, 387
    prevention, 387
    risk factors/associations, 386
    symptoms, 386
    therapy, 387
Desatinib, 378
Desensitization, 320
Desogestrel, 279
Detemir, insulin, 53t, 54
Detoxification, illicit opioid use with, 212
Dexamethasone
    in FGR pregnancies, 424
    FNAIT, 563
    headache, 164t, 165
    HELLP syndrome, 7, 16, 17
    ICP, 107
    ICU setting, 356
    repeated doses of steroids, 380
    septic shock, 360
    SLE, 249, 249t, 251
    thyroid storm, 80, 83, 83t
Dextran, 136
Dextrose saline, 99
Diabetes
    fetal monitoring for, 505, 506
    GDM, *see* Gestational diabetes (GDM)
    LTx, pregnancy after, 125
    management, 433, 434
    mellitus (DM)
        defined, 50
        diagnosis of, 50, 51t
        FGR and, 416
    pregestational, *see* Pregestational
        diabetes
    Rh-isoimmunization and, 525
    screening, 40
Diabetic ketoacidosis, 54, 54t
Diabetic nephropathy, 51
Diabetic retinopathy, 51
Diagnosis
    acute cholecystitis, 120, 120f
    ADP (eczema), 389, 389f
    AFE, 366–369
        cardiac arrest, management, 367–369,
            368t, 370f
        clinical presentation, 366
        differential, 366–367
        laboratory testing, 367
        management of coagulopathy with, 369
    amphetamines, 216
    APS, 254, 255t
    asthma, 225
    benzodiazepines, 217

cancer; *see also* Cancer
  general principles, 381–382
    before pregnancy, 381–382
    during pregnancy, 373–381
CD, 110, 112
chlamydial infection, 312
CHTN, 1, 2t, 3
clinical hypothyroidism, 75, 75t
CMV, 439
cocaine, use, 214
criteria, severe preeclampsia, 15
cutaneous melanoma, 394, 394f
delay in
  acute leukemia, 377
  breast cancer, 374
  invasive cervical cancer, 379
  melanoma, 378
  NHL, 377
  thyroid cancer, 379
DVT, 269, 270, 271–272, 273f
fetal death, 488
FGR, 413–414, 418
FNAIT, 462
GBS, 325, 327–328, 327f
GDM, 59–60, 60t
gonorrhea, 306–307, 307t
hallucinogens, 220
HAV infection, 283
HBV infections
  adults, 285, 286t
  infants, 285
HCV infection
  adults, 291–292
  infants, 292
HD, 375
headache, 162–163, 163t
HELLP syndrome, 16, 17t
herpes, 453
HG, 81, 92, 94t
HIV, 297, 298f
HIV, in infant, 303
hyperthyroidism, 81
hypothyroxinemia, 76
ICP, 103, 104f, 105t
IH (pustular psoriasis of pregnancy),
    392, 393f
influenza, 236, 236t
inherited thrombophilias, 264, 265t
marijuana (cannabis), 209
maternal anemia, 132f, 133f, 134, 135–136
multiple gestation, 399, 400, 400f, 401f
    prenatal, 402
NIH, 478, 478f, 484–485, 484f, 485f
oligohydramnios, 515
opioids, 210
parvovirus, 449, 449f
PCP, 219
PEP, 388, 388f
PFP, 390, 390f
PG, 391–392, 392f
pneumonia, 233
polyhydramnios (hydramnios), 517
postpartum thyroiditis, 77
PP, 390, 391f
preeclampsia, 2t, 8
preeclampsia, prevention, 11
pregestational diabetes, 50, 51t
prolactinoma, 86
pyelonephritis, 156
renal disease, 150
SCI, 173
seizures, 167–168
sepsis, 357, 358t, 359

sickle cell disease, 139
SLE, 246
smoking, 196
subclinical hypothyroidism, 76
superimposed preeclampsia, 2, 2t, 7, 8
syphilis, 319
thyroid nodule, 77
thyroid storm, 83
toxoplasmosis, 444
trauma, pregnancy management with,
    343–345
  admission, 345
  blunt abdominal, 343–344
  coagulation studies, 344–345
  contraction monitoring, 344
  CT, 343, 343t
  DPL, 343–344
  FAST ultrasound, 343, 344
  fetal monitoring, 344
  fetal ultrasound, 344
  KB test, 344
  laparotomy, 344
  open fractures, 344
  penetrating abdominal wound, 344
  Rh status, 344
  spine trauma, 344
  tocodynamometer, 344
  traumatic brain injury, 344
trichomoniasis, 323, 323t
TTTS, 405
tuberculosis, 239
UC, 114, 114t, 115
urinary nephrolithiasis, 157
UTI, 156
VTE, 271–272, 272t
vWD, 145, 146t
VZV infection, 458
Diagnostic peritoneal lavage (DPL),
    343–344
Dialysis, 153–154
  complications, 154
  postpartum care, 154
  pregnancy management, 154
  principles/counseling, 153
Diamniotic (DA) twins, 398, 399t, 400, 401,
    404, 405, 406, 408, 408t, 426
Diazepam, 12, 19, 99, 218, 219
Diazoxide, 5
Dichorionic (DC) twins, 398, 399t, 400, 401,
    403, 404, 404t, 408, 408t, 426
Diclectin, 97
Diclegis, 97
Diclofenac, 155t, 157
Dietary supplements
  FGR, prevention, 416
  for GDM, 61
  pregestational diabetes, 53, 53t
  prepregnancy weight reduction, 38
  proper, hypertensive disorders, 3
  weight loss, 39
Diethylene glycol, 198
Differential diagnosis
  with ACR, 128
  acute hepatitis, 292
  of AFE, 366–367
  CD, 112
  cholelithiasis, 119
  Crohn's disease (CD), 112
  HAV, HBV, HCV, 285
  HELLP syndrome, 16, 17t
  ICP, 103
  microscopic hematuria, 158
  NIH, 479–483, 480t–481t

cardiovascular disorders, 479–481
chromosomal abnormalities, 481
congenital infections, 482
extracardiac anomalies, 481–482
fetal tumors, 483
hematological disorders, 482–483
metabolic diseases, 483
  NVP, 94t
  polyhydramnios (hydramnios), 517
  SLE flare, 248
  UC, 115
DiGeorge syndrome, 24
DIGITAT study, 424, 425
Digoxin, 29, 155t, 479, 486
Dihydroergotamine, 165
Dilantin (phenytoins), 12, 19, 75, 155t, 167,
    169, 169t, 170, 171
Dilated cardiomyopathy, 29
Dilation and evacuation (D&E), 491–492
Diltiazem, 83t, 155t
Dimenhydrinate (Dramamine), 95t, 97
Diphenhydramine (Benadryl), 95t, 97, 380
Diphenoxylate, 492
Dipyridamole, 10
Direct-acting antiviral agents (DAAs), 291,
    294–295
Direct immunofluorescence (DIF) findings,
    in PEP, 388
Discordant growth, multiple gestation, 401
Discordant twins, FGR and, 404
Disseminated intravascular coagulation
    (DIC), 366, 369
Disseminated mycobacterium avium
    complex, 301t
Diuretics, 4, 11, 29
Divalproex sodium, 185t
Dizygotic (DZ) twins
  defined, 398
  etiology, 398, 399t
  incidence, 398
Dobutamine, 360, 368, 368t, 369
Docosahexenoic acid, 419
Domestic violence, 339
Dopamine agonists
  for hyperprolactinemia, 86
  prolactinomas, 86, 87, 88, 88t
Dopamine$_2$ antagonists, for NVP and HG,
    95t, 98
Doppler, color, 514
Doppler evaluation, for FGR
  MCA, 413, 414, 415, 418, 420, 422, 423f,
    425
    limitations, 421
    velocimetry, 421
  UA, 412, 413, 414, 415, 418, 419, 420, 421,
    422, 423f, 424, 425, 426, 426t, 506
    antepartum testing, 496, 499, 501,
    502f, 503, 505, 506, 506f, 508
    limitations, 421
    velocimetry, 420–421
  uterine artery, 418
  venous Doppler (DV) velocimetry,
    421–422, 423f
Doppler of fetal vessels, 501–505, 504f, 505t
  abnormalities, 501, 502f
  application, 501, 503–505, 504f, 505t
  serial MCA Dopplers, 501, 503f
Doppler surveillance, BPS and, 505, 506f
Doppler velocimetry, for FGR, 420–421
Doses
  amoxicillin, 156, 313t
  ampicillin, 157, 328t
  antibiotics, 472

anticoagulation regimens, 276t
anti-D immunoglobulin, 467, 469–470
anti-Xa level, 275
aspirin, 10, 256
azithromycin, 305, 306, 310, 313t
bromocriptine (Parlodel), 88
bupropion HCl, 201
cabergoline (Dostinex), 88
ceftriaxone, 306
cephalexin, 156
cholestyramine, 107
CsA, 393
dalteparin, 275
DDAVP, 146, 148
dependency, of thrombophilia, 264
dopamine agonists, 88t, 89
erythromycin, 313t
folic acid, 402
heparin, 276t
indomethacin, 518
iron, 402
IVIG, 463, 464
lamotrigine, 170, 187
methadone, 212
methimazole, 82
metronidazole, 322, 324
misoprostol, 492, 493
nitrofurantoin, 156
oxytocin, 149, 492
PCP, 219
PGE2 suppositories, 492
prednisone, 249, 393
PTU, 81–82
radiation, 345
steroids, 249
sulindac, 518
thyroxine replacement, 75
trimethoprim-sulfamethoxazole, 156, 157
ursodeoxycholic acid (Ursodiol), 106
vaccination, 333t, 334t–335t
vitamin K, 107
warfarin, 279
Dostinex (cabergoline), 86, 87, 88, 89
Double pigtail stent insertion, 157
Doxepin, 189
Doxorubicin, 374, 375, 377, 378, 381
Doxycycline, 312
Doxylamine, 94, 95t, 97, 98
Dramamine (dimenhydrinate), 95t
D2 receptor antagonists, 96t
Dronabinol (marinol), 209
Droperidol (Inapsine), 95t
Drug abuse, 206–220
    amphetamines, 216–217
        anesthesia, 217
        antepartum testing, 217
        complications, 216–217
        congenital anomalies, 216–217
        defined, 216
        diagnosis, 216
        epidemiology/incidence, 216
        etiology/basic pathophysiology, 216
        fetal/neonatal morphometrics, 217
        historic notes, 216
        long-term neurodevelopmental
            outcome, 217
        neonatal withdrawal, 217
        obstetrical and neonatal
            complications, 217
        postpartum/breast-feeding, 217
        risk factors/associations, 216
        symptoms, signs, and organ toxicity,
            216

        therapy, 217
    background, 206–207, 207t
    benzodiazepines, 217–219
        antepartum testing, 218
        complications, 218
        congenital anomalies, 218
        defined, 217
        diagnosis, 217
        epidemiology/incidence, 218
        etiology/basic pathophysiology, 218
        historic notes, 217
        long-term neonatal outcome, 218
        neonatal withdrawal, 218
        obstetrical and neonatal
            complications, 218
        postpartum/breast-feeding, 219
        risk factors/associations, 218
        symptoms/signs, 218
        therapy, 218
    cessation, 416
    cocaine, 214–215
        anesthesia, 215
        antepartum testing, 215
        congenital anomalies, 214
        diagnosis/definition, 214
        epidemiology/incidence, 214
        etiology/basic pathophysiology, 214
        fetal/neonatal morphometrics, 215
        historic notes, 214
        long-term neonatal outcome, 215
        maternal and perinatal complications,
            214–215
        neonatal withdrawal, 215
        obstetrical complications, 215
        overview, 206
        postpartum/breast-feeding, 215
        risk factors/associations, 214
        symptoms, signs, and
            cardiopulmonary complications,
            214
        therapy, 215
    fetal death, risk factors for, 488, 489
    hallucinogens
        antepartum testing, 220
        complications, 220
        congenital anomalies, 220
        defined, 220
        diagnosis, 220
        epidemiology/incidence, 220
        etiology/basic pathophysiology, 220
        historic notes, 220
        long-term neonatal outcome, 220
        obstetrical and neonatal
            complications, 220
        symptoms, 220
        therapy, 220
    incidence, 207
    key points, 206
    laboratory evaluation, 209, 209t
    management, 208
    marijuana (cannabis), 209–210
        anesthesia, 210
        antepartum testing, 210
        complications, 209–210
        congenital anomalies, 210
        diagnosis/definition, 209
        epidemiology/incidence, 209
        etiology/basic pathophysiology, 209
        fetal/neonatal morphometrics, 210
        historic notes, 209
        long-term neonatal outcome, 210
        neonatal withdrawal, 210
        obstetrical complications, 210

        postpartum/breast-feeding, 210
        risk factors/associations, 209
        symptoms/signs, 209
        therapy, 210
        use during pregnancy, 206
    opioids, 206
    opioids, heroin and prescription opioid
        analgesics, 210–214
        anesthesia, 213
        antepartum testing, 213
        buprenorphine, 212–213
        complications, 211
        congenital anomalies, 211
        delivery, 213
        diagnosis/definition, 210
        epidemiology/incidence, 211
        fetal/neonatal morphometrics, 211
        historic notes, 210
        long-term neonatal outcome, 211–212
        methadone, 212
        neonatal withdrawal, 211
        obstetrical complications, 211
        postpartum/breast-feeding, 213–214
        risk factors/associations, 211
        symptoms, 210–211
        therapy, 212–213
        treatments, 213
    others, 206
    PCP
        antepartum testing, 219
        congenital anomalies, 219
        defined, 219
        diagnosis, 219
        epidemiology/incidence, 219
        etiology/basic pathophysiology, 219
        fetal/neonatal morphometrics, 219
        historic notes, 219
        long-term neonatal outcome, 219
        neonatal withdrawal, 219
        obstetrical complications, 219
        postpartum/breast-feeding, 219
        pregnancy complications, 219
        risk factors/associations, 219
        symptoms, 219
        therapy, 219
    preconception counseling, 208
    prenatal care, 208–209, 209t
    prevention, 208
    risk factors, 207, 207t
    symptoms/signs, 207, 207t
    workup, 207, 208, 208t
Drug Abuse Screening Test (DAST), 207, 208
Drug(s)
    antihypertensive, see Antihypertensive
        drugs
    resistance, 242
    weight loss, 38
Ductus venosus (DV), abnormality, 503
Duloxetine, 183t, 184, 189
DVT, see Deep vein thrombosis (DVT)
Dye-dilution technique, 513
Dysfibrinogenemia, 260
Dysplastic nevus syndrome (DNS), 395

E

Early fetal death, defined, 488
Early goal-directed therapy (EGDT), 359–360
Early latent syphilis, 316
Early-onset neonatal GBS disease, 325, 326,
    326t
Eating disorders, 41
Ebstein's anomaly, 177, 184

Echocardiogram, Marfan syndrome, 29
Echocardiography
    bedside, 366–367
    fetal, 24, 484
    FKCG, 251
Eclampsia, 18–20
    AFE, 366
    complications, 18
    defined, 7, 8, 18
    incidence, 12, 18
    magnesium for, 7
    management, 18–19
        antepartum testing, 19
        delivery, 19
        magnesium sulfate, 19
        postpartum, 19
        principles, 18–19
        therapy, 19
        workup, 19
    reduction in risk, 12
Ecstasy, 216–217; *see also* Amphetamines
Eczema, *see* Atopic dermatitis of pregnancy
    (ADP)
Edinburgh postnatal depression scale
    (EPDS), 177, 178, 179f
Edoxaban, 273
Education, prenatal, 443
Efavirenz, 302t
Effectiveness, antihypertensive drugs, 4–5
    mild-to-moderate HTN, 4–5
    severe HTN, 5
Effexor® and Effexor XR®, 183t
Electroconvulsive therapy (ECT), 188
Electronic cigarettes (e-cigarettes), 198, 201
Electron microscopy (EM), parvovirus, 449
ELISA (enzyme-linked immunosorbent
    assay), 297, 299, 391, 392, 458
Embolectomy, 276, 277
Embryonic death, defined, 488
Embryopathy, risk of, 278
Emtricitabine, 302t
Endocarditis prophylaxis, bacterial, 26–27,
    27t
Endocervical swabs, 306, 312
Endocrine therapy, breast cancer survivors
    on, 382
Endometrium, 33
Endomyometritis, 491
Endoscopic retrograde
    cholangiopancreatography
    (ERCP), 119, 121–122
Endothelin, 365
End-stage liver disease (ESLD)
    defined, 124
    symptoms and signs, 124
End-stage renal disease (ESRD), 150, 153
Engerix-B, 288
Enoxaparin, 41, 256, 257, 266, 275, 279, 493
Entecavir, 289
Enteral nutrition (EN), NVP and HG, 99
Enteric-coated mycopheno-late sodium
    (EC-MPS), 128
Enzyme immunoassays (EIAs), 444
Enzyme-linked immunosorbent assay
    (ELISA), 297, 299, 391, 392, 458
Epidemiology
    acute cholecystitis, 121
    ADP (eczema), 389
    amphetamines, 216
    APS, 254
    benzodiazepines, abuse, 218
    bipolar depression, 178
    cancer, 373

    cardiac disease, 24
    CD, 110
    chlamydia, 310, 311t
    cholelithiasis, 119
    CHTN, 1
    CMV, 436
    cocaine, 214
    cutaneous melanoma, 394
    fetal death, 488
    fetal macrosomia, 432
    FGR, 414
    FNAIT, 460
    GBS, 325, 326f
    gonorrhea, 305
    hallucinogens, 220
    HAV infections, 283, 284f
    HBV infections, 285
    HCV infection, 293
    headache, 162, 163
    HELLP syndrome, 16
    hemolytic disease, 467
    herpes, 451
    HG, 92
    HIV, 298–299
    ICP, 103
    IH (pustular psoriasis of pregnancy),
        392
    influenza, 236
    inherited thrombophilias, 260–261, 261t
    LTx, pregnancy after, 124
    marijuana (cannabis), 209
    multiple gestation, 398
    NIH, 478
    NS, 153
    obesity, 32
    oligohydramnios, 515
    opioids, abuse, 211
    parvovirus, 447
    PCP, 219
    PEP, 388
    PFP, 390
    PG (herpes gestationis), 392
    pneumonia, 234
    polyhydramnios (hydramnios), 517
    PP, 391
    preeclampsia, 8
    pregestational diabetes, 50
    prolactinoma, 86
    renal disease, 150
    SCI, 173
    seizures, 168
    SG, 386
    sickle cell disease, 139
    SLE, 246, 248t
    smoking, 196
    syphilis, 315
    toxoplasmosis, 442
    trichomoniasis, 322
    tuberculosis, 238
    UC, 114
    VTE, 270
    vWD, 145
    VZV infection, 456
Epidural anesthesia
    cardiac disease, 26
    SCI, 175
Epilepsy, defined, 167; *see also* Seizures
Epinephrine, 227t
Epirubicin, 373, 375, 381
Episiotomy, 114
Epstein–Barr virus, 377
Equetro®, 185t
Ergonovine, 225, 233

Ergot alkaloids, 164, 164t
Ergotamine, 165
Ergot (rye fungus) derivative, 220
Erythroblastosis fetalis, defined, 467
Erythromycin, 142, 155t, 235, 310, 312, 313t,
    319, 325, 326, 329
Erythropoietin, 137
Escalate therapy without FBS, 464
Escherichia coli, 121, 156
Escitalopram (Lexapro®), 182t
Eskalith®, 185t
Eslicarbazepine (Aptiom), 169t
Eso-meprazole, 98
Esomeprazole (Nexium), 95t
Estimated date of confinement (EDC), 416
Estimated fetal weight (EFW)
    of acardiac twin, 407
    fetal macrosomia and, 432, 433, 434
Estradiol, 124, 178
Estriol levels, FGR, 424
Estrogens, 163
Etanercept, 249t, 250
Ethambutol, 238, 241, 241t, 242
Ethinyl estradiol, 171
Ethionamide, 242
Ethosuximide, 169t
Etiologies
    acute cholecystitis, 121
    ADP, 389
    amphetamines, 216
    APS, 254
    asthma, 225
    benzodiazepines, abuse, 218
    cardiac disease, 24–25
    cardiac neonatal lupus/CHB, 250
    CD, 111
    chlamydia, 311
    cholelithiasis, 119
    CHTN, 1
    cocaine, 214
    fetal death, 488–489, 489t
    FGR, 414–415
    FNAIT, 460
    GBS, 325
    gonorrhea, 305
    hallucinogens, 220
    HAV infections, 283
    HBV infections, 286, 287f
    HCV infections, 293
    hemolytic disease, 468
    hyperthyroidism, 81
    ICP, 103, 104
    IH (pustular psoriasis of pregnancy),
        393
    influenza, 236
    inherited thrombophilias, 261
    marijuana (cannabis), 209
    maternal anemia, 131, 132, 133, 135t
    multiple gestation, 398–399, 399t
    NIH, 478, 479, 479f
    NVP and HG, 92
    obesity, 33
    oligohydramnios, 515
    PCP, 219
    PEP, 388
    PFP, 390
    PG (herpes gestationis), 392
    pneumonia, 233, 234t
    polyhydramnios (hydramnios), 517
    postpartum thyroiditis, 77
    PP, 391
    preeclampsia, 8–9
    prolactinoma, 86

seizures, 168
SG, 386
SLE, 246
smoking, 196–198
trauma, 339
trichomoniasis, 322
TTTS, 404
tuberculosis, 238
UC, 114
VTE, 270, 271f, 271t
vWD, 145, 147f
Euglycemia, 66, 67
European Association for Study of Liver (EASL), 289
European Centre for Disease Prevention and Control (ECDC), 308
European Gonococcal Antimicrobial Surveillance Programme (Euro-GASP), 307
European prospective cohort on thrombophilia (EPCOT), 264
European Society of Radiology, 164
Euthyroid, 75, 76, 81
Evaluation
    headache, 164
    ICP
        activated charcoal, 107
        cholestyramine, 107
        dexamethasone, 107
        guar gum, 107
        hydroxyzine, 107
        prevention, 106, 106f
        principles, 106
        SAMe, 107
        ursodeoxycholic acid (Ursodiol), 106
        vitamin K, 107
        workup, 106
    trauma, 343–345
        admission, 345
        blunt abdominal, 343–344
        coagulation studies, 344–345
        contraction monitoring, 344
        CT, 343, 343t
        DPL, 343–344
        FAST ultrasound, 343, 344
        fetal monitoring, 344
        fetal ultrasound, 344
        KB test, 344
        laparotomy, 344
        open fractures, 344
        penetrating abdominal wound, 344
        Rh status, 344
        spine trauma, 344
        tocodynamometer, 344
        traumatic brain injury, 344
Exercise
    GDM, management, 61, 66
    preeclampsia, prevention, 11
    pregestational diabetes, 53
    weight loss, 39
Expectant management
    fetal death, 491
    severe preeclampsia, 16
Expedited partner therapy (EPT), 306, 311–312, 313
Extracardiac anomalies, NIH and, 481–482
    gastrointestinal, 480t, 481, 482
    genitourinary, 480t, 481
    skeletal dysplasias, 480t, 482
    thoracic, 480t, 481
    vascular, 480t, 482
Extracorporeal membrane oxygenation (ECMO), 237

Extrahepatic diseases, with HCV infection, 292
Extrapyramidal syndrome, 188
Extreme obesity, defined, 32

F

Factor V Leiden (FVL) mutation, 9, 260, 261–262, 261t, 265t, 266, 277, 279
Fallot, tetralogy of, 28
Famciclovir, 454
Familial hemiplegic migraine (FHM), 163
Famotidine (Pepcid), 95t, 97
FaSTER trial, 40
FazaClo®, 186t
Ferric carboxymaltose, 136, 137
Ferrous sulfate, 75, 142
Fetal and neonatal alloimmune thrombocytopenia (FNAIT), 460–466
    anesthesia, 465
    antenatal management, 460, 461f
    classification, 460, 462, 462t
    counseling, 465
    defined, 460
    delivery, 465
    diagnosis, 462
    epidemiology/incidences, 460
    etiology/basic pathophysiology, 460
    future pregnancy preconception counseling, 466
    genetics/inheritance, 460
    indications for testing, 462
    investigations and consultations, 465
    key points, 460
    management, 463–465
        clinical concerns/issues, 465
        clinical scenarios, 465
        principles, 463–464
        risk-based fetal therapy, 464–465
    monitoring/testing, 465
    natural history/complications, 462
    neonatology management, 465–466
    prevention and screening, 462–463
    risk-based fetal therapy, 464–465
        high risk, 461f, 465
        standard risk, 461f, 464–465
        very high risk, 461f, 465
    routine maternal serologic screening, 463
    serologic testing, 462
Fetal anemia, 142, 447, 448, 449, 467, 470–471, 472, 474, 477, 482, 483, 484, 485, 491, 505, 508
Fetal arrhythmias, 479
Fetal autopsy, 490–491
Fetal blood sampling (FBS), 83, 460, 464–465, 467, 472–473, 472t, 473t
Fetal bradyarrhythmias, 188
Fetal death, 488–493
    associations/risk factors/possible etiologies, 488–489, 489t
    defined, 488
    delivery/anesthesia, 491–493
        D&E, 491–492
        expectant management, 491
        induction, 492–493
    diagnosis, 488
    epidemiology/incidence, 488
    key points, 488
    postpartum, 493
    pregnancy management, 489–491
        counseling, 489, 489t, 490t
        workup, 489, 490–491

prevention, 489, 489t
    recurrence and management in future pregnancy, 493
    trauma and, 340
Fetal demise, defined, 488
Fetal evaluation, after chemotherapy, 380–381
Fetal-echocardiography, 24, 484
Fetal factors, for FGR, 415
Fetal growth restriction (FGR), 412–426
    antepartum testing, 420–424
        AF volume, 422, 424
        BPS, 422, 424
        Doppler velocimetry, 420–421
        estriol levels, 424
        fetal kick counts, 422
        growth assessment, intervals of, 420
        interval of fetal testing, 424
        MCA Doppler velocimetry, 421
        NST/CTG, 422
        ultrasound, 420–422
        venous Doppler (DV) velocimetry, 421–422, 423f
    categorization, 414
    cause, 414
    classification, 414
    complications, 415–416
        overview, 412, 413t
    defined, 412, 413
    delivery, 424–426
        DIGITAT study, 424, 425
        GRIT study, 424–425, 426
        mode of, 426
        multiple gestation and, 426, 426t
        preparation, steroids and magnesium sulfate, 424
        timing, 412, 423f, 424–426
        TRUFFLE study, 424, 425, 426
    diagnosis, 413–414
    epidemiology/incidence, 414
    etiology/basic pathophysiology, 414–415
    fetal factors, 415
    fetal monitoring for, 506
    future pregnancy preconception counseling, 426, 426t
    genetics/inheritance/recurrence, 414
    key points, 412–413
    management, 412, 416–420
        abdominal decompression, 420
        aspirin, 420
        aspirin therapy, 416
        bed rest, 419
        betamimetics, 419
        calcium channel blocker, 419–420
        control of maternal medical disorders, 416
        counseling, 419
        diagnosis, 418
        fundal height, 417
        gestational age determination, 416
        heparin, 420
        interventions, 419–420
        medical conditions, therapy for, 419
        nitric oxide donors, 420
        nutrient therapy, 419
        nutrition, 416
        oxygen therapy, 420
        plasma volume expansion, 420
        pregnancy interval, 416
        prevention, 416
        screening, 416–418
        serum analytes, 416–417
        substance cessation, 416

toxins, discontinuation of, 419
UA Doppler, 418
ultrasonographic growth curve, 417
uterine artery Doppler, 418
workup, 418–419
maternal factors, 415
multiple gestation
discordant growth and, 401
discordant twins, 404
neonatology management, 426
placental factors, 415
risk factors, 412, 413t
severe, 414
workup of, 412, 413t
Fetal heart rate (FHR) testing, 497–498, 497f
Fetal hemorrhage, risk of, 464
Fetal hydrops, defined, 477
Fetal hypothyroidism, 82
Fetal injury, trauma and, 340
Fetal intervention, hemolytic disease, 472–473, 472t, 473t
Fetal kick counts, in FGR pregnancies, 422
Fetal kinetocardiogram/tissue Doppler echocardiography (FKCG), 251
Fetal lung maturity (FLM)
assessment, indications for, 521
characteristics, 522, 523t
determination, 521
on fetal outcome, 525
specific tests for, 522, 524
FSI, 523t, 524
LB counts, 522, 523t, 524
L/S ratio, 522, 523t
PG testing, 522, 523t
SAR test, 522, 523t
Fetal macrosomia, 432–434
complications, 432
defined, 432
epidemiology/incidence, 432
key points, 432
management, 432–434
diabetes, 433, 434
prevention, 432–433
prior cesarean delivery, 434
prior shoulder dystocia, 434
screening, 433
suspected, 433, 433f
uncomplicated, 433
risk factors, 432
Fetal maternal alloimmune thrombocytopenia (FMAIT), defined, 460
Fetal maturity testing, 521–525
AF, techniques for obtaining
amniocentesis, 521–522
vaginal pool collection, 522, 523t
cascade approach, 524
defined, 521
FLM
assessment, indications for, 521
characteristics, 522, 523t
determination, 521
on fetal outcome, 525
FSI, 523t, 524
LB counts, 522, 523t, 524
L/S ratio, 522, 523t
PG testing, 522, 523t
SAR test, 522, 523t
specific tests for, 522, 524
historic notes, 521
key points, 521
multiple tests, 524

pulmonary maturity test
assessment, indications for, 521
clinical conditions, risk of RDS and predictive value, 524–525
vaginal pool specimens, 522, 523t
Fetal monitoring/testing
critical care, 354–355
FNAIT, 465
hemolytic disease, 473–474
methods, 496–509
BPS, 499–501, 499f, 499t, 500t, 501t
condition-specific testing, 505, 506–508, 506t, 507t
CST, 498–499
Doppler of fetal vessels, 501–505, 502f, 503f, 504f, 505t
Doppler surveillance and BPS, 505, 506f
FHR testing (NST/CTG), 497–498, 497f
modified BPS, 501
movement counting in low-risk pregnancy, 496–497
practical antenatal testing, 508–509
NIH, 486
NS, 153
principles, 496
RBC alloimmunized pregnancies, 473–474
trauma and, 344
Fetal movement counting, in low-risk pregnancy, 496–497
Fetal/neonatal complications
acute cholecystitis, 121
amphetamines, use, 217
APS, 255
benzodiazepines, abuse, 218
CD, 111
cholelithiasis, 119
CHTN, 2–3
death, smoking and, 198
GBS, 325
hallucinogens, exposure, 220
HIV infection, 299
multiple gestation
chromosomal and congenital anomalies, 401
FGR and discordant growth, 401
monochorionic gestations, 401
PTB, 401, 402t
single fetal demise in, 401
spontaneous pregnancy loss, 400, 401
NVP and HG, 93
outcomes, trauma and, 340
preeclampsia, 9
prolactinoma, 86–87
seizures, 168–169
SLE, 246–247
toxoplasmosis, 443
UC, 115
VZV infection, 457
Fetal/neonatal morphometrics
amphetamines, use, 217
cocaine, use, 215
marijuana (cannabis), use, 210
opioids, use, 211
PCP, use, 219
Fetal pulmonary maturity tests
assessment
indications for, 521
from vaginal pool specimens, 522, 523t
clinical conditions, risk of RDS and predictive value, 524–525
Fetal surveillance
cancer and, 380

multiple gestation, 407–408
renal transplantation, 155
Fetal syphilis, 317
Fetal testing, interval, 424
Fetal thrombophilias, 263–264
Fetal thyroid physiology, clinical hypothyroidism, 74
Fetal tone, 500
Fetal tumors, NIH and, 483
Fetal ultrasound, 40, 344
Fetal vessels, Doppler of, 501–505, 504f, 505t
abnormalities, 501, 502f
application, 501, 503–505, 504f, 505t
serial MCA Dopplers, 501, 503f
Fetomaternal hemorrhage, 344, 464, 467, 468, 470, 477, 482
Fetoscopic laser coagulation, for TTTS, 406
Fetus
anomalous, 403–404; *see also* Anomalous fetus
hemolytic disease, *see* Hemolytic disease
FGR, *see* Fetal growth restriction (FGR)
Fibrinogen, 369
Fibrosis, radiation-induced cardiac toxicity, 381
Fish oil, for preeclampsia, 11
Five-step assessment (5Rs), for smokers, 197t
Five-step intervention (5As), for patients, 197t
Fixed-drug combination, 232
Flares, SLE, 247
Flecainide, 479, 486
FLM, *see* Fetal lung maturity (FLM)
Floppy infant syndrome, 218
Fluconazole, 155t
Flunisolide, 226t
Fluorescence in situ hybridization (FISH), 485
Fluoroquinolones, 235, 242, 307
Fluorouracil, 382
5-Fluouracil (5FU), 375
Fluoxetine, 165, 182t, 188
Fluphenzinepyridoxine, 98
Fluticasone, 226t, 232
Fluvoxamine (Luvox®, Luvox CR®), 182t
FNAIT, *see* Fetal and neonatal alloimmune thrombocytopenia (FNAIT)
Foam stability index (FSI), for FLM, 523t, 524
Focused abdominal sonogram for trauma (FAST), 343, 344
Foley catheter, 175
Folic acid, supplementation, 39, 170, 187, 402
Folinic acid, 445
Follow-up
after treatment, syphilis, 320
chlamydial infection, 312
of infants, HIV infection, 303
long-term, parvovirus, 450
UTI, 156
Fondaparinux, 274
Forced vital capacity (FVC), 225
Formoterol, 226t
Fragmin, 256, 257
Freud, Sigmund, 214
FRUIT trial, 266
Fundal height, 417
Furosemide, 19

G

Gabapentin (Neurontin), 169t, 171
Gabatril (Tiagabine), 169t
Gadolinium, contrast agent for MRI, 164
Gallbladder disease, 119–122

acute cholecystitis, 120–122
    classification, 120, 121t
    complications, 121
    defined, 120
    diagnosis, 120, 120f
    epidemiology/incidence, 121
    ERCP, 121–122
    etiology/pathogenesis, 121
    fetal complications, 121
    imaging, 121
    labor and delivery considerations, 122
    laboratory investigations, 121
    laparoscopic *vs.* open
        cholecystectomy, 122
    management, 122
    maternal complications, 121
    MRCP, 121
    pregnancy considerations, 121–122
    principles, 121
    risk factors/associations, 121
    surgery, 122
    symptoms, 121
    workup, 121
cholelithiasis, 119–120
    complications, 119
    defined, 119
    diagnosis, 119
    differential diagnosis, 119
    epidemiology/incidence, 119
    etiology/pathophysiology, 119
    fetal complications, 119
    imaging, 120
    labor and delivery issues, 120
    laboratory investigations, 120
    management, 120
    maternal complications, 119
    pregnancy considerations, 120
    principles, 120
    risk factors/associations, 119, 120t
    symptoms, 119
    therapy, 120
    workup, 120
    key points, 119
Gallium scanning, 376
Gamma-hydroxybutyrate (GHB), 216
Ganciclovir, for CMV, 440
Garlic, prevention of preeclampsia, 11
Gastrointestinal anomalies, NIH and, 480t,
        481, 482
GBS, *see* Group B streptococcus (GBS)
GDM, *see* Gestational diabetes (GDM)
Generalized tonic clonic (GTC) seizure, 168
General management, cardiac disease, 25,
        26–27, 27t
Genetic(s)
    cardiac disease, 24
    cutaneous melanoma, 394
    FGR, 414
    FNAIT, 460
    HAV infections, 283
    HBV infections, 285
    HCV infection, 293
    headache, 163
    hemolytic disease, 467
    ICP, 103
    IH (pustular psoriasis of pregnancy), 392
    inherited thrombophilias
        ATIII deficiency, 262
        FVL, 261–262, 261t
        MTHFR/homocysteinemia, 262
        protein C, 262
        protein S, 262
        prothrombin G20210A gene, 262

maternal anemia, 131, 133t, 134t, 135t
    NVP and HG, 92
    obesity, 33
    PEP, 388
    PG (herpes gestationis), 392
    SG, 386
    sickle cell diseases, 139
        counseling for, 141
    smoking, 196
    VTE, 270, 271t, 272t, 275t
    vWD, 145, 146t
Genital herpes, reactivation (recurrent), 452
Genitourinary anomalies, NIH and, 480t, 481
Gentamicin, 155t, 157, 329
Geodon®, 186t
Gestational age determination, 416
Gestational diabetes (GDM), 59–68
    associations, 60
    complications, 60–61
    defined, 59
    incidence, 60
    key points, 59
    multiple gestation, 402
    nephrotic syndrome and, 153
    pathophysiology, 60
    prevention, 61
    risk factors for, 59, 60, 60t
    screening/diagnosis, 59–60, 60t
    treatment, 61–68, 61t, 62t–65t
        anesthesia, 67
        antepartum testing, 67
        delivery, 67
        diet, 61
        exercise, 61, 66
        glucose monitoring, 66
        glyburide, 66
        insulin, 66–67, 66t, 67f
        intrapartum glucose management,
            67, 68f
        metformin (glucophage), 66
        nutritional supplementation, 67
        oral hypoglycemic agents, 66
        postpartum/breast-feeding, 68, 68f
Gestational hypertension (GHTN)
    antenatal management, 5, 6
    complications, 5
    defined, 5
    delivery, 6
    incidence, 5
    risk factors, 5
Gestational thyrotoxicosis
    defined, 80
    Graves' disease from, 81
    transient biochemical thyrotoxicosis, 81
Gestodene, 279
Ghrelin, 33
GHTN, *see* Gestational hypertension (GHTN)
Ginger, 97
Glanzman disease, 149
Glargine, 53t, 54, 55, 66, 67, 67f
Glomerular filtration rate (GFR), 150
Glucagon, for home use, 54
Glucocorticoids, 96t
Glucose
    challenge test, 60
    control, insulin for, 51, 53
    equivalents, 50, 51t
    intrapartum management, 55
    monitoring
        GDM, management, 66
        pregestational diabetes, 53, 53t
Glyburide, 53, 66, 433

Glycoprotein B vaccine, for CMV, 438
Goldenhar syndrome, in children, 382
Gonadotropin-releasing hormone agonists,
        124
Gonococcal Isolate Surveillance Project
        (GISP), 307
Gonorrhea, 305–308
    complications, 306
    epidemiology/incidence, 305
    etiology, 305
    key points, 305
    management, 306–308
        diagnosis, 306–307, 307t
        prevention, 306
        screening, 306, 307t
    pathophysiology/transmission, 305
    symptoms, 305–306
    treatment, 307–308, 308t
G-protein-coupled thyrotropin receptor, 81
Graft rejection, renal, 156
Graves' disease
    defined, 80
    with hyperthyroidism, 81
    neonatal, 81
    overview, 80
    recurrence of, 82
    TSI with, 81
Gray, radiation dose, 345
Group B streptococcus (GBS), 325–330
    classification, 325, 326t
    complications, 326
    defined, 325
    diagnosis, 325
    epidemiology/incidence, 325, 326f
    etiology/basic pathophysiology, 325
    key points, 325
    management, 326–330
        antepartum testing, 330
        collection of screening specimen, 328
        delivery, 330
        detection, 327, 327f
        intrapartum prophylaxis, 328, 328f,
            328t, 329, 330
        intrapartum treatment, 327, 327f
        maternal vaccination, 326
        neonatal (screening and) treatment
            only, 327
        prelabor maternal treatment, 326
        prenatal maternal screening, 326, 327,
            327f
        principles/prevention, 326, 327
        screening/diagnosis, 327–328, 327f
        universal treatment, 326
    neonatal management, 329f, 330
    risk factors/associations, 325, 326
    symptoms/signs, 325
Growth assessment, intervals of, 420
Growth restriction trial (GRIT) study, FGR,
        416, 424–425, 426, 503, 505t
Guanethidine, for thyroid storm, 83t
Guar gum, 107
Guillain–Barré syndrome (GBS), 175
Gummatous syphilis, 317
Gynecologist, Ob-Gyn, 355–356

H

Hallucinogens
    antepartum testing, 220
    complications
        congenital anomalies, 220
        long-term neonatal outcome, 220
        obstetrical and neonatal, 220

defined, 220
diagnosis, 220
epidemiology/incidence, 220
etiology/basic pathophysiology, 220
historic notes, 220
symptoms, 220
therapy, 220
Haloperidol, 187, 188, 189
Handwashing, 436, 438, 448, 454
Harris–Benedict equation, 99
Hashimoto's thyroiditis, hypothyroidism
and, 73, 75
HAV, *see* Hepatitis A virus (HAV) infections
Havrix (Smith Kline Beecham), 283
HBIg therapy, 285, 288, 289
HB therapy, 288, 289
HBV, *see* Hepatitis B virus (HBV) infections
HCV, *see* Hepatitis C virus (HCV) infection
HD, *see* Hodgkin's disease (HD)
Headache, 162–165
background/epidemiology, 162
causes, 162–163, 163t
diagnosis
considerations, 162–163, 163t
epidemiology, 163
genetics, 163
key points, 162
management, 164–165
evaluation, 164
prophylaxis, 165
therapy, 164–165, 164t
microadenoma and, 86
pathophysiology, 163
pregnancy considerations, 163–164
Heart rate testing, fetal, 497–498, 497f
Heart transplantation, pregnancy after, 128t,
129
Helicobacter pylori, 97, 98
HELLP syndrome, 16–18
complications, 16, 17t
diagnoses/definitions, 7, 8
diagnosis, 16, 17t
epidemiology, 16
management, 16, 17, 18f
anesthesia, 17
corticosteroids, 16, 17
delivery, 17, 18
workup, 16
signs and symptoms, 16, 17t
Hemagglutinin (H), 236
Hematological disorders, NIH and, 482–483
hemolysis, 480t, 482
hemorrhage, 480t, 482–483
reduced red blood cell/hemoglobin
production, 480t, 482
TTTS, 480t, 483
Hematology, SCI and, 174
Hematuria, 158
Hemodialysis (HD), 154
Hemodynamic monitoring, preeclampsia
and, 13
Hemoglobin, glycosylated, 53
Hemoglobin E, 144
Hemoglobin production, NIH and, 480t,
482
Hemoglobin S (HbS), 139, 141, 143–144
Hemoglobin S combined with hemoglobin C
(HbSC), 139, 141t, 143
Hemolysis, NIH and, 480t, 482
Hemolytic anemia; *see also* Hemolytic
disease
APS and, 255
fetal, 402

inherited, 132
microangiopathic, 8
mild-to-moderate, 470
pruritus during pregnancy, 104f
sickle cell disease and, 139, 140
Hemolytic disease, of fetus/neonate, 467–474
anti-D immunoglobulin, dosing and
timing, 467, 469–470
"atypical" antibodies
CDE system antigens, 474
Kell alloimmunization, 474
MNS antigen system, 474
defined, 467
epidemiology/incidence, 467
etiology/basic pathophysiology, 468
genetics, 467
key points, 467
management
anesthesia, 474
clinical, 467, 468f
counseling, 470
delivery, 474
fetal intervention, 472–473, 472t, 473t
fetal monitoring/testing, 473–474
long-term outcomes, 474
neonatology, 474
RBC alloimmunized pregnancies,
470–474
workup/investigations, 470–472, 471t
natural history, 468–469, 469t
prevention, 469–470
Hemophilus influenza, 140
Hemorrhages
anemia, 137
cerebral, 1, 2, 7, 9
DDAVP, 148
dot-blot, 51
fetal, risk of, 464
fetomaternal, 344, 464, 467, 468, 470, 477,
482
hypertension, 27, 340, 351, 353, 483
ICH, 9, 340, 460, 461f, 462, 463, 464, 465
intrapartum, 263
liver, 7, 9, 17, 17t
magnesium sulfate and, 12
maternal trauma, 344, 345
mechanical heart valves, 28
NIH and, 480t, 482–483
obesity, 35t, 39, 40
postpartum, 12, 25, 35t, 40, 103, 104, 106,
107, 145, 146, 349
postsphincterotomy, 121
pulmonary hypertension, 27
SCI, 173
subarachnoid, 162, 163, 164
UC and, 110, 114, 115
VTE, 277, 279
Heparin
acute SCI, 174
FGR pregnancies, 420
induced osteoporosis, 274
low-dose, 41
for preeclampsia, 10
therapeutic, 29
therapy
LMWH, 274, 275
UFH, 273, 274
Heparin-induced thrombocytopenia (HIT),
257, 273, 274
Hepatitis A virus (HAV) infections, 283–284
anesthesia, 284
antepartum testing, 284
complications, 283

delivery, 284
diagnosis, 283
epidemiology/incidence, 283
etiology/basic pathophysiology, 283
genetics, 283
key points, 283
postpartum/breast-feeding, 284
pregnancy
considerations, 283
management, 283–284
prenatal care, 283, 284
prevention/preconception counseling,
283
risk factors/associations, 283
symptoms, 283
therapy, 283, 284
vaccination, 334t, 336t
workup, 283
Hepatitis B virus (HBV) infections, 285–289
anesthesia, 289
antepartum testing, 289
classification, 286, 286t
complications, 286
conditions, 289
defined, 285
delivery, 289
diagnosis
adults, 285, 286t
infants, 285
epidemiology/incidence, 285
etiology/basic pathophysiology, 286,
287f
genetics, 285
key points, 285
management, 288–289
prenatal care, 288
prevention/preconception
counseling, 288
principles, 288
workup, 288
postpartum/breast-feeding, 289
pregnancy considerations, 286, 288
rare/related, 289
risk factors/associations, 286
symptoms, 285
therapies, 288–289
nucleoside/nucleotide analogs,
288–289, 289t
vaccines, 288
vaccination, 125, 285, 286t, 288, 289, 301,
332, 333t, 335, 336t
vertical transmission, 125
Hepatitis C virus (HCV) infection, 291–295
anesthesia, 295
antepartum testing, 295
associations, 293
breast-feeding, 295
classification, 291
complications, 293
defined, 291
delivery, 295
diagnosis
adults, 291–292
infants, 292
epidemiology/incidence, 293
etiology/basic pathophysiology, 293
extrahepatic manifestations, 292
genetics, 293
key points, 291
LTx, indication for, 124
management, 294–295
prevention, 294
principles, 294

screening, 294
workup, 294
natural history, 292, 292f
postpartum, 295
preconception/pregnancy counseling, 294
pregnancy considerations, 293–294
mother-to-infant (perinatal) transmission, 293–294, 293t
risk factors, 291, 292t, 293, 294
symptoms, 292
therapy, 294–295
Hepatitis D virus (HDV) infection, 289
Hepatitis virus reactivation, pregnancy after LTx, 125
Herceptin, 375
Heritable thrombophilia, VTEs and, 277
HER2neu expression, 374
Heroin, 210–214
anesthesia, 213
antepartum testing, 213
complications
congenital anomalies, 211
fetal/neonatal morphometrics, 211
long-term neonatal outcome, 211–212
neonatal withdrawal, 211
obstetrical, 211
diagnosis/definition, 210
epidemiology/incidence, 211
historic notes, 210
postpartum/breast-feeding, 213–214
risk factors/associations, 211
symptoms, 210–211
therapy, 212–213
buprenorphine, 212–213
methadone, 212
treatments, 213
use, delivery, 213
Herpes, 451–454
classification/pathophysiology
nonprimary first episode, 452
primary first episode, 452
reactivation (recurrent) genital herpes, 452
complications, 452
gestationis, see Pemphigoid gestationis (PG)
incidence/epidemiology, 451
key points, 451
maternal-fetal transmission, 452
pathogens, 451
pregnancy management, 452–454
antiviral drugs, 453, 454
complicated HSV infection, 454
considerations, 452
counseling/prognosis, 452–453
history of HSV, 454
mode of delivery, 454
postpartum/neonate, 454
prevention, 453, 453f
primary/first episode, 454
screening, 453
therapy, 453, 454
workup/diagnosis, 453
risk factors/associations, 451
symptoms, 452
Herpes simplex virus (HSV), 285, 292, 412, 413t, 418, 419, 484; see also Herpes
Herpes zoster (shingles), 456, 459
Heterotaxy syndrome, 479
HG, see Hyperemesis gravidarum (HG)
Hibiclens, 490
High-dependency unit (HDU), 349

High risk-based fetal therapy, for FNAIT, 461f, 465
High spinal anesthesia, 366
Histamine-1 receptor antagonists, 97
Histamine-2 receptor antagonists, 97–98
Historic notes, ICP, 103
HIV, see Human immunodeficiency virus (HIV)
Hodgkin's disease (HD), during pregnancy, 375, 376–377
diagnosis, 375
hypothyroidism, risk for, 381
pregnancy after, 382
presentation, diagnostic tests, and safety, 375–376
radiotherapy, 377
staging, 376
termination of pregnancy, 376
treatment, 376–377
Hofmann, Albert, 220
Homans' sign, 269
Home uterine activity monitoring, 403
Homocysteine, 266
Homocysteinemia, 9, 261, 262
Hospitalization
pneumonia, treatment, 235
trauma and, 340
H1-receptor antagonists, 95t
H2-receptor antagonists, 95t
HTN, see Hypertension (HTN)
5-HT3 (seratonin) receptor antagonist, 95t–96t, 98
Human chorionic gonadotroponin (HCG), 74, 81
Human immunodeficiency virus (HIV), 297–303
acute HIV infection, 303
aneuploidy screening, 302
antepartum testing, 302
antiretroviral therapy, 300–301, 301t, 302t
breast-feeding, 303
classification, 299, 299t
coinfection with TB and, 242
complications
fetal, 299
maternal, 299
delivery and intrapartum care, 303
diagnosis, 297, 298f
in infant, 303
epidemiology, 298–299
follow-up of infants, 303
historic notes, 297
immunizations, 301, 302
key points, 297
maternal postpartum care, 303
pathophysiology, 299
PPROM, 302
preconception counseling, 300
pregnancy
considerations, 299
management, 299–300
prenatal care
counseling, 300
initial visit history, 300
laboratory investigations, 300
physical examination, 300
principles, 300
prophylaxis for opportunistic infections, 300–301, 301t
risk factors, 299
screening, 299
Trichomonas vaginalis, 323
Human leukocyte antigens (HLAs), 462

Human papilloma virus (HPV), vaccination, 332, 333t, 336t
Human platelet antigens (HPAs), 460, 462t, 465
Humate-P, 148
Hydralazine, 6t, 7, 13, 19, 29, 173, 174, 215
Hydramnios, see Polyhydramnios (hydramnios)
Hydrochlorothiazide, 4
Hydrocodone, 211
Hydrocortisone, 96t, 99, 249
Hydromorphone, 142
Hydroxycarbamide, for sickle cell disease, 141, 142
Hydroxychloroquine (Plaquenil), 246, 248, 249, 249t, 251, 256
Hydroxyethyl starch (HES), 360
Hydroxyurea, for sickle cell disease, 141, 142
Hydroxyzine (Atarax, Vistaril), 95t, 97, 107
Hygiene, prevention of CMV, 438
Hyperbilirubinemia, light therapy for, 474
Hypercapnia, 357
Hypercoagulability, 24–25
Hyperemesis gravidarum (HG)
NVP and, 92–100
antiemetic therapy, 98
benzodiazepines, 99
classification, 92
clonidine, 99
corticosteroids, 99
defined, 80, 92
diagnosis, 81, 92, 94t
EN, 99
epidemiology/incidence, 92
etiology, 92
fetal/neonatal complications, 93
genetics, 92
inpatient assessment and treatment, 98–99
issues, 100
IVF hydration, 99
key points, 92
management, 93–94, 93f
maternal complications, 93
nonpharmacologic interventions, 94, 97
nutritional supplementation, 99–100
pharmacologic interventions, 97–98
PN, 99–100
postpartum management, 100
pregnancy management, 93–94
prevention, 94
risk factors/associations, 92, 93
treatment, 94, 95t–96t
workup, 94
Hyperglycemia, 67
Hyperhomocysteinemia, 261, 264, 265t, 266
Hyperimmune globulin, CMV-specific, 439–440
Hyperprolactinemia, 86, 88
Hypertension (HTN)
amphetamine use, 216, 217
cardiac disease and, 24, 25, 26, 27, 28, 29
cocaine, use, 206, 214, 215
CRI and, 152
disorders, see Hypertensive disorders
FGR and, 412, 413, 415, 416, 418, 419, 424, 426
GDM, 60, 66, 68
gestational, 168, 232, 255
hemorrhage and, 27, 340, 351, 353, 483
inhaled steroids, 232
LTx, pregnancy after, 124, 125, 127

management, 19
mild-to-moderate, 4–5
nephrotic syndrome, 153
obesity, 32, 33, 35
opioids, use, 211
PCP, use, 219
portal, syphilis and, 482
PPHN, 181
pregestational diabetes, 50, 51, 56
pulmonary, 24, 25, 27, 35, 141, 142
renal disease, 150, 152, 153, 154, 155
renal dysfunction and, 393
seizures and, 113, 168
severe, 5
sickle cell disease, 141, 142
sign of ADR, 173, 174
SLE, 246, 247, 248, 249, 250
systemic effects, 214
therapy, 152
VTE, 270
Hypertensive disorders, 1–20
    CHTN, 1–5
        anesthesia, 5
        antepartum testing, 5
        classification, 1, 2
        complications, 2–3
        defined, 1
        delivery, 5
        diagnosis/definition, 1, 2t
        epidemiology/incidence, 1
        etiology/basic pathophysiology, 1
        key points, 1
        management, see Management,
            CHTN
        postpartum/breast-feeding, 5
        risk factors/associations, 2
    GHTN, 5, 6
        antenatal management, 5, 6
        complications, 5
        defined, 5
        delivery, 6
        incidence, 5
        risk factors, 5
    preeclampsia, 6–20
        abnormal uterine Doppler
            ultrasound, prevention, 10
        admission, 12
        anesthesia, 13
        antepartum testing, 13
        antihypertensive therapy, 12–13
        antioxidant therapy, 11
        antiplatelet agents, 13
        aspirin, 10
        calcium, 10–11
        calcium supplementation, 7
        classification, 9
        complications, 9, 14, 15–20
        counseling, 11–12
        definitions, 2, 2t, 6, 8
        delivery, 13
        diagnosis, 2t, 8, 11
        diuretics, 11
        eclampsia, see Eclampsia
        epidemiology/incidence, 8
        etiology/basic pathophysiology, 8–9
        fetal complications, 7
        fetal/neonatal, 9
        fish oil, 11
        garlic, 11
        HELLP syndrome, see HELLP
            syndrome
        heparin, 10
        history, 11

indications for delivery, 7
key points, 6–8
long-term counseling, 20
low-dose aspirin, 7
magnesium, 7, 11
magnesium prophylaxis, 12
management, 9–13, 13t, 14f, 15f
maternal complications, 7, 9
nitric oxide, 11
physical examination, 11
plasma volume expansion, 12
preconception counseling, 11
prediction, 9
prevalence of, 9
prevention, 10–11
principles, 9–10
progesterone, 11
rest/exercise, 11
risk factors/associations, 9
salt intake, 11
severe, see Severe preeclampsia
superimposed, see Superimposed
    preeclampsia
symptoms, 8
vitamin C, antioxidant therapy with, 7
workup, 11
Hyperthyroidism, 80–84
    antepartum testing, 82–83
    complications, 81
    definitions, 80
    etiology, 81
    Graves' disease, 80
    incidence, 80
    key points, 80
    management, 81
    neonatal, 83
    physical examination, 80
    physiology/pathophysiology, 81
    postpartum, 83
    pregnancy considerations, 81
    resources, 84
    screening/diagnosis, 81
    signs/symptoms, 80
    subclinical
        defined, 80
        treatment, 81
    thyroid nodule, 83
    thyroid storm
        defined, 80
        diagnosis, 83
        incidence, 83
        precipitating factors, 83
        signs/symptoms, 83
        treatment, 83, 83t
    thyrotoxicosis
        defined, 80
        gestational, 80
    treatment, 81–82
        beta-blockers, 82
        iodine, 82
        methimazole, 82
        mode of action, 82
        PTU, 80, 81–82
        radioiodine therapy, 82
        side effects, 82
        surgery, 82
        thionamides, 81–82
Hypertrophic cardiomyopathy, 29
Hypertrophic obstructive cardiomyopathy,
    24
Hypnosis, 201
Hypoglycemic agents, oral
    GDM, management

glyburide, 66
for pregestational diabetes, 53
Hypomania, 178, 180
Hypotension, 13, 24, 26, 27, 28, 29, 40, 88, 154,
    173, 210, 213, 214, 215, 217, 249, 340,
    344, 355, 358, 359, 365, 366, 367, 368,
    369, 401, 404
Hypothalamic–pituitary–gonadal
    dysfunction, 124
Hypothyroidism, 73–77
    clinical, 73–76; see also Clinical
        hypothyroidism
    anatomy/radiology, 74
    antepartum management, 76
    complications, 74
    defined, 73, 74f
    fetal thyroid physiology, 74
    incidence, 73
    management, 74
    maternal physiology, 74, 75t
    neonatal, 76
    pathophysiology, 73–74
    placenta physiology, 74–75
    postpartum, 76
    preconception, 74
    pregnancy considerations, 74–75, 75t
    screening/diagnosis, 75, 75t
    signs/symptoms, 73
    treatment, 75–76
    Hashimoto's thyroiditis and, 73, 75
    hypothyroxinemia
        diagnosis, 76
        incidence, 76
        screening and management, 76
    key points, 73
    physiologic changes, 73, 74t
    postpartum thyroiditis
        defined, 77
        diagnosis, 77
        etiology, 77
        incidence, 77
        management, 77
        recurrence risk, 77
        risk factors, 77
        three clinical presentations, 77
    subclinical
        diagnosis, 76
        incidence, 76
        screening and management, 76
    thyroid nodule
        diagnosis, 77
        incidence, 77
        surgery, 77
    TPO-antibodies only, 76–77
Hypothyroxinemia
    defined, 73
    diagnosis, 76
    incidence, 76
    screening and management, 76
Hysterectomy, 340

I

IBD, see Inflammatory bowel disease (IBD)
Ibuprofen, 162, 164t, 165
ICH (intracranial hemorrhage), 9, 340, 460,
    461f, 462, 463, 464, 465
ICP, see Intrahepatic cholestasis of
    pregnancy (ICP)
ICU, see Intensive care unit (ICU)
Idarubicin, 373, 375, 378, 381
Idiopathic hypertrophic subaortic stenosis,
    29

IgA nephropathy, renal disease, 151
IH, *see* Impetigo herpetiformis (IH)
Ileal pouch–anal anastomosis (IPAA), 114, 115–116
Ileostomy, 115
Iliac vein thrombosis, 272
Illicit drugs, use, *see* Drug abuse
Iloperidone, 187
Imaging
    acute cholecystitis, 121
    cholelithiasis, 120
Imatinib, 378
Imipenem, 235
Immunizations, HIV infection, 301, 302
Immunoglobulin (Ig)
    anti-D, 467, 469–470
    IgA
        antibodies, 444
        nephropathy, 151
    IgG, 81, 113, 125, 250, 255, 256, 283, 288, 291, 294, 312, 317, 377, 412, 419, 436, 437, 439–440, 444, 447, 449, 450, 451–453, 456–459, 460, 462, 467–469, 491, 517
    IgM, 125, 155, 255, 256, 283, 285, 312, 412, 419, 436, 437, 439, 444, 447–450, 451, 456, 458, 485, 491, 517
    IVIG, 175, 251, 256, 449, 460, 461f, 463–464, 465
    SLE, 249–250, 249t
Immunomodulators, 112t, 113
Immunosorbent agglutination assay test (IAAT), 444
Immunosuppressive agents, 112t, 113, 125, 127t, 128, 155, 155t, 389
Impetigo herpetiformis (IH)
    complications, 393
    defined, 392
    diagnosis, 392, 393f
    epidemiology/incidence, 392
    etiology/basic pathology, 393
    genetics, 392
    historic notes, 392
    key points, 392
    management
        antepartum testing, 393
        preconception counseling, 393
        prevention, 393
        principles, 393
        therapy, 393
        workup, 393
    overview, 386, 387t
    risk factors/associations, 393
    symptoms, 392
Imuran, 249, 249t
Inapsine (droperidol), 95t
Incentive spirometry, 142
Incidences
    ACS, 143
    acute cholecystitis, 121
    ADP (eczema), 389
    AFE, 365
    amphetamines, 206, 216
    APS, 254
    asthma, 225
    benzodiazepines, abuse, 218
    cancer, in pregnancy, 373
    cardiac disease, 24
    CD, 110
    chlamydia, 310, 311t
    cholelithiasis, 119
    chromosome abnormalities, 481
    CHTN, 1

clinical hypothyroidism, 73
CMV, 436
cocaine, 214
critical care, 349
cutaneous melanoma, 394
drug abuse, 207
eclampsia, 12, 18
fetal death, 488
fetal macrosomia, 432
FGR, 414
FNAIT, 460
GBS, 325, 326f
GDM, 60
GHTN, 5
gonorrhea, 305
hallucinogens, 220
HAV infections, 283, 284f
HBV infections, 285
HCV infection, 293
hemolytic disease, 467
herpes, 451
HG, 92
hyperthyroidism, 80
hypothyroxinemia, 76
ICP, 103, 104
IH (pustular psoriasis of pregnancy), 392
impaired psychomotor function, 74
influenza, 236
inherited thrombophilias, 260–261, 261t
MA twins, 407
marijuana (cannabis), 209
methamphetamine, 216
microscopic hematuria, 158
multiple gestation, 398, 399f
NIH, 478
NODM, 125
NS, 153
obesity, 32
obstetrical complications, 212
oligohydramnios, 515
opioids, abuse, 211
parvovirus, 447
PCP, 219
PEP, 388
PFP, 390
PG (herpes gestationis), 392
polyhydramnios (hydramnios), 517
postpartum thyroiditis, 77
postpartum urinary retention, 157
PP, 391
preeclampsia, 3, 8
pregestational diabetes, 50
prolactinoma, 86
pyelonephritis, 156
renal disease, 150
SCI, 173
seizures, 168
SG, 386
sickle cell disease, 139
SLE, 246, 248t
smoking, 196
subclinical hypothyroidism, 76
syphilis, 315
thyroid nodule, 77, 83
thyroid storm, 83
toxoplasmosis, 442
trauma, 339
trichomoniasis, 322
TTTS, 404
tuberculosis, 238
UC, 114
urinary incontinence, 157
urinary nephrolithiasis, 157

VTE, 270
vWD, 145
VZV infection, 456
Incubation period, syphilis, 316
Indications
    AFV, assessment in singleton pregnancies, 513
    antihypertensive drugs, 5
    colectomy, 115
    for delivery, preeclampsia, 7
    liver transplantation, 124
    prolactinoma
        for neurosurgery in patients, 90t
        therapy, 88t
    for testing, FNAIT, 462
Indocin, 154
Indomethacin, 122, 152, 225, 233, 518
Induction of labor, fetal death, 492–493
Infants, HIV infection and
    diagnosis, 303
    follow-up, 303
Infections
    chlamydia, *see* Chlamydia
    CMV, *see* Cytomegalovirus (CMV)
    HAV, *see* Hepatitis A virus (HAV) infections
    HBV, *see* Hepatitis B virus (HBV) infections
    HCV, *see* Hepatitis C virus (HCV) infection
    HDV infection, 289
    HIV, *see* Human immunodeficiency virus (HIV)
    TB; *see also* Tuberculosis
        coinfection with TB and HIV, 242
        control issues, 242
    UTI, *see* Urinary tract infections (UTI)
    VZV, *see* Varicella zoster virus (VZV) (chickenpox)
Infectious Diseases Society of America (IDSA), 234, 235
Infectious renal disease, 158
Inferior vena cava (IVC) filters, 277
Infertility
    CRI and, 152
    ESLD, women with, 124
    in substance-abusing women, 208
Inflammatory bowel disease (IBD), 110–116
    background, 110
    CD, 110–114
        adalimumab, 112t, 113
        aminosalicylates, 112t, 113
        antepartum testing, 114
        antibiotics, 112t, 113
        certolizumab, 112t, 113
        complications, 111
        corticosteroids, 112t, 113
        cyclosporine, 112t, 113
        defined, 110
        delivery, 114
        diagnosis, 110
        differential diagnosis, 112
        epidemiology/incidence, 110
        etiology/basic pathophysiology, 111
        fetal and neonatal complications, 111
        immunomodulators/immunosuppressants, 112t, 113
        infliximab, 112t, 113
        management, 111–114
        maternal complications, 111
        medications in, 112–113, 112t
        methotrexate, 112t, 113
        naltrexone, 112t, 113–114

natalizumab, 112t, 113
postpartum/breast-feeding, 114
preconception counseling, 112
pregnancy considerations, 111
prenatal care, 112
principles, 111
signs/symptoms, 110, 111t
thalidomide, 112t, 113
UC vs., 111t
workup, 112
defined, 110
key points, 110
pathogenesis, 110
UC, 114–116
antepartum testing, 116
CD vs., 111t
colectomy, 115
complications, 114–115
defined, 110, 114
delivery, 116
diagnosis, 114, 114t
differential diagnosis, 115
epidemiology/incidence, 114
etiology/basic pathophysiology, 114
fetal complications, 115
IPAA, 114, 115–116
management, 115–116
maternal complications, 114
pharmacological therapy, 115
postpartum/breast-feeding, 116
preconception counseling, 115
pregnancy considerations, 115
prenatal care, 115
principles, 115
signs/symptoms, 114
surgery, 115
therapy, 115
workup, 115
Infliximab, 112t, 113, 249t, 250, 393
Influenza, 236–238
antepartum testing, 238
complications, 236–237
delivery, 238
diagnosis, 236, 236t
epidemiology/incidence, 236
etiology/basic pathophysiology, 236
influenza A (H1N1), 236, 237, 356, 358
key points, 236
management, 237
postpartum/breast-feeding, 238
pregnancy considerations, 237
prevention, 237
prophylaxis after suspected exposure, 237
symptoms, 236
therapy, 237–238
vaccination, 139, 140, 142, 234, 236, 237, 301, 332, 333, 333t, 336t
Infrarenal aortic graft, 127
Inhaled corticosteroids, 232
Inhaled steroids, for asthma, 232
Inheritance
FGR, 414
FNAIT, 460
sickle cell disease, 139
Inherited thrombophilias, 260–266
complications, 262–263
adverse pregnancy outcome, 262–263, 263t
VTE, 262
defined, 260
dose dependency, 264
epidemiology/incidence, 260–261, 261t

etiology/basic pathophysiology, 261
fetal thrombophilias, 263–264
genetics/classification
ATIII deficiency, 262
FVL, 261–262, 261t
MTHFR/homocysteinemia, 262
protein C, 262
protein S, 262
prothrombin G20210A gene, 262
historic notes, 260
hyperhomocysteinemia, 261, 264, 265t, 266
key points, 260
management, 264–266
diagnosis, 264, 265t
prevention, 264, 266
prevention of obstetrical complications, 266
screening, 264, 265t
treatment, 264, 265t
risk factors/associations, 262
screening, 260
Initial evaluation, CHTN, 3
Initiation, of smoking, 202
Initiative for Global Elimination of Congenital Syphilis, 315
Inotropes, 365
Inpatient assessment and treatment, NVP and HG, 99
Insulin
detemir, 53t, 54
GDM, 60, 66–67, 66t, 67f
glargine, 53t, 54, 55, 66, 67, 67f
for glucose control, 51, 53
lispro/aspart, 53t, 54, 55, 62t, 65t, 66–67, 67f
long-acting/short-acting, 54
macrosomia and, 433, 434
NPH, 53t, 54, 55, 62t, 64t, 65t, 66, 67
in obese pregnant women, 33
pregestational diabetes
intrapartum glucose management, 55, 56f
prenatal care, 53–54, 53t, 54t
production defect, 50
regular, 53t, 54, 55, 62t, 63t, 65t, 67
resistance, Myoinositol and, 61
Intensive Care Society (ICS), 350
Intensive care unit (ICU)
admission to, 349, 350t, 353, 354t
cesarean delivery in, 355
delivery in, 355
multidisciplinary approach, 354
nursing care in, 352
Ob-Gyn, role, 355–356
obstetrical, 351–352
requirement, specific conditions, 356–361
ARDS and mechanical ventilation, 356–357, 356t
sepsis, 357–361, 358t, 359t
specialized ICU physicians staff, 354
training, 352
undelivered patient, transfer, 354
vaginal delivery in, 355
Intensivist, defined, 352
Interferon gamma-release assay (IGRA), 238, 239, 240, 241
Intermediate fetal death, defined, 488
Intermittent catheterization, SCI and, 174
International Association of Diabetes and Pregnancy Study Groups (IADPSG), 59
International Classification of Adult Underweight, Overweight, and Obesity, 33t

International Headache Society, 162, 163t
International League Against Epilepsy (ILAE), 168
International normalized ratio (INR), 279
Interpersonal psychotherapy, 188
Interpregnancy interval, 416
Interval
of fetal testing, FGR, 424
pregnancy, 416
Interventions
assessment, smoking, 197t, 199
behavioral educational, 188
FGR pregnancies, 419–420
abdominal decompression, 420
aspirin, 420
bed rest, 419
betamimetics, 419
calcium channel blocker, 419–420
heparin, 420
medical conditions, therapy for, 419
nitric oxide donors, 420
nutrient therapy, 419
oxygen therapy, 420
plasma volume expansion, 420
toxins, discontinuation of, 419
NVP and HG, treatment
nonpharmacologic, 94, 97
pharmacologic, 97–98
Intestinal transplantation, pregnancy after, 128t, 129
Intimate-partner violence, 341
Intracondazole, 155t
Intracranial hemorrhage (ICH), 9, 340, 460, 461f, 462, 463, 464, 465
Intrahepatic cholestasis (IC), history of, 103
Intrahepatic cholestasis of pregnancy (ICP), 103–108
antepartum testing, 107
classification, 104
complications (without treatment), 104, 106
defined, 103
delivery, 107–108
dermatoses of pregnancy, 386, 387t
diagnosis, 103, 104f, 105t
epidemiology, 103
etiology/basic pathophysiology, 103, 104
genetics, 103
historic notes, 103
incidence, 103, 104
key points, 103
management/evaluation
activated charcoal, 107
cholestyramine, 107
dexamethasone, 107
guar gum, 107
hydroxyzine, 107
prevention, 106, 106f
principles, 106
SAMe, 107
ursodeoxycholic acid (Ursodiol), 106
vitamin K, 107
workup, 106
pregnancy considerations, 106
risk factors/associations, 104
symptoms, 103
Intrapartum asphyxia, FGR and, 415
Intrapartum care
HIV infection, 303
obesity and, 40
Intrapartum glucose management, 55, 56f
Intrapartum prophylaxis, GBS, 328, 328f, 328t, 329, 330

Intrauterine fetal demise (IUFD), 213, 488
Intrauterine growth restriction (IUGR)
    APS and, 257
    diagnosis, 11
    FGR, 413, 414, 416
    LBW and, 211
    low-dose aspirin, 10
    LTx, pregnancy after, 127
    reduction in, 7
    TG infection, 443
    VAS in, 498
Intravascular volume, increase in, 24
Intravenous fluids (IVFs)
    hydration, NVP and HG, 99
    for sickle cell disease, 142
Intravenous immunoglobulin (IVIG), 175,
        251, 256, 449, 460, 461f, 463–464,
        465
Invasive cervical cancer, see Cervical cancer
Invasive hemodynamic monitoring, 27, 28
Investigations
    CMV, 439
    FNAIT, 465
    hemolytic disease, 470–472, 471t
Iodine supplementation
    childbearing age, women of, 81
    clinical hypothyroidism, management, 76
    hyperthyroidism, management, 82
Ipratropium bromide, 232
Ipratroprium, 227t, 233
Iron
    deficiency, 131, 133, 136
    supplementation, 131, 133, 136, 143, 402
Isoimmunization, defined, 467
Isometheptene caffeine-barbiturate
        combinations, 164, 164t
Isoniazid, 238, 241, 241t, 242
IUGR, see Intrauterine growth restriction
        (IUGR)
IVIG (intravenous immunoglobulin), 175,
        251, 256, 449, 460, 461f, 463–464,
        465
Ixekizumab, 393

J

Japanese encephalitis, 335t
Jarisch–Herxheimer reaction, 320
Jaundice, 50, 51, 59, 103, 105t, 121, 124, 190,
        212, 241, 283, 285, 291, 320, 436, 437,
        454, 469
Jelly beans, 60

K

Kanamycin, 242
Kell alloimmunization, 142, 467, 468, 470, 474;
        see also Hemolytic disease
Keppra (levetiracetam), 169, 169t, 171
Ketanserin, 5
Ketoconazole, 155t
Ketonuria, 81
Ketorolac, 157
Klebsiella spp., 121
Kleihauer–Betke (KB) test, 339, 340, 344, 467,
        469, 470, 482–483, 491
Klippel–Trenaunay syndrome, 173
Kytril, 380

L

L-A-acetylmethadol (LAAM), 213
Labetalol, 1, 4, 5, 6t, 7, 13, 16, 208, 215

Laboratory investigations
    acute cholecystitis, 121
    AFE, 367
    APS, 256
    cholelithiasis, 120
    CHTN, 3
    CRI, 152
    drug abuse, 209, 209t
    GHTN, 5, 6
    HIV infection, 300
    influenza, 236, 236t, 238
    NIH, 484
    pneumonia, 234
    renal transplantation, 155
    for substance use, 208
Labor management
    acute cholecystitis, 122
    cholelithiasis, 120
    LTx, pregnancy after, 129
    NS, 153
    renal transplantation, 155–156
    sickle cell disease, 142
Labor precautions, complications from
        polyhydramnios, 517
Lacosamide (Vimpat), 169t
β-lactam, 233, 235
Lactation, mood disorder management,
        188–190
    antidepressants
        bupropion, 189
        duloxetine, 189
        MAOIs, 189
        mirtazapine, 189
        SSRIs, 188–189
        TCAs, 189
        trazodone, 189
        venlafaxine, 189
    antipsychotics, 189–190
        atypical, 190
    stabilizers
        carbamazepine, 189
        lamotrigine, 189
        lithium, 189
        valproic acid, 189
Lactobacillus GG, 156
Lambda sign, defined, 400
Lamellar body (LB) counts, for FLM, 522,
        523t, 524
Lamictal® and Lamictal XR®, 186t
Lamivudine, 289, 302t
Lamotrigine, 169, 169t, 170, 171, 186t, 187, 189
Lansoprazole (Prevacid), 95t, 97
Laparoscopy, for acute cholecystitis, 122
Laparotomy, 344
Large for gestational age (LGA), risk factor
        for, 35
Laser therapy
    for SG, 387
    for TTTS, 406
Late benign (tertiary) syphilis, 316–317
Late fetal death, defined, 488
Latent syphilis, 316
Latent tuberculosis infection, 238, 239, 241
Late-onset neonatal GBS disease, 325, 326t
Lecithin/sphingomyelin (L/S) ratio, for
        FLM, 522, 523t
Ledipasvir, 291, 295
Leflunomide, 249t, 250
Left ventricular dysfunction, 365
Leptin, 33
Leucovorin, 301t, 445
Leukemia
    acute, 377–378

    delay in diagnosis, 377
    diagnostic tests and safety, 377
    effects, on pregnancy, 377
    termination of pregnancy, 377
    treatment, 377–378
    chronic, 378
    during pregnancy, 377–378
    pregnancy after, 382
Leukotriene receptor antagonists (LTRA),
        226t, 232
Levalbuterol, 227t
Levels, of critical care, 349–350, 350t, 351t
Levetiracetam (Keppra), 169, 169t, 171
Levofloxacin, 235
Levonorgestrel, 279
Levothyroxine, 74, 75, 76, 77
Lexapro® (Escitalopram), 182t
Lidocaine, 472
Lifestyle changes, for CHTN, 3
Light therapy, for hyperbilirubinemia, 474
Limb reduction defects, 220
Linezolid, 235
Liquid ecstasy, defined, 216
Lispro insulin, 53t, 54, 55, 62t, 65t, 66–67, 67f
Lithium, mood stabilizer, 184, 185t, 189
Lithobid®, 185t
Lithotripsy, shock wave, 157
Liver function tests
    isoniazid, use, 241
    pregnancy after LTx, 128
Liver transplantation (LTx), pregnancy after,
        124–129
    antepartum testing, 128
    breast-feeding, 129
    comorbidity and risk factors, 125–127
        ACR rate, 127
        CMV acute infection, 125, 127
        diabetes, 125
        fetal and maternal outcomes, 125, 126t
        hepatitis virus reactivation, 125
        hypertension and renal insufficiency,
                125
        infrarenal aortic graft, 127
    complications, 126t, 127
        abnormal blood chemistry and liver
                function tests, 128
        IUGR, 127
        preeclampsia, 127
        preterm birth and low birth weight,
                126t, 127
    epidemiology, 124
    ESLD, definition/symptoms and signs, 124
    historic notes, 124
    immunosuppression therapy, drugs
            and side effects, 127t, 128
    indications, 124
    key points, 124
    labor and delivery issues, 129
    overview, 124
    pathophysiology, 124
    preconception counseling and timing
            of pregnancy, 125
    workup and management, 127t, 128
LMWH, see Low-molecular weight heparin
        (LMWH)
    adjusted-dose bid, 28, 29
    UFH and, 256–257
    VTE, management, 274, 275, 278, 279
Logistics, critical care, 353, 354–355
Long-acting β-agonist (LABA), 226t, 232
Long-term counseling, preeclampsia, 20
Long-term neonatal outcome
    amphetamines, use, 217

benzodiazepines, abuse, 218
cocaine, use, 215
hallucinogens, exposure, 220
heroin, 211–212
marijuana, use, 210
opioids, use, 211–212
PCP, use, 219
Lovastatin, 155t
Lovenox, 256, 257
Low birth weight (LBW)
CRI and, 152
defined, 414
IUGR and, 211
pregnancy after LTx, 126t, 127
smoking, complication, 198
Low-molecular weight heparin (LMWH)
adjusted-dose bid, 28, 29
UFH and, 256–257
VTE, management, 274, 275, 278, 279
Lumbosacral meningomyelocele, 187
Lupus anticoagulants (LA), 254, 255t, 491
Lupus nephritis, renal disease, 151
Lurasidone, 187
Luvox® and Luvox CR® (Fluvoxamine), 182t
Lymphazurin, for sentinel node, 375
Lymphogranuloma venereum (LGV), 310,
311, 312, 313t
Lynestrenol, 279
Lyrica (pregabalin), 169t
Lysergic acid diethylamide (LSD), 206, 220;
see also Hallucinogens
Lysosomal storage diseases (LSD), 483
Lytic cocktail, magnesium *vs.*, 19

M

Maclobemide, 201
Macroadenomas, 86, 89, 90t
Macrocytic anemia, 133f, 135–136, 135t
Macrolide, 139, 142, 143, 233, 235
Macrosomia
bariatric surgery and, 38
for childhood obesity, 35
diagnosis of, 55
DM and, 51
fetal, *see* Fetal macrosomia
GDM and, 59, 60, 61, 66
prepregnancy obesity, risk factor for, 35
Magic mushrooms, 220; *see also*
Hallucinogens
Magnesium
diazepam *vs.*, 19
for eclampsia, 7, 19
lytic cocktail *vs.*, 19
phenytoin *vs.*, 19
for preeclampsia, 11, 12, 152
preterm labor, 152
supplementation, 402, 416
Magnesium sulfate
cerebral palsy, occurrence, 404
eclampsia, 13, 19
in FGR pregnancies, 424
preeclampsia, 13
severe, 15–16
Magnetic resonance
cholangiopancreatography
(MRCP), 119, 121
Magnetic resonance imaging (MRI), 86, 87,
88, 89, 90, 121, 157, 163, 164, 168,
345, 373, 376, 378, 379, 395, 490, 491
Magnetic resonance urography (MRU), 157
Major depressive disorder (MDD), 177, 180
Maltodextin, 53

Mammography, 374, 375
Management, pregnancy
acute cholecystitis, 122
laparoscopic *vs.* open
cholecystectomy, 122
surgery, 122
ADP (eczema)
therapy, 389
workup, 389
AF assessment in singleton pregnancies,
514–515
AFE, 369, 370f
antenatal, GHTN, 5, 6
APS, 255–257
prevention, 256
principles, 255
screening, 255–256
asthma
preconception care, 228
prenatal care, 228
prevention, 228, 228t
principles, 228
workup, 229
BPS, 500, 500t, 501t
cardiac arrest, 367–369, 368t, 370f
cardiac disease, 25, 26–30
aortic stenosis, 28
coarctation of aorta, 27
coronary artery disease, 29–30
dilated cardiomyopathy, 29
general, 25, 26–27, 27t
hypertrophic cardiomyopathy, 29
Marfan syndrome, 29
mechanical heart valves, 28–29
mitral and aortic insufficiency, 28
mitral stenosis, 28
palpitations, 27
peripartum cardiomyopathy, 29
preconception counseling, 25
prenatal care/antepartum testing, 25
pulmonary hypertension, 27
pulmonic stenosis (PS), 28
specific diseases, 27–30
tetralogy of fallot, 28
CD, 111–114
adalimumab, 112t, 113
aminosalicylates, 112t, 113
antepartum testing, 114
antibiotics, 112t, 113
azathioprine/6-mercaptopurine, 112t,
113
certolizumab, 112t, 113
corticosteroids, 112t, 113
cyclosporine, 112t, 113
delivery, 114
differential diagnosis, 112
immunomodulators/
immunosuppressants, 112t, 113
infliximab, 112t, 113
medications in, 112–113, 112t
methotrexate, 112t, 113
naltrexone, 112t, 113–114
natalizumab, 112t, 113
postpartum/breast-feeding, 114
preconception counseling, 112
prenatal care, 112
principles, 111
thalidomide, 112t, 113
workup, 112
chlamydia
diagnosis, 312
prevention, 311–312
screening, 312

cholelithiasis
imaging, 120
labor and delivery issues, 120
laboratory investigations, 120
pregnancy considerations, 120
principles, 120
therapy, 120
workup, 120
CHTN, 3–5
antihypertensive drugs, 4–5
initial evaluation/workup, 3
lifestyle changes and bed rest, 3
preconception counseling, 3
prenatal care, 3
prevention, 3
principles, 3
screening/diagnosis, 3
therapy, 3
clinical hypothyroidism, 74, 75–76
dose, 75
goal, 75
iodine supplementation, 76
new diagnosis, 75
preexisting hypothyroidism, 75
thyroxine replacement, 75–76
type, 76
CMV, 437–440
CMV-specific hyperimmune
globulin, 439–440
counseling/prognosis, 437–438, 438f,
438t
ganciclovir and valacyclovir, 440
hygiene, 438
investigations/diagnosis/workup,
439
prevention, 438
screening, 439
serum, 439
therapy, 439–440
ultrasound fetal findings, 439
vaccine, 438
CNL/CHB, 251
coagulopathy with AFE, 369
CRI, 152
cutaneous melanoma
preconception counseling, 395
pregnancy, 395
prevention, 395
therapy, 395
workup, 395
diabetic ketoacidosis, 54, 54t
drug abuse, 208
eclampsia, 18–19
antepartum testing, 19
delivery, 19
magnesium sulfate, 19
postpartum, 19
principles, 18–19
therapy, 19
workup, 19
fetal death, 489–491
counseling, 489, 489t, 490t
workup, 489, 490–491
fetal macrosomia, 432–434
diabetes, 433, 434
prevention, 432–433
prior cesarean delivery, 434
prior shoulder dystocia, 434
screening, 433
suspected, 433, 433f
uncomplicated, 433
FGR, 412, 416–420
abdominal decompression, 420

aspirin, 420
aspirin therapy, 416
bed rest, 419
betamimetics, 419
calcium channel blocker, 419–420
control of maternal medical
    disorders, 416
counseling, 419
diagnosis, 418
fundal height, 417
gestational age determination, 416
heparin, 420
interventions, 419–420
medical conditions, therapy for, 419
neonatology, 426
nitric oxide donors, 420
nutrient therapy, 419
nutrition, 416
oxygen therapy, 420
plasma volume expansion, 420
pregnancy interval, 416
prevention, 416
screening, 416–418
serum analytes, 416–417
substance cessation, 416
toxins, discontinuation of, 419
UA Doppler, 418
ultrasonographic growth curve, 417
uterine artery Doppler, 418
workup, 418–419
FNAIT, 463–465
clinical concerns/issues, 465
clinical scenarios, 465
principles, 463–464
risk-based fetal therapy, 464–465
GBS, 326–330
antepartum testing, 330
collection of screening specimen, 328
delivery, 330
detection, 327, 327f
intrapartum prophylaxis, 328, 328f,
    328t, 329, 330
intrapartum treatment, 327, 327f
maternal vaccination, 326
neonatal, 329f, 330
neonatal (screening and) treatment
    only, 327
prelabor maternal treatment, 326
prenatal maternal screening, 326, 327,
    327f
principles/prevention, 326, 327
screening/diagnosis, 327–328, 327f
universal treatment, 326
GDM, 61–68, 61t, 62t–65t
anesthesia, 67
antepartum testing, 67
delivery, 67
diet, 61
exercise, 61, 66
glucose monitoring, 66
glyburide, 66
insulin, 66–67, 66t, 67f
intrapartum glucose management,
    67, 68f
metformin (glucophage), 66
nutritional supplementation, 67
oral hypoglycemic agents, 66
postpartum/breast-feeding, 68, 68f
gonorrhea, 306–308
diagnosis, 306–307, 307t
prevention, 306
screening, 306, 307t
HAV infection, 283–284

HBV infection, 288–289
prenatal care, 288
prevention/preconception
    counseling, 288
principles, 288
workup, 288
HCV infection, 294–295
prevention, 294
principles, 294
screening, 294
workup, 294
headache, 164–165
evaluation, 164
prophylaxis, 165
therapy, 164–165, 164t
HELLP syndrome, 16, 17, 18f
anesthesia, 17
corticosteroids, 16, 17
delivery, 17, 18
workup, 16
herpes, 452–454
antiviral drugs, 453, 454
complicated HSV infection, 454
considerations, 452
counseling/prognosis, 452–453
history of HSV, 454
mode of delivery, 454
postpartum/neonate, 454
prevention, 453, 453f
primary/first episode, 454
screening, 453
therapy, 453, 454
workup/diagnosis, 453
hypertension, 19
hyperthyroidism, 81–82
beta-blockers, 82
iodine, 82
methimazole, 82
mode of action, 82
PTU, 80, 81–82
radioiodine therapy, 82
side effects, 82
surgery, 82
thionamides, 81–82
hypothyroxinemia, 76
ICP
activated charcoal, 107
cholestyramine, 107
dexamethasone, 107
guar gum, 107
hydroxyzine, 107
prevention, 106, 106f
principles, 106
SAMe, 107
ursodeoxycholic acid (Ursodiol), 106
vitamin K, 107
workup, 106
IH (pustular psoriasis of pregnancy)
antepartum testing, 393
preconception counseling, 393
prevention, 393
principles, 393
therapy, 393
workup, 393
influenza, 237
inherited thrombophilias, 264–266
diagnosis, 264, 265t
obstetrical complications, prevention,
    266
prevention, 264, 266
screening, 264, 265t
treatment, 264, 265t
LTx, pregnancy after, 127t, 128

microscopic hematuria, 158
mood disorders
during lactation, 188–190; see also
    Lactation
nonpharmacologic, 188
pharmacologic, 180–188
multiple gestation
low-dose aspirin, 402
nutrition, 402
multiple gestation, complications,
    403–407
anomalous fetus, selective
    termination, 403–404; see also
    Anomalous fetus
FGR/discordant twins, 404
single fetal death, 404, 404t
TTTS, 404, 405–407; see also Twin-twin
    transfusion syndrome (TTTS)
neonatology
FNAIT, 465–466
NIH, 483–486
amniocentesis, 485
cordocentesis and invasive
    procedures, 485
counseling/prognosis, 483
delivery/anesthesia, 486
delivery timing, 486
demographic and clinical history, 484
fetal monitoring/testing, 486
laboratory, 484
neonatology, 486
obstetric, 486
therapeutic approach, 486
treatment, 486
ultrasound, 484
workup/diagnosis, 484–485, 484f, 485f
NS, 153
NVP and HG, 93–94, 93f, 94, 95t–96t
inpatient, 98–99
oligohydramnios, 515, 516f
of oligohydramnios and/or hydramnios,
    518
parvovirus, 448–449
counseling/prognosis, 448
neonate and long-term follow-up, 450
prevention, 448–449
screening, 449
therapy, 449
workup/diagnosis, 449, 449f
PEP, 388–389
preconception counseling, 388–389
workup, 388
PFP, 390
PG (herpes gestationis), 392
pneumonia
prevention, 234
principles, 234
workup, 234
polyhydramnios (hydramnios), 517–518
postpartum; see also Postpartum
    management
thyroiditis, 77
urinary retention, 158
PP, 391
preeclampsia, 9–13, 13t, 14f, 15f
abnormal uterine Doppler
    ultrasound, prevention, 10
admission, 12
antihypertensive therapy, 12–13
antioxidant therapy, 11
antiplatelet agents, 13
aspirin, 10
calcium, 10–11

counseling, 11–12
diagnosis, 11
diuretics, 11
fish oil, 11
garlic, 11
heparin, 10
history, 11
magnesium, 11
magnesium prophylaxis, 12
nitric oxide, 11
physical examination, 11
plasma volume expansion, 12
preconception counseling, 11
prevention, 10–11
principles, 9–10
progesterone, 11
rest/exercise, 11
salt intake, 11
workup, 11
pregestational diabetes, 52, 52t
prolactinoma, 87–89
bromocriptine (Parlodel), 88
cabergoline (Dostinex), 88
dopamine agonists, 88t
indications for therapy, 88t
macroadenomas, 89
microadenomas, 88–89
preconception counseling, 88
principles, 87
workup, 87–88, 87f
pyelonephritis, 156–157
RBC alloimmunized, 470–474
anesthesia, 474
counseling, 470
delivery, 474
fetal intervention, 472–473, 472t, 473t
fetal monitoring/testing, 473–474
long-term outcomes, 474
neonatology, 474
workup/investigations, 470–472, 471t
seizures, 169–170
preconception counseling, 169, 170
prenatal care, 170
prenatal counseling, 170
principles, 169, 169t
severe preeclampsia, 15–16
delivery, timing of, 16
expectant, 16
magnesium sulfate, 15–16
plasma volume expansion, 15–16
SG, 387
SLE, 247–251
CNL/CHB, 251
preconception counseling, 248, 248t
prenatal care, 248, 249
principles, 247–248
workup, 248, 248t
smoking, 199
subclinical hypothyroidism, 76
superimposed preeclampsia, 14
syphilis, 317–320
diagnosis, 319
follow-up, 320
prevention, 317
screening, 317–318, 318t
workup, 319
thyroid storm, 83, 83t
toxoplasmosis, 443, 444–445
prevention, 443, 443t
principles, 443
screening, 443, 444
serum, 443, 444, 444f
therapy, 444–445

ultrasound, 444
workup/diagnosis, 444
trauma, 341–345
care of patient, 341
evaluation and diagnostic studies,
343–345, 343t
prevention, 341
radiation, 345, 345t
stabilization, 342, 343, 343t
workup and management, 342, 342f
trichomoniasis, 323–324
diagnosis, 323, 323t
prevention, 323
screening, 323
treatment, 324
tuberculosis, 241
UC, 115–116
colectomy, 115
differential diagnosis, 115
IPAA, 114, 115–116
pharmacological therapy, 115
postpartum, 116
preconception counseling, 115
prenatal care, 115
principles, 115
surgery, 115
workup, 115
urinary nephrolithiasis, 157
VTE, 271–276
aspirin, 276
clinical scenarios and anticoagulation,
272, 273, 274–276, 275t
diagnosis, 271–272, 272t
LMWH, 274, 275
principles, 271
pulmonary angiography, 272
pulmonary embolism, 272, 274f
UFH, 273, 274
warfarin (Coumadin), 275–276
vWD, 146, 148
preconception counseling, 146
prenatal care, 146
type I, 146, 148
type IIa, 148
type IIb, 148
type III, 148
VZV infection, 457–459
clinical neonatal findings of CVS, 459
considerations, 457
counseling, 457, 458t
maternal shingles (herpes zoster), 459
nonimmune women, 459
prevention, 457
screening, 458
therapy, 458–459
workup/diagnosis, 458
Mania, 178
Marfan syndrome, 24, 27, 29
Marijuana (cannabis), 209–210
anesthesia, 210
antepartum testing, 210
complications, 209–210
congenital anomalies, 210
fetal/neonatal morphometrics, 210
long-term neonatal outcome, 210
neonatal withdrawal, 210
obstetrical complications, 210
diagnosis/definition, 209
epidemiology/incidence, 209
etiology/basic pathophysiology, 209
historic notes, 209
postpartum/breast-feeding, 210
risk factors/associations, 209

symptoms/signs, 209
therapy, 210
use during pregnancy, 206
Marinol (dronabinol), 209
Mask ventilation, obesity and, 41
Mass media campaigns, 199
Maternal anemia, 131–137
antepartum testing, 137
cause, 131, 133
complications, 134
defined, 131
delivery and anesthesia, 137
diagnosis, 132f, 133f, 134, 135–136
etiology/pathophysiology, 131, 132, 133,
135t
genetics, 131, 133t, 134t, 135t
iron
deficiency, 131, 133, 136
supplementation, 131, 133, 136
key points, 131
laboratory tests, 131
macrocytic, 133f, 135–136, 135t
microcytic, 134, 134t, 135–136
normocytic, 133f, 135
postpartum/breast-feeding, 137
prevalence, 131
prevention, 136, 136t
risk factors, 133, 134
symptoms, 131
therapy, 131, 136, 136f
workup, 131, 132f, 133f, 134, 135–136
Maternal bleeding, UFH therapy, 273
Maternal complications
acute cholecystitis, 121
APS, 254–255
autoimmune thrombocytopenia, 255
preeclampsia, 255
venous and arterial
thromboembolism, 254–255
CD, 111
cholelithiasis, 119
CHTN, 2
cocaine, 214–215
congenital anomalies, 214
fetal/neonatal morphometrics, 215
long-term neonatal outcome, 215
neonatal withdrawal, 215
obstetrical complications, 215
HIV infection, 299
multiple gestation, 401, 402
abruptio placentae, 401
acute fatty liver, 402
gestational diabetes, 402
peripartum hysterectomy, 402
preeclampsia, 401
thrombocytopenia, 401–402
NIH, 483
NVP and HG, 93
preeclampsia, 9
prolactinoma, 86
seizures, 168
SLE, 246
UC, 114
VZV infection, 457
Maternal Critical Care Working Group, 350,
355
Maternal death, with trauma, 340
Maternal depression, 177, 178
Maternal echocardiogram, 25
Maternal factors, for FGR, 415
Maternal-fetal transmission
herpes, 452
parvovirus, 448, 448f

toxoplasmosis, 442–443, 443f, 443t
VZV infection, 456, 457
Maternal genital infection, symptoms, 311
Maternal hydration, on AFV, 515, 516
Maternal hypothyroidism, 82
Maternal lifetime complications, smoking, 198
Maternal medical disorders, control of, 416
Maternal morbidity, for ICU, 349, 350t
Maternal mortality, for ICU, 349, 350t
Maternal physiology, clinical hypothyroidism, 74, 75t
Maternal postpartum care, HIV infection, 303
Maternal screening, GBS, 326, 327, 327f
Maternal serum alpha-fetoprotein (MSAFP), 400, 402, 447, 449
Maternal stabilization, after trauma, 342, 343, 343t
Maternal surveillance, cancer and, 380
Maternal treatment, GBS, 326
Maximum vertical pocket (MVP) technique, 407, 513
Measles–mumps–rubella (MMR), 336t
Mechanical heart valves
    pregnancy management, 28–29
    VTE and, 278
Mechanical ventilation, 356–357, 356t
Mechanism of action
    acyclovir, 453
    bromocriptine (Parlodel), 88
    cabergoline (Dostinex), 88
    corticosteroids, 249
    CsA, 393
    DDAVP, 148
    dobutamine, 368t
    indomethacin, 518
    IVIG, 463
    milrinone, 368t
    nitric oxide, 368t
    PCP, 219
    prostacyclin, inhaled/intravenous, 368t
    of PTU, 82
    sildenafil, 368t
    sulindac, 518
    ursodeoxycholic acid (Ursodiol), 106
Meclizine (Bonine, Antivert), 95t, 97
Meconium peritonitis, 481, 482
Medical conditions, morbidity of cardiac disease by, 26
Medical Eligibility Criteria for Contraceptive Use document, 27
Meditation, 201
Medroxyprogesterone acetate, 42
Melanocyte-stimulating hormone (MSH), 378
Melanoma
    cutaneous, see Cutaneous melanoma
    delay in diagnosis, 378
    effects, on pregnancy, 378
    pregnancy after, 382
    staging and sentinel node biopsy, 378
    surgery, 378
    termination of pregnancy, 378
    treatment, 378
Melphalan, 155t
Membranous nephropathy, 153
Meningococcal vaccine, 334t, 336t
Meperidine (Demerol), 19, 164t, 165
6-Mercaptopurine, 112t, 113
Meropenem, 235
Mesalamine, 110, 112t, 113
Mescaline, 220; see also Hallucinogens
Mesoridazine, 189

Metabolic diseases, NIH and, 481t, 483
Metaclopramide, 162
Metformin (glucophage), 53, 66, 433
Methadone, 206, 208, 211, 212, 213, 218
Methamphetamine, 206, 216–217; see also Amphetamines
Methimazole, 80, 82, 83
Methods, fetal monitoring, 496–509
    BPS, 499–501, 501t
        AF volume, 500, 500t
        body movements, 500
        breathing movements, 499, 500
        CTG, 500
        fetal tone, 500
        management, 500, 500t, 501t
        modified BPS, 501
        PNM with, 499, 500t
        prediction of fetal status, 499, 499f
        variables, 499, 499t
    condition-specific testing, 505, 506–508
        advanced maternal age, 508
        diabetes, 505, 506
        fetal anemia, 508
        FGR, 506
        indications for antenatal surveillance, 505, 506t
        nonobstetric procedure monitoring, 508
        obesity, 508
        postdate pregnancy, 508
        PPROM, 508
        preeclampsia, 505
        suggested antenatal surveillance, 505, 507t
    CST, 498–499
    Doppler of fetal vessels, 501–505, 504f, 505t
        abnormalities, 501, 502f
        application, 501, 503–505, 504f, 505t
        serial MCA Dopplers, 501, 503f
    Doppler surveillance and BPS, 505, 506f
    FHR testing (NST or CTG), 497–498, 497f
    movement counting in low-risk pregnancy, 496–497
    practical antenatal testing, 508–509
Methohexital sodium, 188
Methotrexate, 110, 112, 112t, 113, 115, 249t, 250, 378, 382, 389
Methyldopa (Aldomet), 4, 5, 12, 19
Methylene blue dye, 402
3,4-Methylenedioxymethamphetamine, 216–217; see also Amphetamines
Methylenedioxyproalevone, 216
Methylene diphosphonate (MDP), 375
Methylenetetrahydrofolate reductase (MTHFR), 9, 261, 262
Methylergonovine, 233
Methylprednisolone, 96t, 99, 155t, 173, 226t
Methylprednisone, 155t, 227t
Metoclopramide, 95t, 97, 98, 155t, 164t, 165, 380
Metoprolol, 162
Metronidazole, 112t, 113, 212, 322, 324
MI, see Myocardial infarction (MI)
Microadenomas, 86, 88–89
Microcytic anemia, 134, 134t, 135–136
Microscopic hematuria
    defined, 158
    differential diagnosis, 158
    incidence, 158
    management, 158
    risk factors for significant disease, 158
Midazolam, 218

Middle cerebral artery (MCA)
    advantage of, 471
    Doppler
        evaluation, for FGR, 413, 414, 415, 418, 420, 421, 422, 423f, 425
        velocimetry, fetal transfusion, 508
        waveform, 501
    MCA-PSV, 447, 449, 467, 470, 471, 472, 474, 482, 485
Mifepristone, 492
Migraine, see Headache
MIGRA study, 164
Mild intermittent asthma, 230, 232
Mild persistent asthma, 232
Mild preeclampsia, preeclampsia without severe features, 2t, 8
Mild renal insufficiency, 151
Mild-to-moderate HTN, 4–5
Milrinone, 368, 368t, 369
Milton, John Laws, 391
Mirror syndrome, 483
Mirtazapine, 183t, 184, 189
Misoprostol, 488, 492, 493
Mitoxantrone, 381
Mitral insufficiency, 28
Mitral stenosis, 28
MNS antigen system, 474
Mode, of delivery
    CRI, 153
    FGR, 426
    HELLP syndrome, 17, 18
    HSV infection, 454
    IBD, women with, 114
    preeclampsia, 13
    pregestational diabetes, 55
    SCI, 175, 175t
    UC, 116
Moderate persistent asthma, 232
Moderate renal insufficiency, 151
Modified BPS, for fetal monitoring, 501
Monitoring
    ambulatory BP, 3
    contraction, 344
    fetal
        BPS, 499–501, 499f, 499t, 500t, 501t
        condition-specific testing, 505, 506–508, 506t, 507t
        critical care, 354–355
        CST, 498–499
        Doppler of fetal vessels, 501–505, 502f, 503f, 504f, 505t
        Doppler surveillance and BPS, 505, 506f
        FHR testing (NST or CTG), 497–498, 497f
        FNAIT, 465
        hemolytic disease, 473–474
        methods, 496–509
        modified BPS, 501
        movement counting in low-risk pregnancy, 496–497
        NIH, 486
        NS, 153
        practical antenatal testing, 508–509
        principles, 496
        RBC alloimmunized pregnancies, 473–474
        trauma and, 344
    glucose
        GDM, management, 66
        pregestational diabetes, 53, 53t
    hemodynamic, preeclampsia, 13
    home uterine activity, 403

invasive hemodynamic, with pulmonary artery catheter, 27
Monoamine oxidase inhibitors (MAOIs), 184, 189
Monoamniotic (MA) twins, 398, 399t, 404, 407, 408t
Monochorionic (MC) gestations, 401, 402
Monochorionic (MC) twins, 398, 399t, 401, 402, 403, 404, 404t, 405, 407, 408, 408t
Monozygotic (MZ) twins
  defined, 398
  etiology, 399, 399t
  incidence, 398
Montelukast, 226t, 232
Mood disorders, 177–190
  antidepressants, 178, 180, 181–184, 182t–183t
    autism spectrum disorders, 184
    MAOIs, 184
    neonatal toxicity, 181, 182t–183t
    neurodevelopmental effects, 181, 184
    SNRIs, 184
    SSRIs, 181–184, 182t–183t
    TCAs, 184
    teratogenicity, 181, 182t–183t
  behavioral educational interventions, 188
  bipolar depression, 177, 178, 179–180
    complications, 180
    defined, 178
    epidemiology, 178
    pregnancy considerations, 180
    risk factors, 179–180
    screening, 180
  complications, 178
  definitions, 177–178
  depression, see Depression
  ECT, 188
  EPDS, 177, 178, 179f
  epidemiology, 177–178
  key points, 177
  management during lactation, 188–190
    antidepressants, 188–189
    antipsychotics, 189–190
    atypical antipsychotics, 190
    bupropion, 189
    carbamazepine, 189
    duloxetine, 189
    lamotrigine, 189
    lithium, 189
    MAOIs, 189
    mirtazapine, 189
    SSRIs, 188–189
    stabilizers, 189
    TCAs, 189
    trazodone, 189
    valproic acid, 189
    venlafaxine, 189
  MDD, 177, 180
  nonpharmacologic management, 188
  pharmacologic management, 180–188
    antidepressants, 180, 181–184; see also Antidepressants
    antipsychotics, 187–188
    mood stabilizers, 184–187; see also Stabilizers, mood
  postpartum blues, 177
  postpartum depression, 177, 178, 179
  postpartum psychosis, 177–178, 179–180
  risk factors, 178
  screening, 178
  stabilizers, 184–187, 185t–186t

carbamazepine and oxcarbazepine, 187
  lamotrigine, 187
  lithium, 184, 185t
  valproic acid, 187
Mood Disorders Questionnaire (MDQ), 180
Mood swings, 178
Morphine, 142, 164t, 165, 210, 211
Mother-to-infant (perinatal) transmission, HCV infection, 293–294, 293t
Motivational interviewing, defined, 35
Motor vehicle accidents (MVAs), 339, 340, 341, 342f
Movement counting in low-risk pregnancy, fetal, 496–497
Moyamoya disease, 140
MRI (magnetic resonance imaging), 86, 87, 88, 89, 90, 121, 157, 163, 164, 168, 345, 373, 376, 378, 379, 395, 490, 491
MTHFR, 9
Multidrug-resistant (MDR)-TB, 242
Multifetal pregnancy reduction, 403
Multigated equilibrium radionuclide cineangiography (MUGA), 380
Multiple gestation, 398–408
  acardiac twin, 407
  antepartum testing, 407–408
    fetal surveillance, 407–408
    ultrasounds, 407
  complications, 400–402
    abruptio placentae, 401
    acute fatty liver, 402
    chromosomal and congenital anomalies, 401
    fetal, 400, 401
    FGR and discordant growth, 401
    gestational diabetes, 402
    low-dose aspirin, 402
    maternal, 401, 402
    monochorionic gestations, 401
    nutrition, 402
    peripartum hysterectomy, 402
    preeclampsia, 401
    pregnancy considerations, 402
    pregnancy management, 402
    prenatal diagnosis, 402
    prevention and management, 403–407
    PTB, 401, 402t
    PTB, prediction of, 402
    single fetal demise in, 401
    spontaneous pregnancy loss, 400, 401
    thrombocytopenia, 401–402
  conjoined twins, 407
  defined, 398
  delivery
    delayed interval, 408
    route, 408
    timing of, 408, 408t
  diagnosis, 399, 400, 400f, 401f
  epidemiology/incidence, 398, 399f
  etiology, 398–399, 399t
  FGR and, 426, 426t
  key points, 398
  MA twins, 398, 399t, 404, 407, 408t
  MC twins, 398, 399t, 401, 402, 403, 404, 404t, 405, 407, 408, 408t
  neonates, 408
  prevention and management of complications, 403–407
    anomalous fetus, selective termination, 403–404; see also Anomalous fetus

FGR/discordant twins, 404
  single fetal death, 404, 404t
  TTTS, 404, 405–407; see also Twin-twin transfusion syndrome (TTTS)
Multispot testing, for HIV, 297
Multivitamins (MVI)
  before/at conception, 94
  sickle cell disease, 142
MVAs (motor vehicle accidents), 339, 340, 341, 342f
MyATLS app, 342
Mycobacterium tuberculosis, 238, 239, 241, 242, 301t
Myco-phenolate mofetil (MMF), 128, 155t, 249t, 250, 389
Mycophenolic acid, 128
Mycoplasma pneumoniae, 143, 233
Myocardial depression, 27, 28, 210, 365–366
Myocardial fibrosis, 381
Myocardial infarction (MI)
  AFE, 366, 369
  cocaine, effects, 206, 214
  dobutamine, 360
  incidence in pregnancy, 29
  obesity, 42
  during pregnancy, 24
Myocardial ischemia, 367
Myoinositol, 61

N

NAATs (nucleic acid amplification tests), 306–307, 307t, 310, 312, 323
Nalbuphine, 210
Naloxone, 201, 210, 211
Naltrexone, 113–114, 201, 210, 213
Naproxen, 162, 164t, 165
Naratriptan, 165
Narcan (naloxone), 210, 211
Narcolepsy, 216
Narcotics, for sickle cell disease, 142
Natalizumab, 112t
National Asthma Education and Prevention Program (NAEPP), 228, 230, 233
National Birth Defects Prevention study, 181
National Center for Health Statistics (NCHS), 488
National Heart, Lung, and Blood Institute (NHLBI), 227
National Hospital Discharge Survey, 234
National Household Survey on Drug Abuse, 220
National Inpatient Sample (NIS), 339
National Institute for Health and Care Excellence, 289
National Institutes of Health, 150
National Survey on Drug Use and Health (NSDUH), 207
National Teratology Information Service, 217
National Transplantation Pregnancy Registry (NTPR), 124
National Violent Death Reporting System, 340
Natural orifice translumenal endoscopic surgery (NOTES), 122
Nausea and vomiting of pregnancy (NVP)
  bariatric surgery and, 38
  with chemotherapy, 209, 380
  HG and, 92–100
    antiemetic therapy, 98
    benzodiazepines, 99
    classification, 92
    clonidine, 99

complications, 93
corticosteroids, 99
defined, 92
diagnosis, 81, 92, 94t
EN, 99
epidemiology/incidence, 92
etiology, 92
fetal/neonatal complications, 93
genetics, 92
inpatient assessment and treatment, 98–99
issues, 100
IVF hydration, 99
management, 93–94, 93f
maternal complications, 93
nonpharmacologic interventions, 94, 97
nutritional supplementation, 99–100
pharmacologic interventions, 97–98
PN, 99–100
postpartum management, 100
pregnancy management, 93–94
prevention, 94
risk factors/associations, 92, 93
treatment, 94, 95t–96t
workup, 94
signs and symptoms
diabetic ketoacidosis, 54
HELLP syndrome, 16, 17t
Neiman, Albert, 214
Neisseria gonorrhoeae, 305, 306, 307, 308, 311, 322
Neoadjuvant chemotherapy, for invasive cervical disease, 379
Neonatal abstinence syndrome (NAS), 211, 212–213
Neonatal alloimmune thrombocytopenia (NAIT), defined, 460; *see also* Fetal and neonatal alloimmune thrombocytopenia (FNAIT)
Neonatal brachial plexus palsy (NBPP), 432, 433
Neonatal congenital syphilis, 320
Neonatal death, trauma and, 340
Neonatal evaluation, after chemotherapy, 380–381
Neonatal/fetal complications, *see* Fetal/ neonatal complications
Neonatal/fetal morphometrics
amphetamines, use, 217
cocaine, use, 215
marijuana (cannabis), use, 210
opioids, use, 211
PCP, use, 219
Neonatal lupus, SLE, 250
Neonatal management, GBS, 329f, 330
Neonatal respiratory distress syndrome, 521
Neonatal toxicity, SSRIs, 181, 182t–183t
Neonatal withdrawal
amphetamines, use, 217
benzodiazepines, abuse, 218
cocaine, use, 215
marijuana (cannabis), use, 210
opioids, use, 211, 212
PCP, use, 219
Neonates
clinical hypothyroidism, 76
consequences of smoking, reducing, 202
Graves' disease, 81, 83
hemolytic disease of, *see* Hemolytic disease
HSV-infected, 454
hyperthyroidism, 83

hypothyroidism, 82
intensive care unit (NICU), 16
long-term follow-up, parvovirus, 450
multiple gestation, 408
preeclampsia, complications, 9
transient bone marrow suppression of, 380
Neonatology management
FGR, 426
FNAIT, 465–466
hemolytic disease, 474
NIH, 486
Nephrolithiasis
defined, 157
urinary, *see* Urinary nephrolithiasis
Nephropathy, diabetic, 51
Nephrotic syndrome (NS)
causes, 153
complications, 153
defined, 153
epidemiology/incidence, 153
fetal monitoring, 153
labor management, 153
long-term prognosis, 153
management, 153
prenatal care, 153
specific diseases, 153
workup, 153
Neural tube defects (NTDs)
congenital malformations, 168
obesity and, 33
serum screening for, 402
VPA, 187
Neuraminidase, 236
Neurodevelopmental effects, SSRIs, 181, 184
Neurodevelopmental Effects of Antiepileptic Drugs Study, 189
Neurogenic shock, 173
Neurontin (Gabapentin), 169t, 171
Neuropathy, diabetic, 51
Neurosurgery, in patients with prolactinomas, 90t
Neurosyphilis, 317
Neurovegetative symptoms, 177
Neutral protamine Hagedorn (NPH), 53t, 54, 55, 62t, 64t, 65t, 66, 67
New-onset diabetes mellitus (NODM), 125
New York Heart Association (NYHA) system, 25, 25t
Nicardipine, 155t
Nicotine
acetylcholine receptors, 201
agonists, 201
e-cigarettes, 198
gums, 200, 200t
inhalers, lozenges, and nasal spray, 200t, 201
on multiple transmitter pathways, 197
patches, 200–201, 200t
Nicotine replacement therapies (NRT), 196, 200–201, 200t
Nifedipine, 1, 4, 6t, 7, 13, 16, 19, 155t
NIH, *see* Nonimmune hydrops fetalis (NIH)
Nimodipine, 5, 12
Nitric oxide
donors, in FGR pregnancies, 420
inhaled, 27, 368t
preeclampsia, prevention, 11
pulmonary vascular resistances, 368
Nitrofurantoin, 156, 174
Nitroglycerin, 174, 215
Nitroimidazoles, 324
Nitroprusside, 173, 174

Nitrosamines, 198
Nizatidine, 97
N-methyl D-aspartate (NMDA) receptor antagonist, 219
Nolotinib, 378
Non–Hodgkin's lymphoma (NHL), during pregnancy
delay in diagnosis, 377
effects, on pregnancy, 377
treatment, 377
Nonimmune hydrops fetalis (NIH), 477–486
associations/possible etiologies, 479–483
defined, 477, 478
diagnosis, 478, 478f
differential diagnosis, 479–483, 480t–481t
cardiovascular disorders, 479–481
chromosomal abnormalities, 481
congenital infections, 482
extracardiac anomalies, 481–482
fetal tumors, 483
hematological disorders, 482–483
metabolic diseases, 483
epidemiology/incidence, 478
etiology/basic pathophysiology, 478, 479, 479f
key points, 477–478
management, 483–486
amniocentesis, 485
cordocentesis and invasive procedures, 485
counseling/prognosis, 483
delivery/anesthesia, 486
delivery timing, 486
demographic and clinical history, 484
fetal monitoring/testing, 486
laboratory, 484
neonatology, 486
obstetric, 486
therapeutic approach, 486
treatment, 486
ultrasound, 484
workup/diagnosis, 484–485, 484f, 485f
maternal
complications, 483
postpartum, 486
Nonimmune women, VZV infection, 459
Non-nucleoside reverse transcriptase inhibitor (NNRTI), 302t, 303
Nonobstetric procedure monitoring, 508
Nonobstetric sepsis, 358
Nonpharmacologic interventions, NVP and HG, 94, 97
Nonpharmacologic management
headache, 165
mood disorders, 188
Nonprimary first episode, HSV, 452
Nonproteinuric hypertension, bed rest in hospital for, 3
Nonreassuring fetal heart testing (NRFHT), 104, 425, 514, 516
Nonsteroidal anti-inflammatory drugs (NSAIDs), 164, 164t, 165, 233, 249, 249t
Nonstress test (NST), fetal surveillance
APS, 258
drug abuse, 209
FGR, 413, 421, 422, 423f, 424, 425, 426
GDM, 61t, 67
heart rate testing, 497–498, 497f
hyperthyroidism, 82
ICP, 103, 107
multiple gestation, 404, 408
pregestational diabetes, 52, 55

Nontreponemal tests, for syphilis, 318
Norepinephrine, 216, 360, 368
Norepinephrine reuptake inhibitors (NRIs), 184
Noresthisterone, 279
Norgestimate, 279
Normocytic anemia, 133f, 135
North American AED Pregnancy Registry, 187
North American AIDS Cohort Collaboration on Research and Design (NA-ACCORD), 298
North American Antiepileptic Drug (NAAED) Pregnancy Registry, 169, 170
Nortriptyline, 201
NPH (neutral protamine Hagedorn), 53t, 54, 55, 62t, 64t, 65t, 66, 67
NRT (nicotine replacement therapies), 196, 200–201, 200t
NS, *see* Nephrotic syndrome (NS)
NSAIDs (nonsteroidal anti-inflammatory drugs), 164, 164t, 165, 233, 249, 249t
NST, *see* Nonstress test (NST)
Nubain®, 213
Nuchal translucency (NT), 40, 398, 402, 481
Nucleic acid amplification tests (NAATs), 306–307, 307t, 310, 312, 323
Nucleoside analogs, HBV infections, 288–289, 289t
Nucleoside reverse transcriptase inhibitor (NRTI), 302t
Nucleotide analogs, HBV infections, 288–289, 289t
Nursing care, in ICU, 352
Nutritional supplementation, 39
   FGR
      interventions, 419
      prevention, 416
   GDM, management, 67
   multiple gestation, 402
   NVP and HG, 99–100
      EN, 99
      PN, 99–100
NVP, *see* Nausea and vomiting of pregnancy (NVP)

O

Obesity, 32–42
   anesthesia, 40–41
   antepartum fetal testing, 40
   bariatric surgery, 38–39, 38t
   cesarean delivery, 41
   classification, 32, 33t
   complications of, 33–35, 34t–35t
   contraception, 42
   defined, 32
   epidemiology/incidence, 32
   etiology/basic pathophysiology, 33
   extreme, 32
   fetal monitoring and, 508
   FGR and, 416
   folic acid supplementation and vitamins, 39
   future research, 42
   genetics, 33
   health risks associated with, 35t
   intrapartum care, 40
   key points, 32
   long-term maternal and offspring risks, 42

methamphetamine for, 216
postpartum management, 41
   breast-feeding, 41
   complications, 41
   VTE, 41
preconception evaluation, 35–37, 36f, 36t, 37t
preeclampsia and, 33
prenatal care, 39–40
   fetal ultrasound, 40
   general issues, 40
   ideal weight gain, 39, 39t
prepregnancy weight reduction
   behavior therapy, 38
   diet, 38
   pharmacotherapy, 38
   physical activity, 38
preterm birth and, 35
resources, 42
risk factors, 33
super, 32
Ob-Gyn (obstetrician-gynecologist), role, 355–356
Obstetrical complications
   amphetamines, use, 217
   benzodiazepines, abuse, 218
   cocaine, use, 215
   hallucinogens, exposure, 220
   marijuana (cannabis), use, 210
   opioids, use, 211
   PCP, use, 219
Obstetrical ICU, 351–352
Obstetric critical care services, organization, 350, 351, 352–353
Obstetrician-gynecologist (Ob-Gyn), role, 355–356
Obstetric management, NIH, 486
Obstetric sepsis, 358
Obstructive sleep apnea (OSA), obesity and, 35, 40
Odansetron (Zofran), 95t, 380
Offspring, of cancer survivors, 381
Offspring risks, 42
OK-432, sclerosant product, 481
Olanzapine, 186t, 187, 190
Oligohydramnios, 122
   AFI and, 513
   cholecystitis, 122
   CHTN, complications, 1, 2, 4
   color Doppler for, 514
   defined, 425, 515
   FGR and, 425
   herceptin for, 375
   management, 518
   MC/DA gestation with, 405
   NSAIDs, 249
   preeclampsia, complications, 9, 13, 16
   sonographic assessment, of AF, 515–516
      amnioinfusion, 516
      complications, 515
      diagnosis, 515
      epidemiology/incidence, 515
      etiology, 515
      key points, 515
      management, 515, 516f
      maternal hydration, 515, 516
      16 to 22 weeks, 515
      23 to 40 weeks, 515
      40 weeks, 515
   trastuzumab for, 375, 382
   ultrasound, accuracy of, 513–514
Olsalazine, 112t, 113
Ombitasvir, 291, 295

Omega-3 fatty acids, 402
Omeprazole (Prilosec), 95t, 97
Omphalocele, 181
Ondansetron (Zofran), 98, 380
One step screening test, GDM, 59
Open fractures, 344
Opioids, 210–214
   anesthesia, 213
   antepartum testing, 213
   complications
      congenital anomalies, 211
      fetal/neonatal morphometrics, 211
      long-term neonatal outcome, 211–212
      neonatal withdrawal, 211
      obstetrical, 211
   delivery, 213
   diagnosis/definition, 210
   epidemiology/incidence, 211
   headache in pregnancy, 164, 164t, 165
   historic notes, 210
   overview, 206, 208
   postpartum/breast-feeding, 213–214
   risk factors/associations, 211
   in smoking, 201
   symptoms, 210–211
   therapy, 212–213
      buprenorphine, 212–213
      methadone, 212
   treatments, 213
Optimal glucose control, insulin and, 51
Oral contraceptives, 25, 27, 42, 125, 171, 175, 251
Oral hypoglycemic agents
   glyburide, for GDM, 66
   for pregestational diabetes, 53
Oral replacement therapy, for opioid-use disorder, 212
Organization of Teratology Information Specialists (OTIS) Project, 250
Organ toxicity, amphetamines and, 216
Orlistat (Xenical), 38
Oseltamivir, 237–238
Osteoporosis, heparin-induced, 274
Outcomes
   adverse pregnancy, inherited thrombophilias and, 262–263, 263t
   fetal, FLM and, 525
   fetal and maternal, post-LTx pregnancy, 125, 126t
   fetal/neonatal, trauma and, 340
   long-term, hemolytic disease, 474
   long-term neonatal
      amphetamines, 217
      benzodiazepines, 218
      cocaine, 215
      hallucinogens, 220
      heroin, 211–212
      marijuana, 210
      opioids, 211–212
      PCP, 219
   subsequent pregnancy, after delivery of twins, 404
Outpatient setting, chronic treatment in, 5
Ovarian follicles, 33
Overdose, opioid, 211
Oxcarbamazepine, 169t, 171
Oxcarbazepine, 169t, 171, 185t, 187
Oxycodone, 208, 210, 211, 213
Oxygen
   content of fetal blood, 356–357
   therapy in FGR pregnancies, 420
Oxyhemoglobin, 197
Oxymorphone, 210

Oxytocin, 149, 188, 366, 408, 488, 492, 493
Oxytocin contraction test (OCT), 426,
    498–499

P

Pain Medicine Guidelines, 278
Paliperidone, 187
Palpitations, pregnancy management, 27
Pantoprazole (Protonix), 95t, 97
Papillary thyroid cancer, 380
Pap smear, 141, 300, 323
Para-aminosalicylate, 242
Paracetamol, 249t, 250
Parenteral nutrition (PN), NVP and HG,
    99–100
Paritaprevir, 291, 295
Parlodel (bromocriptine), 86, 87, 88, 89, 155t
Paroxetine, 177, 181, 182t
Parvovirus, 447–450
    complications, 448
    incidence/epidemiology, 447
    key points, 447
    maternal-fetal transmission, 448, 448f
    NIH and, 482
    pathogen, 447
    pathophysiology, 447, 448f
    pregnancy management, 448–449
        counseling/prognosis, 448
        neonate and long-term follow-up, 450
        prevention, 448–449
        screening, 449
        therapy, 449
        workup/diagnosis, 449, 449f
    risk factors/associations, 447
    symptoms, 447
    ultrasound fetal findings, 448
Patellar reflexes, monitoring of, 12
Pathogens
    CMV, 436
    herpes, 451
    parvovirus, 447
    toxoplasmosis, 442
    VZV, 456
Pathophysiology
    ACS, 143
    acute cholecystitis, 121
    ADP, 389
    AFE, 365–366
    amphetamines, 216
    APS, 254
    asthma, 225
    benzodiazepines, abuse, 218
    cardiac disease, 24–25
    CD, 111
    chlamydia, 311
    cholelithiasis, 119
    CHTN, 1
    clinical hypothyroidism, 73–74
    CMV, 436–437
        clinical neonatal findings and
            complications, 437
        general, 436–437, 437f, 437t
        primary infection, 437
        recurrent infections, 437
    cocaine, 214
    FGR, 414–415
    FNAIT, 460
    GBS, 325
    GDM, 60
    gonorrhea, 305
    hallucinogens, 220
    HAV infections, 283

HBV infections, 286, 287f
HCV infection, 293
headache, 163
hemolytic disease, 468
herpes
    nonprimary first episode, 452
    primary first episode, 452
    reactivation (recurrent) genital
        herpes, 452
HIV infection, 299
hyperthyroidism, 81
ICP, 103, 104
IH (pustular psoriasis of pregnancy), 393
influenza, 236
inherited thrombophilias, 261
LTx, pregnancy after, 124
marijuana (cannabis), 209
maternal anemia, 131, 132, 133, 135t
NIH, 478, 479, 479f
obesity, 33
parvovirus, 447, 448f
PCP, 219
PEP, 388
PFP, 390
PG (herpes gestationis), 392
pneumonia, 233, 234t
PP, 391
preeclampsia, 8–9
pregestational diabetes, 50
prolactinoma, 86
seizures, 168
SG, 386
sickle cell disease, 140
SLE, 246
smoking, 196–198
syphilis, 315–316
toxoplasmosis, 442
trauma, 339
trichomoniasis, 322
tuberculosis, 238
UC, 114
VTE, 270, 271f, 271t
vWD, 145, 147f
VZV infection, 456, 457f
Patient education, pregnancy with CRI, 152
Patients, "5 As" for, 197t
Pauling, Linus, 139
Paxil® and Paxil CR® (Paroxetine), 182t
PCP, see Phencyclidine (PCP)
PCR (polymerase chain reaction), 442, 443,
    444, 445, 453, 458, 485
Peak expiratory flow (PEF), 227, 229
Peak expiratory flow rate (PEFR)
    measurements, 225
    treatment, 232
Peak systolic velocity (PSV), MCA-PSV, 447,
    449, 467, 470, 471, 472, 474, 482, 485
Pelvic inflammatory disease (PID), 305
Pemphigoid gestationis (PG)
    complications, 392
    defined, 391–392
    diagnosis, 391–392, 392f
    epidemiology/incidence, 392
    etiology/basic pathology, 392
    exclusion of, 388
    genetics, 392
    historic notes, 391
    key points, 391
    management, 392
    overview, 386, 387t
    PEP and, 388
    symptoms, 392
    therapy, 392

workup, 392
Penciclovir, 454
Penetrating abdominal wound, 344
Penicillamine, 249t, 250
Penicillins
    CHD, 27
    GBS, 325, 328, 328t, 329–330
    gonorrhea, 307, 308
    syphilis, 315, 319, 319t, 320
PEP, see Polymorphic eruption of pregnancy
    (PEP)
Pepcid (famotidine), 95t, 97
Peramivir, 237
Percutaneous balloon valvuloplasty, 28
Percutaneous coronary intervention (PCI),
    29
Percutaneous nephrostomy, 157
Percutaneous pulmonary valvuloplasty, 28
Percutaneous umbilical blood sampling
    (PUBS), 439, 449
Pergolide (quinagolide), 88
Pericardial fibrosis, 381
Perihepatitis, 305
Perimortem cesarean delivery (PMCD), 346,
    367
Perinatal complications
    cocaine, 214–215
        congenital anomalies, 214
        fetal/neonatal morphometrics, 215
        long-term neonatal outcome, 215
        neonatal withdrawal, 215
        obstetrical complications, 215
Perinatal mortality (PNM)
    with BPS, 498, 499, 500t
    CRI and, 152
Peripartum cardiomyopathy, 29, 367
Peripartum dilated cardiomyopathy, 367
Peripartum hysterectomy, 402
Peritoneal dialysis (PD), 154
Persistent pulmonary hypertension of
    newborn (PPHN), 181
Pertussis vaccination, 332
Pexeva® (Paroxetine), 182t
Peyote, 220
PFP, see Pruritic folliculitis of pregnancy
    (PFP)
PG, see Pemphigoid gestationis (PG)
PGE2 suppositories, 492
P-glycoprotein, 374
PGM (prothrombin G20210A gene
    mutation), 9, 261, 262, 265t, 279
Pharmacological therapy, UC, 115
Pharmacologic interventions, NVP and HG,
    97–98
Pharmacologic management, mood
    disorders, 180–188
    antidepressants, 180, 181–184; see also
        Antidepressants
    antipsychotics, 187–188
    mood stabilizers, 184–187; see also
        Stabilizers, mood
Pharmacotherapies
    prepregnancy weight reduction, 38
    smoking, 200–201
        bupropion HCl (Zyban®, Wellbutrin®),
            201
        combination therapies, 201
        NOT recommended, 201
        NRT, 200–201, 200t
        varenicline (Chantix®), 201
Phencyclidine (PCP)
    antepartum testing, 219
    defined, 219

diagnosis, 219
epidemiology/incidence, 219
etiology/basic pathophysiology, 219
historic notes, 219
overview, 206
postpartum/breast-feeding, 219
pregnancy complications
  congenital anomalies, 219
  fetal/neonatal morphometrics, 219
  long-term neonatal outcome, 219
  neonatal withdrawal, 219
  obstetrical complications, 219
risk factors/associations, 219
symptoms, 219
therapy, 219
Phenergan, 19, 96t, 98
Phenobarbital
  NAS, 211
  PCP, use, 219
  renal disease, 155t
  seizures, 167, 169, 170, 171
  thyroid storm, 83t
Phenothiazines, 96, 98
Phenylephrine, 360
Phenytoins, 12, 19, 75, 155t, 167, 169, 169t, 170, 171
Phosphatidylglycerol (PG), 67
  testing, for FLM, 522, 523t
Physical activity
  prepregnancy weight reduction, 38
  weight loss, 39
Physical dependence, defined, 207
Physical examination
  CHTN, 3
  HG, diagnosis, 94
  HIV infection, 300
  hyperthyroidism, 80
  preeclampsia, prevention, 11
Physiologic renal changes, 150, 151t
Physiology, hyperthyroidism, 81
Pimecroliums, 389
Pinta, transmission, 318
Piperacillin-tazobactam, 235
Pirbuterol, 227t
Placental abruption, smoking and, 198
Placental pathology, 158
Placental risk factors, for FGR, 415
Placenta physiology, clinical
  hypothyroidism, 74–75
Placenta previa, smoking and, 198
Plaquenil (hydroxychloroquine), 246, 248, 249, 249t, 251, 256
Plasma volume expansion
  in FGR pregnancies, 420
  for preeclampsia, 12, 15–16
Plasminogen-activator inhibitor (PAI), 261
P6 Neiguan point, acupressure at, 94, 97
Pneumatic compression devices, 279
Pneumococcal vaccines, 139, 140, 142, 234, 334t, 335, 336t, 337
Pneumococcus, 125
Pneumocystis carinii pneumonia (PCP), 297, 301t
Pneumonia, 233–235
  anesthesia, 235
  antepartum testing, 235
  antibiotics for, 235
  classification, 233, 234
  complications, 234
  delivery, 235
  diagnosis, 233
  epidemiology, 234
  etiology/basic pathophysiology, 233, 234t

key points, 233
management
  prevention, 234
  principles, 234
  workup, 234
postpartum/breast-feeding, 235
pregnancy considerations, 234
risk factors, 234
symptoms, 234
treatment
  hospitalization, 235
Pneumonia Severity Index (PSI), 234, 235
Pneumovax, 301
Polio vaccine, 301, 334t–335t
Polycystic ovarian syndrome, 66
Polyhydramnios (hydramnios)
  AFE, risk factors for, 366
  defined, 484, 516, 517
  dialysis, complications, 154
  GDM, 59
  management, 518
  NIH and, 483
  pregestational diabetes, 50, 51
  sonographic assessment, of AF, 516–518
    complications, 517
    diagnosis, 517
    etiology, 517
    incidence/epidemiology, 517
    key points, 516–517
    labor precautions, 517
    management, 517–518
    workup (differential diagnosis), 517
  TTTS, 404, 405
Polymerase chain reaction (PCR), 442, 443, 444, 445, 453, 458, 485
Polymorphic eruption of pregnancy (PEP)
  complications, 388
  defined, 388
  diagnosis, 388, 388f
  epidemiology/incidence, 388
  etiology/basic pathology, 388
  genetics, 388
  historic notes, 388
  key points, 388
  management, 388–389
    preconception counseling, 388–389
    workup, 388
  overview, 386, 387t
  PUPPP, 388–389
  symptoms, 388
  therapy, 389
Polysubstance abuse, 216, 219
PORTO trial, 414, 421
Positron emission tomography (PET) scans, 375
Postdate pregnancy, fetal monitoring and, 508
Postnatal morbidities, smoking and, 198
Postpartum blues, 177
Postpartum counseling, recurrence rates of AFE, 369
Postpartum depression, 134, 177, 178, 179, 188
Postpartum management
  amphetamines, use, 217
  anticoagulation, 279
  APS, 258
  asthma, 233
  benzodiazepines, 219
  CD, 114
  CHTN, 5
  clinical hypothyroidism, 76
  cocaine, use, 215
  CRI, 153

dialysis, 154
eclampsia, 19
fetal death, 493
GDM, 68, 68f
HAV infections, pregnancy with, 284
HBV infections, 289
HCV infection, 295
HIV infection, 303
HSV infection, 454
hyperthyroidism, 83
influenza, 238
marijuana (cannabis) abuse, 210
maternal anemia, 137
NIH, 486
NVP and HG, 100
obesity and
  breast-feeding, 41
  complications, 41
  VTE, 41
opioids, use, 213–214
PCP, 219
pneumonia, 235
pregestational diabetes, 55, 56
prolactinoma, 90
renal transplantation, 156
SCI, 175
seizures, 171
sickle cell disease, 143
SLE, 250
smoking, 201–202
trauma, 346
tuberculosis, 242
UC, 116
vWD, 149
Postpartum psychosis, 177–178, 179–180
Postpartum thyroiditis
  defined, 77
  diagnosis, 77
  etiology, 77
  incidence, 77
  management, 77
  recurrence risk, 77
  risk factors, 77
  three clinical presentations, 77
Postpartum urinary retention, 157–158
  defined, 157
  incidence, 157
  management, 158
  risk factors, 158
Potassium chloride, in MC pregnancies, 403
PP, see Prurigo of pregnancy (PP)
PPIs (proton-pump inhibitors), 98
PPROM (preterm premature rupture
  of membranes), 7, 11, 12, 112t, 113, 215, 246, 249, 302, 404, 406, 408, 425, 505, 508, 513, 517, 518
Prazosin, 174
Preconception care, asthma, 228
Preconception counseling
  after bariatric surgery, 38t
  cardiac disease, 25
  CD, 112
  CHTN, 3
  clinical hypothyroidism, 74
  cutaneous melanoma, 395
  drug abuse, 208
  FGR, 426, 426t
  FNAIT, 466
  HAV infections, pregnancy with, 283
  HBV infections, 288
  HCV infection, 294
  HIV infection, 300
  IH (pustular psoriasis of pregnancy), 393

LTx, pregnancy after, 125
PEP, 388–389
preeclampsia, 11–12
pregestational diabetes, 52, 52t
prolactinoma, 88
renal disease, 150, 151
renal transplantation, 154–155
SCI, 173
seizures, 169, 170
sickle cell disease, 140, 141–142
SLE, 248, 248t
UC, 115
VTE, 277
vWD, 146
Preconception evaluation, obesity, 35–37, 36f, 36t, 37t
Prednisolone, 17, 96t, 99, 155t, 226t, 227t, 392
Prednisone, 112t, 113, 129, 155, 155t, 164t, 165, 226t, 227t, 233, 247, 249, 249t, 250, 256, 378, 393, 463, 464, 465
Preeclampsia, 6–20
    ADR vs., 174, 174t
    anesthesia, 13
    antepartum testing, 13
    antihypertensive drugs for, 7
    antioxidant therapy with vitamin C, 7
    calcium supplementation, 7
    CHTN, maternal complications of, 1, 2
    classification, 9
    complications, 9, 14, 15–20
        fetal/neonatal, 9
        maternal, 9
    CRI and, 152
    delivery, 13
        hemodynamic monitoring, 13
        mode, 13
        timing, 13
    diagnoses/definitions, 2, 2t, 6, 8
    eclampsia, 18–20
        antepartum testing, 19
        defined, 7, 8, 18
        delivery, 19
        incidence, 12, 18
        magnesium, 7
        magnesium sulfate, 19
        management, 18–19
        postpartum management, 19
        principles, 18–19
        therapy, 19
        workup, 19
    epidemiology, 8
    etiology/basic pathophysiology, 8–9
    fetal complications, 7
    fetal monitoring for, 505
    HELLP syndrome
        diagnoses/definitions, 7, 8
    hypertensive disorders, 1
    incidence, 3, 8
    indications for delivery, 7
    key points, 6–8
    laboratory tests, 3
    long-term counseling, 20
    low-dose aspirin, 7
    LTx, pregnancy after, 127
    management, 9–13, 13t, 14f, 15f
        abnormal uterine Doppler ultrasound, prevention, 10
        admission, 12
        antihypertensive therapy, 12–13
        antioxidant therapy, 11
        antiplatelet agents, 13
        aspirin, 10
        calcium, 10–11

counseling, 11–12
diagnosis, 11
diuretics, 11
fish oil, 11
garlic, 11
heparin, 10
history, 11
magnesium, 11
magnesium prophylaxis, 12
nitric oxide, 11
physical examination, 11
plasma volume expansion, 12
preconception counseling, 11
prevention, 10–11
principles, 9–10
progesterone, 11
rest/exercise, 11
salt intake, 11
workup, 11
    maternal complications, 7
        APS, 255
    mirror syndrome vs., 483
    multiple gestation and, 401
    obesity and, 33
    prediction, 9
    prevalence of, 9
    recurrence risk of, 20
    risk factors/associations, 9
    screening, 3
    selected clinical risk factors for, 6t
    severe
        defined, 7
        delivery, timing of, 16
        diagnostic criteria, 15
        expectant management, 16
        magnesium sulfate, 15–16
        management, 15–16
        plasma volume expansion, 15–16
        with severe features, 8, 14, 15–16
    smoking, complication, 198
    superimposed
        diagnoses/definitions, 2, 2t, 7, 8
        management, 14
        overview, 14, 14f, 15f
        with severe features, 8
    symptoms, 8
    therapy, 152
    without severe features ("mild preeclampsia"), 2t, 8
    workup for, 1
Preexisting hypothyroidism, 75
Pregabalin (Lyrica), 169t
Pregestational diabetes, 50–56
    anesthesia, 55
    antepartum testing, 55, 55t
    classification, 50
    complications, 51
    defined, 50
    delivery
        intrapartum glucose management, 55
        mode, 55
        timing, 55
    diabetic ketoacidosis, 54, 54t
    diagnosis, 50, 51t
    epidemiology/incidence, 50
    future research, 56
    key points, 50
    management, 52, 52t
    pathophysiology, 50
    postpartum/breast-feeding, 55, 56
    preconception counseling, 52, 52t
    prenatal care, 52, 53–54
        diet, 53, 53t

exercise, 53
glucose monitoring, 53, 53t
insulin, 53–54, 53t, 54t
oral hypoglycemic agents, 53
    risk factors/associations, 50
    symptoms, 50
    very tight vs. tight control, 54
Pregnancy
    ACE inhibitors in, 1, 3, 4, 6t
    AFE, see Amniotic fluid embolism (AFE)
    after chemotherapy, 381
    cancer, see Cancer
    cardiac disease, see Cardiac disease
    chlamydia, see Chlamydia
    CMV, see Cytomegalovirus (CMV)
    complications, see Complications
    considerations
        acute cholecystitis, 121–122
        ADP (eczema), 389
        anatomy/radiology, 74
        APS, 255
        asthma, 228
        bipolar depression, 180
        cardiac disease, 24–25
        CD, 111
        cholelithiasis, 120
        clinical hypothyroidism, 74–75, 75t
        CRI, 152
        cutaneous melanoma, 394–395
        fetal thyroid physiology, 74
        HAV infections, 283
        HBV infections, 286, 288
        HCV infection, 293–294
        headache, 163–164
        HIV, 299
        HSV infection, 452
        hyperthyroidism, 81
        ICP, 106
        influenza, 237
        maternal physiology, 74, 75t
        multiple gestation, 402
        PFP, 390
        placenta physiology, 74–75
        pneumonia, 234
        pregestational diabetes, 51, 51t
        prolactinoma, 87
        SLE, 247
        smoking, 198–199
        trauma, 341
        tuberculosis, 239
        UC, 115
        vWD, 146
        VZV infection, 457
    counseling, HCV infection, 294
    critical care, see Critical care
    dermatoses of, see Dermatoses
    drug abuse, see Drug abuse
    fetal macrosomia, see Fetal macrosomia
    FGR, see Fetal growth restriction (FGR)
    gallbladder disease, see Gallbladder disease
    GBS, see Group B streptococcus (GBS)
    GDM, see Gestational diabetes (GDM)
    gonorrhea, see Gonorrhea
    HAV, see Hepatitis A virus (HAV) infections
    HBV, see Hepatitis B virus (HBV) infections
    HCV, see Hepatitis C virus (HCV) infection
    HIV, see Human immunodeficiency virus (HIV)
    HSV infection, see Herpes

hypertensive disorders, *see* Hypertensive disorders
hyperthyroidism, *see* Hyperthyroidism
hypothyroidism, *see* Hypothyroidism
IBD, *see* Inflammatory bowel disease (IBD)
ICP, *see* Intrahepatic cholestasis of pregnancy (ICP)
inherited thrombophilias, *see* Inherited thrombophilias
interval, 416
loss, smoking and, 198
LTx, *see* Liver transplantation (LTx), pregnancy after
management, *see* Management
maternal anemia, *see* Maternal anemia
mood disorders, *see* Mood disorders
multiple gestation, *see* Multiple gestation
NIH, *see* Nonimmune hydrops fetalis (NIH)
obesity, *see* Obesity
parvovirus, *see* Parvovirus
pregestational diabetes, *see* Pregestational diabetes
prolactinoma, *see* Prolactinoma
renal disease, *see* Renal disease
respiratory diseases, *see* Respiratory diseases
SCI, *see* Spinal cord injury (SCI)
sickle cell disease, *see* Sickle cell disease
SLE, *see* Systemic lupus erythematosus (SLE)
smoking, *see* Smoking
syphilis, *see* Syphilis
transplantations, 128t, 129
trauma, *see* Trauma
trichomoniasis, *see* Trichomoniasis
vaccination, 332, 333; *see also* Vaccination
VZV, *see* Varicella zoster virus (VZV) (chickenpox)
Pregnancy-associated plasma protein-A (PAPP-A), 9, 417
Pregnancy-induced hypertension, defined, 5
Pregnancy-unique quantification of emesis/nausea (PUQE) index, 92
Prelabor maternal treatment, GBS, 326
Premature rupture of membranes (PROM)
    drug abuse, 215
    oligohydramnios, 515, 516, 517, 518
    PPROM, 7, 11, 12, 112t, 113, 215, 246, 249, 302, 404, 406, 408, 425, 505, 508, 513, 517, 518
    preeclampsia, 7, 11, 12, 16
    PTL and, 404
    SLE, 246, 249
    smoking, complication, 198
    vaginal pool specimens in, 522
Prenatal care
    after bariatric surgery, 38t
    asthma, 228
    cardiac disease, 25
    CD, 112
    CHTN, 3
    CRI, 152
    drug abuse, 208–209, 209t
    evaluation, CHB/CNL, 251
    HAV infections, pregnancy with, 283, 284
    HBV infections, 288
    HIV infection, 300
    NS, 153
    obesity, 39–40
        fetal ultrasound, 40
        general issues, 40

ideal weight gain, 39, 39t
pregestational diabetes, 52, 53–54
    diet, 53, 53t
    exercise, 53
    glucose monitoring, 53, 53t
    insulin, 53–54, 53t, 54t
    oral hypoglycemic agents, 53
prolactinoma, 89–90
    macroadenoma, 89, 90t
    microadenoma, 89
renal transplantation, 155, 155t
SCI, 173–174
seizures, 170
sickle cell disease, 140, 141–142
SLE, 248, 249
trauma, 346
UC, 115
vWD, 146
Prenatal counseling, seizures, 170
Prenatal diagnosis, multiple gestation and, 402
Prenatal education, toxoplasmosis, 443
Prenatal exercise, prevention of fetal macrosomia, 433
Prenatal maternal screening, GBS, 326, 327, 327f
Prenatal visits
    CRI, pregnancy with, 152
    HIV infection, pregnancy with, 300
Prepregnancy weight reduction
    behavior therapy, 38
    diet, 38
    pharmacotherapy, 38
    physical activity, 38
Prescription opioid analgesics, *see* Opioids
Preterm birth (PTB), risks
    anomalous fetus, selective termination, 403–404
    APS, 254, 255, 256, 257, 258
    asthma, 225, 228, 232
    cancer and, 380
    chlamydia, 310, 311
    FGR, 415
    GBS, 326
    gonorrhea, 305, 306
    HBV infection, 288
    HIV infection, 299
    influenza, 237
    in multiple gestation, 401, 402t, 403–404
        bed rest, 403
        cerclage, 403
        home uterine activity monitoring, 403
        multifetal pregnancy reduction, 403
        PPROM, 404
        prevention, 403
        progesterone, 403
        prophylactic tocolysis, 403
        PTL, 404
        subsequent pregnancy outcomes, after delivery of twins, 404
        weight gain, 403
    obesity and, 35
    pneumonia, 234
    prediction, multiple gestation, 402
    pregnancy after LTx, 126t, 127
    rate, 211
    SLE, 246
    smoking, complication, 198
    syphilis, 317
    TB, 239
    TG infection, 443
    trauma, 340, 346
    trichomoniasis, 322, 323, 324

Preterm labor (PTL)
    ascertainment and preparation for, 174–175
    CRI and, 152
    multiple gestations and, 404
    therapy, 152
Preterm premature rupture of membranes (PPROM), 7, 11, 12, 112t, 113, 215, 246, 249, 302, 404, 406, 408, 425, 505, 508, 513, 517, 518
Prevacid (lansoprazole), 95t, 97
Prevention
    APS, 256
    asthma, 228, 228t
    chlamydia, 311–312
    CHTN, 3
    clinical hypothyroidism, 74
    CMV, hygiene, 438
    CNL/CHB, 251
    CRI, 152
    cutaneous melanoma, 395
    drug abuse, 208
    fetal death, 489, 489t
    fetal macrosomia, 432–433
    FGR, 416
        aspirin therapy, 416
        control of maternal medical disorders, 416
        gestational age determination, 416
        nutrition, 416
        pregnancy interval, 416
        substance cessation, 416
    FNAIT, 462–463
    GBS, 326, 327
    GDM, 61
    gonorrhea, 306
    HAV infections, pregnancy with, 283
    HBV infections, 288
    HCV infection, 294
    hemolytic disease, 469–470
    herpes, 453, 453f
    ICP, 106, 106f
    IH (pustular psoriasis of pregnancy), 393
    influenza, 237
    maternal anemia, 136, 136t
    multiple gestation, complications, 403–407
        anomalous fetus, selective termination, 403–404; *see also* Anomalous fetus
        FGR/discordant twins, 404
        single fetal death, 404, 404t
        TTTS, 404, 405–407; *see also* Twin-twin transfusion syndrome (TTTS)
    NVP and HG, 94
    obstetrical complications, inherited thrombophilias, 266
    parvovirus, 448–449
    pneumonia, 234
    preeclampsia, 10–11
        abnormal uterine Doppler ultrasound, 10
        antioxidant therapy, 11
        aspirin, 10
        calcium, 10–11
        diuretics, 11
        fish oil, 11
        garlic, 11
        heparin, 10
        magnesium, 11
        nitric oxide, 11
        progesterone, 11
        rest/exercise, 11
        salt intake, 11

pregestational diabetes, 52
of recurrence, fetal death, 493
SG, 387
sickle cell disease, 140
smoking relapse, 202
syphilis, 317
toxoplasmosis, 443, 443t
trauma
air bags, 341
intimate partner violence, 341
seatbelts, 341
trichomoniasis, 323
urinary incontinence, 157
UTI, 156
vaccine-preventable diseases, 332
VTE, 264, 266, 277–278
VZV infection, 457
Prevnar-13, 301
Primary first episode, defined, 452
Primary infection, CMV, 437
Primary syphilis, 316
Primidone, 167, 170
Principles, pregnancy management
acute cholecystitis, 121
APS, 255
asthma, 228
cancer, 381–382
CD, 111
cholelithiasis, 120
CHTN, 3
dialysis, 153
eclampsia, 18–19
fetal monitoring, 496
FNAIT, 463–464
GBS, 326, 327
HBV infections, 288
HCV infection, 294
HG and NVP, 93–94
HIV infection, 300
IH (pustular psoriasis of pregnancy), 393
pneumonia, 234
preeclampsia, 9–10
pregestational diabetes, 52
prolactinoma, 87
renal transplantation, 154
seizures, 169, 169t
sickle cell disease, 140
SLE, 247–248
smoking, 199
toxoplasmosis, 443
tuberculosis, 239
UC, 115
VTE, 271
vWD, 146
Prior cesarean delivery, fetal macrosomia, 434
Prior shoulder dystocia, 434
Prior uterine scar, women with, 492–493
ProCESS trial, for septic shock, 360
Prochlorperazine, 96t, 98, 162, 164t, 165, 492
Prochlorperazine maleate (Compazine; Bukatel), 96t, 98
Proctitis, symptoms, 311, 313t
Proctocolectomy, 115
Proctocolitis, symptoms, 311
Progesterone, 11, 178, 215, 403
Progestins, 251, 279
Prognosis
AFE, survivors, 369
CMV, management, 437–438, 438f, 438t
factors, trauma, 339–340
fetal hydrops, 485
herpes, 452–453
long-term renal

CRI, 153
NS, 153
NIH, 483
parvovirus, 448
TTTS, 405
Prograf (tacrolimus), 125, 155, 155t, 249t, 250, 389
Progressive muscle relaxation, 97
Prolactinoma, 86–90
anesthesia, 90
antepartum testing, 90
breast-feeding, 90
classification, 86
complications, 86–87
fetus, 86–87
mother, 36
delivery, 90
diagnosis/definition, 86
epidemiology/incidence, 86
etiology/basic pathophysiology, 86
key points, 36
management, 87–89
bromocriptine (Parlodel), 88
cabergoline (Dostinex), 88
dopamine agonists, 88t
indications for therapy, 88t
macroadenomas, 89
microadenomas, 88–89
preconception counseling, 88
principles, 87
workup, 87–88, 87f
postpartum, 90
pregnancy
considerations, 87
prenatal care, 89–90
macroadenoma, 89, 90t
microadenoma, 89
symptoms, 86
Proliferative retinopathy, 51
PROM, *see* Premature rupture of membranes (PROM)
Promethazine, 19, 96t, 98, 99, 164t, 165
Prominent pulmonary vascular spasm, 365
Prophylactic tocolysis, in multiple gestation, 403
Prophylaxis effective rate (PER), 288
Propofol, 188
Propranolol
cocaine, use, 215
headache, 162, 165
hyperthyroidism, 82
marijuana abuse, 210
thyroid storm, 80, 83, 83t
Propylthiouracil (PTU), for hyperthyroidism, 80, 81–82, 83, 83t
Prostacyclin, 8, 10, 27, 368, 368t
Prostaglandins, 488, 492
Protease inhibitor (PI), 302t
Protective clothing, 395
Protein C, vitamin K-dependent polypeptide, 262, 264, 265t, 266
Protein S, vitamin K-dependent polypeptide, 262, 264, 265t, 266
Proteinuria, 8, 15, 51, 125, 151, 152, 153, 247
Prothrombin G20210A gene mutation (PGM), 9, 261, 262, 265t, 279
Protonix (pantoprazole), 95t, 97
Proton pump inhibitors (PPIs), 95t, 98
Prozac® and Prozac Weekly® (Fluoxetine), 182t
Prurigo of pregnancy (PP)
complications, 391

defined, 390
diagnosis, 390, 391f
epidemiology/incidence, 391
etiology/basic pathology, 391
historic notes, 390
key points, 390
management, 391
overview, 386, 387t
risk factors/associations, 391
symptoms, 390
therapy, 391
workup, 391
Pruritic folliculitis of pregnancy (PFP)
defined, 390
diagnosis, 390, 390f
epidemiology/incidence, 390
etiology/basic pathology, 390
historic notes, 390
key points, 390
management
therapy, 390
workup, 390
overview, 386, 387t
pregnancy considerations, 390
symptoms, 390
Pruritic urticarial papules and plaques of pregnancy (PUPPP), 388–389
Pruritus, 103, 105t, 106, 107, 128
Pseudohematuria, 158
Psilocin (N, N-dimethyl-4-phosphoryloxytryptamine), 220
Psilocybin, 220; *see also* Hallucinogens
Psychological challenges, ADR, 175
Psychomotor function, impaired, 74
Psychosis, postpartum, 177–178, 179–180
Psychotherapy, 180
PTL, *see* Preterm labor (PTL)
Ptyalism, defined, 93
Pulmacort (budesonide), 232
Pulmonary angiography, 272
Pulmonary artery catheter
invasive hemodynamic monitoring with, 27, 28
utilization of, 353
Pulmonary capillary wedge pressure (PCWP), 28
Pulmonary edema
AFE and, 365, 366, 369
cardiac disease and, 24, 27, 28
CHTN, complications, 1, 2, 6
critical care, requirement, 356, 360
multiple gestations and, 404
opioid overdose, 211
preeclampsia, complications, 7, 8, 9, 13, 15, 16, 18
septic shock and, 360
Pulmonary embolism (PE)
AFE and, 367
treatment of new onset DVT and PE, 276–277, 276f
VTE, management, 272, 274f
Pulmonary function tests, SCI and, 174
Pulmonary hypertension, 24, 25, 27, 35, 141
Pulmonary vascular resistance (PVR), increase in, 27
Pulmonic stenosis (PS), 28
Pulsatility index (PI), 501
Pulsed-wave (PW) Doppler velocimetry, for FGR, 420–421
Pump twin, 407
PUPPP (pruritic urticarial papules and plaques of pregnancy), 388–389
Purified protein derivative (PPD), 238, 239

Pustular psoriasis of pregnancy, *see*
Impetigo herpetiformis (IH)
Pyelonephritis, 156–157
defined, 156
diagnosis, 156
incidence, 156
management, 156–157
Pyrazinamide, 238, 241, 241t, 242
Pyridoxine, 94, 95t, 98, 241, 242, 301t
Pyrimethamine, 301t, 445

Q

Quetiapine, 186t, 187, 190
Quinagolide (Pergolide), 88
Quinolones, 112t, 113
Quitline, 200

R

Rabies vaccine, 334t
Racial differences, prevalence of obesity, 32
Radiation
fear, 345
induced cardiac toxicity due to fibrosis, 381
pregnancy after, 381
in pregnant trauma patient, 345, 345t
Radiographic findings, tuberculosis, 240
Radioiodine therapy, for hyperthyroidism, 80, 82
Radiology
clinical hypothyroidism, in pregnancy, 74
NVP and HG, 94
Radiotherapy, during pregnancy
acute leukemia, 377–378
breast cancer, 375, 376f
cervical cancer, 379
HD, 377
Raltegravir, 302t
Randomized controlled trials (RCTs)
ambulatory BP monitoring, 3
antiemetics and, 98
of BPS, 499
corticosteroids, use of, 99
dextrose *vs.* normal saline, 99
dimenhydrinate, as ginger, 97
doxylamine/vitamin B$_6$, 94
of euthyroid pregnant women, 76–77
FGR pregnancies, 424
ginger, examining, 97
hyperthyroidism, management, 81
insulin requirement in, 61
levothyroxine supplementation, 76
meta-analysis of, 10
mode of delivery in IBD, 110
nausea/symptom relief in, 97
norepinephrine, 360
for NVP or HG, 97–98
ondansetron and metoclopramide, 98
P6 acupressure *vs.* vitamin B$_6$, 97
preconception adjustment, 74
reduction in heroin use, 212
SGA in, 16
TTTS, 406
VTE, prevention, 277
Ranitidine (Zantac), 95t, 97, 155t
Rapid swabs, for trichomoniasis, 323
Rapid testing assays, 297
RCTs, *see* Randomized controlled trials (RCTs)
Reactivation
genital herpes, 452

hepatitis virus, pregnancy after LTx, 125
Recombivax HB, 288
Recurrence, risks
cancer, 381
CMV infections, 437
fetal death, prevention, 493
FGR, 414, 416
postpartum thyroiditis, 77
Recurrence rates of AFE, postpartum
counseling, 369
Red blood cell (RBC) alloimmunization;
see also Hemolytic disease
defined, 467
pregnancies, management of, 470–474
anesthesia, 474
counseling, 470
delivery, 474
fetal intervention, 472–473, 472t, 473t
fetal monitoring/testing, 473–474
long-term outcomes, 474
neonatology, 474
workup/investigations, 470–472, 471t
Reduced red blood cell, NIH and, 482
Reglan (metoclopramide), 95t, 97, 98
Regular insulin, 53t, 54, 55, 62t, 63t, 65t, 67
Relapse, smoking, 201–202
Relaxation training, for headache, 165
Remeron® and Remeron SolTab®
(Mirtazapine), 183t, 184
Renal calculi, *see* Urinary nephrolithiasis
Renal disease, 150–158
classification, 150, 151t
CRI
antenatal testing, 152
complications, 151, 151t
defined, 150
delivery, 153
HTN, 152
laboratory tests, 152
long-term renal prognosis, 153
management, 152
overview, 150, 151t
patient education, 152
postpartum/breast-feeding, 153
preeclampsia, 152
pregnancy considerations, 152
prenatal care, 152
preterm labor, 152
prevention, 152
therapy, 152
workup, 152
defined, 150
diagnosis, 150
dialysis, 153–154
complications, 154
postpartum care, 154
pregnancy management, 154
principles/counseling, 153
epidemiology/incidence, 150
key points, 150
microscopic hematuria
defined, 158
differential diagnosis, 158
incidence, 158
management, 158
risk factors for significant disease, 158
NS
causes, 153
complications, 153
defined, 153
epidemiology/incidence, 153
fetal monitoring, 153
labor management, 153

long-term prognosis, 153
management, 153
prenatal care, 153
specific diseases, 153
workup, 153
physiologic renal changes, 150, 151t
postpartum urinary retention, 157–158
defined, 157
incidence, 157
management, 158
risk factors, 158
pyelonephritis, 156–157
defined, 156
diagnosis, 156
incidence, 156
management, 156–157
risk factors/preconception counseling, 150, 151
specific diseases
IgA nephropathy, 151
insufficiency, mild, moderate, and
severe, 151
lupus nephritis, 151
vasculopathy, 151
stages, 151t
symptoms, 150
transplantation, 154–156
antenatal visits, 155
complications, 154
fetal surveillance, 155
graft rejection, 156
labor management, 155–156
lab work, 155
postpartum/breast-feeding, 156
preconception counseling, 154–155
prenatal care, 155, 155t
principles, 154
resources, 156
urinary incontinence
incidence, 157
prevention, 157
urinary nephrolithiasis
complications, 157
defined, 157
diagnosis, 157
incidence, 157
management, 157
risk factors, 157
UTI
complications, 156
diagnosis, 156
follow-up, 156
prevention, 156
screening, 156
treatment, 156
Renal insufficiency
CRI, *see* Chronic renal insufficiency (CRI)
LTx, pregnancy after, 125
mild, 151
moderate and severe, 151
Renal prognosis, long-term, 153
Renal transplantation, 154–156
antenatal visits, 155
complications, 154
fetal surveillance, 155
graft rejection, 156
labor management, 155–156
lab work, 155
postpartum/breast-feeding, 156
preconception counseling, 154–155
pregnancy after, 129
prenatal care, 155, 155t
principles, 154

resources, 156
Requirement, critical care, 356–361
    ARDS and mechanical ventilation,
        356–357, 356t
    sepsis, 357–361, 358t, 359t
Reserpine, for thyroid storm, 83t
Resistin, 33
Respiratory diseases, 225–242
    asthma, 225–233
        acute treatment, 233
        anesthesia, 233
        antepartum testing, 233
        anticholinergics, 232–233
        β-agonists, 232
        classification, 225–227, 226t, 227t
        complications, 227–228
        cromolyn, 232
        delivery, 233
        diagnosis, 225
        etiology and basic pathophysiology,
            225
        incidence, 225
        inhaled corticosteroids and long-
            acting β-agonists (fixed-drug
            combination), 232
        inhaled steroids, 232
        key points, 225
        LTRA, 232
        management, 228
        mild intermittent, 230, 232
        mild persistent, 232
        moderate persistent, 232
        oral corticosteroids, 233
        postpartum/breast-feeding, 233
        preconception care, 228
        pregnancy considerations, 228
        prenatal care, 228
        prevention, 228, 228t
        severe persistent, 232
        status asthmaticus, 233
        suggested medications, 229–230, 229f,
            230f, 231f
        symptoms, 225
        theophylline, 232
        therapy, 229–233
        workup, 229
    influenza, 236–238
        antepartum testing, 238
        complications, 236–237
        delivery, 238
        diagnosis, 236, 236t
        epidemiology/incidence, 236
        etiology/basic pathophysiology, 236
        key points, 236
        management, 237
        postpartum/breast-feeding, 238
        pregnancy considerations, 237
        prevention, 237
        prophylaxis after suspected exposure,
            237
        symptoms, 236
        therapy, 237–238
    pneumonia, 233–235
        anesthesia, 235
        antepartum testing, 235
        antibiotics, 235
        classification, 233, 234
        complications, 234
        delivery, 235
        diagnosis, 233
        epidemiology, 234
        etiology/basic pathophysiology, 233,
            234t

        hospitalization, 235
        key points, 233
        management, 234
        postpartum/breast-feeding, 235
        pregnancy considerations, 234
        risk factors, 234
        symptoms, 234
        treatment, 235
    tuberculosis, 238–242
        active tuberculosis infection, 241–242,
            241t
        antepartum testing, 242
        coinfection with TB and HIV during
            pregnancy, 242
        delivery, 242
        diagnosis, 239
        drug resistance, 242
        epidemiology/incidence, 238
        etiology/basic pathophysiology, 238
        infection control issues, 242
        key points, 238
        latent tuberculosis infection, 241
        management, 241
        postpartum/breast-feeding, 242
        pregnancy considerations, 239
        pregnancy management, 239
        prevention, 241
        risk factors/associations, 239
        screening, 239–240
        symptoms, 238
        therapy, 241–242
        workup, 240, 241
Respiratory distress syndrome (RDS)
    defined, 521
    risk, predictive value of pulmonary
        maturity tests, 524–525
Retinopathy
    diabetic, 51
    proliferative, 51
Return of spontaneous circulation (ROSC),
    367, 368
Reverse end-diastolic flow (REDF), UA, 404,
    413, 421, 425
Rhabdomyomas, 483
Rh(D) alloimmunization
    for hemolytic disease, 467–474; see also
        Hemolytic disease
    incidence of, 478
Rh disease, 460
Rh status, 344
Ribavirin, 291, 295
Rifabutin, 301t
Rifamixin, 113
Rifampicin, 239, 241t
Rifampin, 75, 155t, 238, 239, 241, 242, 301t
Rimantadine, 238
Risk-based fetal therapy, for FNAIT, 464–465
    high risk, 461f, 465
    standard risk, 461f, 464–465
    very high risk, 461f, 465
Risk factors
    acute cholecystitis, 121
    AFE, 366
    amphetamines, 216
    benzodiazepines, abuse, 218
    bipolar depression, 179–180
    cardiac disease, 25, 26t
    CHDs, 33
    chlamydial infection, 312
    cholelithiasis, 119, 120t
    CHTN, 2
    CMV, 436
    cocaine, 214

    cutaneous melanoma, 394
    drug abuse, 207, 207t
    fetal death, 488–489, 489t
    fetal macrosomia, 432
    FGR, 412, 413t
    GBS, 325, 326, 327
    GDM, 59t, 60
    HAV infections, 283
    HBV infections, 286
    HCV infection, 291, 292t, 293, 294
    herpes, 451
    HIV infection, 299
    ICP, 104
    IH (pustular psoriasis of pregnancy), 393
    inherited thrombophilias, 262
    LTx, pregnancy after, 125–127
        ACR rate, 127
        CMV acute infection, 125, 127
        diabetes, 125
        fetal and maternal outcomes, 125,
            126t
        hepatitis virus reactivation, 125
        hypertension and renal insufficiency,
            125
        infrarenal aortic graft, 127
    marijuana (cannabis), 209
    maternal anemia, 133, 134
    microscopic hematuria, 158
    mood disorders, 178
    NVP and HG, 92, 93
    obesity, 33
    opioids, use, 211
    parvovirus, 447
    PCP, 219
    pneumonia, 234
    postpartum thyroiditis, 77
    postpartum urinary retention, 158
    PP, 391
    preeclampsia, 9
    pregestational diabetes, 50
    renal disease, 150, 151
    seizures, 168
    SG, 386
    smoking, 198
    syphilis, 317
    tuberculosis, 239
    urinary nephrolithiasis, 157
    UTI, 156
    VTE, 270, 272t
    VZV infection, 456
Risk(s)
    associated with obesity, 35t
    chlamydia, 311
    long-term maternal, 42
    offspring, 42
    recurrence
        cancer, 381
        postpartum thyroiditis, 77
    trichomoniasis, 322–323
    VTE, 270
Risperdal® and Risperdal M-Tab®, 186t
Risperidone, 186t, 187, 190
Ristocetin cofactor activity, 145, 148
Ritonavir, 291, 295, 302t
Rituximab, 249t, 250, 377, 392
Rivaroxaban, 273
Routine maternal serologic screening,
    FNAIT, 463
Royal College of Obstetricians and
    Gynaecologists (RCOG)
        guidelines, 39, 40, 143, 417
Rubella vaccination, 301, 303, 332
Rufinamide (Banzel), 169t

S

Sabin–Feldman dye test (SFDT), 444
Sabril (Vigabatrin), 169t
Saccharin, 53
S-adenosylmethionine (SAMe), 107
Salmeterol, 226t, 232
Salt intake, preeclampsia, 11
SAMe (*S*-adenosylmethionine), 107
Sandimmun, 155t
Sarafem® (Fluoxetine), 182t
Saturated solution of potassium iodide (SSKI), 80, 83
SCI, *see* Spinal cord injury (SCI)
Screening
  alpha-fetoprotein, 55
  aneuploidy, HIV infection, 302
  APS, management, 255–256
  bipolar depression, 180
  chlamydial infection, 312
  CHTN, management, 3
  clinical hypothyroidism, 75, 75t
  CMV
    serum, 439
    ultrasound fetal findings, 439
  for depression, 178
  diabetic, 40
  ELISA, 299
  fetal macrosomia, 433
  for FGR, 416–418
    fundal height, 417
    serum analytes, 416–417
    UA Doppler, 418
    ultrasonographic growth curve, 417
    uterine artery Doppler, 418
  FNAIT, 462–463
  GBS, 327–328, 327f
  GDM, 59–60, 60t
  gonorrhea, 306, 307t
  HCV infection, 294
  hemolytic disease, 470–471
  herpes, 453
  HIV, 299
  hyperthyroidism, 81
  hypothyroxinemia, 76
  inherited thrombophilias, 260, 264, 265t
  mood disorders, 178
  parvovirus, 449
  preeclampsia, 3, 9
  for subclinical hypothyroidism, 76
  syphilis, 317–318, 318t
  toxoplasmosis
    serum, 443, 444, 444f
    ultrasound, 444
  trichomoniasis, 323
  TTTS, 405, 405f
  tuberculosis, TST, 239–240, 239t, 240f, 240t
  UTI, 156
  VZV infection, 458
SDPs (single deepest pockets), 513, 514–515, 516, 518
Seatbelts, 341
Secondary syphilis, 316
Seizures, 167–171
  background, 167
  classification, 168
  complications, 168–169
    fetal, 168–169
    maternal, 168
  defined, 167–168
  delivery, 171
  diagnosis, 167–168

epidemiology/incidence, 168
  etiology/basic pathophysiology, 168
  history, 167
  key points, 167
  management, 169–170
    preconception counseling, 169, 170
    prenatal care, 170
    prenatal counseling, 170
    principles, 169, 169t
  postpartum/breast-feeding, 171
  risk factors/associations, 168
  secondarily generalized, 168
  symptoms, 168
  therapy, 170–171
Selective fetocide, for TTTS, 406
Selective serotonin reuptake inhibitors (SSRIs), 165, 177, 180, 181–184, 182t–183t, 188–189
Selective termination, of anomalous fetus, 403–404; *see also* Anomalous fetus
Selenoproteins, as antioxidants, 74
Semi-Fowler (sitting) position, 498
Sentinel node biopsy
  breast cancer, 375
  melanoma, 378, 395
Sepsis, 357–361
  antibiotics, 359
  antimicrobial treatment, 360–361
  betamethasone, 360
  blood cultures, 359
  broad-spectrum antimicrobial therapy, 359
  classification, 357, 358t
  corticosteroids, 360
  dexamethasone, 360
  diagnosis, 357, 358t, 359
  dobutamine, 360
  EGDT, 359–360
  HES, 360
  norepinephrine, 360
  obstetric and nonobstetric, 358
  phenylephrine, 360
  proCESS trial, 360
  recommendations, 361
  SOFA score, 357
  SSC, 359–361, 359t
  vasopressors, 360
Septic shock, 235, 357, 358, 358t, 359, 360
Septostomy, for TTTS, 406
Sequential Organ Failure Assessment (SOFA) score, 357
Serologic screening, for syphilis, 318, 318t, 319
Serologic testing, FNAIT, 462, 463
Seroquel® and Seroquel XR®, 186t
Serotonin, for hallucinogenic effects of amphetamines, 216
Serotonin-norepinephrine reuptake inhibitors (SNRIs), 184
Serotonin reuptake inhibitors, 201
Sertraline (Zoloft®), 182t, 188
Serum, for screening
  analytes, for FGR, 416–417
  CMV, 439
  marker, 402
  toxoplasmosis, 443, 444, 444f
Severe FGR, defined, 414
Severe HTN, 5
Severe persistent asthma, 232
Severe preeclampsia, 14, 15–16
  defined, 7
  diagnostic criteria, 15
  management, 15–16

delivery, timing of, 16
  expectant, 16
  magnesium sulfate, 15–16
  plasma volume expansion, 15–16
  with severe features, 8
Severe renal insufficiency, 151
Severity, asthma, 225, 226t
Sexually transmitted infections (STIs), 299, 306, 310, 312, 313, 322, 323
SG, *see* Striae gravidarum (SG)
SGA (small for gestational age), 4, 211, 413, 414, 415, 416
Shingles (herpes zoster), 456, 459
Shock wave lithotripsy, 157
Shortacting β-agonists (SABA), 230
Short stature, 416
Shoulder dystocia, 35, 433, 434
Sickle cell disease, 139–144
  ACS, 143
    complications, 143
    defined, 143
    incidence, 143
    pathophysiology, 143
    symptoms, 143
    therapy, 143
    workup, 143
  alloimmunization, 142
  anesthesia, 143
  antenatal testing, 142
  complications, 140, 141t
  contraception, 143
  defined, 139
  delivery, 143
  diagnosis, 139
  epidemiology/incidence, 139
  genetics/inheritance, 139
  HBS-/βTHAL, 131, 134t, 139, 141, 143–144
  HBSC disease, 139, 141t, 143
  hemoglobin E, 144
  historic notes, 139
  key points, 139
  pathophysiology, 140
  postpartum, 143
  pregnancy management, 140, 141–142
    folate supplementation, 142
    preconception, 140, 141–142
    prenatal care, 141–142
    preventive care, 140
    principles, 140
    workup, 140
  sickle cell trait, 143
  symptoms, 140
  therapy
    antibiotics, 142
    hydroxyurea (hydroxycarbamide), 142
    incentive spirometry, 142
    intravenous fluids, 142
    iron, folic acid, and multivitamins, 142
    labor and delivery, 142
    narcotics, 142
    transfusions, 142
Sickle cell trait, 143
Side effects
  azathioprine, 155t
  bromocriptine (Parlodel), 88
  cabergoline (Dostinex), 88
  cholestyramine, 107
  cyclosporine, 155t
  dopamine agonists, 88t
  immunosuppressive agents, 127t, 128, 155t
  IVIG, 463

magnesium, 152
mycophenolate mofetil, 155t
prednisone, 155t
sirolimus, 155t
tacrolimus, 155t
thionamides, 82
ursodeoxycholic acid (Ursodiol), 107
SIDS (sudden infant death syndrome), 198, 206, 210
Signs/symptoms, *see* Symptoms/signs
Sildenafil, 368, 368t
Simeprevir, 295
Single deepest pockets (SDPs), 513, 514–515, 516, 518
Single fetal death, multiple gestation and, 401, 404, 404t
Singleton pregnancies, AF assessment in, 513–515
    accuracy of ultrasound, for oligohydramnios, 513–514
    AFV, estimation with SDP or AFI, 514
    background, 513
    color Doppler for AFV, 514
    indications, 513
    key points, 513
    management, 514–515
    techniques, 513
    ultrasound estimates, accuracy, 514
Sirolimus, 155t
Skeletal dysplasias, NIH and, 482
Skin rashes, 316
SLE, *see* Systemic lupus erythematosus (SLE)
Sleep deprivation, 181
Sloane Epidemiology Center Birth Defects Study, 181
Small for gestational age (SGA), 4, 211, 413, 414, 415, 416
Smallpox vaccination, 332, 336t
Smokeless tobacco complications, 198
Smoking, 196–202
    "5 As" for patients, 197t
    bans, 199
    breast-feeding, 201
    carbon monoxide, 197
    carcinogens, 197
    cessation counseling, 197t
    cessation rates, 196, 197t
    complications
        congenital anomalies, 198
        fetal death, 198
        LBW, 198
        maternal lifetime, 198
        placental abruption, 198
        placenta previa, 198
        postnatal morbidities, 198
        preeclampsia, 198
        pregnancy loss, 198
        preterm birth, 198
        PROM, 198
    consequences, reducing, 202
    defined, 196
    diagnosis, 196
    e-cigarettes, 198, 201
    epidemiology/incidence, 196
    etiology/basic pathology, 196–198
    future research, 202
    genetics, 196
    historic notes, 196
    initiation, reducing, 202
    key points, 196
    management, 199
    multiple-choice questionnaire, 197t
    nicotine, 197

pharmacotherapies, 200–201
    bupropion HCl (Zyban®, Wellbutrin®), 201
    combination therapies, 201
    NOT recommended, 201
    NRT, 200–201, 200t
    varenicline (Chantix®), 201
postpartum, 201–202
preeclampsia and, 9
pregnancy
    complications, reducing, 202
    considerations, 198–199
prevention, relapse, 202
principles, 199
risk factors, 198
"5 Rs" for smokers, 197t
smokeless tobacco complications, 198
therapies, 199–201
    alternative treatments, 201
    counseling, 199–200
    intervention, assessment for, 197t, 199
    NRT, 196, 200–201, 200t
    pharmacotherapies, 200–201
Society for Maternal Fetal Medicine (SMFM), 352, 402
Society of American Gastrointestinal and Endoscopic Surgeons (SAGES), 122
Society of Obstetricians and Gynaecologists of Canada (SOGC), 39, 341, 342
Sodium nitroglycerin, 174
Sodium nitroprusside, 13
Sofosbuvir, 291, 295
Sonographic assessment
of AF, 513–518
    accuracy of ultrasound, for oligohydramnios, 513–514
    AFV, estimation with SDP or AFI, 514
    background, 513
    color Doppler for AFV, 514
    indications, 513
    key points, 513, 515
    management, 514–515
    oligohydramnios, 515–516; *see also* Oligohydramnios
    polyhydramnios (hydramnios), 516–518; *see also* Polyhydramnios (hydramnios)
    in singleton pregnancies, 513–515
    techniques, 513
    ultrasound estimates, accuracy, 514
for twin growth, 407
Spectinomycin, 308, 308t
Spinal anesthesia, cardiac disease, 26
Spinal cord injury (SCI), 173–175
    ADR, *see* Autonomic dysreflexia (ADR)
    anesthesia, 175
    classification, 173
    defined, 173
    delivery, 175
    dermatology, 174
    diagnosis, 173
    epidemiology/incidence, 173
    GBS, 175
    hematology, 174
    key points, 173
    postpartum care and breast-feeding, 175
    pregnancy management, 173–175
        preconception counseling, 173
        prenatal care, 173–174
    pulmonary function tests, 174
    resources, 175
    UTI and, 174
    VTE, 174

Spinal shock, 173
Spine trauma, 344
Spiramycin, 444, 445
Splenectomy, 376
Spongiform pustule, of Kogoj, 393
Spontaneous abortion (SAB), 184
Spontaneous pregnancy loss, multiple gestation, 400, 401
Sputum smear, 240–241
SSRIs (selective serotonin reuptake inhibitors), 165, 177, 180, 181–184, 182t–183t, 188–189
Stabilization, maternal, 342, 343, 343t
Stabilizers, mood, 184–187
    carbamazepine and oxcarbazepine, 187
    lamotrigine, 187
    lithium, 184, 185t
    mood disorders, management during lactation
        carbamazepine, 189
        lamotrigine, 189
        lithium, 189
        valproic acid, 187, 189
Stadol®, 213
Staging, during pregnancy
    breast cancer, 375
    cervical cancer, 379
    HD, 376
    laparotomy, 376
    melanoma, 378
    TTTS, 405, 405t
Standard risk-based fetal therapy, for FNAIT, 461f, 464–465
Staphylococcus aureus, 235
Staphylococcus spp., 121, 235
Starzl, Thomas, 124
Status asthmaticus, 233
Stavzor®, 185t
Stent insertion, double pigtail, 157
Sterilization counseling, 25
Steroids
    AFE, management, 369
    in FGR pregnancies, 424
    HELLP syndrome, 7, 17
    IH (pustular psoriasis of pregnancy), 393
    IVIG and, 563, 564
    NODM, 125
    NS, 153
    for PEP, 389
    PG (herpes gestationis), 392
    SLE, 249
Stevens-Johnson syndrome, 189
Stillbirth Collaborative Research Network (SCRN), 488
Stillbirths, risk of
    antimalarial drug, 249
    APAs, 255
    assault during pregnancy, 340
    causes of, 488–489
    CD, 110, 111, 112, 113
    CHTN, 5
    cocaine, effects, 206
    cocaine use, 215
    diabetes, 50
    dialysis, complication, 154
    evaluation of, 490
    FGR, 5, 415, 416, 417, 419, 421
    folate supplementation, 136
    GBS, 325, 326
    headache in pregnancy, 164
    HIV, 299
    ICP, 104, 106, 107–108
    influenza

infection, 333
vaccination, 237
inherited thrombophilias, 260, 263, 264
karyotypic analysis on, 490
marijuana use, 210
multiple gestation, 408
MVAs, 341
obesity, 32, 33, 39
opioids use, 211, 212
by parent groups, 488
prevention, antepartum fetal assessment, *see* Antepartum testing
prior uterine scar, 492–493
radiotherapy, 381
SGA-associated, 415
smokeless tobacco complication, 198
syphilis, 315, 317
TG infection, 443
UC, 110, 115
STIs (sexually transmitted infections), 299, 306, 310, 312, 313, 322, 323
Stones, *see* Urinary nephrolithiasis
Streptococcus agalactiae, 325–330
Streptococcus faecalis, 121
Streptococcus pneumoniae, 140, 233, 235, 334t, 335, 336t, 337
Streptococcus pyogenes, 481
Streptomycin, 242
Stretch marks, *see* Striae gravidarum (SG)
Striae gravidarum (SG), 386, 387
cause of, 386
defined, 386
diagnosis, 386
epidemiology/incidence, 386
etiology/basic pathology, 386
genetics, 386
key points, 386
management, 387
prevention, 387
risk factors/associations, 386
symptoms, 386
therapy, 387
Stroke, 1, 2, 3, 6, 16, 32, 35t, 42, 139, 140, 142, 162, 214, 216, 255, 258, 269, 317, 378, 416, 479
Subclinical hyperthyroidism
defined, 80
treatment, 81
Subclinical hypothyroidism
defined, 73
diagnosis, 76
incidence, 76
screening and management, 76
Subcutaneous insulin pump therapy, 54
Suboxone, 213
Substance abuse, *see* Drug abuse
Substance abuse disorder, defined, 207
Subutex, 213
Succinylcholine, 188
Sucralose, 53
Sudden infant death syndrome (SIDS), 198, 206, 210
Sudden unexpected death in epilepsy (SUDEP), 170
Sulfadiazine, 445
Sulfamethoxazole, 155t, 156, 157
Sulfasalazine, 110, 112, 112t, 113
Sulindac, 518
Sulphonamides, 156
Sumatriptan, 165
Sunscreens, 395
Superimposed preeclampsia
diagnoses/definitions, 2, 7, 8

management, 14
overview, 14, 14f, 15f
with severe features, 8
Super obesity, defined, 32
Suppression, TSH, 81
Surfactant, defined, 521
Surfactant/albumin ratio (SAR) tests, for FLM, 522, 523t
Surgery
acute cholecystitis, 122
bariatric, 38–39, 38t
cesarean delivery, *see* Cesarean delivery
hyperthyroidism, management, 82
during pregnancy
breast cancer, 375
cervical cancer, 379
HD, 376
melanoma, 378
thyroid cancer, 379
thyroid nodule, 77
UC, 115
Surviving Sepsis Campaign (SSC), 359–361, 359t
Survivors
AFE, prognosis, 369
breast cancer, on endocrine therapy, 382
cancer, offspring of, 381
Suspected macrosomia, management, 433, 433f
Sustained virologic response (SVR), 295
Swabs
alcohol, 294
endocervical, 306, 312
rapid, for trichomoniasis, 323
vaginal-perianal, 328
vaginal-rectal, 306, 312, 327, 328
Swan–Ganz catheters, 13
Swedish Medical Birth Registry, 198
Symmetric FGR, 414
Sympathectomy, 217
Symptoms/signs
ACS, 143
acute cholecystitis, 121
ADP (eczema), 389
ADR, 173, 174
amphetamines, 216
APS, 254
asthma, 225
benzodiazepines, 218
cardiac disease, 24
CD, 110, 111t
chlamydia, 310–311
cervicitis/urethritis, 311
chlamydial conjunctivitis, 311
LGV, 311
maternal genital infection, 311
proctitis/proctocolitis, 311
cholelithiasis, 119
clinical hypothyroidism, 73
CMV, 436
cocaine, 214
cutaneous melanoma, 394
depression, 177
drug abuse, 207, 207t
ESLD, 124
GBS, 325
gonorrhea, 305–306
hallucinogens, 220
HAV infections, 283
HBV infections, 285
HCV infection, 292
HELLP syndrome, 16, 17t
herpes, 452

hyperthyroidism, 80, 81
ICP, 103
IH (pustular psoriasis of pregnancy), 392
influenza, 236
marijuana (cannabis), 209
maternal anemia, 131
MDD, 177
opioids, 210–211
parvovirus, 447
PCP, 219
PEP, 388
PFP, 390
PG (herpes gestationis), 392
pneumonia, 234
postpartum depression, 177
PP, 390
preeclampsia, 8
pregestational diabetes, 50
prolactinoma, 86
renal disease, 150
seizures, 168
SG, 386
sickle cell disease, 140
SLE, 246, 247t
syphilis, 316–317
incubation period, 316
late benign (tertiary) syphilis, 316–317
latent, 316
neurosyphilis, 317
primary, 316
secondary, 316
thyroid storm, 83
toxoplasmosis, 442
trichomoniasis, 322
tuberculosis, 238
UC, 114
VTE, 269–270
vWD, 145
VZV infection, 456
Synthetic cannabanoids, *see* Marijuana (cannabis)
Synthetic cathinones, 216–217; *see also* Amphetamines
Syphilis, 315–320
complications, 317
defined, 315
fetal hydrops, cause of, 482
incidence/epidemiology, 315
key points, 315
management, 317–320
diagnosis, 319
follow-up, 320
prevention, 317
screening, 317–318, 318t
workup, 319
neonatal congenital, 320
pathophysiology and transmission, 315–316
risk factors, 317
symptoms and classification, 316–317
incubation period, 316
late benign (tertiary) syphilis, 316–317
latent, 316
neurosyphilis, 317
primary, 316
secondary, 316
testing, 491
treatment, 319–320, 319t
Syphilis Elimination Effort (SEE), 315
SYROCOT study group, 442
Systemic lupus erythematosus (SLE), 246–251
antepartum testing, 250

CNL/CHB, 250–251
  counseling, 250–251
  delivery, 251
  etiology, 250
  management, 251
  prenatal care evaluation, 251
  prevention, 251
  therapy, 251
complications, 246–247
  fetal/neonatal, 246–247
  maternal, 246
contraception, 251
delivery, 250
diagnosis, 246
epidemiology/incidence, 246, 248t
etiology/basic pathophysiology, 246
key points, 246
management, 247–250
  preconception counseling, 248, 248t
  prenatal care, 248, 249
  principles, 247–248
  workup, 248, 248t
neonatal lupus, 250
postpartum/breast-feeding, 250
pregnancy considerations, 247
symptoms, 246, 247t
therapy, 249–250, 249t
  agents, 249t, 250
  azathioprine (Azasan, Imuran), 249, 249t
  corticosteroids, 249, 249t
  cyclosporine, 249t, 250
  hydroxychloroquine sulfate (Plaquenil), 249, 249t
  immunoglobulin, 249–250, 249t
  NSAIDs, 249, 249t
  tacrolimus, 249t, 250
  TNF inhibitors, 249t, 250
Systemic Lupus International Collaborating Clinics (SLICC), 246, 247t
Systemic vascular resistance (SVR), decreased, 24

T

Tachyarrhythmias, 479
Tachycardia, systemic effects, 214
Tacrolimus, 125, 155, 155t, 249t, 250, 389
Tagamet (Cimetidine), 95t, 97, 155t
Talwin®, 213
Tamoxifen, 375, 382
Taxanes, 375
Td (tetanus and diphtheria), vaccination, 301, 333, 333t, 335
Tdap (tetanus toxoid, reduced inactivated diphtheria toxoid, and acellular pertussis), vaccination, 301, 332, 333, 333t, 335, 336t
Technitium-99m (Tc-99m), 375, 378
Tegretol (carbamazepine), 75, 155t, 167, 169, 169t, 170, 185t
Telaprevir, 294
Tenofovir, 289
Tenofovir disoproxil fumarate, 302t
Teratogenicity
  ECT, 188
  methimazole, 82
  SSRIs, 181, 182t–183t
Terbutaline, 227t
Termination, of pregnancy
  acute leukemia, 377
  breast cancer, 374
  HD, 376

invasive cervical cancer, 379
melanoma, 378
selective, of anomalous fetus, 403–404; see also Anomalous fetus
surgery, 374
thyroid cancer, 379
Tertiary (late benign) syphilis, 316–317
Testing
antenatal
  CRI, 152
  sickle cell disease, 142
antepartum, see Antepartum testing
APA, 254, 255t
fetal
  condition-specific, 505, 506–508, 506t, 507t
  critical care, 354–355
  FNAIT, 465
  hemolytic disease, 473–474
  indications for, FNAIT, 462
  NIH, 486
  RBC alloimmunized pregnancies, 473–474
  trauma and, 344
Testosterone, 124
Tetanus and diphtheria (Td), vaccination, 301, 333, 333t, 335, 336t
Tetanus toxoid, reduced inactivated diphtheria toxoid, and acellular pertussis (Tdap), vaccination, 301, 332, 333, 333t, 335, 336t
Tetracyclines, 307
Tetrahydrocannabinol (THC), see Marijuana (cannabis)
Tetralogy of fallot, 28
Thalassemia, 131, 134t, 135t, 139, 143–144, 482
  α-thalassemia, 131, 134t, 482
  β-thalassemia, 131, 134t, 139, 143–144
Thalidomide, 110, 112t, 113
Thebaine, 210
Theophylline, 226t, 232, 233
Therapeutic approach, NIH, 486
Therapeutic hypothermia (TH), 368
Therapies
  ACS, 143
  ADP (eczema), 389
  amphetamines, use, 217
  antiemetic, NVP and HG, 98
  APS, 256–257
    actual therapy, 256–257, 257t
    evidence, 256
    issues, 257
  asthma, 229–233
    anticholinergics, 232–233
    β-agonists, 232
    cromolyn, 232
    general, 229
    goals, 229
    inhaled corticosteroids and long-acting β-agonists (fixed-drug combination), 232
    inhaled steroids, 232
    LTRA, 232
    mild intermittent, 230, 232
    mild persistent, 232
    moderate persistent, 232
    oral corticosteroids, 233
    severe persistent, 232
    suggested medications, 229–230, 229f, 230f, 231f
    theophylline, 232
  behavior, prepregnancy weight reduction, 38

benzodiazepines, use, 218
beta-blockade, Marfan syndrome, 29
cancer
  acute leukemia, 377–378
  breast, 375, 376f
  cervical, 379
  complications, 380
  HD, 376–377
  melanoma, 378
  NHL, 377
  thyroid, 379–380
CD, 112–114, 112t
  adalimumab, 112t, 113
  aminosalicylates, 112t, 113
  antibiotics, 112t, 113
  azathioprine/6-mercaptopurine, 112t, 113
  certolizumab, 112t, 113
  corticosteroids, 112t, 113
  cyclosporine, 112t, 113
  immunomodulators/immunosuppressants, 112t, 113
  infliximab, 112t, 113
  methotrexate, 112t, 113
  naltrexone, 113–114
  natalizumab, 113
  thalidomide, 112t, 113
cholelithiasis, 120
CHTN, 3
CMV
  CMV-specific hyperimmune globulin, 439–440
  ganciclovir and valacyclovir, 440
CNL/CHB, 251
cocaine dependence, 215
CRI
  HTN, 152
  preeclampsia, 152
  preterm labor, 152
CSII, 54
cutaneous melanoma, 395
eclampsia, 19
hallucinogens, 220
HAV, 283, 284
HBV, 288–289
  nucleoside/nucleotide analogs, 288–289, 289t
  vaccines, 288
HCV, 294–295
headache, 164–165, 164t
herpes
  antiviral drugs, 453, 454
  complicated HSV infection, 454
  history of HSV, 454
  primary/first episode, 454
IH (pustular psoriasis of pregnancy), 393
influenza, 237–238
L-Arginine, 19
marijuana (cannabis) abuse, 210
maternal anemia, 131, 136, 136f
mood disorders, 188
opioids, use, 212–213
  buprenorphine, 212–213
  methadone, 212
parvovirus, 449
PCP, 219
PEP, 389
PFP, 390
PG (herpes gestationis), 392
pharmacotherapy, prepregnancy weight reduction, 38
PP, 391
preeclampsia

antihypertensive, 12–13
antioxidant, 7, 11
prolactinoma, 88t
radioiodine, hyperthyroidism, 82
risk-based fetal, for FNAIT, 464–465
    clinical concerns/issues, 465
    high risk, 461f, 465
    standard risk, 461f, 464–465
    very high risk, 461f, 465
seizures, 170–171
SG, 387
sickle cell disease
    antibiotics, 142
    hydroxyurea (hydroxycarbamide), 142
    incentive spirometry, 142
    intravenous fluids, 142
    iron, folic acid, and multivitamins, 142
    labor and delivery, 142
    narcotics, 142
    transfusions, 142
SLE, 249–250, 249t
    agents, 249t, 250
    azathioprine (Azasan, Imuran), 249, 249t
    corticosteroids, 249, 249t
    cyclosporine, 249t, 250
    hydroxychloroquine sulfate (Plaquenil), 249, 249t
    immunoglobulin, 249–250, 249t
    NSAIDs, 249, 249t
    tacrolimus, 249t, 250
    TNF inhibitors, 249t, 250
smoking, 199–201
    alternative treatments, 201
    counseling, 199–200
    intervention, assessment for, 197t, 199
    NRT, 196, 200–201, 200t
    pharmacotherapies, 200–201
subcutaneous insulin pump, 54
thyroxine, 75
toxoplasmosis, 444–445
TTTS, 405, 406–407, 406f
    stage 1, 405, 406
    stages II, III, and IV, 406
    stage V, 406, 407
tuberculosis, 241–242
UC, pharmacological, 115
UTI, 156
vWD, 146, 146t, 148, 148f
VZV infection, 458–459
Thermal biofeedback, for headache, 165
Thiacetazone, 242
Thiamine, 99
Thiazide diuretics, 6t
Thiethylperazine, 98
6-Thioguanine, 377
Thionamides
    dose of, 81
    hyperthyroidism, management, 81–82, 83
        methimazole, 82
        mode of action, 82
        PTU, 80, 81–82
        side effects, 82
Thiothixene, 189
Thoracic extracardiac anomalies, NIH and, 481
Thorazine (chlorpromazine), 19, 189–190
Thrombocytopenia
    autoimmune, 255
    multiple gestation, 401–402
Thromboembolism
    AFE, 366

risks of, 28, 29
    venous, obesity and, 41
Thrombophilia(s)
    fetal, 263–264
    inherited, see Inherited thrombophilias
    testing, 279
    workup, 491
Thromboprophylaxis postpartum, 110, 114
Thromboxane, 8, 10
Thyroglobulin, antithyroid antibodies, 73, 75
Thyroid-binding globulin (TBG), 74
Thyroid cancer, 379–380
    delay in diagnosis, 379
    diagnostic tests and safety, 379
    papillary, 380
    pregnancy after, 382
    surgery, 379
    termination of pregnancy, 379
    treatment, 379–380
Thyroidectomy, 74, 82, 379, 380, 382
Thyroid function tests, 178
Thyroiditis, postpartum
    defined, 77
    diagnosis, 77
    etiology, 77
    incidence, 77
    management, 77
    recurrence risk, 77
    risk factors, 77
    three clinical presentations, 77
Thyroid nodule
    diagnosis, 77
    evaluation, 83
    hyperthyroidism, 83
    incidence, 77, 83
    surgery, 77
Thyroid peroxidase (TPO), antithyroid antibodies, 73, 74, 75, 76–77
Thyroid-stimulating hormone (TSH)
    HG, diagnosis, 94
    levels in pregnancy, 74, 75t
    measurements, 81
    suppression, 74, 81
Thyroid-stimulating hormone-binding inhibitory immunoglobulins (TBIIs), 80, 83
Thyroid-stimulating immunoglobulins (TSIs), 80, 81, 83
Thyroid storm
    defined, 80
    diagnosis, 83
    incidence, 83
    precipitating factors, 83
    signs/symptoms, 83
    treatment, 83, 83t
Thyrotoxicosis
    adrenergic symptoms of, 82
    beta-adrenergic antagonist drug for, 77
    defined, 80
    gestational
        defined, 80
        Graves' disease from, 81
        transient biochemical, 81
    with Graves' disease, 81
Thyrotropin, defined, 73
Thyroxine
    in amniotic fluid, 83
    defined, 73
    replacement, for clinical hypothyroidism, 75–76
        dose, 75
        iodine supplementation, 76
        new diagnosis, 75

preexisting hypothyroidism, 75
    type, 76
    therapy, 75
    for transient hypothyroidism, 77
Tiagabine (Gabatril), 169t
Tight control, very tight vs., 54
Timing
    delivery
        cancer and, 380
        DIGITAT study, 424, 425
        FGR, 412
        FGR pregnancies, 423f, 424–426
        GRIT study, 424–425, 426
        HELLP syndrome, 17
        multiple gestation, 408, 408t
        preeclampsia, 13
        pregestational diabetes, 55
        severe preeclampsia, 16
        TRUFFLE study, 424, 425, 426
    evidence for, anti-D immunoglobulin, 469–470
        after birth (postpartum), 469
        before birth (antepartum), 469–470
        special clinical situations, 470
    pregnancy, LTx and, 125
Tinidazole, 324
TIPPS trial, 266
Tobacco
    complications, smokeless, 198
    dependence, 196
    multiple-choice questionnaire, 197t
Tobramycin, 155t
Tocodynamometer, 344
Tofcitinib, 393
Topical retinoids, 387
Topical tretinoin, 386, 387
Topiramate, 167, 169, 169t, 170–171
Toxemia, 8
Toxins, discontinuation of, 419
Toxoplasma gondii (TG), 442
Toxoplasmic encephalitis, 301t
Toxoplasmosis, 442–445
    complications, 443
    incidence/epidemiology, 442
    key points, 442
    maternal-fetal transmission, 442–443, 443f, 443t
    pathogen, 442
    pathophysiology, 442
    pregnancy management, 443, 444–445
        prevention, 443, 443t
        principles, 443
        screening, 443, 444
        serum, 443, 444, 444f
        therapy, 444–445
        ultrasound, 444
        workup/diagnosis, 444
    symptoms, 442
TRAbs (TSH receptor antibodies), 80
Training, ICU, 352
Trametinib, 395
Tranexamic acid, 145, 369
Transabdominal amnioinfusion, 516
Transaminases, 106
Transcervical amnioinfusion, 516
Transfer, critical illness, 353
Transfusion related acute lung injury (TRALI), 369
Transfusions
    blood
        anemia, 131, 137, 482
        HBV-infection, 286
        HCV infection, 292t, 293

hemolytic disease, 467, 468, 470, 471–473, 472t, 473t, 474
HIV-infection, 299
sickle cell disease, 139, 140, 141, 142, 143
syphilis, 315, 316
FBS, 472–473, 472t, 473t
fetal, 482, 483
intrauterine
antigen-compatible platelets, 464
CMV, 437, 482
fetal anemia with, 471
fetuses with severe hydrops, 486
parvovirus infection, 447, 448, 449, 450
of platelets via FBS, 460, 464, 465
RBC, 360
TRALI, 369
trauma, 340
TTTS, *see* Twin-twin transfusion syndrome (TTTS)
Transient bone marrow suppression, of neonate, 380
Transmission
chlamydia, 311
CMV, 436–437, 437f
gonorrhea, 305
maternal-fetal
herpes, 452
parvovirus, 448, 448f
toxoplasmosis, 442–443, 443f, 443t
VZV infection, 456, 457
syphilis, 315–316
trichomoniasis, 322
Transplantation, pregnancy after
heart, 128t, 129
intestinal, 128t, 129
LTx, *see* Liver transplantation (LTx)
other, 128t, 129
renal, *see* Renal transplantation
Transport, obstetrical patient, 353
Transtheoretical model, of behavior change, 201
Transvaginal ultrasound (TVU), 402
Trastuzumab, 375, 382
Trauma, 339–346
anesthesia, 346
antepartum testing, 346
assault, hospitalization for, 340–341
causes, 341
complications
abruptio placentae, 340
fetal death, 340
fetal injury, 340
fetal/neonatal outcomes, 340
hospitalization, 340
hysterectomy, 340
maternal death, 340
neonatal death, 340
transfusion, 340
CPR, 345–346
defined, 339
delivery, 346
etiology/basic pathophysiology, 339
hematuria and, 158
incidence, 339
key points, 339
postpartum/breast-feeding, 346
pregnancy considerations, 341
pregnancy management, 341–345
admission, 345
blunt abdominal, 343–344
care of patient, 341
coagulation studies, 344–345

contraction monitoring, 344
CT, 343
DPL, 343–344
evaluation and diagnostic studies, 343–345, 343t
FAST ultrasound, 343, 344
fetal monitoring, 344
fetal ultrasound, 344
KB test, 344
laparotomy, 344
open fractures, 344
penetrating abdominal wound, 344
radiation, 345, 345t
Rh status, 344
spine trauma, 344
stabilization, 342, 343, 343t
tocodynamometer, 344
traumatic brain injury, 344
workup and management, 342, 342f
prenatal care, 346
prevention
air bags, 341
intimate partner violence, 341
seatbelts, 341
prognostic factors, 339–340
Traumatic brain injury, 344
Trazodone, 189
Treponema carateum, 318
Treponemal tests, for syphilis, 319
Treponema pallidum, 315–320
Tretinoin, 386, 387
Trial of Umbilical Fetal Flow in Europe (TRUFFLE) study, 421–422, 424, 425, 426, 503
Triamcinolone acetonide, 226t
Trichomonas vaginalis, 322–324
Trichomoniasis, 322–324
complications/risks, 322–323
epidemiology/incidence, 322
key points, 322
management, 323–324
diagnosis, 323, 323t
prevention, 323
screening, 323
treatment, 324
pathophysiology/etiology, 322
symptoms/signs, 322
transmission, 322
Tricyclic antidepressants (TCAs), 184, 189
Trifluoperazine, 189
Triiodothyronine, defined, 73
Trileptal®, 185t
Trimethaphan, 173, 174
Trimethobenzamide (Tigan), 95t
Trimethoprim, 155t, 156, 157, 301t
Trimethoprim-sulfamethoxazole (TMP-SMZ), 301t
Trimethoxypheneylamine, 220
Triplets, vaginal delivery of, 408
Triptans, 164, 164t, 165
Trivalent inactivated vaccine (TIV), 237, 333t
Trofolastin cream, 386, 387
Trophoblastic invasion, 8
TRUFFLE (Trial of Umbilical Fetal Flow in Europe) study, 421–422, 424, 425, 426, 503
TSH receptor antibodies (TRAbs), 80
Tuberculin skin testing (TST), 238, 239–240, 239f, 240t, 241
Tuberculosis, 238–242
active infection, 241–242, 241t
antepartum testing, 242

coinfection with TB and HIV during pregnancy, 242
delivery, 242
diagnosis, 239
drug resistance, 242
epidemiology/incidence, 238
etiology/basic pathophysiology, 238
infection control issues, 242
key points, 238
latent tuberculosis infection, 241
management, 241
postpartum/breast-feeding, 242
pregnancy considerations, 239
pregnancy management principles, 239
prevention, 241
risk factors/associations, 239
screening, TST, 239–240, 239t, 240f, 240t
symptoms, 238
therapy, 241–242
workup, 240, 241
Tumor necrosis factor (TNF) inhibitors
infliximab, 113
for SLE, 249t, 250
TNF-α inhibitors, for IH, 393
Turner and Down syndromes, 481
Twin pregnancies, AF assessment in
background, 518
oligohydramnios/hydramnios, 518
technique, 518
Twin reversal arterial perfusion (TRAP) syndrome, 407, 483
Twinrix, 288
Twin(s)
conjoined, 407
DC/DA, 398, 399t, 401
delivery, subsequent pregnancy outcomes after, 404
DZ
defined, 398
etiology, 398, 399t
incidence, 398
FGR/discordant twins, 404
MA, 398, 399t
MC, 398, 399t, 401
multiple gestation, 408
MZ
defined, 398
etiology, 399, 399t
incidence, 398
peak sign, 400
TRAP syndrome, 407, 483
TTTS, *see* Twin-twin transfusion syndrome (TTTS)
vanishing, defined, 400
Twin-twin transfusion syndrome (TTTS)
diagnosis, 405
etiology, 404
incidence, 404
marker for, 398, 401
NIH and, 480t, 483
overview, 398
prognosis and counseling, 405
screening, 405, 405f
staging, 405, 405t
therapy for, 405, 406–407, 406f
stage 1, 405, 406
stages II, III, and IV, 406
stage V, 406, 407
Two-step screening test, GDM, 60
Typhoid OralTY21a, 335t
Tyrosine kinase inhibitors, 378
Tzanck smear, 453

U

UA, *see* Umbilical artery (UA)
UC, *see* Ulcerative colitis (UC)
UDCA (ursodeoxycholic acid), 103, 106–107, 122
UFH, *see* Unfractionated heparin (UFH)
U.K. Epilepsy and Pregnancy Registry, 168–169
Ulcerative colitis (UC), 114–116
  antepartum testing, 116
  CD *vs.*, 111t
  complications, 114–115
    fetal, 115
    maternal, 114
  defined, 110, 114
  delivery, 116
  diagnosis, 114, 114t
  epidemiology/incidence, 114
  etiology/basic pathophysiology, 114
  management, 115–116
    differential diagnosis, 115
    preconception counseling, 115
    prenatal care, 115
    principles, 115
    workup, 115
  postpartum/breast-feeding, 116
  pregnancy considerations, 115
  signs/symptoms, 114
  therapy, 115
    colectomy, 115
    IPAA, 114, 115–116
    pharmacological, 115
    surgery, 115
Ultrasonographic growth curve, for FGR, 417
Ultrasonography
  compressive, 272
  DVT, 272, 272t
  syphilis, 320
  urinary nephrolithiasis, 157
Ultrasound
  accuracy, for oligohydramnios, 513–514
  acute cholecystitis, 121
  for AFV, 513
  CVS, 458
  diagnosing multiple gestations, 399, 400
  estimates, accuracy, 514
  FAST, 343, 344
  fetal, 40, 344
  fetal death in ICP, 107
  fetal findings
    CMV screening, 439
    parvovirus, 448
  fetal heart rate, thyroid, and growth, 82
  FGR, 420–422
    Doppler velocimetry, 420–421
    growth assessment, intervals of, 420
    MCA Doppler velocimetry, 421
    venous Doppler (DV) velocimetry and sequential changes, 421–422, 423f
  hemolytic disease, 467, 470–471
  HIV infection, 302
  LTx, pregnancy after, 128
  multiple gestation, 407
  NIH, 484
  polyhydramnios (hydramnios), 517
  postpartum urinary retention, 158
  seizures, 170
  sickle cell disease, 142
  toxoplasmosis, 443, 444, 444f
  urinary nephrolithiasis, 157
Umbilical artery (UA)

AEDF, 404, 413, 421, 425, 426
AREDF, 421, 425
Dopplers
  antepartum testing, 496, 499, 501, 502f, 503, 505, 506, 506f, 508
  delivery timing for twins, 408t
  of fetal vessels, 501–505, 502f, 503f, 504f, 505f
  FGR, 412, 413, 414, 415, 418, 419, 420–421, 422, 423f, 424, 425, 426, 426t, 506
  limitations, 421
  velocimetry, 420–421
REDF, 404, 413, 421, 425, 426
Uncomplicated macrosomia, management, 433
Unexplained fetal death, defined, 488
Unfractionated heparin (UFH)
  adjusted-dose, 28, 29
  aspirin and, 256
  VTE, management, 273, 274, 279
    bleeding, 273
    heparin-induced osteoporosis, 274
    HIT, 273, 274
    mechanical heart valves and, 278
United States Preventive Services Task Force, 402
Ureteroscopy, 157
Urethritis, symptoms, 311, 313t
Uric acid, 11
Urinalysis, 208
Urinary incontinence, 157
Urinary nephrolithiasis
  complications, 157
  defined, 157
  diagnosis, 157
  incidence, 157
  management, 157
  risk factors, 157
Urinary retention, postpartum, 157–158
  defined, 157
  incidence, 157
  management, 158
  risk factors, 158
Urinary tract infections (UTI)
  complications, 156
  diagnosis, 156
  follow-up, 156
  prevention, 156
  risk factors for, 156
  SCI and, 174
  screening, 156
  treatment, 156
Urine
  cotinine testing, 199
  drug testing, 208, 208t
  length of time drugs in, 208, 208t
Ursodeoxycholic acid (UDCA), 103, 106–107, 122
Ursodiol (ursodeoxycholic acid), 103, 106–107, 122
U.S. Preventative Services Task Force (USPSTF), 141, 178, 312
Ustekinumab, for IH, 393
Uterine artery Doppler
  FGR, screening, 418
  velocimetry, 9
Uterine artery vasospasm, 214
Uterine Doppler ultrasound, abnormal, 10
Uterine palpation techniques, 175
Uteroplacental perfusion, reduced, 4
Uterotonics, 369
UTI, *see* Urinary tract infections (UTI)

V

Vaccination, 332–337
  anthrax, 335t
  BCG, 239, 240, 241, 242, 302, 332, 336t
  CMV, 438
  contraindications to, 337
  dosing, 333t, 334t–335t
  drug interactions with cyclosporine, 155t
  general guidelines, 332–333, 333t
  HAV, 283–284, 334, 336t
  HBIg, 285, 288, 289
  HBV infections, 125, 285, 286t, 288, 289, 301, 332, 333t, 335, 336t
  HCV, 294, 295
  historical notes, 332
  HIV, 301
  HPV, 332, 333t, 336t
  influenza, 139, 140, 142, 234, 236, 237, 301, 332, 333, 333t, 336t
  Japanese encephalitis, 335t
  key points, 332
  LTx, pregnancy after, 125, 127t
  maternal, against GBS, 326
  meningococcal, 334t, 336t
  mothers with depression, 178
  pertussis, 332
  pneumococcal, 139, 140, 142, 234, 334t, 335, 336t, 337
  polio, 301, 334t–335t
  preconception, 332, 333t
  pregnancy, 332, 333
    vaccine-preventable diseases and, 332
  rabies, 334t
  rubella, 301, 303, 332
  sickle cell disease, 139, 140, 141, 142
  smallpox, 332, 336t
  Td, 301, 333, 333t, 335, 336t
  Tdap, 301, 332, 333, 333t, 335, 336t
  tetanus, 332
  Typhoid OralTY21a, 335t
  varicella, 301t, 302, 332, 336t, 457, 459
  vWD, 146
  yellow fever, 335t
Vaginal birth after cesarean (VBAC) delivery, 40, 434
Vaginal delivery
  AFE, 366, 367, 369
  cardiac diseases, 27
  fetal macrosomia, 432, 433
  FGR, 426
  GHTN, 13
  gonorrhea, 305
  HCV infection, 294
  HELLP syndrome, 17
  HSV infection, 451, 452, 453
  IBD, 110, 114, 115, 116
  in ICU, 355
  NAIT, 464, 465
  NIH, 486
  SCI, 175
  of triplets, 408
  twin delivery, 408
  urinary incontinence, 157
  VTE, 260, 279
  vWD, 149
Vaginal pool collection, 522, 523t
Vaginal-rectal swabs, 327, 328
Valacyclovir (Valtrex)
  CMV, 440
  herpes, 451, 453, 454
  varicella, 459

Valproate, 167, 169, 170, 189
Valproic acid (VPA), 165, 169, 169t, 171, 177, 185t, 187, 189
Valtrex (valacyclovir)
    CMV, 440
    herpes, 451, 453, 454
    varicella, 459
Vancomycin, 155t, 235, 325, 328t, 329
Vanishing twin, defined, 400
Vaqta (Merck), 283
Varenicline (Chantix®), 201
Varicella zoster virus (VZV) (chickenpox), 456–459
    complications
        fetal, 457
        maternal, 457
    HIV infection, 301t, 302
    incidence/epidemiology, 456
    key points, 456
    maternal-fetal transmission, 456, 457
    pathogen, 456
    pathophysiology, 456, 457f
    pregnancy management, 457–459
        clinical neonatal findings of CVS, 459
        considerations, 457
        counseling, 457, 458t
        maternal shingles (herpes zoster), 459
        nonimmune women, 459
        prevention, 457
        screening, 458
        therapy, 458–459
        workup/diagnosis, 458
    risk factors/associations, 456
    symptoms/signs, 456
    vaccine, 301t, 302, 332, 336t, 457, 459
Varivax®, 457
VariZIG™, 456, 458
Vascular tumors, NIH and, 482
Vasculopathy, renal disease, 151
Vasopressors, 360, 365, 367, 368, 369
Veltpatasvir, 295
Vemurafenib, 395
Venereal disease research laboratory (VDRL), 317
Venlafaxine, 181, 183t, 184, 188, 189
Venous Doppler (DV) velocimetry, 421–422, 423f
Venous thromboembolism (VTE), 269–279
    antepartum testing, 278
    anticoagulation, postpartum management of, 279
    APS with, 254
    associations, 270, 272t
    cesarean delivery, 279
    complications, 270
    contraception, 279
    defined, 269
    delivery and anesthesia, 278–279
    diagnosis, 264, 265t
    epidemiology and incidence, 270
    etiology/basic pathophysiology, 270, 271f, 271t
    genetics/classification, 270, 271t, 272t, 275t
        ATIII deficiency, 262
        FVL, 261–262, 261t
        MTHFR/homocysteinemia, 262
        protein C, 262
        protein S, 262
        prothrombin G20210A gene, 262
    key points, 269
    management, 271–276
        aspirin, 276

clinical scenarios and
        anticoagulation, 272, 273, 274–276, 275t
    diagnosis, 271–272, 272t
    LMWH, 274, 275
    principles, 271
    pulmonary angiography, 272
    pulmonary embolism, 272, 274f
    UFH, 273, 274
    warfarin (Coumadin), 275–276
mechanical heart valves, women with, 278
obesity and, 41
overview, 260, 262
preconception counseling, 277
prevention, 264, 266, 277–278
risk of, 260–261, 270, 272t
screening, 264, 265t
symptoms, 269–270
treatment, 264, 265t
treatment of new onset DVT and PE, 276–277, 276f
Ventilation, mechanical, 356–357, 356t
Ventilation/perfusion (V/Q) scan, 269, 272
Ventricular dysfunction, 369
Ventricular septal defects (VSDs)
    decreased SVR, 24
    pregnancy management, 27
Verapamil, 155t, 165, 479, 486
Vertical transmission
    gonorrhea, 305
    HBV, 286, 288, 289
    HCV, 291, 293, 293t
Verum ointment, 386, 387
Very high risk-based fetal therapy, for FNAIT, 461f, 465
Very tight control, tight vs., 54
Vibroacoustic stimulation (VAS), 498, 501
Vigabatrin (Sabril), 169t
Vimpat (Lacosamide), 169t
Vincristine, 375, 377, 378, 381
Violence
    domestic, 339
    intimate-partner, 341
    maternal death and, 340
Visual impairment, prolactinoma and, 86
Vitamin B6, 94, 95, 97, 98
Vitamin C, 7, 202
Vitamin D, 402, 416
Vitamin E, 202
Vitamin K, 28, 29, 103, 107, 168, 187, 275–276
Vitamin K antagonists (VKAs), 275–276
Vitamins, supplementation, 39
Vomiting/nausea, see Nausea and vomiting of pregnancy (NVP)
von Hippel–Lindau syndrome, 173
von Willebrand, Erik, 145
von Willebrand disease (vWD), 145–149
    anesthesia, 149
    antepartum testing, 148
    classification, 145
    complications, 146
    defined, 145
    delivery, 149
    diagnosis, 145, 146t
    epidemiology/incidence, 145
    etiology/basic pathophysiology, 145, 147f
    future research, 149
    genetics, 145, 146t
    historic notes, 145
    key points, 145
    management, 146, 148
        preconception counseling, 146

prenatal care, 146
    type I, 146, 148
    type IIa, 148
    type IIb, 148
    type III, 148
    postpartum/breast-feeding, 149
    pregnancy
        considerations, 146
        management, 146
        principles, 146
    rare/related, 149
    symptoms, 145
    workup (labs), 146, 146t
von Willebrand Factor (vWF), 145
Voucher-based contingency management, 199, 215
VPA (valproic acid), 165, 169, 169t, 171, 177, 185t, 187, 189
VTE, see Venous thromboembolism (VTE)
VWD, see von Willebrand disease (vWD)
VZV, see Varicella zoster virus (VZV) (chickenpox)

W

Warfarin (Coumadin), 29, 275–276, 278, 279
Weight gain
    prenatal care and, 39, 39t
    PTB, in multiple gestation, 403
Weight loss
    drugs, 38
    marijuana, use, 209
Wellbutrin XL®, 183t, 201
Wernicke's encephalopathy, development of, 99
Western blot, 297, 299
Wet mount preparation, of vaginal secretions, 323
Withdrawal
    neonatal
        benzodiazepines, abuse, 218
        cocaine, use, 215
        marijuana (cannabis), use, 210
        opioids, use, 211, 212
    symptoms
        amphetamine, 216
        benzodiazepines, 218
        cocaine, 214, 215
        opioids, 210–211, 213
        PCP, 219
Women's Interagency HIV Study (WIHS), 298
Workup
    ACS, 143
    acute cholecystitis, 121
    ADP (eczema), 389
    asthma control, 229
    CD, 112
    cholelithiasis, 120
    CHTN, 3
    CMV, 439
    CRI, 152
    cutaneous melanoma, 395
    drug abuse, 207, 208, 208t
    eclampsia, 19
    fetal death, 489, 490–491
    FGR, 412, 413t, 418–419
    HAV infections, 283
    HBV infections, 288
    HCV infection, 294
    HELLP syndrome, 16
    hemolytic disease, 470–472, 471t
    herpes, 453

HG and NVP, 94
ICP, 106
IH (pustular psoriasis of pregnancy), 393
LTx, pregnancy after, 127t, 128
maternal anemia, 131, 132f, 133f, 134, 135–136
NIH, 484–485, 484f, 485f
NS, 153
parvovirus, 449, 449f
PEP, 388
PFP, 390
PG (herpes gestationis), 392
pneumonia, 234
polyhydramnios (hydramnios), 517
PP, 391
preeclampsia, 11
pregestational diabetes, 52
prolactinoma, 87–88, 87f

sickle cell disease, 140
SLE, management, 248, 248t
syphilis, 319
thrombophilia, 491
toxoplasmosis, 444
trauma, 342, 342f
tuberculosis, 240, 241
UC, 115
vWD, 146, 146t
VZV infection, 458
Wrist bands
    acupressure, 94, 97
    acustimulation, 97

X

XeCl excimer ultraviolet B (UVB) laser, 387
Xenical (Orlistat), 38

Y

Yaws, transmission, 318
Yellow fever, 335t

Z

Zafirlukast, 226t, 232
Zanamivir, 237
Zidovudine, 297, 298, 300, 302t, 303
Zileuton, 232
Zinc, supplementation, 402
Ziprasidone, 186t, 190
Zoloft® (Sertraline), 182t
Zonegran (Zonisamide), 169t
Zonisamide (Zonegran), 169t
Zyban®, 183t, 201
Zyprexa® and Zyprexa Zydis®, 186t